Peritoneal Surgery

Springer
New York
Berlin
Heidelberg
Barcelona
Hong Kong
London
Milan
Paris
Singapore
Tokyo

Gere S. diZerega, M.D.

Senior Editor
Professor of Obstetrics and Gynecology
University of Southern California School of Medicine
Livingston Research Institute
Los Angeles, California

Peritoneal Surgery

Associate Editors

Alan H. DeCherney, M.D.
Michael P. Diamond, M.D.
Harold Ellis, C.B.E.
Victor Gomel, M.D.
Arthur F. Haney, M.D.
Lena Holmdahl, M.D., Ph.D.
John A. Rock, M.D.
Kathleen E. Rodgers, Ph.D.
Jeremy N. Thompson, M.D.

With a Foreword by Victor Gomel, M.D.

With 178 Illustrations, 22 in Full Color

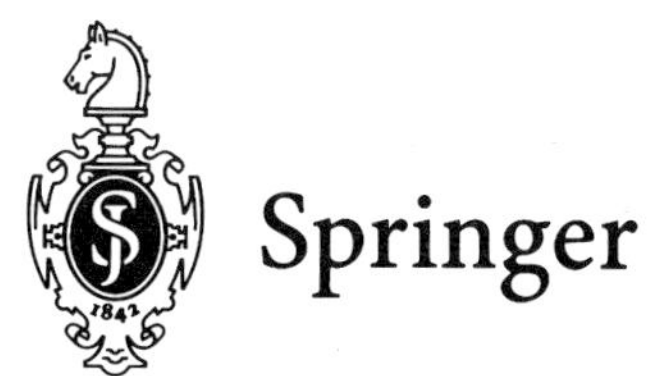

Springer

Senior Editor:
Gere S. diZerega, M.D.
Professor of Obstetrics and Gynecology
University of Southern California School of Medicine
Livingston Research Institute
1321 N. Mission Rd.
Los Angeles, CA 90033
USA

Library of Congress Cataloging-in-Publication Data

Peritoneal surgery / senior editor, Gere S. diZerega : associate editors, Alan DeCherney . . . [et al.].
p. cm.
Includes bibliographical references and index.
ISBN 0-387-98610-3 (hardcover : alk. paper)
1. Peritoneum—Surgery. I. DiZerega, Gere S.
[DNLM: 1. Peritoneum—surgery. 2. Adhesions. 3. Postoperative Complications. WI 575 P4457 1999]
RD548.P47 1999
617.5′58—dc21
DNLM/DLC
for Library of Congress 99-12449

Printed on acid-free paper.

Production coordinated by Impressions Book and Journal Services, Inc. and managed by Terry Kornak; manufacturing supervised by Jeffrey Taub.
Typeset by Impressions Book and Journal Services, Inc., Madison, WI.
Printed and bound by Maple-Vail Book Manufacturing Group, York, PA.
Printed in the United States of America.

9 8 7 6 5 4 3 2 1

ISBN 0-387-98610-3 Springer-Verlag New York Berlin Heidelberg SPIN 10689377

To Laura A. Gillan for
her diligence and dedication in bringing
information to surgical specialists

Foreword

by Victor Gomel, M.D.

There has been increasing appreciation of the deleterious effects of postoperative intraperitoneal adhesions and the importance of prevention or at least reduction of their occurrence. Postoperative adhesions may cause abdominal and pelvic pain, bowel obstruction, and infertility. The commonest cause of bowel occlusion in a woman is a prior hysterectomy. Therefore, prevention of adhesions is important in both conventional and extirpative surgery. This book is a summary of both the science of peritoneal repair as well as a manual of surgical techniques directed to the reduction of postsurgical adhesion and consequently improved surgical outcome. The timing of this book's publication is propitious owing to the recent increase in the understanding of peritoneal adhesion formation and the development in improved surgical techniques especially using a minimal access approach to the peritoneal cavity.

The series or cascade of physiologic or pathophysiologic events that lead to either normal peritoneal healing or formation of postoperative adhesions commences with the initial surgical trauma. Surgical trauma is not confined to the operative site alone; frequently there is significant trauma to adjacent and peripheral tissues. Although the former may be integral to the procedure, the latter should largely be avoidable. For example, in an ovarian cystectomy the incision made on the affected ovary to excise the cyst is an essential part of the procedure. However, undue trauma to the ovarian surface from less than gentle manipulation and from sponging with surgical pads is largely avoidable, as is trauma to adjacent peritoneal surfaces from manipulation, insertion of abdominal pads and introduction of foreign material.

As is evident from other chapters of this book, it is easier to prevent de novo adhesions (adhesions that did not exist before) than adhesions reformed subsequent to adhesiolysis. A situation that is very likely to lead to adhesions, frequently of cohesive type, is the apposition of damaged peritoneal surfaces. This is frequently observed between the posterior surface of the ovary and the peritoneal surface of the fossa ovarica.

The ovary is the organ most frequently involved in adhesions. This propensity is the result of its being covered by a single mesothelial layer that is deprived of the underlying support structures present in the peritoneum. Desiccation of the cells of this single cell layer, even by simple exposure to the atmosphere and lights of the operating room, may be sufficient to cause adhesions. The described propensity and the less than gentle technique frequently used are among the major causes of failure of reconstructive surgery. Recognition of these facts, at a time when reconstructive surgery represented the only treatment option for tubal factor infertility, led to the development and introduction of microsurgical techniques in gynecology. The gynecologist became more acutely aware of tissue trauma and its deleterious effects and began to employ more delicate techniques.

Microsurgical Technique

Microsurgery has been defined as "surgery under magnification." In fact, magnification is only a single facet of microsurgery, which embraces a broad concept of tissue care designed to minimize tissue damage. The principles include the following:

Delicate Handling of Tissues

This concept demands respect for peritoneal surfaces. Every effort must be made not to damage the peritoneum. This requires avoiding the use of traumatic instruments, such as toothed forceps, and laparotomy pads on the peritoneum. Retraction should be achieved with probes rather than by grasping tissues with traumatic instruments. To avoid desiccation, the peritoneum must be kept moistened, at all times, by frequent irrigation with a physiologic solution such as lactated Ringer's. Sponging with pads should be replaced by irrigation, both to clean the operative site and to expose bleeding vessels. Addition of heparin (1000 to 5000 units per liter, depending upon the anticipated total volume of fluid use) to the irrigation solution largely prevents the clotting of extravasated blood, improves the effectiveness of irrigation in keeping the surgical site well exposed and facilitates the removal of blood, soluble fibrin, and debris from the peritoneal cavity at the end of the procedure.

Hemostasis

Good hemostasis is an integral part of good surgical technique. The presence of blood in the peritoneal cavity increases the likelihood of postoperative adhesions. Blood increases the need for fibrinolysis which is limited to the available amounts of plasminogen and plasminogen activator activity (PAA). Blood clots adhere to the traumatized peritoneum and provide the fibrin matrix necessary for the formation of adhesions.

While pedicles must be well secured, the creation of large areas of necrosis must be avoided by limiting the size of the pedicles and the amount of tissue beyond the tie.

Electrosurgery plays an important role in hemostasis; however, it must be used judiciously. Bleeding vessels should be exposed by irrigation and desiccated using the smallest possible caliber electrode or bipolar forceps and with the appropriate power density in order to avoid damage to adjacent tissues and excessive carbonization.

Avoidance of Introduction of Foreign Material into the Peritoneal Cavity

The introduction of foreign bodies into the peritoneal cavity creates an inflammatory reaction that frequently contains giant cells. Powder used in surgical gloves is a major irritant to the peritoneum. For this reason, it is imperative to wash the gloved hands thoroughly prior to entering the peritoneal cavity, especially with open surgery. In open surgery the gloves should be moistened when handling tissues to reduce peritoneal trauma. The use of nonwoven, moistened pads is preferable to that of ordinary pads, which will shed lint into the peritoneal cavity.

Sutures, necessary as they may be, are a foreign body to the peritoneum and thus engender an inflammatory response and not infrequently cause adhesion. For this reason less reactive sutures (synthetic absorbable or when required synthetic permanent) must be selected. In addition, in order to decrease the amount of suture material exposed to the peritoneal cavity the finest caliber suture able to do the task should be used and whenever possible the suture and/or the knot buried.

Complete Excision of Abnormal Tissues

Whenever possible all diseased and necrotic tissues must be excised. For example, in the case of endometriosis it is preferable to remove or ablate all of the lesions. In the case of tubal abortion it is necessary to remove all of the blood, clots, and especially the gestational tissues out of the peritoneal cavity and perform a thorough lavage.

Precise Alignment and Approximation of Tissue Planes

Segments of organs requiring anastomosis must be aligned properly to maintain optimal function. In the case of a tubal or bowel anastomosis it is preferable to approximate the muscular and serosal layers separately.

Adhesiolysis

As a general rule, filmy adhesions are usually avascular and are amenable to sharp dissection. Dense adhesions tend to be vascular but will often have avascular areas that can be used to gain access to the tissue layers to identify and occlude their major blood vessels. Lysis of cohesive adhesions will necessitate development of a dissection plane by sharp and blunt dissection and hydrodissection. Very fibrous and extremely cohesive adhesions, usually secondary to previous pelvic surgery or repeated severe infections, may not be amenable to laparoscopic dissection.

The performance of safe adhesiolysis requires the observation of the following measures: Dissection should always commence in well exposed areas. Each adhesive layer must be clearly identified, grasped, and retracted to achieve optimal exposure. It is essential to recognize what lies behind the adhesion before dissection begins. Transection must be carried out parallel to the organ of interest. Adhesions must be divided one layer at a time. Shallow adhesions are simply transected. Broad adhesions are excised by dividing them both along the organ of interest and at their distal attachments and removed from the peritoneal cavity. Transection can be achieved mechanically using sharp scissors, electrosurgically, or with laser energy. Scissor division can be effected close to vital structures but sufficient distance must be maintained if electrosurgery or laser is being used. The instrument used for division must approach the tissue to be divided at a right angle. Vessels encountered along the transection line should be electrodesiccated prior to division. Filmy shallow adhesions are simply divided, occluding the infrequent blood vessel that will be encountered prior to division. Broad adhesions are divided at both ends and removed. When, as is often the case, these adhesions are multilayered, they should be divided one layer at a time. Hydrodissection is a simple way of developing these layers.

With cohesive adhesions it will be necessary to identify the proper dissection plane. This is achieved by placing a small incision between the two adherent structures and by developing a plane either by spreading the jaws of the scissors, by blunt dissection, or by hydrodissection. No thermal energy should be used in such cases.

Adhesions between loops of bowel are tethered at both ends to a particularly vulnerable structure. The cleavage planes should be developed by using hydrodissection and the adhesions divided at their midpoints using scissors to avoid any potential spread of electrical or laser energy to the bowel wall.

Once the adhesiolysis has been completed, copious lavage is performed and, unless the returning fluid is clear, the areas of division are examined to identify and deal with any residual bleeding points.

Pelvic Lavage

Thorough lavage of pelvic, and, when indicated, of the whole abdominal cavity, with a buffered irrigating solution (lactated Ringer's solution), is designed to remove from the peritoneal cavity substances such as blood, fibrin, lint, and other foreign bodies. A buffered irrigating solution is preferred over normal saline in order to remove the hydrogen ions which form during surgery and thereby return the pH of peritoneal fluid to physiologic condition. To suction all of the fluid out of the peritoneal cavity it is essential to place the patient in reverse Trendelenburg position; This applies to both laparotomy and laparoscopy.

When laparoscopic access is used for the procedure, underwater examination of the operative site may be performed. When the irrigation fluid remains clear, the pneumoperitoneum pressure is reduced and the regions inspected with the distal end of the laparoscope under the surface of the fluid. This permits prompt recognition of any small bleeding vessels, which can be desiccated with use of a microbipolar forceps.

Magnification

Magnification may be used when necessary or when performing microsurgical procedures. Magnification enables prompt identification of abnormal morphologic changes, recognition and avoidance of surgical injury and application of the preceding principles with the use of fine microsurgical instruments and suture materials.

Mode of Access

The microsurgical principles outlined above are applicable irrespective of the mode of access, be it abdominal, laparoscopic, or vaginal. Many procedures can be performed through any one of these access routes. The selection of the specific access is dependent upon the lesion, the procedure required, and the skill of the surgeon. The aim would be to select the access that will yield the best outcome for the patient.

Operating within a closed peritoneal cavity largely prevents desiccation of the peritoneal surfaces, especially if the insufflation gas has been moistened and warmed to body temperature. Working within a closed environment eliminates the need to use pads and prevents the introduction of foreign materials such as lint and talcum powder. Laparoscopy permits intraoperative irrigation for lavage and to expose bleeding vessels. Fine electrodes may also be used to achieve precise electrosurgical hemostasis. As in microsurgery, laparoscopic procedures are performed with a limited number of instruments. The laparoscope provides a degree of magnification that can be enhanced further by the monitor and special cameras. The laparoscope provides excellent coaxial illumination. The visibility can be enhanced by bringing the distal end of the scope close to the area of interest.

Abdominal Incision

Most reproductive surgical procedures can be performed through a small (minilaparotomy) suprapubic transverse or vertical (if a midline or paramedian sear is present) incision. We have successfully used this approach since 1986. The length of the incision is usually 5 to 6 cm, but is dependent upon the prior pelvic findings and especially the depth of the patient's subcutaneous adipose layer. The site of the proposed incision is infiltrated with a long-acting anesthetic agent such as 0.25% bupivacaine (Marcaine) solution. A transverse suprapubic incision is made and extended down to the fascia. The subcutaneous fat is dissected over the fascia, in the midline upward and downward. The fascia is then incised vertically in the midline. The recti muscles are separated in the midline, and the peritoneum incised vertically, with the incision curbed laterally at the lower end to avoid the bladder. The subcutaneous tissues are reinfiltrated with the same solution before closure of the skin incision. Thereafter, a bilateral inguinal nerve block is established. The small size of the incision, the lack of bowel manipulation along with gentle handling of tissues during the procedure, and the use of local anesthesia reduce postoperative discomfort and analgesia requirements. This approach permits prompt mobilization of the patient and discharge from the hospital within 24 hours. These patients return to normal activity almost as rapidly as those in whom the procedures were performed laparoscopically.

Further Reading

Gomel V. Reconstructive Tubal Surgery. In: Rock JA, Thompson JD, editors. TeLinde's Operative Gynecology, 8th edition. 1997:549–584.

Gomel V, Taylor P. Principles of Gynecologic Laparoscopy. In: Gomel V, Taylor P, editors. Diagnostic and Operative Gynecologic Laparoscopy. St. Louis: Mosby 1995:71–88.

Preface

The mission of this book is to provide the thoughtful surgeon a user-friendly path to deliver a better clinical outcome to his patients. In fulfillment of this mission, the leading investigators currently contributing to this rapidly expanding field summarized recent advances in peritoneal surgery. As their contributions are in both basic science and clinical arenas, the text is authoritative and detailed yet broad enough in scope to benefit the practicing surgeon, surgeon-in-training, and basic science investigator.

The science of mesothelial repair and its clinical application to surgical practice provides practitioners with progressive surgical tools and advanced techniques that benefit surgical patients. Scientists are continuing to uncover the complex interplay of inter- and intracellular messengers that orchestrate mesothelial regeneration, fibrogenesis, and inflammation.

Today, surgical therapeutics includes utilization of adhesion prevention adjuvants and techniques—a development of the last two decades with resultant improvements in surgical outcomes. This book summarizes these recent advances in peritoneal surgery from the leading investigators actively contributing to this rapidly expanding field. The editors have endeavored to incorporate an understanding of the peritoneal membrane, its response to surgical trauma, and adhesion-formation biology with a full spectrum of surgical procedures and discussion of appropriate clinical adjuvants, thus providing the surgeon and surgeon-in-training with the knowledge necessary to minimize tissue response to injury and maximize benefit of surgical therapy. Adhesion formation and the challenge to surgical therapy in their reduction are considered by integrating the science of fibrinolysis together with new considerations of surgical technique. The contribution adhesions make to the morbidity of our patients as well as to the cost of healthcare is reviewed across surgical disciplines. Adjuvants available to reduce formation of postsurgical adhesions are critically evaluated to identify ways to maximize their efficacy in surgical practice as well as understand their limitations. The direction of ongoing research is presented with an eye toward identifying questions for future study.

The editorial board would like to thank Ginger Mayerson and her colleagues Leticia Corona and Alec DeCherney for maintaining throughout creation of this text a high quality of professionalism, which is evident on every page; Susan Kreml for a thorough copyediting, which often led to creative rewrites; and Claire Huismann and Terry Kornak for production that exceeded unrealistic expectations.

Gere S. diZerega, M.D.
Los Angeles
New York

Contents

Contributors

Florence Alexandre, M.D., Department of Obstetrics, Gynecology and Reproductive Medicine, Polyclinique de l'Hôtel Dieu, Université Clermont-Ferrand, 13, boulevard Charles-De-Gaulle, 63003 Clermont-Ferrand, Cedex 1 France

Stig Bengmark, M.D., Ph.D., Lund University, Ideon Research Center, Box 73X, S-22007 Lund, Sweden

Revaz Botchorishvili, M.D., Department of Obstetrics, Gynecology and Reproductive Medicine, Polyclinique de l'Hôtel Dieu, Université Clermont-Ferrand, 13, boulevard Charles-De-Gaulle, 63003 Clermont-Ferrand, Cedex 1 France

Marie Claude Anton Bousquet, M.D., Department of Obstetrics, Gynecology and Reproductive Medicine, Polyclinique de l'Hôtel Dieu, Université Clermont-Ferrand, 13, boulevard Charles-De-Gaulle, 63003 Clermont-Ferrand, Cedex 1 France

Ivo A. Brosens, M.D., Ph.D., Leuven Institute for Fertility and Embryology, Medisch Centrum, Tiensevest 168, B-3000, Leuven, Belgium

Maurice Bruhat, M.D., Department of Obstetrics, Gynecology and Reproductive Medicine, Polyclinique de l'Hôtel Dieu, Université Clermont-Ferrand, 13, boulevard Charles-De-Gaulle, 63003 Clermont-Ferrand, Cedex 1 France

Rudi Campo, M.D., Leuven Institute for Fertility and Embryology, Medisch Centrum, Tiensevest 168, B-3000, Leuven, Belgium

Michel Canis, M.D., Department of Obstetrics, Gynecology and Reproductive Medicine, Polyclinique de l'Hôtel Dieu, Université Clermont-Ferrand, 13, boulevard Charles-De-Gaulle, 63003 Clermont-Ferrand, Cedex 1 France

Charles Chapron, Department of Gynecologic Surgery, University Rene Descartes, Hospital Baudelocque 123, boulevard Port Royal, 75014 Paris, France

Mark A. Damario, M.D., Section of Reproductive Endocrinology, Department of Obstetrics and Gynecology, Mayo Clinic, 200 First Street SW, Rochester, MN 55905-0001, USA

Alan H. DeCherney, M.D., Department of Obstetrics and Gynecology, UCLA School of Medicine, 10833 LeConte Avenue, 27-117 CHS, Mailcode 174017, Los Angeles, CA 90095-2828, USA

William C. Parks, Ph.D., Division of Dermatology, Department of Medicine, Washington University School of Medicine at the Jewish Hospital, St. Louis, MO 63110, USA

Lynn S. Peck, D.V.M., M.S., Biomaterials Center, Department of Materials Science and Engineering, University of Florida, 306-MAE, Gainesville, FL 32611-6400, USA

Jean-Luc Pouly, M.D., Department of Obstetrics, Gynecology and Reproductive Medicine, Polyclinique de l'Hôtel Dieu, Université Clermont-Ferrand, 13, boulevard Charles-De-Gaulle, 63003 Clermont-Ferrand, Cedex 1 France

Andrew T. Raftery, B.Sc., M.D., Department of Surgery, Sheffield Kidney Institute, Northern General Hospital, Herries Road, Sheffield S5 7AU, United Kingdom

John A. Rock, M.D., Department of Gynecology and Obstetrics, Emory University School of Medicine 1639 Pierce Dr., Room 4208 WMB, Atlanta, GA 30322, USA

Kathleen E. Rodgers, Ph.D., Department of Obstetrics and Gynecology, University of Southern California, Livingston Research Institute, 1321 N. Mission Road, Los Angeles, CA 90033, USA

Luk Rombauts, M.D., Ph.D., Leuven Institute for Fertility and Embryology, Medisch Centrum, Tiensevest 168, B-3000, Leuven, Belgium

David M.B. Rosen, M.D., Sydney Women's Endosurgery Center, Sydney, Australia, and Royal Surrey County Hospital, Guildford Surrey, GU12AW, United Kingdom

Gregory S. Schultz, Ph.D., Department of Obstetrics and Gynecology, University of Florida, 1600 S. Archer Road, Box 100294, Gainesville, FL 32610-3001, USA

Sonteara Seak-San, M.D., Department of Obstetrics, Gynecology and Reproductive Medicine, Polyclinique de l'Hôtel Dieu, Université Clermont-Ferrand, 13, boulevard Charles-De-Gaulle, 63003 Clermont-Ferrand, Cedex 1 France

John F. Steege, M.D., Department of Obstetrics and Gynecology, University of North Carolina, CB 7570, MacNider Building, Chapel Hill, NC 27599-7570, USA

Christopher J.G. Sutton, M.D., Department of Gynecology, Chelsea and Westminster Hospital, Waterden Road Clinic 8, Waterden Road, Guildford Surrey, GU12AW, United Kingdom

Salli Tazuke, M.D., Department of Obstetrics and Gynecology, Stanford University Medical Center, 300 Pasteur Drive, H333, Stanford, CA 94305, USA

Jeremy Thompson, M.D., Department of Surgery, Chelsea-Westminster Hospital, Westminster Ward, 369 Fulham Road, London, SW10-9NH, United Kingdom

Nicholas Topley, Ph.D., Institute of Nephrology, University of Wales College of Medicine, Cardiff Royal Infirmary, Newport Road, Cardiff, CF2 15Z, United Kingdom

Togas Tulandi, M.D., Division of Reproductive Endocrinology and Infertility, Department of Obstetrics and Gynecology, McGill University, Royal Victoria Hospital, Women's Pavilion, 687 Pine Avenue, West Montreal, P.Q., H3A 1A1, Canada

Arnaud Wattiez, M.D., Department of Obstetrics, Gynecology and Reproductive Medicine, Polyclinique de l'Hôtel Dieu, Université Clermont-Ferrand, 13, boulevard Charles-De-Gaulle, 63003 Clermont-Ferrand, Cedex 1 France

Steven D. Wexner, M.D., Department of Colorectal Surgery, Cleveland Clinic Florida, 3000 West Cypress Creek Road, Fort Lauderdale, FL 33309-1743, USA

David M. Wiseman, Ph.D., Synechion, 6757 Arapaho Road, Suite 711, Dallas, TX 75248, USA

Section 1
Peritoneum and Peritoneal Repair

1

Peritoneum, Peritoneal Healing, and Adhesion Formation

Gere S. diZerega

CONTENTS

The Peritoneum

Peritoneum is the most extensive serous membrane in the body. The surface area of the peritoneum is generally equal to that of the skin (Table 1.1).[1] It forms a closed sac in the male and an open sac in the female because the ends of the fallopian tubes are not covered by peritoneum. The peritoneum lines the walls of the abdomen (parietal peritoneum) and is reflected over the viscera (visceral peritoneum). It consists of two layers, a loose connective tissue and a mesothelium. The connective tissue is arranged into loose bundles that interlace in a plane parallel to the surface. There are numerous elastic fibers, especially in the deeper layer of the parietal peritoneum, and comparatively few connective tissue cells. The peritoneum serves to minimize friction, facilitating free movement between abdominal viscera, to resist or localize infection, and to store fat, especially in the greater omentum.

The intraabdominal surface of the peritoneum is a continuous sheet of mesothelial cells attached to the abdominal wall and viscera by areolar tissue (subserous fascia). Where the peritoneum is freely mobile, loose connective or "subserous" tissue, rich in elastin and containing varying numbers of fat cells, connects the peritoneum with the underlying tissue. The peritoneum is well supplied with blood vessels and lymphatics, which give rise to a rich capillary network. The mesothelial cells form a continuous layer that rests upon loose mesenchymal connective tissue, a basal lamina, and basement membrane. The mesentery contains a loose network of collagenous and elastic fibers, scattered fibroblasts, macrophages, mast cells, and a varying number of fat cells.[2]

TABLE 1.1. Peritoneal surface area (cm^2)

	Adult	Infant
Intestine	4,815	665
Liver	624	139
Anterior abdominal wall	411	79
Diaphragm	424	35
Stomach	631	32
Omentum	1,581	29
Mesentery	1,469	32
Spleen	149	25
Pelvic organs	275	29
Total peritoneal area	10,379	1,065
Weight (kg)	59.3	2.743
Peritoneal area (cm^2)/body weight (kg)	177	383

From Esperanca and Collins.[1]

Histology

Omentum is covered by mesothelium on both sides, which is folded over the loose connective tissue. The membrane is pierced by numerous holes or fenestrations to form collagenous bundles covered by mesothelial cells that supply the blood vessels. Thicker areas of omentum contain many macrophages, small lymphocytes, plasma cells, a few eosinophils, and mast cells. In areas where macrophages accumulate in large numbers the omentum appears grossly to contain "milky spots."[3]

The mesothelium that covers the peritoneum consists of a single layer of flattened cells with microvilli, peripheral vesicles, and discrete bundles of cytoplasmic microfilaments (Fig. 1.1). The cells are attached to one another by desmosomes. The diaphragmatic surface is covered by a single layer of mesothelial cells that contain regional variations. Dome-shaped cells with microvillous projections are arrayed in bands that extend from the

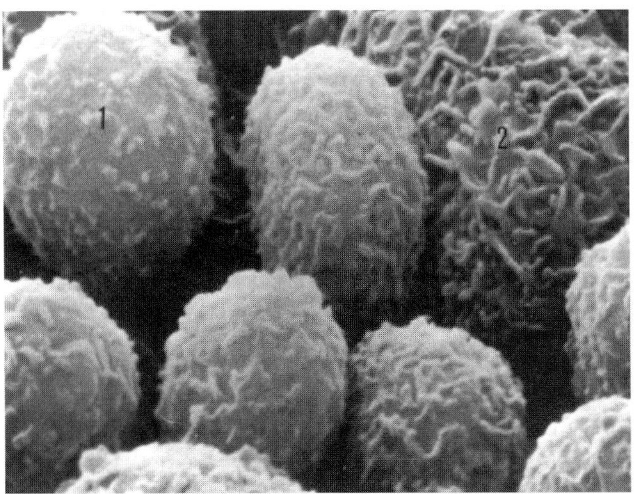

FIG. 1.1. Features of mesothelial cells on the peritoneal surface. Cell *1* has numerous microvilli, while cell *2* has thin folds of the membrane. These cells are loosely attached; as a result, they can be readily detached during peritoneal mobilization during surgery. ×6200.[4]

musculotendinous junction toward the rib cage. Adjacent cell margins are separated to form mesothelial pores located over lymphatic vessels. Lymphatic endothelial cells form a channel extending from the peritoneal cavity directly into the diaphragmatic lymphatics. The second type of cell, which constitutes the peritoneal covering of the diaphragm, is a flat cell that contains numerous microvilli on its apical surfaces and overlies a thin layer of connective tissue. The cell margins of the flattened cell are in close apposition and do not form pores.[4]

The mesothelial covering of the peritoneum may account for the formation of mesenteric cysts occasionally found in the parietal peritoneum or within supporting structures (mesentery or ligaments). These cysts are thought to arise from embryonic nests of either mesothelium, gut, or urogenital ridge. These cysts can be filled with serous fluid or blood and can range from 1 to 2 or from 15 to 20 cm in diameter. The cysts occur either in a single cyst or in multiple clusters. Most neoplasms of the peritoneum are metastatic, including ovarian, pancreatic, or other gastrointestinal carcinomas. Primary peritoneal neoplasms are rare and present as mesotheliomas.

Ultrastructure of Peritoneum

Pfeiffer et al.[5] described the ultrastructure of the visceral peritoneum covering the stomach, small intestine, and colon of the immature pig using the scanning electron microscope. The peritoneal surface was composed of a single layer of loosely attached squamous epithelial cells that contained scant microvilli. The outer surface contained an undulating surface with a cobblestone appearance.

This monolayer is loosely attached to the underlying connective tissue. At high magnification, an abundance of long, widely spaced microvilli cover the apical surface of the mesothelial cells (see Fig. 1.1). Adjacent mesothelial cells are either joined by desmosomes or are loosely connected at their peripheral edges. The mesothelium is separated from underlying collagenous bundles by basement membrane. The serosal connective tissue base, upon which the mesothelium of the small intestine rests, is less compacted than that of the stomach.

The apical surface of mesothelial cells contains an abundance of long microvilli that increase the functional surface area of the peritoneum (2.5 μm long × 0.08 μm in diameter).[6] Microvilli projecting from the mesothelial cells dramatically increase the functional surface area of both parietal and visceral peritoneum for absorption and secretion. Most of the mesothelial cells contain motile cilia.[6] A role for mesothelial microvilli in transport function is supported by the absorptive and exudative ability of the mesothelium.[7–11] Transport functions of gastrointestinal mesothelium utilize several pathways, including pinocytosis, transmembrane diffusion,[9] and excursion between cell boundaries.[11]

Basement Membrane

The peritoneum is supported by a basement membrane supporting both visceral and parietal surfaces (Fig. 1.2). A thin layer of loose areolar tissue some 2 to 3 mm in thickness underlies both parietal and visceral mesothelium. It contains bundles of collagen fibers oriented in different layers of variable complexity according to anatomic site.[12] The basement membrane over the stomach is 8 to 10 μm thick. It consists of a delicate fibrillar plexus and interwoven reticulum fibers. The orientation of the reticulum and fibroblasts in longitudinal to the plane of expansion appropriate for the anatomic site. Connection with the underlying network of elastin involves collagen and mucopolysaccharides. The deep longitudinal elastin network is closely connected with underlying collagen. The elastin fibers from the lower surface of the longitudinal network penetrate into the more deeply located collagen, forming a collagen–elastin lattice.

Blood and Lymphatic Vessels

Blood and lymphatic vessels of the peritoneum are found in the deep collagenous layer. Above this are layers of collagen, mucopolysaccharides, elastin, connective or mesenchymal tissue, superficial collagen, and mesothelial cells. In some areas, for instance, in intestinal peritoneum, fatty lobules are situated under the elastin within the deep collagen lattice.

Blood vessels of the mesentery or intestinal peritoneum contain adventitial sheaths: elastin for the arteries,

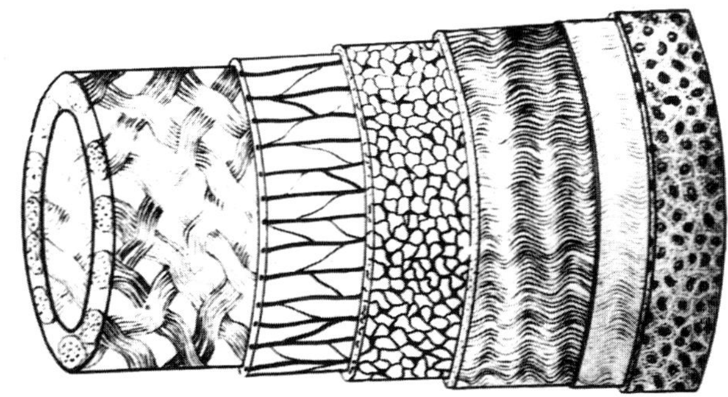

FIG. 1.2. General scheme of construction of the peritoneum of the small intestine in humans and the fibroarchitecture of the various layers. The innermost layer is a collagen lattice surrounded by rich microcirculation. A layer of glycosaminoglycans or mucopolysaccharide proteins is covered by elastin. The surface mesothelial cells rest upon a connective tissue matrix of proteins including collagen.[12]

collagen for the veins. The sheaths extend onto the capillaries. The deepest vessels of the peritoneum are parallel with the musculature underlying the peritoneum. More superficial vessels, penetrating to the thickness of the deep collagenous layer, are parallel with the spiral arterioles that prevent overextension of the vessels which may occur during peritoneal stretching.

Numerous lymphatic channels lead from the peritoneal cavity, especially from the lower surface of the diaphragm. With each diaphragmatic excursion, relatively large quantities of lymph flow out of the peritoneal cavity into the thoracic duct. If these ducts become occluded (i.e., cancer, inflammation), the return of protein to the circulation is blocked. As a result, intraperitoneal osmotic pressure rises and ascites ensues.[13]

Free cells including erythrocytes and epithelial cells enter stomata that underlie the accumulated cells. Likewise, fluids, large molecules, and particulate materials are able to enter the diaphragmatic lymphatics through stomata.[14] This movement is indicated by the rapid removal of trypan blue dye and colloidal carbon injected intraperitoneally from this cavity into the mediastinal lymphatic vessels and lymph nodes. The importance of the structural integrity of the stoma as a continuous passageway from the peritoneal cavity into the lymphatic lumen is underscored by the loss of this passageway when the diaphragmatic surface is completely occluded by chemical or surgical abrasions that prevent fluid and cellular removal from the peritoneal cavity.[15]

Mesothelial Histology

The diaphragmatic mesothelium contains two morphologically distinct cell types: flattened and dome-shaped cells.[16–18] Flattened cells are in close apposition to occluded junctions. In contrast, margins of the dome-shaped cells are often separated by stomata that open into lymphatic vessels.[19] Many of the cells migrate over the mesothelial surface, whereas others enter submesothelial lymphatic vessels via stomata (mesothelial pores). These pores may provide a passageway for the removal of fluids as well as large molecules and cells from the peritoneal cavity.[14,20,21]

Stomata are present at sites where margins of several lymphatic endothelial cells span the submesothelial connective tissue. This arrangement creates a passageway between the peritoneal cavity and lymphatic lumen. To account for the increased number of stomata observed after peritoneal stimulation, mesothelial cells may respond by retracting their cell margins. Contraction and relaxation of the diaphragmatic muscles during inhalation and exhalation probably leads to widening and narrowing of stomatal orifices. Therefore, a number of passageways would be maintained for a constant removal of fluids and cells by the diaphragmatic lymphatics under normal physiologic conditions.

Peritoneal Fluid

The peritoneal cavity of the human usually contains 5 to 20 mL of serous exudate, which varies widely depending on the physiologic condition. In the female, this volume changes during the menstrual cycle to reach maximal levels after ovulation (Fig. 1.3). When pressure in the hepatic sinusoids rises more than 5 to 10 mmHg, fluid containing large amounts of protein transudes through the liver surface into the abdominal cavity. Excess fluid in the peritoneal cavity is either a transudate (specific gravity, <1.010), which accumulates (ascites) from peritoneal obstruction or circulatory differences (cardiac failure, portal hypertension, hypofibrinogenemia, etc.), or an exudate (specific gravity, >1.020), which arises from inflammation. The hepatic resistance to portal blood flow induces a capillary pressure in the visceral peritoneum that is higher than elsewhere in the body.

The pH of peritoneal fluid ranges between 7.5 and 8.0 and contains significant buffering capacity. Because of the hydrostatic pressure gradient between plasma and the peritoneal compartment, normal peritoneal fluid also contains many of the plasma proteins in about 50% of the plasma concentration. Plasma that accumulates in the peritoneal cavity provides a source of fibrinogen. The resultant fibrin may play an important role in the aggregation of peritoneal cells on the diaphragmatic surface and over the visceral or parietal surfaces. The amounts of peritoneal fluid and plasma greatly increase in the peritoneal cavity during postsurgical repair or following an inflammatory insult.[22]

Human peritoneal fluid contains at least four types of differentiated cells: macrophages, mesothelial cells, lym-

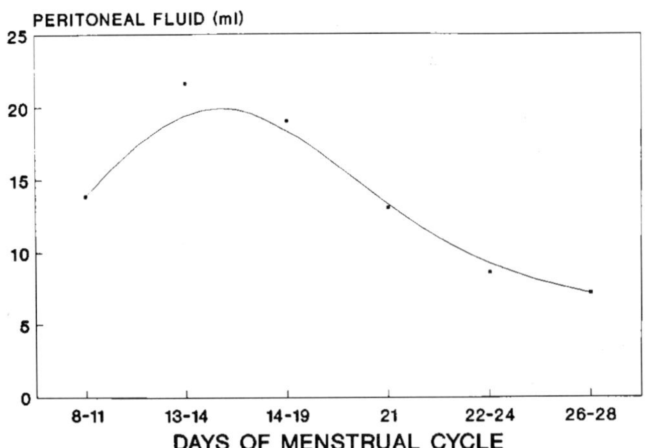

FIG. 1.3. The volume of fluid recovered from the peritoneal cavity of patients undergoing laparoscopy at various days of the menstrual cycle peaks around the time of ovulation and declines to approximately 7 mL at the end of the menstrual cycle. These data are the mean volume from three to six patients per time point.[22]

phocytes, and polymorphonuclear leukocytes.[22] The macrophages and mesothelial cells represent the two major types of cells, each group constituting about 36% of the population, while the lymphocytes and polymorphonuclear cells comprise 18% and 7% of the population, respectively. A similar distribution of cellular elements was identified in cul-de-sac aspirates of women during the menstrual cycle, pregnancy, post partum, and menopause.[23–25] Cellular content of fluids from women 35 years or older consists of mesothelial cells (25%), lymphocytes (23%), erythrocytes (15%), polymorphonuclear cells (8%), histiocytes (4%), and squamous cells.[23]

It is well known that postsurgical macrophages play an important role in the repair of injured peritoneum.[26] Following stimulation, macrophages produce factors that modulate the proliferation of fibroblasts by both stimulation (macrophage-derived growth factor, interleukin-1, prostaglandin F_2, and transforming growth factor-β) and inhibition (prostaglandin E_2, fibroblast growth inhibitor, and interferon-α).[27,28] The secretory products of macrophages at various times after surgery initially suppress (during the initial 48 hours) and later enhance (following 48–54 hours) the proliferation of mesothelial cells.[29] Macrophages are also critical in the formation of connective tissue matrix and mesothelial syncytium.[30] Thus, macrophages stimulate the secretion of connective tissue protein, such as fibronectin, porteoglycans, collagen, and proteases such as collagenase and elastase.

Macrophages are also known to modulate fibroblast proliferation and stimulation.[29–31] Surgical trauma to the peritoneum, in the absence of infection, elicits a rapid and transient influx of polymorphonuclear leukocytes (PMNs) into the peritoneal cavity, followed by accumulation of large mononuclear cells, mainly macrophages.[31,32] These recruited macrophages may also secrete cytokines.

A number of cytokines and hormones that can be found in peritoneal fluid correlate with ongoing clinical events of the reproductive organs or gastrointestinal systems. Prorennin in large concentrations can be found in the peritoneal fluid of patients with ruptured luteal cysts or hyperstimulation (see also Chapter 2).[33]

Endometriosis

A significant body of information has been assembled concerning the contents, volume, and characteristics of peritoneal fluid in patients with endometriosis.[34,35] Secretory products of macrophages such as tumor necrosis factor-α (TNF-α),[36] growth factors,[37] interleukin-1 (IL-1),[38] interleukin-8 (IL-8), and a chemoattrachant cytokine for neutrophils[39] are also found in increased quantities in the peritoneal fluid of women with endometriosis.[40]

Peritoneal fluid in women with endometriosis is proinflammatory. Numbers of macrophages, as well as their activation level, are increased with endometriosis.[41] Activation of macrophages involves changes in size, rate of spread, adherence, enzyme production, oxygen consumption, prostaglandin release, and increased secretory activity.[42] Hill et al.[43] found peritoneal leukocyte concentrations to be the highest in stage I endometriosis versus stage IV. Akoum et al.[44] reported increased levels of monocyte chemotactic factor-1 (MCP-1) in the peritoneal fluid of patients with endometriosis. MCP-1 is secreted by activated macrophages and by stimulated epithelial cells.

The levels of IL-1β and TNF in peritoneal fluid and production of IL-1β and TNF by peritoneal macrophages were determined in patients with benign gynecologic disease.[45] The level of IL-1β was elevated in acute pelvic inflammatory disease (PID) and stages I and II endometriosis groups compared with normals. The level of TNF was elevated in peritoneal fluid from patients with PID and endometriosis (stages III and IV). Peritoneal macrophages produce IL-1β and TNF in vitro in the absence of stimulants. The levels of IL-1β and TNF are presumably linked to the activation of peritoneal macrophages.

Contradictory data have been reported regarding immunoglobulins (Ig) in the peritoneal fluid. Some authors found increased concentrations of IgG, IgM, and IgA,[46] an increased production of IgG and IgA in the culture of B lymphocytes obtained from peritoneal fluid,[47] and elevated titers of antibodies against endometrial antigens in endometriosis patients compared with controls.[48] However, other authors reported similar[49] or significantly lower concentrations of IgG, IgA, and IgM in peritoneal fluid from endometriosis patients compared with controls[50,51] or differences in the peritoneal fluid antibodies to autologous endometrial and implant antigens.[52] One group showed significant amounts of autoantibodies to endometrium in only 5 of 22 patients with mild forms of endometriosis.[52] Another group showed that antiendometrial antibodies are more common in serum from women with endometriosis than in controls without the disease.[53] Whether these apparently conflicting results reflect biologic differences or variation in assay, methodology, or disease states is unclear.

Inflammatory Disease

In the peritoneal fluid of women with laparoscopically confirmed PID, plasminogen activator inhibitor antigen (PAI-1-Ag), tissue PA-Ag (tPA-Ag), and urokinase-Ag (uPA-Ag) are elevated[54] (Tables 1.2A and B). Because the tPA activity was not elevated, the bulk of the tPA-Ag may be complexed to PAI, thereby quenching tPA activity. Parallel with the increase in tPA-Ag in the peritoneal fluid of patients with PID, Dorr et al. found that the peri-

TABLE 1.2A. Parameters of fibrinolytic activity in peritoneal fluid of patients with pelvic inflammatory disease (PID) and control group

Peritoneal fluid	PID group[a] ($n = 10$)		Control group[a] ($n = 9$)		p
PAI-1-Ag (ng/mL)	296	105–332	13.4	11–12.1	0.0003
tPA-Ag (ng/mL)	74.2	36.7–123.3	4	2.3–6.2	0.0002
tPA-act (mLU/mL)	13	0.5–212	98	23–134	>0.05
uPA-AG (ng/mL)	19.0	9.6–33.7	5.1	4.1–7.6	0.0015
scu-PA (ng/mL)	1.65	1.4–2.7	1.5	1.2–1.8	>0.05
tcu-PA (ng/mL)	<0.1		<0.1		
TDP (μg/mL)	585	390–750	27	15–48	0.0002
FbDP (μg/mL)	497.5	320–660	13	9.6–24	0.0002

PAI, plasminogen activator inhibitor; tPA, tissue plasminogen activator, uPA, urokinase plasminogen activator; scu-PA, single-chain uPA; tcu-PA, two-chain uPA; TDP, total fibrin and fibrinogen degradation products; FbDP, fibrin degradation products; Ag, antigen; act, activity.
[a]Median and interquartile ranges.

TABLE 1.2B. Parameters of fibrinolytic activity in plasma of patients with PID and control group

Plasma	PID group[a] ($n = 10$)		Control group[a] ($n = 9$)		p
PAI-1-Ag (ng/mL)	24.05	14.7–34.9	12.9	9.2–19.8	>0.05
tPA-Ag (ng/mL)	2.6	1.4–9.8	4.8	3.9–8.2	>0.05
tPA-act (mLU/mL)	42.5	8–122	28	15–93	>0.05
uPA-Ag (ng/mL)	3.6	3.2–4.2	2.7	2.4–2.9	0.0101

PAI-Ag, plasminogen activator inhibitor antigen; tPA-Ag, tissue plasminogen activator antigen; tPA-act, tissue plasminogen activator activity; uPA-Ag, urokinase plasminogen activator antigen.
[a]Median and interquartile ranges.
From Dorr et al.[54]

toneal fluid uPA-Ag concentration was significantly higher in the PID group than in the control group.[54] The combination of an increase in tPA and an increase in uPA is consistent with different sources of the two plasminogen activators: uPA from inflamed tissue is endothelial cells (with leakage to the peritoneal fluid) and tPA either from the peritoneum, peritoneal macrophages, or an exudate from the fallopian tubes.

The proinflammatory nature of peritoneal fluid after surgery as well as endometriosis led a number of clinicians to evaluate the utility of corticosteroids in reducing adhesion formation after surgery. Their reports are generally negative,[55–57] although other clinical trials showed decreased adhesion scores[58] and increased pregnancy rates.[59]

Embryology

During embryonic and fetal life, the mesentery and visceral ligaments expand or fuse. The greater omentum is an expanded sacculation of the dorsal mesentery of the stomach. During development, its surfaces fuse with each other and drape the anterior aspect of the intestine. After 4.5 to 5 months of fetal life, the peritoneum can be identified as a layer of mesothelium with a thin mesenchymal lining. Both lymphatic and blood vessels within these tissues are in close contact because of the absence of intervening fibrous layers. Through months 6 and 7 in utero, the peritoneum develops a deep latticed collagenous layer that forms the basement membrane. Although visceral peritoneum covering the intestine does not contain elastin fibers at this time, the parietal peritoneum of the subdiaphragm is richly endowed with an elastin network. By 6 to 7 months of fetal life, the deep collagenous layer begins to appear at the time the fetal peritoneum consists primarily of mesothelium and basement membrane. At this time, the elastic fibers are absent. At 8 months of fetal life, fibroblasts align adjacent to the basement membrane, which elongate in the axis of greatest physiologic tension. The elastin network becomes apparent at about 9 months of fetal life.

In between the mesothelial linings, mesenchyme is still present to a greater or lesser extent. This mesenchyme is relatively broad in the younger stages, but diminishes with maturation. With respect to the intraperitoneal organs it is referred to as "meso," bounded by mesothelial linings and containing vessels and nerves that supply the organ.

In later developmental stages, the visceral peritoneum is firmly attached to the capsule of the adjoining organs. It is vascularized, innervated, and lymphatically drained via vessels and nerves that also supply these organs and can therefore be considered a part of the body wall. It is attached to a submesothelial layer of loose connective tissue, which in turn adheres to the deep body fascia. The parietal peritoneum contains nerves possessing thermo-, chemo-, and mechanoreceptors, whereas the nerves of the visceral peritoneum do not possess such specialized receptors but instead form networks that respond to tension.[60]

Anatomy

Subdivisions of Greater Sac

The peritoneal cavity is the potential space between the parietal and visceral peritoneum. In general, the parietal and visceral peritoneum are in direct contact with one another (Fig. 1.4). The peritoneal cavity is divided into two distinct compartments: (1) the greater sac is the peritoneal cavity per se and (2) the lesser sac or omental bursa comprises the dorsal surface of the stomach. The two sacs are distinguished by a constriction between the liver and duodenum, named the epiploic foramen or foramen of Winslow.[61]

The greater sac is subdivided by the greater omentum, transverse colon, and transverse mesocolon into an upper, anterior part, the supramesocolic compartment, and a lower, posterior part, the inframesocolic compartment. These compartments form channels or recesses that determine how or where peritoneal fluid gravitates or spreads. The supramesocolic compartment is subdivided by the liver into subphrenic and subhepatic spaces. The inframesocolic compartment is further divided by the mesentery of the small intestine into right (upper) and left (lower) parts. The latter drains into the pelvis. The paracolic grooves or gutters are longitudinal depressions lateral to the ascending and descending colon.

In some instances the peritoneum constricts to form bands that lead to abnormal intestinal fixation. These bands are considered to be congenital and are typically attached to the duodenum, jejunum, or transverse colon.[62]

Ligaments or Folds

The term mesenteris refers to the peritoneal suspension of the small intestine; "entery" indicates intestine and the prefix "meso," a general prefix for peritoneum, is used to identify the suspending folds of other organs in the peritoneal cavity, for example, mesocolon and mesovarium. When these connective tissues are condensed into a distinct bundle they are referred to as ligaments. Most ligaments contain blood vessels and nerves. In contrast, viscera more tightly attached to the abdominal wall having only the exposed surface covered by peritoneum are referred to as retroperitoneal viscera. Accordingly, many retroperitoneal structures are also covered at least in part by parietal peritoneum. A large portion of the dorsal aspect of the diaphragmatic surface of the liver is not covered by peritoneum. In the adult human, a 15-cm area of the liver bordered anteriorly by the anterior leaf of the coronary ligament is termed the bare area of the liver. The posterior boundary of this area is the posterior leaf of the coronary ligament where the peritoneum is reflected from the liver to the diaphragm. Although the bare area of the liver is not covered by visceral peritoneum, this site is not directly exposed to the peritoneal cavity because of the communications of the anterior and posterior coronary ligaments with reflections of the adjacent parietal peritoneum.

Innervation

The parietal peritoneum is supplied by nerves from the adjacent body wall, the subdiaphragmatic part by the

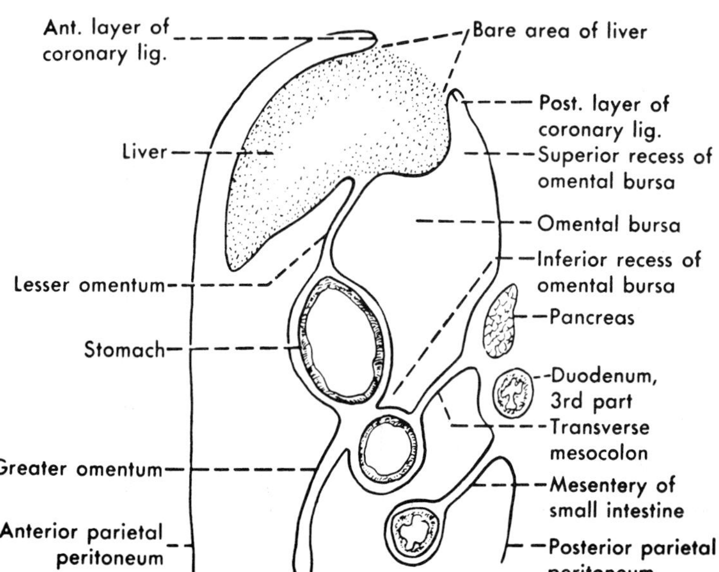

FIG. 1.4. The disposition of the peritoneum in a sagittal section through the abdominal cavity.[61] All the abdominal pelvic viscera are covered by peritoneum, except for the ovaries and the diaphragmatic aspect of the liver (bare area of liver).

phrenic nerves and the remainder by the thoracoabdominal and subcostal nerves and by branches of the lumbosacral plexus.[61] Both sensory and vasomotor nerves supply the peritoneum. Most of the parietal peritoneum is sensitive to pain. Painful stimuli to the anterior and lateral regions are localized to the point of stimulation. By contrast, painful stimuli to the central part of the diaphragmatic peritoneum are referred to the shoulder. Painful stimuli to the peripheral part of the diaphragmatic peritoneum are felt in an intercostal space. The roots of mesenteries contain pain fibers that are sensitive to stretch. Sensory supply to the parietal peritoneum covering the diaphragm involves the phrenic nerves as well as the intercostals. Thus, diaphragmatic pain may be perceived either at the base of the neck or shoulder (from C-3, C-4, and C-5 via the phrenic nerves) or in the abdominal wall. Because the parietal peritoneum is innervated by branches of the spinal nerves that supply the abdominal wall, peritoneal involvement in visceral disease provides pain sensation through the lower intercostal nerves. Pain fibers have not been clearly demonstrated for visceral peritoneum; rather, visceral pain is perceived via the viscus itself or by stretch or spasm of smooth muscles of the viscus.[61]

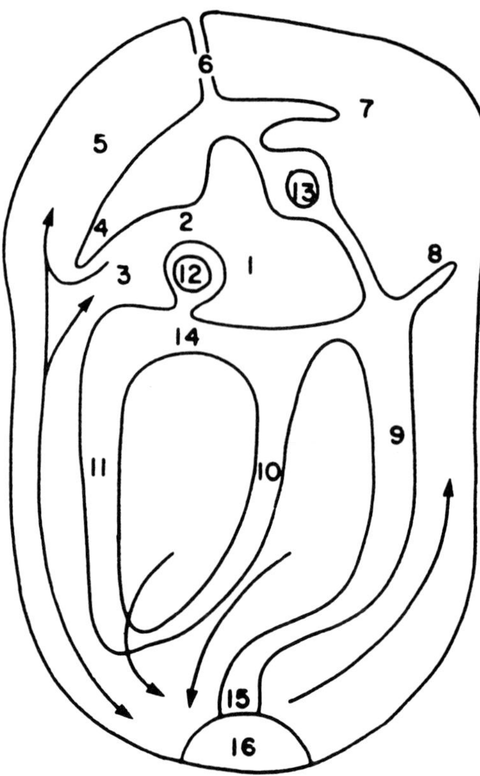

FIG. 1.5. Circulation of fluid in the peritoneal cavity. *Solid arrows* indicate the flow generated by diaphragmatic movement and absorption of material from the diaphragmatic lymphatics. *1,* lesser sac; *2,* foramen of Winslow; *3,* Morison's pouch; *4,* right triangular ligament; *5,* right subphrenic space; *6,* falciform ligament; *7,* left subphrenic space; *8,* phrenocolic ligament; *9,* bare area of the descending colon; *10,* root of the small-bowel mesentery; *11,* bare area of ascending colon; *12,* duodenum; *13,* esophagus; *14,* root of the transverse mesocolon; *15,* bare area of rectum; *16,* bladder.[64]

Peritoneal Circulation

The intraperitoneal circulation follows the pattern shown in Fig. 1.5. The routes by which intraperitoneal effusions spread and the spaces in which they accumulate have been studied in surgical patients. Radiographic contrast medium was injected at selected intraperitoneal sites at the conclusion of operations for removal of the gallbladder or appendix. The spread of the contrast medium was followed by roentgenographic examinations taken from 3 to 87 hours after operation.[63] In roentgenograms taken from 3 to 8 hours after surgery, contrast material was widely disseminated into several of the peritoneal spaces, whether it was introduced into the upper or the lower abdomen.

In general, the distance a material spreads depends upon its volume, viscosity, and specific gravity. Movement both from Morison's pouch downward and from the cecal region upward was primarily along the right paracolic gutter and upward from the pelvic space along the left paracolic gutter. The mobility of the small bowel tends to limit the accumulation of fluid in the central portion of the peritoneal cavity under normal circumstances.[64] The most dependent recess is the cul-de-sac that lies between the rectum and the body of the uterus. The perirectal circulation favors unilateral spread of exudate because the phrenocolic ligament, which spans the diaphragm, spleen, and splenic flexure of the colon, interrupts the flow into the left subphrenic space during respiration.[64]

Peritoneal Reepithelialization

It was shown in 1919 that peritoneal healing differs from that of skin. Hertzler[65] observed that when a defect is made in the parietal peritoneum "the entire surface becomes epithelialized simultaneously and not gradually from the borders as in epidermidalization of skin wounds." Multiplication and migration of mesothelial cells from the margin of the wound may play a small part in the regenerative process but cannot play a major part because new mesothelium develops in the center of a large wound at the same time as it develops in the center of a smaller one. The granulation and contraction that occur around the edges of skin wounds do not occur during peritoneal healing. The morphologic organization of new blood vessels after peritoneal trauma was evaluated in Wistar rats at deperitonealized sidewall sites covered with Silastic.[66] Peritoneal angiogenesis was evident on day 4 in 20% of the rats and progressively increased to 100% by day 12.

General agreement exists between investigators on the time required for regeneration of the mesothelial layer. Ellis et al.[67] and Hubbard et al.[68] reported that healing occurs in 5 to 6 days in the case of parietal peritoneum. Peritoneal defects of 2 × 2 cm and 0.5 × 0.5 cm were both entirely covered by a continuous sheet of mesothelium 3 days after wounding.[67] Glucksman[69] reported that the visceral mesothelium covering the terminal ileum heals in 5 days, and Eskeland[70] demonstrated that regeneration of the mesothelial layer of parietal peritoneum is not complete until 8 days. Raftery[71] confirmed that parietal peritoneum of the rat is healed within 8 days.

Mesothelial Regeneration

Eskeland[70] described the cellular sequence of repair in the parietal peritoneum of rats after either burning or stripping of the peritoneum off the body wall (Fig. 1.6). Both small and large wounds contained a continuous layer of mesothelial cells by day 8 after injury. Wounds that measured 36 mm in diameter were completely covered with new mesothelium at day 8. The intact peritoneum adjacent to the wound (1–3 mm) formed the second day after injury until completion of mesothelial regeneration contained mitotic figures and evidence of migratory activity. Differences between intact mesothelial cells peripheral to the wound and the cytology of the cells on the wound surface were distinct at day 3 after injury. Thereafter, the cytologic differences between the cell types became less evident as the cells on the wound surface became more like mature mesothelial cells.

Raftery[71] studied the regeneration of parietal and visceral peritoneum using scanning electron microscopic evaluation of healing peritoneal defects in the rat. Twelve hours after injury, numerous polymorphonuclear leukocytes (PMNs) were seen intangled in fibrin strands. Very little cellular infiltrate was found in the depths of the wound compared to the wound surface. At 24 to 36 hours after wounding, the number of cells in the superficial part of the wound was greatly increased; most of the increase in cell number resulted from infiltration by macrophages. The macrophages were intertwined with the filaments of fibrin projecting from the wound surface. The base of the wound remained relatively acellular.

At 2 days most of the wound surface was covered with a single layer of macrophages supported by a fibrin scaffold. Two additional cell types were also seen on the wound surface: a cell that looked like a primitive mesenchymal cell, which was also seen in small numbers at the base of the wound, and islets of mesothelial cells that were interconnected by desmosomes and tight junctions. No basement membrane was evident beneath these cells.

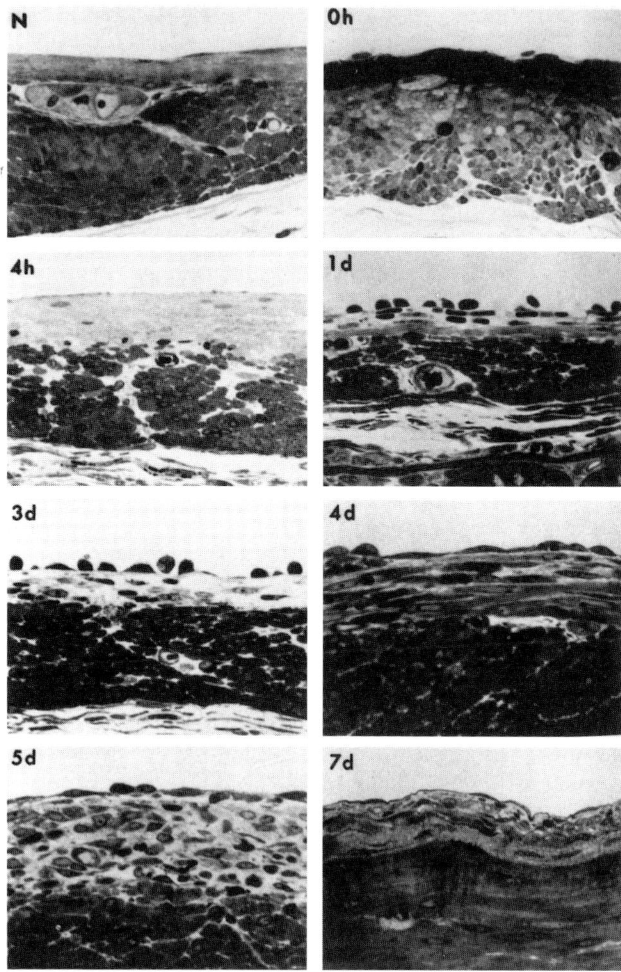

FIG. 1.6. Histology of cecum showing various stages of damage and recovery after drying injury of surface: normal cecum (*N*); immediately after drying (*0h*); 4 hours (*4h*); 1 day (*1d*); 3 days (*3d*); 4 days (*4d*); 5 days (*5d*); 7 days (*7d*). ×400.[70]

Three days after injury the number of primitive mesenchymal cells on the wound surface increased, although macrophages were still the most prevalent cell type. The base of the wound contained scattered mesenchymal cells and some proliferating fibroblasts. The cells on the wound surface at 3 days were similar in appearance to cells in the deeper layers of the wound and were similar to primitive mesenchymal cells.

At 4 days, cells resembling primitive mesenchymal cells or proliferating fibroblasts on the wound surface were in contact with one another. In some areas healing appeared complete at 5 days, as a single layer of mesothelial cells was present on the wound surface interconnected by desmosomes and tight junctions. No basement membrane was found beneath the mesothelial cells of parietal peritoneum or cecum at this stage, although one was often present beneath those covering the liver. Thus, peritoneal healing of parietal peritoneum was associated with basement membrane formation at this time, in contrast to visceral peritoneum which although similar in appearance on the surface did not contain a basement membrane.

In other areas healing was far less advanced. Primitive mesenchymal cells were present both on the surface and in the base of the wound. At days 5 to 6, the number of macrophages was clearly decreased from the wound surface while most of the wound surface was covered by mesothelial cells. At day 7 after surgery, the appearance of the wound resembled that of day 6 except that a discontinuous basement membrane was now evident beneath the mesothelial cells lining the parietal peritoneum and covering the cecum. At day 8 a continuous layer of mesothelial cells was present over the wound surface.

A single layer of mesothelial cells resting on a continuous basement membrane was seen at day 10. Fibroblasts in the base of the wound were arranged with their long axis parallel to the wound surface, and bundles of collagen were present between the fibroblasts.

Watters and Buck[4] studied peritoneal repair after removal of only the surface layer of mesothelium. Special attention was given so as not to damage the underlying connective tissues. The denuded areas were examined by scanning electron microscopy through 7 days. Normal parietal mesothelial surface of the rat peritoneal cavity contained a mat of microvilli that obscured the contour of the cells to which they were attached. New cells were seen in the surface at 30 minutes after injury; at 8 hours most of the surface contained new cells with a variety of forms. These authors found a more rapid recovering of the damaged peritoneal surface than other investigators, perhaps because the depth of the injury was less. These new cells were scattered over the entire surface of the injured site. At 3 days after surgery many of the surface cells contained short microvilli, which increased in length by 4 days. A virtually normal appearance via scanning electron microscopy (SEM) was apparent at 7 days.

Visceral Versus Parietal Peritoneum

Visceral peritoneum appears to differ little in its healing properties from the parietal peritoneum. Light microscopy indicates that the liver acquires a new mesothelial covering 1 day earlier than either cecum or parietal peritoneum.[71] A discontinuous basement membrane is present beneath mesothelial cells covering the liver at 5 days. In contrast, discontinuous basement membrane does not form beneath the mesothelial cells of the parietal peritoneum or cecum until 7 days after surgery. Raftery hypothesized that the liver (viscera) provides a firmer substrate for development of a new mesothelium than either the parietes or the cecum, both of which are subject to greater distension.

By the fifth day after injury, differences between parietal and visceral peritoneal repair are evident. On the surface of wounds in the parietal peritoneum, cells appear to be uniform, containing many microvilli resembling proliferating fibroblasts connected by tight junctions. On the surface of the visceral peritoneal wounds, a continuous layer of mesothelial cells forms, joined together by tight junctions or desmosomes. Although a basement membrane is present beneath some of the mesothelial cells covering the liver at this stage, frequent breaks in the basement membrane occur. Basement membrane can be found beneath the mesothelial cells of the new visceral peritoneum but not beneath the parietal peritoneum.

Seven days after injury, continuous layers of mesothelial cells cover the surface of both the visceral and parietal peritoneum. A basement membrane forms beneath the mesothelial cells in most areas but gaps are still visible. Dense bundles of collagen are present at the basement membrane formed primarily by fibroblasts. By the eighth day, the basement membrane beneath the mesothelial cells of both types of peritoneum is continuous.

Neonate

Intestinal obstruction caused by adhesion formation was reported to be more prevalent after abdominal surgery in the infant or neonate in comparison to the adult.[72] Peritoneal repair occurs more rapidly in the immature rat than in mature animals.[67] Accordingly, peritoneal healing in the neonate or pediatric patient manifests a clinically different response to injury in comparison to reperitonealization in the adult.

Raftery[73] described the healing of visceral and parietal peritoneum in the immature rat at various times after standardized surgical injury to the liver capsule and parietal peritoneum. Although the wounds looked hemorrhagic and uneven 24 hours after injury, they were smooth and glistening at 3 days, and usually indistinguishable from the normal surrounding parietal peritoneum at 5 days. The cellular changes that accompanied these gross morphologic changes were the same as those described for the adult rat except that mesothelial regeneration occurred more rapidly. By 2 days after injury, the acute inflammatory response had subsided, leaving primarily macrophages and fibroblasts on the wound surface.

Active fibroblast proliferation occurred at the base of the wound. By 5 days the number of macrophages had diminished, leaving only fibroblasts. These fibroblasts came together to form the new mesothelium by 7 days, compared with 8 days in the adult. In the case of visceral peritoneum, mesothelial regeneration was complete by 5 days compared to 7 days in the adult rat. Again, there was no difference in the rate of healing between large and small peritoneal defects.

Source of New Mesothelial Cells

Difficulties of tissue preparation and identification of primitive cell types, as well as availability of vascular and peritoneal fluid and adjacent tissue, have caused the healing of peritoneal defects (i.e., the cytology or histology of peritoneal repair or mesothelial regeneration) to remain a controversial subject (Table 1.3; Fig. 1.7A–D). Some investigators have suggested that cells detach from the adjacent intact peritoneum and become implanted on the wound surface where they proliferate to form a continuous layer of mesothelium.[74,75]

Ellis et al.[67] assessed the origin of the cells that form the surface of healed peritoneal defects by staining the cells which remained with trypan blue after excision of parietal peritoneum in rats. On day 3, the entire defect was covered by a sheet of cells. Trypan blue was not detected by microscopy in any of the cells covering the wound. By day 5, the new surface mesothelium achieved continuity with the surrounding edges of the previously undamaged mesothelium. By 7 to 10 days, no evidence of mitosis was evident within the wound base or surface nor along the margins of the previous uninjured peritoneum. A similar experiment was performed on another group of rats in which a polythene sheet was placed over the peritoneal defect after injury and sutured in place. Up to 2 weeks after injury, the surface of the polythene was covered by macrophages without appreciable numbers of fibroblastic or mesothelial cells. The cells that did cover the polythene were separated by large areas of fibrin. At 3 to 4 weeks after injury the wound surface became covered with mesothelium.

Thus, new peritoneal cells do not arise to any significant degree by the centripetal spreading of the mesothelial cells surrounding the wounded area as they are distributed rather uniformly at an early stage over the wound surface.[76] Cells are scattered over the entire surface as early as 30 minutes after injury. Initially, these cells are morphologically distinct from normal mesothelial cells at the time of their first appearance. After several days they appear to develop the characteristics of mesothelium. The mesothelial cell is capable of contributing to the repair process by the release of local factors including prostaglandin E_2 (PGE_2).[77]

TABLE 1.3. Five possible methods of mesothelial regeneration

1. Transformation of underlying mesenchymal stem cells into a new peritoneal membrane[67,68,78,79,149]
2. Growth from cells at the periphery of the defect[67,68,70,74]
3. Transformation of blood cells into a new peritoneal membrane[67,74]
4. Transplantation of cells from peritoneal surfaces of adjacent viscera[70]
5. Transformation of cells from the peritoneal fluid to peritoneal cells[70]

Some investigators consider that metaplasia of fibroblasts within the loose connective tissue beneath the surface of the peritoneum leads to mesothelial regeneration.[67,78,79] Electron microscopic observations identify undifferentiated primitive mesenchymal cells in the perivascular connective tissue, suggesting that these cells may also contribute to the new mesothelial cells. Further experimental evidence for this hypothesis was provided by Ellis et al.,[67] who postulated that peritoneal reformation results from transformation of subperitoneal fibroblasts into an intact mesothelial layer. This idea supported the work of Robbins et al.,[78] who theorized that new peritoneum arose from the transformation of underlying connective tissue cells. Ellis' work was confirmed by Raftery,[71,73] who further noted that peritoneum appears to arise by metaplasia of subperitoneal fibroblasts.

Direct support for the role of mesenchymal stem cells (MSC) arising from within the adjacent peritoneum to form mature mesothelial cells was provided by transplantation of MSCs into the abdominal cavity of rats at different times after surgery. MSCs given 4 to 5 hours after surgery increased formation of postoperative adhesions, perhaps by means of direct implantation on preexisting fibrin strands.[79] However, when MSCs were injected immediately after surgery, a significant reduction in adhesion formation occurred with half the rats remaining adhesion free (Fig. 1.8). These results suggest that stem cells contribute to postsurgical remesothelialization as well as to adhesions once fibrin bridges are available for their implantation.

Still others favor the concept that mesothelial regeneration results from differentiation of peritoneal cells: such cells settle on the denuded surface where they spread out and attach to one another. Evidence also exists that free peritoneal cells provide a source of regenerated mesothelium: denuded parietal mesothelial surfaces were very quickly (within 4 hours) covered with new cells initially; at 24 hours after peritoneal injury, flattened cells (with both microvilli and folds) became progressively more plentiful; and by 3 days, many cells were extremely flat and were studded with short microvilli, which elongated over the next few days.[4] Johnson and Whitting[74] suggested that implantation of free cells from the peritoneal cavity may give rise to new mesothelium. They observed islands of proliferating surface cells on wounds of the liver surface, and concluded that these were mesothelial cells that had detached from adjacent areas of peritoneum.

Summary

New mesothelial cells may have multiple sources: (1) transformed peritoneal cells, (2) metaplasia of subperi-

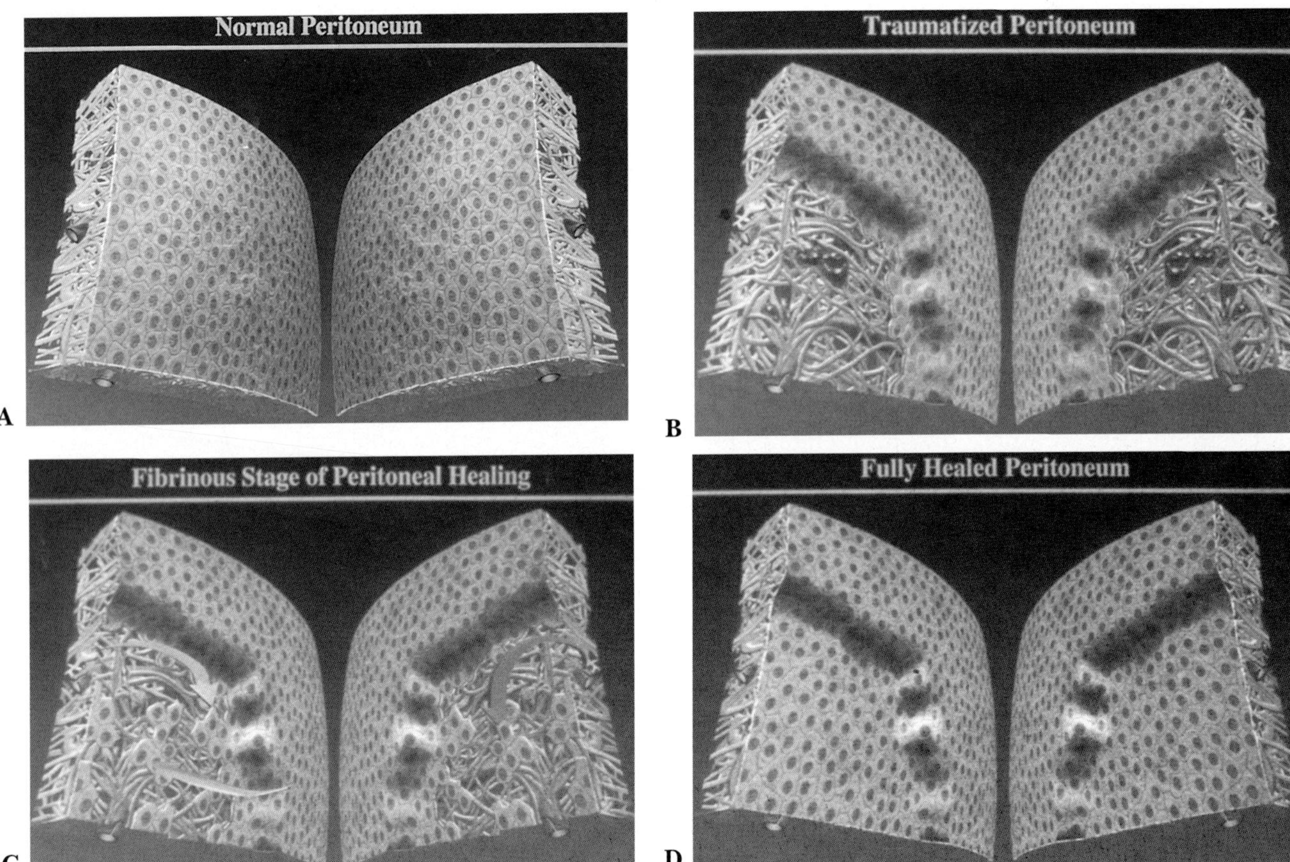

FIG. 1.7. **A.** Representation of the peritoneum, as it covers the pelvic sidewall. All pelvic and abdominal organs, except the ovary, are covered by a true peritoneum. The surface of the peritoneum is composed of mesothelial cells, which are supported by a scaffold of connective tissue (*white strands*). The rich microcirculation supplying the peritoneum is shown in *red*. Scattered within the connective tissue are mesothelial stem cells (*green*), which may be progenitors of the mature mesothelial cells. **B.** After a localized trauma to the peritoneum occurs, the injured mesothelial cells desquamate, leaving a denuded area. The border of this damaged site contains dying cells. This process of reepithelialization is initiated by the local production of chemotactic messengers that arise from the coagulation process. **C.** Healing of the peritoneum occurs primarily by reepithelialization of the damaged site. New mesothelial cells are attracted to the site of injury by chemotactic messengers released by platelets, blood clots, or leukocytes within the injured tissue. At this point, healing of the peritoneum differs from that of skin. With skin, healing occurs at the periphery of the injury. As a result, the duration of healing directly correlates with the size of the injury; larger injuries take longer to heal than smaller ones. In contrast, reepithelialization of peritoneal injuries occurs by the formation of multiple "islands" of new mesothelial cells scattered upon the surface of the peritoneum. The source of these epithelial cells, which is controversial, includes adjacent normal mesothelial cells and mesothelial stem cells. The mesothelial cells in each "island" continue to divide until the surface of the entire site of injury is covered by new mesothelium. **D.** Under conditions in which normal fibrinolytic activity occurs, mesothelial cell proliferation results in reepithelialization of the injured site. The surface of peritoneal injuries is typically reepithelialized 5–7 days after surgical injury. Beneath the surface, remodeling of collagen and other connective tissue proteins continues for a few months. *Please see insert for color reproduction of this figure.*

toneal connective tissue cells, (3) maturation of mesenchymal stem cells, or (4) adjacent normal peritoneum. Primitive mesenchymal cells identified on the wound surface in the early stages of healing may differentiate into mesothelial cells. Whether these cells are differentiated fibroblasts or undifferentiated multipotential mesenchymal stem cells is unclear. However, cells that comprise the surface of the new peritoneum are probably neither macrophages nor cells from the peritoneal fluid or adjacent to the surface edge of the injury which have migrated, become adherent to the wound site, and then differentiated into mesothelium. Thus, the origin of new mesothelium remains circumspect because of difficulty in distinguishing between primitive mesenchymal cells and proliferating fibroblasts in the later stages of healing. It is possible that the former give rise to the latter, but definitive evidence for this is lacking. Substantial evidence exists of a role for a variety of cell adhesion molecules including integrins and other fibronection-interacting proteins in the

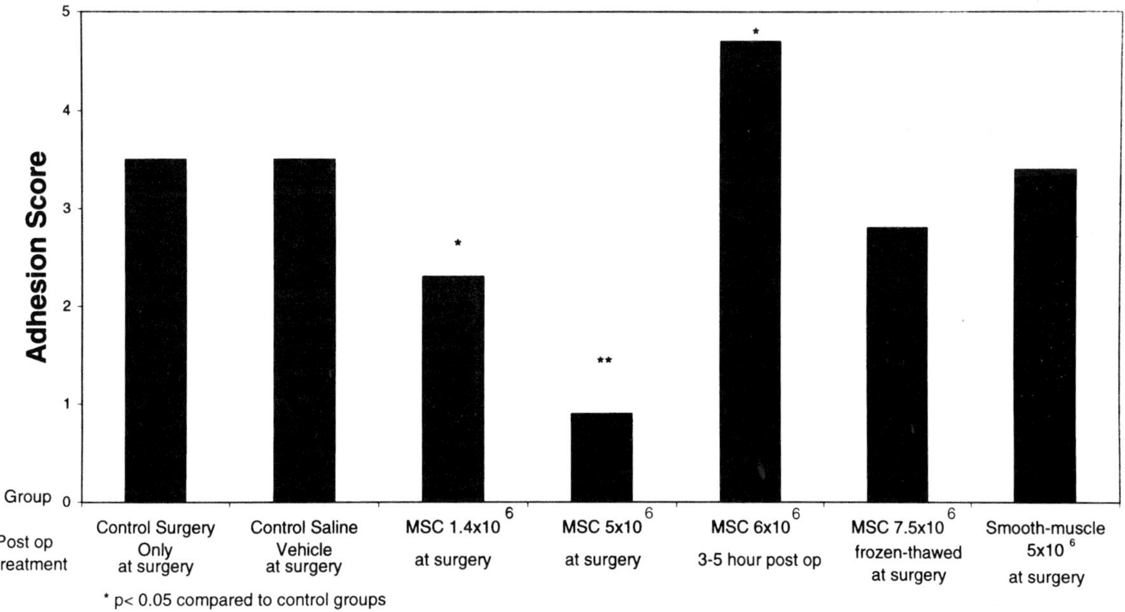

FIG. 1.8. Role of mesenchymal stem cells (MSC) in reduction of formation of postoperative intraperitoneal adhesions.[79] At different times after standardized trauma to the peritoneum, varying numbers of MSCs or smooth muscle cells were placed in the peritoneal cavity of animals. Subsequent determination of adhesion scores showed that MSCs are associated with adhesion formation if added 3–5 hours postoperatively, consistent with the hypothesis of MSC implantation onto preexisting fibrin bridges as an early determination of adhesion formation.

process of peritoneal repair and adhesion formation.[80] These subjects are addressed in detail in Chapters 3 and 4. Cytokines, integrins, fibrin, and proteases are also an integral part of peritoneal repair and adhesion formation. As such, their role in peritoneal repair is reviewed in Chapters 5, 6, and 7.

Surgical Injury and Electrocautery

Elkins et al.[81] compared the response of rabbit peritoneum to a variety of injuries: excision, abrasion, electrocautery, linear incision (with 2-0 polyglycolic acid), and without suture closure. Throughout the first 12 hours after injury, all four peritoneal injury sites contained polymorphonuclear leukocytes, surface fibrin deposit, white cell exudate, and both muscle and mesothelial tissue necrosis. Surface fibrin disappeared by 24 hours post surgery and the other reactions slowly diminished. In contrast, the electrocautery or burn injuries persisted throughout the 3-week study period.

The area of peritoneal excision without suture closure contained tissue necrosis by 24 hours and at 48 hours was the first injury site to contain fibroblasts and consistent mesothelial reepithelialization. Secondary cellular infiltrates of macrophages and plasma cells were noted by 48 hours, and collagen formation was present at 5 days. Gross healing was present at 5 days. By 7 days, tissue necrosis was resolved, and at 21 days after surgery this injury site was the only one with abundant fibroblasts and subepithelial collagen. Healing appeared to occur by proliferation and metaplasia of mesothelial cells. The peritoneal excision site showed less inflammatory reaction and more prompt reepithelialization than the other peritoneal injury sites.

Where sutures were used to close the peritoneal incision, early inflammatory changes were similar to those observed after other peritoneal injuries. At 24 hours after surgery, there were some early signs of reestablished mesothelial integrity, although this was not a consistent finding until 48 hours after surgery. Collagen formation became apparent at 5 days post surgery. The major difference between this site and the peritoneal excision site without repair was the presence of an intense foreign-body reaction surrounding the sutures. This ongoing tissue reaction persisted at 5 days, as evidenced by a foreign-body granuloma, and at 3 weeks postoperatively, as seen by the presence of fat necrosis. Gross healing was present at 2 to 3 weeks.

Elkins et al.[81] and Bellina et al.[82] both noted, at the sites of peritoneal cautery and suture repair, deep submesothelial hemorrhage and necrosis that prolonged the duration of inflammation and associated delay in collagen deposition. The sites of cauterization contained tissue necrosis and inflammation 3 weeks after surgery. Cauterization of peritoneal injury induced more tissue damage than other types of wounding. Early collagen deposition was noted at 5 days after surgery. However, at 3 weeks these lesions contained PMNs, tissue necrosis, and granulation tissue, with no fibroblasts and minimal collagen formation. Thus, healing at the cauterized site was not completed by 3 weeks after surgery. Elkins et al.[81] found that mesothelial regeneration was also delayed after peritoneal damage by electrocautery. Peritoneal repair after cauterization by electrical current or laser is complicated by carbonization: the black-brown tissue rests in the area of the wound. Carbon induces an inflammatory reaction, leading to giant cell formation that is required to phagocytize the foreign body, thereby further delaying mesothelial repair.

Filmar et al.[83] compared the histology of uterine horn repair in rats after incision with the carbon dioxide laser or microcautery. Incisions were reapproximated with 10-0 nylon sutures. Although the general appearance of the scars and the amount of collagen that accumulated during a 21-day observation period were similar, foreign-body reaction as measured by histocyte and giant cell infiltration was significantly greater in the electrocautry group. Carbon particles that formed in response to cautery may lead to formation of foreign-body granulomas. Cutting with the carbon dioxide laser caused significantly more necrosis and foreign-body reaction than cutting with microscissors. Sharp mechanical transection was followed by the least amount of tissue reaction or necrosis and an absence of particulate carbon. Montgomery et al.[84] compared the healing pattens of canine uterine peritoneum and myometrium after injury by CO_2 laser, scalpel, or an electric knife standardized to a 3-cm incision. Their observations confirmed those of other investigators in that necrosis was less with the scalpel than either the CO_2 laser or electric knife.

Adhesion Formation

A major clinical problem relating to peritoneal repair is the formation of intraabdominal and pelvic adhesions. Although the term "adhesions" is used in reference to ophthalmic, orthopedic, central nervous systems, cardiovascular, and intrauterine repair processes, the formation of peritoneal adhesions is unique and specific to the peritoneal response to injury.

Incidence

The most common cause of peritoneal adhesions is prior surgery.[85] Perry et al.[86] found that of the 388 patients with abdominal adhesions whom he surveyed, 79% had a history of surgery, 18% had a history of inflammatory disease, and 11% had congenital adhesions. In a further analysis of patients with adhesions related to inflammatory disease, Perry reported that 42% had acute appendicitis, 14.5% had diverticulitis, and the remaining patients had pelvic inflammatory disease, cholecystitis, and Crohn's disease. Raf[87] reported that 86% of patients with adhesions had a history of peritoneal surgery. In a survey of 142 patients with obstruction of the small intestine caused by adhesions, Nemir[88] reported that 73% had prior surgery, 20% had inflammatory disease, and 6% had congenital adhesions. In a prospective analysis of 210 patients undergoing laparotomy who previously underwent 1 or more abdominal operations, 93% had intraabdominal adhesions, compared with 115 first-time laparotomies in which only 10% of patients had adhesions.[89] Bowel obstruction from adhesion is most prevalent in the pediatric age group, where 8% of neonates undergoing abdominal surgery were shown in one study to require a future laparotomy for this complication.[90]

Adhesions occur in 55%–100% of fertility-enhancing procedures as determined by second-look laparoscopy performed in a number of large, multicenter studies[91,92] (Table 1.4). Diamond et al.[93] used second-look laparoscopy to evaluate the location of adhesions in 161 infertility patients after reproductive pelvic surgery. Of the pelvic sites that did not contain adhesions at the time of the initial procedure, 50% developed adhesions following this procedure. In a prospective study of 955 patients undergoing laparoscopic sterilization, Szigetvari et al.[94] confirmed that significant adhesions were more frequent among patients with prior pelvic or abdominal surgery (28% versus 2% in the no-prior-surgery group). DeCherney and Mezer[95] found that 75% of the 61 infertile females they evaluated after salpingostomy contained adhesions on follow-up laparoscopy. An adhesion

TABLE 1.4. Occurrence of adhesions at second-look laparoscopy (SSL) in patients undergoing fertility-enhancing procedures

Reference	Time from initial procedure	Total no. of patients	Total no. with adhesions	% with adhesions
Diamond et al. (1987)[93]	1–12 weeks	106	91	86
DeCherney and Mezer (1984)[95]	4–16 weeks	20	17	75
	1–3 years	41	31	76
Surrey and Friedman (1982)[175]	6–8 weeks	31	22	71
	>6 months	6	5	83
Pittaway et al. (1985)[124]	4–6 weeks	23	2	100
Trimbos-Kemper et al. (1985)[178]	8 days	188	104	55
Daniell and Pittaway (1983)[173]	4–6 weeks	25	24	96

TABLE 1.5. Comparison of adhesiolysis hospitalizations in the United States in 1988 and 1994

Year	Adhesiolysis hospitalization	Hospitalization rate (per 100,000 persons)	Expenditures (1994, $million)[a]		
			Hospitalization	Surgeon	Total
1988	Primary procedure	22.16	769.8	45.3	815.1
	Secondary procedure	93.35	431.3	190.7	622.0
	Total	115.51	1,201.1	236.0	1,437.1
1994	Primary procedure	22.49	715.2	48.7	764.0
	Secondary procedure	94.85	356.3	205.6	561.9
	Total	117.34	1,071.5	254.3	1,325.9

[a]Expenditures were calculated based on inpatient cost per day of $1,226 and surgeon cost of $837.[98,99]

formation rate of 54% after cesarean section was reported in a retrospective study in which adhesion assessment was made via laparoscopy at the time of tubal sterilization.[96] Most of these adhesions occurred in the anterior pelvis. Repeat cesarean sections are associated with adhesion formation in the majority of cases, with the bladder and omentum the most commonly involved anatomic sites.[97] Appendectomy and gynecologic surgery are the surgical procedures most frequently implicated in the formation of clinically significant adhesions.[87]

Health Care Cost of Adhesions

Adhesiolysis procedures in the United States associated with the female reproductive system, hepatobiliary system, and pancreas accounted for $166.9, $25.4, and $332.2 million, respectively, in 1988 (Table 1.5).[98] Using prevalence-based cost-of-illness methods, a cross-sectional study was designed to estimate inpatient expenditures associated with adhesiolysis for all persons in the United States in 1994. Although representing only 1% of all hospitalizations, lysis of adhesions was found to contribute $1.33 billion to health care expenditures in 1994, of which 58% was hospitalizations precipitated by adhesiolysis and 42% was for adhesiolysis performed as a secondary procedure.[99] Similar reports from Sweden[100,101] and Holland (see Chapters 27 and 30) confirm the substantial cost of adhesions to health care.

Diagnosis

In general, diagnosis of adhesion is made either under consciousness sedation via small-diameter laparoscopy or under general anesthesia (laparoscopy, laparotomy). Adhesions cannot definitively be diagnosed by noninvasive means. Workers have used ultrasound to assess the movement of viscera against the parietal peritoneum (visceral slide test) to predict the presence of adhesion to the anterior abdominal wall.[102] Viscera slide either occurs spontaneously as a result of respiratory movement or may be induced by manual ballottement (Fig. 1.9). Adhesions between the abdominal contents and the anterior abdominal wall often tether the viscera to the wall, resulting in viscera slide restriction (Fig. 1.10). During longitudinal ultrasound scanning, normal spontaneous viscera slide (produced by respiratory movement) ranges from 2 to 5 cm or more in distance. During either longitudinal or transverse scanning, normal induced viscera slide (produced by manual compression) can exceed 1 cm in distance. Restricted viscera slide is an ultrasonically detected reduction in viscera slide excursion of less than 1 cm for both spontaneous and induced viscera slide.[102,103]

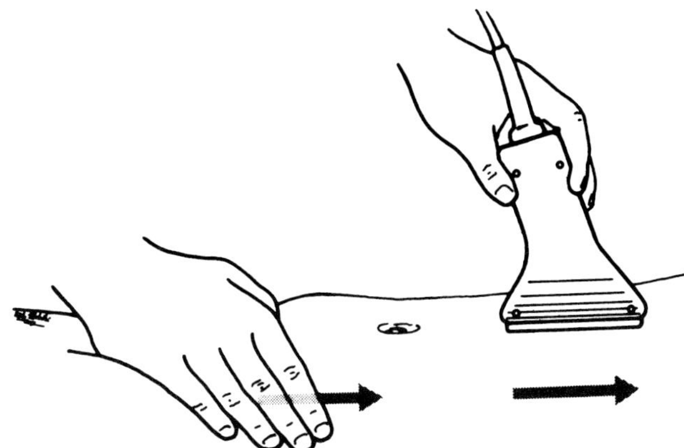

FIG. 1.9. Manual compression (*left arrow*) of the abdominal wall produces induced viscera slide (*right arrow*) beneath the transducer. The direction of the compressive force lies along the scan path of the transducer (linear axis of the transducer).[102]

Morphogenesis of Adhesion Formation

Adhesion formation typically occurs when two injured peritoneal surfaces are apposed.[104,105] The initiation of adhesion formation begins with formation of a fibrin matrix, which typically occurs during coagulation (Fig. 1.11) in the presence of suppressed fibrinolysis. Surgical injury of tissue reduces or eliminates blood flow, thereby

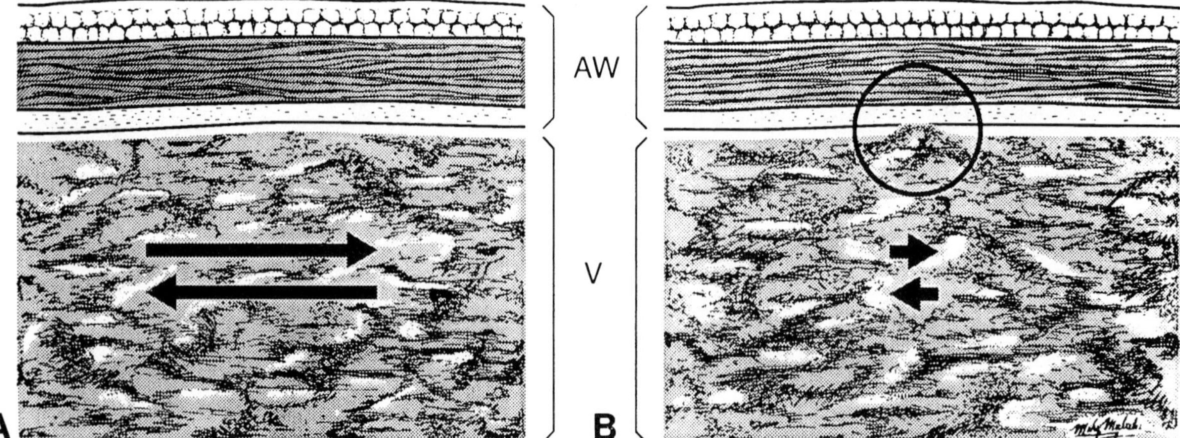

FIG. 1.10. Schematic drawing of viscera slide (*AW*, abdominal wall; *V*, viscera). **A.** Normal viscera slide showing a wide excursion (*long arrows*) of the viscera. **B.** Restricted viscera slide caused by an adhesion to the abdominal wall (*within circle*) that is characterized by a shorter excursion of viscera (*short arrows*).[102]

producing ischemia, which leads to local persistence of fibrin matrix (Fig. 1.12). This matrix is gradually replaced by vascular granulation tissue containing macrophages, fibroblasts, and giant cells. The clots are slow to achieve complete organization. In the process, they consist of erythrocytes separated by strands or condensed masses of fibrin, which are covered with two or three layers of flattened cells and contain a patchy infiltrate of mononuclear cells (Fig. 1.13). Eventually the adhesion matures into a fibrous band, often containing small nodules of calcification. The adhesions are often covered by mesothelium and contain blood vessels and connective tissue fibers, including elastin. Even at 6 months, collections of hemosiderin-filled macrophages are present in many adhesions.

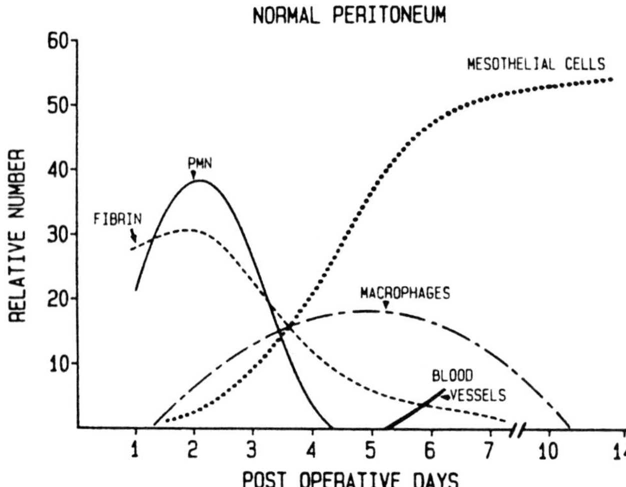

FIG. 1.11. Change in the relative number of cellular elements and fibrin deposition at the site of peritoneal injury in mature rats during the course of reepithelialization.[67,73,74]

Nerve fibers were found in pelvic adhesions from 17 patients, 10 of whom had a history of pelvic pain.[106] There was no significant correlation of pelvic pain with the number of adhesions containing nerve fibers or in the presence of mesothelial proliferation, calcification, edema, vascularization, inflammation, fibroblastic proliferation, or collagenization. These results were confirmed and extended by Tulandi et al.,[107] who additionally noted the presence of inflammatory cells in adhesions concomitant with endometriosis but not in adhesions associated with other disease states.

Milligan and Raftery[108] described the histologic and morphologic features of postsurgical adhesion formation in rats using light and electron microscopic techniques. They compared adhesions arising from the liver, cecum, and ileocecal junction using both peritoneal abrasion and stripping techniques to create petechial bleeding or a clear, well-demarcated peritoneal defect. Rats were killed at 7 or 14 days or at 1 or 2 months after the initial trauma. At days 1 to 3, the adhesion was characterized by a variety of cellular elements encased in a fibrin matrix. The cells were primarily PMNs but also included macrophages, eosinophils, red blood cells (RBC), and tissue debris as well as necrotic cells presumably desquamated from the peritoneal injury. By 4 days, macrophages were the predominant leukocyte in the fibrin mesh, which primarily contained large strands of fibrin associated with a few fibroblasts. A few mast cells were seen at day 5, and unorganized fibrin was not apparent. In contrast, many fibroblasts were lying together, assuming the formation of a syncytium together with macrophages. Distinct bundles of collagen were evident as were scattered foreign-body granulomas. At 7 days,

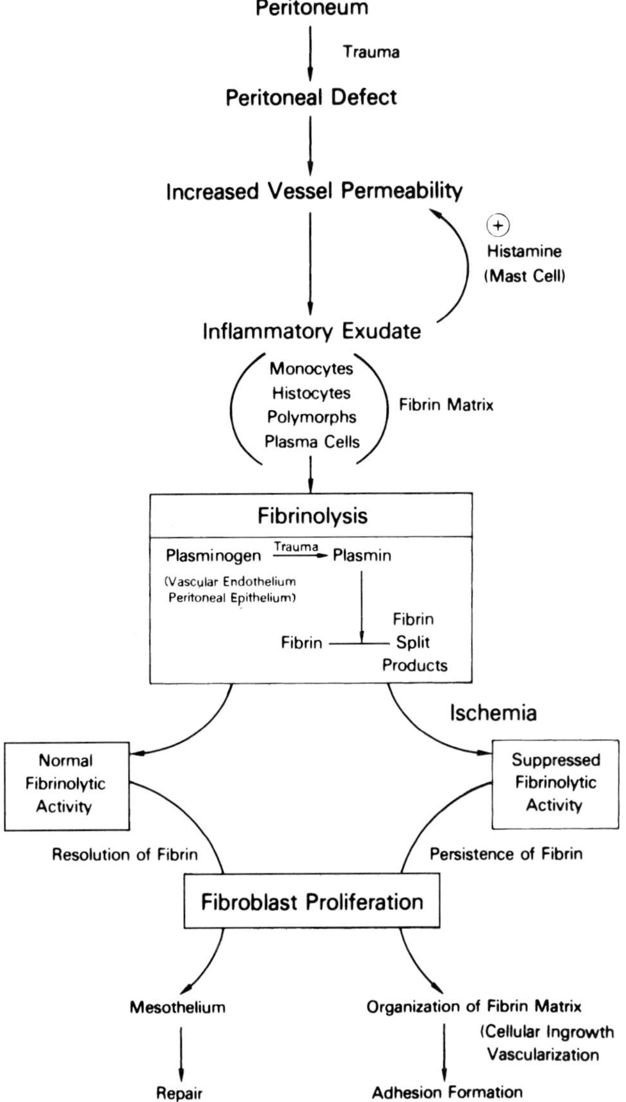

FIG. 1.12. Summary of normal tissue repair and adhesion formation following surgical trauma. After trauma to the peritoneum, increased vascular permeability, mediated by histamine, produces an inflammatory exudate and formation of fibrin matrix. As with other parts of the body, this fibrin matrix is normally removed by fibrinolysis. Under normal conditions, where fibrinolytic activity is allowed to occur, fibroblast proliferation results in remesothelialization. However, under the ischemic conditions present in surgical trauma, fibrinolytic activity is suppressed and fibrin is allowed to persist. Once the fibrin bands are infiltrated with fibroblasts, they become organized into adhesions.

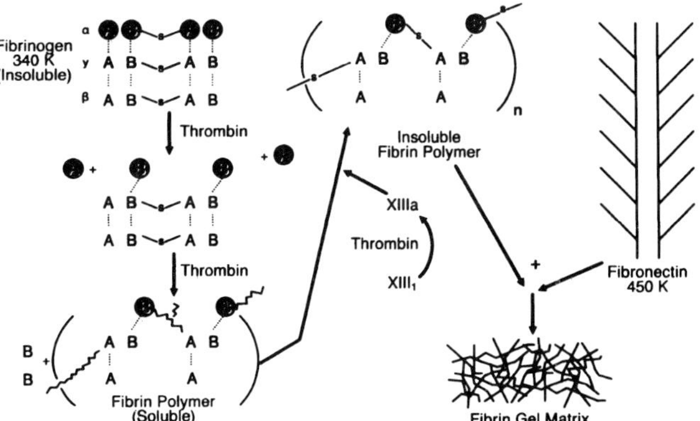

FIG. 1.13. Schematic representation of fibrin gel matrix formation. Fibrinogen deposited on the surface of injured peritoneum interacts with thrombin to become the soluble polymer fibrin, which is further modified to an insoluble form. Together with fibronectin, the insoluble fibrin polymer and cellular debris form the fibrin gel matrix, which provides the scaffolding for intraperitoneal adhesion formation. Frequent irrigation during surgery can remove the soluble polymer; delays in irrigation reduce the removal of deposited fibrin because it is converted into an insoluble form.

collagen and fibroblasts were the predominant components of the adhesion. However, small vascular channels containing endothelial cells were present. The number of mast cells slightly increased between 2 weeks and 2 months. During this interval the cellularity of the adhesion was replaced almost entirely by collagen fibrils associated with macrophages. Occasional macrophages and lymphocytes persisted for about 2 weeks.

The minimum postoperative interval required for the use of an impermeable barrier to prevent adhesion formation was established.[109] By removing a Silastic sheet 6, 12, 18, 24, 30, 36, 72, or 96 hours after peritoneal injury, the incidence of adhesions dropped from 100% to 0% during the first 36 hours (Fig. 1.14).

Electron Microscopy

A wide heterogeneity exists among adhesions when examined by electron microscopy.[108] Two days after injury, fibrin appears as fibrils. The number of macrophages exceeds the number of PMNs, and a scattering of eosinophils is present throughout the damaged peritoneum. Fibroblasts and collagen are found; however, fibroblasts appear in areas not associated with eosinophils. Early on there is no evidence of mesothelial cell attachment to the surface of the adhesion. By 4 days, most of the fibrin is gone and larger numbers of fibroblasts and collagen are present. Through days 5 to 10, fibroblasts become aligned and collagen deposition and organization advance (Fig. 1.14). The other cells involved at this time include macrophages and eosinophils. Similar studies performed by Abe and diZerega also identified the presence of eosinophils in adhesions that formed in the peritoneal cavity of rabbits after surgical injury.[110] At 2 weeks the relatively few cells present are predominantly fibroblasts, and 1 to 2 months after injury the collagen fibrils are organized into discrete bundles inter-

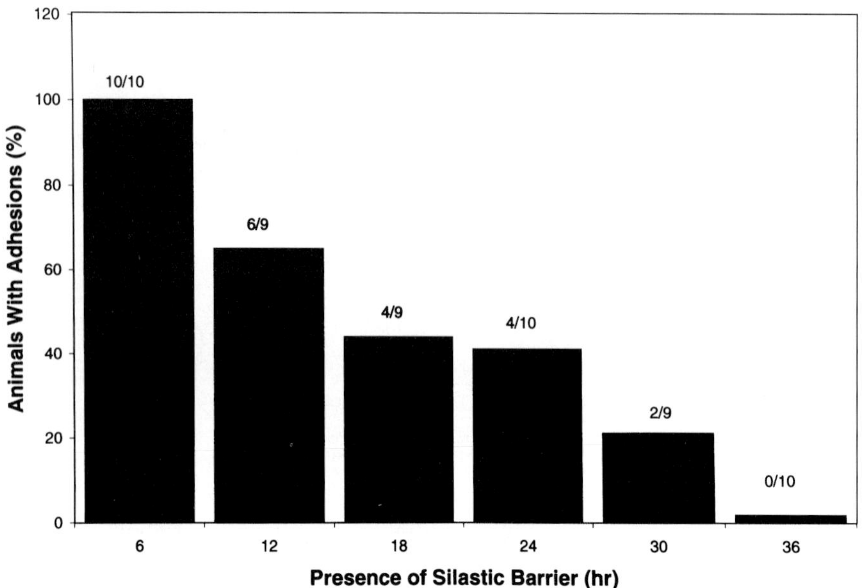

FIG. 1.14. Kinetics of adhesion formation. Removal of silastic barrier from between two wounded surfaces at various times after injury documented the susceptibility of wounds to form adhesions as a function of time.[110]

posed by spindle-shaped fibroblasts and a rare macrophage.

Mast Cells and Adhesion

Mast cells are involved in peritoneal inflammation resulting from either immunologic stimulation[111] or chemical irritation.[112] In addition, mast cell degranulation has been documented after simple handling of the intestine.[113,114] The effects of perioperative mast cell stabilization on the formation of intraabdominal adhesions and on mast cell degranulation were assessed in the rat.[115] The rats were treated with saline or one of two mast cell stabilizers, disodium cromoglycate (DSCG) or nedocromil sodium (NED), intraperitoneally 30 minutes before laparotomy and at the time of abdominal closure. The adhesions were assessed blindly 1 week later using a standardized scale. When the results in rats treated with DSCG were compared with those obtained in rats treated with saline, the DSCG-treated rats had significant attenuation of adhesion formation. The application of NED decreased adhesions in a dose–response fashion. Histologic analysis using toluidine blue staining was performed to assess the effect of DSCG on mast cell degranulation in the same adhesion model. DSCG significantly decreased the number of degranulated mast cells in the bowel wall when compared with saline. Thus, mast cells may play a role in the inflammatory process leading to adhesion formation.

Fibrin

Fibrinous exudate is a necessary precursor for adhesions (Fig. 1.15). Highly mobile intraperitoneal structures will

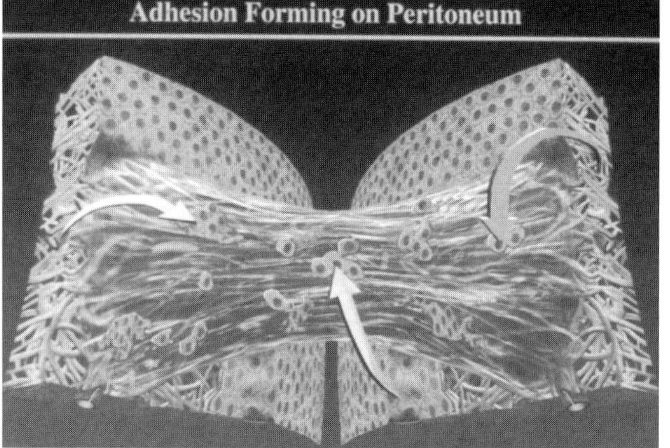

FIG. 1.15. After trauma to the peritoneum, there is increased vascular permeability, medicated by histamine, which often produces an inflammatory exudate and the formation of a fibrin matrix. Frequently, this fibrin matrix interconnects two adjacent pelvic structures, leading to the formation of fibrin bands. These fibrin bands are usually resolved by fibrinolysis, converting the large fibrin molecules into small fibrin-split products that are readily removed from the peritoneal cavity. Under the ischemic conditions present after surgical trauma, fibrinolytic activity is suppressed, which results in persistence of the fibrin bands. Once the fibrin bands are infiltrated with fibroblasts, they become organized to form what are clinically identified as adhesions. *Please see insert for color reproduction of this figure.*

not permanently adhere to each other unless held in continuous, close apposition until fibroblast invasion leads to collagen deposition, beginning on the third postoperative day. Thus, the crucial consideration is the factor which determines whether the fibrin bridge is absorbed, or persists and is organized.[116–119]

Further evidence for the role of fibrin in the formation of adhesions comes from the observation that use of defibrinated blood or blood products is less frequently associated with adhesion formation. Serosal injury, although relatively innocuous per se, readily leads to adhesions if combined with blood products. Peritoneal injury sufficient to produce adhesions requires removal of the mesothelial surface: not only drying but even prolonged moistening is sufficient to denude the surface of peritoneal mesothelium.[120] Plasma alone on dried areas creates fibrinous attachments, most of which disappear within a few days. Fibrin provides the initial bridge between two surfaces; when the bridge is made of fibrin only, it is amenable to lysis by fibrinolytic mechanisms, but when it contains cellular elements (erythrocytes, leukocytes, platelets, etc.) within the fibrin it will likely undergo organization into an adhesion. Under these experimental conditions, (1) desquamation of mesothelial cells appears to be the critical event in adhesion formation and (2) adhesions apparently develop only when two denuded surfaces are involved.

Foreign Body

The most common foreign body that leads to adhesion formation is starch or other particulate from glove powder, suture, and lint from drapes[121] (see also Chapter 11). Schade and Williamson[122] evaluated the temporal course of adhesion formation in rats after the addition of foreign body (colloidal silica oxide) into the peritoneal cavity. Three phases were discernible in adhesion induced by foreign body. The first phase (0 time–7 hours) involved degeneration and desquamation of mesothelial cells. In the second phase (7 hours–10 days), fibrin deposition on exposed basement membrane led to formation of fibrinous adhesions. This transformation of fibrinous exudate into fibrous adhesions occurred over an extended period of time (10 days–1 month).

Predisposing Factors

In two large surveys, postsurgical adhesion formation did not appear to be age dependent[85,86]; however, no prospective evaluation of the effect of age on adhesion formation is available. Weibel and Majno[85] reported a slightly higher frequency of "spontaneous" adhesions (i.e., those adhesions that form without any apparent cause) after 60 years of age.

There does not appear to be a sex bias in the development of postoperative adhesions. Weibel and Majno[85] reported a slightly higher frequency of adhesions among male patients. After excluding adhesions resulting from gynecologic procedures, Raf[87] reported that the incidence of intraperitoneal adhesions was 47% in male patients and 53% in female patients.

The omentum is particularly susceptible to adhesion formation (Table 1.6). In Weibel and Majno's studies,[85] the omentum was involved in 92% of patients with postoperative adhesions. The omentum was also the predominant organ involved in "spontaneous" adhesions (i.e., those with no prior history of surgery); 100% of the 126 spontaneous adhesions examined by Weibel and Majno involved the omentum. These reports raise the question of omentectomy during pelvic surgery where postoperative adhesion formation is likely to occur. With the exception of the omentum, the internal organs involved in postoperative adhesions may vary as a function of the surgical procedure. The small intestine was involved in 21% of the adhesions present after appendectomy but in only 6% of those formed following gynecologic laparotomy; 47% and 19% of adhesions that form after appendectomy and gynecologic laparotomy, respectively, involve the colon.[123] The ovary, because of its close proximity to the other peritoneal surfaces and the fragility of the coelomic epithelium that covers the ovarian surface, is the most common site for adhesions to form after reconstructive surgery of the female pelvis (Fig. 1.16; Table 1.6).[91–93] Ovarian adhesions were found at second-look laparoscopy in more than 90% of cases after ovarian surgery.[124]

Blood

The role of blood in the peritoneal cavity in the formation of adhesions is controversial. Hertzler[65] reported that large volumes of clotted blood could be completely absorbed by a normal peritoneum within 48 hours. Jackson[125] found that 100 mL of free blood and a well-formed clot were absorbed from the peritoneal cavity within 8 days. Nissell and Larsson[55] suggested that trauma to the serosa rather than blood was the instigator of adhesion formation. Bronson and Wallach,[126] on the other hand, finding no etiologic factor in 46% of their infertile patients with pelvic adhesions, suggested that

TABLE 1.6. Incidence of adhesions at initial surgery and follow-up laparoscopy

	Initial surgery[a]		Follow-up laparoscopy[b]	
Tissue	No.	%	No.	%
Ovaries	303/387	78	207/376	55
Fimbria	244/384	64	135/372	36
Cul-de-sac	87/208	42	42/208	20
Omentum	32/208	15	39/208	19
Colon	63/208	30	30/204	15
Small intestine	30/208	14	30/208	14
Pelvic sidewall	124/208	60	84/208	40

[a]Initial surgery performed using CO_2 laser plus 35% Dextran 70 or nonlaser surgical technique with or without Dextran. Results are pooled over three initial surgical procedure groups.
[b]Within 12 weeks of initial surgery.
Adapted from Diamond et al.[93]

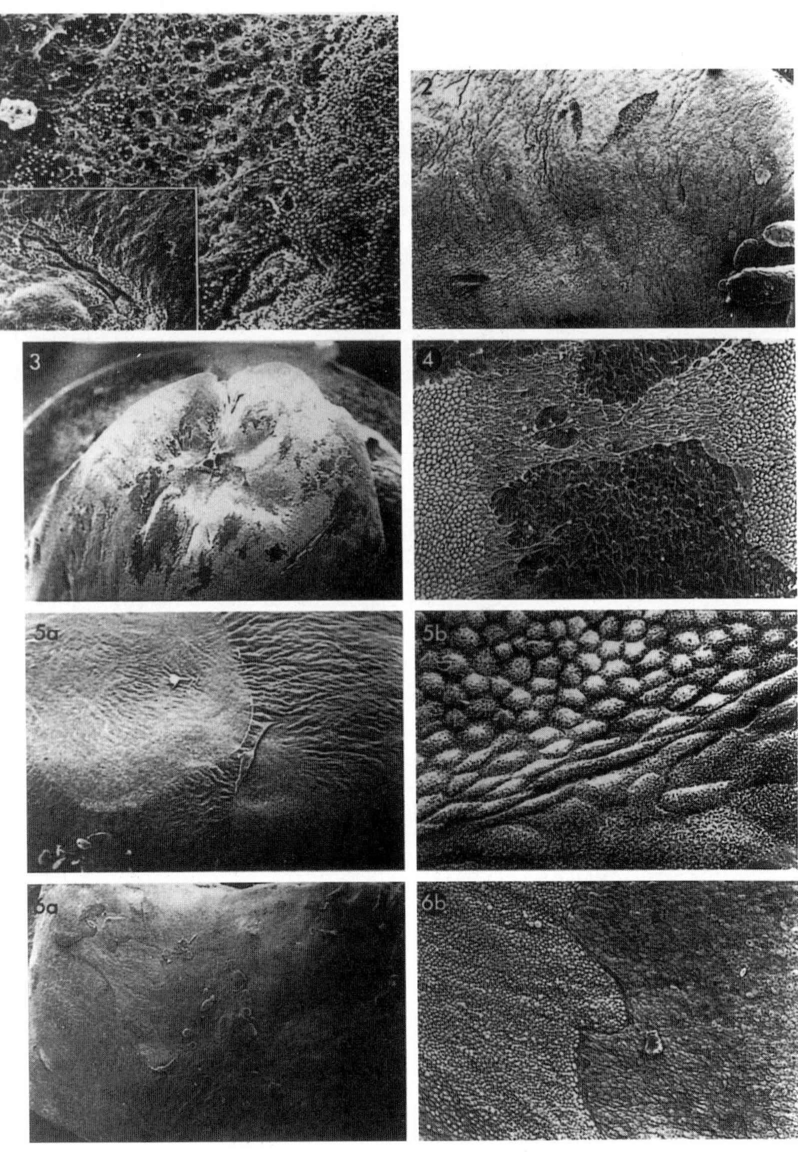

FIG. 1.16. Scanning electron photomicrograph of the junction between wiped and unwiped surfaces of a human ovary (×150). *Inset* **1.** Cells retained in a surface cleft (×55). **2.** Scanning electron photomicrograph of the ovarian surface over a 20-mm follicle (×48). Note the small patch of lost cells. **3.** Scanning electron photomicrograph of the ovarian surface over an old corpus luteum (×9). Note the bridges over the central healed stigma. Reepithelialization is complete, but because of difficulty in retrieving this ovary at minilaparotomy, the surface around the healed stigma lost cells. **4.** Scanning electron photomicrograph of the surface of an ovarian capsule (×170). Note the lost cells and the migrating epithelial cells. **5.** Scanning electron photomicrographs of the wall of a 16-mm follicle: (*a*) note the different cell zones (*darker regions* indicate flattened cells) (× 25); (*b*) junction between the zones (×640). *6.* Scanning electron photomicrographs of an ovarian capsule: (*a*) the whole surface is covered with an epithelial layer (×140); (*b*) junction between different cell zones (×90).[199]

ovarian bleeding associated with follicle rupture at the time of ovulation may produce significant adhesion formation.

Ryan et al.[127] showed that blood may play an important part in the pathogenesis of adhesions. Addition of fresh blood to an otherwise uninjured peritoneal cavity resulted in omental adhesions, and preformed clots produced widespread adhesions even without peritoneal injury. When 0.2 to 2 mL of fresh blood was dripped onto a dried peritoneal surface and allowed to clot, adhesions formed at the site of injury. If peritoneum was excised, the degree to which clot induced adhesion formation was markedly enhanced. When addition of fresh blood was delayed, adhesions formed if blood was added to the injured site. The addition of blood alone without cecal drying led to more limited adhesion formation. Serosal damage, no matter how mild, may lead to adhesions in the presence of blood. Clotted blood may constitute a fibrinous network upon which fibroblasts may proliferate, resulting in adhesions.[5] Golan and Winston[128] confirmed the findings of Ryan et al.,[127] reporting that blood in conjunction with trauma to the serosa is more important in adhesion formation than either trauma alone or trauma plus serum.

Fibrinolysis

The importance of fibrin disposition and fibrinolysis in adhesion formation is discussed in detail elsewhere (Chapters 8 and 9). In brief, functional fibrinolytic activity of peritoneum is present on all mesothelial surfaces (Fig. 1.17) and is dependent primarily on the balance of tPA and PAIs (tissue plasminogen activator and plasminogen activity inhibitors).[129,130] The plasminogen-activating activity of the peritoneal exudate is reduced as early as 6 hours after surgery and disappears at 24 to 48

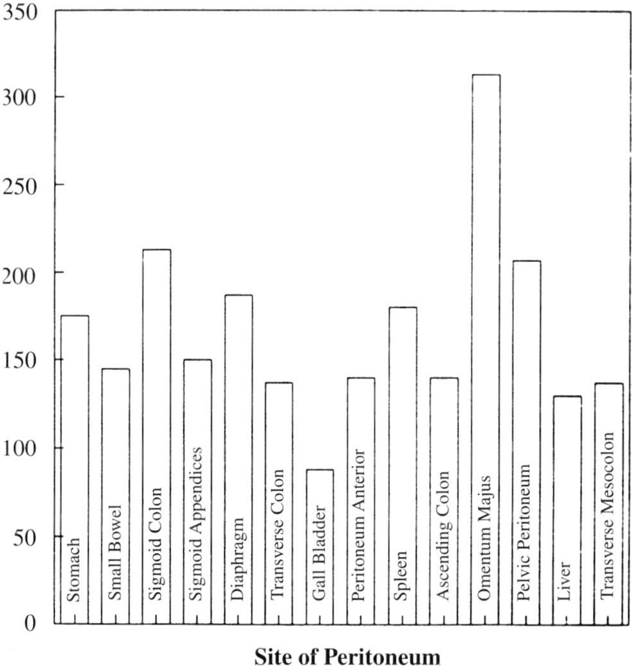

FIG. 1.17. The level of fibrinolytic activity of the human peritoneum from biopsies.[200] Biopsies of serosal peritoneum were obtained from various sites during peritoneal surgery. Fibrinolytic activity of human serosal peritoneum is primarily caused by plasminogen activator.

hours. Although there is a transient reduction in the concentration of tPA following surgery, the principal cause of reduced fibrinolytic activity appears to be an increase in concentration of both PAI-1 and PAI-2. The levels of PAI-1 and PAI-2 in cell lines, including cultured human mesothelial cells, can be increased by the presence of bacterial lipopolysaccharide and inflammatory mediators such as IL-1 and tumor necrosis factor (TNF). Such molecules are present in the peritoneum following inflammation and may stimulate PAI-2, thereby inhibiting lysis of fibrinous deposits within the abdominal cavity and promoting adhesion formation.[131]

There is a wide variation in the volume of peritoneal exudate among patients, which may affect the concentrations of individual fibrinolytic parameters and lead to a reduction in functional fibrinolytic activity. Concentrations of both PAI-1 and PAI-2 are increased in inflamed peritoneum during appendicitis, in association with a reduction in peritoneal plasminogen-activating activity. Thus, there appears to be a biphasic response to surgery by the peritoneum; the early reduction in peritoneal plasminogen-activating activity may be secondary to a reduction in tPA levels, whereas the subsequent loss of fibrinolytic activity probably arises from the dramatic increase in PAI-1 and PAI-2 concentrations.[130,132] Further, differences in endogenous PAI (especially PAI-2) may lead to individual differences in tPA activity, resulting in individual susceptibility to adhesion formation.

The recent availability of recombinant tissue plasminogen activator (rtPA) has led to several studies demonstrating that the administration of rtPA into the peritoneal cavity in excess of the inhibitor activity will correct the deficit in fibrinolytic activity and reduce or eliminate adhesion formation.[89] However, there is a significant reduction of both bursting strength and hydroxyproline content in wounds from rats treated with intraperitoneal rtPA. The levels of rtPA required to alter or prevent intraabdominal adhesion formation in animals also produce a significant impairment of the early phase of wound healing, as measured by the wound content of hydroxyproline, and are close to the LD_{50} level because of hemorrhage from disruption of coagulation.

TNF is a proinflammatory cytokine produced primarily by macrophages following their activation. It has been shown to increase the synthesis of PAI-1 by endothelial cells in culture and to increase plasma PAI-1 levels following administration to rats and human volunteers. TNF is present in human peritoneal drain fluid following surgery. TNF production can be stimulated by bacterial endotoxin (lipopolysaccharide) and other cytokines. Such stimulants may be present during abdominal surgery, often in large amounts. The time course of TNF changes in human peritoneal fluid after surgery is analogous to that seen in ascites after intraperitoneal administration of endotoxin.[131] The evidence is overwhelming that transforming growth factor-β (TGF-β) is involved in fibrosis[133] and adhesion formation.[134]

Peritoneal Closure

Adhesions, delayed healing, and wound breakdown are often attributed to failure of peritoneal suturing or the presence of deperitonealized areas within the abdomen. To reconstruct the pelvis after removal of viscera and peritoneum seems a logical procedure for good surgical practice. However, examination of the data indicates that approximation of peritoneum by sutures to cover vascularized areas denuded by the previous dissection may not facilitate repair. After resection of peritoneal tissue, natural healing is associated with less adhesion formation than occurs after reapproximation with staples or sutures.[135] There is no difference in adhesions to the previous laparotomy incisions after closure with or without peritoneal suturing.[136]

Animal Studies

The effects of peritoneal suturing on the healing of abdominal wounds have been evaluated in a number of

TABLE 1.7. Comparison of the use of suture on the finding of adhesions

Reference	Group	Study method	Suture	Adhesions		
				Suture	%	No. of suture
Chester et al.[149]	Dogs	Peritoneal graft to bowel anastomosis	Cotton	12/16	75.0	N/A
Thomas and Rhoads[150]	Albino rats	Oversew denuded	Silk	20/27	74.1	8/28
	Guinea pigs	Bowel serosa		18/21	85.7	7/19
Trimpi and Bacon[144]	Dogs	Deperitonization	Chromic	3/10	30.0	NA
		Deperitonization plus colon anastomosis		10/10	100.0	NA
Tulandi et al.[155]	Infertility patients	Anterior peritoneal closure	Plain catgut	14/63	22.2	9/57

prospective clinical trials (Table 1.7). Ellis and Heddle[137] observed no significant difference in wound dehiscence or incisional hernia rates between groups in which the peritoneum was sutured with chromic catgut or left unsutured during closure of paramedian and midline wounds. Milewczyk[138] found that adhesion formation in the anterior peritoneum of rabbits occurred in 17 of 50 wounds that were sutured but in only 3 of 50 wounds not sutured. Likewise, Swanwick et al.[139] noted that 50% of peritoneal closures in the horse developed adhesions but in contrast only 27% of the unclosed peritoneums developed adhesions. This significant difference indicates that parietal peritoneum that has not been sutured heals with fewer adhesions than sutured parietal peritoneum. Similar results were reported by McDonald et al.[135] Resection of peritoneal tissue followed by natural healing is preferable to reapproximation of free peritoneal edges with either staples or sutures.[140] In addition, Hugh et al.[140] demonstrated that peritoneal suture or nonsuture produced no significant difference in postoperative pain scores or analgesic requirements. Long-term follow-up (beyond 1–2 years) and hence late incisional hernia rates were not reported in any studies.

The effects of suturing and stapling peritoneal edges or excising, cauterizing, and abrading areas of peritoneum on adhesion formation were evaluated by McDonald in rabbits.[135] Two weeks after peritoneal injury, the amount of adhesion formation was noted. Resection of peritoneal tissue with natural healing was preferable to reapproximation of free peritoneal edges with either staples or sutures. Ling et al.[141] assessed adhesion formation after peritoneal closure with absorbable staples and found that absorbable staples were associated with increased adhesion formation when compared to the other methods of injury. The amount of adhesion formation correlates with the presence and quantity of suture material.[142] Sutured peritoneum is twice as likely to be associated with adhesion formation that is associated with postoperative bowel obstruction.[143]

Clinical Studies

Clinical reports after oncologic surgery demonstrate normal healing of unsutured peritoneum.[75,78] No instance of bowel obstruction occurred, and at later reoperation the surgical sites were covered by a smooth, glistening peritoneal surface. Trimpi and Bacon[144] reported 49 cases of abdominoperineal resection of the rectum. In 18 patients the peritoneal floor was closed and there were 4 instances of intestinal obstruction; in 28 patients no reperitonealization was performed and there were no instances of obstruction. Ulfelder and Quinby[145] found that, after combined abdominoperineal resection, 50% of postoperative intestinal obstructions were caused by incarceration of small bowel between sutures of the newly constructed peritoneal floor. All experimental evidence indicates that areas denuded of peritoneum will heal satisfactorily[78,146–148] and that suturing of peritoneum actually increases the incidence of adhesions.[65,75,78,144,148–151]

The value of peritoneal closure at the time of cesarean birth was evaluated prospectively. Hull and Varner[151] as well as Pietrantoni et al.[152] compared the clinical outcome of postcesarean section patients who did or did not undergo peritoneal closure. Closure of the peritoneum extended the duration of the surgical procedure by 5 minutes. There were no differences between groups in the incidence of postoperative wound infection, dehiscence, endometritis, ileus, or length of hospital stay. Nonclosure of the visceral and parietal peritoneum after low transverse cesarean section had no adverse effects on recovery and decreased operating time. Similar studies were conducted with abdominal hysterectomy[153–155] with the same conclusions. Thus, leaving the parietal peritoneum unsutured is an acceptable way to manage patients at cesarean delivery.

The effect of peritoneal closure after reproductive surgery through a Pfannenstiel incision was studied by second-look laparoscopy.[152] No difference was found in the length of hospital stay, incidence of wound complications, or other postoperative complications after abdominal closure with or without peritoneal suturing. In other clinical studies, no difference was found in postoperative complications, wound healing, and adhesions to previous laparotomy incisions after closure with or without peritoneal suturing. These observations were reported for midline wounds by Hugh et al.[140] and for closure of lateral paramedian by Gilbert et al.[156] In summary, pre-

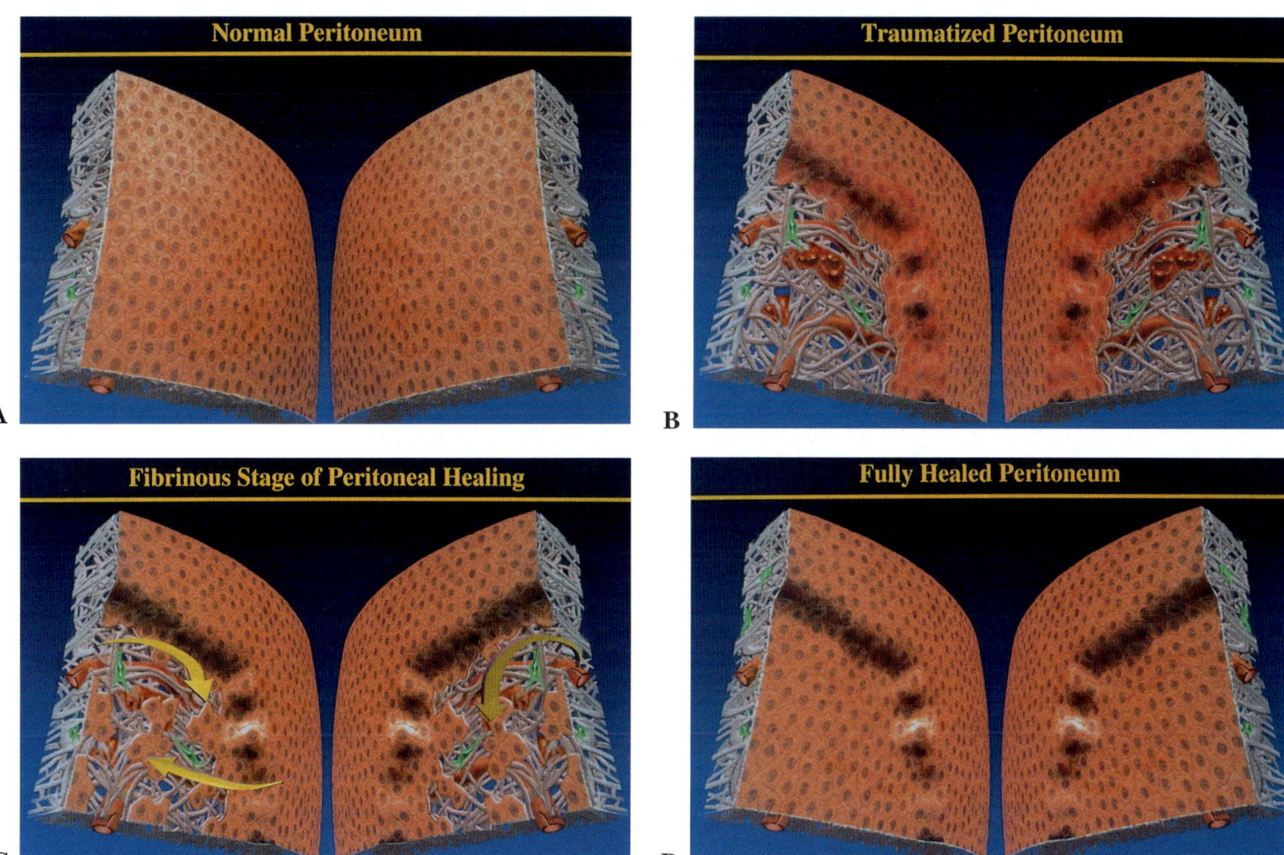

FIG. 1.7. **A.** Representation of the peritoneum, as it covers the pelvic sidewall. All pelvic and abdominal organs, except the ovary, are covered by a true peritoneum. The surface of the peritoneum is composed of mesothelial cells, which are supported by a scaffold of connective tissue (*white strands*). The rich microcirculation supplying the peritoneum is shown in *red*. Scattered within the connective tissue are mesothelial stem cells (*green*), which may be progenitors of the mature mesothelial cells. **B.** After a localized trauma to the peritoneum occurs, the injured mesothelial cells desquamate, leaving a denuded area. The border of this damaged site contains dying cells. This process of reepithelialization is initiated by the local production of chemotactic messengers that arise from the coagulation process. **C.** Healing of the peritoneum occurs primarily by reepithelialization of the damaged site. New mesothelial cells are attracted to the site of injury by chemotactic messengers released by platelets, blood clots, or leukocytes within the injured tissue. At this point, healing of the peritoneum differs from that of skin. With skin, healing occurs at the periphery of the injury. As a result, the duration of healing directly correlates with the size of the injury; larger injuries take longer to heal than smaller ones. In contrast, reepithelialization of peritoneal injuries occurs by the formation of multiple "islands" of new mesothelial cells scattered upon the surface of the peritoneum. The source of these epithelial cells, which is controversial, includes adjacent normal mesothelial cells and mesothelial stem cells. The mesothelial cells in each "island" continue to divide until the surface of the entire site of injury is covered by new mesothelium. **D.** Under conditions in which normal fibrinolytic activity occurs, mesothelial cell proliferation results in reepithelialization of the injured site. The surface of peritoneal injuries is typically reepithelialized 5–7 days after surgical injury. Beneath the surface, remodeling of collagen and other connective tissue proteins continues for a few months.

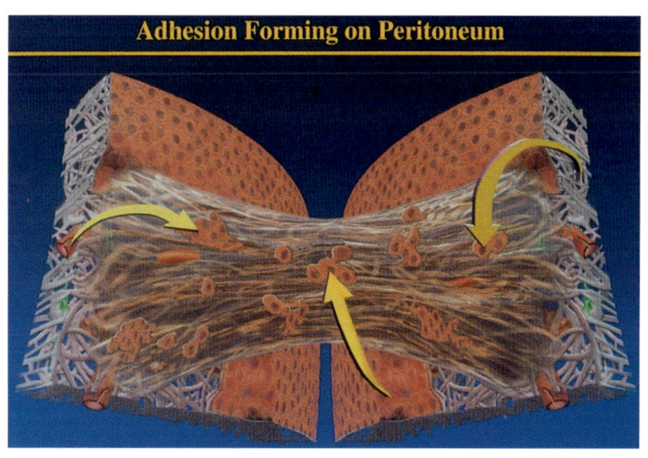

FIG. 1.15. After trauma to the peritoneum, there is increased vascular permeability, medicated by histamine, which often produces an inflammatory exudate and the formation of a fibrin matrix. Frequently, this fibrin matrix interconnects two adjacent pelvic structures, leading to the formation of fibrin bands. These fibrin bands are usually resolved by fibrinolysis, converting the large fibrin molecules into small fibrin-split products that are readily removed from the peritoneal cavity. Under the ischemic conditions present after surgical trauma, fibrinolytic activity is suppressed, which results in persistence of the fibrin bands. Once the fibrin bands are infiltrated with fibroblasts, they become organized to form what are clinically identified as adhesions.

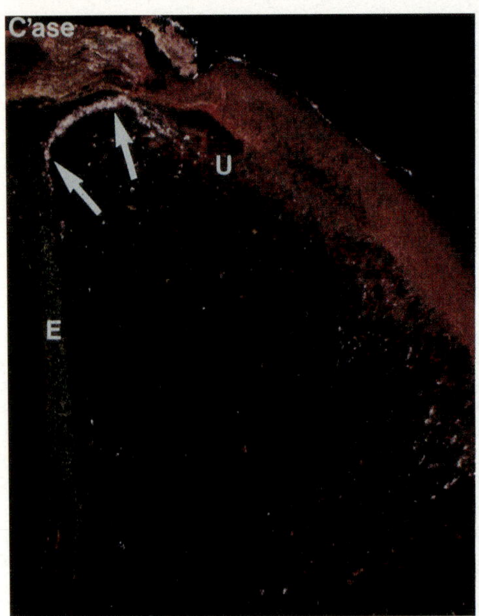

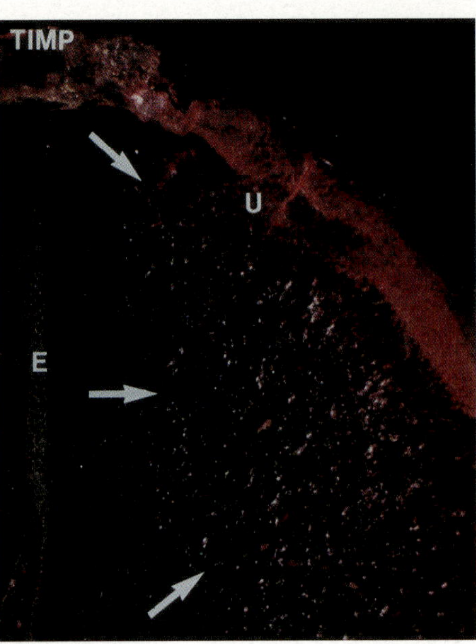

FIG. 7.1. Distinct localization of collagenase-1 and tissue inhibitor of metalloproteinase (TIMP-1) expression. Serial sections of ulcerated pyogenic granuloma were hybridized for collagenase-1 (C'ase) or TIMP-1 mRNAs. An ulceration (*U*) is indicated with underlying inflammatory cells; the adjacent epidermis (*E*) has formed an epithelial tongue to cover the defect. Collagenase-positive basal keratinocytes (*left*) are detected only at the migrating front of epithelium (*arrows*). In contrast, TIMP-positive cells (*right*) are found within the underlying granulation tissue (*bordered by arrows*), but not in epidermis.

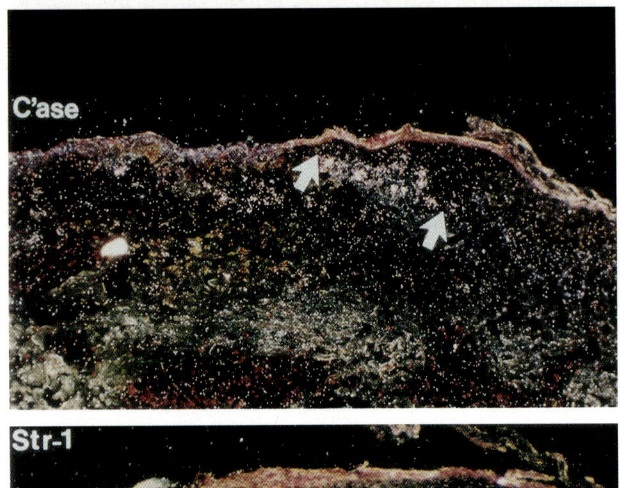

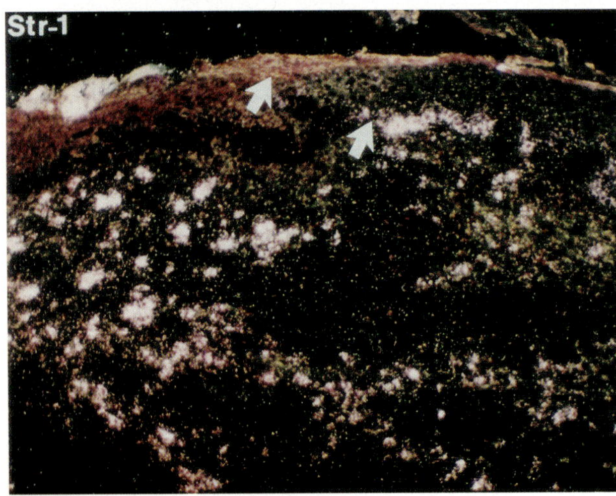

FIG. 7.2. Collagenase-1 (*top*) and stromelysin-1 (*bottom*) are expressed in distinct areas of the healing epidermis. Serial sections of a nonspecific ulcer were hybridized with ^{35}S-labeled antisense RNA probes for collagenase-1 (C'ase) and stromelysin-1 (Str-1) mRNAs. The migrating front of the epidermis, adjacent to an ulceration (*U*) in the upper left corner, is indicated by *large arrows*. Signal for collagenase-1 mRNA was detected only in basal keratinocytes within the migrating front. In contrast, signal for stromelysin-1 mRNA was seen in the epidermis away from the migrating front of epithelium and in many dermal fibroblasts.

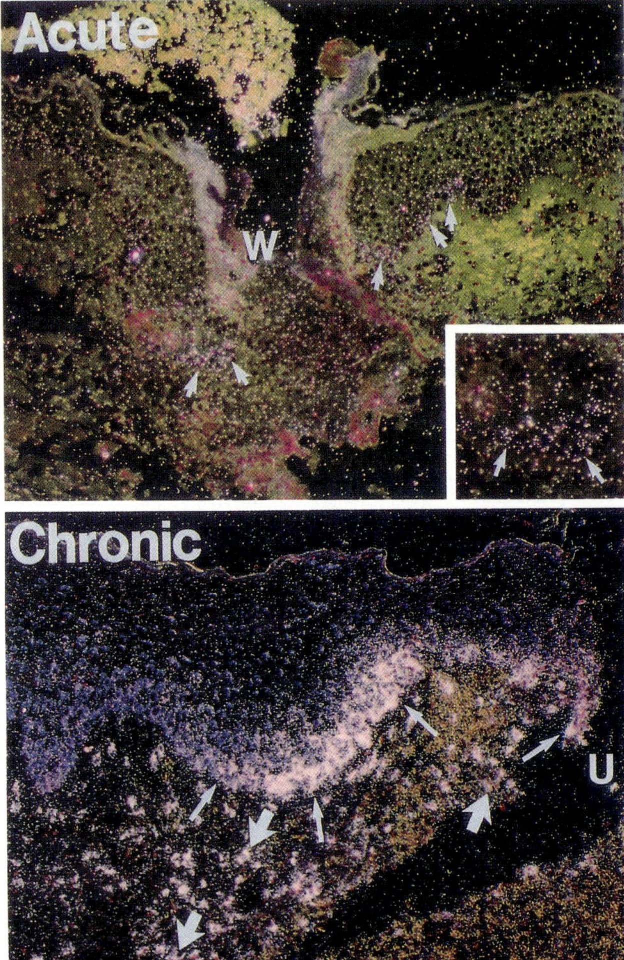

FIG. 7.4. Expression of collagenase-1 is elevated in chronic ulcers. For further details, please see text, p. 109.

clinical and clinical evidence indicates that normal peritoneal repair occurs in the absence of reperitonealization.

Sepsis and Suturing

Surgical trauma and peritonitis each depress peritoneal fibrinolytic activity.[118,130,157,158] The net results of these interactions might be increased adhesion formation if the peritoneum is sutured in the presence of sepsis. This possibility was tested in rats undergoing laparotomy after intraperitoneal inoculation with bacterial cultures or saline. In 10 animals that received saline inoculum, the peritoneum was sutured with nylon, and adhesions to the laparotomy scar formed in 3 animals. In contrast, in the presence of intraperitoneal infection, adhesion to the laparotomy scar formed in 8 of 9 animals when the peritoneum was sutured with nylon but in only 2 of 10 when it was left unsutured.[158] Intraperitoneal infection, independent of a particulate or chemical irritant, proved to be a potent cause of adhesions. Moreover, suturing the peritoneum and sepsis appeared to act synergistically to promote adhesions to the scar.

Surgical Techniques and Adhesion Formation

Incision Location

Brill et al.[159] correlated the location and frequency of skin incision with subsequent adhesion formation (Fig. 1.18). Adhesions to the omentum and bowel were found in 70 women (27%) in the Pfannenstiel group, in 48 women (55%) in the midline group when incision was above the umbilicus, and in 10 women (67%) in the midline group when incision was below the umbilicus. The distribution of adhesions to the omentum and bowel varied for each type of incision. In the Pfannenstiel group, 87% had adhesions to the omentum and 13% had adhesions to the omentum and bowel. In the midline below the umbilicus group, 72 of 87 (83%) had adhesions to the omentum and 15 patients (17%) had adhesions to the omentum and bowel. In the midline above the umbilicus group, 60% had adhesions to the omentum and 40% had adhesions to the omentum and bowel.

After a single incision, 25% in the Pfannenstiel group had adhesions, whereas 31% had adhesions after two to five incisions. In the midline below the umbilicus group, 53% had adhesions after a single incision, whereas 59% had adhesions after two to six incisions. In the midline above the umbilicus group, 5 of 10 patients had adhesions after a single incision, and all 5 patients had adhesions after two to four incisions. When subjects with all types of incisions were combined, adhesions were present in 22% in the obstetric group, a finding that was significantly different from 42% of patients in the gynecologic group.[159]

Levrant et al.[160] determined the incidence of adhesions to the anterior abdominal wall peritoneum to assess the risk of umbilical trocar insertion in patients with previous surgery. No anterior wall adhesions were present in 91 patients with no previous surgery; 33 (36%) had pelvic adhesions. Of 45 patients with a previous laparoscopy (12 had more than one laparoscopy), 22 had pelvic adhesions and none had anterior wall adhesions. Of 29 patients with a previous midline vertical incision, 12 had pelvic adhesions and 17 (59%) had anterior wall adhesions. Of 39 patients with a previous suprapubic

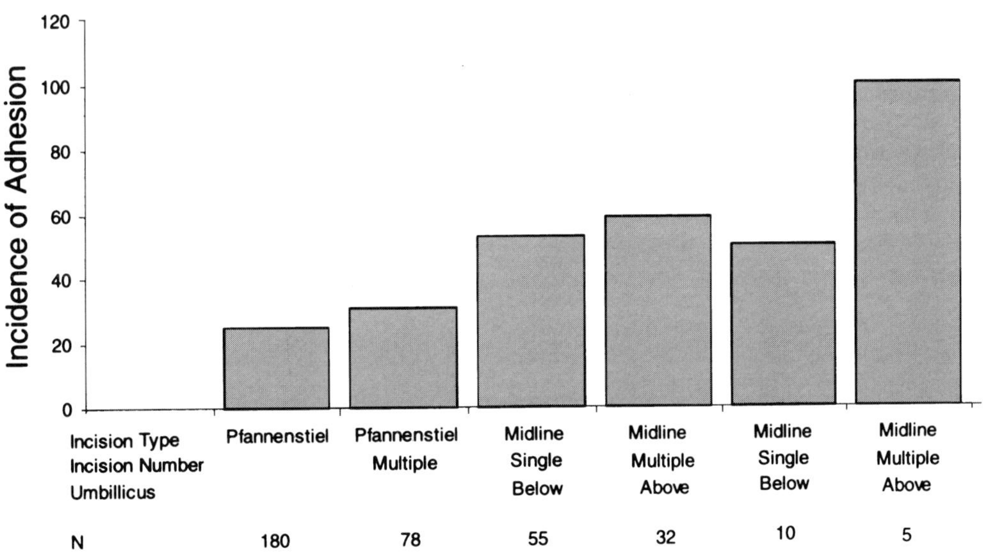

FIG. 1.18. Correlation between skin incision, prior surgery, and subsequent adhesion formation.[159]

transverse incision, 32 had pelvic adhesions, and 11 (28%) had anterior wall adhesions. The anterior wall adhesions were all close enough to the umbilicus to interfere with the safe placement of a laparoscopic umbilical trocar (96% of the adhesions involved omentum and 29% included bowel). The incidence of anterior wall adhesion was significantly higher in the previous midline vertical versus suprapubic transverse incision group. The incidence of pelvic adhesions did not differ significantly between the previous laparoscopy and previous laparotomy groups.

Sutures

In a rat adhesion model, suture material, volume, and diameter, as well as knot configuration of commonly used sutures, were evaluated quantitatively for extent and type of adhesion that formed.[161] Prolene showed a significantly smaller mean adhesion percentage compared to the Vicryl- and catgut-treated peritoneal defects, which confirmed previous studies.[162] The adhesion type differed significantly from the catgut-treated defects. Catgut created the most severe and extensive adhesion of every subgroup of the study. Thus, suture material seems to be a significant factor in the induction of adhesion formation (see Chapter 15).

Laser

It has been suggested that the carbon dioxide (CO_2) laser, by virtue of its hypothetical capabilities for precise incisions, minimization of tissue handling and bleeding, and shortened operating time, may improve the success rate of gynecologic infertility surgery.[163] To assess this hypothesis, a multicenter prospective study was performed to assess adhesion formation at early second-look laparoscopy after intraabdominal laser surgery.[164] Procedures performed included salpingoneostomy, fimbrioplasty, lysis of adhesions, vaporization of endometriosis, and ovarian wedge resection. Adhesions present at the time of the second-look procedure were reduced from initial presentation at most sites by both CO_2 laser and standard surgical procedures; however, nonlaser infertility surgery appeared to have equal or greater efficacy in the prevention of adhesion formation. When tested in animals, the number of adhesions was found to be significantly higher after vaporization using the CO_2 laser and the YAG (yttrium-aluminum-garnet) contact laser than after thermal coagulation using bipolar current.[165] Some authors recommended the laser for cutting to avoid postoperative adhesions. These findings could not be confirmed by others.[166] Use of laser vaporization to achieve hemostasis was more adhesiogenic than bipolar coagulation when the area and depth of the injured site were controlled in an animal study (Table 1.8).[163] Thus, from a peritoneal repair or adhesion reduction perspective, the use of laser remains controversial.

Irrigation Fluids

The most commonly used distending medium in laparoscopic surgery is carbon dioxide (CO_2) gas. The most commonly used irrigation solutions are normal saline or lactated Ringer's solution. Although irrigation facilitates visualization, Sahakian showed that the mixture of CO_2 and normal saline yields carbonic acid, which produces an acidic medium.[167] Lactated Ringer's solution contains a larger buffering capacity than normal saline when saturated with CO_2. The pH drop in normal saline is from a baseline of pH 6.6 to pH 4.1; the drop in lactated Ringer's solution is from a baseline of pH 6.0 to pH 5.0. This acidity may be potentially harmful to tissue surfaces, leading to adhesion formation. When tested in rabbits there was no significant difference in adhesion formation between the CO_2-only group and the normal saline with CO_2 group. However, the mean adhesion score of rabbits treated with lactated Ringer's solution with CO_2 was significantly less than that of those which received normal saline with CO_2 and CO_2 alone.

Abdominal Distension

Air quality is affected by production of particulates and gaseous materials produced during surgery by use of laser, electrosurgical, and mechanical devices. The chemicals and potentially infectious materials are produced by combustion, mechanical, or vibratory mechanisms interacting with tissue. Aerosols contain poten-

TABLE 1.8. Formation of adhesions on the rat abdominal wall provoked in animal experiments 1 to 10 days after the procedure, depending on the technique employed: coagulation or vaporization

	Coagulation		Vaporization	
	Endocoagulation	Bipolar high-frequency current	CO_2 laser	YAG contact laser
Number of lesions	52	48	80	108
Number of lesions with adhesions	1 (2.0%)	6 (12.5%)	50 (62.5%)	73 (67.6%)
Number of lesions without adhesions	51 (98.0%)	42 (87.5%)	30 (37.5%)	35 (32.4%)

Note: Mencke[163] indicated that the surface inflammatory reaction is greater after vaporization when compared with coagulation.

tially hazardous carcinogenic, mutagenic, and infectious particles in various concentrations. Identification qualitatively or quantitatively of the products and by-products of tissue combustion requires critical evaluation. A study was designed to evaluate components of tissue pyrolysis.[168] Smoke from tissue combustion at pelvic surgery was evaluated. Mass spectral chemical analysis of combusted human tissue particle-size analysis was performed. Carbon monoxide (CO), free radicals, hydrogen cyanide, benzene, acrolein, and polyaromatic hydrocarbons (PAH) are a few of the more than 27 toxic materials produced by human tissue pyrolysis. Each 50 mg of tissue pyrolyzed caused production of 12.8 μg of benzene, 3.6 μg PAH, 4.3 μg of acrolein, and 3.4 μg of formaldehyde. Each gram of tissue combustion resulted in 284 mg of particulates. The mean distribution of particle size was 0.3 to 0.5 μm. Experimental measurements showed there are 5.4×10^9 0.3-μm particles per milliliter. CO levels were increased to levels of 2100 part per million. Chemical and particulate production are consequences of tissue combustion, and studies are in progress to evaluate their effects on pelvic surgery and adhesion formation. Until these are completed, minimalization of coagulation with evacuation of these materials is advised.

Ultrasonic Scalpel

The ultrasonic scalpel is an instrument that potentially causes minimal tissue injury and good hemostasis. Ultrasonically activated, the scalpel blade moves longitudinally at 55,000 vibrations per second in cutting the tissue. Use of the ultrasonic scalpel is associated with reduced bleeding compared to a traditional scalpel. It causes tissue blanching without charring and with minimal smoke production. It is believed that the vibration of the ultrasonic scalpel generates low heat at the incision site, and that the combination of the vibration and the heat causes the proteins to denature. The denatured proteins form a coagulum that seals the bleeding vessels. Previous investigators[83] demonstrated that the use of a traditional scalpel produces less tissue destruction than the ultrasonic scalpel and that both modalities are superior to the CO_2 laser and electrocautery with regard to tissue destruction.

Tulandi et al.[169] evaluated the histologic changes and subsequent adhesion formation in rat uterine tissue after a standard incision with an ultrasonic scalpel or with a traditional scalpel. Incisions of the uterine horn using a regular scalpel resulted in bleeding that stopped easily with mild pressure. No bleeding was encountered after incisions with the ultrasonic scalpel. The tissue appeared to blanch when in contact with the activated ultrasonic scalpel blade. At repeat laparotomy, adhesions to the incision site were found in both groups of rats. The adhesions were mild, and no significant difference was found in adhesion score between the ultrasonic scalpel and the regular scalpel group on day 7 and on day 14 after the initial surgery. On day 21, distal uterine dilatation was seen in eight of nine tubes in the ultrasonic scalpel group, and no dilatation was encountered in nine uterine horns in the regular scalpel group. However, the degree of coagulation necrosis was significantly higher at 7 and 14 days after incision with an ultrasonic scalpel than with a regular scalpel.

Second-Look Laparoscopy

In 1967, second-look laparoscopy (SLL) was used to evaluate the results of certain surgical techniques.[170] Multicenter collaborative studies show that the majority of adhesions reform after lysis and that the severity of the reformed adhesion often becomes worse[197] (Fig. 1.19). More recently, the potential role of SLL in assessing the outcome of infertility surgery and in lysing postoperative adhesions was investigated.[91,171–177] Many authors agreed that SLL performed within 4 to 6 weeks (short interval) of the original surgery appears to be more advantageous because adhesions are less dense and easier to lyse at that time.[174–177] Evaluation of pelvic adhesions after laparoscopic lysis in an in vitro fertilization program supports the use of this approach except in the case of severe, dense adhesions.[171] However, little information is available to establish indications and the criteria for patient selection for a short-interval SLL.

Although the effect on pregnancy rates of "second-look" laparoscopy to lyse adhesions that form after reproductive surgery was examined, generalized use of SLL remains controversial. Tables 1.9 and 1.10 summarize the overall pregnancy rates and rates of ectopic pregnancy in five studies employing SLL during which adhesions were separated or lysed. Daniell et al.[171] described intrauterine pregnancy in 9 of 25 infertility patients within 6 months after adesiolysis was performed at SLL at 4 to 6 weeks after the initial laparotomy. Trimbos-Kemper et al.[178] reported success with SLL as early as 8 days after surgery. After SLL, intrauterine pregnancy rates (40%) were the same with or without SLL although a decrease in ectopic pregnancies was noted (Fig. 1.20).[18]

Many studies directly evaluated the rate of adhesion reformation after adhesiolysis. Adhesiolysis by SLL was effective in preventing adhesion reformation in 52% of 64 patients who underwent a second follow-up laparoscopy (i.e., third-look procedure).[180] Furthermore, in this study, significantly more of the adnexa evaluated at the time of the third-look laparoscopy had no adhesions present when adhesiolysis was performed at the second-look procedure (63%) than when no adhesiolysis was performed via second-look laparoscopy (39%). Similar findings using third-look laparoscopy were reported by

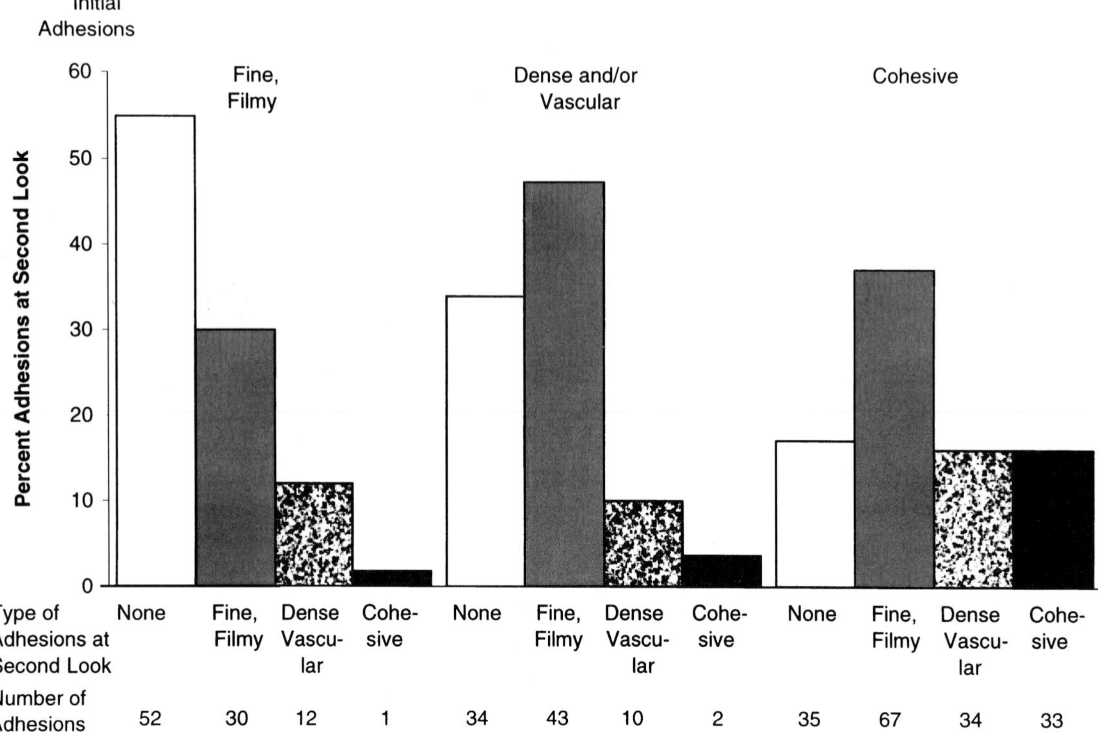

Fig. 1.19. Frequency and type of adhesion observed at early second-look procedures after laparoscopic adhesiolysis of fine, filmy adhesions, dense and/or vascular adhesions, or cohesive adhesions.[197]

Jansen[179] (Fig. 1.20) and Osada (personal communication). Diamond et al.[93] reported significant reductions in the incidence of adhesion involving the ovaries, fimbria, cul-de-sac, colon, and pelvic sidewall at the time of second-look laparoscopy following reproductive surgery. The overall reduction in adhesions involving these tissues at the time of the second-look procedure ranged from 30% to 50% (Tables 1.11, 1.12). Swolin,[58] Osada (personal communication), Trimbos-Kemper et al.,[178] Jansen,[179] and Serour et al.[180] all reported success with early second-look laparoscopy (Fig. 1.21). Not all reports are favorable. Mecke et al.[181] found that 50% of the ipsilateral adnexa still contained adhesions at third look after their resection following laparoscopic removal of an ectopic pregnancy.

The interval between the initial surgery and the SLL varied in these studies. In those studies in which the interval between the initial surgery and SLL varied among patients,[174,175] the benefits of SLL appear to be greater the shorter the postoperative interval before the procedure. Many clinicians believe that adhesion density and organization increase as the duration of the postoperative interval increases.[94,174,175] DeCherney and Mezer[177] found a 75% incidence of adhesion formation at the time of SLL at both 4 to 16 weeks and 16 to 19 months after laparotomy in infertility patients. There was, how-

Table 1.9. Summary of pregnancy rates following second-look laparoscopy (SLL)

Reference	Interval between original surgery and SLL	No. of patients	Percent of patients: Pregnant	Ectopic pregnancy
Raj and Hulka[a] (1982)[174]	4–8 weeks	51	20%	14%
Surrey and Friedman (1982)[175]	6–8 weeks	31	52%	0%
	≥ 6 months	6	17%	17%
Trimbos-Kemper et al. (1985)[178]	8 days	188	30%	10%
Tulandi et al.[b] (1989)[155]	12 months	19	67%[b]	47%[b]

[a]Originally, 60 patients were evaluated, 9 of whom had no postoperative adhesion and were excluded. Most of the 60 patients (83%) had SLL after 4–8 weeks; 3 patients had SLL at ≤2 weeks, and 7 patients had SLL >12 weeks postoperatively.
[b]Cumulative probability at 36 months using life table analysis.

TABLE 1.10. Results of early and late second-look laparoscopy (SLL) following reproductive surgery

Reference	Early[a]	Late[a]	Study design	Results
Swolin (1967)[58]	—	1 year	Cohort	Introduction to the use of SLL
Raj and Hulka (1982)[174]	1–8 weeks (53)	Up to 2 years (7)	Cohort	Optimal time of SLL appears to be 4–8 weeks after a reproductive surgery
Surrey and Friedman (1982)[175]	6 weeks (31)	6 months (6)	Cohort	Pregnancy rate after early SLL (52%) was higher than after late SLL (16.67%)
Daniell and Pittaway (1983)[173]	4–6 weeks (25)	—	Cohort	Early SLL may improve pregnancy rates
DeCherney and Mezer (1984)[95]	4–6 weeks (20)	16–19 months (41)	Cohort	60% of early SLL patients had filmy adhesions; 63% of the late SLL patients had thicker adhesions
Trimbos-Kemper et al. (1985)[178]	8 weeks (188)	—	Historical control	SLL reduced the occurrence of ectopic pregnancy
Diamond et al. (1987)[93]	1–12 weeks (161)	—	Cohort	Reproductive surgery by laparotomy is frequently complicated by de novo adhesion formation
Jansen (1988)[179]	8–21 days (256)	—	Cohort	Early SLL is safe and effective in reducing adhesion formation
Tulandi et al. (1989)[155]	—	1 year (74)	Randomized control	Late SLL does not increase the pregnancy rate or decrease the incidence of ectopic pregnancy

[a]Numbers in parentheses are numbers of patients.
From Tulandi et al. (1989).[155]

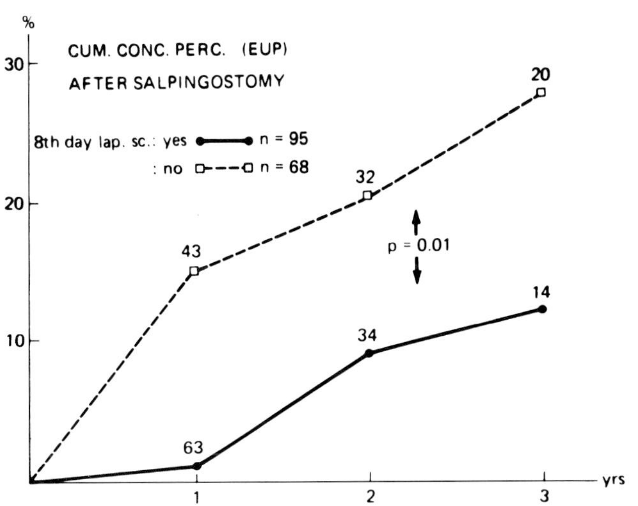

FIG. 1.20. *Left:* cumulative conception percentages of ectopic pregnancies in patients with and without second-look laparoscopy on the 8th day after salpingostomy. *Right:* cumulative conception percentage of intrauterine pregnancies in patients with and without second-look laparoscopy on the 8th day after salpingostomy, fimbrioplasty, or adhesiolysis.[178]

TABLE 1.11. Results of adhesiolysis

Reference	No. of patients	Live births (%)	Ectopic pregnancies (%)	ESLL
Conventional technique				
Wallach et al. (1983)[201]	94	45.7	2.1	No
Young et al. (1970)[202]	47	32.0	4.0	No
Trimbos-Kemper et al. (1985)[178]	N/A	48.0	N/A	Yes
Microsurgical technique				
Frantzen and Schlosser (1982)[203]	49	38.8	4.1	No
Diamond (1979)[204]	140	57.1	0.7	No
Luber et al. (1986)[205]	13	62.0	7.7	Yes
Hulka (1982)[206]	47	25.5	2.1	No
Laparoscopic lysis only				
Gomel (1983)[207]	92	58.7	5.4	—

ESLL, early second-look laparoscopy; N/A, not available.

TABLE 1.12. Preoperative GnRH treatment and adhesion formation after myomectomy

	No treatment		
	GnRH ($n = 21$)	No GnRH ($n = 36$)	p
Sites to uterus	7.2 ± 3.0	7.8 ± 3.3	0.60
Severity	2.7 ± 0.6	2.3 ± 0.9	0.03
Extent	1.8 ± 0.9	1.6 ± 0.9	0.32
Area	18.7 ± 13.2	19.0 ± 14.6	094

Use of gonadotropin-releasing hormone (GnRH) agonists during myomectomy did not reduce postoperative adhesion formation irrespective of barrier use.[197]
Area, cm^2.

ever, a relative enhancement in the adhesion grades that were present between the two groups (Fig. 1.22). In a case-control study, Raj and Hulka[174] found that the optimal time for a SLL and adhesiolysis is 4 to 8 weeks after a reproductive surgery. A randomized study with a clinical outcome is required to clarify this matter. Clearly, late SLL 1 year following a reproductive surgery does not lead to a significant increase in pregnancy rates.[155] Steege reported adhesion reduction by repeated adhesiolysis (four times in 2 weeks) in a small group of patients undergoing minilaparoscopy under conscious sedation.[182] Use of this technology may significantly alter both the time and route of "second-look" procedures in the future.

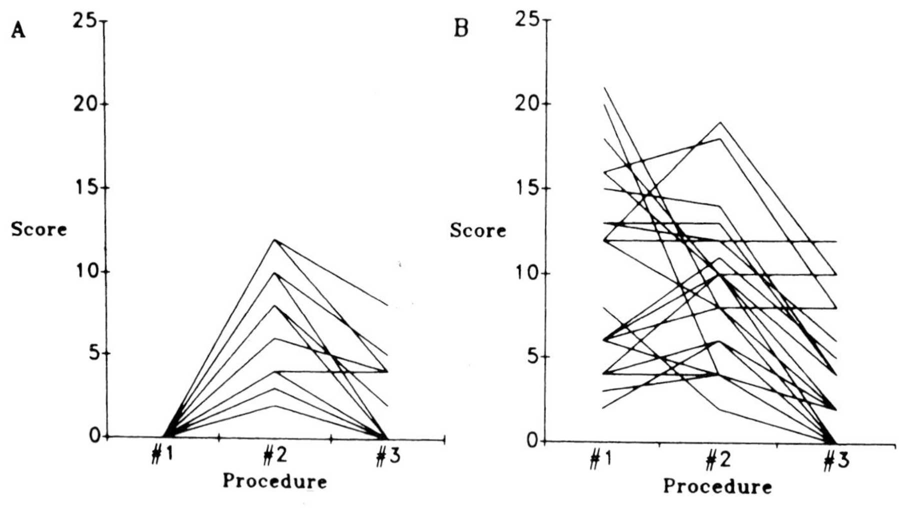

FIG. 1.21. Effect of postoperative laparoscopy on adhesion scores in patients with no initial adhesions **(A)** and with initial adhesions **(B)**. Procedures: initial infertility operation (#*1*), postoperative laparoscopy (#*2*), and subsequent evaluation (#*3*).[179]

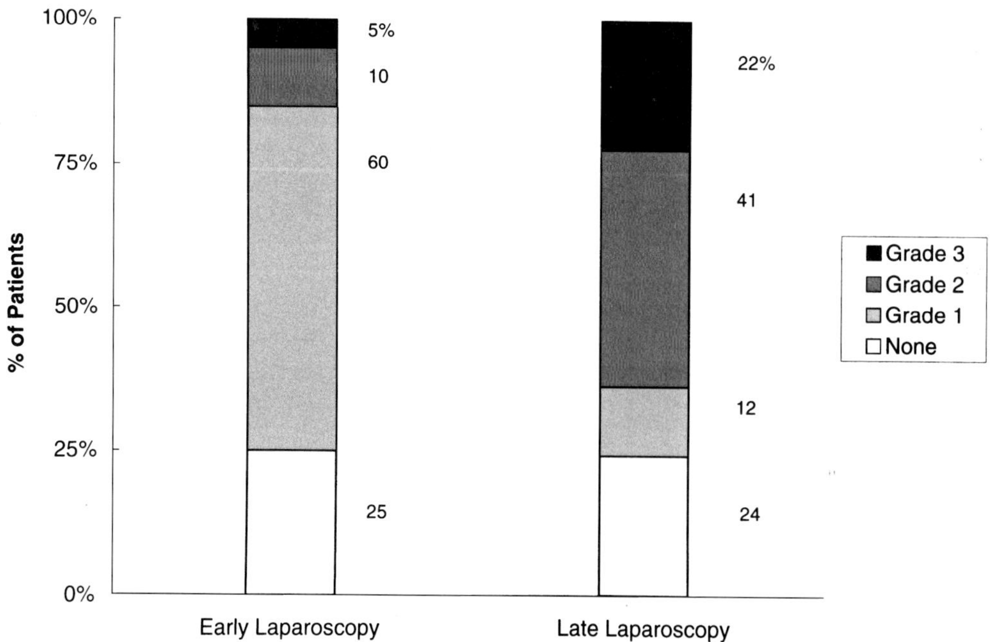

FIG. 1.22. Type of adhesion at second-look laparoscopy after tubal surgery. A relative enhancement in the grade of adhesions was noted between early (4–16 weeks after surgery) and late (16–19 months after surgery) laparoscopy.[95]

Hypoestrogenism

Estrogen may play a role in the formation of postoperative pelvic adhesions because estrogen may facilitate angiogenesis in uterine tissue production of uterine growth factors and possibly proliferation of mesothelial cells and fibroblasts.[57,183–187] Estrogen-dependent growth factors and growth modulators could play a role in adhesion formation. Insulin-like growth factors (IGF) stimulate mitosis in a wide variety of tissues. Regulation of IGF in the uterus has been studied extensively in rats, in which the predominant stimulator of IGF is estrogen.[186] Keratinocyte-derived growth factor is steroid responsive and is mitogenic for epithelial cells. In addition, estrogen-sensitive growth factors (epidermal growth factor [EGF] and platelet-derived growth factor [PDGF]) enhance the growth of cultured peritoneal mesothelial cells.[187] Montanino-Oliva et al.[188] found that both GnRH-α (gonadotropin-releasing hormone-alpha) and medroxyprogesterone acetate reduce adhesion formation in the rat uterine horn model when compared with controls. They considered the antiinflammatory and immunosuppressive actions of progestins as potential mechanisms behind the observed adhesion prevention. Fibroblast growth factor (FGF), EGF, PDGF, and TGF-β directly increase the mitogenic activity of peritoneal repair cells.[30,189,190] Chegini et al.[190] reported that intraperitoneal adhesions contained immunoreactive EGF, EGF receptor, and tranforming growth factor-alpha (TGF-α). These growth factors are modulated by estrogen in the female reproductive tract. Although the mesothelium covering the normal human peritoneum is reported to be negative for both estrogen receptor (ER) and progesterone receptor (PR), positive reactivity for ER and PR has been identified in a small portion of the underlying mesenchymal cells.[191–193] However, unlike normal mesothelium, mesothelium adjacent to endometriotic lesions is reported to contain focal positivity for ER and PR.[193] Several groups have presented animal data suggesting that a hypoestrogenic state causes a decrease in postoperative adhesion formation.[185,190]

To evaluate the possible role of estradiol in adhesion formation, 36 oophorectomized New Zealand white rabbits that had undergone a standardized adhesiogenic stimulus 2 weeks previously were randomized to receive 5 mg estradiol valerate or vehicle 2 days before adhesiolysis.[194] Animals receiving estradiol replacement showed an increased adhesion score following adhesiolysis, while nonreplaced animals demonstrated a decreased adhesion score. Preoperative GnRH-α therapy was shown to reduce adhesion formation in rats with surgically induced endometriosis or adhesions. Combined pre- and postoperative GnRH-α therapy, but not postoperative GnRH-α therapy, reduced adhesion reformation after adhesiolysis.[183]

In contrast, Lamorte et al.[195] evaluated the effects of physiologic estrogen levels upon de novo adhesion formation in a rat uterine horn model. Twenty-one adult Sprague-Dawley rats underwent bilateral oophorectomy and were then randomized to receive 17-β-estradiol (1.5-mg pellets) or vehicle. Two weeks later each animal underwent abrasion of the right uterine horn. Adhesion extent measured 2 weeks following the adhesiogenic stimulus was not different for the estrogen-treated animals. These data suggest that high levels of estradiol may be associated with increased adhesion formation and that regulation of estradiol at the time of surgery may be a means of preventing adhesion formation.

Grow et al.[196] reported on a prospective, randomized crossover study for the prevention of pelvic adhesions using surgical barriers or careful surgical technique alone with and without suppressions of estrogen production by preoperative GnRH-α therapy. Monkeys were assigned to either chronic GnRH-α (depot), chronic mifepristone (RU486), or vehicle control (saline). The adhesion scores were twofold greater and significantly higher in cycling controls than for primates treated with either GnRH-α or mifepristone. However, this observation was inconsistent with the clinical results of perioperative GnRH-α therapy on adhesion formation after myomectomy performed in patients with and without adhesion prevention barriers applied to the uterus.[197] Irrespective of the use of adhesion prevention barriers, no difference in adhesion formation rates was noted based on GnRH therapy (see Table 1.12). Limited animal studies with progesterone have not reported any reduction in postoperative adhesions.[198]

Conclusion

The special complexity of peritoneal morphology, including surface covering by mesothelial cells, a vascularized connective tissue underpinning laced by extracellular matrix proteins and mesenchymal stem cells, leads to a unique response to injury (see Fig. 1.7). Large peritoneal injuries reepithelialize as quickly as small peritoneal injuries. Virtually all types of surgical injury including cutting, coagulation, drying, and abrasion induce an inflammatory reaction that may lead to adhesion formation. Clean excision of peritoneal tissue without suture placement to reapproximate edges provides the best opportunity for rapid reperitonealization. Peritoneal repair is not accelerated with reapproximation of incised peritoneal edges. Reapproximation of peritoneal edges increases tissue necrosis and foreign-body reactions, which may slow the healing process. The prolonged presence of an acute inflammatory reaction in areas of extensive thermal injury disrupts healing and makes adhesion formation beyond 72 hours of postoperative injury a likely event. Frequent irrigation with buffered solutions like lactated Ringer's solution provides the best method of preventing tissue desiccation and removing soluble fibrin during the surgical procedure. Nevertheless, the majority of patients develop postoperative adhesions following peritoneal surgery, and the majority of adhesions that are lysed reform.

References

1. Esperanca JM, Collins DL. Peritoneal dialysis efficiency in relation to body weight. J Pediatr Surg 1966;1:162–169.
2. Bloom W, Fawcett DW. A Textbook of Histology, 9th Ed. Philadelphia: Saunders, 1968:186–187.
3. Robbins SL. A Textbook of Histology, 3rd Ed. Philadelphia: Saunders, 1967:891–896.
4. Watters WB, Buck RC (1972) Scanning electron microscopy of mesothelial regeneration in the rat. Lab Invest 26:604–609.
5. Pfeiffer CJ, Pfeiffer DC, Misra HP. Enteric serosal surface in the piglet. A scanning and transmission electron microscopic study of the mesothelium. J Submicrosc Cytol 1987; 19:237–246.
6. Dobbie JW. New concepts in molecular biology and ultrastructural pathology of the peritoneum: their significance of peritoneal dialysis. Am J Kidney Dis 1990;15:97–109.
7. Berndt WO, Gosselin RE. Rubidium and creatinine transport across isolated mesentery. Biochem Pharmacol 1961; 8:359–366.
8. Gosselin RE, Berndt WO. Diffusional transport of solute through mesentery and peritoneum. J Theor Biol 1962; 3:487–495.
9. Fukata H. Electron microscopic study on normal rat peritoneal mesothelium and its changes in absorption of particulate iron dextran complex. Acta Pathol Jpn 1963;13: 309–325.
10. Shear J, Harvey JD, Barry KG. Peritoneal sodium transport; enhancement by pharmacologic and physical agents. J Lab Clin Med 1966;67:181–188.
11. Cotran RS, Karnovsky JJ. Ultrastructural studies on the permeability of the mesothelium to horseradish peroxidase. J Cell Biol 1968;37:123–137.
12. Baron MA. Structure of the intestinal peritoneum in man. Am J Anat 1941;69:439–497.
13. Atkinson M, Losowsky MS. Mechanism of ascites formation in chronic liver disease. Clin Sci 1962;22:383–389.
14. Leak LV, Rahil K. Permeability of the diaphragmatic mesothelium: the ultrastructural bases for "stomata." Am J Anat 1978;151:557–569.
15. Lill SR, Parsons RH, Buchac I. Permeability of the diaphragm and fluid resorption from the peritoneal cavity in the rat. Gastroenterology 1979;76:997–1002.
16. MacCallum WG. On the mechanism of absorption of granular material from the peritoneum. Johns Hopkins Hosp Bull 1903;14:105–112.
17. Allen L. The peritoneal stomata. Anat Rec 1936;67:89–99.
18. French JE, Florey HW, Morris B. The absorption of particles by the lymphatics of the diaphragm. J Exp Physiol 1960;45:88–93.
19. Leak LV. The adhesion of peritoneal cells to the diaphragmatic mesothelium. Bibl Anat 1979;17:115–124.
20. Murphy MJ, Morris B. A study of the peritoneal surface of the diaphragm by steroscan electron microscopy. In: Grenoble FP (ed) Microscopie Electronique, Vol. 3. Paris, France: Société française de Microscopie électronique, 1970:587–592.
21. Tsilibury EC, Wissig SL. Absorption from the peritoneal cavity: SEM study of the mesothelium covering the peritoneal surface of the muscular portion of the diaphragm. Am J Anat 1977;149:127–133.
22. diZerega GS, Rodgers K. Peritoneal fluid. In: The Peritoneum. New York: Springer-Verlag, 1990:26–52.
23. Bercovici B, Gallily R. The cytology of the human peritoneal fluid. Acta Cytol 1978;22:197–207.
24. McGowan L, Davis RH, Stein DB, et al. The cytology of the pelvic peritoneal cavity in normal women. Am J Clin Pathol 1968;49:506–511.
25. McGowan L, Davis RH. Peritoneal fluid cellular patterns in obstetrics and gynecology. Am J Clin Gynecol 1970; 106:979–995.
26. Diegelmann RF, Cohen IK, Kaplan AM. The role of macrophages in wound repair: a review. Plast Reconstr Surg 1981;68:107–113.
27. ArRajab A, Dawidson I, Sentementes J, et al. Enhancement of peritoneal macrophages reduces postoperative peritoneal adhesion formation. J Surg Res 1995;58:307–312.
28. Rodgers KE, diZerega GS. Modulation of peritoneal reepithelialization by postsurgical macrophages. J Surg Res 1992;53:542–548.
29. Fukasawa M, Yanagihara D, Rodgers KE, diZerega GS. The mitogenic activity of peritoneal tissue repair cells: control by growth factors. J Surg Res 1989;47:45–51.
30. Orita H, Campeau JD, Gale J, et al. Modulation of fibroblast proliferation and transformation by activated macrophages during postoperative peritoneal reepithelialization. Am J Obstet Gynecol 1986;155:905–911.
31. Leibovich SJ, Ross R. A macrophage-dependent factor that stimulates the proliferation of fibroblasts in vitro. Am J Pathol 1976;84:501–514.
32. diZerega GS. The peritoneum and its response to surgical injury. In: diZerega GS, Malinak LR, Diamond MP, Linsky CB, eds. Treatment of Post Surgical Adhesions. Prog Clin Biol Res 1990;358:1–11.
33. Itskovitz-Eldor J, Kol S, Lewit N, Sealey JE. Ovarian origin of plasma and peritoneal fluid prorenin in early pregnancy and in patients with ovarian hyperstimulation syndrome. J Clin Endocrinol Metab 1997;82:461–464.
34. Chacho K, Chacho S, Andersen P, Scommegna A. Peritoneal fluid in patients with and without endometriosis: prostanoids and macrophages and their effect on the spermatozoa penetration assay. Am J Obstet Gynecol 1986;154: 1290–1297.
35. DeLeon F, Vijayakumar R, Brown M, Rao C, Yussman M, Schultz G. Peritoneal fluid volume, estrogen, progesterone, prostaglandin, and epidermal growth factor concentrations in patients with and without endometriosis. Obstet Gynecol 1986;68:189–193.
36. Halme J. Release of tumor necrosis factor-alpha by human peritoneal macrophages in vivo and in vitro. Am J Obstet

Gynecol 1989;161:1718–1725.
37. Oosterlynck DJ, Meuleman C, Waer M, Koninckx PR. Transforming growth factor-β activity is increased in peritoneal fluid from women with endometriosis. Obstet Gynecol 1994;83:287–292.
38. Fakih H, Bagget B, Holtz G, Tsang KY, Lee J, Williamson H. Interleukin-1: possible role in the infertility associated with endometriosis. Fertil Steril 1987;47:213–217.
39. Arici A, Tazuke SI, Attar E, Kilman HJ, Olive DL (1996) Interleukin-8 concentration in peritoneal fluid of patients with endometriosis and modulation of interleukin-8 expression in human mesothelial cells. Mol Hum Reprod 2:40–45.
40. Oral EP, Arici A. Peritoneal growth factors and endometriosis. Semin Reprod Endocrinol 1996;14:257–267.
41. Halme J, Becker S, Haskill S. Altered maturation and function of peritoneal macrophages: possible role in pathogenesis of endometriosis. Am J Obstet Gynecol 1987;136: 783–789.
42. Werb Z. Phagocytic cells: chemotaxis and effector functions of macrophages and granulocytes. In: Daniel S, Stobo J, Wells V, eds. Basic and Clinical Immunology, Vol. 6. Norwalk: Appleton & Lange, 1987:96–113.
43. Hill JA, Faris H, Schiff I, Anderson D. Characterization of leukocyte subpopulations in the peritoneal fluid of women with endometriosis. Fertil Steril 1988;50:216–222.
44. Akoum A, Lemay A, McColl S, Turcot-Lemay L, Maheux R. Elevated concentration and biologic activity of monocyte chemotactic protein-1 in the peritoneal fluid of patients with endometriosis. Fertil Steril 1996;66:17–23.
45. Mori H, Swairi M, Nakagawa M, Itoh N, Wada K, Tamaya T. Peritoneal fluid interleukin-1 beta and tumor necrosis factor in patients with benign gynecologic disease. Am J Reprod Immunol 1991;26:62–67.
46. Liu J, Lian LJ, Wang YF, et al. The immunological study of patients with endometriosis. Contrib Gynecol Obstet 1987;16:66–72.
47. Badawy SZ, Cuenca V, Stitzel A, et al. The regulation of immunoglobulin production by B cells in patients with endometriosis. Fertil Steril 1989;51:770–773.
48. Badawy SZ, Cuenca V, Kaufman L, et al. The regulation of immunoglobulin production by B cells in patients with endometriosis. Fertil Steril 1989;51:770–773.
49. Badawy SZ, Cuenca V, Marshall L, et al. Cellular components in peritoneal fluid in infertile patients with and without endometriosis. Fertil Steril 1984;42:701–708.
50. Meek SC, Hodge DD, Musich JR. Autoimmunity in infertile patients with endometriosis. Am J Obstet Gynecol 1988;158:1365–1373.
51. Confino E, Harlow L, Gleicher N. Peritoneal fluid and serum autoantibody levels in patients with endometriosis. Fertil Steril 1990;53:242–245.
52. Garza D, Mathur S, Dowd MM, et al. Antigenic differences between the endometrium of women with and without endometriosis. J Reprod Med 1991;36:177–182.
53. Fernandez-Shaw S, Hicks BR, Judkin PL, et al. Anti-endometrial and anti-endothelial auto-antibodies in women with endometriosis. Hum Reprod (Oxf) 1993;8:310–315.
54. Dorr PJ, Brommer EJP, Dooijewaard G, et al. Peritoneal fluid and plasma fibrinolytic activity in women with pelvic inflammatory disease. Thromb Haemostasis 1992;68: 102–105.
55. Nissell H, Larsson B. Role of blood and fibrinogen in development of intraperitoneal adhesions in rats. Fertil Steril 1978;30:470–473.
56. Larsson B. Prevention of postoperative formation and reformation of pelvic adhesions. In: Treutner KH, Schumpleck V, eds. Peritoneal Adhesions. Berlin: Springer, 1997.
57. Rosenberg L. Tronstad SE, Sponland G, et al. Results of electromicrosurgery in 78 women for correction of infertility. A two-center comparative study. Infertility 1982;5: 35–41.
58. Swolin K. Die einwirkung von grossen, intraperitoneal en dusen glukortikiod auf die bildung von postoperative adhesionen. Acta Obstet Gynecol Scand 1967;46:204–209.
59. Querleu D, Vankeerberghen-Deffense F, Boutteville C. Traitement adjuvant des plasties tubaires. J Gynecol Obstet Biol Reprod 1989;18:935–940.
60. Williams PL, Warwick R, Dyson M, Bannister LH, eds. Gray's Anatomy. Edinburgh: Churchill Livingstone, 1989.
61. Hollinshead HW. The thorax, abdomen, and pelvis. In: Anatomy for Surgeons, Vol. 2. New York: Harper & Row, 1978:78–161.
62. Wakefield EG, Mayo CW. Intestinal obstruction produced by mesenteric bands in association with failure of intestinal rotation. Arch Surg 1936;33:47–67.
63. Mitchell GAG. The spread of acute intraperitoneal effusions. Br J Surg 1941;28:291–296.
64. Ahrenholz DH, Simmons RL. Peritonitis and other intraabdominal infections. In: Howard RF, Simmons RL, eds. Surgical Infectious Disease, 2nd Ed. Norwalk: Appleton & Lange, 1988:605–646.
65. Hertzler AE. The Peritoneum. St. Louis: Mosby, 1919.
66. Bigatti G. Neoangigogenesis in Adhesion Formation and Peritoneal Healing. Berlin: Springer, 1997.
67. Ellis H, Harrison W, Hugh TB. The healing of peritoneum under normal and pathological conditions. Br J Surg 1965;52:471–476.
68. Hubbard TB, Khan MZ, Carag VR, Albites VE, Hricko GM. The pathology of peritoneal repair: its relation to the formation of adhesions. Ann Surg 1967;165:908–916.
69. Glucksman DL. Serosal integrity and intestinal adhesions. Surgery (St. Louis) 1966;60:1009–1011.
70. Eskeland G. Regeneration of parietal peritoneum in rats. I. A light microscopical study. Acta Pathol Microbiol Scand 1966;68:355–378.
71. Raftery AT. Regeneration of parietal and visceral peritoneum: an electron microscopical study. J Anat 1973;115: 375–392.
72. Devens K. Recurrent intestinal obstruction in the neonatal period. Arch Dis Child 1963;38:118–119.
73. Raftery AT. Regeneration of parietal and visceral peritoneum. A light microscopical study. Br J Surg 1973;60: 293–299.
74. Johnson FR, Whitting HW. Repair of parietal peritoneum. Br J Surg 1962;49:653–660.
75. Brunschwig A, Robbins GF. Regeneration of peritoneum: experimental observations and clinical experience in radical resections of intra-abdominal cancer. In: XVth Con-

gress of the Society of International Chirurgie, Lisbonne, 1953. Bruxelles: Henri de Smedt, 1954:756–765.

76. diZerega GS, Rodgers K. Fibroblasts and tissue repair cells. In: The Peritoneum. New York: Springer-Verlag, 1990: 122–144.
77. Hott JW, Godbey SW, Antony VB. Mesothelial cell modulation of pleural repair: thrombin stimulated mesothelial cells release prostaglandin E2. Prostaglandins Leukot Essent Fatty Acids 1994;51:329–335.
78. Robbins GF, Brunschwig A, Foote FW. Deperitonealization: clinical and experimental observations. Ann Surg 1949;130:466–479.
79. Lucas PA, Warejcka DJ, Young HE, et al. Formation of abdominal adhesion is inhibited by antibodies to transforming growth factor-β1. J Surg Res 1996;65:135–138.
80. Witz CA, Montoya-Rodriguez IA, Bena BS, et al. Mesothelium expression of integrins in vivo and in vitro. J Soc Gynecol Invest 1998;5:87–93.
81. Elkins TE, Stovall TG, Warren J, Ling FW, Meyer NL. A histologic evaluation of peritoneal injury and repair: implications for adhesion formation. Obstet Gynecol 1987;70: 225–228.
82. Bellina JH, Hemmings R, Voros JI, Ross LF. Carbon dioxide laser and electrosurgical wound study with an animal model: a comparison of tissue damage and healing patterns in peritoneal tissue. Am J Obstet Gynecol 1984;148: 327–334.
83. Filmar S, Jeta N, McComb P, et al. A comparative histologic study on the healing process following tissue transection: Part I. CO_2 laser and electromicrosurgery. Am J Obstet Gynecol 1989;160:1068–1072.
84. Montgomery TC, Sharp JB, Bellina H, Ross LF. Comparative gross and histological study of the effects of scalpel, electric knife and carbon dioxide laser on skin and uterine incisions in dogs. Lasers Surg Med 1983;3:9–22.
85. Weibel MA, Majno G. Peritoneal adhesions and their relation to abdominal surgery. A postmortem study. Am J Surg 1973;126:345–353.
86. Perry JF Jr, Smith GA, Yonehiro EG. Intestinal obstruction caused by adhesions. A review of 388 cases. Ann Surg 1955;142:810–816.
87. Raf LE. Causes of abdominal adhesion in cases of intestinal obstruction. Acta Chir Scand 1969;135:73–76.
88. Nemir P. Intestinal obstruction; ten year survey at the Hospital of the University of Pennsylvania. Ann Surg 1952; 135:367–375.
89. Menzies D, Ellis H. Adhesion formation: the role of plasminogen activator. Surg Gynecol 1991;172:362–366.
90. Wilkins BM, Spitz L. Incidence of postoperative adhesion obstruction following neonatal laparotomy. Br J Surg 1986;73:762–764.
91. Adhesion Study Group. Reduction of postoperative pelvic adhesions with intraperitoneal 32% dextran 70: a prospective, randomized clinical trial. Fertil Steril 1983;40: 612–619.
92. Interceed (TC7) Adhesion Barrier Group. Prevention of postsurgical adhesions by Interceed (TC7), an absorbable adhesion barrier: a prospective randomized multicenter clinical study. Fertil Steril 1989;51:933–938.
93. Diamond MP, Daniell JF, Feste J. Adhesion reformation and de novo adhesion formation after reproductive pelvic surgery. Fertil Steril 1987;47:864–866.
94. Szigetvari I, Feinman M, Barad D, et al. Association of previous abdominal surgery and significant adhesions in laparoscopic sterilization patients. J Reprod Med 1989;34: 465–498.
95. DeCherney AH, Mezer HC. The nature of posttuboplasty pelvic adhesions as determined by early and late laparoscopy. Fertil Steril 1984;41:643–646.
96. Ali V, Newton E, Miller I, Sri I. Frequency of abdominal and pelvic adhesion after Cesarean section (abstract S63). J Am Assoc Gynecol Laparosc 1997;4(suppl 4):563.
97. Browne AH, Hynes T. Multiple repeat caesarean section. J Obstet Gynaecol Br Commonw 1965;72:693–699.
98. Ray NF, Larsen JW, Stillman RF, Jacobs RF. Economic impact of hospitalization for lower abdominal adhesiolysis in United States in 1988. Surg Gynecol Obstet 1993;176: 271–276.
99. Ray NF, Denton WG, Thamer M, et al. Adbominal adhesiolysis: inpatient care and expenditures in the United States in 1994. J Am Coll Surg 1998;186:1–9.
100. Ivarsson ML, Holmdahl L, Franzjen G, Reisbert B. Cost of bowel obstruction resulting from adhesions. Eur J Surg 1997;163:679–684.
101. McGuire A. The economic impact of post-operative adhesions. Clinical and epidemiological perspectives on post-operative adhesions. Abstract presented at the annual scientific meeting of the Association of Surgeons Great Britain and Ireland, 13–15 May, Edinburgh Scotland, 1998.
102. Sigel B, Golub M, Loiacono LA, et al. Technique of ultrasonic detection and mapping of abdominal wall adhesions. Surg Endosc 1991;5:161–165.
103. Kodama I, Loiacono LA, Sigel B, et al. Ultrasonic detection of viscera slide as an indicator of abdominal wall adhesion. J Clin Ultrasound 1992;20:375–801.
104. Lamont PM, Menziers D, Ellis H. Intra-abdominal adhesion formation between two adjacent deperitonealised surfaces. Surg Res Commun 1992;13:127–130.
105. Haney AF, Doty E. The formation of coalescing peritoneal adhesions requires injury to both contacting peritoneal surfaces. Fertil Steril 1994;61:767–775.
106. Kligman I, Drachenberg C, Papadimitriou J, et al. Immunohistochemical demonstration of nerve fiber in pelvic adhesions. Obstet Gynecol 1993;82:566–568.
107. Tulandi T, Chen MF, Sundus A, et al. A study of nerve fibers and histopathology of postsurgical, postinfectious, and endometriosis-related adhesions. Obstet Gynecol 1998;92:766–768.
108. Milligan DW, Raftery AT. Observations on the pathogenesis of peritoneal adhesions: a light and electron microscopical study. Br J Surg 1974;61:270–280.
109. Harris ES, Morgan RF, Rodeheaver GT. Analysis of the kinetics of peritoneal adhesion formation in the rat and evaluation of potential antiadhesive agents. Surgery (St. Louis) 1995;117:663–669.
110. Abe H, Rodgers KE, Campeau JD, et al. The effect of intraperitoneal administration of sodium tolmetin-hyaluronic acid on the postsurgical cell infiltration in vivo. J Surg Res 1990;49:322–327.
111. Ramos BF, Qureshi R, Olsen KE, Jakschik BA. The importance of mast cells for the neutrophil influx in immune complex-induced peritonitis in mice. J Immunol 1990; 145:1868–1873.

112. Qureshi R, Jakschik BA. The role of mast cells in thioglycollate-induced inflammation. J Immunol 1988;141: 2090–2096.
113. Collins SM, Marzio L, Vermillion DL, Blennerhassett P, Chiverton S. The immunomodulation of gut motility: factors that determine the proliferation of mast cells in the sensitized gut. Gastroenterology 1988;94:A74.
114. Moriwaki K, Jujii K, Yuge O. Protein exudation induced by manipulation of the intestines and mesentery during laparotomy in rat: a study of the mechanism of 'third space' loss. In Vivo 1997;11:325–327.
115. Liebman SM, Langer JC, Marshall JS, et al. Role of mast cells in peritoneal adhesion formation. Am J Surg 1993; 165:127–130.
116. Ellis H. The cause and prevention of postoperative intraperitoneal adhesions. Surg Gynecol 1971;133:497–511.
117. Ellis H. Prevention and treatment of adhesions. Infect Surg 1983;11:803–807.
118. Buckman RF, Buckman PD, Hufnagel HV, et al. A physiologic basis for the adhesion-free healing of depertonealized surfaces. J Surg Res 1976;21:67–76.
119. Bridges JB, Johnson FR, Whitting HW. Peritoneal adhesion formation. Acta Anat (Basel) 1965;261:203–212.
120. Richardson EH. Studies on peritoneal adhesions: with a contribution to the treatment of denuded surfaces. Am Surg 1911;54:758–797.
121. Holmdahl L, Risberg B. Surgical glove powder: an overlooked risk. Severe adverse effects are well-documented. Lakartidningen 1993;90:2047–2049.
122. Schade DS, Williamson JR. The pathogenesis of peritoneal adhesions: an ultrastructural study. Ann Surg 1968; 167:500–510.
123. Turunen AOI. Ueber die postoperativen verwachs ungen und deren verhutung speziell im anschluss an gynakologische laparotomien. Duodecim Ser B 1933;18:1–9.
124. Pittaway DE, Daniell JF, Maxson WS. Ovarian surgery in an infertility patient as an indication for short-interval second-look laparoscopy: a preliminary study. Fertil Steril 1985;44:611–614.
125. Jackson BB. Observations on intraperitoneal adhesions, an experimental study. Surgery (St. Louis) 1958;44: 507–518.
126. Bronson RA, Wallach EE. Lysis of periadnexal adhesions for correction of infertility. Fertil Steril 1977;28:613–619.
127. Ryan GB, Grobety J, Majno G. Postoperative peritoneal adhesions: a study of the mechanisms. Am J Pathol 1971; 65:117–148.
128. Golan A, Winston RML. Blood and intraperitoneal adhesion formation in the rat. J Obstet Gynaecol 1989;9: 248–252.
129. Thompson JN, Scott-Coombes DM, Whawell SA. Peritoneal fibrinolysis and adhesion formation. In: diZerega GS, ed. Pelvic Surgery. New York: Springer-Verlag, 1997.
130. Holmdahl L, Eriksson E, Eriksson B, Risberg B. Depression of peritoneal fibrinolysis during operation is a local response to trauma. Surgery (St. Louis) 1998;123: 539–544.
131. Whawell SA, Scott-Coombes DM, Vipond MN, Tebbutt SJ, Thompson JN. Tumor necrosis factor mediated release of plasminogen activator inhibitor-1 by human peritoneal mesothelia cells. Br J Surg 1994;81:214–216.
132. Scott-Coombes DM, Whawell SA, Vipond MN, Thompson JN. The human intraperitoneal fibrinolytic response to elective surgery. Br J Surg 1995;160:471–477.
133. Bordes WA, Noble NA. Transforming growth factor β in tissue fibrosis. N Engl J Med 1994;331:1286–1292.
134. Williams RS. Rossi AM, Chegini N, et al. Effect of transforming growth factor-β on postoperative adhesion formation and intact peritoneum. J Surg Res 1992;51: 65–70.
135. McDonald MN, Elkins TE, Wortham GF, et al. Adhesion formation and prevention after peritoneal injury and repair in the rabbit. J Reprod Med 1988;33:436–439.
136. Tulandi T. Adhesion formation after reproductive surgery with and without the carbon dioxide laser. Fertil Steril 1987;47:704–706.
137. Ellis H, Heddle R. Does the peritoneum need to be closed at laparotomy? Br J Surg 1977;64:733–736.
138. Milewczyk M. Experimental studies on the development of peritoneal adhesions in cases of suturing and nonsuturing of the parietal peritoneum in rabbits. Ginekol Pol 1989;60:1–6.
139. Swanwick RA, Stockdale PH, Milne FJ. Healing of parietal peritoneum in the horse. Br Vet J 1963;129:29–35.
140. Hugh TB, Nankivel C, Meagher AP, et al. Is closure of the peritoneal layer necessary in the repair of midline surgical abdominal wounds? World J Surg 1990;14: 231–234.
141. Ling FW, Stovall TG, Meyer NL, et al. Adhesion formation associated with the use of absorbable staples in comparison to other types of peritoneal injury. Int J Gynaecol Obstet 1989;30:361–366.
142. Luciano AA, Hauser KS, Benda J. Evaluation of commonly used adjuvants in the prevention of postoperative adhesion. Am J Obstet Gynecol 1983;146:88–92.
143. Connolly JE, Stephens FO. Factors influencing the incidence of intra-peritoneal adhesions: an experimental study. Surgery (St. Louis) 1968;63:976–979.
144. Trimpi HD, Bacon HE. Clinical and experimental study of denuded surfaces in extensive surgery of the colon and rectum. Am J Surg 1952;34:596–602.
145. Ulfelder H, Quinby WC Jr. Small bowel obstruction following combined abdominoperitoneal resection of the rectum. Surgery (St. Louis) 1951;30:174–177.
146. Glucksman DL. Warren WD. The effect of topically applied corticosteroids in the prevention of peritoneal adhesions: an experimental approach with a review of the literature. Surgery (St. Louis) 1966;60:352–360.
147. Rhoades JE, Schwegman CW. One-stage combined abdominoperineal resection of the rectum (Miles) performed by two surgical teams. Surgery (St. Louis) 1965; 58:600–606.
148. Singelton AO Jr, Rowe EB, Moore RM. Failure of reperitonealization to prevent abdominal adhesions in the dog. Am J Surg 1952;18:789–792.
149. Chester J, Zimmer CH, Hoffman LD. The use of free peritoneal grafts in intestinal anastomosis. Surg Gynecol Obstet 1948;89:605–608.
150. Thomas JW, Rhoads JE. Adhesion resulting from removal of serosa from an area of bowel: failure of oversewing to lower incidence in the rat and the guinea pig. Arch Surg 1950;61:565–576.

151. Hull DB, Varner MW. A randomized study of closure of the peritoneum at cesarean delivery. Obstet Gynecol 1991;77:818–821.
152. Pietrantoni M, Parsons MT, O'Brien WF, et al. Peritoneal closure or non-closure at cesarean section. Obstet Gynecol 1991; 77:2–6.
153. Nagele F, Husslein P. Visceral peritonealization after abdominal hysterectomy—a retrospective pilot study. Geburtsh Frauenheilkd 1991;51:925–928.
154. Gupta JK, Dinas K, Kahn KS. To peritonealize or not to peritonealize? A randomized trial at abdominal hysterectomy. Am J Obstet Gynecol 1968;178:796–800.
155. Tulandi T, Falcone T, Kafka I. Second-look operative laparoscopy 1 year following reproductive surgery. Fertil Steril 1989;52:421–424.
156. Gilbert JM, Ellis H, Foweraker S. Peritoneal closure after lateral paramedian incision. Br J Surg 1987;74:113–115.
157. Vipond MN, Whawell SA, Thompson JN, et al. Peritoneal fibrinolytic activity and intra-abdominal adhesions. Lancet 1990;335:1120–1122.
158. O'Leary D, Coakley JB. The influence of suturing and sepsis on the development of postoperative peritoneal adhesions. Ann R Coll Surg Engl 1992;74:134–137.
159. Brill AI, Farr MD, Nezhat MD, et al. The incidence of adhesions after prior laparotomy: a laparoscopic appraisal. Obstet Gynecol 1995;85:269–272.
160. Levrant SG, Bieber EJ, Barnes RB. Anterior abdominal wall adhesions after laparotomy or laparoscopy. J Am Assoc Gynecol Laparosc 1997;4:353–356.
161. Bakkum EA, Trimbor-Kemper GCM. Natural course of postsurgical adhesions. Microsurgery 1995;16:650–654.
162. DeCherney AH, Laufer N. The use of a new synthetic absorbable monofilament suture, polydioxanone (PDS) for surgery. Fertil Steril 1983;39:401–405.
163. Mencke H, Schünke M, Schultz S, Semm K. Incidence of adhesions following thermal tissue damage. Res Exp Med 1991;191:405–412.
164. Diamond MP, Daniell JF, Martin DC, et al. Tubal patency and pelvic adhesions at early second-look laparoscopy following intraabdominal use of the carbon dioxide laser: initial report of the intraabdominal laser study group. Fertil Steril 1984;42:717–723.
165. Filmar S, Gomel V, McComb P. The effectiveness of CO_2 laser and electromicrosurgery in adhesiolysis: a comparative study. Fertil Steril 1986;45:407–411.
166. Luciano AA, Maier DB, Kock EI, et al. A comparative study of postoperative adhesions following laser surgery by laparoscopy in the rabbit model. Obstet Gynecol 1989; 74:220–224.
167. Sahakian V, Rogers R, Halme J, et al. Effects of carbon dioxide-saturated normal saline and Ringer's lactate on postsurgical adhesion formation in the rabbit. Obstet Gynecol 1993;82:851–853.
168. Ott DE. Pollutants resulting from intraabdominal tissue combustion. In: diZerega GS, ed. Pelvic Surgery. New York: Springer-Verlag, 1997:251–252 (abstract 11).
169. Tulandi T, Chan KL, Arseneau J. Histopathological and adhesion formation after incision using ultrasonic vibrating scalpel and regular scalpel in the rat. Fertil Steril 1994;61:548–550.
170. Operative Laparoscopy Study Group. Postoperative adhesion development after operative laparoscopy: evaluation at early second-look procedures. Fertil Steril 1991;44: 700–704.
171. Daniell JF, Pittaway DE, Maxson WE. The role of laparoscopic adhesion lysis in an in vitro fertilization program. Fertil Steril 1983;40:49–52.
172. Diamond MP, Daniell JF, Martin DC, et al. Tubal patency and pelvic adhesions at early second-look laparoscopy following intraabdominal use of the carbon dioxide laser: initial report of the intraabdominal laser study group. Fertil Steril 1984;42:717–723.
173. Daniell JF, Pittaway DE. Short interval second-look laparoscopy after infertility surgery: a preliminary report. J Reprod Med 1983;28:281–283.
174. Raj SG, Hulka JF. Second-look laparoscopy in infertility surgery; therapeutic and prognostic value. Fertil Steril 1982;38:325.
175. Surrey MW, Friedman S. Second-look laparoscopy after reconstructive pelvic surgery for infertility. J Reprod Med 1982;27:658–660.
176. McLaughlin DS. Evaluation of adhesion reformation by early second-look laparoscopy following microlaser ovarian wedge resection. Fertil Steril 1984;42:531–537.
177. DeCherney AH, Mezer HC. The nature of posttuboplasty pelvic adhesions as determined by early and late laparoscopy. Fertil Steril 1984;41:643–646.
178. Trimbos-Kemper TCM, Trimbos JB, van Hall EV. Adhesion formation after tubal surgery: results of the eighth-day laparoscopy in 188 patients. Fertil Steril 1985;43: 395–398.
179. Jansen RP. Early laparoscopy after pelvic operations to prevent adhesions: safety and efficacy. Fertil Steril 1988; 49:26–31.
180. Serour GI, Badraoui MH, el Agizi HM, et al. Laparoscopic adhesiolysis for infertile patients with pelvic adhesive disease. Int J Gynaecol Obstet 1989;30:249–252.
181. Mencke H, Semm K, Freys I, et al. Incidence of adhesions in the true pelvis after pelviscopic operative treatment of tubal pregnancy. Gynecol Obstet Invest 1989;28:202–204.
182. Steege JF. Repeated clinic laparoscopy for the treatment of pelvic adhesions: a pilot study. Obstet Gynecol 1994; 83:276–279.
183. Wright JA, Sharpe-Timms KL. Gonadotropin-releasing hormone agonist therapy reduces postoperative adhesion formation and reformation after adhesiolysis in rat models for adhesion formation and endometriosis. Fertil Steril 1995;63:1094–1100.
184. Smith SK. Vascular endothelial growth factor and the endometrium. Hum Reprod (Oxf) 1996;11:56–61.
185. Grow DR, Coddington CC, Hsiu JG, Mikich Y, Gidgeb GD. Role of hypoestrogenism or sex steroid antagonism in adhesion formation after myometrial surgery in primates. Fertil Steril 1996;66:140–147.
186. Murphy LJ, Ghahary A. Uterine insulin-like growth factor. I: Regulation of expression and its role in estrogen induced uterine proliferation. Endocr Rev 1990;11: 443–453.
187. Iwamoto I, Imada A. Effects of growth factors on proliferation of cultured mesothelial cells. Nippon Jinzo Gakkai Shi 1992;34:1201–1208.

188. Montanino-Oliva D, Metzerga DA, Luciano AA. Use of medroxyprogesterone acetate in the prevention of postoperative adhesions. Fertil Steril 1996;65:650–654.
189. Rodgers KE, Ellefson DD, Girgis W, et al. Modulation of postsurgical cell infiltration and fibrinolytic activity by tolmetin in two species. J Surg Res 1994;56:314–325.
190. Chegini N, Simms J, Williams S, Materson BJ. Identification of epidermal growth factor, transforming growth factor-α, and epidermal growth factor receptor in surgically induced pelvic adhesions in the rat and intraperitoneal adhesions in the human. Am J Obstet Gynecol 1994; 17:321–328.
191. Hill JA, Muldoon TG, Gallup DG, Turner WA, Loy RA, Talledor OE. Cytosol estrogen receptor content of female parietal peritoneum. Am J Obstet Gynecol 1986;154: 943–944.
192. Prentice A, Randall BJ, McGill A, et al. Ovarian steroid receptor expression in endometriosis and in two potential parent epithelia: endometrium and peritoneal mesothelium. Hum Reprod (Oxf) 1992;7:1318–1325.
193. Nakayama K, Masuzawa H, Ki SF, et al. Imunohistochemical analysis of the peritoneum adacent to endometriotic lesions using antibodies for Ber-EP4 antigen, estrogen receptors, and progesterone receptors: implication of peritoneal metaplasia in the pathogenesis of endometriosis. Int J Gynecol Pathol 1994;4:348–358.
194. Metzger DA, Breault DT, Chaffkin L, et al. The role of estrogen in adhesion reformation. Soc Gynecol Invest 1993;292:347 (abstract).
195. Lamorte A, Gutmann JN, Carcangiu ML, et al. The role of estrogen in adhesion formation. Soc Gynecol Invest 1993;292:238 (abstract).
196. Grow DR, Seltman HJ, Coddington CC, Hodgen GD. The reduction of postoperative adhesions by two different barrier methods versus control in cynomolgus monkeys: a prospective, randomized, crossover study. Fertil Steril 1994;61:1141–1146.
197. Diamond MP, Seprafim Adhesion Group. Reduction of adhesions after uterine myomectomy by Seprafilm® membrane (HAL-F®): a blinded, prospective, ramdomized, multicenter clinical study. Fertil Steril 1996;66: 904–910.
198. Blauer KL, Collins RL. The effect of intraperitoneal progesterone on postoperative adhesion formation in rabbits. Fertil Steril 1988;49:144–149.
199. Gillett WR. Artefactual loss of human ovarian surface epithelium: potential clinical significance. Reprod Fertil Dev 1991;3:93–98.
200. Merlo G, Fausone G, Barbero C, et al. Fibrinolytic activity of the human peritoneum. Eur Surg Res 1980;88: 623–630.
201. Wallach EE, Manara LR, Eisenberg E. Experience with 143 cases of tubal surgery. Fertil Steril 1983;39:609–617.
202. Young PE, Egan JE, Barlow JJ, et al. Reconstructive surgery for infertility at the Boston Hospital for Women. Am J Obstet Gynecol 1970;108:1092–1097.
203. Frantzen C, Schlosser HW. Microsurgery and postinfectious tubal infertility. Fertil Steril 1982;38:397–420.
204. Diamond E. Lysis of postoperative pelvic adhesions in infertility. Fertil Steril 1979;31:287–295.
205. Luber K, Beeson CC, Kennedy JF, et al. Results of microsurgical treatment of tubal infertility and early second-look laparoscopy in the post-pelvic inflammatory disease patient: implication for in vitro fertilization. Am J Obstet Gynecol 1986;154:1264–1270.
206. Hulka JF. Adnexal adhesions: a prognostic staging and classification system based on a five-year survey of fertility surgery results at Chapel Hill, North Carolina. Am J Obstet Gynecol 1982;144:141–148.
207. Gomel V. Microsurgery in Female Infertility. 1st Ed. Boston: Little, Brown 1983:225–244.

2

Peritoneal Fluid

Arthur F. Haney

CONTENTS

The lining of the abdominal cavity is composed of a single layer of mesothelial cells overlying a basement membrane and a large layer of extracellular matrix (ECM) proteins.[1] A unique feature of this histologic architecture is that these surface mesothelial cells are in constant contact with the peritoneal fluid (PF), which is contained within the abdominal cavity. Although the function of the PF is not typically given much emphasis in physiology textbooks, it undoubtedly facilitates mobility of the viscera within the peritoneal cavity. This movement is required for normal function of (1) the gastrointestinal tract, for example, peristalsis and defecation, (2) the bladder, for example, voiding, and (3) the female genital tract, for example, tubal motility for oocyte pickup. This function of PF is similar to that of the pleural fluid, which allows unrestricted sliding movement between the chest wall and the pleural surface of the lung during respiration, as well as that of the pericardium, which allows efficient contraction of the heart within the fluid environment of the pericardial sac. Not surprisingly, the peritoneal mesothelial cells not only share functional similarities with the pleural and pericardial mesothelial layers but a common embryology as well.[2,3]

In some functional ways, the peritoneal cavity can be considered analogous to the vascular system. The blood vessels are lined by a single layer of endothelial cells, wherein biologically active molecules in the blood are carried to distant sites, altering the function of the vascular bed. These molecules can be secreted by the vascular endothelium, leukocytes, or other cells or bacteria at sites of inflammation or injury. In an analogous fashion, soluble or particulate material that enters the peritoneal cavity is disbursed in the PF and thus throughout the peritoneum with the potential to affect the entire mesothelial layer. Although the PF does not actually circulate via the action of a pump as does the vascular system, PF circulates within the peritoneal cavity and is in continuity, via lymphatics, with the pleural fluid within the thoracic cavity and the vascular system.[4] Biologically active molecules can enter the peritoneal cavity via transudation, exudation, facilitated transport, or the lymphatics, or can be secreted by the leukocytes in the PF. These anatomic and functional features allow the PF to influence the behavior of the mesothelial cells throughout the entire peritoneum. Likewise, the reconstitution of the peritoneal membrane after surgical trauma occurs while it is in continuous contact with the PF, with the potential for bioactive molecules within the PF, such as cytokines and eicosanoids, to modulate the pattern of the healing response.

Similarly, the constituents of the PF reflect the events that are occurring at the wound surface during healing.[5] By studying the molecular environment at the injury site, we can learn more about the mechanism of peritoneal wound healing and potentially manipulate these events pharmacologically in a beneficial manner. Thus, it is important to understand the constituents as well as the function of the PF that may shed light on the molecular and cellular events critical to normal and pathologic wound healing so that we can therapeutically intervene.

Peritoneal Fluid Volume

The volume of the PF represents primarily a transudate across the peritoneal membrane, with a disproportionate contribution in women, originating from the surface of the cycling ovary.[6,7] In men, the volume of the peritoneal fluid is rarely greater than 5 mL in normal circumstances, whereas in women the volume varies with the menstrual cycle. PF for women is typically between 5 and 18 mL, with the greatest volume observed in the middle of the menstrual cycle at the time of ovulation.[8,9] Based on the correlation between PF volume and the ovarian steroid concentrations within the PF of women, an exudate from the ovary accounts for the majority of the difference between the sexes, suggesting that 5 mL is the minimum volume of PF required for normal function of the abdominal viscera. Whether the larger volume present in women at ovulation plays a physiologic role in reproduction or is simply an incidental response to cyclic ovarian function remains unclear.

When women go through spontaneous menopause, or their ovaries are removed before menopause, or if ovulation is suppressed with oral contraceptives, the observed volume of PF more closely approximates that of men.[6,7] When the uterus is removed but the ovaries remain in place and continue to cycle, the volume of the PF does not change appreciably from that of women with the uterus in place.[6,7] These data support the conclusion that ovarian function is the critical determinant of the differences in PF volume between women and men.

Pathologically high volumes of PF can be observed (1) when venous outflow of the abdominal viscera is mechanically impeded, such as with ovarian fibromas (Meigs' syndrome), bowel cancers metastasizing to the ovaries, ovarian torsion, and pedunculated uterine leiomyomata; (2) when the ovaries are therapeutically hyperstimulated and multiple corpora lutea are present (the severe ovarian hyperstimulation syndrome); (3) when reduced venous outflow of the portal system of the liver occurs, with cirrhosis; and (4) when an intraperitoneal inflammatory process is present in the peritoneal cavity, either a benign process such as endometriosis or miliary tuberculosis or a malignant process such as advanced epithelial cancer of the ovary with extensive metastasis throughout the peritoneum.

Soluble Factors in the Peritoneal Fluid

The soluble factors in the PF are likely a combination of a transudation of plasma, with a relative barrier to molecules above 20,000 kDa and facilitated transport.[10,11] The result is a concentration gradient from the PF to the plasma of large molecules in the PF, while those molecules of less than 20,000 kDa are close to being isotonic with plasma. Notable exceptions are the steroids secreted by the dominant cyclic structure of the ovary in women, where the concentrations are several orders of magnitude higher than plasma, reflecting the passage of the steroids from the ovarian cyclic structures across the ovarian surface epithelium.[8,9] As the fluid volume varies with the menstrual cycle in women, the evaluation of the importance of the various biologically active molecules as a concentration may be misleading unless the stage of the menstrual cycle is taken into consideration.

When larger molecules are secreted into the PF by the intraperitoneal leukocytes, such as cytokines, proteolytic enzymes, and protease inhibitors, they can be preferentially retained in the PF because of their size, resulting in higher concentrations than those observed in the peripheral circulation. This difference allows high local concentrations at the mesothelial surface during wound healing, amplifying the potential for an impact on the cellular events at the healing peritoneal surface. These cytokines are secreted by macrophages in response to a variety of inflammatory stimuli under complex control, which necessitates the removal of these bioactive molecules by either active transport or enzymatic degradation. The reverse situation is encountered in patients with renal failure undergoing peritoneal dialysis, where high molecular weight molecules in plasma, such as prolactin, are excluded from the peritoneal cavity on a weight basis and thus are not cleared by using the abdominal cavity as a dialysis membrane.[12,13]

Eicosanoids have been observed in the PF,[14–19] particularly in women with endometriosis. Because macrophages can secrete prostaglandins and the number of macrophages is elevated in women in various clinical situations such as endometriosis,[14,15] they are likely the source of the PF prostaglandins. A variety of cytokines, including enzymes, extracellular matrix proteins, growth factors, and other molecules, have been observed in the

TABLE 2.1. Potential modulating soluble factors present in the peritoneal fluid

Class	Factor
Cytokines	IL-1[20–27]
	IL-1β[20]
	IL-2[20,24]
	IL-5[20–22]
	IL-6[25,26]
	IL-10[25]
	Tumor necrosis factor-α[21,26–29]
	Interferon-γ[21,30]
Enzymes	Lysozyme[31]
	Lipid peroxides[32]
Extracellular matrix proteins	Glycosaminoglycans[33]
	Fibronectin[34]
Growth factors	Macrophage colony-stimulating factor[35,36]
	Vascular endothelial growth factor[37]
	Macrophage-derived growth factor[38]
	Transforming growth factor-β[39–41]
	Uncharacterized T-lymphocyte growth promoters that activate macrophages[42]
Others	α_2-macroglobulin[43]
	Heat shock protein, hsp60[30]
	CA 125[44]
	Monocyte chemotactic protein-1[45]

PF under varying clinical circumstances (Table 2.1). Although these cytokines are not unique to the PF, their concentrations may be higher than in plasma if they are secreted by PF macrophages, leading to a concentration gradient from the PF to the plasma.

Cellular Constituents of the Peritoneal Fluid

Cytopathologists have long described the cells present in the PF as "reactive mesothelial cells" without any objective scientific evidence as to their character or origin. There was no clinical need to distinguish the specific cell types; rather, a premium was placed on the ability to distinguish malignant cells from the resident benign population. However, this designation as "reactive mesothelial cells" is inaccurate as there appear to be few if any free-floating mesothelial cells in the PF.[46] The peritoneal mesothelial cells remain firmly adherent both to the basement membrane and to each other and are only dislodged as large sheets of adherent cells by mechanical abrasion during surgery. In reality, the cell population in the PF is composed overwhelmingly of leukocytes, with the vast majority being mononuclear phagocytes, typical tissue-differentiated macrophages (Fig 2.1). The remainder are lymphocytes with a small number of polymorphonuclear leukocytes (PMN), eosinophils, and basophils. Significant numbers of PMNs are not normally observed in the PF unless a bacterial infection is present.[31,46–52]

A resident population of PF macrophages is present in both sexes with higher numbers of cells in women with regular menstrual cycles and patent fallopian tubes.[46] The oviducts provide continuity with the lower genital tract, for example, the endometrial cavity, as well as the external environment through the cervix. The regurgitation of menstrual debris during menstruation appears to represent a significant stimulus to increase the number of these macrophages because the number of PF leukocytes is dramatically reduced if the continuity of the female genital tract is interrupted when the fallopian tubes are ligated or the uterus is removed. Similarly, if ovulation is hormonally suppressed, the PF cell number also declines, verifying the contribution of retrograde menstruation, a nearly universal event in ovulatory women with patent fallopian tubes, as an eliciting stimulus.[46] Not surprisingly, the PF leukocyte number varies throughout the menstrual cycle, with higher numbers being present in the follicular phase immediately following menses.[53] The finding that iron levels are elevated in the PF of women with endometriosis,[54] a clinical situation in which higher numbers of PF leukocytes are pre-

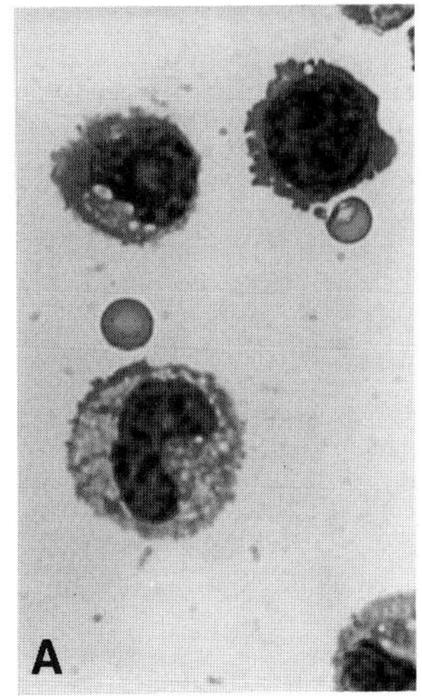

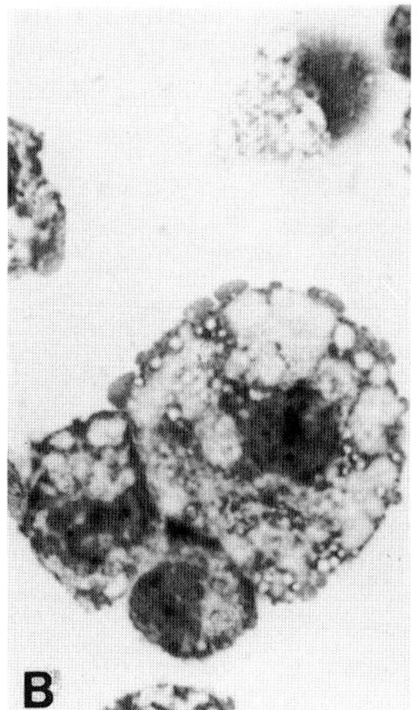

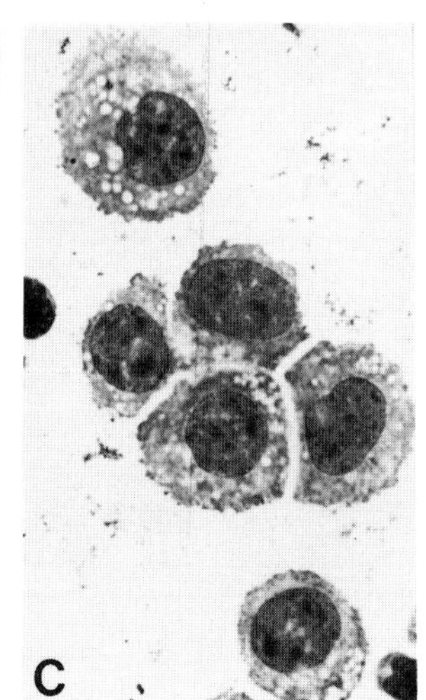

FIG. 2.1. This is a series of photomicrographs of cytospin preparations of peritoneal fluids from mice. The resident population of peritoneal macrophages of control mice is shown in (**A**). Three days after insertion of oxidized regenerated cellulose barrier material in the peritoneal cavity, the macrophages increase in number and are morphologically altered, suggesting activation (**B**). After insertion of expanded polytetrafluoroethylene barriers the macrophages are also morphologically altered (**C**), although not to the same extent as with oxidized regenerated cellulose. These preparations were stained with Wright's stain (original magnification × 1000).

sent, is also consistent with this conclusion. Infertile women with endometriosis and women with unexplained infertility, presumably with incessant ovulation and menstrual regurgitation, have a higher number of PF leukocytes and the increase is primarily in activated macrophages.[31,46–49,52] Thus, retrograde menstruation appears to be the major factor responsible for eliciting PF leukocytes.[55–57]

The physiologic function of these resident PF macrophages is likely to prevent ascending infection through the female genital tract and to remove any inert debris entering the peritoneal cavity via the fallopian tubes by phagocytosis. Examples include regurgitated menstrual debris, sperm, bacteria, and inert detritus, which can be transported via estrogen-stimulated genital tract secretions that flow out the fimbrial end of the fallopian tube. Because there is no physiologic access to the peritoneal cavity of men under normal circumstances, it is not surprising that the number of PF macrophages in men is significantly less than that observed in normally cycling women with patent fallopian tubes.

Circulating immature monocytes derived from the bone marrow serve as the reservoir for the tissue macrophages, which are differentiated only after leaving the vascular system and entering the tissue, when they take on the specific characteristics required by their site of residence; examples include pulmonary alveolar macrophages and von Kupffer's cells in the liver. Thus, entry into the PF is a normal process, and they develop their functional characteristics only after entering the peritoneal cavity. Under pathologic circumstances, increased numbers of PF macrophages may be elicited by specific stimuli or chemoattractants leading to an altered PF cell population, both numerically and functionally. For example, women with endometriosis, where the volume of regurgitated menstrual debris is high, have up to 100 fold the number of macrophages present in the PF.[31,46–49,52] Furthermore, phagocytosis of the menstrual debris appears to activate the macrophages both morphologically and functionally, as measured by phagocytosis, adherence to plastic and phytohemagglutin- (PHA-) stimulated hydrogen peroxide production as well as increased cytokine production. Similar increases in the PF macrophage number and state of activation are observed in patients with renal failure undergoing peritoneal dialysis, with the frequent surgical peritoneal entry representing the eliciting and activating stimulus.

Whether there is a single dominant chemoattractant primarily responsible for the entry of leukocytes into the PF or if several factors are involved in specific clinical circumstances remains to be determined. However, a potent attractant for mononuclear phagocytes, monocyte chemotactic protein-1 (MCP-1), has been identified in the PF, and higher levels of this protein have been observed in the PF of women with adhesions.[45] As macrophages themselves secrete MCP-1, once they initially infiltrate the wound healing site they have the potential to amplify the stimulus for entry of additional macrophages. Other soluble factors known to elicit leukocytes have been identified in the PF, including transforming growth factor-β,[39–41] known to be associated with amplification of scar formation. Further work is necessary to fully characterize the factors responsible for the diapedesis of circulating monocytes into the peritoneal cavity and to determine if these differ from those attracting leukocytes to other tissue sites from the vascular system.

Peritoneal Wound Healing

The initial event after a surgical injury to the peritoneum is deposition of fibrin at the wound surface. As normal peritoneum has fibrinolytic activity,[58–62] the deposited fibrin will be quickly degraded if the wound site comes into contact with uninjured normal peritoneum. This clearance of fibrin matrix occurs even if a clot is present at the wound surface, and blood clots per se have not been associated with adhesion formation. The injured peritoneum in contact with the PF is quickly reconstituted, with mesothelial cells completely resurfacing the injury site and the basic relationship between mesothelial surfaces reestablished. This process typically takes 5 to 7 days[63–65] and will occur in this time frame regardless of the size of the injury. Beneath this surface, the fibrin matrix is rapidly infiltrated by fibroblasts with collagen and ECM deposition, tissue remodeling, and neovascularization occurring over a much longer time scale.[66,67]

If an injured peritoneal surface with its fibrin deposit is in contact with another injured peritoneal surface, it is more economical for the two fibrin matrices to combine into a single matrix, converting the two sites into a single wound healing site. This combined fibrin scaffold facilitates fibroblast infiltration and proliferation and collagen deposition, increasing the tensile strength of the coalescing adhesion between the two wound sites. The mesothelial cells recover the exterior aspects of the adhesion, isolating the ECM from the peritoneal cavity and reconstituting an intact peritoneal mesothelial surface. This process results in the development of a coalescing adhesion that, over time, gains tensile strength with the deposition of additional ECM proteins and neovascularization, resulting in a permanent adhesion.[68]

Independent of whether there is an isolated peritoneal injury or two injury sites, the PF is constantly in contact with the injury site and it is at this stage that the preexisting constituents of the PF have the potential to influence the wound healing process. Little is known of the magnitude of influence, which may be exerted by alterations in PF. In elective surgery, therapeutic interventions may be able to favorably influence the PF and alter the nature of the peritoneal wound healing process as well as correct abnormal PF constituents.

Peritoneal Fluid Volume During Wound Healing

Although this has not been carefully studied, the volume of the PF is generally believed to increase immediately following an abdominal surgery as a normal physiologic response to the abdominal entry. This idea is consistent with the observations of increased PF volume at "second-look" laparoscopies, designed to assess the results of therapeutic interventions to reduce the rate of postoperative adhesion formation.

There has been an attempt to increase the volume of PF during the postoperative interval with the intent of providing a "hydroflotation" effect and to mechanically separate the surfaces of the abdominal viscera during the immediate postoperative interval, the critical period for the restitution of the mesothelial layer. This intervention was accomplished by instilling 32% dextran 70 (high molecular weight dextran, averaging 75,000 kDa) at the termination of surgery.[69] Because high molecular weight dextran is well above the molecular size that can easily pass through the peritoneum, the dextran molecules are retained in the peritoneal cavity, creating an osmotic gradient. This gradient increases the amount of fluid within the cavity for a number of days postoperatively until the dextran molecules are metabolized to smaller molecules and excreted. An initial clinical trial suggested efficacy,[69] but a subsequent study did not,[70] and the use of 32% dextran 70 to reduce postoperative adhesions has largely been abandoned.

Interestingly, intraperitoneal dextran is also internalized by the PF leukocytes and alters their functional capabilities in vitro.[71] Thus, any purported impact on peritoneal wound healing by instilling 32% dextran 70 may be the result of the intended "hydroflotation" effect or potentially a functional alteration in the PF macrophage population. An effect on PF macrophage function has also been reported with the use of radiographic contrast material used for hysterosalpingography, which spills into the PF, demonstrating tubal patency.[72,73] Understanding the mechanism of any effect of intraperitoneal instillates is important in interpreting the results of both clinical and laboratory experiments.

Cellular Constituents of the Peritoneal Fluid During Wound Healing

The first cell type that appears in the PF after a surgical injury is the PMN.[66,67] While elective surgery does not represent an infection, this initial response reflects the role of the PMN in defense of bacterial contamination of the peritoneal cavity. Once it is apparent that the injury is surgical and not the result of a bacterial infection, the PMNs promptly disappear from the PF because their continued presence requires molecular signals emanating from bacteria. Lymphocytes are mediators of the adaptive immune response, and this type of response is not typically involved in either the immediate response to injury or in wound healing, unless immunogenic epitopes are present. As a result, low numbers of lymphocytes are present in the PF and this number does not change with injury or repair, making it unlikely that lymphocytes play an active role in healing of the peritoneum.

The predominant leukocyte to appear in the PF is the mononuclear phagocyte or tissue macrophage,[66,67] a participant in both the innate and adaptive immune responses as well as phagocytosis of debris and tissue repair. There is little evidence to suggest that PF macrophages are involved in any adaptive immune responses initiated in the peritoneal cavity. However, wound healing is remarkably similar to the innate immune response involved in the removal of dead and dying cells, production of cytokines and ECM proteins, stimulation of neovascularity, and, over a longer time scale, remodeling of the wound. Soluble factors secreted into the PF by macrophages may be critical participants in these events with the potential for aberrant responses leading to an increased risk of adhesion formation.

Immediately after the surface mesothelial cells are denuded, resident macrophages temporarily replace the mesothelial layer and cover the exposed ECM, which normally is not in contact with other peritoneal surfaces. Over the next several days, proliferating mesothelial cells rapidly displace these macrophages and cover the entire surface area of the injury. The overriding principle seems to be to reconstitute the mesothelial surface as promptly as possible and thereby prevent the ECM and fibrin at an injury site from coming into direct contact with other injured sites with similar fibrin and exposed ECM. Once the mesothelial surface is reconstituted, the risk of development of coalescing adhesions is past, despite the continued proliferation of fibroblasts within the wound but below the surface. Therefore a critical step in the repair of the peritoneum without the formation of coalescing adhesions, the proliferation of the mesothelial cells, is susceptible to influence by the constituents of the PF.

Soluble Factors in the Peritoneal Fluid During Wound Healing

The cytokines secreted by PF macrophages and mesothelial cells are likely to be involved in or at least reflect the events occurring during peritoneal wound healing. Additionally, granulocyte-macrophage colony-stimulating factor (GM-CSF), a mitogen and differentiation factor that accelerates wound healing, also is increased in the PF after injury.[74–76] Because of the number of potent cytokines present in PF (see Table 2.1), these soluble PF constituents have the clear potential to modulate the cellular events involved in reconstituting the peritoneal membrane after surgical trauma. For example, alterations in soluble factors present in the PF may influence the development of coalescing adhesions by their effect on tissue repair cells at the site of the wound by affecting either cell numbers or function.[77–82] Experimental evidence to support this concept comes from observations that cytokines can influence the proliferation and secretion of tissue repair cells in vitro, harvested from the site of a peritoneal injury.[83–86] The interpretation of these experiments is somewhat limited as they are unable to distinguish the various cell types present (such as fibroblasts from mesothelial cells) within the overall population of tissue repair cells.

As noted earlier with cellular constituents, little information is available regarding the influence of soluble PF products on wound healing in vivo in humans. The experimental design must take into consideration the fact that normal wound healing alters the soluble products in the PF, complicating the identification of aberrant responses. However, in intact animal models, the administration of transforming growth factor-beta$_1$ (TGF-β_1) has been observed to increase adhesion formation, and when specific neutralizing antibodies to the TGF-βs are administered, the rate of adhesion formation is reduced.[78,79,82,87] Similarly, when either the antiinflammatory cytokine IL-10 is administered or eicosanoid production is inhibited,[88–94] the rate of adhesion formation is decreased.

Immunomodulation of Peritoneal Fluid Cells

There is a suggestion from experiments utilizing intact animals that suppression of gonadal steroid production during wound healing might alter the likelihood of postoperative adhesion formation.[95] Presumably, this might result from the impact of gonadal steroids on either the tissue repair cells themselves or the leukocytes attracted into the site of the wound. Pituitary suppression of gonadotropins with a gonadotropin hormone-releasing hormone (GnRH) agonist provides virtual complete suppression of ovarian steroidogenesis and the marked depression of circulating sex steroids. Based on the observations of the high gonadal steroid concentrations in the PF of cycling women, this should dramatically reduce the PF concentrations of gonadal steroids as well. As macrophage function is known to be influenced by estrogen, an effect might be mediated by the alteration in function of the PF macrophage by the change in the steroid environment within the PF. Comparable studies utilizing GnRH agonists have not been reported in humans, so the clinical utility of inducing hypogonadism preoperatively has yet to be demonstrated.

The use of glucocorticoids or progesterone, both of which are generally considered to be immunosuppressive and thus to alter the immune response and by inference the PF immune cells, has been advocated. No credible data demonstrating efficacy in humans have been reported. Experimental demonstration of efficacy with immunosuppressive steroids is hampered by the difficulty in maintaining high concentrations of these steroids at the site of the wound or within the PF. The small molecular size of steroids coupled with their lipid solubility virtually guarantees uniform body distribution and will undoubtedly make this approach a daunting technical feat. Administering large enough doses to ensure a high PF concentration simply has too many systemic side effects to be useful on a clinical basis without the clear demonstration of a very high degree of efficacy.

Attempts at specifically altering PF macrophage function have also been considered. Results of experiments using the immunomodulator pentoxyfine[96] and calcium channel blockers[97–101] have not yielded a benefit of sufficient magnitude in animal models to embark on large-scale human trials. As noted earlier, the use of nonsteroidal antiinflammatory drugs (NSAIDs) (ibuprofen and meclofenamate) in animal models to reduce eicosanoid production[88–94] has proven effective in lowering the rate of postsurgical adhesions. However, these agents have not yet been adequately tested for efficacy in large-scale clinical trials. A similar problem of being unable to maintain an adequately high local concentration of the NSAID at the site of tissue repair without systemic toxic effects is likely a major stumbling block.

Attempts to simply reduce the numbers of macrophages drawn into the wound have also been carried out. Neutralizing antibodies to MCP-1 have been noted to reduce adhesion formation in an animal model.[45] It is too early to know whether these experiments will lead to a treatment option in humans, but the focus on the cellular constituents of the PF during wound healing response appears to be a worthwhile avenue of inquiry, based on these animal experiments.

Modulating Hemostasis in the Peritoneal Fluid

Attempts to interrupt the initial event in the wound healing process, the deposition of fibrin at the wound surface during the postoperative interval, have not been promising. The use of the anticoagulant heparin both systematically and within the peritoneal cavity has been advocated without supporting experimental or clinical data demonstrating efficacy in controlled clinical trials.[70] Similarly, increasing fibrinolytic activity by using intraperitoneal or systemic tissue plasminogen activator (tPA) has not yet been demonstrated to be of value. Given the serious hazards of anticoagulation in surgical patients and the expense of tPA, these therapeutic strategies will require rigorous proof of efficacy before introducing them for routine use on a clinical basis.

Does Peritoneal Fluid Inflammation Influence Postoperative Adhesions?

The general assumption has been that when the peritoneum is required to heal in the midst of an inflammatory exudate, the process is adversely influenced, favoring the formation of adhesions. However, on closer inspection, the process of wound healing closely resembles an inflammatory response, at least in terms of the tissue repair cells and cytokines involved.[18] Furthermore, in the midst of an inflammatory process, tissues not surgically injured, especially the subcutaneous tissue, are regularly reconstituted without excessive adhesion formation, such as occurs after the drainage of a subcutaneous abscess or a surgical wound infection. Retrospective observations are complicated by the fact that a surgical procedure performed to drain an abscess may itself represent a stimulus for any observed postoperative adhesions. For example, the procedure to drain an appendiceal abscess may be responsible for any adhesions at the site, quite independent of the impact of the abscess itself. This issue will remain unresolved until appropriate experimental designs are utilized to separate the impact of the inflammation itself from the surgical procedures designed to treat the inflammatory process.

Impact of Surgical Barrier Material in the Peritoneal Fluid

Because peritoneal injuries reconstitute normal peritoneum without coalescing adhesions when healing occurs without the injured site coming into direct contact with another injured site, a therapeutic barrier strategy has evolved. Simply put, surgically injured peritoneal surfaces are prevented from apposition with other injured surfaces during the healing interval by covering the injured site with a surgical barrier. The ideal antiadhesion barrier would be composed of a material that (1) is not injurious to the peritoneum in its own right, (2) does not elicit PF leukocytes, (3) is removed from the peritoneum by simple hydrolysis and not by degradation, (4) remains intact for 5 to 7 days, (5) is not thrombogenic, (6) adheres to peritoneal surfaces without sutures, (7) has the flexibility to conform to the contours of the pelvic viscera, and (8) can be used at both laparotomy and laparoscopy. Not surprisingly, there are no ideal surgical barriers clinically available, but the greater the number of characteristics of the biomaterial that are favorable, the more attractive the barrier. The impact of the various biomaterials on the PF becomes a critical issue when evaluating clinical usefulness (Table 2.2).

One currently available barrier is composed of oxidized regenerated cellulose (ORC, Interceed®). ORC certainly acts as a temporary mechanical barrier between surgically injured peritoneal surfaces, but its removal requires degradation by PF peritoneal leukocytes.[102] ORC, in fact, elicits and activates large numbers of PF macrophages[5] for this purpose. As it is currently commercially manufactured, ORC is extremely acidic, injuring any cells that come into direct contact with the barrier. Further complicating this picture is the fact that ORC is thrombogenic and actually increases the postoperative adhesion risk if meticulous hemostasis is not attained. Not surprisingly, although ORC has been found to reduce adhesion formation in multicenter randomized clinical trials at specific pelvic sites, the magnitude of the benefit is relatively small,[103,104] and this material is actually adhesiogenic in some animal models.[105] Whether the efficacy of ORC as a barrier material could be improved by manufacturing it with characteristics less evocative of a degrading inflammatory response or with less directly injurious effects on tissues remains to be determined.

A second currently available barrier material is composed of expanded polytetrafluoroethylene (PTFE, Preclude® Surgical Membrane), a nonreactive permanent

TABLE 2.2. Impact of surgical barrier material on the peritoneal fluid leukocyte population

Barrier material	Leukocyte number	Leukocyte activation
Oxidized regenerated cellulose (Interceed®)[5]	Increased	Increased
Expanded polytetrafluoroethylene (Preclude Surgical Membrane®)[5]	Normal	Increased
Hyaluronic acid-carboxymethylcellulose (Seprafilm®)	Not yet evaluated	Not yet evaluated
Chemically modified hyaluronic acid (Incert®)[111]	Normal	Normal

material. PTFE does not elicit large numbers of PF leukocytes although it does have some impact on the activation of PF leukocytes, albeit less than that of ORC.[5] While it has been demonstrated to reduce postoperative adhesions in both animal models[105] and humans,[106,107] its major drawback is that it is a permanent material and pelvic surgeons are understandably reluctant to leave it in place. In cardiac surgery, where PTFE is used to replace the pericardial membrane, and in other surgical applications, it has been left in place permanently without complications.[108]

Concerns regarding the characteristics of the initial biomaterials utilized in clinical surgical barriers have led to interest in constructing barriers of naturally occurring extracellular matrix molecules such as hyaluronic acid (HA). A solid barrier composed of HA coupled with carboxymethylcellulose (Seprafilm®) has been shown to be clinically efficacious in reducing postoperative adhesion formation in both gynecologic and general surgery.[109,110] Another barrier composed of chemically cross-linked HA (Incert®), which is efficacious in animal models, has been demonstrated to have minimal impact on the cellular constituents of PF.[111] Interpreting these data from the various barriers remains difficult, but there seems little doubt that developing surgical barrier materials that have the desired rapid disappearance and tissue response characteristics while simultaneously minimally impacting the PF constituents remains the goal (see also Chapters 34, 40, and 41).

Summary

PF is a biologically important fluid critical to the normal function of the intraabdominal viscera. Soluble and cellular constituents of the PF both reflect the events occurring during wound healing in the peritoneal cavity and have the potential to modulate the outcome of tissue response to injury. The basic question as to whether greater numbers of PF leukocytes with higher levels of activation enhance or retard development of postoperative adhesion formation is not known. However, a more thorough understanding of the impact of macrophages and macrophage-derived cytokines on the wound healing process will undoubtedly help in developing more effective therapeutic strategies to reduce the risk of postoperative adhesion formation.

References

1. diZerega GS, Rodgers KE. Peritoneum. In: The Peritoneum. New York: Springer-Verlag, 1992:1–25.
2. Filatow D. Uber die Bildung des Anfangstadium bie der extremitatenentwhchlung. Roux's Arch Entwicklungsmech Org 1933;127:776.
3. Maximow A. Uber der Mesothel Deckzellen der serosen Exudate: Untersuchungen an entzundetem Gewebe und Gerwebskulturen. Arch Exp Zellforsch 1927;4:1.
4. Levinson ME, Pontzer RE. Peritonitis and other intra-abdominal infections. In: Mandel GL, Douglas RG Jr, Bennett JE, eds. Principles and Practice of Infectious Diseases, 2nd Ed. New York: Wiley, 1979:476–503.
5. Haney AF, Doty E. Comparison of the peritoneal cells elicited by oxidized regenerated cellulose (Interceed®) and expanded-polytetrafluoroethylene (Gore-Tex® Surgical Membrane) in a murine model. Am J Obstet Gynecol 1992;166:1137–1149.
6. Maathuis JB, Van Look PFA, Michie EA. Changes in volume, total protein and ovarian steroid concentrations of peritoneal fluid throughout the human menstrual cycle. J Endocrinol 1978;76:123–133.
7. Koninckx PR, Renaer M, Brosens IA. Origin of peritoneal fluid in women: an ovarian exudation product. Br J Obstet Gynaecol 1980;87:177–183.
8. Brosens IA, Koninckx PR, Corveleyn PA. A study of plasma progesterone, oestradiol-17β, prolactin and LH levels, and of the luteal phase appearance of the ovaries in patients with endometriosis and infertility. Br J Obstet Gynaecol 1978;85:246–250.
9. Dhont M, Serreyn R, Duvivier P, et al. Ovulation stigma and concentration of progesterone and estradiol in peritoneal fluid: relation with fertility and endometriosis. Fertil Steril 1984;41:872–877.
10. Flessner MF, Dedrick RL, Schultz JS. A distributed model of peritoneal-plasma transport: analysis of experimental data in the rat. Am J Physiol 1985;248 (Renal Fluid Electrolyte Physiol 17):F413–F424.
11. Flessner MF, Dedrick RL, Schultz JS. Exchange of macromolecules between peritoneal cavity and plasma. Am J Physiol 1985;248 (Heart Circ Physiol 17):H15–H25.
12. Olgaard K, Hagen C, McNeilly AS. Pituitary hormones in women with chronic renal failure: the effect of chronic intermittent haemo- and peritoneal dialysis. Acta Endocrinol 1975;80:237–246.
13. Ross RJ, Goodwin FJ, Hougghton BJ, Boucher BJ. Alteration of pituitary-thyroid function in patients with chronic renal failure treated by haemodialysis or continuous ambulatory peritoneal dialysis. Ann Biochem 1985;22: 156–160.
14. Drake TS, O'Brien WF, Ramwell PW, et al. Peritoneal fluid thromboxane B_2 and 6-keto-prostaglandin F_{2a} in endometriosis. Am J Obstet Gynecol 1981;140:401.
15. Badawy SZA, Marshall L, Gabal AA, et al. The concentration of 13,14-dihydro-15-keto-prostaglandin F_{2a} and prostaglandin E_2 in peritoneal fluid of infertile patients with and without endometriosis. Fertil Steril 1982;38: 166–170.
16. Rock JA, Dubin NH, Ghodganokar RB, et al. Cul-de-sac fluid in women with endometriosis: fluid volume and prostanoid concentration during the proliferative phase of the cycle—days 8 to 12. Fertil Steril 1982;37:747–750.
17. Dawood MY, Khan-Dawood FS, Wilson L Jr. Peritoneal fluid prostaglandins and prostanoids in women with endometriosis, chronic pelvic inflammatory disease and pelvic pain. Am J Obstet Gynecol 1984;148:391–395.

18. Rodgers KE. Biochemical messengers in postsurgical repair and adhesion formation. In: diZerega GS, DeCherney AH, Diamond MP, et al., eds. Pelvic Surgery: Adhesion Formation and Prevention. New York: Springer-Verlag, 1997;1:11–25.
19. Chegini N, Rossi MJ, Holmdahl L. Cellular distribution of 5-lipoxygenase and leukotriene receptors in postsurgical wound repair. Wound Repair Regen 1997;5:235–242.
20. Fakih H, Baggett B, Holtz G, et al. Interleukin-1: a possible role in the infertility associated with endometriosis. Fertil Steril 1987;47:213–215.
21. Ho N-H, Wu M-Y, Chao K-H, et al. Decrease in interferon gamma production and impairment of T lymphocyte proliferation in peritoneal fluid of women with endometriosis. Am J Obstet Gynecol 1996;175:1236–1241.
22. Koyama N, Matsuura K, Okamura H. Cytokines in the peritoneal fluid of patients with endometriosis. Int J Gynaecol Obstet 1993;43:45–50.
23. Ueki M, Tsurunaga T, Ushiroyama T, et al. Macrophage activation factors and cytokines in peritoneal fluid from patients with endometriosis. Asia-Oceania J Obstet Gynaecol 1994;20:427–431.
24. Ho N-H, Wu M-Y, Chao K-H, et al. Peritoneal interleukin-10 increases with decrease in activated CD4+ T lymphocytes in women with endometriosis. Hum Reprod 1997; 12:2528–2533.
25. Punnonen J, Teisala K, Ranta H, et al. Increased levels of interleukin-6 and interleukin-10 in the peritoneal fluid of patients with endometriosis. Am J Obstet Gynecol 1996; 174:1522–1526.
26. Harada T, Yoshioka H, Yoshida S, et al. Increased interleukin-6 levels in the peritoneal fluid of infertile women with active endometriosis. Am J Obstet Gynecol 1997;176: 593–597.
27. Halme J. Release of tumor necrosis factor-alpha by human peritoneal macrophages in vivo and in vitro. Am J Obstet Gynecol 1989;61:1718–1725.
28. Liang XS, Hu LN, Wu P. Tumor necrosis factor in peritoneal fluid of infertile women with endometriosis and its relation to sperm motility. Chin J Obstet Gynecol 1994;29: 524–526.
29. Vercellini P, De Benedetti F, Rossi E, et al. Tumor necrosis factor in plasma and peritoneal fluid of women with and without endometriosis. Gynecol Obstet Invest 1993;36: 39–41.
30. Kligman I, Grifo JA, Witkin SS. Expression of the heat shock protein in peritoneal fluids from women with endometriosis: implications for endometriosis-associated infertility. Hum Reprod 1996;11:2736–2738.
31. Olive DL, Haney AF, Weinberg JB. The nature exudate associated with infertility: peritoneal fluid and serum lysozyme activity. Fertil Steril 1987;48:802–806.
32. Arumugam K, Dip KC. Endometriosis and infertility: the role of exogenous lipid peroxides in the peritoneal fluid. Fertil Steril 1995;63:198–199.
33. Kucera E, Presl J, Uher J, et al. Glycosaminoglycans in the peritoneal fluid of infertile women with endometriosis. Cesk Gynekol 1994;59:59–61.
34. Kauma S, Clark MR, White C, et al. Production of fibronectin by peritoneal macrophages and concentration of fibronectin in peritoneal fluid from patients with or without endometriosis. Obstet Gynecol 1988;72:13–18.
35. Weinberg JB, Haney AF, Xu FJ, et al. Peritoneal fluid and plasma levels of human macrophage colony-stimulating factor in relation to peritoneal fluid macrophage content. Blood 1991;78:513–516.
36. Fukaya T, Sugawara J, Yoshida H, et al. The role of colony stimulating factor in the peritoneal fluid in infertile patients with endometriosis. Tohoku J Exp Med 1994; 172:221–226.
37. McLaren J, Prentice A, Charnock-Jones DS, et al. Vascular endothelial growth factor (VEGF) concentrations are elevated in peritoneal fluid of women with endometriosis. Hum Reprod 1996;11:220–223.
38. Halme J, White C, Kauma S, et al. Peritoneal macrophages from patients with endometriosis release growth factor activity in vitro. J Clin Endocrinol Metab 1988;66: 1044–1049.
39. Mizumoto Y. Changes in NK activities and TGF-beta concentrations in the peritoneal cavity in endometriosis and their interaction related to infertility. Acta Obstet Gynaecol Jpn 1996;48:379–385.
40. Rong H, Tang X-M, Zhao Y, et al. Intraperitoneal exposure to surgical glove powders differentially modulate inflammatory and immune related cytokine production during surgically induced peritoneal adhesion formation. Wound Repair Regen 1997;5:85–96.
41. Osterlynek DJ, Meuleman C, Waer M, et al. Transforming growth factor-β activity is increased in peritoneal fluid from women with endometriosis. Obstet Gynecol 1994; 83:287–292.
42. Hill JA, Anderson DJ. Lymphocyte activity in the presence of peritoneal fluid from fertile women and infertile women with and without endometriosis. Am J Obstet Gynecol 1989;161:861–864.
43. Hoffman M, Haney AF, Weinberg JB. Reduced trypsin-binding capacity of alpha$_2$-macroglobulin in the peritoneal fluid of women with endometriosis: possible relevance to alterations in macrophage function. Fertil Steril 1988;50:39–47.
44. Eisermann J, Collins JL. Enzyme immune assay determination of CA-125 in serum, peritoneal fluid, and follicular fluid from women with minimal endometriosis and ovarian hyperstimulation. Fertil Steril 1989;51:344–347.
45. Zeyneloglu HB, Senturk LM, Seli E, Oral E, Olive DL. The role of monocyte chemotactic protein-1 in intraperitoneal adhesion formation. Hum Reprod 1998;13:1194–1199.
46. Haney AF, Muscato JJ, Weinberg JB. Peritoneal fluid cell populations in infertility patients. Fertil Steril 1981;35: 696–698.
47. Halme J, Becker S, Hammond MG, et al. Increased activation of pelvic macrophages in infertile women with endometriosis. Am J Obstet Gynecol 1983;145:333–337.
48. Badawy SZA, Cuenca V, Marshall L, et al. Cellular components in peritoneal fluid in infertile women with and without endometriosis. Fertil Steril 1984;42:704–708.
49. Olive DL, Weinberg JB, Haney AF. Peritoneal macrophages and infertility: the association between cell number and pelvic pathology. Fertil Steril 1985;44:772–777.
50. Haney AF, Weinberg JB. Reduction of the intraperitoneal inflammation associated with endometriosis by treatment

with medroxyprogesterone acetate. Am J Obstet Gynecol 1988;159:450–454.

51. Haney AF, Jenkins SJ, Weinberg JB. The stimulus responsible for the peritoneal fluid inflammation observed in infertile women with endometriosis. Fertil Steril 1991;56: 408–413.

52. Jha P, Farooq A, Agarwal N, et al. In vitro sperm phagocytosis by human peritoneal macrophages in endometriosis-associated infertility. Am J Reprod Immunol 1996;36: 235–237.

53. Syrop CH, Halme J. Cyclic changes of peritoneal fluid parameters in normal and infertile patients. Obstet Gynecol 1987;69:416–418.

54. Arumugam K. Endometriosis and infertility: raised iron concentration in the peritoneal fluid and its effect on the acrosome reaction. Hum Reprod 1994;9:1153–1157.

55. Blumenkrantz MJ, Gallagher N, Bashore RA. Retrograde menstruation in women undergoing chronic peritoneal dialysis. Obstet Gynecol 1981;57:667–670.

56. Halme J, Hammond MG, Hulka JF. Retrograde menstruation in healthy women and in patients with endometriosis. Obstet Gynecol 1984;64:141–144.

57. Liu DTY, Hitchcock A. Endometriosis: its association with retrograde menstruation, dysmenorrhea and tubal pathology. Br J Obstet Gynaecol 1968;93:859–863.

58. Myhre-Jensen O, Larsen SB, Astrup T. Fibrinolytic activity in serosal and synovial membranes. Arch Pathol 1969;88: 623–630.

59. Porter JM, McGregor FH, Mullen DC, Silver D. Fibrinolytic activity of mesothelial surfaces. Surg Forum 1969; 20:80–82.

60. Porter JM, Ball AP, Silver D. Mesothelial fibrinolysis. J Thorac Cardiovasc Surg 1971;62:725–730.

61. Raftery AT. Regeneration of peritoneum: a fibrinolytic study. J Anat 1979;129:659–664.

62. Merlo G, Fausone G, Barbero C, et al. Fibrinolytic activity of the human peritoneum. Eur Surg Res 1980;12: 433–438.

63. Ellis H, Harrison W, Hugh TB. The healing of peritoneum under normal and pathological conditions. Br J Surg 1965;52:471–476.

64. Ryan GB, Grobety J, Majino G. Mesothelial injury and recovery. Am J Pathol 1973;71:93–113.

65. Eskland G. Regeneration of parietal peritoneum (brief report). Acta Pathol Microbiol Scand 1964;62:459–460.

66. Ellis H, Harrison W, Hugh TB. The healing of peritoneum under normal and pathological conditions. Br J Surg 1965;52:471–476.

67. Raftery AT. Regeneration of parietal and visceral peritoneum in the immature animal: a light and electron microscopical study. Br J Surg 1973;60:969–975.

68. Haney AF, Doty E. The formation of coalescing peritoneal adhesions requires injury to both contacting peritoneal surfaces. Fertil Steril 1994;61:767–775.

69. Adhesion Study Group. Reduction of postoperative pelvic adhesions with intraperitoneal 32% Dextran-70: a prospective, randomized clinical trial. Fertil Steril 1983;40: 612–619.

70. Jansen RPS. Failure of intraperitoneal adjuncts to improve the outcome of pelvic operations in young women. Am J Obstet Gynecol 1985;153:363–371.

71. Rein MS, Hill JA. 32% dextran 70 (Hyskon) inhibits lymphocyte and macrophage function in vitro: a potential new mechanism for adhesion prevention. Fertil Steril 1989;52:953–957.

72. Boyer P, Territo MC, de Ziegler D, et al. Ethiodol inhibits phagocytosis by pelvic peritoneal macrophages. Fertil Steril 1986;46:715–717.

73. Goodman SB, Rein MS, Hill JA. Hysterosalpingography contrast media and chromotubation dye inhibit peritoneal lymphocyte and macrophage function in vitro: a potential mechanism of fertility enhancement. Fertil Steril 1993;59:1022–1027.

74. Vyalov S, Desmouliere A, Gabbiani G. GM-CSF-induced granulation tissue formation: relationships between macrophages and myofibroblast accumulation. Virchows Arch B Cell Pathol 1993;63:231–239.

75. Jyung RW, We L, Pierce GF, et al. Granulocyte macrophage stimulating factor and granulocyte colony-stimulating factor: differential action on incisional wound healing. Surgery (St. Louis) 1994;115:325–334.

76. Rong H, Tang X-M, Zhao Y, et al. Intraperitoneal exposure to surgical glove powders differentially modulate inflammatory and immune related cytokine production during surgically induced adhesion formation. Wound Repair Regen 1997;5:85–96.

77. Hershlag A, Otterness IG, Bliven ML, et al. The effect of interleukin 1 on adhesion formation in the rat. Am J Obstet Gynecol 1991;165:771–774.

78. Williams RS, Rossi AM, Chegini N, et al. Effect of transforming growth factor-β on postoperative adhesion formation and intact peritoneum. J Surg Res 1991;52:65–70.

79. Chengi N, Gold LI, Williams RS, et al. Localization of transforming growth factor beta isoforms TGF-β1, TGF-β2, and TGF-β3 in surgically induced pelvic adhesions in the rat. Obstet Gynecol 1994;83:449–454.

80. Chengi N, Ross MJ, Holmdahl L. Cellular distribution of 5-lipoxygenase and leukotriene receptors in postsurgical peritoneal wound repair. Wound Repair Regen 1997;5: 235–242.

81. Holschneider CH, Cristoforoni PM, Ghosh K, et al. Endogenous versus exogenous IL-10 in postoperative adhesion formation in a murine model. J Surg Res 1997; 70:138–144.

82. Holmdal L, Bergstrom M, Duo Q, et al. Over-expression of TGF-β is associated with adhesion formation and fibrinolytic impairment. Wound Repair Regen 1998;6:A487.

83. Fukasawa M, Yanagihara DL, Rogers KE, et al. The mitogenic activity of peritoneal tissue repair cells: control by growth factors. J Surg Res 1987;47:45–51.

84. Fukasawa M, Bryant SM, Orita H, et al. Modulation of proline and glucosamine incorporation into tissue repair cells by peritoneal macrophages. J Surg Res 187;46: 166–171.

85. Fukasawa M, Bryant SM, Nakamura RM, et al. Modulation of fibroblast proliferation by postsurgical macrophages. J Surg Res 1987;43:513–520.

86. Fukasawa M, Campeau JD, Yanagihara DL, et al. Mitogenic and protein synthetic activity of tissue repair cells: control by the postsurgical macrophage. J Invest Surg 1989;2: 169–180.

87. Lucas PA, Warejcka DJ, Young HE, et al. Formation of abdominal adhesions is inhibited by antibodies to transforming growth factor-β_1. J Surg Res 1996;135–138.
88. Grow DR, Coddington CC, Hsiu JG, Mikich Y, Hodgen GD. Role of hypoestrogenism or sex steroid antagonism in adhesion formation after myometrial surgery in primates. Fertil Steril 1996;66:140–147.
89. Steinleitner A, Lambert H, Kazensky C, Danks P, Roy S. Pentoxyfilline, a methylxanthine derivative, prevents postsurgical adhesion reformation in rabbits. Obstet Gynecol 1990;75:926–928.
90. Siegler AM, Kontopoulos V, Wang CE. Prevention of postoperative adhesions in rabbits with ibuprofen, a nonsteroidal anti-inflammatory agent. Fertil Steril 1980;34: 46–49.
91. Nishimura K, Nakamura RM, diZerega GS. Biochemical evaluation of postsurgical wound repair: prevention of intraperitoneal adhesion formation with ibuprofen. J Surg Res 1983;34:219–226.
92. Kapur BML, Talwar JL, Gulati SM. Oxyphenbutazone—anti-inflammatory agent in prevention of peritoneal adhesions. Arch Surg 1969;98:301–302.
93. Larsson B, Svanberg SG, Swolin K. Oxybutazone—an adjuvant to be used in the prevention of adhesions in operations for fertility. Fertil Steril 1977;28:807–808.
94. Golan A, Bernstein T, Wexler S, et al. The effect of prostaglandins and aspirin: an inhibitor of prostaglandin synthesis on adhesion formation in rats. Hum Reprod 1991;6:251–254.
95. Cofer KF, Himebaugh KS, Gauvin JM, et al. Inhibition of adhesion formation in the rabbit model by meclofenamate: an inhibitor of both prostaglandin and leukotriene production. Fertil Steril 1994;62:1262–1265.
96. LeGrand KE, Rodgers KE, Girgis W, et al. Comparative efficacy of nonsteroidal anti-inflammatory drugs and antithromboxane agents in a rabbit adhesion-prevention model. J Invest Surg 1995;8:187–194.
97. Steinleitner A, Lambert H, Montoro L, et al. The use of calcium channel blockade for the prevention of postoperative adhesion formation. Fertil Steril 1988;50:818–821.
98. Steinleitner A, Lambert H, Montoro L, et al. Use of diltiozem for preventing postoperative adhesions. J Reprod Med 1988;33:891–894.
99. Steinleitner A, Kazensky C, Lambert H. Calcium channel blockade prevents postsurgical reformation of adnexal adhesions in rabbits. Obstet Gynecol 1989;74:796–798.
100. Steinleitner A, Lambert H, Kazensky C, Sanchez I, Sueldo C. Reduction of primary postoperative adhesion formation under calcium channel blockade in the rabbit. J Surg Res 1990;48:42–45.
101. Dunn RC, Steinleitner AJ, Lambert H. Synergistic effect of intraperitoneally administered calcium channel blockers and recombinant tissue plasminogen activator to prevent adhesion formation in an animal model. Am J Obstet Gynecol 1991;164:1327–1330.
102. Dimitrijevich SD, Tatarko M, Gracy RW, et al. *In vivo* degradation of oxidized regenerated cellulose. Carbohydr Res 1990;198:331–341.
103. INTERCEED®(TC7) Adhesion Barrier Study Group. Prevention of postsurgical adhesions by INTERCEED® (TC7), an absorbable adhesion barrier: a prospective randomized multicenter clinical study. Fertil Steril 1989; 51:933–938.
104. Sekiba K, Obstetrics and Gynecology Adhesion Prevention Committee. Use of Interceed®(TC7) absorbable adhesion barrier to reduce postoperative adhesion reformation in infertility and endometriosis surgery. Obstet Gynecol 1992;79:518–522.
105. Haney AF, Doty E. Murine peritoneal injury and de novo adhesion formation caused by oxidized regenerated cellulose (Interceed®) but not expanded-polytetrafluoroethylene (Gore-Tex® Surgical Membrane). Fertil Steril 1992;57:202–208.
106. The Myomectomy Adhesion Multicenter Study Group. An expanded-polytetrafluoroethylene barrier (Gore-Tex® Surgical Membrane) reduces post-myomectomy adhesion formation. Fertil Steril 1995;63:491–493.
107. Haney AF, Hesla J, Hurst BS, et al. Expanded-polytetrafluoroethylene (Gore-Tex® Surgical Membrane) is superior to oxidized regenerated cellulose (Interceed® TC7) in preventing adhesions. Fertil Steril 1995;63:1021–1026.
108. Harada Y, Imai Y, Kurozawa H, et al. Long-term results of the clinical use of an expanded polytetrafluoroethylene surgical membrane as a pericardial substitute. J Thorac Cardiovasc Surg 1988;96:811–815.
109. Diamond M, Seprafilm® Adhesion Study Group. Reduction of adhesions after uterine myomectomy by Seprafilm® membrane (HAL-F): a blinded, prospective, randomized multi-center clinical study. Fertil Steril 1996; 66:904–910.
110. Becker JM, Dayton MT, Fazio VW, et al. Prevention of postoperative abdominal adhesions by a sodium hyaluronate-based bioresorbable membrane: a prospective, randomized, double-blind multi-center study. J Am Coll Surg 1996;183:297–306.
111. Haney AF, Doty E. A barrier composed of chemically cross-linked hyaluronic acid (Incert) reduces postoperative adhesion formation. Fertil Steril 1998;70:145–151.

3

Peritoneal Tissue Repair Cells

Kathleen E. Rodgers

CONTENTS

The function of two types of cells (peritoneal leukocytes and tissue repair cells [TRC] or mesothelial cells) in the repair of peritoneal injury has been extensively studied. The contribution of these cells to the process of peritoneal repair and studies on the functional alterations of these cells following surgical trauma and exposure to various growth factors are reviewed as part of this chapter.

Inflammation

In response to the initiation of inflammatory and coagulatory responses, numerous cytokines and lipid mediators are released that modulate and orchestrate cellular function. After the acute release of mediators by the cells resident in the peritoneum, their continued production is dependent on the cell type present and the activation state of the cells. Cytokines or growth factors are proteins that work as paracrine or autocrine regulators of cell functions. The actions of some of these factors are described further here with specific reference to modulation of function of postsurgical TRCs (cells harvested from the site of injury in rabbits after abrasion of the sidewall) or mesothelial cells and leukocytes (in the exudative fluid after surgery). One of the essential events for the development of inflammation is the recruitment of inflammatory cells to the sites of tissue injury. This phase involves the release of mobile effector cells (polymorphonuclear neutrophils, PMNs), monocytes, and eosinophils) from storage sites and modulation of their response by extracellular matrix, plasma, and factors.

The kinetics of cellular infiltration observed at the site of injury are similar to those observed in the peritoneal cavity after surgical trauma. The earliest cells to appear on the damaged peritoneum are predominantly PMNs, which persist in large numbers for 1 to 2 days and then rapidly disappear if infection is absent. This PMN influx is followed by an increase in the number of monocytes, which rapidly differentiate into macrophages. This influx of monocytes is greater than local macrophage production during the first 6 to 48 hours, depending upon the stimulus employed. The contribution of stimulated local production, if any, is not evident until the second day after initiation of inflammation.[1] On days 4 and 7, the predominant cells on the peritoneal surface are mesothelial cells. After postoperative day 5, the predominant cells in the peritoneal fluid are macrophages, which are critical to the resolution of surgical injury. TRCs, which secrete connective tissue matrix, proliferate throughout the wound base.[2] The activity of TRCs, as measured by protein and collagen synthesis, also increases after surgery, reaching peak levels on postsurgical days 5 to 7. These cells are not "fibroblasts" as they respond to a variety of stimuli, including monokines, in a manner distinct from established cell lines.

Peritoneal Leukocytes

It has become evident that leukocytes are essential in the repair of peritoneal injury. Cells composing the mononuclear phagocyte system include bone marrow precursors, monocytes, and macrophages and share a similar morphology, bone marrow origin, and avid phagocytic capacity. The macrophage has received considerable attention in studies of peritoneal repair because of the multitude of functions this cell performs. Healing after peritoneal surgery involves a complex process of cellular

TABLE 3.1. Ligands for macrophage receptors

- Immunoglobulin and complement
  - IgG-1, IgG-2b
  - IgG-2a
  - IgG-3
  - IgG-1, IgG-3 monomers
  - IgG complexes
  - IgE
  - C3b, C4b, C3bi, C3d, C5a
- Other proteins
  - Mannosyl-, fucocyl-, *N*-acetylglucosaminyl-terminal glycoproteins
  - Alpha$_2$-macroglobulin-protease complex
  - Fibronectin
  - Fibrin
  - Lactoferrin
  - Colony-stimulating factors
  - Migration inhibitory and macrophage activation factors
  - Insulin
  - Factors VII, VIIa
  - Interferons
- Peptides
  - Neuropeptides (enkephalins, endorphins)
  - Arginine vasopressin
  - *N*-Formylated peptides from bacteria, mitochondria
- Polysaccharides
  - Lipopolysaccharide endotoxin
  - Carbohydrates on certain cells
  - Hyaluronic acid
- Others
  - Adrenergic agents
  - Cholinergic agents
  - Phorbol diesters
  - Histamine

Modified from Nathan and Cohn.[3]

TABLE 3.2. Secretory products of macrophages

- Enzymes
  - Lysozyme
  - Plasminogen activator
  - Collagenase
  - Elastase
  - Angiotensin convertase
  - Acid proteases
  - Acid lipases
  - Acid nucleases
  - Acid phosphatases
  - Acid glycosidases
  - Acid sulfatases
  - Arginase
  - Lipoprotein lipase
  - Phospholipase A_2
- Enzyme inhibitors
  - Alpha$_2$-macroglobulin
  - Alpha$_1$-antiprotease
  - Lipocortin
  - Alpha$_1$-antichymotrypsin
- Coagulation factors
  - Factors X, IX, VII, V
  - Protein kinase
  - Thromboplastin
  - Prothrombin
  - Thrombospondin
  - Fibrinolysis inhibitor
- Complement cascade components
  - C1, C2, C3, C4, C5
  - Factors B, D
  - Properdin
  - C3b inactivator
  - Beta-1H
- Additional proteins
  - Transferrin
  - Transcobalamin II
  - Fibronectin
  - Apolipoprotein E
  - Tumor necrosis factor
    - Interleukin-1
    - Colony-stimulating factor
    - Erythropoietin
  - Thymosin-β_4
  - Serum amyloid A, P
  - Haptoglobin
  - Interferons alpha, beta
    - Platelet-derived growth factors
  - Transforming growth factor-β
- Reactive oxygen intermediates
  - O_2^-
  - H_2O_2
  - OH•
- Hypohalous acids
  - Lipids
  - PGE_2, $PGF_{2}\alpha$
    - Prostacyclin
    - Thromboxane A_2
  - Leukotrienes B, C, D, E
    - Mono-HETES and di-HETES
  - Platelet-activating factor
- Small molecules
  - Purines
- Pyrimidines
  - Glutathione

migration, proliferation, differentiation, interaction, and secretion of extracellular matrix, and macrophages play a pivotal role in these events. In addition to the regulation of wound healing, macrophages are involved not only in the elimination of bacteria, tissue debris, and fibrin deposits. The macrophage surface is endowed with a variety of proteins that allow it to maintain continual contact with its environment (Table 3.1).

Macrophages are able to secrete at least 80 different products (Table 3.2); these include various components of the complement cascade, coagulation factors, proteases and antiproteases, and arachidonic acid metabolites.[5] Regulation of the macrophage's secretory ability differs from molecule to molecule, with most of the secretion being stimulated by receptor–ligand interaction. The secreted material is released via different routes, such as fusion of the vesicles with the membrane or by opening of the phagolysome to the surface.

A summary of the effects of surgery on the function of peritoneal macrophages can be found in Table 3.3.[6] After peritoneal surgery, macrophages are recruited into the site of injury and differentiate. The function of peritoneal macrophage changes as healing progresses. The functional alterations of peritoneal macrophages have been assessed by examination of the respiratory burst capacity (superoxide anion release), arachidonic acid (AA) metabolism, cytokine production, the production of proteases and protease inhibitors, and tumoricidal activity.

Respiratory Burst

Macrophages are a major defense against a variety of microorganisms, such as viruses, bacteria, fungi, and protozoa. Microorganisms are recognized by macrophages primarily through the bindings of opsonins. A variety of opsonins exist, including immunoglobulin and complement fragments. Once recognition occurs, the major antimicrobial activity of the macrophage is the production and intracellular release of reactive oxygen intermediates (ROI), such as O_2^-, H_2O_2, and OH^-.[7,8] There is a close correlation between the antimicrobial activity of a macrophage population and its ability to secrete ROIs as well as between the ability of a microorganism to trigger ROI secretion during its ingestion and its susceptibility to macrophage destruction.[9]

The release of ROIs increases rapidly after surgery, peaking at 6 hours and decreasing by day 1.[10,11] Thereafter, the production of superoxide anion increases to a peak on days 4 and 7 after surgery and returns to control levels by day 15. This suggests that resident peritoneal macrophages are primed by operative injury and function as antimicrobial agents in conjunction with PMNs during the first few hours after operative injury.[11] Newly infiltrating macrophages or resident macrophages may interact with PMNs, secretory factors from PMNs, or other factors from an acute inflammatory response to be functionally altered. Studies of the interaction of early postoperative macrophages with conditioned media from postsurgical PMNs support this hypothesis.[11] In the absence of infection, this early priming stimulus will abate.

Arachidonic Acid Metabolites

AA metabolites are potent mediators of inflammatory responses and may therefore regulate many events that occur in wound repair, such as leukocyte chemotaxis. Prostaglandin E_2 (PGE_2) is proinflammatory and mediates events such as edema formation, endothelial cell procoagulant activity, and vasodilation.[12] Thromboxane (TxB_2) is a potent stimulator of platelet aggregation and is chemotactic for PMNs.[13] Hydroxyeicosatetraenoic acid (HETE) metabolites inhibit the formation of AA metabolites and lead to PMN infiltration.[14] Therefore, an increase in AA metabolism by peritoneal exudate cells

TABLE 3.3. Alterations in peritoneal exudate cell (PEC) functions as a function of postoperative time (increased or decreased activity compared to resident, nonoperative controls)

	Time after surgery (hours)				
PEC function	6	24	48	72	120
Cell PMNs	↑	↑↑↑	↑↑	↑	No change
Cell macrophages	No change	↑	↑	↑↑	↑↑↑
Superoxide anion stimuli	↑↑↑	↑	↑	↑↑	↑↑
No stimuli	No change	No change	No change	No change	↑
Interleukin-1 stimuli	NA	No change	NA	↑↑	No change
No stimuli	NA	No change	NA	↑	↑↑
Tumor necrosis factor stimuli	NA	↑	NA	↑↑	↑
No stimuli	NA	↑↑	NA	↑↑	↑
Plasminogen activator	NA	↓↓	↓	↓	No change
Plasminogen activator inhibitor	NA	↑↑	↑	↑	No change

PMNs, polymorphonuclear neutrophils; NA, not applicable. ↑, increased; ↓, decreased.

(PEC) from postoperative rabbits may contribute to the ongoing inflammatory and wound healing processes. Studies of postsurgical leukocytes have revealed a selective increase in synthesis of 15-HETE and diHETE beginning 24 hours after operative injury was observed along with a diminution of 5-HETE, suggesting a reduction in PMN number. Thereafter, an additional increase in TxB_2 (the stable end product of TxA) and PGE_2 on days 2 to 10 after operation was observed.[15]

Cytokine Production

Interleukin-1 (IL-1) and tumor necrosis factor (TNF) are two of several soluble proteins produced by macrophages in response to a variety of stimuli. These cytokines alter many of the biological activities of cells involved in peritoneal postoperative repair (Table 3.4). IL-1 was shown to stimulate the production of collagen, collagenase, and prostaglandins (PGs) by fibroblasts as well as endothelial cells in vitro.[14–51] The treatment of endothelial and mesothelial cells with IL-1 resulted in decreased production of tissue plasminogen activator (tPA), an increase in cell-associated activity, and an increase of a tissue plasminogen activator inhibitor (PAI) (Table 3.4). Thus, exposure to IL-1 could result in a significant reduction in the fibrinolytic activity of endothelial and mesothelial cells.[52–56] These complementary actions of IL-1 on procoagulant and fibrinolytic activities may, in turn, enhance the production and maintenance of fibrin. This idea is supported by in vivo studies which have shown that postoperative and postirradiation administration of IL-1 increased adhesion formation.[57,58]

Secretion of IL-1 by peritoneal macrophages from postoperative rabbits changes as a function of postoperative time.[59,60] In conditioned culture media from unstimulated macrophages harvested from postoperative rabbits, IL-1 levels are increased on postoperative day 14 compared with the level of IL-1 secreted on postoperative days 3 and 7. Secretion of TNF, which can modulate mesothelial cell function, by unstimulated macrophages from postoperative rabbits peaks on days 1 and 14. Therefore, the levels of TNF and IL-1 secreted from peritoneal macrophages of postoperative rabbits are elevated during the later phases of peritoneal healing and may be involved in the remodeling phase rather than the healing phase of peritoneal repair. IL-1 and TNF also stimulate the release of PGE_2, which inhibits fibroblast replication and macrophage activation, both of which are important in the remodeling phase.[61,62] Korn et al.[63] reported that supernatants of monocytes or macrophages suppressed fibroblast proliferation and that this inhibition of growth parallels the increase in PGE_2 synthesis by the fibroblast. In addition, this inhibition is reversed by inhibitors of PGE_2 synthesis (e.g., indomethacin) and is reproduced by addition of exogenous PGE_2 to fibroblast cultures. Thus, IL-1 and TNF secretion by macrophages from postoperative animals may play a role in the later phase of repair after peritoneal operation through several different mechanisms.

Tumoricidal Activity

In certain stages of activation, macrophages have the ability to cytolyse tumor cells in the absence of a specific antitarget cell antibody.[64,65] Such cytolysis occurs over 1 to 3 days and is contact dependent, selective for neoplastic cells, and does not involve phagocytosis.[66] Cytolysis involves two clearly definable steps: selective capture of tumor cells and binding to the macrophage surface, and secretion of toxic substances.[67] The lytic substance appears to be secreted into the limited space formed between the junction of the macrophage and the bound tumor cell. There is some evidence that a novel serine protease as well as TNF may serve as lytic substances.[68]

The effect of peritoneal surgery on the tumoricidal activity of leukocytes was examined in the rat.[69] As early as 24 hours after surgery, there was a slight increase in the tumoricidal activity of PEC. This elevation in tumoricidal activity was maximal by day 7 after surgery and had begun to return to control levels by day 14. This study also showed that acute administration of a cyclooxygenase inhibitor, tolmetin, at the time of surgery further elevated the tumoricidal activity of postsurgical macrophages.

Macrophage-Mediated Regulation of Extracellular Matrix Degradation and Deposition

Macrophages have been implicated in the degradation of the extracellular connective tissue matrix at inflammatory sites. Degradation of rat vascular smooth muscle cell matrix by thioglycollate-elicited macrophages was shown to be dependent on both the length of incubation and the number of macrophages plated.[70,71] The ability of the macrophage to degrade is related to the secretion of neutral proteinases, including plasminogen activator, elastase, and collagenase. Each of these proteinases digests a different component of the extracellular matrix. Plasmin, the result of an interaction between plasminogen activator (PA) and plasminogen, is a potent proteinase that degrades the insoluble glycoprotein components of the extracellular matrix and is a primary fibrinolytic enzyme. The matrix components, elastin and collagen, are principally degraded by the enzymes elastase and collagenase, respectively.

The ability of various macrophage populations to digest collagen was augmented by the addition of fibroblasts to the macrophage culture.[72] The extent of colla-

TABLE 3.4. Effect of cytokines and various intraperitoneal agents on mesothelial cell function

	High glucose	Antibiotics	IL-1	TNF	TGF-β	LPS	IFN-γ	MØ	PDGF	IL-6	Crystalloid osmotic	Oncotic osmotic	EGF	Amino acids	Insulin	FGF
Proliferation	↓[16,17]	↓[16,22]	NE[23], ↑[2,4]	NE[23,24]			↓[35]	↑[23,24]	↑[24]				↑[29]	↓[17]		↑[24]
Viability	↓[18]		↓[18]	↓[18]	↓[18]	↓[18]										
Antioxidant enzymes			NE[18]	NE[18]	NE[18]	NE[18]										
PG synthesis	↓[19]		↑[25]	↑[25]	↑[25]											
PMN adherence			↑[26]	↑[28]		↑[44]										
IL-8 secretion			↑[26,27]	↑[27]		↑[45]										
ICAM-1 expression			↑[26,28]	↑[28]	NE[42]	↑[44]	↑[46]						NE[42]			
PAI-1 secretion	↑[20]		↑[29,30]	↑[29,30,40]	↑[29]	↑[30]				↑[47]						
TGF-β secretion			↑[31]	NE[31]			NE[44]									
IL-1α/β secretion			↑[32]	↑[32]		↑[32]										
HA secretion	↑[20,21]		↑[33,34]	↑[33,34]	↑[33,34]				↑[33]	↑[33]	↓[21]	↑[21]				
IL-6 secretion	↑[20]		↑[35]	↑[35]			↑[35]									
Collagen				NE[41]												
TPA secretion	↑[20]		↓[29,30]	↓[29,30]	↓[29]	↓[30]										
Fibrinolysis	↓[17]		↓[29,48]	↓[29,48]	↓[29,45]									↓[17]		
CD44 expression				NE[42]	NE[42]								NE[42]			
Monocyte adhesion			NE[36]	↑[42]	↓[42]								↑[42]			
Phospholipid	↓[17]													↓[17]	↓[17]	
TNF shedding			↑[37]	NE[37]		↓[37]										
TNF RNA			NE[37]	NE[37]		NE[37]										
Self-adherence				NE[43]												
Chemokine secretion			↑[38,39]	↑[38,39]		↑[43]	↑[39]									

MØ, macrophage-conditioned medium; TNF, tumor necrosis factor; TGF-β, transforming growth factor-beta; LPS, lipopolysaccharides; IFN, interferon; PDGF, platelet-derived growth factor; EGF, epidermal growth factor; FGF, fibroblast growth factor; PG, prostaglandin; ICAM, intracellular adhesion molecule; PAI, plasminogen-activation inhibitor; HA, hyaluronic acid; NE, no effect.

gen degradation in coculture of macrophages and fibroblasts was greater than the sum of degradation observed with either two cell populations alone. Enhanced collagen degradation was observed when only a small number of fibroblasts (≤1% of total cell number) were cultured with macrophages. Synergy between fibroblasts and macrophages with respect to glycoprotein depletion was also demonstrated by these researchers, but this effect was less obvious because of the high rate of glycoprotein digestion achieved by either cell type alone.

There are two types of PA, tissue PA (tPA) and urokinase (uPA). Macrophages secrete uPA, which interacts with cellular receptors and mediates cell-associated fibrinolysis.[73] PECs from postoperative rabbits secrete increasing levels of PA 3 to 7 days after operation, reaching peak values on day 10 and thereafter decreasing to control levels by day 21.[74] The levels of PA produced by macrophages from postoperative rabbits, however, are lower during the first 5 days after operation than the levels expressed by peritoneal macrophages from nonoperative rabbits.

Decreased release of PA by postoperative macrophages early after operation may be caused by the release of an inhibitor (PAI) by these cells.[75] The early secretion of an inhibitor of fibrinolysis may be instrumental in facilitating the deposition of fibrin during early stages (postoperative days 1 to 5) of vascular hemostasis and peritoneal repair. Later, an increase in the fibrinolytic activity in the healing wound, through an increase in PA and a decrease in PAI activity, may be important in promoting deposition of the tissue matrix and resolving fibrin deposits.

Peritoneal macrophages secrete an inhibitor of uPA that is most prevalent at 1 to 3 days after peritoneal operation and thereafter gradually decreases to nonoperative levels by day 10.[75] Macrophage-mediated inhibition of PA is partially acid sensitive, suggesting that at least two types of PAIs are secreted. Macrophage-conditioned medium suppresses the enzymatic activity of both small (33-kDa) and large (54-kDa) uPA. Secretion of PA and PAI activities by macrophages from postoperative rabbits was elevated by exposure to IL-1 in culture.[76] Therefore, macrophages from postoperative rabbits may directly modulate fibrinolytic activity during peritoneal reepithelialization by inhibiting fibrinolysis during postoperative days 1 to 5 and, later, by decreasing inhibition of fibrinolysis as well as increasing the level of PA activity to resident (nonoperative) macrophage levels.

In addition to its indirect facilitatory effect on elastase and collagenase activity, plasmin appears to influence the activation of collagenase to its active form.[77] The collagenase synthesized by the macrophage is in a latent form and must be activated before it is capable of digesting collagen. Plasmin is among the molecules that are capable of activating latent collagenase.

Tissue Repair Cells

Reepithelialization of peritoneal defects was shown to occur over the entire surface simultaneously.[78,79] Therefore, a relatively large injury will reepithelialize as rapidly as a smaller wound. The proliferation of cells found at the site of peritoneal trauma and the modulation of their proliferation by macrophage secretory products and growth factors is reviewed.

To study the role of macrophages in the repair of injured peritoneum, the influence of peritoneal macrophages on activity of TRCs (tissue repair cells) was examined. TRCs are morphologically transformed and activated to proliferate when cocultured with postsurgical macrophages. An alteration in the morphology of a TRC from a flat-oval shape to a more spindly appearance occurs together with the macrophage-induced inhibition of TRC proliferation. Alterations in the morphology of TRC cultures upon exposure to medium from postsurgical macrophage cultures indicate a complex change in cell metabolism to maximize the potential for migration. This dissociation between basal proliferation and responsiveness to stimuli might be related to a time constraint for the cell to return to the original nonmigratory state before division at the site of injury.

Mesothelial and other epithelial cells collected from the site of peritoneal injury at various times after trauma are referred to in this chapter as TRCs. To study the reepithelialization of peritoneal injury and the changing character of these cells, a standardized excision of rabbit parietal peritoneum was used to initiate peritoneal repair.[80–84] At 4 days after peritoneal injury, the surface of the healing peritoneum contains proliferating mesothelial cells that actively secrete connective tissue matrix.[78,79] The cells on the surface of the parietal defect are harvested and grown in culture for 4 to 8 days to allow for the generation of a confluent layer of adherent cells. This layer is essentially devoid of leukocytes. The activity of TRCs, as measured by protein and collagen synthesis, increases after surgery, reaching peak levels on postsurgical days 5 to 7.[81] These TRCs respond to a variety of stimuli including monokines in a manner distinctly different from that of established fibroblast cell lines.[82,84]

Cell-to-Cell Response

Macrophages are critical in the final resolution of tissue debris and completion of healing, a process that ends in the formation of the connective tissue matrix and mesothelial syncytium.[85,86] In nonsurgical systems, macrophages provide the primary stimulus for proliferation of fibroblasts.[87–90] Factors secreted by activated macrophages in nonsurgical systems can stimulate fibroblast proliferation (macrophage-derived fibroblast growth factor [FGF], IL-1, and tumor necrosis factor [TNF]). As a direct or indirect response to these factors, fibroblasts proliferate and secrete connective tissue proteins including fibronectin, proteoglycans, collagen, and proteases such as collagenase and elastase. Proper coordination of these fibroblast-mediated functions leads to the repair and remodeling of tissue. In addition, the rate and extent to which these factors regulate wound healing may be amenable to modulation by extrinsic intervention.

Fibroproliferative activity in TRCs is increased on postsurgical days 4 and 7 and decreases to resident levels on day 28.[83] TRC proliferation is generally suppressed in situ when compared to TRC cultured in medium supplemented with only fetal bovine serum.[80,83] Candidates for mediators of this suppression of proliferation include prostaglandins,[91,92] interferons,[93] arginase,[94] and complement cleavage products.[95,96] The manifestation of these complex signals appears to be a function of (1) the period of time after surgery and (2) the length of preincubation of the cells.

Effect of Culture Time

Proliferative and functional activities of TRCs collected directly from injured peritoneum were determined in vitro to study activation and differentiation of TRCs in vivo. Although TRCs rapidly proliferate after recovery from injured peritoneum, this activity gradually decreases during culture. In addition, collagen production (as measured by ^{3}H-proline incorporation) by TRCs also decreases during culture.[81] Because sulfate is found mainly in glycosaminoglycans, ^{35}sulfate was used to monitor the production of glycosaminoglycans by TRCs. Interestingly, ^{35}S-sulfate incorporation into TRCs gradually increases during culture.[81]

The secretory products of macrophages recovered from peritoneal exudate at various times after surgery initially suppress (during the initial 48 hours of culture) and later enhance (following 48 to 54 hours of incubation) the incorporation of thymidine into fibroblasts.[83] This suppression by postsurgical macrophages is significantly less than that observed with resident (nonsurgical) macrophages.[80,83] Therefore, modulation of TRC proliferation by macrophages appears to be a complex process involving elements of both suppression and stimulation. There may be a lag time during which TRCs are either refractory to proliferative signals from postsurgical macrophages or are controlled by inhibitors of proliferation. Alternatively, TRCs may not be initially responsive to macrophage-derived growth factor(s), but the inhibitory signal(s), which is presumably also macrophage derived, initially predominates. Because the inhibition of TRC proliferation is reduced at later times in culture, the inhibitory signals (1) may be short lived (as prostaglandins are thought to be) or (2) may be overcome (or inactivated) by fibroproliferative factor(s), or (3) changes in TRC responsiveness to inhibitory factors may occur during culture.

Macrophages produce soluble mediators that modulate TRC growth during peritoneal repair. Interaction between TRCs and regulatory proteins from surgically elicited macrophages is important for peritoneal reepithelialization. Maximal stimulation of TRC proliferation can be achieved by an extract of macrophage-spent media. Macrophages are potent secretory cells, and spent medium contains many soluble mediators for peritoneal repair including growth factors, prostaglandins (PGs), and uPA.[87,97–103] PGE_2 inhibits the proliferation of fibroblasts, whereas PGF_{2a} is usually stimulatory.[104–106] Although resident (nonactivated) macrophages may function as negative modulators of fibroblast proliferation, a facilitation of TRC proliferation and protein secretion may occur after interaction between TRCs and macrophages elicited and subsequently activated by surgical injury. In this way, macrophages may function in many aspects of peritoneal tissue repair after surgery.[107–109]

At day 5 after peritoneal surgery in rabbits, TRCs incorporate greater amounts of thymidine compared to day 2 TRCs.[82] Thereafter, mitogenic activity decreases during extended postsurgical times. Day 2 TRCs might not be fully capable of mitogenesis, whereas day 5 TRCs are more active in vivo. At postsurgical day 7 and day 10, TRCs differentiate, allowing for production of extracellular matrix. TRCs are morphologically transformed and activated to proliferate when cocultured with postsurgical macrophages.[110] The mitogenic activity of TRCs cocultured with postsurgical macrophages or spent media from postsurgical macrophages is greater than that measured when they are cultured with nonsurgical macrophages.

The effect of postsurgical macrophages on TRC proliferation changes as a function of postsurgical time. Postsurgical macrophages alter the composition of their secretory products as a function of time.[56,60,82] Initially, macrophages may stimulate the proliferation of TRCs; later macrophages modulate differentiation of TRCs to produce extracellular matrix.[83,86]

The net effect result of macrophage growth factor secretion is TRC proliferation in an appropriate ratio during peritoneal reepithelialization. Transforming growth Factor-β (TGF-β) enhances the anchorage-independent proliferation of fibroblasts but does not stimulate anchorage-dependent growth.[82,111] However, stimulation of extracellular matrix production may be a more specific activity of TGF-β rather than enhancement of cell proliferation.

From the foregoing observation, the following hypothesis was developed: the mobilization and proliferation of TRCs are responsive to factors secreted by postsurgical macrophages. Although resident macrophages may function as negative modulators of TRC proliferation, the postsurgical macrophage secretes substances that induce migration and proliferation of TRCs. The effect of postsurgical macrophages on TRC function may thus be dependent upon (1) the responsiveness of TRCs to these substances and (2) the populations of macrophages present. This concept is supported by the observation that, after surgical trauma in vivo, migration and proliferation of TRCs are accelerated and then stop once tissue repair is complete. In addition, postsurgical macrophages can modulate the proliferation, morphology, and secretory products of postsurgical TRCs in vitro. Accordingly, peritoneal wound healing may be controlled by the regulation of macrophage migration or TRC proliferation.

Growth Factors

A large number of factors contribute to the growth of fibroblasts.[99,112–116] At the injured site, TRCs are involved with other cell types (i.e., lymphocytes, PMNs, platelets) that may modulate the in situ proliferative and functional activities of TRCs via cell-to-cell interactions or secretion of cytokines.[117,118] Platelet-derived growth factor (PDGF), isolated from platelets, stimulates the proliferation of normal skin and established fibroblast cell lines. PDGF also functions as a chemoattractant for fibroblasts.[119] Shimakado and his colleagues reported the production of a PDGF-like factor by macrophages.[120] Many factors occur in several compartments involved in tissue repair: serum, wound fluid, platelets, macrophages, and TRCs. FGF, readily produced by macrophages,[115] stimulates the proliferation of fibroblasts and endothelial cells.[63,116] Epidermal growth factor (EGF), initially isolated from the submaxillary gland, is present in serum.[121] Insulin-like growth factor-1 (IGF-1)/somatomedin-C was isolated from fibroblasts.[122] TGF-β is found in platelets, wound fluid, and macrophages.[123–125] Following stimulation in vivo or in vitro, macrophages produce "factors" that stimulate the proliferation and expression of differentiated functions of a variety of cell types.[51,109,126] IL-1, which is produced by stimulated macrophages, has the potential to enhance the proliferation and differentiation of fibroblasts.[49,50,106,127]

A large number of factors were shown to modulate the proliferation of fibroblasts. Because TRCs are not fibroblasts, however, the effects of some of these factors on the proliferation of TRC were examined (Table 3.5). At the site of peritoneal injury, TRCs are in contact with other types of cells that may modulate the proliferative and functional activities of TRCs through cell-to-cell interaction or the secretion of cytokines, such as PDGF, IL-1, TNF, fibroblast growth factor (FGF), EGF, and TGF-β.

EGF and FGF stimulate the incorporation of thymidine into TRCs.[82] Interestingly, TRC responsiveness to EGF increases during the postsurgical period, with TRCs on postsurgical day 10 demonstrating the greatest response to EGF. PDGF also stimulates the incorporation of thymidine into TRCs, but the stimulation is only 30% of control values for postsurgical day 10 TRCs.[82,128] PDGF stimulates the proliferation of fibroblasts, especially under conditions of confluent culture. The effect of PDGF on proliferation is thought to induce the entry of G_0-arrested cells into the proliferative phase of the cell cycle.[129] TRCs may be undergoing a mitotic cycle and, therefore, do not manifest as great a response to the addition of PDGF as established fibroblasts. EGF and FGF, which affect the proliferation of TRC, may function as competence factors involved in the transition of cells from the G_0 to the S phase.[129,130]

Proliferation and production of prostaglandin E_2, collagen, collagenase, and hyaluronic acid are all stimulated by IL-1α and IL-1β.[49,109,131] (see Table 3.4). Although IL-1 does not stimulate proliferation of TRCs, IL-1 stimulates protein synthesis by TRCs.[82] IL-1 may function as an initiation factor, similar to the role played by PDGF, or may be more important for the production of extracellular matrix.

IL-2 stimulates the healing of skin wounds[132]; however, IL-2 does not affect proliferation of fibroblasts or TRCs.[82] IL-2 may indirectly affect the growth of TRCs in vivo through stimulation of other cellular elements. For example, macrophages have cell-surface receptors for

TABLE 3.5. Summary of effects of growth factors on rabbit tissue repair cells (TRCs)

	Growth factors						
Postsurgical day	EGF	PDGF	FGF	TGF-β	IL-2	IL-1	IGF-1
Proliferation							
Day 2	↑	↑	↑↑↑	↓↓↓	NC	NC	NC
Day 5	↑	↑	↑↑↑	↓↓↓	NC	NC	NC
Day 7	↑↑	↑	↑↑↑	↓↓↓	NC	NC	NC
Day 10	↑↑↑	↑	↑↑↑	↓↓↓	NC	NC	NC
Protein synthesis							
Day 10	ND	ND	ND	↑↑	ND	↑	ND

IGF, insulin-like growth factors; NC, no change; ND, not done (not assessed).
From diZerega and Rodgers.[148]

IL-2 and IL-2 that can stimulate the respiratory burst of macrophages in the absence of other stimuli.

IGF-I does not affect the incorporation of tritiated thymidine into TRCs.[82] IGF-I/somatomedin-C stimulates the proliferation of fibroblasts by effecting the transition from the S–G_2 phase to the M phase.[129] As IGF-I affects the M phase, and because this factor may be produced by fibroblasts, the growth factors involved in the G_1–S phase of the cell cycle may be more important for the enhancement of TRC proliferation.[133,134]

TGF-β stimulates the anchorage-independent proliferation of fibroblasts but not anchorage-dependent growth.[111,123,135] TGF-β inhibits the incorporation of thymidine into TRCs[82,128] and stimulates the production of extracellular matrix (collagen and fibronectin) by fibroblasts.[116,135–140] Incubation of TRC with TGF-β enhances the incorporation of radiolabeled proline (to measure protein synthesis); in contrast, TGF-β inhibits the proliferation of TRCs.[82] In this context, TGF-β may function as a modulator of TRC differentiation in that it may induce these mesothelial cells to enter a functional (secretory) stage rather than to proliferate. Cromack et al.[125] reported that increase in TGF-β levels in wound fluid occurs late after surgery, not during the early phase of tissue repair.

Further studies showed that after dialysis and lyophilization, conditioned medium from macrophage cultures (postsurgical day 10) is more potent at stimulating the proliferation of TRCs than the purified growth factors. These results suggest postsurgical macrophages are capable of secreting a combination of stimulatory and inhibitory factors that may act in an additive or synergistic fashion in appropriate proportions to maximize the proliferation of TRC.

Effect of Growth Factors on Mesothelial Cell Proliferation and Cytokine Production

Several publications have discussed the effect of cytokines and growth factors on human mesothelial cell formation after in vitro exposure (see Table 3.4). Factors to which the abdominal cavity (and hence mesothelial cells) are exposed during chronic peritoneal dialysis, such as high concentrations of glucose, antibiotics, or amino acids, have been shown to inhibit cell growth and induce the release of inflammatory mediators.[16,17,19–22] On the other hand, cytokines have been shown to upregulate cell function including increased chemokine secretion, increased prostaglandin secretion, increased cytokine secretion, and reduced fibrinolytic activity in several studies.[23–36,38,39] Lipopolysaccharide, TNF, and TGF-β were shown to have actions similar to IL-1.

Fibrin Deposition and Removal by Mesothelial Cells

Fibrin deposition occurs during the early acute inflammatory process that is initiated by surgical injury. Further, the process of injury and inflammation modifies the ability of the deposited fibrin to be removed. As discussed, macrophages will contribute to the fibrolytic process. The mesothelial lining of the peritoneal cavity also contains fibrinolytic activity and contributes to fibrin removal. Surgical injury and exposure to the proinflammatory cytokines, such as TNF, IL-1, and IL-6, may modulate the level of the fibrinolytic activity of mesothelial cells.[141,142]

The fibrinolytic activity of canine serosa from various parts of the gastrointestinal tract (including the descending colon, ileum, stomach, and omentum) after different types of surgical injuries was assessed.[143] After abrasion, a 20% to 100% decrease in fibrinolytic activity was noted. A 50% decrease in the fibrinolytic activity of the midportion of the ileum was accompanied by severe adhesions. In later studies, Raferty[144] determined the changes in peritoneal fibrinolytic activity in rats following four types of trauma. Immediately after each procedure there was a reduction in fibrinolytic activity that was further reduced over the next 24 hours. The unsutured peritoneal defects showed the smallest reduction in fibrinolytic activity and were associated with the lowest incidence of adhesion formation. Free peritoneal grafting, electrocoagulation, and ischemic bowel resulted in a significant reduction in fibrinolytic activity compared with the unsutured defect and were associated with a significantly higher incidence of adhesion formation. A general correlation was apparent between suppression of peritoneal fibrinolytic activity by abrasion and the extent of subsequent adhesion formation.

Further studies by Buckman et al.[145] compared the fibrinolytic activity of normal peritoneum with that of peritoneal defects or peritoneal grafts. Activity in rat cecal peritoneum was suppressed for 48 and 96 hours after crush and abrasion injuries, respectively. PA was more severely suppressed after ischemia produced by an avascular graft. This suppression persisted for the entire 96-hour study interval, although partial recovery became measurable after 48 hours. Incubation of normal peritoneum with a biopsy from a peritoneal defect resulted in significantly elevated fibrinolytic activity. However, a biopsy of a peritoneal graft with normal peritoneum resulted in reduced fibrinolytic activity. These studies support a role for alterations in fibrinolytic activity in the formation of adhesions.

The fibrinolytic activity of human peritoneum is modulated by proinflammatory cytokines or inflammation. The PA activity of the inflamed peritoneum was much lower than control tissue because of an increase in PAI-1 production rather than a decrease in tPA antigen.

Mesothelial cells from human peritoneum produce tPA along with PAI-1 and PAI-2.[146] PAI-1 antigen was present in the culture medium of mesothelial cells, whereas PAI-2 antigen was cell associated. Upon exposure of the mesothelial cultures to TNF, the level of tPA antigen was reduced, whereas levels of both PAI-1 and PAI-2 antigens were elevated (see Table 3.3). In addition, exposure of human mesothelial cells to IL-1, IL-6, TGF-β, and lipopolysaccharide (LPS) also increased the production of PAI.[29,30,40,47] In general, inflammation, surgery, or cytokine exposure suppresses intraperitoneal cell-associated or cell-secreted fibrinolytic activity.[29] In addition, induction of fibrinopurulent peritonitis by the creation of an ischemic portion of the ileum has been shown to abolish fibrinolytic activity.[147] Because peritoneal infection is known to lead to adhesion formation, these data are consistent with the finding that adhesion formation is inversely correlated with fibrinolytic activity. The fibrinolytic activity of rat sidewall biopsies was shown to be modulated by in vitro exposure to tolmetin.

Summary

In conclusion, peritoneal repair is a complex process that requires the appropriate interaction of multiple cell types which undergo differentiation during the healing process, as well as inflammatory mediators and cytokines. In response to surgical injury, the function of peritoneal exudate cells is modified (Table 3.3). During the early postoperative phase, the number of PMNs increases and then normalizes with a concomitant increase in respiratory burst activity. At later time points, the level of cytokines and PAI that can be produced is elevated.

These alterations suggest that, during the early postoperative interval, these cells act to remove microbial agents and to maintain hemostasis. At later times, peritoneal exudate cells may be involved in tissue remodeling. Alterations in the function of the cells that line the peritoneal surface in response to mediators released by macrophages and platelets is also observed (see Tables 3.4 and 3.5). IL-1, a cytokine released by postoperative macrophages, is a potent modifier of mesothelial cell functions, including the release of inflammatory mediators and regulators of fibrinolytic activity.

Alterations in the balance of these processes may result in adhesion formation. For example, prolongation of the inflammatory process by a foreign body may reduce the fibrinolytic activity of mesothelial cells, a major contributor to removal of fibrin, prolonging fibrin deposition and allowing adhesion formation. Understanding of the processes of postoperative healing should allow the development of rational therapeutics for the reduction of adhesion formation.

References

1. van Furth R, Cohn ZA. The origin and kinetics of mononuclear phagocytes. J Exp Med 1968; 128:415–435.
2. Orita H, Nakamura RM, diZerega GS. Kinetic analysis of postoperative peritoneal healing: incorporation of proline and glucosamine by exudative and tissue repair cells. Surg Forum 1985;36:467–468.
3. Nathan CF, Cohn ZA. Cellular components of inflammation: monocytes and macrophages. In: Kelley W, Harris E, Ruddey S, Hedge R, eds. Textbook of Rheumatology. Philadelphia: Saunders, 1980:144–169.
4. Adams DO, Hamilton TA. Phagocytic cells: cytotoxic activities of macrophages. In: Gallin JI, Goldstein IM, Synderman R, eds. Inflammation: Basic Principles and Clinical Correlates. New York: Raven Press, 1988:471–492.
5. Unanue ER. Secretory function of mononuclear phagocytes. Am J Pathol 1986;83:396–417.
6. Rodgers KE, diZerega GS. Function of peritoneal exudate cells after abdominal surgery. J Invest Surg 1993;6:9–13.
7. Clark RA, Klebanoff SJ. Neutrophil-mediated tumor cell cytotoxicity: role of the peroxidase system. J Exp Med 1975;141:1442–1457.
8. Klebanoff SJ. Antimicrobial mechanisms of neutrophilic polymorphonuclear-leukocytes. Semin Hematol 1975;12: 117–124.
9. Nathan CF, Root KA. Hydrogen peroxide release from mouse peritoneal macrophages: dependence on sequential activation and triggering. J Exp Med 1977;146: 1648–1662.
10. Fukasawa M, Bryant SM, diZerega GS. Superoxide anion production by postsurgical macrophages. J Surg Res 1988; 45:382–388.
11. Kuraoka S, Campeau JD, Nakamura RM, et al. Modulation of postsurgical macrophage function by early postsurgical polymorphonuclear neutrophils. J Surg Res 1992;53: 245–250.
12. Randall RW, Eakins KE, Higgs GA. Inhibition of arachidonic acid cyclooxygenase and lipo-oxygenase activities by indomethacin and compound BW755. Agents Actions 1980;10:553–555.
13. Schnyder J, Dewald B, Baggiolini M. Effects of cyclooxygenase inhibitors and prostaglandin E2 on macrophage activation in vitro. Prostaglandins 1981;22:411–419.
14. Vanderhock JY, Bailey JM. Activation of a 15-lipoxygenase/leukotriene pathway in human polymorphonuclear leukocytes by the anti-inflammatory agent ibuprofen. J Biol Chem 1984;259:6752–6755.
15. Shimanuki T, Nakamura RM, diZerega GS. A kinetic analysis of peritoneal fluid cytology and arachidonic acid metabolism after abrasion and reabrasion of rabbit peritoneum. J Surg Res 1986;41:245–251.
16. Tsai TJ, Yen CJ, Fang CC, et al. Effect of intraperitoneally administered agents on human peritoneal mesothelial cell growth. Nephron 1995;71(1):23–28.
17. Witowski J, Brebowicz A, Knapowski J, et al. In vitro culture of human peritoneal mesothelium for investigation of mesothelial dysfunction during peritoneal dialysis. J Physiol Pharmacol 1994;45(2):271–284.

18. Chen JY, Yang AH, Lin YP, et al. Absence of modulating effects of cytokines on antioxidant enzymes in peritoneal mesothelial cells. Perit Dial Int 1997;17(5):455–466.
19. Rooney OB, Odd PD, Gokal R, et al. Dialysis fluid cytotoxicity and inhibition of host defense in cultured human mesothelial cells are neutralized rapidly with incubation in the peritoneum. Nephrol Dial Transplant 1996;11(12): 2472–2477.
20. Berborowicz A, Rodela H, Karon J, et al. In vitro simulation of the effect of peritoneal dialysis solution on mesothelial cells. Am J Kidney Dis 1997;29(3):404–449.
21. Kumano K, Ma P, Hyodo T, et al. Effects of osmotic agents on hyaluronan synthesis in human peritoneal mesothelial cells and fibroblasts. Adv Perit Dial 1997;13:58–63.
22. Yen CJ, Tsai TJ, Chen HS, et al. Effects of intraperitoneal antibiotics on human peritoneal mesothelial cell growth. Nephron 1996;74(4):694–700.
23. Bachus KE, Doty E, Haney AF, et al. Differential effects of interleukin-1 alpha, tumor necrosis factor-alpha, indomethacin, hydrocortisone, and macrophage co-culture on the proliferation of human fibroblasts and peritoneal mesothelial cells. J Soc Gynecol Invest 1995;2(4):636–642.
24. Beavis MJ, Williams JD, Hoppe J, et al. Human peritoneal fibroblast proliferation in 3-dimensional culture: modulation by cytokines, growth factors and peritoneal dialysis effluent. Kidney Int 1997;51(1):205–215.
25. Topley N, Petersen MM, Mackenzie R, et al. Human peritoneal mesothelial cell prostaglandin synthesis: induction of cyclooxygenase mRNA by peritoneal macrophage-derived cytokines. Kidney Int 1994;46(3):900–909.
26. Zeillemaker AM, Mul FP, Hoynck van Papendrect AA, et al. Neutrophil adherence to and migration across monolayers of human peritoneal mesothelial cells. The role of mesothelium in the influx of neutrophils during peritonitis. J Lab Clin Med 1996;127(3):279–286.
27. Arici A, Tazuke SI, Attar E, et al. Interleukin-8 concentration in peritoneal fluid of patients with endometriosis and modulation of interleukin-8 expression in human mesothelial cells. Mol Hum Reprod 1996;2(1):40–45.
28. Liberek T, Topley N, Luttmann W, et al. Adherence of neutrophils to human peritoneal mesothelial cells: role of intercellular adhesion molecule-1. J Am Soc Nephrol 1996;7(2):208–217.
29. Zang Y, Hou F, Zhang X. Effects of epidermal growth factor (EGF) on proliferation of human peritoneal mesothelial cells. Chung-Hua Nei K'o Tsa Chih 1996;35(2):92–94.
30. Sitter T, Spannagl M, Schiffl H, et al. Imbalance between intraperitoneal coagulation and fibrinolysis during peritonitis of CAPD patients: the role of mesothelial cells. Nephrol Dial Transplant 1995;10(5):677–683.
31. Offner FA, Feichtinger H, Stadlmann S, et al. Transforming growth factor-beta synthesis by human peritoneal mesothelial cells. Induction by interleukin-1. Am J Pathol 1996;148(5):1679–1688.
32. Douvdevani A, Raport J, Konforty A, et al. Human peritoneal mesothelial cells synthesize IL-1 alpha and beta. Kidney Int 1994;46(4):993–1001.
33. Yung S, Coles GA, Davies M. IL-1 beta, a major stimulator of hyaluronan synthesis in vitro of human peritoneal mesothelial cells: relevance to peritonitis in CAPD. Kidney Int 1996;50(4):1337–1343.
34. Breborowicz A, Korybalska K, Grzybowski A, et al. Synthesis of hyaluronic acid by human peritoneal mesothelial cells: effect of cytokines and dialysate. Perit Dial Int 1996;16(4):274–278.
35. Offner FA, Obrist P, Stadlmann S, et al. IL-6 secretion by human peritoneal mesothelial and ovarian cancer cells. Cytokine 1995;7(6):542–547.
36. Zeillemaker AM, Mul FP, van Papendrecht AA, et al. Limited influence of the mesothelium on the influx of monocytes into the peritoneal cavity. Inflammation 1996;20(1): 87–95.
37. Douvdevani A, Einbinder T, Ylzari R, et al. TNF-receptors on human peritoneal mesothelial cells: regulation of receptor levels and shedding by IL-1 alpha and TNF alpha. Kidney Int 1996;50(1):219–228.
38. Arici A, Oral E, Attar E, et al. Monocyte chemotactic protein-1 concentration in peritoneal fluid of women with endometriosis and its modulation of expression in mesothelial cells. Fertil Steril 1997;67(6):1065–1072.
39. Visser CE, Tekstra J, Brouwer-Steenbergen JJ, et al. Chemokines produced by mesothelial cells: huGRO-alpha, IP-10, MCP-1 and RANTES. Clin Exp Immunol 1998; 112(2):270–275.
40. Whawell SA, Scott-Coombes DM, Vipond MN, et al. Tumor necrosis factor-mediated release of plasminogen activator inhibitor 1 by human peritoneal mesothelial cells. Br J Surg 1994;81(2):214–216.
41. Perfumo F, Altieri P, Degl'Innocenti ML, et al. Effects of peritoneal effluents on mesothelial cells in culture: cell proliferation and extracellular matrix regulation. Nephrol Dial Transplant 1996;11(9):1903–1909.
42. Muller J, Yoshida T. Interaction of murine peritoneal leukocytes and mesothelial cells: in vitro model system to survey cellular events on serosal membranes during inflammation. Clin Immunol Immunopathol 1995;75(3): 231–238.
43. Toh H, Torisu M, Shimura H, et al. In vitro analysis of peritoneal adhesions in peritonitis. J Surg Res 1996;61(1): 250–255.
44. Gibson FC III, Onderdonk AB, Kasper DL, et al. Cellular mechanism of intraabdominal abscess formation by *Bacteroides fragilis.* J Immunol 1998;160(10):5000–5006.
45. Zeillemaker AM, Hoynck van Papendricht AA, Hart MH, et al. Peritoneal interleukin-8 in acute appendicitis. J Surg Res 1996;62(2):263–277.
46. Valle MT, Degl'Innocenti ML, Bertelli R, et al. Antigen-presenting function of human peritoneum mesothelial cells. Clin Exp Immunol 1995;101(1):172–176.
47. Whawell SA, Thompson JN. Cytokine-induced release of plasminogen activator inhibitor-1 by human mesothelial cells. Eur J Surg 1995;161(5):315–318.
48. Tietze L, Elbrecht A, Schauerte C, et al. Modulation of pro- and antifibrinolytic properties of human peritoneal mesothelial cells by transforming growth factor beta 1 (TGF-beta 1), tumor necrosis factor alpha (TNF-alpha) and interleukin 1 beta (IL-1 beta). Thromb Haemostasis 79:362–370.

49. Postlethwaite AE, Lachman LB, Mainadri CL, et al. Interleukin-I stimulation of collagenase production by cultured fibroblasts. J Exp Med 1983;157:801–806.
50. Matsushima K, Bano M, Kidwell WR, et al. Interleukin-1 increases collagen type IV production by murine mammary epithelial cells. J Immunol 1985;134:904–909.
51. Bronson RE, Bertiolami CN, Siebert EP. Modulation of fibroblast growth and glycosaminoglycan synthesis by interleukin-1. Collagen Relat Res 1987;7:323–332.
52. Bevilacqua MP, Pober JS, Majeau GR, et al. Interleukin-1 (IL-1) induces biosynthesis and cell surface expression of procoagulant activity in human vascular endothelial cells. J Exp Med 1984;160:618–623.
53. Bevilacqua MP, Schleef RR, Gimbrone MA, et al. Regulation of fibrinolytic system of cultured human vascular endothelium by interleukin 1. J Clin Invest 1986;73:587–591.
54. Emeis JJ, Kooestra J. Interleukin-1 and lipopolysaccharide induce an inhibitor of tissue-type plasminogen activator in vivo and in cultured endothelial cells. J Exp Med 1986; 163:1260–1266.
55. Nachman RL, Hajjar KA, Silverstein RL, et al. Interleukin-1 induces endothelial cell synthesis of plasminogen activator inhibitor. J Exp Med 1986;163:1545–1547.
56. Nawroth PP, Stem DM. Modulation of endothelial cell hemostatic properties by tumor necrosis factor. J Exp Med 1986;163:740–745.
57. McBride WH, Mason K, Withers HR, et al. Effect of interleukin-1, inflammation, and surgery on the incidence of adhesion formation after abdominal irradiation in mice. Cancer Res 1988;49:169–173.
58. Herschlag A, Herness IGO, Wimberly HC, et al. The effect of interleukin-1 on adhesion formation in the rat. Am J Obstet Gynecol 1991;165:771–774.
59. Abe H, Rodgers KE, Ellefson D, et al. Kinetics of interleukin-1 and tumor necrosis factor by rabbit macrophages recovered from the peritoneal cavity after surgery. J Invest Surg 1991;4:141–151.
60. Abe H, Rodgers KE, Ellefson D, et al. Kinetics of interleukin-1 secretion by murine macrophages recovered from the peritoneal cavity after surgery. J Surg Res 1989;47: 178–182.
61. Ko SD, Page RC, Narayanan AS. Fibroblast heterogeneity and prostaglandin regulation of subpopulation. Proc Natl Acad Sci USA 1977;74:3429–3440.
62. Phan SH, McGarry BM, Loeffler KM, et al. Regulation of macrophage derived fibroblast growth factor release by arachidonate metabolites. J Leukocyte Biol 1987;42: 106–113.
63. Korn JH, Halushka PV, LeRoy EC. Mononuclear cell modulation of connective tissue function: suppression of fibroblast growth by stimulation of endogenous prostaglandin production. J Clin Invest 1980;65:543–554.
64. Alexander P, Evans R. Endotoxin and double stranded RNA render macrophages cytotoxic. Nature (Lond) 1971; 232: 76–79.
65. Hibbs JB, Lambert LH, Remington JS. In vitro nonimmunologic destruction of cells with abnormal characteristics by adjuvant activated macrophages. Proc Soc Exp Biol Med 1972;139:1049–1055.
66. Adams DO, Marino P. Activation of mononuclear phagocytes for destruction of tumor cells as a model for the study of macrophage development. In Gordon AS, Silver R, LoBue J, eds. Contemporary Topics in Hematology Oncology. New York: Plenum Press, 1984:69–136.
67. Adams DO, Johnson WJ, Marino PJ. Mechanisms of target recognition and destruction in macrophage mediated tumor cytotoxicity. Fed Proc 1982;41:2212–2221.
68. Adams DO, Nathan CF. Molecular mechanisms in tumor-cell killing by activated macrophages. Immunol Today 1983;4:166–170.
69. Rodgers KE, Ellefson D, Girgis W, et al. Effects of tolmetin sodium dehydrate on normal and postsurgical cell function. Int J Immunopharmacol 1988;10:111–120.
70. Jones PA, Werb Z. Degradation of connective tissue matrices by macrophages. III. Influence of matrix composition on proteolysis of glycoprotein, elastin and collagen by macrophages in culture. J Exp Med 1980;152: 1527–1536.
71. Werb Z, Banda MJ, Jones PA. Degradation of connective tissue matrices by macrophages. I. Proteolysis of elastin, glycoproteins and collagen by proteinases isolated from macrophages. J Exp Med 1980;152:1340–1357.
72. Laub R, Huybrechts-Godin G, Peeters-Joris C, et al. Degradation of collagen and proteoglycan by macrophages and fibroblasts. Biochim Biophys Acta 1982;721:425–433.
73. Unkeless J, Gordon S, Reich E. Secretion of plasminogen activator by stimulated macrophages. J Exp Med 1974; 139:834–850.
74. Orita H, Campeau JD, Gale JA, et al. Differential secretion of plasminogen activator activity by postsurgical activated macrophages. J Surg Res 1986;41:569–573.
75. Fukasawa M, Campeau JD, Girgis W, et al. Production of protease inhibitors by postsurgical macrophages. J Surg Res 1989;46:256–261.
76. Kuraoka S, Campeau JD, Rodgers KE, et al. Effects of interleukin 1 on postsurgical macrophage secretion of protease and protease inhibitor activates. J Surg Res 1992; 52:71–78.
77. Diegelmann RF, Cohen IK, Kaplan AM. The role of macrophages in wound repair: a review. Plast Reconstr Surg 1981;68:107–113.
78. Raftery AT. Regeneration of parietal and visceral peritoneum. Br J Surg 1973;60:293–299.
79. Raftery AT. Regeneration of parietal and visceral peritoneum in the immature animal. Br J Surg 1973;60: 969–975.
80. Fukasawa M, Bryant SM, Nakamura RM, et al. Modulation of fibroblast proliferation by postsurgical macrophages. J Surg Res 1987;43:513–520.
81. Fukasawa M, Campeau JD, Yanagihara DL, et al. Mitogenic and protein synthetic activity of tissue repair cells: control by the postsurgical macrophage. J Invest Surg 1989;2: 169–180.
82. Fukasawa M, Yanagihara DL, Rodgers KE, et al. The mitogenic activity of peritoneal tissue repair cells: control by growth factors. J Surg Res 1989;47:45–51.
83. Fukasawa M, Bryant SM, diZerega GS. Incorporation of thymidine by fibroblasts: evidence for complex regulation by postsurgical macrophages. J Surg Res 1988;45:460–466.
84. Rodgers KE, diZerega GS. Modulation of peritoneal re-epithelialization by postsurgical macrophages. J Surg Res 1992;53:542–548.

85. Ryan GG, Grobety J, Majno G. Mesothelial injury and recovery. Am J Pathol 1973;71:93–112.
86. Bryant SM, Fukasawa M, Orita H, et al. Mediation of postsurgical wound healing by macrophages. In: Growth Factors and Other Aspects of Wound Healing. Biological and Clinical Implications. New York: Liss, 1988:263–290.
87. Martin BM, Gimbrone MA Jr, Unanue ER, et al. Stimulation of nonlymphoid mesenchymal cell proliferation by a macrophage-derived growth factor. J Immunol 1981;126: 1510–1515.
88. Tsukamoto Y, Helsen WE, Wahl SM. Macrophage production of fibronectin. A chemoattractant for fibroblast. J Immunol 1981;127:673–678.
89. Postlethwaite AE, Kang AH. Induction of fibroblast proliferation by human mononuclear derived proteins. Arthritis Rheum 1983;26:22–27.
90. Gosline JM, Rosenbloom J. Elastin. In: Piez KA, Reddi AH, eds. Extracellular Matrix Biochemistry. New York: Elsevier, 1984:191–227.
91. Samuelson B, Branstrom E, Greek K, et al. Prostaglandins. Annu Rev Biochem 1971;44:669–692.
92. Opitz HG, Niethammer D, Lemk H, et al. Inhibition of ^{3}H-thymidine incorporation of lymphocytes by a soluble factor from macrophages. Cell Immunol 1975;16:379–388.
93. Gresser J, Brouty-Boye K, Thomas MG, et al. Interferon and cell division I. Inhibition of the multiplication of mouse leukemia C12 106/B in vitro by interferon preparations. Proc Natl Acad Sci USA 1970;66:1052–1058.
94. Kung JT, Brooks SB, Jakway JB, et al. Suppression of in vitro cytotoxic response by macrophage due to induced arginase. J Exp Med 1977;146:665–680.
95. Harris A, Dunn G. Centripetal transport of attached peptides on both surfaces of moving fibroblasts. Exp Cell Res 1972;73:519–523.
96. Prydze HA, Allison AC, Schlorlemner HU. Further link between complement activation and coagulation. Nature (Lond) 1977;270:173–178.
97. Abercrombie M, Heaysman JEM, Pegrum SM. The locomotion of fibroblasts in culture. IV. Electron microscopy of the leading lamella. Exp Cell Res 1971;67:359–367.
98. Lemke H, Huget R, Flad HD. Biochemical characterization of a factor released by macrophages. Cell Immunol 1975;18:70–75.
99. Leibovich SJ, Ross R. A macrophage-dependent factor that stimulates the proliferation of fibroblast in vitro. Am J Pathol 1976;84:501–508.
100. Leibovich SJ. Production of macrophage-dependent fibroblast-stimulating activity (M-FSA) by murine macrophages. Exp Cell Res 1978;113:47–53.
101. Bitterman PB, Rennard SI, Hunninghake GW, et al. Human alveolar macrophage growth factor regulation and partial characterization. J Clin Invest 1982;70:806–822.
102. Takemura R, Werb Z. Secretory products of macrophages and their physiological functions. Am J Physiol 1984;246: C1–C9.
103. Bleiberg I, Harvey AK, Smale G, et al. Identification of a PDGF-like chemoattractant produced by NIH/3T3 cells after transformation with SV40. J Cell Biol 1985;123: 161–166.
104. Jimenez de Asua L, Clingan D, Rudland PS. Initiation of cell proliferation in cultured mouse fibroblasts by prostaglandin Fα. Proc Natl Acad Sci USA 1975;72: 2724–2728.
105. Jimenez de Asua LL, Otto AM, Lingren J, et al. The stimulation of the initiation of DNA synthesis and cell division in Swiss mouse 3T3 cells by prostaglandin Fα requires specific functional groups in the molecule. J Biol Chem 1983;258:8774–8777.
106. Mizel SB, Dayer JM, Krane SM, et al. Stimulation of rheumatoid synovial cell collagenase and prostaglandin production by partially purified lymphocyte activating factor. Proc Natl Acad Sci USA 1981;78:2474–2477.
107. Calderon J, Williams RT, Unanue ER. An inhibitor of cell proliferation related by cultures of macrophages. Proc Natl Acad Sci USA 1974;71:4273–4277.
108. Carpenter G. Vanadate epidermal growth factor and the stimulation of DNA synthesis. Biochem Biophys Res Commun. 1981;102:1115–1121.
109. Schmidt JA, Mizel SB, Cohen D, et al. Interleukin-1, a potential regulator of fibroblast proliferation. J Immunol 1982;128:2177–2192.
110. Orita H, Campeau JD, Nakamura RM, et al. Modulation of fibroblast proliferation by post-surgical macrophages: a time and dose-response study during postsurgical peritoneal re-epithelialization. Am J Obstet Gynecol 1986;155: 905–911.
111. Roberts AB, Anzano MA, Wakefield LM, et al. Type β transforming growth factor: a bidirectional regulation of cell growth. Proc Natl Acad Sci USA 1985;82:119–123.
112. Cohen S, Carpenter G. Human epidermal growth factor: isolation and chemical and biological properties. Proc Natl Acad Sci USA 1975;72:1317–1323.
113. Ross R, Bowen-Pope DF. Platelet derived growth factor. J Clin Endocrinol Metab 1984;13:191–199.
114. Baird A, Esch F, Mormede P, et al. Molecular characteristics of fibroblast growth factors distribution and biological activities in various tissues. Recent Prog Horm Res 1986;42:143–205.
115. Baird A, Mormede P, Bohlen P. Immunoreactive fibroblast growth factor in cells of peritoneal exudate suggest its identity with macrophage derived growth factor. Biochem Biophys Res Commun 1985;126:358–364.
116. Ignotz RA, Massaque J. Transforming growth factor β stimulates the expression of fibronectin and collagen and their incorporation into the extracellular matrix. J Biol Chem 1986;261:4337–4345.
117. Simpson DM, Ross R. The neutrophilic leukocyte in wound repair. A study with anti-neutrophil serum. J Clin Invest 1972;51:2009–2023.
118. Leibovich SJ, Ross R. The role of macrophages in wound repair. A study with hydrocortisone and anti-macrophage serum. Am J Pathol 1975;78:71–100.
119. Seppae H, Grotendorst G, Seppae S, et al. Platelet derived growth factor is chemotactic for fibroblasts. J Cell Biol 1982;92:584–588.
120. Shimakado K, Raines EW, Madtes DK, et al. A significant part of macrophage derived growth factor consists of at least two forms of PDGF cell. Cell 1985;43:277–286.
121. Cohen S. Isolation of a mouse submaxillary gland protein accelerating incisor eruption and eyelid opening in the newborn animal. J Biol Chem 1962;237: 1555–1568.

122. Clemmons DR, Underwood LE, Van Wyk JJ. Hormonal control of immunoreactive somatomedin production by cultured human fibroblasts. J Clin Invest 1981;64:10–19.
123. Assoian RK, Kornoriya A, Meyers CA, et al. Transforming growth factor-β in human platelets. J Biol Chem 1983; 258:7155–7160.
124. Assoian RK, Fleurdelys BE, Stevenson HC, et al. Expression secretion of type β transforming growth factor by activated human macrophage. Proc Natl Acad Sci USA 1987;84:6020–6024.
125. Cromack DT, Spom MB, Roberts AB, et al. Transforming growth factor β levels in rat wound chambers. J Surg Res 1987;42:622–628.
126. Dinarello CA, Cannon JG, Mier JW, et al. Multiple biological activities of human recombinant interleukin 1. J Clin Invest 1986;77:1734–1739.
127. Postlethwaite AE, Lachman LB, Kang AH. Induction of fibroblast proliferation by interleukin-I derived from human monocytic leukemia cells. Arthritis Rheum 1984; 27:1001–1011.
128. Fukasawa M, Campeau JD, Yanighihara DL, et al. Regulation of proliferation of peritoneal tissue repair cells by peritoneal macrophages. J Surg Res 1990;49:81–87.
129. Pledger WJ, Stiles CD, Antoniades HN, et al. An ordered sequence of events is required before BALB/c-3T3 cells have become committed to DNA synthesis. Proc Natl Acad Sci USA 1987;74:2839–2848.
130. Abercrombie M, Heaysman JEM, Pegrum SM. Locomotion of fibroblasts in culture. V. Surface marking with concanavilin A. Exp Cell Res 1972;3:536–539.
131. Postlethwaite AE, Keski-Oja J, Moses HL, et al. Stimulation of the chemotactic migration of human fibroblasts by transforming growth factor. J Exp Med 1987;165: 251–256.
132. Barbul A, Knud-Hansen J, Wasserkrug HL, et al. Interleukin-2 enhances wound healing in rats. J Surg Res 1986; 40:315–319.
133. Kleinman HK, McGoodwin EB, Klebe RJ. Localization of the cell attachment region in types I and II collagen. Biochem Biophys Res Commun 1976;72:426–432.
134. Kleinman HK, Klebe RJ, Martin GR. Role of collagenous matrices in adhesion and growth of cells. J Cell Biol 1981; 88:473–485.
135. Assoian RK. Biphasic effect of type β transforming growth factor on epidermal growth factor receptors in NRK fibroblasts: functional consequences for epidermal growth factor stimulated mitosis. J Biol Chem 1986;260: 9613–9617.
136. Sporn MB, Roberts AB, Shull JH, et al. Polypeptide transforming growth factors isolated from bovine sources and used for wound healing in vivo. Science 1983;219: 1329–1331.
137. Mensing H, Czametozki BM. Leukotriene B induces in vitro fibroblast chemotaxis. J Invest Dermatol 1984;82: 9–12.
138. Thalacker FW, Nilsen-Hamilton M. Specific induction of secreted proteins by transforming growth factor and 12-O-tetra-decanoyl phorbol-13-acetate. J Biol Chem 1987; 262:2288–2290.
139. Varga J, Jimenez SA. Stimulation of normal human fibroblast collagen production and processing by transforming growth factor-β and 12-O-tetradecanoyl phorbol-I 3-acetate. J Biol Chem 1987;262:2283–2287.
140. Wahl SM, McCartney-Francis N, Mergenhagen SE. Inflammatory and immunoregulatory roles of TGF-β. Immunol Today 1989;10:258–261.
141. Vipond MN, Whawell SA, Thompson JN, et al. Peritoneal fibrinolytic activity and intra-abdominal adhesions. Lancet 1990;335:1120–1122.
142. van der Poll T, Levi M, Buller HR, et al. Fibrinolytic response to tumor necrosis factor in healthy subjects. J Exp Med 1991;175:729–732.
143. Gervin AS, Puckett CL, Silver D. Serosal hypofibrinolysis. A cause of postoperative adhesions. Am J Surg 1973; 125:80–88.
144. Raftery AT. Effect of peritoneal trauma on peritoneal fibrinolytic activity and intraperitoneal adhesion formation. Eur Surg Res 1981;13:397–401.
145. Buckman RF Jr, Maj MC, Buckman PD, et al. A physiologic basis for the adhesion-free healing of deperitonealized surfaces. J Surg Res 1976;21:67–76.
146. van Hinsbergh VWM, Kooistra T, Scheffer MA, et al. Characterization and fibrinolytic properties of human omental tissue mesothelial cells. Comparison with endothelial cells. Blood 1990;75:1490–1497.
147. Hau T, Payne D, Simmons RL. Fibrinolytic activity of the peritoneum during experimental peritonitis. Surg Gynecol Obstet 1979;148:415–418.
148. diZerega GS, Rodgers KE. Tissue repair cells In: The Peritoneum. New York: Springer-Verlag, 1992:58.

4

The Biology of Peritoneal Tissue Repair

Andrew T. Raftery

CONTENTS

Intraabdominal fibrous adhesions are a major cause of intestinal obstruction.[1] By far the most common cause of intraabdominal adhesions is previous surgical intervention. Most surgeons regard intraabdominal adhesions as a problem, because reoperation on the abdomen is made difficult by prolonged dissection of fibrous adhesions with the risk of visceral damage. Because adhesions may have such serious consequences, it is not surprising that a very large number of techniques have been devised with the aim of preventing their development. Many of these however have been shown to be unreliable.[1,2] Many of the techniques used have been of an empirical nature, and little improvement can be expected unless the underlying pathogenesis is understood because a clear understanding of pathogenesis is a prerequisite to rational prophylaxis and therapy.

The relationship between the frequency of abdominal operations and the production of adhesions, with the possibility of resulting intestinal obstruction, led to the concept that adhesion formation occurred as a result of serosal injury. On the basis of this, it was considered good surgical practice to avoid peritoneal injury, that raw, damaged, serosal surfaces should be eliminated within the peritoneal cavity, and that these defects should be oversewn, patched, or covered by grafts. The concept that damaged peritoneum healed by fibrous adhesions was the result of theory rather than clinical observation or laboratory experimentation. It has become clear over the years that adhesions do not necessarily follow serosal damage. Knowledge of the healing of peritoneum is fundamental to the practice of abdominal and pelvic surgery. This chapter reviews the literature on peritoneal repair and its relation to peritoneal adhesions.

Peritoneal Healing

As early as 1919, Hertzler[3] showed that when a defect was created in the parietal peritoneum of an experimental animal, 'the entire surface becomes endothelialised simultaneously and not gradually from the border as in epidermitization of skin wounds.' Hertzler added 'that the endothelium of the surrounding surface of the peritoneum has any direct part in the covering of these surfaces cannot be demonstrated.' These observations have since been confirmed by several workers.[4-7] However, there has been disagreement over the exact origin of the cells that form the new mesothelium. Some workers[4,5,8,9] considered that mesothelial regeneration took place by metaplasia of subperitoneal fibroblasts. Other workers[10-12] considered that mesothelial cells became detached from the adjacent intact peritoneum and became implanted on the wound surface, proliferating and eventually giving rise to a continuous sheet of mesothelial cells. Johnson and Whitting[11] also suggested that monocytes and macrophages that were present in the wound exudate could become transformed into mesothelial cells, a suggestion which received support from Eskeland[6,13] and Eskeland and Kjaerheim.[14,15]

The early work on peritoneal regeneration was blighted by the difficulty of identification of mesothelial cells in histologic sections cut perpendicular to the wound surface. Because many of the cells were flat with attenuated cytoplasm, it was extremely difficult to identify the different types of cells. This limitation was overcome by the use of Häutchen preparations, which permit examination of the surface cells en face. This technique involves stripping off the surface layer of the cells on a sheet of celloidin. The surface cells are then more easily identified when viewed en face, and it is possible to identify cell-to-cell contact by impregnating the sections with silver nitrate (Fig. 4.1).

A study involving the use of Häutchen preparations[7] demonstrated that unsutured peritoneal defects in the rat healed rapidly and, for the most part, without adhesion formation. Parietal peritoneal defects in the rat healed completely in 8 days. Following wounding of the parietal peritoneum, the majority of cells seen on the wound surface during the first 48 hours were inflammatory cells, consisting of macrophages, monocytes, polymorphs, eosinophils, lymphocytes, and occasional mast cells (Fig. 4.2). At 3 days after wounding there were marked changes on the wound surface. Polymorphs, lymphocytes, eosinophils, and mast cells were rarely seen, and the only cells of the initial inflammatory reaction that remained were monocytes and macrophages. At this stage, a further type of cell was seen on the wound surface that had a poorly defined cell boundary, was larger than a monocyte, and possessed a large, round, or oval nucleus containing one or more prominent nucleoli (Fig. 4.3). These cells resembled subperitoneal fibro-

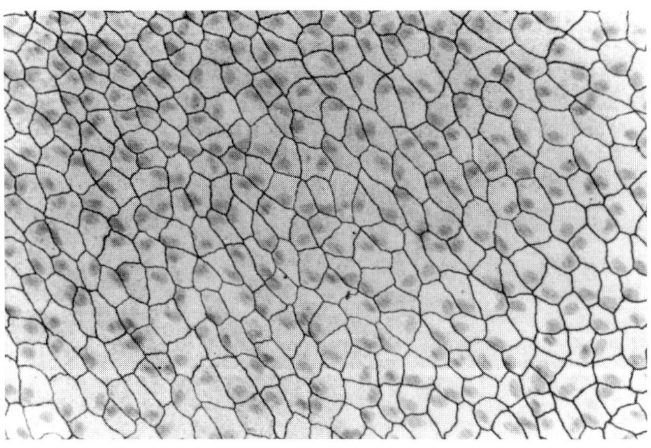

Fig. 4.1. Normal parietal peritoneum. Note the single layer of mesothelial cells with the intercellular substance stained with silver. Häutchen preparation, ×180.

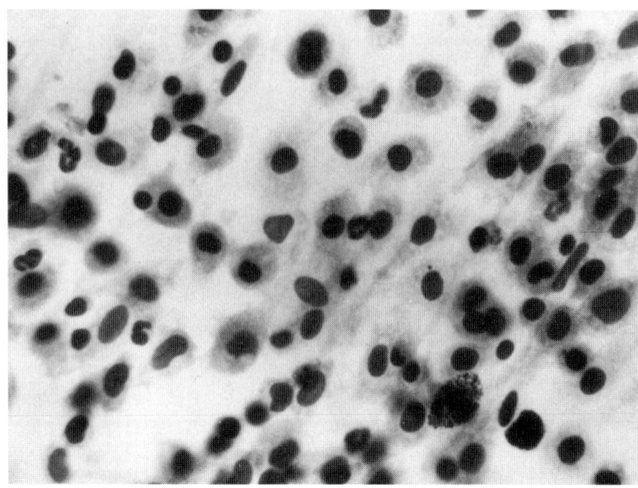

Fig. 4.2. Parietal peritoneum at 1 day. Macrophages, monocytes, polymorphs, eosinophils, lymphocytes, and an occasional mast cell are seen on the wound surface. Most cells are of the monocyte/macrophage type. Häutchen preparation, ×220. (Reproduced from the British Journal of Surgery[7] by permission of Blackwell Science Ltd.)

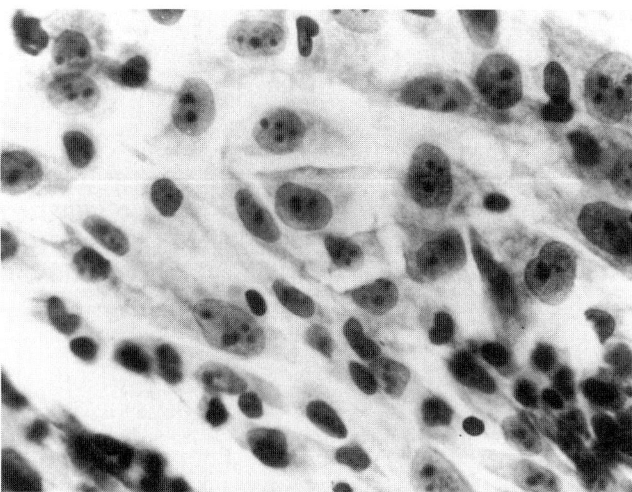

Fig. 4.3. Parietal peritoneum at 3 days. Two types of cells are seen on the wound surface: one resembles a monocyte and the other is a large cell with indistinct boundary and many prominent nucleoli. Häutchen preparation, ×220. (Reproduced from the British Journal of Surgery[7] by permission of Blackwell Science Ltd.)

blasts. This type of cell gradually came to occupy more and more of the wound surface, such that at 6 days these cells occupied most of the wound surface; in those sections impregnated with silver nitrate, silver lines were seen between most cells, although they were broader than in normal mesothelium. By 8 days the surface was lined by a continuous layer of flattened cells, which resembled normal mesothelium except that a few mitotic figures were seen.

Raftery[7] concluded that the new mesothelium probably developed from subperitoneal fibroblasts. To test the previous theory that monocytes and macrophages became transformed into mesothelial cells,[6,13–15] peritoneal macrophages were labeled with polystyrene spheres.[7,16] Although the macrophages remained full of polystyrene spheres, no such spheres were subsequently present in fibroblasts or the reconstituted mesothelium. This finding was put forward as strong evidence against the theory that peritoneal macrophages become transformed into mesothelial cells either directly or via fibroblasts.

On the basis of a light microscopic study, however, it was not possible to discount the theory that mesothelial cells become detached from adjacent normal peritoneal surfaces and give rise to a new mesothelium. The reason for this was that it was impossible to accurately identify isolated mesothelial cells in peritoneal fluid by light microscopy. A subsequent study[17] searched for detached mesothelial cells in peritoneal fluid by examining pellets of mesothelial cells, prepared for electron microscopy, both by toluidine blue staining under high-power light microscopy and by examination under electron microscopy. This study revealed that a few detached mesothelial cells were present in the peritoneal fluid of rats that had undergone abdominal surgery, involving excision of areas of peritoneum, but most of these cells were injured or dying. Subsequent electron microscopic investigation of peritoneal regeneration[16] failed to show any contribution from detached mesothelial cells in the healing process. The electron microscopic study also confirmed the findings of the light microscopic study, namely, that there was no evidence to support the theory that new mesothelium arose from transformation of peritoneal macrophages.

Sequence of Cellular Events

The sequence of events following creation of peritoneal defects was as follows: 12 hours after wounding, numerous cells were seen entangled in fibrin strands. At this stage polymorphs predominated, but a large number of macrophages and a few eosinophils and mast cells were also seen. Polystyrene spheres used for labeling were seen in macrophages and polymorphs. At 24 to 36 hours after wounding, the number of cells in the superficial part of the wound was greatly increased and the majority of cells were macrophages. By 2 days there were marked changes both on the surface and on the base of the wound; in most areas, the wound surface was covered by a single layer of macrophages resting on a fibrin base. Macrophages contained polystyrene spheres (Fig. 4.4.) By 2 days after wounding, two additional cell types had appeared on the wound surface. The first type of cell possessed all the characteristics of a perivascular primitive mesenchymal cell. The second type of cell was extremely rare, being seen on only two occasions in numerous sections, and these were identified as islets of mesothelial cells. Because of their rarity in the many animals examined, it was thought that they did not make a significant contribution to peritoneal healing. By 3 days, the majority of cells on the wound surface were macrophages but cells of the primitive mesenchymal type were becoming more common. Cells on the wound surface at 3 days were similar in appearance to cells in the deeper layers of the wound and possessed all the characteristics of primitive mesenchymal cells.

By 4 days, cells resembling primitive mesenchymal cells or proliferating fibroblasts came to the wound surface and were in contact with one another (Fig. 4.5). Cells appearing in stages between primitive mesenchymal cells and fibroblasts were seen, and it was considered that primitive mesenchymal cells either developed into mesothelial cells directly or via cells of the fibroblast type. In some areas of the wound, healing appeared complete at 5 days because there was a single layer of mesothelial cells present on the wound surface connected by desmosomes and tight junctions. No basement membrane could be identified beneath the mesothelial

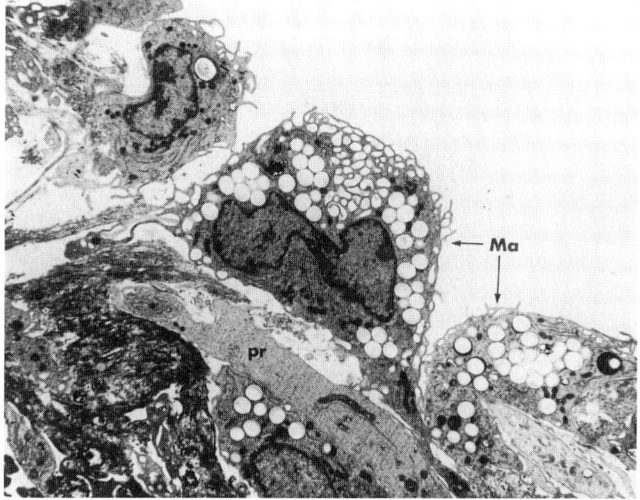

FIG. 4.4. Parietal peritoneum at 2 days. Macrophages (*Ma*) containing polystyrene spheres (*white 'empty' spheres*) rest on a fibrin base. A process (*pr*) of a primitive mesenchymal cell extends toward the wound surface. Electron photomicrograph, ×4250. (Reproduced from the British Journal of Surgery[25] by permission of Blackwell Science Ltd.)

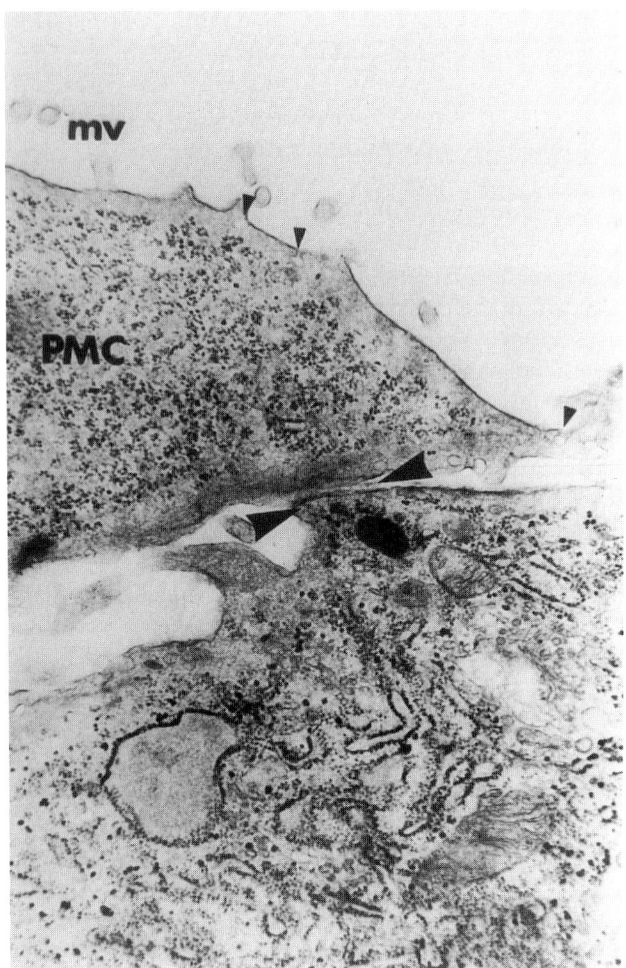

Fig. 4.5. Parietal peritoneum at 4 days. A primitive mesenchymal cell (*PMC*) and a cell that has features common to both PMC and fibroblast are in close contact (*large arrowheads*) on the wound surface. No junctional complexes are visible. Note the microvilli (*mv*) and pinocytic vesicles (*small arrowheads*) in relation to the primitive mesenchymal cell. Electron photomicrograph, ×4000.

cells at this stage. In other areas of the wound surface, healing was less advanced with primitive mesenchymal cells present both on the surface and in the base of the wound. At 7 days after wounding, the appearance of the wound showed a layer of cells that now resembled mesothelial cells except that there was a discontinuous basement membrane. By 8 days there was a continuous layer of mesothelial cells over the wound, although the basement membrane was not complete, and completeness of the basement membrane did not occur until 10 days. At 10 days, fibroblasts in the base of the wound were arranged with their long axis parallel to the wound surface and bundles of collagen were present between the fibroblasts. At no time were any polystyrene spheres seen in primitive mesenchymal cells, subperitoneal fibroblasts, or mesothelial cells.

Electron Microscopic Studies

On the basis of light and electron microscopic studies, it was concluded that the new mesothelium arose from subperitoneal connective tissue cells, but it was not possible to determine conclusively whether these were primitive mesenchymal cells or fibroblasts. Watters and Buck[18] studied peritoneal repair by scanning electron microscopy after removing only the surface layer of mesothelium on a film of gelatin. The peritoneal surface was completely devoid of mesothelial cells immediately following the stripping procedure. Transmission electron microscopy showed that the basement membrane remained in situ following stripping of the mesothelium using gelatin film. New cells were seen on the surface as early as 30 minutes after injury, and at 8 hours most of the surface contained new cells of a variety of types. By 1 hour after stripping of the mesothelium, the cells were evenly spaced from each other and covered about 50% of the denuded surface. Some of them were starting to flatten against the basement membrane.

By 4 hours after wounding, the denuded area was virtually covered with cells. Some of these were rounded and others were starting to flatten. By 24 hours, the proportion of rounded cells had started to decrease while the flattened cells were plentiful. By 3 days, many of the cells were extremely flat and studded with short microvilli. Very few of the rounded cells were seen. By 4 days, the microvilli of the cells had increased in length and in many places they obscured the cell outline as in the normal mesothelium. A virtually normal appearance was present in the 7-day specimens.

The experiments of Watters and Buck inflicted little injury on the underlying connective tissue. On the basis of this, Watters and Buck suggested that the cells seen on the wound surface were derived from macrophages or lymphocytes of the peritoneal fluid, which tended to support the contention of Eskeland[6,13] and Eskeland and Kjaerheim.[14,15] However, Watters and Buck did consider that another possible source of the cells was the blood vessels underlying the wound area. They admitted that it was obviously difficult, if not impossible, to determine from the static images whether the cells that had adhered to the surface were the same as those which eventually flattened and covered the surfaces as normal-appearing mesothelium. They considered that it was possible that subsequent to the attachment of the rounded cells from the peritoneal fluid, certain cells from the underlying connective tissue differentiated into mesothelium, the round cells being lost and having served only as a temporary covering. They also thought it was possible that the ultimate covering cells might have been derived from preexisting surrounding mesothelial cells that detached themselves from the wound surface and implanted on the wound.

A subsequent study by Watters and Buck[19] showed that if a wound was placed in the parietal peritoneum so that it contacted the visceral peritoneum of the liver, mitotic activity was seen in the liver mesothelium. Although the wound was covered with macrophages and lymphocytes at an early stage, the cells that finally repaired the wound appeared to be new mesothelial cells, many of which migrated from the opposing stimulated peritoneum of the liver.

Immunohistochemical Studies

In an attempt to further elucidate which particular cell was responsible for the development of new mesothelium, Raftery[20] applied enzyme histochemical techniques. A previous study had demonstrated[21] that peritoneal mesothelial cells were extremely active metabolically, as judged by the presence of various enzymes. The enzyme histochemical study showed that it was possible to identify histochemically on the wound surface, in the early stages of healing, two main types of cell which corresponded with those previously described on the basis of examination of Häutchen preparations stained with hematoxylin.[7] One was a macrophage and the other a fibroblast-like cell. The larger, fibroblast-like cell differed from the macrophages histochemically in that (i) it gave a negative reaction for nonspecific esterase; (ii) it gave a negative reaction for adenosine triphosphatase in the early stages of healing; and (iii) it showed only scattered punctate deposits of acid phosphatase reaction products as compared with a concentrated strongly positive reaction in the macrophage.

The large fibroblast-like cells seen on the wound surface in the early stages of healing resembled subperitoneal fibroblasts in that (i) they contained no alkaline phosphatase; (ii) they contained no adenosine triphosphatase in the early stages of healing; (iii) they contained no nonspecific esterase; and (iv) they possessed the same scattered punctate deposits of acid phosphatase reaction product. Further, the new mesothelial cells possessed the following histochemical characteristics in common with the subperitoneal fibroblasts in the later stage of healing: (i) they contained no alkaline phosphatase; (ii) they contained no nonspecific esterase; and (iii) they possessed the same scattered punctate deposits of acid phosphatase activity. The enzyme histochemical study does not clearly indicate whether the new mesothelial cells arose from primitive mesenchymal cells or from subperitoneal fibroblasts. It does, however, lend further weight to the view that the new mesothelium is derived from subperitoneal connective tissue cells and not by transformation of macrophages.

Bolen et al.[22] further studied peritoneal healing using electron microscopy and immunocytochemical studies. They showed that following loss of surface mesothelium there was a striking proliferation of stromal cells, which they designated as subserosal multipotential cells. Although these cells possessed the ultrastructural features of myofibroblasts, they also exhibited from an early stage the immunocytochemical markers of epithelium. Active subserosal multipotential cells showed peripherally arranged myofilaments, focal investment by basal lamina, and abundant rough surface endoplasmic reticulum. Immunocytochemical studies demonstrated the presence of low molecular weight cytokeratins, coexpression of vimentin, and the absence of desmin. These cells were therefore distinct from connective tissue myofibroblasts, which shared only vimentin. As the cells rose to cover the denuded wound surface, they progressively acquired high molecular weight cytokeratins and lost vimentin. Bolen et al. considered therefore that there was a mesenchymal stem cell responsible for the regeneration of mesothelium.

Healing of Visceral Peritoneum

The healing of visceral peritoneum was found to differ little from the healing of parietal peritoneum. Raftery[7] studied the healing of the visceral peritoneum covering the liver and the visceral peritoneum covering the cecum. The liver acquired a new mesothelial layer 1 day earlier than either the cecum or the parietal peritoneum. There were two possible reasons for this. First, the liver provides a fairly firm substrate for healing while the peritoneum of the anterior abdominal wall and more so that of the cecum are subject to distension. Second and less likely, the cecum and parietal peritoneum may have been damaged by stretching when they were removed and prepared for histologic examination.

Peritoneal Healing in Infancy

Intestinal obstruction caused by peritoneal adhesions is more common following abdominal surgery in early life,[23,24] especially in the neonatal period. The greater incidence and severity of adhesions in the infant compared with the adult may reflect a difference in the nature of healing of the peritoneum. Ellis et al.[5] have shown that peritoneal regeneration occurred more rapidly in immature experimental animals than in mature ones, but flattening of the surface layer cells as seen in paraffin sections cut perpendicular to the wound surface was used as a criterion for assessing complete mesothelial regeneration. Raftery[25] studied the regeneration of parietal and visceral peritoneum in the immature animal using Häutchen preparations and electron microscopy and confirmed that regeneration of peritoneum occurred more rapidly in the immature animal. The parietal peritoneum was covered by a new mesothelial layer in 7 days whereas the liver was covered in 5 days. The study again lent support to the fact that new mesothelium had developed from subperitoneal perivascular connective tissue cells, but it was not possible to determine whether these were primitive mesenchymal cells or fibroblasts. Again, there was no difference in the rate of healing between large and small peritoneal defects.

Factors Affecting Peritoneal Regeneration

Surprisingly, there has been little work done on factors affecting peritoneal regeneration, particularly in recent years. Most of these studies were carried out using paraffin sections examined by light microscopy, and therefore the identification of mesothelial cells was not ideal. It was demonstrated that protein deficiency,[26] uremia,[27] vitamin C deficiency,[5] and local irradiation[28] all impaired fibroblast proliferation in peritoneal defects and the subsequent healing process. However, the administration of cytotoxic drugs had no overall effect on the rate or quality of healing peritoneum.[29] The presence of malignant disease is also known to delay wound healing, but in an experimental study in the rat of the effect of malignant disease on peritoneal healing, no difference could be shown in the rate or quality of healing between control and tumor-bearing animals.[30]

The precise effect of all these factors on mesothelial healing is not clear because of the difficulty of identifying mesothelial cells in paraffin sections cut perpendicular to the wound surface. A study of the role of infection in would healing[31] showed that distant sterile inflammation, distant bacterial infection, and transient bacteremia had a marked inhibitory affect on the healing of peritoneum. This study used Häutchen preparations, and the effect on mesothelial healing was clear. The authors concluded that this was a systemic effect that was not related to low plasma protein level or early colonization of the wounds with bacteria.

Peritonitis

Despite the surgical importance of peritonitis, there have been few studies of the structural changes occurring in the peritoneum as the result of the various forms of peritonitis. Cleaver et al.[32] using Häutchen preparations, showed disruption of the mesothelium with islets of inflammatory cells occurring on the peritoneal surface 3 hours after induction of fecal peritonitis in rats. Following peritoneal lavage, surviving animals were examined 8 days after induction of fecal peritonitis; inflammatory cells were still found to occupy most of the peritoneal surface and there was no sign of healing.

Walker[33] studied the effect of blood, bile, and starch in the peritoneal cavity of rats. Intraperitoneal injection of blood caused no change but sterile human bile provoked a severe peritonitis with purulent exudate. Five days after injection of bile, the peritoneum was heavily infiltrated with inflammatory cells. Mitotic figures were prominent in mesothelial cells and by 14 days, as studied in Häutchen preparations, the peritoneum had returned to normal. Intraperitoneal injection of starch, which at the time the study was carried out was used to lubricate surgical gloves, caused a dense inflammatory response around the starch granules, but the peritoneum remained intact. The addition of starch to blood and bile enhanced the peritonitis and delayed healing. Raftery[34] studied the effect of blood, bile, and urine on the peritoneal mesothelium. Blood caused no change in peritoneal structure but urine caused a mild peritonitis. Bile caused a moderately severe peritonitis with disruption of cell-to-cell contact, as seen in Häutchen preparations, together with patches of inflammatory cells.

There has been little interest in ultrastructural studies of the peritoneum mesothelium in the various forms of clinical peritonitis, for example, perforated peptic ulcer, perforated diverticular disease, or biliary peritonitis. All recent ultrastructural studies relate to continuous ambulatory peritoneal dialysis- (CAPD-) associated peritonitis, which tends to be less severe than that associated with perforation of a hollow viscus.

Source of New Mesothelial Cells

It is apparent from the foregoing discussion that controversy exists so far as the source of the new mesothelial cells is concerned. It is clear, because small wounds heal as rapidly as larger wounds and areas of new mesothelium are seen in the center of the wound at the same time they occur at the periphery, that growth of cells from the periphery of the defect contributes little to the healing of peritoneal defects. A major source of difficulty in the early days of the study of peritoneal wound healing was the inability to identify mesothelial cells in paraffin sections cut perpendicular to the wound surface. This was particularly so when trying to study the time sequence of complete mesothelial healing. The development of Häutchen preparations helped clarify the picture but did little to help decide on the origin of the new mesothelium. Even following studies by transmission and scanning electron microscopy, the controversy regarding the origin of the new mesothelial cell was not completely solved.

The following represent potential methods of peritoneal repair:

1. Metaplasia of subperitoneal fibroblasts
2. Transformation of underlying undifferentiated primitive mesenchymal cells
3. Transformation of monocytes and macrophages present on the wound surface
4. Detachment of cells from adjacent intact peritoneum with subsequent implantation and proliferation on the wound surface
5. Centripetal growth of cells at the periphery of the wound

Some investigators have suggested that cells detach from the adjacent peritoneum and become implanted on the wound surface, where they proliferate to produce a continuous layer of mesothelium.[10–12] These studies were carried out by light microscopy, examining paraffin sections cut perpendicular to the surface, and therefore it is impossible to tell with any certainty whether the cells had detached from the wound surface. Also, this rather begs the question of how the adjacent surfaces repair, although the work of Watters and Buck[19] has suggested that this may occur by mitotic activity of adjacent cells. Some investigators consider that metaplasia of subperitoneal fibroblasts is responsible for the development of the new mesothelium.[4,5,8,9] Again, these were light microscopic studies, but the work of Raftery[7,16] using the electron microscope tended to support this contention. However, it was not clear from this work whether the cells arose directly from subperitoneal fibroblasts or indirectly from subperitoneal perivascular cells, which resemble primitive mesenchymal cells. The work of Raftery has received support from the studies of Bolen et al.,[22] who believe on the basis of electron microscopic studies that there is a mesenchymal stem cell responsible for the regeneration of mesothelium.

Others believe that transformation of cells from the peritoneal fluid is responsible for the new mesothelium.[6,13–15] They believe that peritoneal macrophages are transformed into mesothelial cells, but this is based on the identification of intermediate forms between the two cells. It is of course difficult to interpret a dynamic process on the basis of a series of static electron photomicrographs. The work of Raftery[7,16] did not support the contention of Eskeland. Raftery labeled peritoneal macrophages with polystyrene spheres, and at no time were any polystyrene spheres seen in developing mesothelial cells. It was Raftery's contention that, had transformation from peritoneal macrophages to mesothelial cells taken place, then these polystyrene spheres would have been seen in developing mesothelial cells at some time during the process. It would appear at the present time that the weight of evidence suggests that the new mesothelium arises from perivascular primitive mesenchymal cells, which proliferate in the wound base. It is likely that a small contribution is made from the normal adjacent peritoneum.

Role of Mesothelium in the Prevention of Intraperitoneal Adhesions

Injury or inflammation in the peritoneal cavity produces a fibrinous exudate, and as a result of this, the involved surfaces adhere to one another. This fibrinous exudate may be absorbed or may be invaded by fibroblasts to become a permanent fibrous adhesion.

Fibrinous Exudate

It has been argued that absorption of a fibrinous exudate depends upon the presence of an intact mesothelium. It was argued that if the mesothelium remained intact, fibrin disappeared; if it was destroyed, adhesions would develop. It has been shown that large peritoneal defects will heal without adhesions in most cases,[8,35,36] but when attempts were made to oppose the edges by sutures as recommended in standard surgical textbooks, adhesions were formed to the wound[9,36,37] Robbins et al.[4] discovered that large peritoneal defects, left unsutured in the pelvic peritoneum after radical pelvic clearance, healed smoothly and without adhesion. Ellis[36] found that large defects created by excising areas of parietal peritoneum in rats healed within days to produce a glistening smooth peritoneum, with no adhesions in most animals.

Damage to the peritoneum, whatever the cause, results in a fibrinous exudate causing adjacent surfaces to stick together to form a fibrinous adhesion. Removal of this fibrin before it is invaded by fibroblasts prevents the formation of a permanent fibrous adhesion. Hartwell[38] considered that mesothelial cells prevented adhesions 'by combining their fibrinolytic power with their epithelial-like function of extending themselves as solid sheets to cover any raw surface.' At the time that Hartwell wrote this statement, there was no hard evidence to suggest that mesothelial cells had fibrinolytic activity, but subsequently such activity was demonstrated.[39,40] However, the supposed epithelial-like ability of mesothelial cells to cover a raw surface is now known to be erroneous. Raftery[41] subsequently showed that fibrinolytic activity was absent from a peritoneal wound surface during the first 48 hours of the healing process, after which there was a gradual increase; thus, 8 days after wounding, when healing was complete, the fibrinolytic activity was greater than that in normal mesothelium. The method used was not sensitive enough to localize fibrinolytic activity to any one particular type of cell. However, the absence of fibrinolytic activity during the first 48 hours after wounding, when cells on the wound surface were largely of the inflammatory type, together with the gradual increase of activity as definitive mesothelial cells came to occupy more and more of the wound surface, strongly suggested that the activity was confined to the definitive mesothelial cells.

A method was subsequently developed for measuring fibrinolytic activity in a single layer of cells removed from the surface on a gelatin disk.[42] Using this method it was shown that peritoneal fibrinolytic activity was depressed immediately following peritoneal trauma and declined further during the first 24 hours postoperatively. Furthermore, free grafting of peritoneum, diathermy of peritoneal wounds, and intestinal ischemia were accompanied by a significant reduction in peritoneal fibrinolytic activity when compared with unsutured peritoneal defects, and all were also associated with a significant increase in adhesion formation when compared with unsutured peritoneal defects.[43]

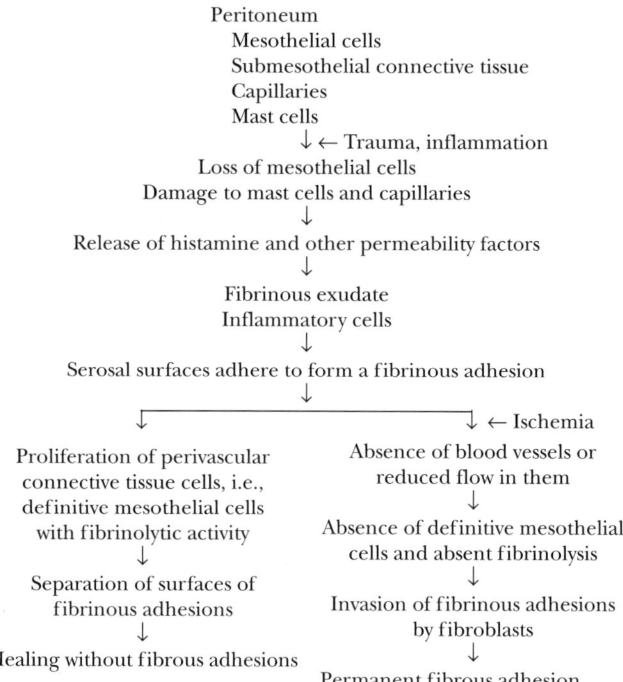

FIG. 4.6. Summary of mesothelial repair and the pathogenesis of adhesion formation. The absence of definitive mesothelial cells with their associated fibrinolytic activity allows a fibrinous adhesion to become organized, resulting in a permanent fibrous adhesion.

Ischemia

On the basis of the foregoing observations, it was argued that fibrinolytic activity of the definitive mesothelial cells allowed them to penetrate and lyse fibrinous adhesions before fibroplasia led to the formation of a permanent fibrous adhesion. A summary of the stages of peritoneal repair and adhesion formation is shown in Fig. 4.6. The argument in the past was that absorption of a fibrinous exudate depended upon an intact mesothelium. If it was destroyed, adhesions would develop. However, it is now clear that large peritoneal defects can heal without adhesion formation in the majority of cases, but when attempts are made to oppose the edges of wounds with sutures, adhesions form. Ellis[36] concluded that it was not the peritoneal defect itself that stimulated adhesion formation, but the presence of ischemic tissue, which probably resulted from pulling the wound edges together under tension. The effect of ischemia on the mesothelium is not clear. In ischemia associated with strangulating obstruction of the small intestine in dogs, it has been demonstrated by scanning electron microscopy[44] that mesothelium is lost in the first hour following ischemia and is almost complete at 6 hours.

It therefore appears that the loss of mesothelium is a prerequisite of adhesion formation and that regeneration of the mesothelium without adhesion formation depends upon the rapid invasion of a fibrinous exudate by definite mesothelial cells with their associated fibrinolytic activity. Ellis[36] attributed adhesions to ischemia, and Raftery[25] argued that this ischemia could result either from inadequate ingrowth of vessels in the base of the wound or, if adequate ingrowth did occur, from an inadequate blood flow in such vessels. In either case, perivascular connective tissue cells may not proliferate because of ischemia, leading to delay in the appearance of definitive mesothelial cells. The absence of these cells and their associated fibrinolytic activity would facilitate adhesion formation by allowing fibroplasia to occur before definitive mesothelial cells grew between and separated the apposed surfaces of a fibrinous adhesion. It would appear, therefore, that fibrinolytic activity of the mesothelium is of great importance in ensuring adhesion-free healing of the peritoneum.

Summary

An understanding of the healing of the peritoneum is fundamental to the understanding of the pathogenesis of peritoneal adhesions and a logical approach at attempts at their prevention. Peritoneal defects heal rapidly, large defects healing as rapidly as small ones. Centripetal growth from the wound margins contributes little to the healing process. Healing occurs for the most part without adhesion formation, which may reflect the fibrinolytic properties of mesothelial cells. Although several theories have been put forward to explain the source of new mesothelial cells, the weight of evidence suggests that they are derived from metaplasia of subperitoneal perivascular connective tissue cells which resemble primitive mesenchymal cells.

References

1. Ellis H. The cause and prevention of post-operative intraperitoneal adhesions. Surg Gynecol Obstet 1971;133: 497–511.
2. Connolly JE, Smith JW. The prevention and treatment of intestinal adhesions. Surg Gynecol Obstet 1960;110: 417–431.
3. Hertzler AE. The Peritoneum, Vol. 1. St. Louis: Mosby, 1919.
4. Robbins GF, Brunschwig A, Foote FW. Deperitonealization; clinical and experimental observations. Ann Surg 1949;130:466–479.
5. Ellis H, Harrison W, Hugh TB. The healing of peritoneum under normal and pathological conditions. Br J Surg 1965;52:471–476.
6. Eskeland G. Regeneration of parietal peritoneum. 1. A light microscopical study. Acta Pathol Microbiol Scand 1966;68:355–378.
7. Raftery AT. Regeneration of parietal and visceral peritoneum. A light microscopical study. Br J Surg 1973;60: 293–299.
8. Williams DC. The peritoneum. A plea for a change in attitude towards this membrane. Br J Surg 155;42:401–405.
9. Hubbard TB, Khan MZ, Carag VR, et al. The pathology of peritoneal repair: its relation to the formation of adhesions. Ann Surg 1967;65:908–916.
10. Cameron GR, Hassan SM, De SN. Repair of Glisson's capsule after tangential wounds of the liver. J Pathol Bacteriol 1957;73:1–10.
11. Johnson FE, Whitting HW. Repair of parietal peritoneum. Br J Surg 1962;49:653–660.
12. Bridges JC, Whitting HW. Parietal peritoneal healing in the rat. J Pathol Bacteriol 1964;87:123–130.
13. Eskeland G. Growth of autologous peritoneal fluid cells in intraperitoneal diffusion chambers in rats. A light microscopical study. Acta Pathol Microbiol Scand 1966;68: 481–500.
14. Eskeland G, Kjaerheim A. Regeneration of parietal peritoneum in rats. 2. An electron microscopical study. Acta Pathol Microbiol Scand 1966;68:379–395.
15. Eskeland G, Kjaerheim A. Growth of autologous peritoneal fluid cells in intraperitoneal diffusion chambers in rats. 2. An electron microscopical study. Acta Pathol Microbiol Scand 1966;68:501–516.
16. Raftery AT. Regeneration of parietal and visceral peritoneum; an electron-microscopical study. J Anat 1973;115: 375–392.
17. Raftery AT. Mesothelial cells in peritoneal fluid. J Anat 1973;115:237–253.
18. Watters WB, Buck RC. Scanning electron microscopy of mesothelial regeneration in the rat. Lab Invest 1972;26: 604–609.
19. Watters WB, Buck RC. Mitotic activity of peritoneum in contact with a regenerating area of peritoneum. Virchows Arch Abt B Zellpathol 1973;13:48–54.
20. Raftery AT. Regeneration of parietal and visceral peritoneum: an enzyme histochemical study. J Anat 1976;121: 589–597.
21. Raftery AT. An enzyme histochemical study of mesothelial cells in rodents. J Anat 1973;115:365–373.
22. Bolen JW, Hammer SP, McNutt MA. Serosal tissue: reactive tissue as a model for understanding mesotheliomas. Ultrastruct Pathol 1987;11:251–262.
23. Devens K. Recurrent intestinal obstruction in the neonatal period. Arch Dis Child 1963;38:118–119.
24. Replogle RL, Johnson R, Gross RE. Prevention of post-operative intestinal adhesions with combined promethazine and dexamethazone therapy: experimental and clinical studies. Ann Surg 1966;163:580–588.
25. Raftery AT. Regeneration of parietal and visceral peritoneum in the immature animal: a light and electronmicroscopical study. Br J Surg 1973;60:969–975.
26. Mott TJ, Ashby EC, Flannery BP, et al. The effect of protein deficiency upon peritoneal healing and peritoneal wound contraction in the rat. Br J Nutr 1969;23: 497–504.
27. Mott TJ, Ellis H. A method of producing experimental uraemia in the rabbit, with some observations on the influence of uraemia on peritoneal healing. Br J Urol 1967; 39:341–346.
28. Venables C, Ellis H, Burns JE. The effects of X-radiation on peritoneal healing: an experimental study. Br J Radiol 1967;40:275–279.
29. Gordon JA, Smith GMR, Ellis H. The effect of cytotoxic drugs on the healing of peritoneal wounds in the rat. Br J Cancer 1967;21:763–767.
30. Jagelman DG, Stoker TAM, Ellis H. The effect of malignant disease on peritoneal healing in the rat. Br J Cancer 1972;26:226–229.
31. deHaan BB, Ellis H, Wilks M. The role of infection on wound healing. Surg Gynecol Obstet 1974;138:693–700.
32. Cleaver CLT, Hopkins AD, Kee Kwong KC Ng, Raftery AT. The effect of postoperative peritoneal lavage on survival, peritoneal wound healing and adhesion formation following fecal peritonitis: an experimental study in the rat. Br J Surg 1974;61:601–604.
33. Walker DM. Effects of blood, bile and starch in the peritoneal cavity of the rat. J Anat 1978;126:495–507.
34. Raftery AT. The effect of urine and bile in the peritoneal cavity: a histological and fibrinolytic study in the rat. Ann R Coll Surg Engl 1980;62:380.
35. Trimpi HD, Bacon HE. Clinical and experimental study of denuded surfaces in extensive surgery of the colon and rectum. Am J Surg 1952;84:596–602.
36. Ellis H. The aetiology of post-operative abdominal adhesions. An experimental study. Br J Surg 1962;50:10–16.
37. Thomas JW, Rhoads JE. Adhesions resulting from removal of serosa from an area of bowel; failure of 'over sewing' to lower incidence in the rat and guinea pig. Arch Surg 1950;61:565–567.
38. Hartwell SW. The Mechanics of Healing in Human Wounds. Springfield: Thomas, 1955:109.
39. Myrhe-Jensen O, Larsen SB, Astrup T. Fibrinolytic activity in serosal and synovial membranes. Arch Pathol 169;88: 623–630.

40. Gervin AS, Puckett CL, Silver D. Serosal hypofibrinolysis. A cause of postoperative adhesions. Am J Surg 1973;125: 80–88.
41. Raftery AT. Regeneration of peritoneum: a fibrinolytic study. J Anat 1979;129:659–664.
42. Raftery AT. A method for measuring fibrinolytic activity in a single layer of cells. J Clin Pathol 1981;34:625–629.
43. Raftery AT. Effect of peritoneal trauma on peritoneal fibrinolytic activity and intraperitoneal adhesion formation. An experimental study in the rat. Eur Surg Res 1981;13: 397–401.
44. Booth WV, Zimny M, Kaufman HJ, et al. Scanning electron microscopy of small bowel strangulation obstruction. Am J Surg 1973;125:129–133.

5

Cytokine Responses to Peritoneal Inflammation: The Role of the Mesothelium

Nicholas Topley

CONTENTS

During the past 20 years, our understanding of the process of peritoneal inflammation and the key role played by mediators (cytokines and prostaglandins) released from both infiltrating and resident cells has increased significantly. In humans, the process of peritoneal infection and inflammation is best understood in peritoneal dialysis (PD), a form of renal replacement therapy that is used to treat more than 100,000 patients yearly worldwide.

The frequency of, and morbidity associated with, peritoneal infection inevitably led research in this area into examination of the host response following bacterial contamination of the peritoneum and subsequent infection. These studies focused on peritoneal "host defense" mechanisms and in particular on the function, maturity, and reactivity of the resident and infiltrating leukocyte populations as well as the host's humoral response to infection.[1–3] More recently it has become apparent that, in addition to leukocytes that reside within or migrate to the peritoneal cavity, the resident cells within it, the mesothelial cells lining the visceral and parietal peritoneum, and the fibroblasts which reside within the submesothelial interstitium make a significant and pivotal contribution to peritoneal inflammation.[4–6] Thus, a more contemporary view of the peritoneum response to infection is one in which both resident as well as infiltrating cells contribute through the secretion of inflammatory mediators as well as the expression of surface proteins (e.g., adhesion molecules) to a network of events that initiate, amplify, and eventually control the inflammatory response.

Although many of the in vivo findings described in this review are derived from data on peritoneal inflammation in the scenario of PD, many of the cellular processes have been delineated in cell culture or animal models of peritoneal inflammation, and as such probably represent some of the basic cellular processes that occur in the normal peritoneal cavity following infection or surgical trauma.

Scope of This Review

This chapter focuses on the role of cytokines and other inflammatory mediators, secreted by resident (mesothelial cells, peritoneal macrophages and peritoneal fibroblasts) and infiltrating leukocytes, in the initiation, amplification, and subsequent control of peritoneal inflammation. Latterly, we examine how these processes if uncontrolled might lead to fibrotic alterations in the submesothelial interstitium that might be the hallmark of peritoneal sclerosis or contribute to peritoneal adhesion formation.

Initially, we examine how bacterial activation of mesothelium might contribute to the induction of the inflammatory cascade (or peritoneal cytokine network). Subsequently, we discuss how the interaction of peritoneal macrophages (PMØ) with mesothelial cells acts to amplify peritoneal inflammation and examine how the influx of leukocytes into the peritoneal cavity is controlled by mesothelial cell-derived directed chemokine secretion and by bacterial products. Finally, we examine how intraperitoneal inflammation is controlled and examine which cytokines might be important in the processes that lead to its resolution.

Ex Vivo Characterization of Peritoneal Inflammation

Peritoneal infection is characterized by pain, followed by a massive influx of leukocytes (initially, predominantly polymorphonuclear neutrophils [PMNs] but also significant numbers of mononuclear cells) into the peritoneal cavity. A considerable amount of the information available about cytokine activation within the peritoneal cavity has been derived from studies in which inflammatory mediator and cytokine levels as well as the phenotype of infiltrating leukocytes have been measured in peritoneal effluent during peritonitis and stable PD. This so-called ex vivo approach not only has allowed the definition of the time courses of leukocyte infiltration and mediator elaboration within the peritoneum, but also has provided important information about the contribution of the various resident cell populations to the inflammatory process. These data suggest that both peritoneal macrophage (PMØ) and mesothelial cell products potentially contribute to peritoneal inflammation.[7–18]

Examination of the intraperitoneal levels of inflammatory mediators (prostaglandins, interleukin-6 [IL-6], tumor necrosis factor-α [TNF-α], interleukin-1β [IL-1β]), their soluble receptors or antagonists (interleukin receptor antagonist [IL-1 RA], TNF-soluble receptors [p55 and p75]), and other immunomodulatory cytokines (interferon-α [IFN-α], interleukin-10 [IL-10], and others) during and after episodes of peritonitis[8,11–13,15,16,19,20] has identified that the levels of all are increased during acute infection and subsequently returned to control levels. In fact, intraperitoneal cytokine levels (at least proinflammatory cytokines IL-1β and TNF-α) are probably increased before overt clinical signs of infection,[12] suggesting that activation of the inflammatory cascade occurs before the symptoms. All these studies demonstrated local synthesis within the peritoneal cavity, identifying that secretion of pro- or antiinflammatory mediators by resident cells was an important component in the process. In addition, these studies identified that the elaboration of the various mediators proceeded with unique time courses, suggesting that different cytokines and mediators play specific roles during the course of inflammation. In this respect, both the major PMØ-derived proinflammatory cytokines and drivers of inflammatory processes were elevated at the beginning of the inflammatory episode (before clinical symptoms) and rapidly subsided,[21] while other mediators including IL-6, IL-1 RA, and the soluble TNF receptors reached peak levels at later periods. These latter data were the first to suggest that mediators important in the control of inflammation were elaborated within the peritoneal cavity.[12]

The Process of Peritoneal Inflammation

For the sake of convenience, our understanding of the series of events that characterize cytokine activation in peritoneal inflammation allows us to divide it into three main phases: (i) activation phase, (ii) amplification phase, and (iii) resolution phase. To a large degree these definitions are arbitrary, because the events described overlap and certain features (such as leukocyte recruitment) occur throughout the process. Key events during each phase, however, allow us to make these definitions in time.

Initiation of Inflammation: The Role of the Mesothelium

The initial view on peritoneal host defense suggested that the PMØ controlled the peritoneum response to bacterial invasion and did not identify a role for the mesothelium in the process. While PMØ are known to produce a number of inflammatory mediators, over the past decade, since methods were established for the isolation and in vitro culture of mesothelial cells, it has become apparent that this reactive monolayer may be the key player in peritoneal inflammation. As we discuss later, it may have other facets that make it responsible for maintaining peritoneal homeostasis and membrane architecture.[22–41]

The mesothelial cell lines the surface of the visceral and parietal peritoneal surface. The peritoneal membrane is composed of a mesothelial monolayer resting on a basal lamina beneath which is a submesothelial stroma consisting of interstitial fibroblasts interspersed in a collagenous extracellular matrix.[42,43] Observations made on cultured human peritoneal (and pleural) mesothelial cells suggest that many of the inflammatory mediators locally produced within the peritoneal cavity during inflammation are potentially of mesothelial cell origin. In this respect, mesothelial cells secrete prostaglandins, interleukin-6, interleukin-1, and chemotactic cytokines (e.g., interleukin-8, MCP-1, and RANTES).[18,27–29,33,44,45] These observations suggest that the mesothelium has significant potential to contributing to a "cytokine network" via its secretion of inflammatory and immunomodulatory mediators and is thus a prime candidate for a central role in initiating, amplifying, and potentially controlling peritoneal inflammation.[4–6,46,47]

Several lines of argument suggest that mesothelial cell activation by invading microorganisms might be a key process that initiates the peritoneum response to infection.

1. The mesothelial cell is the major resident cell within the peritoneal cavity ($\sim 10^{10}$ cells/1.73 m^2).
2. The number of PMØ in the normal peritoneal cavity is small ($\sim 10^3$–10^4).[48]
3. PMØ phagocytosis is ineffective at low bacteria/PMØ ratios.[49]
4. The likelihood of bacteria–PMØ interaction in such a large area is small.

These observations are not definitive evidence of the role of the mesothelium in the initiation process, but they do suggest that bacterial activation of mesothelium is a more likely occurrence than their interaction with PMØ. To add to this argument, recent data indeed suggest that peritoneal pathogens (both *Staphylococcus aureus* and *S. epidermidis* and gram-negative organisms) can attach to and in some cases be ingested by cultured mesothelial cells.[50,51] This attachment process results in the activation of mesothelial cell IL-8, secretion, an observation suggesting that direct bacterial activation of mesothelium may be one mechanism whereby inflammation and leukocyte recruitment are initiated at the onset of infection. Our own observations suggest that *Staphylococcus spp.* supernatants (derived from nonproliferating cultures[52–55]) are potent activators of human peritoneal mesothelial cell (HPMC) IL-8 synthesis at both the mRNA and the protein level.[56] These supernatants contain bacterial toxins or superantigens and type 5 and type 8 capsular polysaccharides[57] that are known to be capable of activating cytokine synthesis; the precise nature of the activating capacity however remains to be fully identified.[58–62] Using an in vitro transmigration system, we have demonstrated that the migration of leukocytes across mesothelial cell monolayers is dependent on the creation of an IL-8 gradient and that these bacterial supernatants contain their own intrinsic chemotactic activity.[63]

Taken together, these data suggest that following bacterial invasion of the peritoneal cavity mesothelial cell activation might play a key role in the activation of inflammation and the initiation of leukocyte recruitment. These data do not exclude the possibility that bacterial activation of PMØ does occur; indeed, staphylococcal species and gram-negative bacteria are potent activators of PMØ prostaglandin, leukotriene, and cytokine synthesis.[52–55]

Amplification of Peritoneal Inflammation: The Role of Peritoneal Macrophage–Mesothelial Cell Interaction

Another process that appears to be crucial in the amplification of peritoneal inflammation is the activation of the mesothelium by PMØ-derived inflammatory cytokines.[64] Although many of the inflammatory mediators present in the peritoneal cavity may be of mesothelial origin, the initial activation of their synthesis is thought at least partly to be initiated by proinflammatory cytokines secreted from resident or invading PMØ.

The normal peritoneal cavity contains a small resident population of peritoneal macrophages (PMØ).[48] The largest amount of information about the function of these cells derives from studies performed on peritoneal inflammation in PD. During PD the numbers of PMØ in the peritoneal cavity are increased, presumably as a result of constant removal during fluid exchange and possibly as a result of subclinical inflammation. In vitro observations suggest that following isolation and secondary stimulation they have significant potential to generate IL-1β and TNF-α.[65,66]

Culture supernatants from PMØ are potent activators of mesothelial cell prostaglandin and cytokine synthesis.[27,33,64] Blocking experiments using specific antibodies, receptor antagonists (IL-1 RA), or soluble receptors (TNF-p55/75) have demonstrated that the stimulatory capacity of these conditioned media is largely related to their IL-1 and TNF-α content.[27,33,64] As mentioned previously, ex vivo data suggest that PMØ–mesothelial cell interaction may indeed occur in vivo. During the initiation phase of peritoneal infection, the levels of IL-1 and TNF-α protein are significantly elevated at time points when their natural inhibitor levels are low[11,17,21]; this suggests that at least part of the signals to activate this phase of the inflammatory cascade originate from PMØ because mesothelial cells do not make TNF-α. The data of Moutabarrik et al. suggest that the same may be true for IL-1, although mesothelial cells themselves do synthesize low amounts of IL-1α and IL-1β. Autocrine as well as paracrine activation processes may well therefore be involved.[17,29]

One of the features that has been identified in mesothelial cells which might also contribute to the amplification of inflammatory episodes is their ability, in common with other isolated cell populations (e.g., glomerular mesangial cells), to superinduce the expression of certain cytokine genes under appropriate stimulation.[28,67,68] This feature was first identified when examining mesothelial cell interleukin-8 (IL-8) synthesis following proinflammatory cytokine stimulation but has more recently been delineated for interleukin-6 (IL-6) secretion.[28,67] As is discussed later, both these cytokines appear to play a key role in peritoneal inflammation and thus the ability to dramatically increase their concentration (which correlates with that which occurs in vivo) might represent an important facet of the peritoneum response to infection.[10,69]

Recruitment of Leukocytes into the Peritoneum

Leukocyte influx following peritoneal infection is characterized by increases in both neutrophil and mononuclear cells (mononuclear phagocytes [MNC] and lymphocytes).[8,14,70] Initially, PMNs predominate, and these are subsequently replaced by mononuclear cells as the main cell population as infection resolves.[8] Mechanisms therefore exist by which both neutrophils and mononuclear cells are specifically recruited into the peritoneal cavity. As mentioned previously, bacterial products can themselves recruit leukocytes both in an in vitro transmigration system and in animal models of peritoneal inflammation[56,63] (Wilkinson and Topley, unpublished data). The magnitude of these responses is small, however, and the key element that controls the majority of leukocyte infiltration is the intraperitoneal secretion of chemotactic cytokines.[13,18,28,33,39] Central in this process appears to be the ability of the mesothelial cell not only to secrete chemotactic cytokines, but to do so in a directed manner such that a chemotactic gradient is created from their basolateral to apical aspects and to express adhesion molecules on their surface that facilitate the migration process.[18,34,39–41,44,45,71] The chemokines are a superfamily of cytokines structurally characterized by four conserved cysteine residues in their amino acid sequence. Two subfamilies can be distinguished according to the position of the first two cysteines, which are either separated by one amino acid (C-X-C chemokines) or are adjacent (C-C chemokines). IL-8, a prototype C-X-C or α-chemokine, has more specific action on neutrophils while MCP-1[72–75] and RANTES,[76] both C-C or β-chemokines, are involved in the recruitment of mononuclear cells.

Initial in vitro studies identified the ability of mesothelial cells to secrete IL-8 and these cells have subsequently been shown to secrete many of the other described α- and β-chemokines.[45] In common with other secreted products, PMØ-derived proinflammatory cytokines are the major activators of mesothelial cell chemokine secretion, although following activation with live bacteria or their secreted products biologically relevant quantities are generated.[28,33,45,51,56]

Using mesothelial cells grown as a monolayer (on porous supports), it has been demonstrated that the secretion of all chemokines measured occurs in a directed manner such that a gradient of chemotactic activity is generated across the cells.[44,71] The migration of neutrophils across the mesothelium was dependent on IL-8 secretion while the migration of mononuclear cells occurred in response to both MCP-1 and RANTES. These observations parallel those made in vivo that have correlated leukocyte subset numbers in the PD peritoneum with the levels of specific α- and β-chemokine levels.[8,13,18,33] Dissipation of the chemokine gradient in vitro with specific antibodies confirmed its importance in directing leukocyte trafficking.[44]

In addition to the secretion of chemokines, the expression of adhesion molecules on the surface of mesothelial cells is important in the process of leukocyte (PMNs, mononuclear phagocytes, and lymphocytes) attachment and migration.[28,33,34,39–41,77] Initial studies identified that mesothelial cells constitutively expressed both intercellular adhesion molecule-1 (ICAM-1) and vascular cell adhesion molecule-1 (VCAM-1/2).[34,39–41] Following activation with inflammatory cytokines, their expression was induced and this correlated in monolayer culture with increased leukocyte adherence or in insert cultures with increased transmigration.[34,39–41,44] Blocking experiments with soluble ICAM-1 or specific antibody confirmed the functionality of this expression.

Taken together, these results suggest that the mesothelium has the capacity not only to direct leukocyte influx via the directed and upregulated secretion of chemokines (and thus the formation of a chemotactic gradient)[71] but also (as we discuss later) to control the phenotype of recruited leukocytes by the expression of specific chemokines. These processes are facilitated by adhesion molecule expression on the surface of the mesothelium that in turn can control the phenotype of recruited leukocytes. These factors together with the ability of mesothelial cells to superinduce IL-8 secretion following defined stimulation suggest that these cells play a key and controlling role in the leukocyte recruitment process in vivo.[28,78]

Resolution of Inflammation

Once the process of inflammation begins, mechanisms must be in place whereby its level is controlled and by which inflammation response is switched off. In the peritoneal cavity, there is increasing evidence that the mesothelial cell plays a critical role in both these processes. The activation of inflammation is accompanied by a massive increase in the intraperitoneal levels of locally secreted IL-6.[10,11] Our previous in vitro data identified the mesothelial cell as its potential source and subsequently demonstrated that its levels could be superinduced under conditions mimicking peritoneal inflammation.[27,67,79] These in vitro observations paralleled the massive increases seen in vivo.[10] Although IL-6 levels were massively elevated, the precise role of this cytokine in the peritoneal cavity was unclear as data in other organ systems and inflammation models had ascribed to it both pro- and antiinflammatory functions.[80–83] Our preliminary observations in IL-6-deficient mice, however, suggest that in peritoneal inflammation at least IL-6 serves to control the level of inflammation because neutrophil influx in IL-6-deficient mice is three- to fivefold higher than in wild-type animals (Wilkinson and Topley, in manuscript).

During peritonitis, the switch from neutrophil infiltrate during acute inflammation to a predominately mononuclear cell phenotype as inflammation progresses is thought to represent the normal process of resolution.[84] Our recent data suggest that the mesothelium, through its ability to differentially express the α-chemokine (IL-8) and the β-chemokines MCP-1 and RANTES, controls the phenotype of leukocytes recruited across mesothelial cell monolayers.[85] The mechanism by which this process occurs appears to be related to the ability of the Th-2 cytokine IFNγ, which is present in the peritoneal cavity during infection,[86,87] to simultaneously downregulate IL-1-driven mesothelial cell IL-8 synthesis while upregulating MCP-1 and RANTES synthesis.[85] The result is a reduction in neutrophil migration across mesothelial cell monolayers. Preliminary observations using an intraperitoneal inflammation model suggest that a similar mechanism is operative in vivo (Wilkinson, Robson, and Topley, unpublished data).

Taken together these data suggest that the mesothelium not only is capable of contributing to the induction of inflammation (see earlier) but also plays a significant role in its control and resolution. Clearly, this is an area of significant research interest because understanding how inflammation is resolved would provide significant therapeutic potential.

Negative Consequences of Peritoneal Inflammation: Preservation of Mesothelial Cell Integrity and Function

Although inflammation in any organ system is a necessary and normal response to tissue invasion, when it is repeated or uncontrolled it can have negative consequences on tissue function. In the peritoneal cavity there is significant evidence of inflammation-associated changes in the structure and function of the peritoneal membrane.[88,89] Peritonitis is a frequent complication in PD patients, and its occurrence correlates with loss of membrane function as evidenced by loss of ultrafiltration and increased small molecular weight solute clearance.[90] There is increasing evidence that these functional changes are accompanied by ultrastructural changes within the peritoneal membrane, including in some cases altered morphology or loss of mesothelium, submesothelial cell fibrosis, and angiogenic changes within the peritoneal capillaries.[43,88,89,91–98]

At present it is not known which factors contribute to the development of the fibrotic and angiogenic process, although it is known that upon appropriate stimulation mesothelial cells can synthesize both extracellular matrix components and growth factors and enzymes important in extracellular matrix turnover.[24,25,32,99–108] One might hypothesize that following inappropriate activation the normal balance of extracellular matrix turnover potentially controlled by mesothelial cells might be altered, resulting in matrix deposition. In this respect, mesothelial cell phenotype and secretory capacity are altered during long-term PD.[109,110] Whether the same inappropriate modulation of mesothelial cell function contributes to surgical adhesion formation remains to be determined.

It is becoming increasingly clear that preservation of mesothelial cell integrity may be important in maintaining peritoneal homeostasis. Clearly an intact and functional mesothelium is important if these cells play a pivotal role in host defense. What is also clear is that, given that these cells synthesize and secrete a large number of other bioactive molecules, preserving mesothelial integrity (and by definition reducing damage to it) is key in maintaining the normal peritoneal environment. One of the facets of mesothelial cells is their ability to regenerate following injury; in a recently described model, the remesothelialization process occurred as a result of cell migration and appeared to be the result of mediators released by the cells themselves.[22] These observations on the recovery of mesothelial cells following mechanical injury may be of great significance both to peritoneal dialysis and to peritoneal injury following surgery as they provide a model system within which the efficacy of therapeutic agents at promoting remesothelialization can be tested.

Many of the data that suggest the importance of maintaining mesothelial cell integrity come from observations made in PD.[110–114] During PD, there is continuous loss of mesothelial cells as evidenced by exfoliated cells in dialysis effluent, which is exacerbated during episodes of peritonitis,[114] and also evidence of phenotypic changes in both the structure and secretory ability of these cells. This evidence includes both ultrastructural changes, as shown by direct observation both in animal models and in peritoneal biopsies from PD patient cells,[43,95,96,112,113,115,116] and changes in peritoneal effluent levels or ratios of molecules such as phospholipids and members of the fibrinolytic cascade that may be exclusively or predominantly of mesothelial cell origin.[30,37,109,117] In long-term PD, there is some evidence that complete loss of mesothelium precipitates the end stages of peritoneal sclerosis (also described as sclerosing peritonitis),[118] suggesting its importance in maintaining normal tissue architecture.

These data suggest that the preservation of an intact and normally functioning mesothelium is important in maintaining both the function and the structure of the peritoneal membrane. Disturbance of its integrity or function as occurs in long-term PD or following mechanical or surgical trauma may have detrimental consequences and might contribute to structural or fibrotic alterations within the peritoneal cavity.

Conclusions and Future Perspectives

This review has focused on the importance of cytokines and other inflammatory mediators in the activation and control of intraperitoneal inflammation and has identified the potential of the mesothelium, in conjunction with resident and infiltrating PMØ, to initiate and control inflammatory processes within the peritoneum (Fig. 5.1). Based on current data it is reasonable to hypothesize that the mesothelium to some extent contributes to the following processes:

1. The initial response of the peritoneum to bacterial infection
2. The amplification of that response
3. The recruitment of leukocytes to control infection
4. The control of inflammation severity and its resolution
5. The control of peritoneal fibrinolysis
6. The control of peritoneal homeostasis and maintenance of peritoneal membrane structure and function

While the mesothelium does not achieve these effects alone and is acted upon by products derived from resident and infiltrating leukocytes as well as potentially other peritoneal membrane cell populations (peritoneal fibroblasts), it does appear to contribute to many processes. As such, preservation of its normal function would appear to be important in preserving peritoneal homeostasis and its controlled response to inflammation. Loss of mesothelium as occurs in long-term PD or following mechanical injury clearly has negative consequences that we are only beginning to understand.

Future work in this area will concentrate on increasing our understanding of how mesothelial cell injury contributes to peritoneal fibrosis or adhesion formation as well as increasing our knowledge of the process of remesothelialization following injury. In this respect, recent data using ex vivo mesothelial cell gene therapy to deliver therapeutic or antiinflammatory proteins into the peritoneal cavity will provide the potential to modulate the process of inflammation, increasing its benefits and

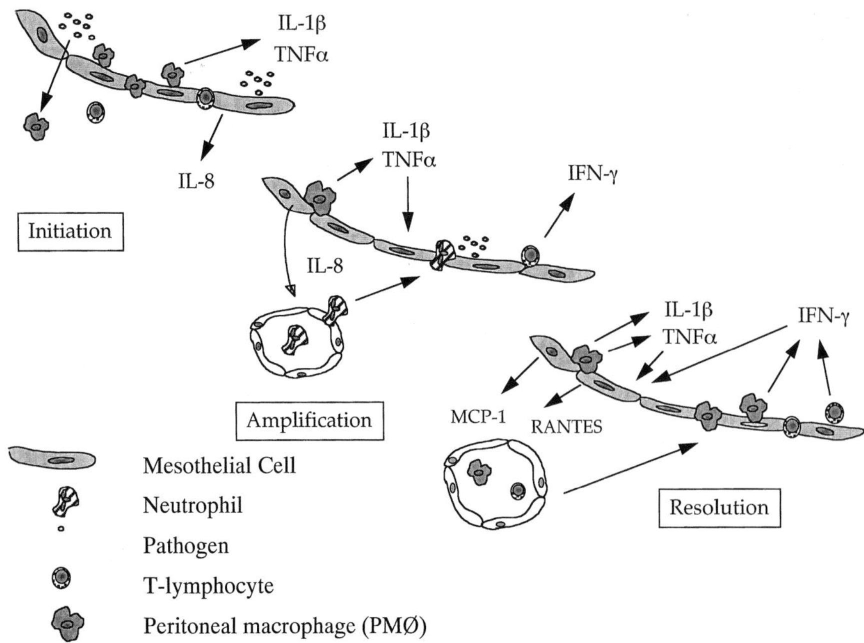

FIG. 5.1. Schematic representation of the role of the mesothelium in the initiation, amplification, and resolution phases of peritoneal inflammation.

potentially reducing its negative consequences.[119-121] Only by having a more complete understanding of how inflammation contributes to peritoneal membrane damage will we have the potential to design therapeutic strategies to limit its negative consequences.

Acknowledgments

This work has included contributions by many individuals in the peritoneal inflammation research group: Professor Gerald Coles, Professor John Williams, Dr. Tomasz Liberek, Dr. Janusz Witowski, Dr. Andrew Davenport, Dr. Rachel Robson, Dr. Felix Li, Dr. Huw Fear, and Mr. Tom Wilkinson. It would not have been possible without the surgical teams at East Glamorgan Hospital (Mr. Mike Lewis) and the University Hospital of Wales (Mr. Ian Lane, Mr. Philip Matthews, and Mr. Tim Stephenson). This work was supported by the Kidney Research Unit Foundation and grants from the Medical Research Council, Welsh Scheme for the Development of Health and Social Research, and the Baxter Extramural Grant Program.

References

1. Holmes CJ. Peritoneal host defense mechanisms in peritoneal dialysis. Kidney Int 1994;46:S58–S70.
2. Holmes C, Lewis S. Host defense mechanisms in the peritoneal cavity of continuous ambulatory peritoneal dialysis patients, II: humoral defenses. Perit Dial Int 1991;11: 112–117.
3. Lewis S, Holmes C. Host defense mechanisms in the peritoneal cavity of continuous ambulatory peritoneal dialysis patients. Perit Dial Int 1991;11:14–21.
4. Topley N, Mackenzie R, Jörres A, Coles GA, Williams JD. Cytokine networks in CAPD: interactions of resident cells during inflammation in the peritoneal cavity. Perit Dial Int 1993;13:S282–S285.
5. Topley N, Williams JD. The role of the peritoneal membrane in the control of inflammation in the peritoneal cavity. Kidney Int 1994;46:S71–S78.
6. Topley N, Davenport A, Li F-K, Fear H, Williams JD. Activation of inflammation and leukocyte recruitment into the peritoneal cavity. Kidney Int 1996;50:S17–S21.
7. Bagby GJ, Plessala KJ, Wilson LA, Thompson JJ, Nelson S. Divergent efficacy of antibody to tumor necrosis factor-α in intravascular and peritonitis models of sepsis. J Infect Dis 1991;163:83–88.
8. Brauner A, Hylander B, Wretlind B. Interleukin-6 and interleukin-8 in dialysate and serum from patients on continuous ambulatory peritoneal dialysis. Am J Kidney Dis 1993;22:430–435.
9. Brauner A, Hylander B, Wretlind B. Tumor necrosis factor-α, interleukin-1β, and interleukin-1 receptor antagonist in dialysate and serum from patients on continuous ambulatory peritoneal dialysis. Am J Kidney Dis 1996; 27:402–408.
10. Goldman M, Vandenabeele P, Moulart J, et al. Intraperitoneal secretion of interleukin-6 during continuous ambulatory peritoneal dialysis. Nephron 1990;56:277–280.
11. Zemel D, Koomen GCM, Hart AAM, ten Berge RJM, Struijk DG, Krediet RT. Relationship of TNFα, interleukin-6, and prostaglandins to peritoneal permeability for macromolecules during longitudinal follow-up of peritonitis in continuous ambulatory peritoneal dialysis. J Lab Clin Med 1994;122:686–696.
12. Zemel D, Imholz ALT, de Wart DR, Dinkla C, Struijk DG, Krediet RT. The appearance of tumor necrosis factor-α and soluble TNF-receptors I and II in peritoneal effluent during stable and infectious CAPD. Kidney Int 1994; 46:1422–1430.
13. Zemel D, Krediet RT, Koomen GCM, Kortekaas WMR, Geertzen HGM, ten Berge RJM. Interleukin-8 during peritonitis in patients treated with CAPD: an *in vivo* model of acute inflammation. Nephrol Dial Transplant 1994;9: 169–174.
14. Betjes MGH, Tuk CW, Visser CE, et al. Analysis of peritoneal cellular immune system during CAPD shortly before clinical peritonitis. Nephrol Dial Transplant 1994;9: 684–692.
15. Steinhauer HB, Schollmeyer P. Prostaglandin mediated loss of proteins during peritonitis in continuous ambulatory peritoneal dialysis. Kidney Int 1986;29:584–590.
16. Steinhauer HB, Günter B, Schollmeyer P. Stimulation of peritoneal synthesis of vasoactive prostaglandins during peritonitis in patients on continuous ambulatory peritoneal dialysis. Eur J Clin Invest 1985;15:1–5.
17. Moutabarrik A, Nakanishi I, Namiki M, Tsubakihara Y. Interleukin-1 and its naturally occurring inhibitor in peritoneal dialysis patients. Clin Nephrol 1995;43:243–248.
18. Tekstra J, Visser CE, Tuk CW, et al. Identification of the major chemokines that regulate cell influxes in peritoneal dialysis patients. J Am Soc Nephrol 1996;7:2379–2384.
19. Zemel D, ten Berge RJM, Stuijk, DG, Bloemena E, Koomen GCM, Krediet RT. Interleukin-6 in CAPD patients without peritonitis: relationship to the intrinsic permeability of the peritoneal membrane. Clin Nephrol 1992;37: 97–103.
20. Zemel D, ten Berge RJM, Koomen GCM, Struijk DG, Krediet RT. Serum interleukin-6 in continuous ambulatory peritoneal dialysis patients. Nephron 1993;64:320–321.
21. Zemel D, Betjes MGH, Dinkla C, Struijk DG, Krediet RT. Analysis of inflammatory mediators and peritoneal permeability to macromolecules shortly before the onset of overt peritonitis in patients treated with CAPD. Perit Dial Int 1994;15:134–141.
22. Yung S, Davies M. Response of the human peritoneal mesothelial cell to injury: an in vitro model of peritoneal wound healing. Kidney Int. 1998;54:2160–2169.
23. Yung S, Coles GA, Davies M. IL-1β, a major stimulator of hyaluronan synthesis in vitro of human peritoneal mesothelial cells: relevance to peritonitis in CAPD. Kidney Int 1996;50:1337–1343.
24. Yung S, Thomas GJ, Stylianou E, Williams JD, Coles GA, Davies M. Source of peritoneal proteoglycans: human peritoneal mesothelial cells synthesize and secrete mainly small dermatan sulphate proteoglycans. Am J Pathol 1995;146:520–529.
25. Yung S, Coles GA, Williams JD, Davies M. The source and possible significance of hyaluronan in the peritoneal cavity. Kidney Int 1994;46:527–533.

26. Stylianou E, Jenner LA, Davies M, Coles GA, Williams JD. Isolation, culture, and characterisation of human peritoneal mesothelial cells. Kidney Int 1990;37:1563–1570.
27. Topley N, Jörres A, Luttmann W, et al. Human peritoneal mesothelial cells synthesize IL-6: induction by IL-1β and TNFα. Kidney Int 1993;43:226–233.
28. Topley N, Brown Z, Jörres A, et al. Human peritoneal mesothelial cells synthesize IL-8: synergistic induction by interleukin-1β and tumor necrosis factor α. Am J Pathol 1993;142:1876–1886.
29. Douvdevani A, Rapoport J, Konforty A, Argov S, Ovnat A, Chaimowitz C. Human peritoneal mesothelial cells synthesize IL-1α and β. Kidney Int 1994;46:993–1001.
30. Beavis MJ, Harwood JL, Coles GA, Williams JD. Synthesis of phospholipids by human peritoneal mesothelial cells. Perit Dial Int 1994;14:348–355.
31. Beavis MJ, Topley N. Isolation, culture, and characterisation of human peritoneal mesothelial cells. In: Griffiths JB DA, Newell Doyle G, eds. Cell and Tissue Culture: Laboratory Procedures. Specialised Vertebrate Cultures—Integumentary Systems and Muscular Tissue. Chichester, UK: John Wiley, 1995. Section 11B:10.1–10.13.
32. Bermudez E, Everitt J, Walker C. Expression of growth factor and growth factor receptor RNA in rat pleural mesothelial cells in culture. Exp Cell Res 1990;190:91–98.
33. Betjes MGH, Tuk CW, Struijk DG, et al. Interleukin-8 production by human peritoneal mesothelial cells in response to tumor necrosis factor α, interleukin-1, and medium conditioned by macrophages co-cultured with *Staphylococcus epidermidis.* J Infect Dis 1993;168:1202–1210.
34. Cannistra SA, Ottensmeier C, Tidy J, DeFranzo B. Vascular cell adhesion molecule-1 expressed by peritoneal mesothelium partly mediates the binding of activated human T lymphocytes. Exp Haematol 1994;22:996–1002.
35. Coene MC, Solheid C, Claeys M, Herman AG. Prostaglandin production by cultured mesothelial cells. Arch Int Pharmacodyn 1981;249:316–318.
36. Coene MC, C. vH, Claeys M, Herman AG. Arachidonic acid metabolism by cultured mesothelial cells. Biochim Biophys Acta 1982;710:437–445.
37. Dobbie JW, Pavlina T, Lloyd J, Johnson RC. Phosphatidylcholine synthesis by peritoneal mesothelium: its implication for peritoneal dialysis. Am J Kidney Dis 1988;12: 31–36.
38. Lanfrancone L, Boraschi D, Ghiara P, et al. Human peritoneal mesothelial cells produce many cytokines (granulocyte colony-stimulating factor [CSF], granulocyte-monocyte-CSF, macrophage-CSF, interleukin-1 [IL-1], and IL-6) and are activated and stimulated to grow by IL-1. Blood 1992;80:2835–2842.
39. Jonjic N, Peri G, Bernasconi S, et al. Expression of adhesion molecules and chemotactic cytokines in cultured human mesothelial cells. J Exp Med 1992;176:1165–1174.
40. Liberek T, Topley N, Luttmann W, Williams JD. Adherence of neutrophils to human peritoneal mesothelial cells: role of intercellular adhesion molecule-1. J Am Soc Nephrol 1996;7:208–217.
41. Andreoli SP, Mallett C, Williams K, McAteer JA, Rothlein R, Doerschuk CM. Mechanisms of polymorphonuclear leukocyte mediated peritoneal mesothelial cell injury. Kidney Int 1994;46:1100–1109.
42. Gotloib L, Digenis GE, Rabinovich S, Medline A, Oreopoulos DG. Ultrastructure of normal rabbit mesentery. Nephron 1983;34:248–255.
43. Gotloib L, Shostack A. Ultrastructural morphology of the peritoneum: new findings and speculations on transfer of solutes and water during peritoneal dialysis. Perit Dial Bull 1987;7:119–129.
44. Li F-K, Davenport A, Robson RL, et al. Leukocyte migration across human peritoneal mesothelial cells (HPMC) is dependent on directed chemokine secretion and ICAM-1 expression. Kidney Int 1998;54:2170–2183.
45. Visser CE, Tekstra J, Brouwer-Steenbergen JJE, et al. Chemokines produced by mesothelial cells: huGRO-α, IFN-γ inducible protein-10, monocyte chemotactic protein-1, and RANTES. Clin Exp Immunol 1998;112: 270–275.
46. Topley N, Jörres A, Mackenzie R, Coles GA, Williams JD. Interactions of macrophages and mesothelial cells in peritoneal host defence. Nieren-Hochdruckkr 1994;23: S88–S91.
47. Topley N, Davenport A, Li F-K, Fear H, Williams JD. Peritoneal defence in peritoneal dialysis. Nephrology 1996; 2:S167–S172.
48. Cichocki T, Hanicki Z, Sulowicz W, Smolenski O, Kopec J, Zembala M. Output of peritoneal cells into peritoneal dialysate. Nephron 1983;35:175–182.
49. Verbrugh HA, Keane WF, Conroy WE, Peterson PK. Bacterial growth and killing in chronic ambulatory peritoneal dialysis fluids. J Clin Microbiol 1984;20:199–203.
50. Visser CE, Brouer-Steenbergen JJE, Schadee-Eestermans IL, Meijer S, Krediet RT, Beelen RHJ. Ingestion of *Staphylococcus aureus, Staphylococcus epidermidis,* and *Escherichia coli* by human peritoneal mesothelial cells. Infect Immun 1996; 64:3425–3428.
51. Visser CE, Steenbergen JJE, Betjes MGH, et al. Interleukin-8 production by human mesothelial cells after direct stimulation with staphylococci. Infect Immun 1995; 10:4206–4209.
52. Mackenzie RK, Coles GA, Williams JD. Eicosanoid synthesis in human peritoneal macrophages stimulated with *S. epidermidis.* Kidney Int 1990;37:1316–1324.
53. Mackenzie RK, Coles GA, Williams JD. The response of human peritoneal macrophages to stimulation with bacteria isolated from episodes of continuous ambulatory peritoneal dialysis-related peritonitis. J Infect Dis 1991;163: 837–842.
54. Mackenzie R, Coles GA, Topley N, Powell WS, Williams JD. Down regulation of cyclooxygenase product generation by human peritoneal macrophages. Immunology 1992;76: 648–654.
55. Mackenzie R, Topley N, Neubauer A, Coles GA, Williams JD. Staphylococcal exoproducts down-regulate cyclooxygenase 1 and 2 in peritoneal macrophages. J Lab Clin Med 1997;129:23–34.
56. Williams JD, Fear H, Topley N. Staphylococcal exoproducts direct neutrophil passage across mesothelium via chemokine dependent and independent mechanisms. J Am Soc Nephrol 1997;8:275.
57. Lee JC, Michon F, Perez NE, Hopkins CA, Pier GB. Chemical characterization and immunogenicity of capsular polysaccharide isolated from mucoid *Staphylococcus aureus.* Infect Immun 1987;55:2191–2197.

58. Trede NS, Castigli E, Geha RS, Chatila T. Microbial superantigens induce NF-kB in the human monocytic cell line THP-1. J Immunol 1993;150:5604–5613.
59. Trede NS, Chatila T, Geha RS. Activator protein-1 (AP-1) is stimulated by microbial superantigens in human monocytic cells. Eur J Immunol 1993;23:2129–2135.
60. Zumla A. Superantigens, T cells, and microbes. Clin Infect Dis 1992;15:313–320.
61. Heumann D, Barras C, Severin A, Glauser MP, Tomasz A. Gram-positive cell walls stimulate synthesis of tumor necrosis factor and interleukin-6 by human monocytes. Infect Immun 1994;62:2715–2721.
62. Stout RD, Li Y, Miller AR, Lambe DW Jr. Staphylococcal glycocalyx activates macrophage prostaglandin E2 and interleukin-1 production and modulates tumor necrosis factor alpha and nitric oxide production. Infect Immun 1994;62:4160–4166.
63. Fear H, Williams JD, Topley N. Staphylococci direct leukocyte recruitment across mesothelium via IL-8-dependent and independent mechanisms. Kidney Int 1997;52: 1117–1118.
64. Topley N, Petersen MM, Mackenzie R, et al. Human peritoneal mesothelial cell prostaglandin synthesis: induction of cyclooxygenase mRNA by peritoneal macrophage derived cytokines. Kidney Int 1994;46:900–909.
65. Fieren MWJA, van den Bemd GJ, Bonta IL. Peritoneal macrophages from patients on CAPD show an increased capacity to secrete interleukin-1 beta during peritonitis. Adv Perit Dial 1990;6:120–122.
66. Fieren MWJA, van den Bemd GJCM, Bonta IL. Endotoxin-stimulated peritoneal macrophages obtained from continuous ambulatory peritoneal dialysis patients show increased capacity to release interleukin-1beta in vitro during peritonitis. Eur J Clin Invest 1990;20:453–457.
67. Witowski J, Jörres A, Williams JD, Topley N. Superinduction of IL-6 synthesis in human peritoneal mesothelial cells is related to induction and stabilization of IL-6 mRNA. Kidney Int 1996;50:1212–1223.
68. Topley N, Floege J, Wessel K, et al. Prostaglandin E2 production is synergistically increased in cultured human glomerular mesangial cells by combinations of IL-1 and tumor necrosis factor-alpha. J Immunol 1989;143:1989–1995.
69. Betjes MGH, Visser CE, Zemel D, et al. Intraperitoneal interleukin-8 and neutrophil influx in the initial phase of a CAPD peritonitis. Perit Dial Int 1996;16:385–392.
70. Betjes MGH, Tuk CW, Struijk DG, et al. Immuno-effector characteristics of peritoneal cells during CAPD treatment: a longitudinal study. Kidney Int 1993;43:641–648.
71. Zeillemaker AM, Mul FPJ, Hoynck van Papendrecht AAGM, et al. Polarized secretion of interleukin-8 by human mesothelial cells: a role in neutrophil migration. Immunology 1995;84:227–232.
72. Yoshimura T, Robinson EA, Tanaka S, Appella E, Leonard EJ. Purification and amino acid analysis of two human monocyte chemoattractants produced by phytohemagglutinin-stimulated human blood mononuclear leukocytes. J Immunol 1989;142:1956–1962.
73. Yoshimura T, Robinson EA, Tanaka S, Appella E, Kuratsu J, Leonard EJ. Purification and amino acid analysis of two human glioma-derived monocyte chemoattractants. J Exp Med 1989;169:1449–1459.
74. Rollins BJ, Walz A, Baggiolini M. Recombinant human MCP-1/JE induces chemotaxis, calcium flux, and the respiratory burst in human monocytes. Blood 1991;78: 1112–1116.
75. Sozzani S, Luini W, Molino M, et al. The signal transduction pathway involved in the migration induced by a monocyte chemotactic cytokine. J Immunol 1991;147: 2215–2221.
76. Schall TJ, Bacon K, Toy KJ, Goeddel DV. Selective attraction of monocytes and T lymphocytes of the memory phenotype by cytokine RANTES. Nature (Lond) 1990;347: 669–671.
77. Suassuna JHR, Das Neves FC, Hartley RB, Ogg CS, Cameron JS. Immunohistochemical studies of the peritoneal membrane and infiltrating cells in normal subjects and in patients on CAPD. Kidney Int 1994;46:443–454.
78. Holmes CJ, Topley N. Adhesion molecules in the defense of the peritoneum. In: Paul LC, Issekutz T, eds. Adhesion Molecules in Health and Disease. New York: Dekker, 1997: 709–733.
79. Witowski J, Williams JD, Topley N. Mechanism of IL-6 superinduction in human peritoneal mesothelial cells (HPMC): potential role of interferon-γ. J Am Soc Nephrol 1996;7:1750.
80. Xing Z, Gauldie J, Cox G, et al. IL-6 is an anti-inflammatory cytokine required for controlling local and systemic acute inflammatory responses. J Clin Invest 1998;101: 311–320.
81. Romano M, Sironi M, Toniatti C, et al. Role of IL-6 and its soluble receptor in induction of chemokines and leukocyte recruitment. Immunity 1997;6:315–325.
82. van der Poll T, Keogh CV, Guirao X, Buurmann WA, Kopf M, Lowry SF. Interleukin-6 gene-deficient mice show impaired defence against pneumococcal pneumonia. J Infect Dis 1997;176:439–444.
83. Karkar AM, Smith J, Tam FWK, Pusey CD, Rees AJ. Abrogation of glomerular injury in nephrotoxic nephritis by continuous infusion of interleukin-6. Kidney Int 1997;52: 1313–1320.
84. Bellingan GJ, Caldwell H, Howie SEM, Darnsfield I, Haslett C. *In vivo* fate of the inflammatory macrophage during the resolution of inflammation. J Immunol 1996;157:2577–2585.
85. Robson RL, Witowski J, Loetscher P, Topley N. Differential regulation of C-C and C-x-C chemokine synthesis in cytokine-activated human peritoneal mesothelial cells by IFN-γ. Kidney Int 1997;52:1123.
86. Lu Y, Hylander B, Brauner A. Interleukin-10, interferon gamma, interleukin-2, and soluble interleukin-2 receptor alpha detected during peritonitis in the dialysate and serum of patients on continuous ambulatory peritoneal dialysis. Perit Dial Int 1996;16:607–612.
87. Dasgupta MK, Larabie M, Halloran PF. Interferon-gamma levels in peritoneal dialysis effluents: relation to peritonitis. Kidney Int 1994;46:475–481.
88. Rubin J, Herrara GA, Collins D. An autopsy study of the peritoneal cavity from patients on continuous ambulatory peritoneal dialysis. Am J Kidney Dis 1991;17:97–102.
89. Pollock CA, Ibels LS, Eckstein RP, et al. Peritoneal morphology on maintenance dialysis. Am J Nephrol 1989;9: 198–204.
90. Davies SJ, Bryan J, Phillips L, Russell GI. Longitudinal changes in peritoneal kinetics: the effects of peritoneal

dialysis and peritonitis. Nephrol Dial Transplant 1996;11: 498–506.

91. Honda K, Nitta K, Horita H, Yumura W, Nihei H. Morphological changes in the peritoneal vasculature of patients on CAPD with ultrafiltration failure. Nephron 1996;72: 171–176.

92. Slingeneyer A, Canaud B, Mion C. Permanent loss of ultrafiltration capacity of the peritoneum in long term peritoneal dialysis: an epidemiological study. Nephron 1983;33: 133–138.

93. Dobbie JW, Lloyd JK, Gall CA. Categorization of ultrastructural changes in peritoneal mesothelium, stroma, and blood vessels in uremia and CAPD patients. Adv Perit Dial 1990:63–12.

94. Di Paolo N, Sacchi G. Peritoneal vascular changes in continuous ambulatory peritoneal dialysis (CAPD): an in vivo model for the study of diabetic microangiopathy. Perit Dial Int 1989;9:41–45.

95. Di Paolo N, Sacchi G, De Mia M, et al. Morphology of the peritoneal membrane during continuous ambulatory peritoneal dialysis. Nephron 1986;44:204–211.

96. Di Paolo N, Sacchi G, Buoncristiani V. The morphology of the human peritoneum in CAPD patients. In: Maher J, ed. Frontiers in Peritoneal Dialysis. New York: Field Rich, 1985:11–19.

97. Gotloib L, Bar-Sella P, Shostak A. Reduplicated basal lamina of small venules and mesothelium of human parietal peritoneum: ultrastructural changes of reduplicated peritoneal basement membrane. Perit Dial Bull 1985;5: 212–214.

98. Gotloib L, Shostak A, Jaichenko J. Loss of mesothelial electronegative fixed charges during murine septic peritonitis. Nephron 1989;51:77–83.

99. Cantor J, Willhite M, Bray B, Keller S, Mandl I, Turino G. Synthesis of crosslinked elastin by a mesothelial cell culture. Proc Soc Exp Biol Med 1986;181:387–391.

100. Whitaker D, Papadimitriou JM, Walters MN. The mesothelium and its reactions: a review. Crit Rev Toxicol 1982;10:81–144.

101. Ryan GB, Grobety J, Majno G. Mesothelial injury and recovery. Am J Pathol 1973;71:93–113.

102. Rennard SI, Jaurand M-C, Bignon J, et al. Role of pleural mesothelial cells in the production of the submesothelial connective tissue matrix of lung. Am Rev Respir Dis 1984; 130:267–274.

103. Renvall S, Lehto M, Penttinen R. Development of peritoneal fibrosis occurs under the mesothelial cell layer. J Surg Res 1987;43:407–412.

104. Offner A, Feichtinger H, Stadlmann S, et al. Transforming growth factor-β synthesis by human peritoneal mesothelial cells. Am J Pathol 1996;148:1679–1688.

105. Marshall BC, Santana A, Xu Q-P, et al. Metalloproteinases and tissue inhibitor of metalloproteinases in mesothelial cells: cellular differentiation influences expression. J Clin Invest 1993;91:1792–1799.

106. Kumano K, Schiller B, Hjelle JT, Moran J. Effect of osmotic solutes on fibronectin mRNA expression in rat peritoneal mesothelial cells. Blood Purif 1996;14: 165–169.

107. Harvey W, Amlot PL. Collagen production by human mesothelial cells *in vitro*. J Pathol 1983;139:337–347.

108. Davilla RM, Crouch EC. Role of mesothelial and submesothelial stromal cells in matrix remodeling following pleural injury. Am J Pathol 1993;142:547–556.

109. Sitter T, Spannagl M, Schiffl H, van Hinsburgh VWM, Kooistra T. Imbalance between intraperitoneal coagulation and fibrinolysis during peritonitis of CAPD patients: the role of the mesothelial cells. Nephrol Dial Transplant 1995;10:677–683.

110. Gotloib L, Shostack A, Bar-Sella P, Cohen R. Continuous mesothelial injury and regeneration during long term peritoneal dialysis. Perit Dial Bull 1987;7:148–155.

111. Gotloib L, Waisbrut V, Shostak A, Kushnier R. Biocompatibility of dialysis solutions evaluated by histochemical techniques applied to mesothelial cell imprints. Perit Dial Int 1993;13:201–207.

112. Gotloib L, Waisbrut V, Shostak A, Kushnier R. Acute and long-term changes observed in imprints of mouse mesothelium exposed to glucose-enriched, lactated, buffered dialysis solutions. Nephron 1995;70:466–477.

113. Gotloib L, Wajsbrot V, Shostak A, Kushnier R. Population analysis of mesothelium in situ and in vivo exposed to bicarbonate-buffered peritoneal dialysis fluid. Nephron 1996;73:219–227.

114. Bos HJ, Struijk DG, Tuk CW, et al. Peritoneal dialysis induces a local sterile inflammatory state and the mesothelial cells in the effluent are related to the bacterial peritonitis incidence. Nephron 1991;59:508–509.

115. Slater ND, Raftery AT, Cope GH. The ultrastructure of human abdominal mesothelium. J Anat 1989;167:47–56.

116. Slater ND, Cope GH, Raftery AT. Mesothelial hyperplasia in response to peritoneal dialysis fluid: a morphometric study in the rat. Nephron 1991;58:466–471.

117. Beavis J, Harwood JL, Coles GA, Williams JD. Intraperitoneal phosphatidyl choline levels in patients on continuous ambulatory peritoneal dialysis do not correlate with adequacy of ultrafiltration. J Am Soc Nephrol 1993;3: 1954–1960.

118. Nomoto Y, Kawaguchi Y, Kubo H, Hirano H, Sakai S, Kurokawa K. Sclerosing encapsulating peritonitis in patients undergoing continuous ambulatory peritoneal dialysis: a report on the Japanese sclerosing encapsulating peritonitis study group. Am J Kidney Dis 1996;28: 420–427.

119. Nagy JA, Shockley TR, Masse EM, Harvey VS, Hoff CM, Jackman RW. Systemic delivery of a recombinant protein by genetically modified mesothelial cells reseeded on the parietal peritoneal surface. Gene Ther 1995;2:402–410.

120. Nagy JA, Schockley TR, Masse EM, Harvey VS, Jackman RW. Mesothelial cell-mediated gene therapy: feasibility of an ex vivo strategy. Gene Ther 1995;2:393–401.

121. Hoff CM, Cuisick JL, Masse EM, Jackman RW, Nagy JA, Shockley TR. Modulation of transgene expression in mesothelial cells by activation of an inducible promoter. Nephrol Dial Transplant 1998;13:1420–1429.

6

The Role of Integrins in Peritoneal Healing

Kathleen E. Rodgers

CONTENTS

Integrins are a large family of heterodimeric transmembrane glycoproteins that were initially identified as receptors for components of the extracellular matrix (ECM).[1,2] Integrins are obligate heterodimers, composed of noncovalently associated α- and β-subunits, each of which spans the plasma membrane and, typically, possesses a short (40–60 amino acids) cytoplasmic domain. Both the α- and β-subunits of integrins consist of a relatively large extracellular domain (~1000 residues for the α- and ~750 for the β-subunit), a transmembrane domain, and a short cytoplasmic tail.[3-6] Receptor diversity and specificity of ligand binding are determined by the extracellular domains through the regulated pairing of at least 9 β-subunits and 16 α-subunits, forming a family of more than 20 functional heterodimers including receptors for fibronectin, laminin, vitronectin, and collagens. In vitro, integrins have been shown to mediate cell adhesion to at least 12 different matrix proteins, and to several receptors that mediate cellular interactions, including members of the immunoglobulin and cadherin families.[7] During mammalian development the ECM directs cellular motility and influences the growth and differentiation of epithelial and mesenchymal tissues.

Integrin–ECM interactions are mediated primarily by an Arg-Gly-Asp (RGD) tripeptide, which functions as a core cell-binding sequence in many matrix proteins. In addition to mediating cell adhesion, integrins function as signaling receptors, participating in a diverse array of cellular effects including spreading, migration, proliferation, differentiation, and survival.[3,8,9] Furthermore, integrin ligation can have profound effects on expression of a number of other genes, including those encoding metalloproteinases,[10] milk proteins,[11] and cytokines.[12]

Members of the integrin family are expressed in virtually every cell of most multicellular organisms. In adult mammals, most cells constitutively express multiple integrins.[13-16] However, the expression of certain integrins is tissue restricted, for example, the leukocyte expression of β_2 integrins such as $\alpha_L\beta_2$ (LFA-1) and $\alpha_M\beta_2$ (Mac-1), and platelet-specific expression of the $\alpha_{IIb}\beta_3$ integrin (gpIIb-IIIa). The leukocyte integrins mediate interactions with membrane-bound ligands, such as intercellular adhesion molecule-1 (ICAM-1), and in activated platelets, $\alpha_{IIb}\beta_3$ binds fibrogen and von Willebrand factor, indicating the extreme versatility of integrin receptors in mediating an array of biological responses.[2,4,17–21] Many cells simultaneously express more than one receptor for the same ligand and the same integrins are often expressed on cells with markedly divergent functions. It is thus likely that different integrins can direct divergent cellular responses to a single ligand, and that specific integrins perform different functions in different cells.

Some integrins are very narrow in their binding specificity. In contrast, many integrins can bind to multiple ligands such as the ECM proteins fibrinogen and fibronectin. This complexity may at least in part occur because integrins can recognize the short amino acid sequences present in many proteins, for example, the amino acid sequence RGD. Nearly one-half of the members of the integrin family are known to interact with RGD sequences in their ligands.[21] The α-subunit contains three to four putative divalent cation-binding sites that have homology to the helix-loop-helix Ca^{2+}-binding structure ("EF-hand") found in proteins such as calmodulin, troponin C, and parvalbumin.[22] These cation-binding domains are contained within a larger stretch of seven homologous repeated domains (Fig. 6.1). Those integrins with only three divalent cation-binding sites in the α-subunit have an additional inserted domain (I) between the second and third repeats. The I domain is about 200 amino acid residues long and is homologous to the A domain of von Willebrand factor.[23] Recently, it has also been shown to bind divalent cation through a novel cation-binding motif.[24,25]

This chapter discusses both the possible sites of integrin interaction in the complex process of peritoneal repair and adhesion formation and data from animal studies that evaluated the effect of soluble, inhibitory RGD-containing peptides on adhesion formation.

Adhesion Formation

Adhesion formation is a major source of postoperative morbidity and mortality.[26,27] General and gynecologic surgery are the most frequent surgical procedures implicated in clinically significant adhesion formation. The most serious complication of intraperitoneal adhesions is intestinal obstruction.[28–32] The surgical procedure most frequently associated with intestinal obstruction, following adhesion formation, is hysterectomy.[33,34] Adhesions are also associated with chronic or recurrent pelvic pain and secondary infertility in females.[35–40] Most re-

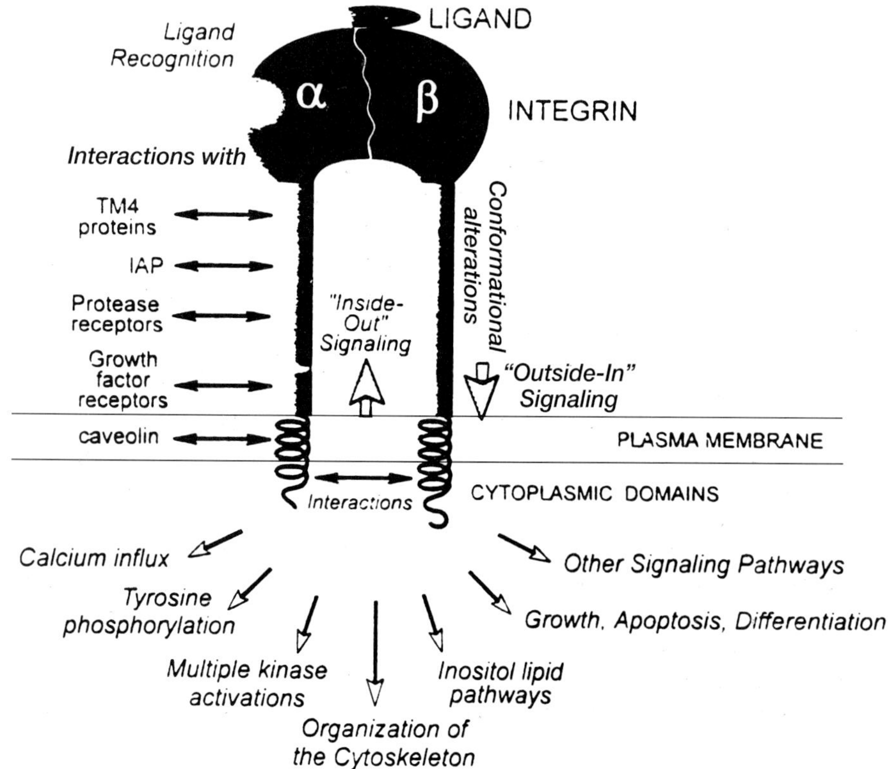

FIG. 6.1. Schematic overview of integrin signaling. Integrins, using bidirectional signaling mechanisms, provide communication between these cell-surface proteins and their ligands.

cently, intraoperative complications and prolonged operative time have been recognized as serious consequences arising from postoperative adhesion formation.

Integrins may mediate some events that occur during postsurgical peritoneal repair and adhesion formation. Within the integrin superfamily, at least three families of adhesion receptors can be distinguished on the basis of their β-subunits. Members of each of these families could potentially be involved in the formation of adhesions through the regulation of a variety of events, such as fibrin deposition and inflammatory processes.

Sites of Integrin Interaction in Adhesion Formation

One family of receptors belong to the fibronectin receptor class. This family may regulate the interaction of various cell types, including fibroblasts, keratinocytes, and potentially mesothelial cells with their ECM.[1,2,41] Through blocking the binding of cells to the fibrin clot, one could envision several points of blocking adhesion formation. For example, if mesothelial cells could not bind to the fibrin scaffold, reorganization into a permanent adhesion may not take place.

Fibronectins

Fibronectins have been most extensively studied among the many extracellular proteins identified so far as being adhesive for cells.[41–46] Fibronectins found in body fluids, loose connective tissues, basement membranes, and granulation tissues (~300 μg/mL in plasma, lesser amounts in other fluids) are multifunctional ECM and plasma proteins, and have been implicated in a wide variety of cellular properties. These properties include cell adhesion, morphology, cytoskeletal organization, migration, differentiation, phagocytosis, and hemostasis. There are at least two types of fibronectins, termed plasma and cellular fibronectin. These two kinds of fibronectins, although distinguishable, are very similar in structure and properties. One major source of plasma fibronectin appears to be hepatocytes,[47] although endothelial cells[48] and macrophages[49] could also contribute.

Recent studies have demonstrated the structure of the fibronectin molecule and the localization of the various binding sites within the molecule.[50–52] One of the most important findings was demonstration that its cell attachment site consisted essentially of a tetrapeptide of Arg-Gly-Asp-Ser (RGDS) in the cell binding of fibronectin.[53] Other cell adhesion-promoting regions in fibronectin, with one active site based on an RGD-type motif and a second site apparently unrelated, are also shown within an alternatively spliced segment designated IIICS[54–56] and within the C-terminal heparin-binding domain of fibronectin.[51,57–61]

Fibronectin binds to fibrin or to fibrinogen both via its N-terminal domain and through site(s) near the C-terminus of the molecule.[46,62] The binding of fibronectin to fibrin from blood may be important in the initial stages of wound healing. Fibroblasts involved in the healing process adhere particularly well to fibronectin cross-linked to fibrin by factor XIIa transglutaminase. The second site in fibronectin involved in matrix assembly includes the first type I repeats.[63–66] A recent study has shown that the N-terminal fragment of fibronectin binds to fibroblasts that are coated with integrin.[67] These results are in accordance with the view that cell-mediated binding of the N-terminus of fibronectin is closely coupled to a complex formed by specific high-affinity interactions between RGD and synergistic sites in fibronectin and $\alpha_5\beta_1$ integrin receptor. Through binding to fibronectin and fibrin, the scaffold for mesothelial cell implantation and adhesion formation, mesothelial cells anchor during the healing process and form the immature fibrin bands that organize into adhesions.

Platelet Aggregation and Activation

The second family of adhesion receptors that may be blocked by RGD-containing peptides include the platelet glycoprotein IIb/IIIa receptor.[42,43] Inhibition of the binding of this receptor to its ligand will inhibit platelet aggregation and activation. Because these events accelerate clotting and presumably increase fibrin deposition, a blockade of this integrin with its ligand may reduce fibrin deposition and subsequent adhesion formation. $\alpha_{IIb}\beta_3$ consists of a two-chain α-subunit bound noncovalently to a single-chain β-subunit. Each subunit spans the platelet membrane once. The N-terminus and most of the remainder of each subunit are extracellular, and the membrane-spanning domain is connected to a short C-terminal cytoplasmic tail consisting of 20 amino acid residues in α_{IIb} and 47 residues in β_3. Electron microscopy of heterodimers shows an N-terminal globular head connected to two C-terminal stalks.[68,69] Although the atomic structure of $\alpha_{IIb}\beta_3$ is not known, biochemical, genetic, and molecular modeling studies indicate that ligand binding is primarily a function of the globular heads.[70] Because ligand binding is regulated by signals from within the platelet and also triggers platelet responses, mechanisms must exist to propagate information back and forth between the cytoplasmic tails and the globular heads. The mechanism of information transmission is termed inside-out signaling.

Inflammatory Responses

The third adhesion receptor family that could be involved in the formation of adhesions between organs is the family of integrins found on leukocytes (leukocyte antigen receptor family).[71–73] Through inhibition of the interactions between these integrins and their ligands, inflammatory processes that occur in the early postoperative interval, such as leukocyte infiltration and phagocytosis, may be reduced by postoperative administration of RGD-containing peptides.

Early events in inflammation enhance expression of adhesion molecules such as selectins and integrins on endothelial cells. Selectins are molecules that share structural domains including (1) a calcium-dependent lectin domain; (2) an epidermal growth factor-like domain; (3) tandem repeats; (4) a transmembrane domain; and (5) a cytoplasmic tail. Among the mediators that can increase P-selection expression rapidly (in the absence of transcription) are thrombin and platelet-activating factor, both generated early in response to injury. The first step in this process is the tethering of polymorphonuclear leukocytes (PMNs) to the endothelium. P-selectin on endothelium and L-selectin on PMNs act sequentially in the initial tethering of PMNs to the endothelium, a process that leads to PMN margination and increased contact with the endothelium. PMN interaction with the endothelium is enhanced by flow conditions, as would occur in a blood vessel.[74] The mechanism of flow-enhanced avidity is not completely clear, but strain on the bond between selection and ligand may lead to a conformational change in one or both molecules, enhancing interaction. In the presence of shear stress, this leads to PMNs rolling along the endothelial surface. All selectins have the ability to mediate cell rolling on a ligand under flow conditions.

The second step in PMN transmigration is integrin activation. Leukocyte integrins can exist in two states with respect to adhesion. In circulating unactivated cells, the integrins are of low avidity and will not mediate adhesion, even if ligand is expressed on the endothelium. On activation, the integrin avidity for ligand is markedly increased. The mechanism of this regulation remains uncertain and probably represents a combination of conformational change in the extracellular domain of the integrins to enhance affinity of individual receptors and alterations in interaction with cytoplasmic proteins to affect integrin clustering and association with cytoskeleton. When PMNs are rolling on endothelium because of selectin interactions, the chance of exposure to potential integrin-activating agents such as chemokines, formulated bacterial peptides, or complement fragments is increased. Binding of PMNs with increased integrin avidity to endothelium-expressing ligand leads to arrest of the rolling leukocytes, with close and stable cell–cell adhesion between the PMN and endothelial cell. This is the third step in PMN transmigration.

Two molecules whose neutralization will block PMN transmigration are platelet-endothelial cell adhesion molecule (PECAM; CD31) and integrin-associated protein (IAP; CD47). Both molecules are expressed on PMNs as well. Treating either endothelium or PMNs with antibodies to these molecules can block transmigration, although treating both cells is required for optimal inhibitory effect. PECAM can mediate homophilic binding, but IAP does not (Fig. 6.1). Rather, IAP is closely associated with functions of the integrin $\alpha_v\beta_3$, found on both endothelium and PMNs.

PMNs express low levels of a number of integrins ($\alpha_2\beta_1$, $\alpha_3\beta_1$, $\alpha_4\beta_1$, $\alpha_6\beta_1$, $\alpha_6\beta_1$, $\alpha_6\beta_1$) that bind a large number of ECM proteins. $\alpha_M\beta_2$ also is important in PMN interaction with both protein and glycosaminoglycan components of the ECM. Further, monocytes and macrophages contain numerous integrin-binding sites that can mediate inflammatory events including monocyte chemotaxis, macrophage activation, and phagocytosis. Prolonged inflammatory responses, resulting from deposition of foreign bodies or cellular debris from tissue necrosis, can contribute to adhesion formation through increased fibrin deposition and prolonged inhibition of fibrinolysis.

Leukocyte Interactions with Laminins

As described, integrin expression on leukocytes has been shown to regulate many cell-to-cell interactions and processes involved in the inflammatory response. The role of the laminins in leukocyte biology has been of particular interest. The laminins are structurally related glycoproteins found predominantly in basement membranes.[75–79] Laminins stimulate cell adhesion and migration, as well as influence gene expression, which underlies their critical importance in development, differentiation, and tissue homeostasis. All the seven known laminins are composed of three subunits, designated α, β, and γ.[80] Structural isoforms exist for each of these subunits, and the association of these isoforms into heterotrimers gives rise to the different laminins.[80] Numerous studies have revealed that the expression of specific laminin isoforms is tissue specific and that this expression pattern is often altered in disease.

The $\alpha_6\beta_1$ integrin is the major leukocyte laminin receptor in macrophages,[81,82] neutrophils,[83] and T cells.[84] However, this integrin when expressed on the surface of these cells is unable to mediate laminin interactions unless activated by physiologic or pharmacologic stimuli. This regulation of function may provide a mechanism for controlling leukocyte interactions with basement membranes and other laminin-containing matrices. This process of activation by physiological stimuli, which is often referred to as inside-out signaling, is now described further.

As described, physiologic processes such as leukocyte transmigration through endothelium involve the regulated and sequential activation of a spectrum of adhesion molecules, including integrins. Recent studies on chemokine-mediated activation of the $\alpha_6\beta_1$ integrin in monocytes have provided insight into the nature of this process.[85] In these cells, the integrin $\alpha_6\beta_1$ binds to VCAM-1 on the endothelial cell surface and both $\alpha_4\beta_1$ and $\alpha_5\beta_1$ bind to fibronectin in the matrix. In vitro adhesion to these ligands under static flow conditions stimulated by the CC (Cys–Cys bond) class of chemokines resulted in the early activation of subsequent deactivation of $\alpha_4\beta_1$, whereas activation of $\alpha_5\beta_1$ occurred later and persisted. Because these two integrins share the same β-subunit and differ only in their α-subunit, these data suggest that the differential regulation of $\alpha_4\beta_1$, and $\alpha_5\beta_1$ by CC chemokines may result from their differential interaction with putative regulatory molecules through their α-subunits. A similar mechanism for the differential regulation of the $\alpha_6A\beta_1$ and $\alpha_6B\beta_1$ integrins in macrophages may exist. The actual mechanism by which chemokines influence integrin avidity is unclear, but it appears that integrin redistribution and reorganization of actin cytoskeleton are required because the effects of chemokine activation of $\alpha_4\beta_1$ can be abolished by cytochalasin B.[85]

Integrins in Mesothelial Repair

Histologic description of the peritoneum originated more than 100 years ago.[86,87] As described elsewhere in this volume, the peritoneum is seen as a single layer of mesothelial cells over a continuous basement membrane that overlies connective tissue consisting of fibroblasts, collagen fibers, adipocytes, leukocytes, and an abundant supply of lymphatics and microvessels. The first electron photomicrographs revealing the ultrastructure of human mesothelium were published in 1981.[86] The mesothelium is seen as a continuous sheet of flattened cells joined by tight junctions and desmosomes (maculae adherens).[86,87] Hence, the mesothelium may be viewed as an ultrathin epithelial barrier separating the contents of the peritoneum from the underlying connective tissue of the peritoneal membrane.

Integrin–ligand interactions are thought to play a vital role in such processes as adhesion formation, endometrial receptivity, placentation, embryonic development, and tumor invasion. In disease states, such as metastatic ovarian endometrial cancer, endometriosis, and adhesion formation, the mesothelium may function not as a barrier but as a substrate for tissue or cellular implantation. Ovarian tumors can metastasize by direct extension into the peritoneal cavity through firm attachment to the underlying stroma. Although the etiology is not precisely known, endometriosis may result from the seeding of viable endometrial fragments into the peritoneal cavity via retrograde menstruation. After initial attachment, there is evidence suggesting early endometriosis lesions invade the ECM of the peritoneum.[88]

Integrin Expression on Mesothelial Cells

Studies were conducted to assess integrin expression in the peritoneum of normal women and in disease states. Mesothelium from the abdominal wall and uterine serosa expressed α_2, α_3, and α_6 integrins. The intensity of mesothelial expression of α integrin subunits was identical for these two anatomic sites. The mesothelium strongly expressed α_2 and α_3 and weakly expressed α_6.[89] Others have reported the expression of integrins in peritoneal biopsies and in epithelial cells recovered from peritoneal fluid in women with and without endometriosis. In patients without endometriosis, α_2, α_3, α_4, α_5, and α_6 are expressed. However, it is unclear whether the staining in the peritoneum biopsy samples was limited to the mesothelium.[90]

Kurk et al.[91] reported similar integrin subunit expression of mesothelial monolayers derived from ovarian surface epithelium (OSE). These investigations found that these cells express α_2, α_3,α_5, α_v, and β_1 subunits. Expression of α_1 and α_4 was not investigated. In this study, OSE cells were grown on plastic, Matrigel, collagen, and fibrin. Cell morphology, growth, protease production, and integrin expression were modulated by the composition of the ECM. In addition, mesothelial cell cultures derived from omentum have been shown to express β_1 and β_3 integrin subunits.[92] In this study, these cells did not express α_4, nor did they express β_2 or β_4. Cultured human mesothelial cells also express two integrin ligands, intercellular adhesion molecule-1 (ICAM-1) and vascular cell adhesion molecule-1 (VCAM-1).[92,93] Expression of these adhesion molecules in vitro was increased by exposure to the cytokines tumor necrosis factor-α and γ-interferon.[93]

In Vivo Versus In Vitro Expression of Integrins by Mesothelial Cells

Importantly, differential expression of mesothelial integrins was found in vivo and in vitro. In vivo, the mesothelium expressed α_2 and α_3, and variably expressed α_6. In monolayer culture, the mesothelial cells expressed α_2, α_3, α_5, and α_v. The additional expression of α_5 and α_v, both fibronectin receptors, could be a result of cellular binding to fibronectin that is interposed between the cell and the glass slide as a result of serum in the culture medium or production of fibronectin by mesothelial cells.[94] In contrast, the absence of α_6 expression, a laminin receptor, in vitro could be the result of cell growth in the absence of a laminin-rich basement membrane found in vivo.

To examine the possibility that the altered integrin expression of mesothelial monolayers was caused by adhesion to fibronectin, mesothelial integrin subunit expression in peritoneal explants was examined. That the mesothelium expression of α_5 and α_v subunits was also found in explants suggested that differential integrin expression in monolayers is not caused by the dissociation of mesothelium from the ECM. Furthermore, exposure to fibronectin present in the culture media did not alter this expression.

Influence of Integrin Expression on Cellular Morphology

Mesothelium from abdominal wall and uterine serosa was found, using electron microscopy, to have distinct ultrastructural morphology. Similar ultrastructural differences have been reported between the mesothelium of the abdominal wall and the ovarian germinal epithelium. Unique characteristics of mesothelium in different locations, including morphology and differential expression of cell adhesion molecules (ligands for integrins), could explain the predilection of tumor metastases and endometriotic implants for specific locations in the peritoneal cavity. However, despite ultrastructural differences in mesothelium, the integrin expression did not differ and thus cannot explain these anatomic differences in disease processes.

Cellular Distribution of Integrins

As can be seen from the foregoing, integrins are involved in the interaction of the mesothelial cell and its surrounding ECM and may be involved in mesothelial cell-to-cell adhesion. Immunoelectron microscopy revealed that the integrin subunits were not limited to plasma membrane but were distributed throughout the cytoplasm. However, the identification of integrins along the surface of the mesothelium suggests that mesothelial integrins could play a role in the initial attachment of tumor cells and ectopic endometrium.

Many studies reporting immunohistochemical localization of integrins have reported cytoplasmic immunoreactivity.[95,96] The nature of this immunoreactivity is not clear. In most cells the β-subunit is expressed in excess. Appearance on the cell surface depends on heterodimerization of the integrin subunits. The expression of integrins on the plasma membrane seems to be regulated by the production of α-subunit.[96] This method of regulation of expression of heterodimeric proteins on plasma membranes is consistent with that in other systems, for example, expression of the class II heterodimer of the major histocompatability complex.

Localization of Ligand-Binding Sites

Significant progress has been made in the identification of potential sites for ligand–integrin interactions using the platelet-specific integrin $\alpha_{IIb}\beta_3$ as the prototype. $\alpha_{IIb}\beta_3$ binds to multiple ligands, including fibrinogen,[97,98] fibronectin,[99,100] von Willebrand factor,[101] and vitronectin.[102] Fibrinogen binding to $\alpha_{IIb}\beta_3$ plays an essential role in platelet aggregation. A tripeptide sequence common to all these ligands, RGD, has been shown to function as a recognition sequence for ligand binding to $\alpha_{IIb}\beta_3$.[53] Similarly, many other integrins bind to ligands via this motif. Fibrinogen contains two RGD sequences located on its Aα-chain (residues 95–97 and 572–574). However, some studies indicate that the RGD sequence at position 572–574 may play only a minor role in fibrinogen binding to $\alpha_{IIb}\beta_3$.[103,104] Fibrinogen contains an additional recognition site (HHLGGAKQAGDV) for $\alpha_{IIb}\beta_3$ found at the C-terminal end of its γ-chain. This region (γ400–411) also plays an important role in fibrinogen binding to $\alpha_{IIb}\beta_3$.[105,106]

The importance of the amino-terminal portion of $\alpha_{IIb}\beta_3$ in ligand binding is highlighted by the proteolytic production of amino-terminal 55-kDa α_{IIb} and 85-kDa β_3 fragments, which form a calcium-dependent heterodimer that binds fibrinogen in a RGD-dependent manner.[107] Further evidence for the role of this region in ligand binding comes from epitope mapping of inhibitory monoclonal antibodies to the amino-terminal region of β_3.[108] Similarly, the use of neutralizing monoclonal antibodies also indicated that the amino-terminal region of the integrin $\alpha_{IIb}\beta_3$ was expressed and functionally active.[109] More specifically, ligand recognition specificity for the integrin $\alpha_{IIb}\beta_3$ has been mapped to the first 334 residues in the α_{IIb} chain.[110]

Signal Transduction: In Brief

Recent research has focused on the process by which integrin–ligand interations regulate cellular function. Figure 6.2 summarizes some of the key issues in integrin signaling. The molecular basis of integrin recognition and binding of ligands is now understood at the level of specific key residues and binding domains in the ligand and the integrin receptor. The conformation and binding affinity of an integrin can be changed markedly by "inside-out" signaling, and novel insights into the nature of this process have come from studies of integrin-specific proteins that bind to a cytoplasmic domain and activate the integrin. In addition, cytoskeletal mechanisms of regulation have also been postulated. The process of ligand binding results in conformational changes in inte-

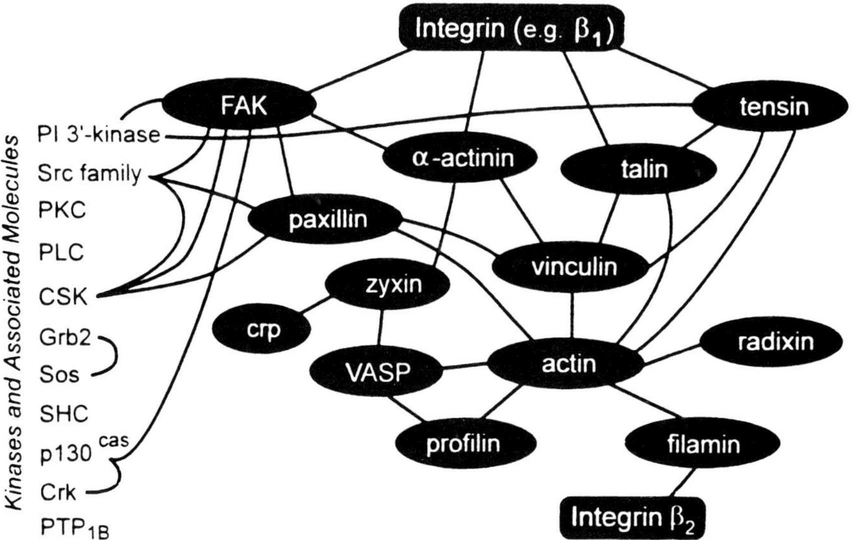

FIG. 6.2. Through interactions between integrins and their ligands, clustering of the receptor allows the formation of cytoskeletal proteins and proteins that transduce signals. This schematic demonstrates some of the interactions currently defined.

grins, with alterations observed in the globular head region and in the β-subunit stalk domain, as detected by the appearance of new epitopes. Information associated with this conformational change is thought to be transmitted in some fashion across the membrane.

Inside-Out Signaling

Inside-out signaling denotes those reactions initiated by the binding of one or more agonists to their plasma membrane receptors, leading to the conversion of the $\alpha_{IIb}\beta_3$ receptor on platelets from a low-affinity/avidity receptor to a high-affinity/avidity receptor (see Fig. 6.1). This conversion has consequences in that it determines whether $\alpha_{IIb}\beta_3$ can engage soluble adhesive ligands, such as fibrinogen and vWF, which contain the integrin recognition sequence RGD. These multivalent ligands can function as bridges between receptors on adjacent platelets, thus allowing platelet aggregation.[96] Because $\alpha_{IIb}\beta_3$ can diffuse laterally within the plasma membrane, inside-out signaling can have two distinct components: (1) affinity modulation, which implies a structural change intrinsic to the heterodimer that results in a greater strength of ligand binding; and (2) avidity modulation, which implies a change in the functional affinity of the interaction between receptor and ligand.[111] One plausible way that the latter could occur is through integrin clustering within the plane of the plasma membrane.

Outside-in signaling denotes reactions initiated by integrin ligation and clustering, and coordinated with signals resulting from other plasma membrane receptors (e.g., growth factor, cytokine, and G-protein-linked receptors).[112–114] Integrin signals help to regulate a host of postligand-binding events, the particular pattern varying with the cell and the integrin. Postligand-binding events regulated by $\alpha_{IIb}\beta_3$ in platelets include the stabilization of large platelet aggregates, platelet spreading, granule secretion, clot retraction, and possibly platelet postcoagulant activity.[115]

Second-Messenger Systems in Signal Transduction by Integrins

Besides signaling pathways, integrins have dramatic effects on the actin-containing cytoskeleton. Nevertheless, integrins regulate the interactions of cytoskeletal proteins including talin, α-actinin, and tensin (see recent review[116]). However, integrin-induced adhesion complexes also include multifunctional docking molecules such as focal adhesion kinase (FAK).[117,118] The interactions within adhesion complexes involves both cytoskeletal and signaling molecules. As indicated in Figs. 6.1 and 6.2, the binding interactions between these molecules appear remarkably complex and interconnected as they form three-dimensional molecular complexes such as the focal contact.

The membrane-proximal portions of integrin cytoplasmic domains are highly conserved. Truncations that disrupt the most membrane-proximal five to seven residues of either the α_{IIb} or β_3 cytoplasmic tail markedly increase ligand-binding affinity, most likely because of disruption in intersubunit interactions that normally maintain a default low-affinity state.[119,120] Selected point mutations in this region induce ligand binding and initiate spontaneous tyrosine phosphorylation of FAK.[120] Accordingly, the membrane-proximal integrin hinge region regulates bidirectional integrin signaling.

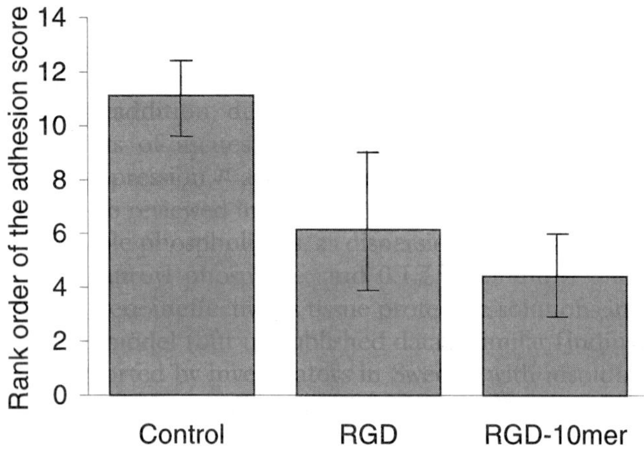

FIG. 6.3. Rank order analysis of the overall adhesion score given to rabbits in which placebo (saline), RGD, or a 10-amino-acid peptide containing RGD was administered to the site of injury throughout the postsurgical interval. Results are the mean ± SD of data from four to eight rabbits per group. A p value of less than 0.05 was considered significant.

Integrins have been shown to play a role in regulating gene expression and cell growth, differentiation, and survival.[121–123] They accomplish these tasks by a process of outside-in signaling whereby ligand-occupied and clustered integrins control cell shape and the organization of the cytoskeleton and generate a variety of biochemical signals. Many integrin-triggered reactions, for example, activation of protein tyrosine kinases, such as pp60^{Src}, pp125^{FAK}, and pp72^{Syk}, and activation of phosphatidylinositol 3-kinase and mitogen-activated protein (MAP) kinases, are shared with those generated by more traditional agonist receptors, such as those for growth factors and cytokines.

A plethora of proteins has recently been identified that can bind directly to integrin cytoplasmic tails, at least in vitro. Some of these proteins can bind to integrin α- or β-subunit, others to only a single type. In the case of one of these, β_3-endonexin, selective binding to the β_3 tail, but not to the β_1 or β_2 tail, is the result of an NITY (Asn-Ile-Thr-Tyr amino acid sequence) motif that is specific for the β_3 tail.[124] In most cases, identification of these binding proteins has outstripped the characterization of their biologic functions, and further analyses of their roles in vivo are required. Nonetheless, there are complex relationships between integrin tail-binding proteins and integrin signaling. For example, some of these proteins are cytoskeletal structural proteins (α-actinin, fiamin, talin), while possessing kinase activity (pp125^{FAK}, ILK) or guanine necleotide exchange activity (cytohesin-1), or function as adapters (e.g., paxillin). Overexpression of two different tail-selective binding proteins, cytohesion-1 and β_3-endonexin, results in specific activation of the adhesive function of $\alpha_L\beta_2$ and $\alpha_{IIb}\beta_3$, respectively.[125,126] Finally, calreticulin can bind to the membrane-proximal portion of α-cytoplasmic tails.[127] Although this protein can be found in more than one subcellular location and may have several functions even with respect to adhesion receptors and cytoskeletal proteins,[128,129] it is noteworthy that calreticulin-null embryonic stem cells are deficient in integrin-mediated cell adhesion and calcium influx.[130]

Reduction of Adhesion Formation by RGD-Containing Peptides

As described, many of the processes that lead to adhesion formation could involve integrin–ligand interac-

TABLE 6.1. Alterations in cell function associated with peptides

RGD-containing peptides	Amino acid sequence	Effect of RGD peptides on cell binding to ECM	Effect of RGD peptides on ECM binding to platelets
RGD	Arg-Gly-Asp	↓ Cell binding to ECM	↓ Fg, FN, VN, vWF binding to platelets
RGDSPASSKP	Arg-Gly-Asp-Ser-Pro-Ala-Ser-Ser-Lys-Pro	↓ Cell binding to ECM	↓ Fg, FN, VN, vWF binding to platelets
GRDGdSP	Gly-Arg-Gly-Arg-*d*-Ser-Pro	↓ Cell binding to fibronectin No change in cell binding to vitronectin	↓ Fg, FN, VN, vWF binding to platelets Resistant to carboxypeptidase
GdRGDSP	Gly-*d*-Arg-Gly-Arg-Ser-Pro	↓ Cell binding to fibronectin and vitronectin	Resistant to carboxypeptidase and trypsin
GRGDS	Gly-Arg-Gly-Arg-Ser	↓ Cell binding to fibronectin	↓ Fg, FN, VN, vWF binding to platelets
NMe-GRGDSP	*n*Me-Gly-Arg-Gly-Arg-Ser-Pro	↓ Cell binding to fibronectin and vitronectin	↓ Fg, FN, VN, vWF binding to platelets Resistant to carboxypeptidase and aminopeptidase
GRGDNP	Gly-Arg-Gly-Arg-Asn-Pro	↓ Cell binding to fibronectin (superior) ↓ Cell binding to vitronectin (weak)	↓ Fg, FN, VN, vWF binding to platelets Resistant to carboxypeptidase
GRGDSP	Gly-Arg-Gly-Arg-Ser-Pro	↓ Cell binding to fibronectin and vitronectin	Resistant to carboxypeptidase
GRGDTP	Gly-Arg-Gly-Arg-Thr-Pro	↓ Cell binding to fibronectin and vitronectin ↓ Cell binding to collagen	↓ Fg, FN, VN, vWF binding to platelets

RGD, arginine-glycine-aspartic acid; ECM, extracellular matrix; Fg, fibrinogen; FN, fibronectin; VN, vitronectin; vWF, von Willebrand factor; ↓, decrease.

TABLE 6.2. Effect of continuous administration of RGD-containing peptides on the overall adhesion score in the rabbit double uterine horn model

	Control	GRGDdSP (0.13 mg/mL)	GdRGDSP (0.14 mg/mL)	GRGDS (0.13 mg/mL)	n-MeGRGDSP (0.122 mg/mL)	GRGDNP (0.133 mg/mL)	GRGDSP (0.135 mg/mL)	GRGDTP (0.132 mg/mL)
	3.0	1.0	1.0	1.5	1.0	1.5	1.5	1.5
	2.5	2.0	1.5	1.0	1.5	2.0	1.0	
	3.5	1.0	1.5	1.5	1.5	1.5	0.5	1.5
	3.0	2.5	1.0	1.0	1.5	1.0	2.0	1.5
	2.5							
	2.0							
Rank ± SD	29.9 ± 2.4	19.13 ± 9.1	11.0 ± 5.5	11 ± 5.5	13.8 ± 54.8	16.0 ± 7.1	12.1 ± 9.6	16.5 ± 0.0
p value		0.022	0.000	0.000	0.000	0.002	0.002	0.000

Each number in a column denotes the number given to an individual animal.

tions. These interactions include (1) platelet aggregation and activation leading to accelerated coagulation and fibrin deposition, (2) inflammatory processes such as neutrophil transmigration and macrophage activation, and (3) implantation of mesothelial cells on the fibrin-fibronectin scaffold of the immature adhesion. Because of these numerous sites of potential intervention by blockers of integrin–ligand interactions, RGD-containing peptides, which have been shown to act in this manner, were tested for their ability to reduce adhesion formation in the animal model described in Chapter 37 (this volume).

Administration of RGD Peptides via Alzet Pump

Initial studies were conducted in which the 3-amino-acid peptide, RGD, and a 10-amino-acid peptide containing RGD were administered to the site of injury for 7 days after abrasion and devascularization of both uterine horns. Administration of both RGD-containing peptides resulted in a significant reduction in the overall adhesion scores (Fig. 6.3). The effect of administration of several of five to six amino acid peptides containing RGD with a variety of biological activities (Table 6.1) on adhesion formation was then evaluated. All peptides tested reduced adhesion formation score in this model (Table 6.2). In Table 6.3, the percentage of the uterine horns involved in adhesions to various organs is shown. Administration of these peptides to the site of injury significantly reduced the extent of adhesion formation to various sites. Further, the number of sites without adhesions was increased by administration of these RGD-containing peptides (Fig. 6.4).

RGD Peptides in an Instillate at the End of Surgery

The efficacy of several viscous formulations (CREMOPHORE [BASF, Ludwigshafen]) containing RGD peptides in the reduction of adhesion formation when administered at the end of surgery was also tested in the rabbit double uterine horn model. The overall score given to the rabbits and the rank order analysis of these data are shown in Fig. 6.5. The extent of adhesion formation at the individual organ sites and the percentage of the sites adhesion free can be seen in Table 6.4 and Fig. 6.6, respectively. Administration of several formulations containing RGD peptides at the end of surgery significantly reduced adhesion formation in this model.

TABLE 6.3. Effect of continuous administration of RGD-containing peptides on the extent of adhesion formation in the rabbit double uterine horn model

	Control	GRGDdSP	GdRGDSP	GRGDS	n-MeGRGDSP	GRGDNP	GRGDSP	GRGDTP
Right horn								
Bowel	35.0 ± 6.2	10.0 ± 5.8*	12.5 ± 7.5	7.5 ± 4.8*	2.5 ± 2.5*	10.0 ± 4.1*	12.5 ± 2.5*	0.0 ± 0.0*
Bladder	45.0 ± 8.1	22.5 ± 7.5	10.0 ± 5.8*	15.0 ± 5.0*	10.0 ± 7.1*	7.5 ± 4.8*	7.5 ± 4.8*	16.7 ± 3.3
Itself	30.0 ± 3.7	22.5 ± 4.8	25.0 ± 2.9	25.0 ± 2.9	12.5 ± 2.5*	17.5 ± 2.5*	15.0 ± 6.5	23.3 ± 3.3
Left horn	30.0 ± 2.6	15.0 ± 6.5*	5.0 ± 5.0*	17.5 ± 2.5*	12.5 ± 2.5*	12.5 ± 7.5*	2.5 ± 2.5*	0.0 ± 0.0*
Left horn								
Bowel	35.0 ± 6.2	10.0 ± 5.8*	12.5 ± 7.5*	5.0 ± 5.0*	2.5 ± 2.5*	10.0 ± 4.1*	10.0 ± 4.1*	0.0 ± 0.0*
Bladder	45.0 ± 8.1	22.5 ± 7.5	10.0 ± 5.8*	15.0 ± 5.0*	7.5 ± 7.5*	7.5 ± 4.8*	10.0 ± 5.8*	16.7 ± 3.3
Itself	33.3 ± 3.3	20.1 ± 4.1*	25.0 ± 2.9	20.0 ± 4.1*	20.0 ± 0.0*	15.0 ± 2.9*	12.5 ± 2.5*	20.0 ± 0.0*
Right horn	30.0 ± 2.6	15.0 ± 6.5*	5.0 ± 5.0*	17.5 ± 0.5*	12.5 ± 2.5*	12.5 ± 7.5*	2.5 ± 2.5*	0.0 ± 0.0*

Values are expressed as percentages ± S.D.
*Significantly different from control ($p \leq 0.05$).

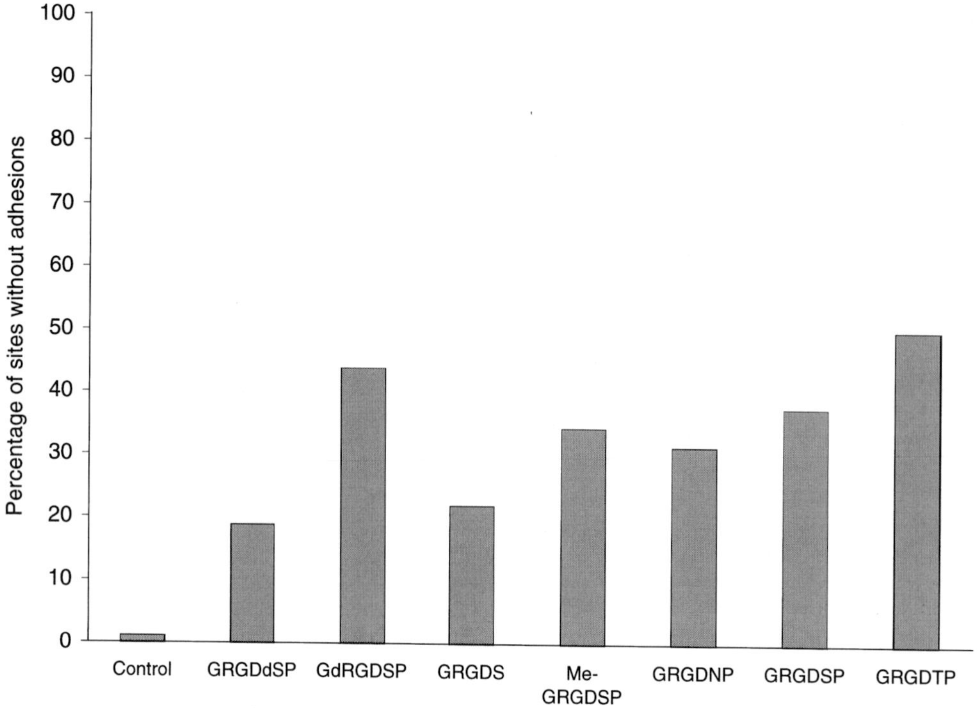

FIG. 6.4. Percentage of sites evaluated that did not form adhesions to the uterine horns after surgery.

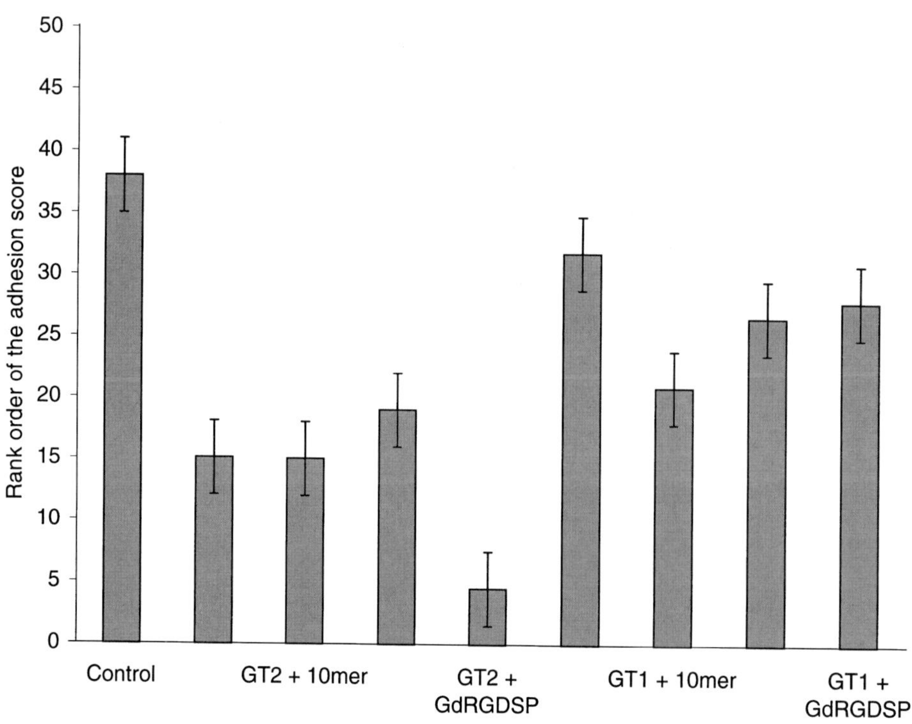

FIG. 6.5. Rank order analysis of the overall adhesion score given to rabbits treated at the end of surgery with nothing (control), vehicle, or vehicle-containing RGD peptides at the end of surgery. Results are the mean and SE of data from six to seven rabbits per group.

TABLE 6.4. Effect of administration of RGD-containing peptides in a viscous gel at the end of surgery on the extent of adhesion formation in the rabbit double uterine horn model

	Control	GT2	GT2 + 10mer	GT2 + nMeGRGDSP	GT2 + GdRGDSP	GT1	GT1 + 10mer	GT1 + nMeGRGDSP	GT1 + GdRGDSP
Right horn									
Bowel	24.0 ± 8.1	6.0 ± 4.0*	6.0 ± 4.0*	0.0 ± 0.0*	0.0 ± 0.0*	24.0 ± 2.5	14.0 ± 6.8	12.0 ± 5.8	24.0 ± 10.3
Bladder	12.0 ± 12.0	6.0 ± 2.5	6.0 ± 4.0	12.0 ± 3.7	5.0 ± 2.0	8.0 ± 5.8	10.0 ± 5.5	6.0 ± 4.0	12.0 ± 4.9
Itself	34.0 ± 4.0	24.0 ± 4.0	16.0 ± 2.5*	20.0 ± 2.3*	12.5 ± 2.5*	18.0 ± 2.9*	20.0 ± 4.5*	30.0 ± 0.0	24.0 ± 2.5
Left horn	34.0 ± 4.0	10.0 ± 5.5	10.0 ± 3.2*	10.0 ± 3.2*	2.5 ± 2.5*	24.0 ± 4.0	18.0 ± 8.0	18.0 ± 5.7*	22.0 ± 5.8
Left horn									
Bowel	24.0 ± 8.1	6.0 ± 4.0*	6.0 ± 4.0*	2.0 ± 2.0*	0.0 ± 0.0*	22.0 ± 3.7	14.0 ± 6.8	12.0 ± 5.8	12.4 ± 10.3
Bladder	12.0 ± 12.0	6.0 ± 2.5	6.0 ± 4.0	10.0 ± 3.2*	50.0 ± 2.0	8.0 ± 5.8	10.0 ± .5	6.0 ± 4.0	12.0 ± 4.9
Itself	34.0 ± 4.0	24.0 ± 4.0	24.0 ± 4.0	16 ± 6.0*	2.5 ± 2.5*	20.0 ± 5.5	24.0 ± 4.0	26.0 ± 2.5	24.0 ± 5.1
Right horn	34.0 ± 4.0	10.0 ± 5.5*	10.0 ± 3.2*	10.0 ± 3.2	2.5 ± 2.5*	24.0 ± 4.0	18.0 ± 8.0	18.0 ± 5.7*	22.0 ± 5.8

*Significantly different from control ($p \leq 0.05$).

The most efficacious formulation was a viscous gel containing the peptide n-MeGRGDSP.

These studies showed that postoperative administration of RGD-containing peptides, which block a variety of integrin–ligand interactions, reduced adhesion formation in this animal model.

Conclusions

The field of integrin biology has been emerging and rapidly progressing during the past 15 years. Only recently has the contribution of these molecules to reproduction function (e.g., embryo implantation), gynecologic disease states (e.g., implantation of endometrium in endometriosis and metastatic tumors), and adhesion formation been recognized. As an example, recent work has indicated that administration of soluble RGD-containing peptides will reduce adhesion formation.[131] The complexity and promiscuity of these systems is only now being fully understood. A full appreciation of the contribution of this field of cellular biology to mesothelial healing is still in its infancy.

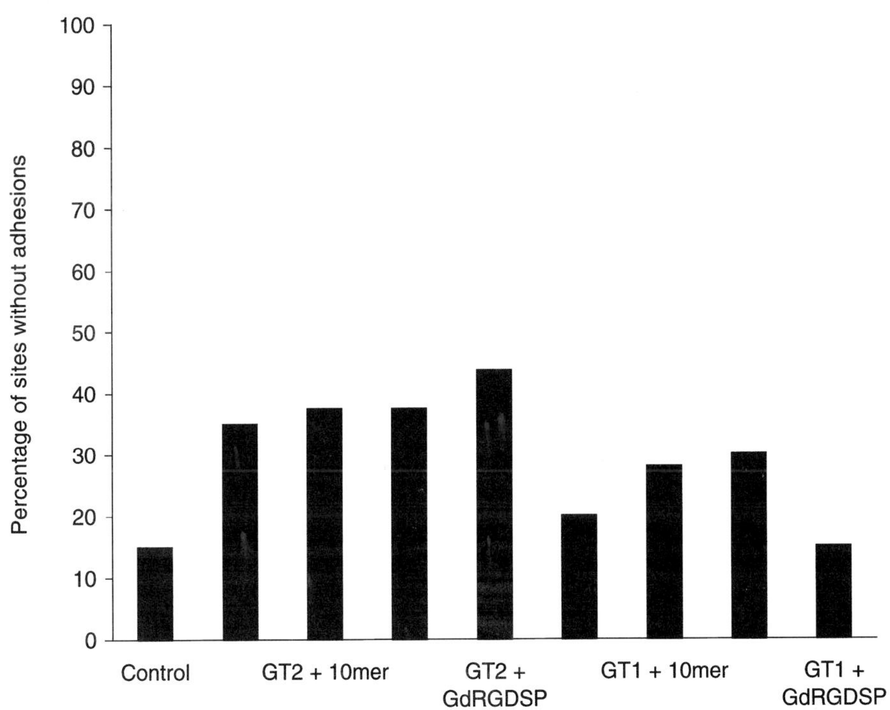

FIG. 6.6. Percentage of sites evaluated that did not form adhesions to the uterine horns after surgery.

References

1. Hynes RO. Integrins: a family of cell surface receptors. Cell 1987;48:549–554.
2. Ruoslahti E, Pierschabacher MD. New perspectives in cell adhesion: RGD and integrins. Science 1987;238:491–497.
3. Hynes R. Integrins: versatility, modulation, and signaling in cell adhesion. Cell 1992;69:11–25.
4. Helmer ME, Weitzman JB, Pasqualini R, et al. Structure, biochemical properties and biological functions of integrin cytoplasmic domains. In: Takada Y, ed. Integrins: The Biological Problem. Boca Raton: CRC Press, 1994:1–36.
5. Loftus JC, Smith JW, Ginsberg MH. Integrin-mediated cell adhesion: the extracellular face. J Biol Chem 1994;269: 325–338.
6. Williams MJ, Hughes PE, O'Toole TE, et al. The inner world of cell adhesion: integrin cytoplasmic domains. Trends Cell Biol 1994;4:109–112.
7. Cepek KL, Shaw SK, Parker CM, et al. Adhesion between epithelial cells and T lymphocytes mediated by E-cadherin and the alpha E beta 7 integrin. Nature (Lond) 1994; 372:190–193.
8. Juliano RL, Haskill S. Signal transduction from the extracellular matrix. J Cell Biol 1993;120:577–585.
9. Ruoslahti E, Reed JC. Anchorage dependence, integrins and apoptosis. Cell 1994;77:477–478.
10. Werb Z, Tremble PM, Behrendtsen O, et al. Signal transduction through the fibronectin receptor induces collagenase and stromelysin gene expression. J Cell Biol 1989; 109:877–889.
11. Streuli CH, Bailey N, Bissell MJ. Control of mammary epithelial differentiation: basement membrane induces tissue-specific gene expression in the absence of cell-cell interaction and morphological polarity. J Cell Biol 1991;115: 1383–1395.
12. Miyake S, Yagita H, Maruyama T, et al. Beta 1 integrin-mediated interaction with extracellular matrix proteins regulates cytokine gene expression in synovial fluid cells of rheumatoid arthritis patients. J Exp Med 1993;177: 863–868.
13. Damjanovich L, Albelda SM, Mette SA, et al. Distribution of integrin cell adhesion receptors in normal and malignant lung tissue. Am J Respir Cell Mol Biol 1992;6: 197–206.
14. Mette SA, Pilewski J, Buck CA, et al. Distribution of integrin cell adhesion receptors on normal bronchial epithelial cells and lung cancer cells in vitro and in vivo. Am J Respir Cell Mol Biol 1993;8:562–572.
15. Paallysaho T, Tervo T, Virtanen I, et al. Integrins in the normal and healing corneal epithelium. Acta Ophthalmol Suppl 1992;202:22–25.
16. Stepp MA, Spurr-Michaud S, Gipson IK. Integrins in the wounded and unwounded stratified squamous epithelium of the cornea. Invest Ophthalmol Visual Sci 1993;34: 1829–1844.
17. Stewart M, Thiel M, Hogg N. Leukocyte integrins. Curr Opin Cell Biol 1995;7:690–696.
18. Helmer ME. Structures and functions of VLA proteins and related integrins. In: Mecham RP, McDonald JA, eds. Receptors for Extracellular Matrix. New York: Academic Press, 1991:255–299.
19. Hogg N, Landis RC, Bates PA, et al. The sticking point: how integrins bind to their ligands. Trends Cell Biol 1994;4:379–382.
20. Huttenlocher A, Sandborg RR, Horwitz A. Adhesion in cell migration. Curr Opin Cell Biol 1995;7:697–706.
21. Adams JC, Watt FM. Regulation of development and differeniation by the extracellular matrix. Development (Camb) 1993;117:1183–1198.
22. Tuckwell DS, Brass A, Humphries MJ. Homology modelling of integrin EF-hands. Evidence for widespread use of conserved cations-binding site. Biochem J 1992;285: 325–231.
23. Colombatti A, Bonaldo P. The superfamily of proteins with von Willebrand factor type A-like domains: one theme common to components of extracellular matrix, hemostasis, cellular adhesion, and defense mechanisms. Blood 1991;77:2305–2325.
24. Lee JO, Bankston LA, Arnaout MA, et al. Two conformations of the integrin A-domain (I-domain): a pathway for activation. Structure (Lond) 1995;3:1333–1340.
25. Qu A, Leahy DJ. Crystal structure of the I-domain from the CD11a/CD18(LFA-1.$\alpha_L\beta_2$) integrin. Proc Natl Acad Sci USA 1995;92:10277–10281.
26. diZerega GS, Rodgers KE. Intraperitoneal adhesions. In: The Peritoneum. New York: Springer-Verlag, 1992: 274–306.
27. Thornton M, diZerega GS. The use of barriers in adhesion prevention. Contemp Obstet Gynaecol 1996;41:201–214.
28. Menzies D, Ellis H. Intestinal obstruction from adhesions—how big is the problem? Ann R Coll Surg Engl 1990;72:62–63.
29. DeCherney AH, diZerega GS. Clinical problem of intraperitoneal postsurgical adhesion formation following general surgery and the use of adhesion prevention barriers. Surg Clin North Am 1997;77:671–688.
30. Blanco J. Bowel obstruction related to prior gynecologic surgery. In: Pelvic Surgery—Adhesion Formation and Prevention. New York: Springer-Verlag, 1997:160.
31. Federmann G, Walenzyk J, Schneider A, Scheele C, Bauermeister G. Efficacy of laparoscopy in treatment of acute small bowel obstruction caused by adhesions. In: Peritoneal Adhesions. New York: Springer-Verlag, 1997: 291.
32. Treutner KH, Bertram P, Latzsch G, Schumpelick V. Causes of intestinal obstruction—a retrospective study of 550 surgical cases. In: Peritoneal Adhesions. New York: Springer-Verlag, 1997:1991.
33. Ratcliff JB, Kapernick P, Brook GG, et al. Small bowel obstruction of gynecologic surgery. S Med J 1983;76: 1349–1360.
34. Strickler B, Blanco J, Fox HE. The gynecologic contribution to intestinal obstruction in females. J Am Coll Surg 1994;178:617–623.
35. Stout AL, Steege JF, Dodson WC, Hughes CL. Relationship of laparoscopic findings to self-report of pelvic pain. Am J Obstet Gynecol 1991;146:73–79.
36. Peters AAW, Trimbos-Kemper TCM, Admiraal C, et al. A randomized clinical trial on the benefit of adhesiolysis in patients with intraperitoneal adhesions and chronic pelvic pain. Br J Obstet Gynaecol 1992;99:59.

37. Trimbos-Kemper TCM, Trimbos JB, van Hall EV. Adhesion formation after tubal surgery: results of the eight-day laparoscopy in 188 patients. Fertil Steril 1985;43:396.
38. Marana R, Rizzi M, Ludovico M. Adhesions and infertility. In: Pelvic Surgery—Adhesion Formation and Prevention. New York: Springer-Verlag, 1997:126.
39. Lundorff P. Infertility and ectopic pregnancy. In: Pelvic Surgery—Adhesion Formation and Prevention. New York: Springer-Verlag, 1997:144.
40. Bakkum E, Peters AAW. Clinical significance of adhesion in patients with chronic pelvic pain. In: Pelvic Surgery—Adhesion Formation and Prevention. New York: Springer-Verlag, 1997:150.
41. Yamada KM. Cell surface interactions with extracellular materials. Annu Rev Biochem 1983;52:761–799.
42. Hynes RO. Molecular biology of fibronectin. Annu Rev Cell Biol 1985;1:67–90.
43. Hynes RO, Yamada KM. Fibronectin: multifunctional modular glycoproteins. J Cell Biol 1982;95:369–377.
44. Mohri H. Fibronectin and integrin interaction. J Invest Med 1996;44:3429–3441.
45. Mosher DF. Physiology of fibronectin. Annu Rev Med 1984;35:561–575.
46. Petersen TE, Skorstengaard K. Fibronectins. In: McDonagh J, ed. Hematology, Vol. 5. New York: Dekker, 1985: 7–30.
47. Voss B, Allah S, Rauterberg J, et al. Primary cultures of rat hepatocytes synthesize fibronectin. Biochem Biophys Res Commun 1979;90:1348–1354.
48. Macarak EJ, Kirby E, Kirk T, et al. Synthesis of cold-insoluble globulin by cultured calf endothelial cells. Proc Natl Acad Sci USA 1978;75:3273–3277.
49. Villiger B, Kelly DG, Engleman W, et al. Human alveolar macrophage fibronectin—synthesis, secretion and ultrastructural localization during gelatin-coated latex particle binding. J Cell Biol 1981;90:711–720.
50. Schwarzbauer JE, Paul JI, Hynes RO. On the origin of species of fibronectin. Proc Natl Acad Sci USA 1985;82: 1424–1428.
51. Kornblihtt AR, Umezawa K, Vibe-Pederson K, et al. Primary structure of human plasma fibronectin: differential splicing may generate at least 10 polypeptides from a single gene. EMBO J 1985;4:1755–1759.
52. Skorstengaard K, Jensen MS, Petersen TE, et al. Purification and complete primary structures of the heparin-, cell-, and DNA-binding domains of bovine plasma fibronectin. Eur J Biochem 1986;154:15–29.
53. Pierschbacher MD, Rouslahti E. Cell attachment activity of fibronectin can be duplicated by small synthetic fragments of the molecule. Nature (Lond) 1984;309:30–33.
54. Humphries MJ, Komoriya A, Akiyama SK, et al. Identification of two distinct regions of the type III connecting segment of human plasma fibronectin that promote cell type-specific adhesion. J Biol Chem 1987;262:6886–6892.
55. Mould AP, Komiyama A, Yamada KM, et al. The CS5 peptide is a second site in the IIICS region of fibronectin recognized by the integrin $\alpha_4\beta_1$. J Biol Chem 1991;266: 3579–3585.
56. Wayner E, Garcia-Pardo A, Humphries MJ, et al. Identification and characterization of the T lymphocyte adhesion receptor for an alternative cell attachment domain (CS-1) in plasma fibronectin. J Cell Biol 1989;109:1321–1330.
57. Fujita H, Mohri H, Kanamori H, et al. Binding site in human plasma fibronectin to HI-60 cells localizes in the C-terminal heparin-binding region independently of RGD and CSI. Exp Cell Res 1995;217:484–489.
58. McCarthy JB, Chelberg MK, Mickelson DJ, et al. Localization and chemical synthesis of fibronectin peptides with melonoma adhesion and heparin binding activities. Biochemistry 1988;75:3273–3277.
59. McCarthy JB, Hagen ST, Furcht LT. Human fibronectin contains distinct adhesion and motility promoting domains for metastatic melanoma cells. J Cell Biol 1986;102:179–188.
60. McCarthy JB, Skubitz APN, Shao Q, et al. RGD-independent cell adhesion to the carboxy-terminal heparin-binding fragment of fibronectin involves heparin-dependent and -independent activities. J Cell Biol 1990;110:777–787.
61. Mugnai G, Lewandowska K, Carnemolla B, et al. Modulation of matrix adhesive responses of human neuroblastoma cells by neighboring sequence in the fibronectin. J Cell Biol 1988;106:931–943.
62. Hormann H, Seidl M. Affinity chromatography on immobilized fibrin monomer III; the fibrin affinity center of fibronectin. Hoppe-Seyler's Z Chem 1980;361:1449–1452.
63. McKown-Longo PJ, Mosher DF. Interaction of the 70,000-mol-wt amino-terminal fragment of fibronectin with the matrix-assembly receptor of fibroblasts. J Cell Biol 1985; 100:364–374.
64. Quade B, McDonald JA. Fibronectin's amino-terminal matrix assembly site is located within the 29-kDa amino-terminal domain containing five type I repeats. J Biol Chem 1988;253:19602–19609.
65. Schwarzbauer JE. Identification of the fibronectin sequences required for assembly of a fibrillar matrix. J Cell Biol 1991;113:1463–1473.
66. Dzamba BJ, Bultmann H, Akiyama SK, et al. Substrate specific binding of the amino terminus of fibronectin to an integrin complex in focal adhesions. J Biol Chem 1994; 269:19646–19652.
67. Sottile J, Schwarzbauer J, Selegue J, et al. Five type 1 modules of fibronectin form a functional unit that binds to fibroblasts and *Staphylococcus aureus*. J Biol Chem 1991;266: 12840–12843.
68. Parise LV, Phillips DR. Reconstitution of the purified platelet fibrinogen receptor. Fibrinogen binding properties of the glycoprotein IIb-IIIa complex. J Biol Chem 1985;160:10698–10707.
69. Weisel JW, Nagaswami C, Vilaire G, et al. Examination of the platelet membrane glycoprotein IIb-IIIa complex and its interaction with fibrinogen and other ligands by electron microscopy. J Biol Chem 1992;267:16637–16643.
70. Plow EF, D'Souza SE, Ginsberg MH. Ligand binding to GP IIb–IIIa: a status report. Semin Thromb Hemostasis 1992; 18:324–332.
71. Niessen CM, Hogervorst F, Jaspars LH, et al. The alpha-6 beta-4 integrin is a receptor for both laminin and kalinin. Exp Cell Res 1994;211:360–367.
72. Lee EC, Lotz MM, Steele GD Jr, Mercurio AM. The integrin alpha-6 beta-4 is a laminin receptor. J Cell Biol 1992; 117:671–678.

73. Sepp NT, Cornelius LA, Romani LJ, et al. Polarized expression and basic fibroblast growth factor-induced down regulation of the alpha-6 beta-4 integrin complex on human microvascular endothelial cells. J Invest Dermatol 1995;104:266–270.
74. Furie MB, Cramer EB, Naprstek BL, et al. Cultured endothelial cell monolayers that restrict the transendothelial passage of macromolecules and electrical current. J Cell Biol 1984;98:1033–1041.
75. Springer TA. Traffic signals on endothelium for lymphocyte recirculation and leukocyte emigration. Annu Rev Physiol 1995;57:827–872.
76. Martin GR, Timpl R. Laminin and other basement membrane components. Annu Rev Cell Biol 1987;3:57–85.
77. Beck K, Hunter I, Engel J. Structure and function of laminin: anatomy of a multidomain glycoprotein. FASEBJ 1990;4:148–160.
78. Yurchenco PD, O'Rear JJ. Basal lamina assembly. Curr Opin Cell Biol 1994;6:674–681.
79. Mercurio AM. Laminin receptors—achieving specificity through cooperation. Trends Cell Biol 1995;5:419–423.
80. Burgeson RE, Chiquet M, Deutzmann R, et al. A new nomenclature for the laminins. Matrix Biol 1994;14: 209–211.
81. Shaw LM, Messier JM, Mercurio AM. The activation dependent adhesion of macrophages to laminin involves cytoskeletal anchoring and phosphorylation of the α_6 β_1 integrin. J Cell Biol 1990;110:2167–2174.
82. Shaw LM, Lotz MM, Mercurio AM. Inside-out integrin signaling in macrophages. Analysis of the role of the $\alpha_6 A\beta_1$ and $\alpha_6\beta_1$ integrin variants in laminin adhesion by cDNA expression in an α_6 integrin-deficient macrophage cell line. J Biol Chem 1993;268:11401–11408.
83. Bohnsack JF, Akiyama SK, Damsky CH, et al. Human neutrophil adherence to laminin in vitro. Evidence for a distinct neutrophil integrin receptor for laminin. J Exp Med 1990;171:1221–1237.
84. Shimizu Y, Van Seventer GA, Horgan KJ, et al. Regulated expression and binding of three VLA (β1) integrin receptors on T cells. Nature (Lond) 1990;345:250–253.
85. Weber C, Alon R, Moser B. Sequential regulation of α4β1 and α5β1 integrin avidity by CC chemokines in monocytes—implications for transendothelial chemotaxis. J Cell Biol 1996;134:1063–1073.
86. Dobbie JW. Morphology of the peritoneum in CAPD. Curr Concepts CAPD Blood Purif 1989;7:74–85.
87. Di Paolo N, Sacchi G. Anatomy and physiology of the peritoneal membrane. Contrib Nephrol 1990;84:10–26.
88. Spuiijbroek M, Dunselman G, Menheere P, et al. Early endometriosis invades the extracellular matrix. Fertil Steril 1992;58:929–933.
89. Witz CA, Montoya-Rodriguez IA, Miller BS, et al. Mesothelium expression of integrins in vivo and in vitro. J Soc Gynecol Invest 1998;5:87–93.
90. van der Linden P, de Goeij A, Dunselman G, et al. Expression of integrins and E-cadherin in cells from menstrual effluent, endometrium, peritoneal fluid, peritoneum and endometriosis. Fertil Steril 1994;51:85–90.
91. Kurk PA, Uitto VJ, Firth JD, et al. Reciprocal interactions between human ovarian surface epithelial cells and adjacent extracellular matrix. Exp Cell Res 1994;215:97–108.
92. Gardner MJ, Jones LMH, Catterall JB, et al. Expression of cell adhesion molecules on ovarian tumour cell lines and mesothelial cells, in relation to ovarian cancer metastasis. Cancer Lett 1995;91:229–234.
93. Jonjic N, Peri G, Bernasconi S, et al. Expression of adhesion molecules and chemotactic cytokines in cultured human mesothelial cells. J Exp Med 1992;176:1165–1174.
94. Cannistra SA, Ottensmeier C, Niloff J, et al. Expression and functions of β1 and αvβ3 integrins in ovarian cancer. Gynecol Oncol 1995;58:216–225.
95. Tabibzadeh S. Evidence of T-cell activation and potential cytokine action in human endometrium. J Clin Endocrinol Metab 1990;71:645–649
96. Bosman FT. Integrins: cell adhesives and modulators of cell function. Histochem J 1993;25:469–477.
97. Bennett JS, Vilaire G. Exposure of platelet fibrinogen receptors by ADP and epinephrine. J Clin Invest 1979; 64:1393–1401.
98. Marguerie GA, Plow EF, Edgington TS. Human platelets possess an inducible and saturable receptor specific for fibrinogen. J Biol Chem 1979;254:5357–5363.
99. Haverstick DM, Cowan JF, Yamada KM, et al. Inhibition of platelet adhesion to fibronectin, fibrinogen, and von Willebrand factor substrates by a synthetic tetrapeptide derived from the cell-binding domain of fibronectin. Blood 1985;66:946–952.
100. Plow EF, McEver RP, Coller BS, et al. Related binding mechanisms for fibrinogen, fibronectin, von Willebrand factor, and thrombospondin on thrombin-stimulated human platelets. Blood 1985;66:724–727.
101. Ruggeri ZM, De Marco L, Gatti L, et al. Platelets have more than one binding site for von Willebrand factor. J Clin Invest 1983;72:1–12.
102. Pytela RP, Pierschbacher MD, Ginsberg MH, et al. Platelet membrane glycoprotein IIb/IIa: member of a family of Arg-Gly-Asp-specific adhesion receptors. Science 1986; 231:1559–1562.
103. Peerschke EIB, Galanakis DK. The synthetic RGDS peptide inhibits the binding of fibrinogen lacking intact alpha chain carboxy terminal sequences to human blood platelets. Blood 1987;69:950–952.
104. Plow EF, Pierschbacker MD, Ruoslahti E, et al. Arginyl-glycyl-aspartic acid sequences and fibrinogen binding to platelets. Blood 1987;70:110–115.
105. Hawiger J, Timmons S, Kloczewiak M, et al. Gamma and alpha chains of human fibrinogen possess sites reactive with human platelet receptors. Proc Natl Acad Sci USA 1983;79:2068–2071.
106. Farrell DH, Thiagarajan P, Chung DW, et al. Role of fibrinogen α and γ chain sites in platelet aggregation. Proc Natl Acad Sci USA 1992;89:10729–10732.
107. Lam SC-T. Isolation and characterization of a chymotryptic fragment of platelet GOIIb-IIIa retaining Arg-Gly-Asp binding activity. J Biol Chem 1992;267:5649–5655.
108. Calvete JJ, Rivas G, Mauri M, et al. Tryptic fragment of human glycoprotein IIIa. Isolation and biochemical characterization of the 23-kDa N-terminal glycopeptide carrying the antigenic determinant for a monoclonal antibody (P37) which inhibits platelet aggregation. Biochem J 1988;250:697–704.

109. Wippler J, Kouns WC, Schlaeger EJ, et al. The integrin $\alpha_{IIb}\beta_3$, platelet membrane glyco-protein IIb-IIIa, can form a functionally active heterodimer complex without the cysteine rich repeats of the β_3 subunit. J Biol Chem 1994;89:7890–7894.
110. Loftus JC, Halloran CE, Ginsberg MH, et al. The amino-terminal one-third of α_{IIb} defines the ligand recognition specificity of integrin $\alpha_{IIb}\beta_3$. J Biol Chem 1996;271: 2033–2039.
111. Neri D, Monigiani S, Kirkham PM. Biophysical methods for the determination of antigen-antibody affinities. Trends Biochem Sci 1996;14:465–470.
112. Sastry SK, Horwitz AF. Adhesion-growth factor interactions during differentiation: an integrated biological response. Dev Biol 1996;180:455–467.
113. Miyamoto S, Teramoto H, Gutkind JS, et al. Integrins can collaborate with growth factors for phosphorylation of receptor tyrosine kinases and MPA kinase activation: roles of integrin aggregation and occupancy of receptors. J Cell Biol 1996;135:1633–1642.
114. Juliano R. Cooperation between soluble factors and integrin-mediated cell anchorage in the control of cell growth and differentiation. Bioassays 1996;18:911–917.
115. Peerschke EI. Regulation of platelet aggregation by post-fibrinogen binding events. Thromb Haemostasis 1995; 73:862–867.
116. Yamada KM, Geiger B. Molecular interactions in cell adhesion complexes. Curr Opin Cell Biol 1997;9:76–85.
117. Parsons JT, Schaller MD, Hildebrand J, et al. Focal adhesion kinase: structure and signalling. J Cell Sci Suppl 1994;18:109–113.
118. Hanks SK, Polte TR. Signaling through focal adhesion kinase. Bioassays 1997;19:137–145.
119. O'Toole TE, Katagiri Y, Faull RJ, et al. Integrin cytoplasmic domains mediate inside-out signaling. J Cell Biol 1994;135:1047–1059.
120. Hughes PE, O'Toole TE, Ylanne J, et al. The conserved membrane-proximal region of an integrin cytoplasmic domain specifies ligand-binding affinity. J Biol Chem 1995;270:12411–12417.
121. Schwartz MA, Schaller MD, Ginsberg MH. Integrins: emerging paradigms of signal transduction. Annu Rev Cell Biol 1995;11:549–599.
122. Assoian RK, Zhu XY. Cell anchorage and the cytoskeleton as partners in growth factor dependent cell cycle progression. Curr Opin Cell Biol 1997;9:93–98.
123. Boudreau N, Myers C, Bissell MJ. From laminin to lamin-regulation of tissue-specific gene expression by the ECM. Trends Cell Biol 1995;5:1–4.
124. Eigenthaler ML, Hofferer SJ, Shattil SJ, et al. A conserved sequence motif in the integrin $\beta3$ cytoplasmic domain is required for its specific interaction with $\beta3$-endonexin. J Biol Chem 1997;272:7693–7698.
125. Kolanus W, Nagel W, Schiller B, et al. Alpha-$_L$-beta-2 integrin/LFA-1 binding to ICAM-1 induced by cytohesin-1, a cytoplasmic regulatory molecule. Cell 1996;86:233–242.
126. Kashiwagi H, Schwartz MA, Eigenthaler MA, et al. Affinity modulation of platelet integrin α_{IIb} β_3 by β_3-endonexin, a selective binding partner of the β_3 integrin cytoplasmic tail. J Cell Biol 1997;137:1433–1443.
127. Copponlino M, Leung-Hagesteijn C, Dedhar S, et al. Inducible interaction of integrin $\alpha_2\beta_1$ with calreticulin—dependence on the activation state of the integrin. J Biol Chem 1995;135:1913–1923.
128. Opas M, Szewczenko-Pawlikowski M, Jass GJ, et al. Calreticulin modulates cell adhesiveness via regulation of vinculin expression. J Cell Biol 1996;135:1913–1923.
129. Zhu Q, Zlinka P, White T, et al. Calreticulin-integrin bidirectional signaling complex. Biochem Biophys Res Commun 1997;232:354–358.
130. Coppolino MG, Woodside MJ, Demaurex N, et al. Calreticulin is essential for integrin-mediated calcium signalling and cell adhesion. Nature (Lond) 1997;386: 843–847.
131. Rodgers KE, Girgis W, Campeau J, et al. Reduction of adhesion formation by intraperitoneal administration of Arg-Gly-Asp-containing peptides. Fertil Steril 1998; 70(6): 1131–1138.

7

Proteases and Protease Inhibitors in Tissue Repair

William C. Parks and Gregory S. Schultz

CONTENTS

Healing of wounds in the peritoneum and the skin may seem to be quite different, but at the molecular level they share many common aspects. For example, both peritoneal and skin wound healing involve inflammation, chemotactic migration, mitosis and differentiation of wound cells, and synthesis or remodeling of extracellular matrix. In this chapter, we describe the roles of matrix metalloproteinases and their tissue inhibitors in normal and abnormal wound healing in the skin.

Matrix Metalloproteinases in Wound Healing

The matrix metalloproteinases (MMPs) comprise a gene family of enzymes that share important common properties.[1] Their catalytic mechanism requires an active site Zn^{2+}; they are secreted as inactive zymogens; they can degrade various components of the extracellular matrix;

and their proteolytic activity is inhibited by tissue-derived inhibitors, called TIMPs (tissue inhibitors of metalloproteinases). In addition, the various metalloproteinases share a high degree of structural similarity, reflected by about 40% amino acid homology among all members of the family. To date, more than 17 different MMPs, each representing distinct gene products, have been characterized and additional members of this gene family continue to be identified. Detailed information about the MMP family can be found in recent reviews.[2,3]

Classification of Matrix Metalloproteinases

Five major classes of matrix metalloproteinases are involved in wound repair: collagenases, gelatinases, stromelysins, membrane-type metalloproteinases, and other matrix metalloproteinases. MMPs are categorized by their capacity to degrade various extracellular matrix substrates, a property that is conferred by constituent structural domains.

Collagenases

The best characterized, and historically oldest, subgroup of MMPs are the interstitial collagenases, which possess the unique ability to cleave native type I, II, and III collagens.[4] These types of collagen molecules are designated as fibrillar collagens because they are rigid rods formed by the triple helix of three collagen protein chains. The fibrillar collagen molecules associate in a head-to-tail and side-by-side arrangement to form a fibril, and multiple fibrils associate to form a collagen fiber that has extremely high tensile strength (resistance to breaking). Intact collagen fibrils are very resistant to proteolytic destruction by most enzymes except collagenases. Three interstitial collagenases have been identified, all of which cleave native type I collagen at a single locus (at Gly775-Ile776 in the α_1 chain and at Gly775-Leu776 in α_2), which is located about three-fourths of the distance from the N-terminus of the collagen molecule. At physiologic temperature (37°C), the three-fourths and one-fourth length fragments of collagenase digestion denature spontaneously into randomly coiled gelatin peptides and can be further attacked by a variety of enzymes, including the gelatinases. However, the single cleavage of the collagen triple helix catalyzed by interstitial collagenases is the rate-limiting step of collagen degradation, and these enzymes are believed to be uniquely capable of initiating type I collagen degradation in vivo at neutral pH.[5]

Of the three known human metallocollagenases, collagenase-1 (MMP-1) seems to be the enzyme that is principally responsible for collagen turnover in most tissues. In a variety of normal and disease-associated tissue remodeling events, collagenase-1 may be expressed by epithelial cells, fibroblasts, endothelial cells, chondrocytes, and macrophages.[6–11] Collagenase-2 (MMP-8) is found only in neutrophils and chondrocytes,[12,13] and collagenase-3 (MMP-13), originally cloned from a breast carcinoma line,[14] is also expressed in articular cartilage[15,16] and developing bone.[17,18]

Gelatinases

There are two metallogelatinases, of M_r 72,000 and 92,000, which possess virtually identical substrate specificity, but are expressed in different tissues and are subject to distinct regulation.[19,20] The 72-kDa gelatinase (gelatinase A, MMP-2) is produced by most mesenchyme-derived cell types, including fibroblasts, osteoblasts, and smooth muscle cells, but unlike other metalloproteinases, its expression is not markedly regulated by cytokines, growth factors, or hormones, with the exception of transforming growth factor-β (TGF-β).[21] This paucity of regulatory modification most likely reflects the lack of an AP-1 sequence in its promoter, a unique property of 72-kDa gelatinase as compared to all other MMPs. The 92-kDa gelatinase (gelatinase B, MMP-9) is actively expressed by eosinophils,[22,23] monocytes/macrophages, and epithelial-derived cells (e.g., keratinocytes) and is stored by neutrophils.[12,22] The MMP-9 promoter contains two AP-1 sites, and its expression is subject to modification by a variety of physiologic signals.[24] Both gelatinases are able to degrade all types of denatured collagens to small fragments, but are able to degrade type I collagen only after the initial cleavage of intact collagen by MMP-1. In addition, MMP-2 and MMP-9 also degrade intact fibronectin and insoluble elastin, and the gelatinases can attack and degrade intact basement membranes containing native type IV collagen, which is the major type of collagen found in basement membranes.[25] Type IV collagen molecules are not straight, rigid rods like the fibrillar collagen molecules, but have bends in the triple helical region. This structure causes type IV collagen molecules to aggregate together into a sheet-like meshwork of polygonal shapes that ultimately form a multilayered network.

Stromelysins

The stromelysins are so designated because of their broad substrate specificity. Three stromelysins have been characterized, and two of these, stromelysin-1 (MMP-3) and stromelysin-2 (MMP-10), possess very similar catalytic activity but exhibit quite different gene regulation.[26] Stromelysin-1 and -2 are strong proteoglycanases and can also degrade basement membranes, laminin, fibronectin, and the nonhelical telopeptides of some collagens (e.g., types IV and IX).[25] Proteoglycans are large molecules that contain a core protein which is linked to many long carbohydrate chains. Proteoglycans bind large amounts of water because of their enormous carbohydrate content and provide compressibility to the extracellular matrix. The third stromelysin, stromelysin-3 (MMP-11), appears to exhibit only weak and limited proteolytic activity[27] and on the basis of structural distinctions may not be a true MMP.[1]

Membrane-Type Metalloproteinases

A group of four novel MMPs (MMP-14, MMP-15, MMP-16, and MMP-17) possess a transmembrane domain that directs these enzymes to the cell surface where they may activate the pro-forms of other MMPs, such as 72-kDa gelatinase and collagenase-3, or function as proteinases during cell migration.[28] The MMPs are called membrane-type MMPs or MT-MMPs and are often designated MT1-MMP, MT2-MMP, MT3-MMP, and MT4-MMP.

Other Matrix Metalloproteinases

Matrilysin (MMP-7) is the smallest matrix metalloproteinase (M_r 28,000) but possesses broad and potent catalytic activity against extracellular matrix (ECM) substrates and nonmatrix proteins.[29] Matrilysin is a stronger proteoglycanase than stromelysin-1,[30] and also degrades basement membranes, insoluble elastin, laminin, fibronectin, gelatin, and entactin.[25,31] Matrilysin appears to be produced only by a select population of cell types, most prominent of which are the glandular epithelium of a variety of tissues including the endometrium, breast, prostate, pancreas, and parotid, and sweat glands of the skin.[29] Macrophage metalloelastase (MMP-12) possesses high specific activity against insoluble elastin but can also degrade many other matrix proteins.[32] Metalloelastase may have the most limited cellular expression of MMPs, being essentially only produced by tissue macrophages.

Tissue Inhibitors of Metalloproteinases

The overall activities of MMPs in a wound environment are determined by several parameters including the rate of synthesis of MMPs, the activation of latent MMPs, and the levels of specific inhibitor proteins of MMPs, the tissue inhibitors of metalloproteinases or TIMPs. To date, four such TIMPs have been characterized and are designated TIMP-1, TIMP-2, TIMP-3, and TIMP-4. TIMPs block the catalytic activity of MMPs but have no efficacy against serine, sulfhydryl, or acid proteases. In addition to their metalloproteinase inhibitory effects, the TIMPs have been reported to possess growth-promoting activities for a wide range of cells.[33] TIMP-1 forms a strong complex with activated MMP-1, MMP-2, and MMP-3. TIMP-2 binds and inhibits both active and latent forms of MMP-2.

Synthesis of MMPs and TIMPs is extensively regulated by growth factors and cytokines, and frequently there is coordinated synthesis of the MMPs, TIMPs, and ECM proteins by growth factors and cytokines. For example, interleukin-1 (IL-1), epidermal growth factor (EGF), and basic fibroblast growth factor (bFGF) upregulate the expression of MMP-1, MMP-3, TIMP-1, and collagen. TGF-β_1, which is a very powerful inducer of scar formation, upregulates collagen synthesis while downregulating MMP expression and upregulating TIMP-1 production by fibroblasts. These examples demonstrate how growth factors, cytokines, MMPs, and TIMPs regulate key processes of normal healing.

Domain Structure of Matrix Metalloproteinases

The MMPs are organized into structural domains that impart their specific biologic functions. All MMPs have a catalytic domain of 21 kDa that binds the active site Zn^{2+}. The Zn-coordinating region is highly conserved with three histidine residues representing three of four Zn-interactive ligands.[34] Single amino acid mutations introduced into this sequence render the enzyme catalytically inactive. This catalytic domain is also the site of TIMP interaction with active metalloenzyme and contributes to determining the substrate specificity of MMPs.[25,35] All MMPs also contain an N-terminal pro-domain of 8 kDa that maintains the enzymes in an inactive, or zymogen, state. This propeptide is characterized by the invariant sequence PRCGVPD, with the cysteine residue representing the fourth interactive ligand of the active site Zn^{2+}. Enzyme latency is conferred by this Cys–Zn interaction.[36] MMP zymogens can be activated by exposure to proteases, chaotropes, or sulfhydryl chelators, all of which disrupt the Cys–Zn association, causing the enzymes to cleave themselves by an intramolecular process at the start of their catalytic domain. Matrilysin, the smallest, and perhaps primordial MMP, contains only the pro-domain and the catalytic domain.

Other than matrilysin, all MMPs contain a 22-kDa C-terminal domain that has structural homology to the heme-binding protein, hemopexin. This domain has been implicated, at least partially, in two major MMP functions: determining their substrate specificity and modulating their interactions with TIMPs. The contribution of the hemopexin-like domain to substrate specificity is variable, but is most clearly illustrated in the case of interstitial collagenase. Here, truncation of the hemopexin-like domain yields an enzyme that can nonspecifically attack casein but is incapable of degrading type I collagen.[35] Furthermore, substitution of the hemopexin-like domain of stromelysin onto the collagenase catalytic domain fails to restore collagenolytic activity. For other enzymes, such as stromelysin[37] and the metallogelatinases,[35,38] however, C-terminal truncation does not appear to alter substrate specificity. The metallogelatinases are unique among the MMPs in the capacity of their zymogen forms to bind TIMPs. This TIMP-binding capacity of the metallogelatinase zymogens is conferred entirely by their hemopexin-like domains.[35,38] Furthermore, this domain also participates, in addition to the catalytic domain, in the binding of TIMP to all active MMPs.[39] The collagenases, stromelysins, and macrophage metalloelastase are composed of a catalytic domain, a pro-domain, and a hemopexin-like domain.

The metallogelatinases both contain three head-to-tail repeats of the Fn-2 domain of the cell adhesion protein, fibronectin. These Fn-2 repeats divide the catalytic domain of both gelatinases and are specifically responsible for the strong gelatin-binding affinity of these enzymes.[40] The 92-kDa gelatinase, in addition, contains a unique collagen-like domain, the function of which is unknown.

Roles of Matrix Metalloproteinases in Wound Repair

Collagenase-1 Expression in Skin Wounds: A Paradigm of the Role of Metalloproteinases in Tissue Repair

Tissue repair involves an orderly progression of events to reestablish the integrity of the injured tissue. The initial injury sets off a programmed series of interdependent yet separate responses, such as reepithelialization and epithelial proliferation, inflammation, angiogenesis, fibroplasia, matrix accumulation, remodeling, and eventually resolution. During each stage in this process, proteinases are needed to remove or remodel ECM components in both the epithelial and interstitial compartments, in part to accommodate cell migration and other ongoing events. Much of the knowledge of the patterns, function, and regulation of MMPs in tissue repair has been obtained from studies of cutaneous wounds and ulcers.

Reepithelialization of Skin Wounds

As shown in Fig. 7.1, collagenase-1 is prominently and invariably expressed by basal keratinocytes at the migratory front in all forms of cutaneous wounds with an injury that breaches the basement membrane, including normally healing wounds, burns in humans and animals, various forms of blisters, and chronic ulcers.[6–8] When detected in the dermis, the expression of collagenase-1 is typically low and confined to a few cells. Furthermore, collagenase mRNA or protein is always confined to the basal layer of the epidermis and diminishes progressively away from the wound edge. It is not detected in any cell in intact healthy skin. In wounded skin, collagenase-1 is not expressed by the hyperproliferative cells just behind the wound front that are residing on basement membrane or by suprabasal cells in intact or wounded skin. This restricted pattern of collagenase-1 expression suggests that the activity of collagenase-1 serves a beneficial role in reepithelialization. Indeed, keratinocyte migration on native collagen is completely blocked by treatment with a synthetic hydroxamate inhibitor of collagenase-1.[41]

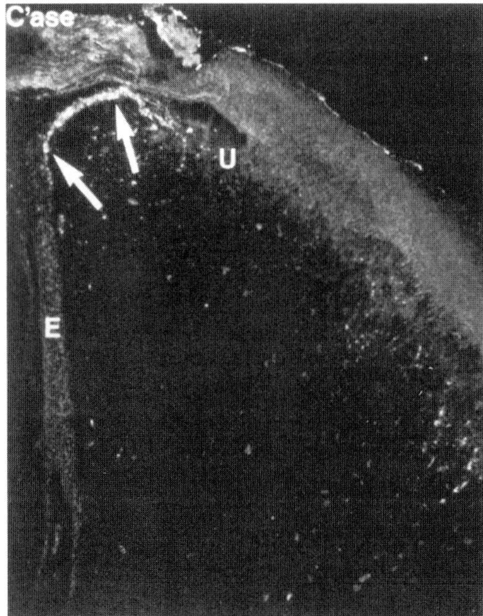

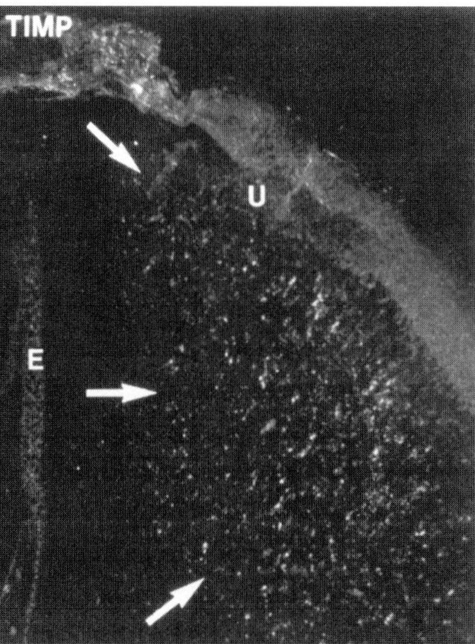

FIG. 7.1. Distinct localization of collagenase-1 and tissue inhibitor of metalloproteinase (TIMP-1) expression. Serial sections of ulcerated pyogenic granuloma were hybridized for collagenase-1 (C'ase) or TIMP-1 mRNAs. An ulceration (*U*) is indicated with underlying inflammatory cells; the adjacent epidermis (*E*) has formed an epithelial tongue to cover the defect. Collagenase-positive basal keratinocytes (*left*) are detected only at the migrating front of epithelium (*arrows*). In contrast, TIMP-positive cells (*right*) are found within the underlying granulation tissue (*bordered by arrows*), but not in epidermis. *Please see insert for color reproduction of this figure.*

Expression of collagenase-1 by migrating epithelial cells is specific to the skin. During repair of mucosal surfaces, such as in the colon and the airways, migrating epithelial cells do not express collagenase-1 but rather produce and release matrilysin (MMP-7), which is not produced in skin wounds.[42,43] Although the pattern of the expression of these two MMPs among tissues is similar, that is, both are expressed by migrating epithelium, the precise function of the enzymes and the events controlling their production are likely to be distinct.

Collagen Induces Collagenase-1 Expression

Because collagenase-1 was not detected in intact epidermis, disruption of the basement membrane and subsequent exposure of keratinocytes to the underlying dermal stroma may be a critical determinant for the induction of epidermal collagenolytic activity. Basal keratinocytes normally rest on a basement membrane composed of laminins, entactin/nidogen, proteoglycans, and type IV collagen. During wound healing, keratinocytes migrate from the edge of the wound under a provisional matrix of fibrin and fibronectin and over or through the viable dermis, which includes structural macromolecules, such as type I collagen, microfibrils, and elastin, distinct from those in the basement membrane. Thus, loss of contact with the basement membrane and establishment of new cell–matrix interactions with components of the dermal and provisional matrices may be a critical determinant that alters keratinocyte phenotype and induces collagenase-1 production.

Native type I collagen, the most abundant protein in the body, found in essentially all interstitial spaces, induces expression of collagenase-1 in keratinocytes, and this induction is mediated by high-affinity contact via the $\alpha_2\beta_1$ integrin.[41,44] Other molecules with which keratinocytes may interact include laminin-1, laminin-5, elastin, fibrinogen/fibrin, fibronectin, and type III collagen.[44] Gelatin, generated by heat denaturation, does not influence collagenase-1 expression. These findings support the idea that contact with native type I collagen is an important, if not the principal, determinant regulating the invariant expression of collagenase-1 by migrating keratinocytes during wound repair. Furthermore, these results imply that interaction with a matrix substrate influences the expression and release of a specific metalloproteinase. In turn, the product of proteolysis, gelatin, may repress MMP expression, thereby providing a feedback signal to accurately control the site and duration of proteinase release. This paradigm implies that the pericellular environment, and the matrix in particular, regulates the pattern and level of MMP expression.

Expression of Matrix Metalloproteinases in Other Epithelial Tissues

Matrilysin is expressed by migrating airway and colon epithelial cells that have migrated off a basement membrane and onto the underlying interstitium.[42,43] Collagenase-1 is not expressed in the injured epithelia of these other tissues, and matrilysin is not expressed by keratinocytes in skin wounds. Thus, the pattern of MMPs expressed in response to injury differs among tissues. Collagenase-1 facilitates migration of keratinocytes over the collagen-rich matrix of dermis, whereas matrilysin would be a more appropriate proteinase to remodel airway wall matrix components, which include elastin, adhesive glycoproteins, and proteoglycans that are substrates for matrilysin but not collagenase-1.

Inhibition of Collagen-Mediated Induction of Collagenase-1

As epithelial wounds heal, collagenase-1 production ceases. Two major processes promote the downregulation of collagenase-1. One is cell–cell contact. Even though confluent epithelial cells are in contact with type I collagen, they do not express collagenase-1. The second is contact with specific basement membrane proteins such as laminin. Laminin-1 is deposited in the newly formed basement membrane just behind the migrating front of epidermis and inhibits keratinocyte migration. As reepithelialization progresses, the mass of laminin-1 deposited under the previously migrating keratinocytes accumulates, providing a site-specific mechanism to downregulate collagenase-1 expression. Consistent with this idea, relatively small concentrations of laminin-1 can block the inductive effect of native type I collagen.[44] Assuming one binding event per molecule, one laminin-1 molecule effectively blocked the induction of collagenase-1 mediated by about 3000 collagen molecules. Because type I collagen is so abundant in the dermis, it is not surprising that the inhibitory effect of laminin-1 is so potent.

Tissue Inhibitor of Metalloproteinase-1 in Wounds

Although dermal collagen induces collagenase-1 expression, other factors in the wound environment may affect collagenase-1 expression and activity. Keratinocytes are capable of secreting TIMP-1 in vitro, but TIMP-1 mRNA seldom colocalizes with collagenase-1 mRNA in migrating keratinocytes in wounds.[6,8] The distinct localization of enzyme and inhibitor suggests that keratinocyte-derived collagenase-1 acts without impedance from TIMP-1, and this actually makes sense. As for most biologic processes, matrix degradation is a precise event. Proteinases are produced and released on demand from cells activated to degrade matrix proteins. By means of specific cell-surface receptors, the cell recognizes a particular matrix molecule and is instructed to produce the appropriate metalloproteinase, which is then released into the pericellular space where it degrades its specific substrate. It is possible that sites of matrix degradation are isolated by reorganization of the cell membrane, analogous to the ruffled border of osteoclasts. As the cell moves beyond the site of matrix degradation, excess or spent proteinase would spill into the open extracellular space. Thus, TIMPs may act in the tissue environment to neutralize 'spent' proteinases, thereby preventing excessive and unwanted degradation away from the sites of metalloproteinase production. The presence of TIMP-1 beneath the epidermis may provide a mechanism to contain collagenolytic activity to the epidermal front.

Expression of Cytokines and Collagenase by Keratinocytes

Expression of collagenase-1 is also regulated by many soluble factors, and these may have a role in modulating expression in normal wounds and in overexpression of proteinase in chronic wounds.[24,45] Collagenase-1 expression is upregulated by hepatocyte growth factor (HGF), but interestingly, this stimulation was seen only in keratinocytes plated on collagen, not in cells on gelatin.[43] Furthermore, basic fibroblast growth factor (bFGF or FGF-2) and keratinocyte growth factor (KGF) repress collagenase-1 production in keratinocytes but stimulate enzyme production in mesenchymal cells.[41] TGF-β_1 is considered to be a fibrogenic factor because it stimulates production of structural matrix proteins and TIMP-1, while repressing expression of collagenase-1 in fibroblasts.[45] In keratinocytes, however, TGF-β_1 stimulates collagenase-1 production.[45] Similarly, interferon-γ upregulates collagenase-1 production in keratinocytes but inhibits expression in dermal fibroblast. Collectively, these findings indicate that the regulation of collagenase-1 in keratinocytes is unique compared to that in other cell types.

Expression of Stromelysin in Wound Repair

Other MMPs are expressed by human keratinocytes during wound repair. For example, stromelysin-2 (MMP-10) is produced by the same basal keratinocytes that express collagenase-1, whereas stromelysin-1 (MMP-3) is seen in a spatially distinct population of basal keratinocytes adjacent to but removed from the wound edge. Unlike collagenase-1 and stromelysin-1, expression of stromelysin-2 is confined strictly to the epidermis. Because stromelysins can activate procollagenase, stromelysin-2 may have a role in regulating collagenolytic activity at the migratory front of the epidermis.[26] Similar to collagenase-1, stromelysin-2 may facilitate keratinocyte migration by degrading noncollagenous matrix molecules or by removing damaged basement membrane.

As shown in Fig. 7.2, stromelysin-1 is also expressed in the basal epidermis, but the keratinocytes expressing this metalloproteinase are removed from the migrating front and are in contact with an intact basement

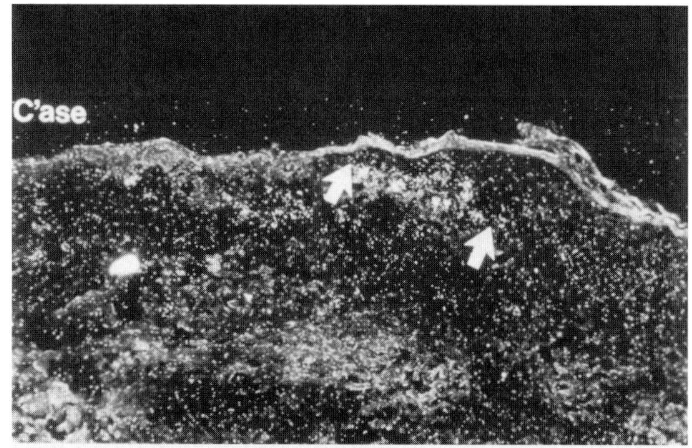

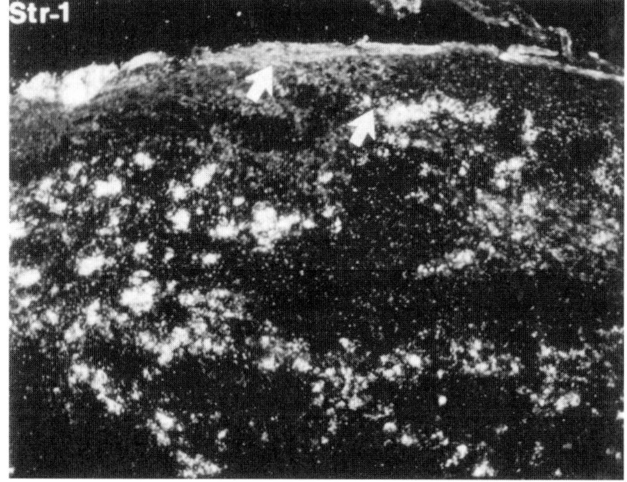

FIG. 7.2. Collagenase-1 (*top*) and stromelysin-1 (*bottom*) are expressed in distinct areas of the healing epidermis. Serial sections of a nonspecific ulcer were hybridized with ^{35}S-labeled antisense RNA probes for collagenase-1 (C'ase) and stromelysin-1 (Str-1) mRNAs. The migrating front of the epidermis, adjacent to an ulceration (*U*) in the upper left corner, is indicated by *large arrows*. Signal for collagenase-1 mRNA was detected only in basal keratinocytes within the migrating front. In contrast, signal for stromelysin-1 mRNA was seen in the epidermis away from the migrating front of epithelium and in many dermal fibroblasts. *Please see insert for color reproduction of this figure.*

membrane. Because it is produced by proliferating keratinocytes, stromelysin-1 is probably not involved in reepithelialization per se but rather is needed for restructuring the newly formed basement membrane. In further contrast to stromelysin-2, stromelysin-1 is abundantly expressed by dermal fibroblasts in the granulation tissue associated with wounds. The promoter regions of stromelysin-1 and stromelysin-2 genes are quite separate. Thus, although stromelysin-1 is synthesized by many cell types and is stimulated by a variety of cytokines, stromelysin-2 production is seemingly limited to epithelial cells. Furthermore, although expression of both enzymes is induced by tumor necrosis factor-α (TNF-α), epidermal growth factor (EGF), keratinocyte growth factor (KGF), and TGF-β_1, stromelysin-2 production is not influenced by IL-1, IL-6, or platelet-derived growth factor (PDGF). Because of its broad substrate specificity, stromelysin-1 may be an important enzyme in remodeling the dermal matrix during wound repair and may function with collagenase-3, which is expressed in the same location at the same stage of repair.

Expression of Gelatinases in Wound Repair

Other matrix metalloproteinases with broad catalytic activity, such as the 72-kDa and 92-kDa gelatinases, may be important in releasing keratinocytes from the basement membrane before lateral movement at the beginning of epithelial wound healing, and both gelatinases are transiently seen in epidermal cells shortly after wounding. Gelatinase-B is produced by human keratinocytes plated on plastic, and its expression is stimulated by growth on collagen and by TGF-β_1. In addition, upregulation of 92-kDa gelatinase is seen in the epithelial layer of healing rabbit corneal wounds, and hence the healing response in the cornea may be distinct from that in the skin.[24] Because neutrophils store 92-kDa gelatinase but do not actively make it, this enzyme may be involved in a wound healing response when these cells are present.[22]

Collagenase-1 in Wound Fibroblasts

In addition to the epidermis, collagenase-1 (MMP-1) is expressed by dermal fibroblasts in normally healing wounds and chronic ulcers.[6,7] Typically, however, only a few scattered positive cells are seen, and the signal per cell is much less than that detected in keratinocytes. Dermal expression of collagenase-1 may be limited to certain stages of wound repair, such as resolution of granulation tissue. In contrast to the idea that cell–matrix interactions are required for collagenase-1 induction in keratinocytes, enzyme expression in stromal cells may be more dependent on cytokines. Stimulation of collagenase-1 gene expression by fibroblasts is mediated by an IL-1 autocrine loop and is augmented by other factors, such as TNF-α, EGF, and PDGF. Supportive of the requirement of inflammatory mediators for expression of collagenase-1 by stromal cells, no expression of collagenase-1 is seen in samples of fibrotic ulcers lacking any inflammation or in acute wounds made ex vivo, which are also devoid of an inflammatory infiltrate.[7]

Cell–matrix interactions may also influence metalloproteinase production in dermal fibroblasts. Collagenase-1 expression is markedly increased in dermal fibroblasts grown in collagen, and as for keratinocytes, this induction is mediated by $\alpha_2\beta_1$ integrin. However, because fibroblasts, unlike keratinocytes, normally reside in a collagen-rich environment, the cells must possess a mechanism to repress collagenase-1 expression in resting tissue where they likely contact collagen. Indeed, many studies have indicated that changes in cell shape are required for expression of collagenase-1 by fibroblasts in collagen gels, and thus factors that control fibroblast movement, shape, and contractility may also regulate the expression of MMP-1 in activated cells. In addition, matrix fragments that may be generated and encountered in the wound environment can induce collagenase-1 expression in fibroblasts. Collagenase-1 is not expressed by synovial fibroblasts plated on intact fibronectin, but elevated levels of the enzyme are produced by cells grown on a 120-kDa, RGD-containing fragment of fibronectin. The inductive effect of this fibronectin fragment is mediated by cooperative signaling through $\alpha_5\beta_1$ and $\alpha_4\beta_1$ integrins. Interestingly, this effect is markedly enhanced by exposure to tenascin, an abundant and early deposited component of the wound bed matrix (see also Chapter 6).

Thus, as in keratinocytes, the regulation of collagenase-1 production in fibroblasts is seemingly complex, being affected by multiple and diverse stimuli. Importantly, the degradative activity of collagenase-1 in the epidermis and dermis may be involved in distinct processes related to healing that are accomplished by the different cellular compartments. Whereas keratinocytes may cleave dermal collagen at the surface to aid migration and promote reepithelialization, stromal collagenolytic activity may be needed for tissue remodeling associated with granulation and scar formation. The diagram shown in Fig. 7.3 summarizes the localization and differences in MMPs and TIMPs between normal and chronic wound healing conditions.

Metalloproteinase in Chronic Wounds

The failure of wounds to heal represents a major health care problem, and because cytokines, growth factors,

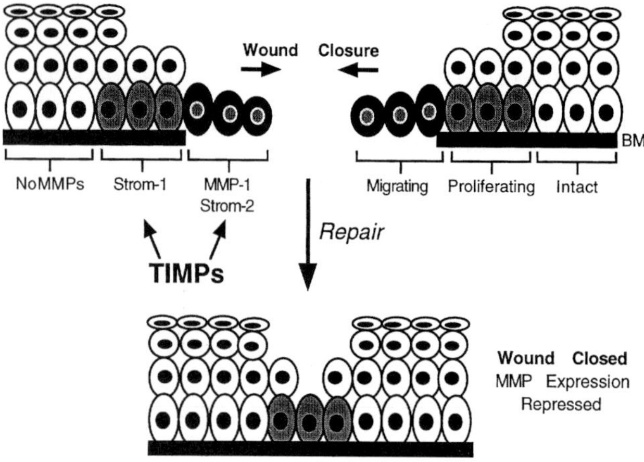

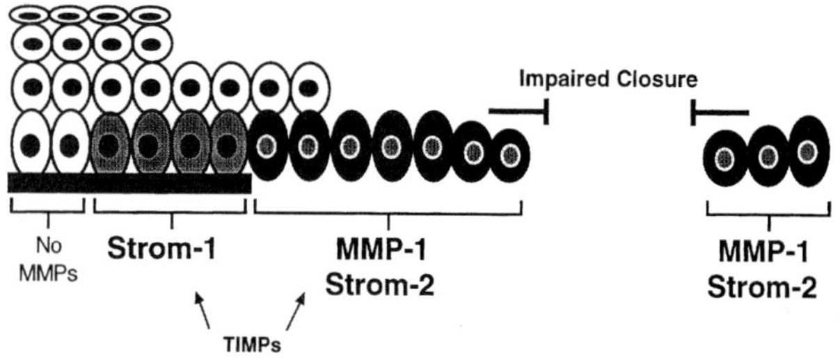

FIG. 7.3. Balance of matrix metalloproteinases (MMPs) and TIMP-1 in normal and chronic wounds may affect repair. A. In normally healing wounds, collagenase-1 is expressed by migrating basal keratinocytes that have moved beyond the edge of the disrupted basement membrane (*BM*). Stromelysin-2 (Strom-2) is also expressed by this same population of migrating cells. Stromelysin-1 (Strom-1) is also expressed in the wounded epidermis but by a functionally distinct population of basal keratinocytes. The stromelysin-1-expressing keratinocytes are hyperproliferative cells whose daughters maintain the migratory front as well as differentiate to reestablish the suprabasal layers. Further removed from the wound site, no metalloproteinase is produced in intact epidermis. As reepithelialization progresses, these spatial relationships are maintained. That is, migrating cells stop migrating and become hyperproliferative once they contact a newly formed basement membrane (which they produce), and in turn, proliferating keratinocytes assume the phenotype of cells in intact skin. At the completion of reepithelialization, expression of all metalloproteinases is turned off. Natural antiproteinases, such as TIMP-1, produced in the underlying wound would neutralize metalloproteinase activity after remodeling, thereby preventing excess degradation. B. In chronic ulcers, the same spatial patterns of metalloproteinases are maintained, but quantitative differences of enzyme expression may contribute to the inability of these lesions to close. In ulcers many more cells express collagenase-1, and the stromelysins and the expression levels of these metalloproteinases are much greater than seen in normal wounds. In addition, TIMP-1 levels are markedly reduced. The overproduction of MMPs coupled with continued inflammation and the underproduction of TIMP-1 may lead to excess matrix degradation and impaired healing.

proteases, and endocrine hormones play key roles in regulating acute wound healing, it is possible that alterations in the actions of these molecules could contribute to the failure of wounds to heal normally. Several methods have been used to assess differences in molecular environments of healing and chronic wounds. Homogenates of wound biopsies can be used to measure levels of mRNAs and proteins. Histologic sections of biopsies can be used to immunolocalize proteins in wounds. Fluids that spontaneously collect in acute surgical wounds and chronic skin ulcers also can be used to analyze the molecular environment of healing and chronic wounds. Several important concepts have emerged from the molecular analyses of acute and chronic wound environments.

The first major concept to emerge from analysis of wound fluids is that the molecular environments of chronic wounds have reduced mitogenic activity compared to the environments of acute wounds. For example, when fluids collected from acute mastectomy wounds are added to cultures of normal human skin fibroblasts, keratinocytes, or vascular endothelial cells, the acute wound fluids consistently stimulate DNA synthesis of the cultured cells. In contrast, addition of fluids collected from chronic leg ulcers typically does not stimulate DNA synthesis of the cells in culture. Also, combining acute and chronic wound fluids inhibited the mitotic activity of acute wound fluids. Similar results were reported by several groups of investigators, who found that acute wound fluids promote DNA synthesis although chronic wound fluids do not.[46–48]

The second major concept to emerge from analysis of wound fluids is that the cytokine environment of chronic wounds is substantially more proinflammatory than the molecular environment of acute wounds. For example, the ratios of two key inflammatory cytokines, TNF-α and IL-1β, and their natural inhibitors, P55 and IL-1 receptor antagonist in mastectomy fluids are significantly higher in mastectomy wound fluids than in chronic wound fluids (Table 7.1). At the 1994 meeting of the European Tissue Repair Society, Trengove and colleagues also reported high levels of the inflammatory cytokines IL-1,

TABLE 7.1. Ratios of cytokine inhibitor to cytokines in fluids from healing and chronic wounds

Wound fluids	P55/TNF-α	IL-1 RA/IL-1β
Healing wounds	12:1	480:1
Chronic ulcers	4:1	7:1

Fluids from acute healing wounds or chronic wounds were measured by ELISA for levels of cytokine agonists and their selective inhibitors. Molar ratio of TNF-α and its inhibitor, P55 protein which is a soluble form of the TNF-α receptor, are approximately 3 fold higher in healing wounds compared to chronic wound fluids. Similarly, the molar ratio of IL-1β and its natural inhibitor, IL-1 receptor antagonist (IL-1 RA), is approximately 70 fold higher in healing wounds.

IL-6, and TNF-α in fluids collected from venous ulcers of patients admitted to hospital. More importantly, levels of the cytokines significantly decreased in fluids collected 2 weeks after the chronic ulcers had begun to heal. Harris et al.[48] also found cytokine levels were generally higher in wound fluids from nonhealing ulcers than healing ulcers. These data suggest that chronic wounds typically have elevated levels of proinflammatory cytokines, and that the molecular environment changes to a less proinflammatory cytokine environment as chronic wounds begin to heal.

A third important concept that has emerged from analysis of wound biopsies and wound fluids is that protease activity in chronic wounds is significantly elevated compared to acute wounds. In our examination of many samples of pyogenic granuloma, pyoderma gangrenosum, and decubitus and stasis ulcers, the levels of collagenase-1 mRNA were markedly higher and the transcripts were seen over much longer distances of the basal epidermis than the levels and pattern seen in normally healing wounds.[7] (Figure 7.4) Also, analyses of wound fluids have shown the average level protease activity in mastectomy fluids determined using a general substrate for MMPs, Azocoll, is low (0.75 μg collagenase equivalents per milliliter; $n = 20$) with a range of 0.1 to 1.3 μg collagenase equivalents per milliliter. This finding suggests that protease activity is tightly controlled during the early phase of wound healing. In contrast, the average level of protease activity in chronic wound fluids (87 μg collagenase equivalents per milliliter, $n = 32$) is approximately 116 fold higher ($p < 0.05$) than in mastectomy fluids. Also, the range of protease activity in chronic wound fluids is rather large (from 1 to 584 μg collagenase equivalents per milliliter). More importantly, the levels of protease activity tend to decrease in chronic venous ulcers 2 weeks after the ulcers begin to heal (Fig. 7.5). Yager and colleagues[49] also found 10-fold-higher levels of MMP-2 protein, 25-fold-higher levels of MMP-9 protein, and 10-fold-higher collagenase activity in fluids from pressure ulcers compared to surgical wound fluids, using gelatin zymography and cleavage of a radioactive collagen substrate. Using immunohistochemical localization, Rogers et al.[50] observed elevated levels of MMPs in granulation tissue of pressure ulcers along with elevated levels of neutrophil elastase and cathepsin G. Bullen et al.[51] reported that levels of TIMP-1 were decreased while levels of MMP-2 and MMP-9 were increased in fluids from chronic venous ulcers compared to mastectomy wound fluids.

Other classes of proteases also appear to be elevated in chronic wound fluids. Rao et al.[52] reported that fluids from skin graft donor sites or breast surgery patients contained intact α_1-antitrypsin, a potent inhibitor of serine proteases, very low levels of neutrophil elastase activity, and intact fibronectin. In contrast, fluids from the chronic venous ulcers contained degraded α_1-anti-

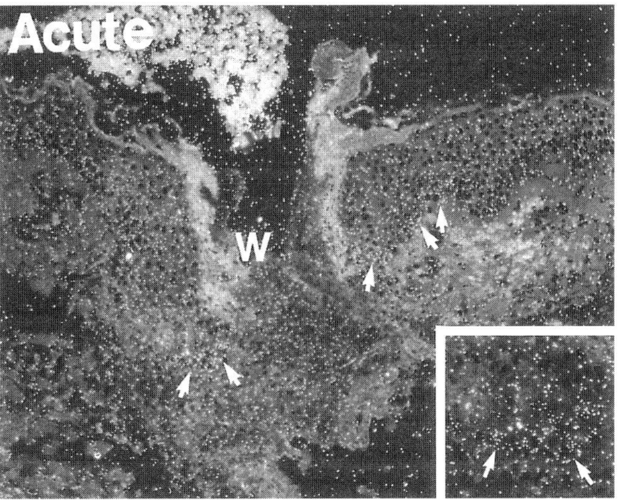

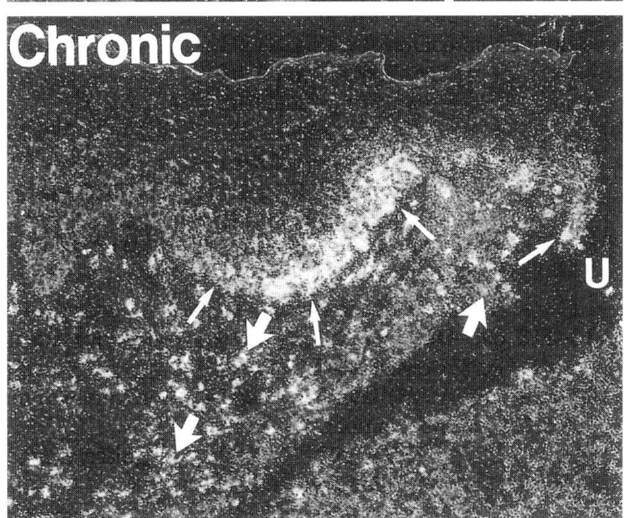

FIG. 7.4. Expression of collagenase-1 is elevated in chronic ulcers. In situ hybridization for collagenase-1 mRNA was performed on sections of an acute wound (*upper panel*) and a nonspecific ulcer (*bottom panel*) using an ^{35}S-labeled RNA probe. Partial thickness wounds were made under aseptic conditions on the ventral forearm of normal subjects, and one day later, a 4-mm punch biopsy was obtained. In the dark-field photomicrograph, two epidermal fronts are seen migrating into the wound bed (*W*). Weak signals for collagenase-1 mRNA are seen in basal keratinocytes at the forward extent of the wound edge (*arrows*). Inset: higher-magnification view of the epidermal front seen to the left of the wound bed. In the chronic wound section (*lower panel*), strong signals for collagenase-1 are seen in several basal keratinocytes (*small arrows*) at the ulcer edge (*U*). Signal for collagenase-1 mRNA in keratinocytes is much stronger in the ulcer than in the acute wound. Because the autoradiographic exposure for the acute wound was 21 days and only 10 days for the ulcer, the difference in signal per cell is even greater than that seen in these photomicrographs. In addition, many more keratinocytes express collagenase-1 in the chronic ulcer than in the normally healing wound, and collagenase-1 is also expressed by many cells in the dermal space, which in this specimen are macrophages. Thus, collagenase-1 can be markedly upregulated in nonhealing lesions. *Please see insert for color reproduction of this figure.*

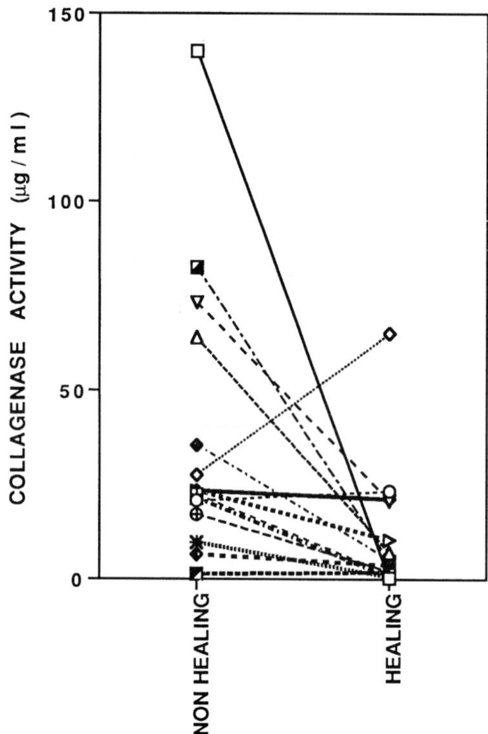

FIG. 7.5. Protease levels in fluids collected from nonhealing and healing chronic venous leg ulcers of 15 patients at the start of hospitalization (nonhealing) and 2 weeks later after the ulcers had clinical evidence of healing (healing). Protease activities were measured using Azocoll as the substrate. *Lines* connect the protease levels measured in the two samples from each patient (nonhealing and healing).

trypsin, 10- to 40-fold more neutrophil elastase activity, and degraded fibronectin. Wysocki and colleagues[53] also found that chronic leg ulcers contained elevated MMP-2 and MMP-9, and Grinnell and Zhu[54] reported that fibronectin degradation in chronic wounds depended on the relative levels of elastase, α_1-proteinase inhibitor, and α_2-macroglobulin. Besides being implicated in degrading essential extracellular matrix factors like fibronectin, proteases in chronic wound fluids also have been reported to degrade exogenous growth factors in vitro such as EGF, TGF-β_1[55] or PDGF.[55,56] In contrast, exogenous growth factors were stable in acute surgical wound fluids in vitro.

Supporting this general concept of increased degradation of endogenous growth factors by proteases in chronic wounds, the average immunoreactive levels of some growth factors such as EGF and TGF-β_1 were found to be lower in chronic wound fluids than in acute wound fluids, while PDGF-AB, TGF-α, and insulin-like growth factor (IGF-1) were not.[55,57,58] In general, these results suggest that many chronic wounds contain elevated levels of MMP and neutrophil elastase activities. The physiologic implications of these data are that elevated protease activities in some chronic wounds may directly contribute to the failure of wounds to heal by degrading proteins that are necessary for wound healing such as extracellular matrix proteins, growth factors, their receptors, and protease inhibitors. Interestingly, Steed and colleagues[59] reported that extensive debridement of diabetic foot ulcers improved healing in patients treated with placebo or with recombinant human PDGF. It is possible that frequent sharp debridement of diabetic ulcers helps to convert the detrimental molecular environment of a chronic wound into a pseudoacute wound molecular environment.

Biologic Response of Chronic Wound Cells

Biochemical analyses of fluids and biopsies from healing and chronic wounds suggest that there are some important molecular differences in the wound environments. However, these data describe only half the picture. The other essential component of the chronic wound environment is the capacity of the cells in a chronic wound to respond to these molecular regulators. Interesting new data are emerging which suggest that fibroblasts in

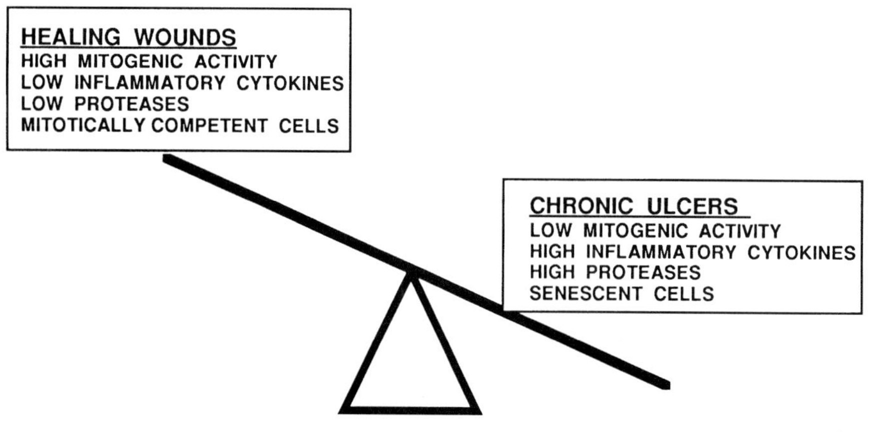

FIG. 7.6. Diagram of the relationships of factors in the environment of healing wounds and chronic ulcers. Analyses indicate that healing wounds (*left*) generally have high levels of mitogenic activity, low levels of inflammatory cytokines, low levels of proteases, high levels of growth factors, and mitotically competent fibroblasts. In contrast, chronic wounds (*right*) tend to have low levels of mitotic activity, high levels of inflammatory cytokines, high levels of proteases, low levels of growth factors, and nearly senescent fibroblasts.

skin ulcers which have failed to heal for many years may not be capable of responding to growth factors and extensively dividing as fibroblasts do in healing wounds. Data presented by Dr. Magnus Ågren at the 1998 meeting of the European Tissue Repair Society indicated that fibroblasts cultures established from chronic venous leg ulcers grew to lower densities than fibroblasts cultures established from acute wounds or from uninjured dermis. Also, fibroblasts from venous leg ulcers that had been present for more than 3 years grew more slowly and responded more poorly to PDGF than fibroblasts from venous ulcers that had been present for less than 3 years. These results suggest that fibroblasts in ulcers of long duration may have decreased ability to respond to exogenous growth factors and may have reduced capacity to divide (premature senescence).

Future Concepts for the Treatment of Chronic Wounds

Based on these biochemical analyses of the molecular environments of acute and chronic human wounds, it is possible to propose a general model of differences between healing and chronic wounds. As shown in Fig. 7.6, the molecular environment of healing wounds promotes mitosis of cells, has low levels of inflammatory cytokines, has low levels of proteases, and has high levels of growth factors and cells capable of rapid division. In contrast, the molecular environments of chronic wounds generally have the opposite characteristics, that is, these do not promote mitosis of cells, have elevated levels of inflammatory cytokines, have high levels of proteases and low levels of growth factors, and have cells that are approaching senescence. If these general concepts are correct, then it may be possible to develop new treatment strategies reestablishing in chronic wounds the balance of cytokines, growth factors, proteases, their natural inhibitors, and competent cells found in healing wounds.

New treatment strategies could be designed to reduce the elevated protease levels. Fortunately, new potent synthetic inhibitors of MMPs as well as naturally occurring protease inhibitors such as TIMP-1 and α_1-antitrypsin, are available by recombinant DNA technology. The use of a recombinant growth factor, PDGF-BB, was recently approved by the FDA for diabetic foot ulcers. Treatment of chronic wounds with engineered tissue replacements such as Dermagraph® and Apligrapf® has proven to be effective in selected types of ulcers. The cells that populate the synthetic skin substitutes probably do not survive long term in the wound, but probably secrete important cytokines, growth factors, matrix proteins, and protease inhibitors that eventually recruit healthy cells around the wound to migrate into the chronic wound. In the future, treatment of chronic wounds with combinations of selective inhibitors of proteases, growth factors, and tissue replacements may synergistically promote healing and provide an adjuvant for traditional treatment of chronic skin ulcers.

References

1. Woessner JF Jr. The matrix metalloproteinase family. In: Parks WC, Mecham RP, eds. Matrix Metalloproteinases. San Diego: Academic Press, 1998:1–14.
2. Parks WC, Mecham RP. Matrix metalloproteinases. In: Mecham RP, ed. Biology of the Extracellular Matrix. San Diego. Academic Press, 1998:1–362.
3. Shapiro SD. Matrix metalloproteinase degradation of extracellular matrix: biological consequences. Curr Opin Cell Biol 1998;10:602–608.
4. Jeffrey JJ. Interstitial collagenases. In: Parks WC, Mecham RP, eds. Matrix Metalloproteinases. San Diego: Academic Press, 1998:15–42.
5. Welgus HG, Jeffrey JJ, Eisen AZ. The collagen substrate specificity of human skin fibroblast collagenase. J Biol Chem 1981;256:9511–9515.
6. Saarialho-Kere UK, Chang ES, Welgus HG, Parks WC. Distinct localization of collagenase and TIMP expression in wound healing associated with ulcerative pyogenic granuloma. J Clin Invest 1992;90:1952–1957.
7. Saarialho-Kere UK, Kovacs SO, Petland AP, Olerud J, Welgus HG, Parks WC. Cell-matrix interactions modulate interstitial collagenase expression by keratinocytes actively involved in wound healing. J Clin Invest 1993;92: 2858–2866.
8. Stricklin GP, Li L, Jancic V, Wenczak BA, Nanney LB. Localization of mRNAs representing collagenase and TIMP in sections of healing human burn wounds. Am J Pathol 1993;143:1657–1666.
9. Wolfe GC, MacNaul KL, Beuchel FF, et al. Differential in vivo expression of collagenase messenger RNA in synovium and cartilage. Arthritis Rheum 1993;36:1540–1557.
10. Fisher C, Gilbertson-Beadling S, Powers EA, Petzold G, Poorman R, Mitchell MA. Interstitial collagenase is required for angiogenesis in vitro. Dev Biol 1994;162: 499–510.
11. Galis ZS, Sukhova GK, Lark MW, Libby P. Increased expression of matrix metalloproteinases and matrix degrading activity in vulnerable regions of human atherosclerotic plaques. J Clin Invest 1994;94:2493–2503.
12. Hasty KA, Pourmotabbed TF, Goldberg GI, et al. Human neutrophil collagenase. A distinct gene product with homology to other matrix metalloproteinases. J Biol Chem 1990;265:11421–11424.
13. Chubinskaya S, Huch K, Mikecz K, et al. Chordrocyte matrix metalloproteinase-8: up-regulation of neutrophil collagenase by interleukin-1 beta in human cartilage from knee and ankle joints. Lab Invest 1996;74:232–240.
14. Freije JM, Diez-Itza I, Balbin M, et al. Molecular cloning and expression of collagenase-3, a novel human matrix metalloproteinase produced by breast carcinomas. J Biol Chem 1994;269:16766–16773.
15. Mitchell PG, Magna HA, Reeves LM, et al. Cloning, expression, and type II collagenolytic activity of matrix met-

alloproteinase-13 from human osteoarthritic cartilage. J Clin Invest 1996;97:761–768.

16. Reboul P, Pelletier JP, Tardif G, Gloutier JM, Martel-Pelletier J. The new collagenase, collagenase-3, is expressed and synthesized by human chondrocytes but not by synoviocytes. A role in osteoarthritis. J Clin Invest 1996;97: 2011–2019.
17. Gack S, Vallon R, Schmidt J, et al. Expression of interstitial collagenase during skeletal development of the mouse is restricted to osteoblast-like cells and hypertrophic chondrocytes. Cell Growth Differ 1994;6:759–767.
18. Knauper V, Murphy G. Collagenase-3 (MMP-13) is expressed by hypertrophic chondrocytes, periosteal cells, and osteoblast during human fetal bone development. Dev Dyn 1997;208:387–397.
19. Vu TH, Werb Z. Gelatinase B: structure, regulation, and function. In: Parks WC, Mecham RP, eds. Matrix Metalloproteinases. San Diego: Academic Press, 1998:115–149.
20. Yu AE, Murphey AN, Stetler-Stevenson WG. 72-kDa gelatinase (gelatinase A): structure, activation, regulation and substrate specificity. In: Parks WC, Mecham RP, eds. Matrix Metalloproteinases. San Diego: Academic Press, 1998: 85–114.
21. Overall CM, Sodek J. Concanavalin A produces a matrix-degradative phenotype in human fibroblasts. Induction and endogenous activation of collagenase, 72-kDa gelatinase, and PUMP-1 is accompanied by the suppression of the tissue inhibitor of matrix metalloproteinases. J Biol Chem 1990;256:21141–21151.
22. Stahle-Backdahl M, Parks WC. 92-kDa gelatinase is actively expressed by eosinophils and secreted by neutrophils in invasive squamous cell carcinoma. Am J Pathol 1993;142: 995–1000.
23. Stahle-Backdahl M, Inoue M, Giudice GJ, Parks WC. 92-kDa gelatinase is produced by eosinophils at the site of blister formation in bullous pemphigoid and cleaves the extracellular domain of the 180-kDa bullous pemphigoid autoantigen. J Clin Invest 1994;93:2202–2230.
24. Fini ME, Cook JR, Mohan R, Brinckerhoff CE. Regulation of matrix metalloproteinase gene expression. In: Parks WC, Mecham RP, eds. Matrix Metalloproteinases. San Diego: Academic Press, 1998:300–356.
25. Murphy G, Cockett MI, Ward RV, Docherty AJP. Matrix metalloproteinase degradation of elastin, type IV collagen and proteoglycan. A quantitative comparison of the activities of 95-kDa and 75-kDa gelatinases stromelysins-1 and-2 and punctuated metalloproteinase (PUMP). Biochem J 1991;277:277–279.
26. Nagase H. Stromelysins 1 and 2. In: Parks WC, Mecham RP, eds. Matrix Metalloproteinases. San Diego: Academic Press, 1998:43–84.
27. Pei D, Weiss SJ. Furin-dependent intracellular activation of the human stromelysin-3 zymogen. Nature (Lond) 1995;375:244–247.
28. Knauper V, Murphy G. Membrane-type matrix metalloproteinases and cell surface-associated activation cascades for matrix metalloproteinases. In: Parks WC, Mecham RP, eds. Matrix Metalloproteinases. San Diego: Academic Press, 1998:199–218.
29. Wilson CL, Matrisian LM. Matrilysin. In: Parks WC, Mecham RP, eds. Matrix Metalloproteinases. San Diego: Academic Press, 1998:149–184.
30. Halpert I, Roby JD, Sires UI, et al. Matrilysin is expressed by lipid-laden macrophages at sites of potential rupture in atherosclerotic lesions and localizes to areas of versican deposition, a proteoglycan substrate for the enzyme. Proc Natl Acad Sci USA 1996;93:9748–9753.
31. Sires UI, Griffin GL, Broekelmann T, et al. Degradation of entactin by matrix metalloproteinases. Susceptibility to matrilysin and identification of cleavage sites. J Biol Chem 1993;268:2069–2074.
32. Shapiro SD. Macrophage elastase (MMP-12). In: Parks WC, Mecham RP, eds. Matrix Metalloproteinases. San Diego: Academic Press, 1998:185–198.
33. Hayakawa T, Yamashita K, Uchujima E, Iwata K. Growth promoting activity of tissue inhibitor of metalloproteinase-1 (TIMP-1) for a wide range of cells. FEBS Lett 1992; 298:29–32.
34. Goldberg GI, Wilhelm SM, Kronberger A, Bauer EA, Grant GA, Eisen AZ. Human fibroblast collagenase. Complete primary structure and homology to an oncogene transformation-induced rat protein. J Biol Chem 1986; 261:6600–6605.
35. Murphy G, Allan JA, Willenbrock F, Cockett MI, O'Connell JP, Docherty AJP. The C-terminal domain in collagenase and stromelysin specificity. J Biol Chem 1992; 267:9612–9618.
36. Van Wart HE, Birkedal-Hansen H. The cysteine switch: a principle of regulation of metalloproteinase activity with potential applicability to the entire matrix metalloproteinase gene family. Proc Natl Acad Sci USA 1990; 87:5578–5582.
37. Murphy G, Willenbrock F, Ward RV, Cockett MI, Eaton D, Docherty AJP. The C-terminal domain of 72-kDa gelatinase A is not required for catalysis, but is essential for membrane activation and modulates interactions with tissue inhibitors of metalloproteinases. Biochem J 1992; 283:637–641.
38. O'Connell JP, Willenbrock F, Docherty AJP, Eaton D, Murphy G. Analysis of the role of the COOH-terminal domain in the activation, proteolytic activity, and tissue inhibitor of metalloproteinase interactions of gelatinase B. J Biol Chem 1994;269:14967–14973.
39. Baragi VM, Fliszar CJ, Conroy MC, Ye QZ, Shipley JM, Welgus HG. Contribution of the C-terminal domain of metalloproteinases to binding by tissue inhibitor of metalloproteinases. C-terminal truncated stromelysin and matrilysin exhibit equally compromised binding affinities as compared to full-length stromelysin. J Biol Chem 1994;269: 12692–12697.
40. Murphy G, Nguyen Q, Cockett ML, et al. Assessment of the role of the fibronectin-like domain of gelatinase A by analysis of a deletion mutant. J Biol Chem 1994;269: 6632–6636.
41. Pilcher BK, Dumin JA, Sudbeck BD, Krane SM, Welgus HG, Parks WC. The activity of collagenase-1 is required for keratinocyte migration on a type I collagen matrix. J Cell Biol 1997;137:1445–1457.

42. Saarialho-Kere UK, Vaalamo M, Karjalainen-Lindsberg ML, Airola K, Parks WC, Puolakkainen P. Enhanced expression of matrilysin, collagenase, and stromelysin-1 in gastrointestinal ulcers. Am J Pathol 1996;148:519–526.
43. Dunsmore SE, Saarialho-Kere UK, Roby JD, et al. Matrilysin function and expression in airway epithelium. J Clin Invest 1998;102:1321–1331.
44. Sudbeck BD, Pilcher BK, Welgus HG, Parks WC. Induction and repression of collagenase-1 by keratinocytes is controlled by distinct components of different extracellular matrix compartments. J Biol Chem 1997;272:22103–22110.
45. Mauviel A, Uitto J. The extracellular matrix in wound healing: role of the cytokine network. Wounds 1993;5: 137–152.
46. Bucalo B, Eaglstein WH, Falanga V. Inhibition of cell proliferation by chronic wound fluid. Wound Repair Regen 1993;1:181–186.
47. Katz MH, Alvarez AF, Kirsner RS, Eaglstein WH, Falanga V. Human wound fluid from acute wounds stimulates fibroblast and endothelial cell growth. J Am Acad Dermatol 1991;25:1054–1058.
48. Harris IR, Yee KC, Walters CE, et al. Cytokine and protease levels in healing and non-healing chronic venous leg ulcers. Exp Dermatol 1995;4:342–349.
49. Yager DR, Zhang L, Liang H, Diegelmann RF, Cohen IK. Wound fluids from human pressure ulcers contain elevated matrix metalloproteinase levels and activity compared to surgical wound fluid. J Invest Dermatol 1996; 107:743–748.
50. Rogers AA, Burnett S, Moore JC, Shakespeare PG, Chen WYJ. Involvement of proteolytic enzymes, plasminogen activators and matrix metalloproteinases in the pathophysiology of pressure ulcers. Wound Repair Regen 1995;3: 273–283.
51. Bullen EC, Longaker MT, Updike DL, Benton R, Ladin D, Hou Z. Tissue inhibitor of metalloproteinases-1 is decreased and activated gelatinases are increased in chronic wounds. J Invest Dermatol 1995;104:236–240.
52. Rao CN, Ladin DA, Liu YY, Chilukuri K, Hou ZZ, Woodley DT. α1-Antitrypsin is degraded and non-functional in chronic wounds but intact and functional in acute wounds: the inhibitor protects fibronectin from degradation by chronic wound fluid enzymes. J Invest Dermatol 1995;105:572–578.
53. Wysocki AB, Staiano-Coico L, Grinnell F. Wound fluid from chronic leg ulcers contains elevated levels of metalloproteinases MMP-2 and MMP-9. J Invest Dermatol 1993;101:64–68.
54. Grinnell F, Zhu M. Fibronectin degradation in chronic wounds depends on the relative levels of elastase, 1-proteinase inhibitor, and α_2-macroglobulin. J Invest Dermatol 1996;106:335–341.
55. Yager DR, Chen SM, Ward SI, Olutoye OO, Diegelmann RF, Cohen IK. Ability of chronic wound fluids to degrade peptide growth factors is associated with increased levels of elastase activity and diminished levels of proteinase inhibitors. Wound Repair Regen 1997;5:23–32.
56. Wlaschek M, Pees D, Achterberg V, Meyer-Ingold W, Scharfetter-Kochanek K. Protease inhibitors protect growth factor activity in chronic wounds. Br J Dermatol 1997;137:646–647.
57. Bennett NT, Schultz GS. Growth factors and wound healing: Part II. Role in normal and chronic wound healing. Am J Surg 1993;166:74–81.
58. Cooper DM, Yu EZ, Hennessey P, Ko F, Robson MC. Determination of endogenous cytokines in chronic wounds. Ann Surg 1994;219:688–692.
59. Steed DL, Donohoe D, Webster MW, Lindsley L. Effect of extensive debridement and treatment on the healing of diabetic foot ulcers. J Am Coll Surg 1996;183:61–64.

Section 2
Adhesion Formation

urokinase) and is upon activation by plasmin converted to the active two-chain urokinase.[10]

Plasminogen Activator Inhibitors

Plasminogen-activator inhibitor-1 (PAI-1) is the main inhibitor of tPA and uPA. Endothelial cells produce PAI-1 as do a variety of cells including macrophages, fibroblasts, synovial endometrial, and mesothelial cells.[15,19,23,33,34,47–54] Platelets contain large amounts of PAI-1,[55] which they release upon activation. PAI-1 is released from cells to the ECM in response to various stimuli including endotoxin, trauma, or infection.[56–60] More recent studies have demonstrated that the secretion of PAI-1 from a variety of cultured cell types increased after exposure to transforming growth factor-beta (TGF-β)[33,52,61,62]; (Falk et al., in manuscript). Extracellularly, PAI-1 is deposited bound to vitronectin.[63,64] The half-life of tPA in plasma resulting from inactivation of PAI-1 is about 100 seconds.[65] PAI-1 is unusual in that it spontaneously converts to an inactive (latent) form.[66] Active PAI-1 forms inactive complexes with both uPA and tPA.

Initially found in human placenta,[67] PAI-2 has later been identified in plasma[68] and in several cell types including human omental mesothelial cells, macrophages, and pulmonary epithelial cells.[20,47,50,70] It is also produced by peritoneal mesothelial cells in culture.[34] In the peritoneum, PAI-2 expression in mesothelial cells was considerably increased in peritonitis when it is, in addition, expressed by inflammatory cells (Holmdahl et al., in manuscript). PAI-2 is a relatively poor inhibitor of tPA, and it has been proposed that PAI-1 and PAI-2 have different biologic functions.[70] PAI-2 forms inactive complexes with both uPA and tPA. Although present in inflamed human peritoneum, the role of PAI-2 in peritoneal tissue repair is not well defined.

Protease nexin 1 is a broad-spectrum inhibitor of trypsin-like serine proteases (including PAs) produced by a number of anchorage-dependent cells, as has been reviewed.[65] It is not detectable in plasma, and the role of protease nexin 1 in peritoneal fibrinolysis is to be determined. PAI-3 is a relatively unspecific heparin-dependent serine protease inhibitor present in plasma and urine. It is less well characterized than the other PA inhibitors. PAI-3 is identical to the protein C inactivator, and has a considerably reduced inhibiting efficiency compared to the other PA inhibitors.[71] It has also been suggested to be identical to kallikrein-binding protein.[72] It is not known if PAI-3 is present in peritoneal tissue.

Plasmin Inhibitors

There are at least three kinds of plasmin inhibitors (α_2-macroglobulin, α_2-antiplasmin, α_1-antitrypsin), of which α_2-antiplasmin is specifically directed against plasmin. Because the plasmin inhibitors act much more slowly than plasminogen activator inhibitors, it has been suggested that they have diverse biologic functions.[65] A common feature of plasmin inhibitors is that they do not inactivate receptor-bound plasmin, which is protected from inactivation.[73] Because plasmin typically binds to fibrin or to cell-membrane receptors, both of which are likely to occur in peritoneal tissue repair and adhesion development, the role of plasmin inhibitors in peritoneal biology is not well defined.

The Plasmin System in Peritoneal Repair

The mesothelium is perceived to have a barrier function regulating molecular traffic to and from the peritoneal cavity. Typically the mesothelium is a flat, continuous layer without distinct cell boundaries. In addition to the direct surgical injury, an abdominal operation elicits a local inflammatory reaction. Recent morphologic studies of human inflamed peritoneum revealed that in inflammation the mesothelial cells rounded up, lost contact with each other, and occasionally detached, exposing the edematous submesothelium (Holmdahl et al., in manuscript). This reaction constitutes a barrier breach, probably of importance in the pathogenesis of intraabdominal fibrin deposition. Inflammation typically produces extravasation of plasma proteins including fibrinogen, which then could ooze into the peritoneal cavity. Considering the vascularity and the surface area of peritoneum, the exudation could be substantial. The ballooning of mesothelial cells, also noticed in conjunction with surgically induced peritoneal injuries in animals (Jakobsson et al., in manuscript), is likely to indicate that the cells are activated in response to a challenge.

Several lines of evidence indicate that the plasmin system, especially PAs, are key factors in the different stages of tissue repair including inflammation, cellular migration, matrix formation, and reepithelialization. PAs are produced by several cell types of importance in peritoneal tissue repair (Holmdahl et al., in manuscript): (1) mesothelial cells, (2) fibroblasts and capillary endothelium in the submesothelial tissue, (3) inflammatory cells that have migrated into the wounded area, and (4) free-floating intracavitary cells. The PAs released by these cells conceivably have a concerted action in tissue repair including the removal of the fibrin clot, degradation of ECM, growth factor mobilization and activation, angiogenesis, and reepithelialization.[11]

Fibrin

Fibrin is an endogenous polymer. During coagulation it polymerizes from monomers that are cleaved from fibrinogen by thrombin. Fibrinogen is soluble but forms an insoluble gel on conversion to fibrin. During polymerization, fibrin is very tacky and adheres to a moist or even wet surface. After polymerization, it loses its tackiness and becomes a semirigid, fluid-tight sealant.[74] These biochemical insights might explain observations on the tendency of peritoneal surfaces to stick to each other after abdominal surgery. In an experimental animal model, it was demonstrated that the susceptibility for adhesion formation was significantly decreased or eliminated after the first 36 hours and that the magnitude of adhesion prevention was directly proportional to the agent's ability to remain at the site of injury during that critical period of adhesion development.[75] A likely explanation for this is that intraabdominal fibrin polymerization and stabilization took place within that time frame, and once the fibrin deposit is mature, surfaces no longer need to be separated.

The formation of a blood clot is facilitated by the binding of fibrinogen to an integrin receptor in the cell membrane of activated platelets. This binding apparently aids in the initial stabilization of the clot and may also greatly enhance the establishment of the clot by release of thrombin and PAI-1 from the entrapped, activated platelets.[55] Finally, the fibrin mesh is stabilized by intermolecular cross-linking of adjacent fibrin monomers by Factor VIII. Although platelet activation and aggregation are of paramount importance in thrombus formation in the vasculature,[76] the contribution of platelets in the formation of fibrin deposits in the peritoneal cavity is obscure. If intraperitoneal bleeding has occurred, platelets are obviously around, but otherwise not. Nonetheless, platelets are not essential in the formation of a clot, and fibrin polymerizes in the absence of platelets,[77] although the clot structure and mechanical properties are different.[74] Interestingly, some proteins interact with fibrin, altering clot structure and properties.[74] Some macromolecules including dextrans may also affect fibrin polymerization.[77] It is well established that clot structure and stability have profound impact on its resistance to fibrinolysis, as reviewed by Falk.[76] It might therefore be that this was a mode of action of dextrans, once frequently used to reduce postoperative adhesion formation in pelvic surgery.

Tissue Markers of Peritoneal Injury

tPA

Early on it was proposed that there was a central common pathway in the early development of adhesions.[78–82] During this initial phase of peritoneal tissue repair (0–3 days post injury) the adhesive attachment consists of a fibrin network infiltrated by inflammatory cells.[83] Biologically, this phase is similar to intravascular thrombus formation post injury. In analogy with intravascular clotting, where the thrombus must be lysed to restore vascular patency, intraabdominally deposited fibrin has to be lysed to free attached structures and restore the patency of the cavity. Investigations on the potential fibrin degradation capacity intraperitoneally revealed that peritoneum possesses plasminogen-activating activity (PAA)[84–88] as well as an inhibitor of fibrinolysis.[89] Based on these observations and in support of the hypothesis, it was demonstrated that a reduction in peritoneal PAA was associated with an increased formation of adhesions.[81,82,90] In animals, typical intraoperative trauma including diathermy coagulation, ischemia, free peritoneal grafting, or infection reduced peritoneal PAA perioperatively.[82,90] Furthermore, it was noted that the PAA was not maximally depressed at the time of operation, but further declined during the first 24 hours postoperatively, and that there was a relationship between the magnitude of PAA depression and adhesion development.[82] Thus there seemed to be a relationship between peritoneal PAA and trauma.

From animal work using diverse species, it is well established that ischemia is a powerful stimulator of adhesion development.[79,91–99] It has also been demonstrated that ischemia causes a significant reduction in PAA.[81,82,100] The clinical relevance of these findings was verified by Thompson and coworkers, who were able to demonstrate reduced PAA in peritoneum from ischemic bowel in humans.[17] Using a human model, a reduction of peritoneal PAA, paralleled by a decline in tPA, was noted.[101] The reduction in peritoneal PAA during surgery was caused by a reduced tPA activity, accounting for about 95% of the PAA.[22] The reduction in tPA activity was observed in noninflamed as well as in inflamed peritoneum, indicating that it was caused by the operative trauma.[22]

It is well established that surgery affects the systemic fibrinolytic response,[102,103] and the changes in intraperitoneal PAA could thus be a part of a generalized response. To clarify this, a study was undertaken in which paired peritoneal samples and peripheral blood were sampled every 30 minutes during surgery.[25] This study revealed that systemically there was a transient and significant immediate increase in tPA activity, followed by an increase in the total levels of tPA (tPA antigen). A corresponding decrease in PAI-1 activity was noted during an operation that lasted up to 90 minutes. It was not until the very end of the operation that signs of a systemic fibrinolytic shutdown occurred. None of the parameters investigated correlated with time (Fig. 8.3).

Locally, in the peritoneal cavity, the response was different. There was an immediate and ongoing reduction in tPA activity, significantly correlating with a decline in total levels of tPA ($p < 0.001$), indicating that the reduced tPA activity was, to a significant degree, caused by a reduced expression of tPA locally. The decline of tPA

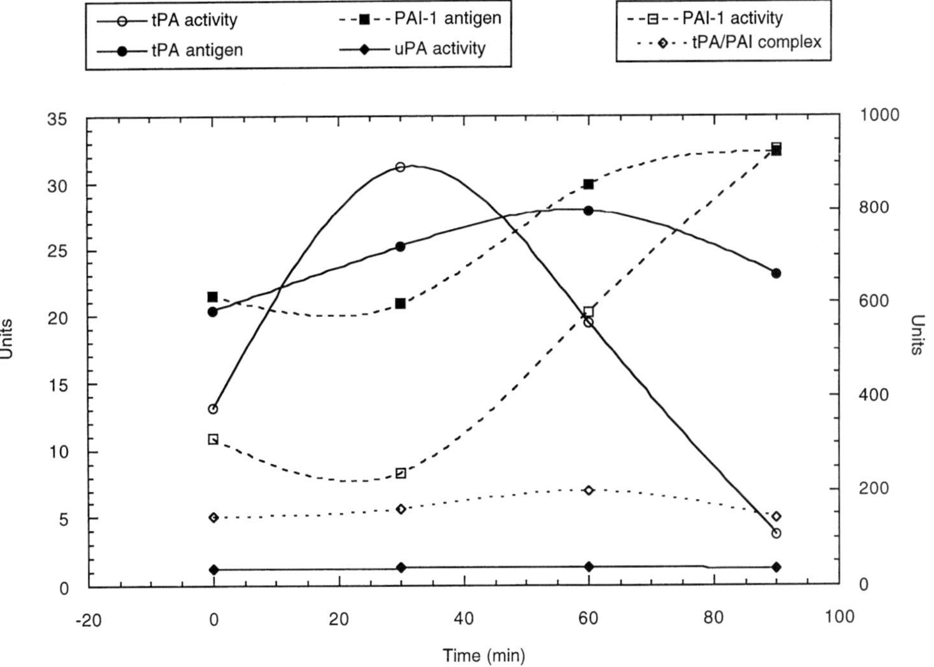

FIG. 8.3. Intraoperative changes in components of the plasmin system in peripheral blood. Note that there was an early peak in tPA activity ($p < 0.05$) followed by a later increase in tPA antigen ($p < 0.05$). After 90 min, PAI-1 activity had increased significantly ($p < 0.05$) compared with values at the opening of the abdominal cavity. The inactive complex between tPA and PAI-1 seemed to be dependent of tPA concentration (tPA antigen) rather than PAI-1 concentration. uPA did not change significantly. The tPA activity (IU/mL), tPA antigen (ng/mL), PAI-1 antigen (ng/mL), and uPA activity (ng/mL) refer to the *left* y-axis, whereas PAI-1 activity (IU/mL) and tPA–PAI complex (pmol/L) refer to the *right* y-axis. (Redrawn from Holmdahl et al.[25])

antigen and activity correlated significantly with time ($p < 0.05$ and $p < 0.01$, respectively). Obviously, tPA disappeared from the peritoneum during the operation. Interestingly, the decline in peritoneal tPA antigen and activity was more profound at the wound site where there typically is an ongoing trauma (i.e., from retractors), compared to a remote site ($p < 0.05$) where the trauma was less intense (Fig. 8.4). This finding combined with the differential expression of tPA systemically led to the conclusion that the reduced fibrinolytic activity was a local response to trauma and provided an explanation for the frequent involvement of the wound site in adhesion development.[25] Moreover, it indicated that measurement of peritoneal tPA activity could be used as a marker of peritoneal injury.

Although detectable in samples obtained from patients with peritonitis, in none of these studies was PAI-1 detectable in normal peritoneum, and the role of PAI-1 was unclear. Mesothelial cells in culture produced large amounts of PAI-1,[15] and by using immunohistochemistry it was shown that mesothelial cells expressed PAI-1 in vivo.[23]

PAI-1

Using a more efficient extraction technique, PAI-1 was detectable in peritoneal samples.[24] This method enabled a more thorough analysis of the kinetics of the plasmin system expression systemically and in peritoneal tissue during surgery,[26] which revealed dramatic intraoperative changes in peritoneal expression of the plasmin system. The initial event was a significant decline in tPA activity within the first hour of surgery, followed by an increase in PAI-1, uPA, and tPA–PAI complex detected during the second hour of surgery. These changes persisted throughout the operation. The kinetics was not reflected in peripheral blood samples, and there was no significant correlation between local and systemic expression, confirming the previous observation. Because of this, sampling of peripheral blood as done in these studies cannot be utilized as a means to predict peritoneal expression. Because tPA is readily absorbed from the abdominal cavity to systemic circulation,[104] it was suggested that the increase in systemic expression might reflect a transperitoneal absorption.[26]

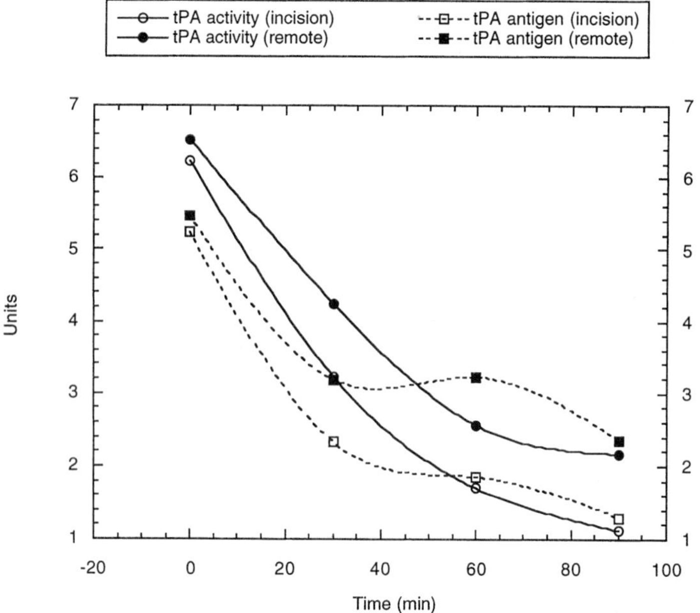

FIG. 8.4. Peritoneal expression of tPA during abdominal surgery at the wound where retractors had been placed and at a remote site, away from the incision. There was a rapid and parallel decline in tPA activity and the total levels of tPA (tPA antigen). However, the decline was more pronounced at the wound sites where retractors had been placed compared with a remote site where the trauma was less intense ($p < 0.05$ at 90 min). The unit for tPA activity is IU/mg protein, and for tPA antigen, pg/μg protein. (Redrawn from Holmdahl et al.[25]).

Although the initial tPA activity was significantly lower in inflamed peritoneum, the reduction was proportionally equal in inflamed and noninflamed tissue, indicating that the operative trauma elicited a similar response in tPA expression irrespective of the inflammatory status in the abdominal cavity. Apparently the local depletion of tPA empties the peritoneum of its main stimulator of fibrinolysis, at least temporarily. The secretion of tPA is regulated,[105,106] suggesting that abdominal surgery triggers a signaling pathway leading to tPA release from the mesothelium. Several possible factors that downregulate tPA expression are identified, including tumor necrosis factor-alpha (TNF-α), endotoxin (LPS), interleukin 1-beta (IL-1β), and TGF-β[15,107] (Falk et al., in manuscript), at both the protein and gene levels.[108] Of these, TGF-β, released from platelets[109] during surgery, is likely to be the first one at the scene.

PAI-1 is produced by the mesothelium, but also by cells in the submesothelial tissue, especially in peritonitis, where it partly colocalizes with macrophages as does the expression of uPA.[23] Considering the timing, it seems unlikely that macrophages accumulate and produce significant amounts of PAI-1 within 2 hours. Indeed, a preliminary study investing the density of macrophages in peritoneum did not reveal any substantial accumulation during surgery.[22] This result suggests that other cell types present including the mesothelium and fibroblasts[52] are likely sources in noninflamed conditions. The increase in PAI-1 was proportionally higher in noninflamed tissue, but the tissue levels were still less than in inflamed peritoneum, being four times greater in peritonitis. This discrepancy might be caused by a greater amount of tissue macrophages releasing PAI-1.[26]

Growth factors and cytokines that decrease the secretion of tPA also tend to increase the secretion of PAI-1 from human mesothelial cells[15,107,110] (Falk et al., in manuscript), an increase that is transcriptionally regulated.[108] However, because transcriptionally regulated processes require some time before the corresponding protein is secreted, typically several hours, transcriptionally regulation is unlikely to contribute to the intraoperative changes in protein expression. Indeed, an in vitro study showed that a transcriptionally regulated increase in PAI-1 from mesothelial cells might require considerable time, because increased PAI-1 m-RNA concentrations was not observed until after 12 hours.[108] How the intraoperative change in PAI-1 expression is regulated and what are the key players thus remains to be determined, especially in patients without preexisting peritonitis.

uPA

Contradictory to the decline in tPA activity, there was a 1.5-fold increase in uPA in noninflamed tissue during surgery; this was not observed in samples from patients with peritonitis. It may be that the expression of uPA was already increased in inflamed tissue and the potential for further expression exhausted. uPA has been demonstrated to be produced by a variety of cell types including mesothelium,[23] fibroblasts,[52] and macrophages.[111] Typically, uPA has been associated more with tissue remodeling than fibrin degradation.[1] tPA is much more fibrin specific than uPA[27] and is the main PA in peritoneum.[22] It therefore seems reasonable to assume that tPA expression has a greater impact on fibrin degradation in the peritoneal cavity than uPA. On the other hand, fibrin deposits in tissues have been observed to correlate with the expression of uPA.[43] Because of this, the lack of peroperative increase of uPA in inflamed peritoneum may contribute to the propensity to form adhesions.

Differential Expression of the Plasmin System in Inflammation

The PAA of human peritoneum has been found to be reduced during inflammatory conditions,[17,18,22] a reduction that has been attributed to the presence of PAI-1[18] and PAI-2,[20] as concluded from tissue extracts from inflamed appendices. Gene expression for PAI-1 was detected in the mesothelium and the submesothelial capillary endothelium.[19]

Immunohistochemistry of noninflamed and inflamed human peritoneum showed that the increase of PAI-1 in peritonitis was primarily caused by an increased protein expression in the submesothelial matrix, where it partly colocalized with macrophages.[23] Another cell type that might contribute to PAI-1 production submesothelially is fibroblasts.[52] The seemingly divergent results when investigating PAI-1 gene and protein expression might be explained by that PAI-1 gene expression was transitional in the inflammatory process and not present at the time of sampling, although the resulting protein was. This notion is supported by the observation that PAI-1 is known to be stored extracellularly in conjunction with vitronectin.[63,64]

In a recent study using a refined extraction technique comparing the expression of components of the plasmin system in peritoneum during surgery, previous observations were confirmed and extended. The tPA activity was reduced in inflamed peritoneum, in part caused by an overexpression of active PAI-1 that resulted in a quenching of tPA. The intraoperative changes in the peritoneum were similar but attenuated in peritonitis, possibly reflecting that the inflammation had partly exhausted or was counteracting the mechanisms involved. There was no significant correlation between peritoneal expression and concentrations in peripheral blood.[26]

Tissue Markers of the Propensity to Develop Adhesions

It is well documented that almost all patients form adhesions after an abdominal or pelvic operation. To some extent, the adhesion formation is related to the magnitude of the previous surgery. A postmortem study investigating the relationship between surgery and adhesion formation showed that the incidence of adhesions after minor, major, and multiple operations was 51%, 72%, and 93%, respectively.[112] A more recent multicenter study investigating adhesion development after previous laparotomies confirmed that the more extensive the previous surgery, the more adhesions developed.[113]

Clinically, it is well known that the propensity to form adhesions varies greatly among patients. Following seemingly equivalent operative procedures, some patients develop extensive, dense, fibrous adhesions tethering organs, whereas some have limited, filmy adhesions, mainly to the site of the previous surgery as assessed at relaparotomy or laparoscopy. Although many intraoperative factors might influence the development of adhesions, it thus appears that there is an inborn variability in the predilection to form adhesions. Because of the previously demonstrated reduced peritoneal fibrinolytic capacity in conditions associated with the development of adhesions (surgery, peritonitis), it was hypothesized that reduced peritoneal fibrin degradation capacity might be a significant pathogenetic factor in those who developed extensive adhesions.

To address this possibility, 21 patients who had previously undergone abdominal surgery were investigated.[114] At a scheduled subsequent laparotomy for a clinical reason, peritoneal samples were taken and adhesion development assessed. Thirteen patients were categorized as having moderate adhesions, and 8 formed severe adhesions, of whom 3 had previously had been operated because of bowel obstruction resulting from adhesions. Men and women were equally distributed in the groups. Although the peritoneal tPA activity in patients with severe adhesions was about 70% of that of the peritoneal tPA activity of those who had moderate adhesions in the beginning of surgery and 35% at the conclusion of surgery, these differences did not reach statistical significance ($p = 0.18$ and $p = 0.07$, respectively). Peritoneal uPA tended to be higher in severe adhesion formers both at the beginning and at the conclusion of surgery, but these differences also were not statistically significant ($p = 0.3$ and $p = 0.08$, respectively) (Fig. 8.5).

In contrast, the peritoneal concentration of PAI-1 was more than 10 fold higher ($p = 0.009$) in severe adhesion formers at the beginning and almost twice as high ($p = 0.04$) at the end of the abdominal procedure. If the PAI-1 present was in its active form, this result indicates that once tPA was released it would be quenched, by PAI-1 inhibiting the generation of plasmin and fibrin clearing. That this actually occurred in peritoneum is evident from the determinations of tPA–PAI-1 complex. In peritoneum from severe adhesion formers, the tPA–PAI-1 complex was 3 fold higher as soon as the abdomen was opened ($p = 0.008$), and remained at that level at abdominal closure ($p = 0.01$), compared to patients who had formed moderate adhesions (Fig. 8.6). None of the patients with less severe adhesion formation had a PAI-1 level exceeding 60 ng/g, whereas the majority of those with severe adhesions did have such a level. If the cutoff level was set to 60 ng/g tissue, thus most of those with a greater propensity to form adhesions would be identified. Systemically, there were no significant differences between the patient groups. Peripheral blood samples

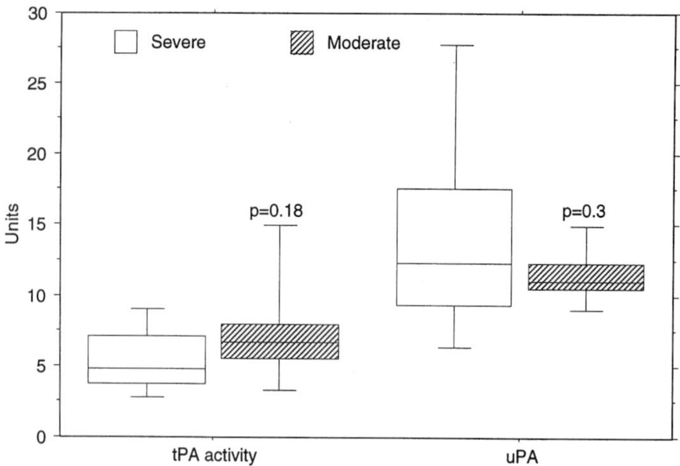

Fig. 8.5. Peritoneal expression of tPA activity and uPA in patients who had formed severe compared to moderate adhesions at opening of the abdominal cavity. There was no significant differences between the two patient populations. The unit for tPA activity is pmol/g tissue and for uPA, ng/g. (Redrawn from Ivarsson et al.[114])

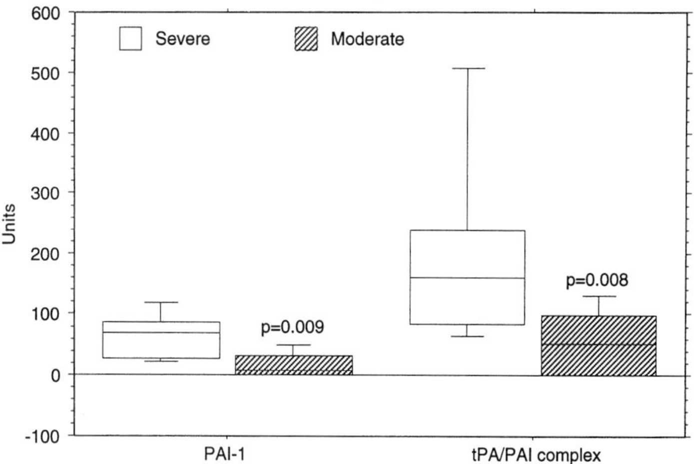

Fig. 8.6. Peritoneal expression of PAI-1 and the inactive tPA–PAI complex in patients who had formed severe compared to moderate adhesions at opening of the abdominal cavity. PAI-1 was overexpressed in peritoneum from patients that had developed severed adhesions which had resulted in an increased quenching of tPA, thereby reducing the fibrinolytic capacity. The unit for PAI-1 is ng/g tissue and for tPA–PAI complex, fmol/g. (Redrawn from Ivarsson et al.[114])

thus seem not to be useful in identifying patients at high risk for severe adhesions.

Additional support for the concept that components of the plasmin system could be used as tissue markers of the tendency to form adhesions was gained from investigations on adhesion tissue. Adhesions, once divided, typically reform.[115] This reformation is of clinical importance, not only in reproductive surgery but also in abdominal surgery with a high frequency of recurrence of bowel obstruction once lysis of the bowel because of adhesive obstruction has been performed.[116] Therefore, adhesions seem to represent a tissue exhibiting a high predilection to develop adhesions. Similar investigations were therefore carried out using adhesion tissue and the tissue concentrations were compared with adjacent, unaffected peritoneum from the same patients ($n = 10$). Similar to the results obtained comparing patients with a varying propensity to form adhesions,[114] the tPA activity in adhesion tissue was less than 40% of that in adjacent peritoneum ($p = 0.005$; Fig. 8.7). In contrast, uPA antigen was more than fourfold higher in the adhesions ($p = 0.008$; Fig. 8.8). PAI-1 was more than threefold higher in adhesion tissue ($p = 0.01$; Fig. 8.9), and the increased PAI-1 expression had resulted in more than tripled levels of tPA–PAI complex in adhesions compared with peritoneal biopsies ($p = 0.008$), reflecting a quenching of tPA (Fig. 8.10). Furthermore, it showed that PAI-1 was in its active form.

PAI-1 is an unusual molecule in that it can adopt any of four different forms: active, latent, substrate, or cleaved.[117] Depending on the antibody used, detection of PAI-1 does not necessarily mean that the molecule is capable of inhibiting tPA (i.e., in the active conformation). By measuring tPA–PAI-1 complex, it could be demonstrated that PAI-1 was functionally active and present at sites where tPA was available.

The peritoneum is an active organ, as deduced from ultrastructural observations, immunohistochemistry, tissue extraction, and cell culture experiments, expressing or secreting a vast array of compounds,[26,33,34,118–169] many of which are elevated systemically during diseases affecting the abdominal cavity. It seems therefore reasonable to assume that synthesis and release of compounds from the mesothelium may have a profound im-

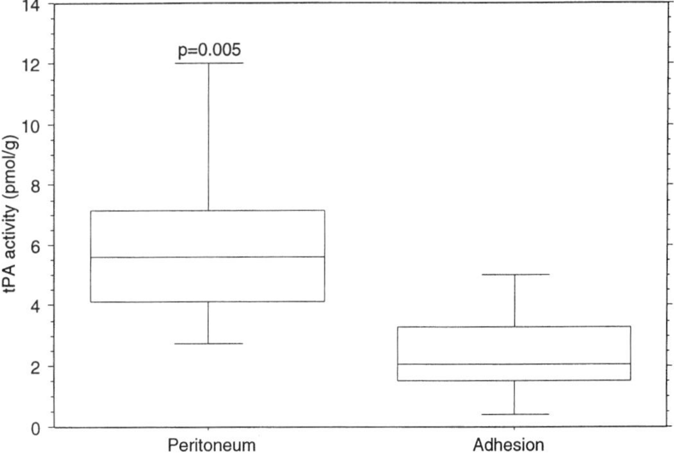

FIG. 8.7. Peritoneal expression of tPA activity compared with adhesion tissue from the same patient. tPA activity was significantly lower in adhesion tissue, demonstrating a reduced capacity to degrade fibrin. (Redrawn from Ivarsson et al.[114])

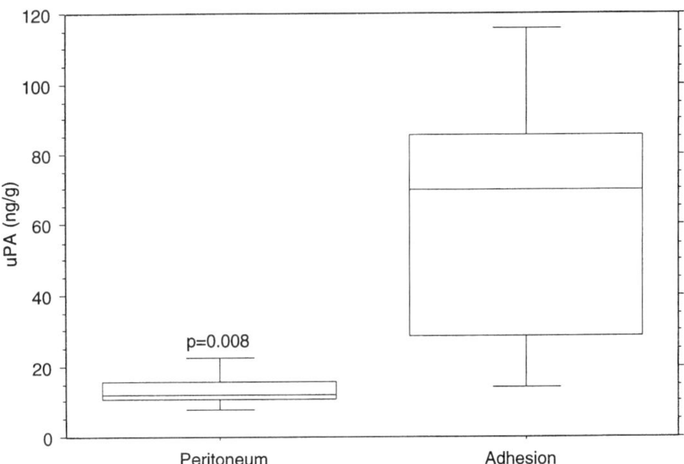

FIG. 8.8. Peritoneal expression of uPA compared with adhesion tissue from the same patient. uPA expression was significantly higher in adhesion tissue, probably reflecting a comparatively higher density of macrophages and ongoing tissue remodeling. (Redrawn from Ivarsson et al.[114])

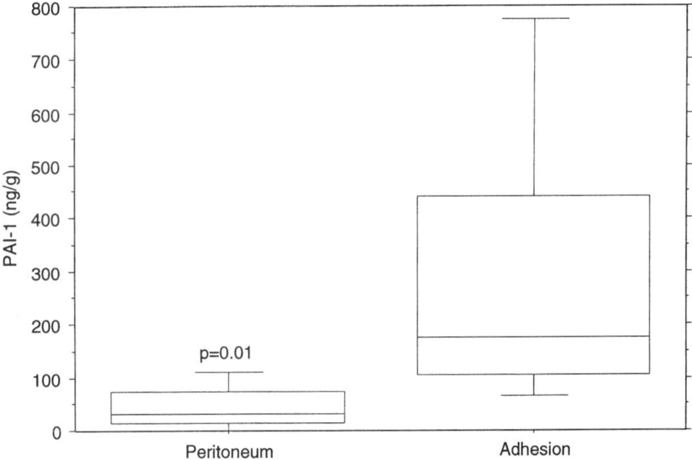

FIG. 8.9. Peritoneal expression of PAI-1 compared with adhesion tissue from the same patient. PAI-1 expression was significantly higher in adhesion tissue, indicating that the decline in fibrin degradation capacity in adhesion tissue was, at least in part, caused by an overexpression in PAI-1. (Redrawn from Ivarsson et al.[114])

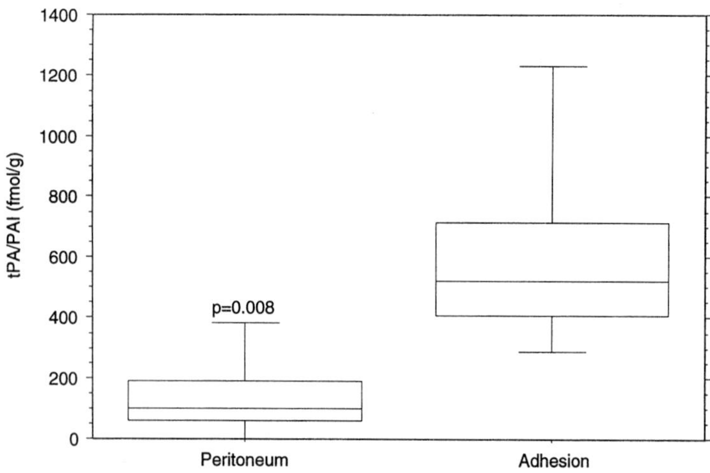

FIG. 8.10. Peritoneal expression of tPA–PAI complex compared with adhesion tissue from the same patient. The inactive complex was elevated in adhesion tissue, reflecting a quenching of the main peritoneal plasminogen activator tPA by PAI-1. (Redrawn from Ivarsson et al.[114])

pact, not only on abdominal adhesion formation, but on the entire organism, and that the significance of this is grossly underestimated.

Acknowledgments

This work has been supported by the Göteborg University and The Swedish Medical Research Council (K98-17X-12650-01A).

References

1. Vassalli J-D, Pepper MS. Membrane proteases in focus. Nature (Lond) 1994;370:14–15.
2. Mignatti P, Rifkin DB. Biology and biochemistry of proteinases in tumor invasion. Physiol Rev 1993;73:161–195.
3. Huber R, Carrell RW. Implication of the three-dimensional structure of alpha 1-antitrypsin for structure and function of serpins. Biochemistry 1989;34:15872–15879.
4. Wong AP, Cortez SL, Baricos WH. Role of plasmin and gelatinase in extracellular matrix degradation by cultured rat mesangial cells. Am J Physiol 1992;263:F1112–F1118.
5. Saksela O, Rifkin DB. Release of basic fibroblast growth factor-heparan sulfate complexes from endothelial cells by plasminogen activator-mediated proteolytic activity. J Cell Biol 1990;110:767–775.
6. Sato Y, Rifkin DB. Inhibition of endothelial cell movement by pericytes and smooth muscle cells: activation of a latent transforming growth factor-beta 1-like molecule by plasmin during co-culture. J Cell Biol 1989;109:309–315.
7. Sato Y, Tsuboi R, Lyons R, Moses H, Rifkin DB. Characterization of the activation of latent TGF-beta by co-cultures of endothelial cells and pericytes or smooth muscle cells: a self-regulating system. J Cell Biol 1990;111:757–763.
8. Murphy G, Ward R, Gavrilovic J, Atkinson S. Physiological mechanisms for metalloproteinase activation. Matrix Suppl 1992;1:224–230.
9. Murphy G, Atkinson S, Ward R, Gavrilovic J, Reynolds JJ. The role of plasminogen activators in the regulation of connective tissue metalloproteinases. Ann NY Acad Sci 1992;667:1–12.
10. Petersen LC, Lund LR, Nielsen LS, Danø K, Skriver L. One-chain urokinase-type plasminogen activator from human sarcoma cells is a proenzyme with little or no intrinsic activity. J Biol Chem 1988;263:11189–11195.
11. Mignatti P, Rifkin DB, Welgus HG, Parks WC. Proteinases and tissue remodelling. In: Clark RAF, ed. The Molecular and Cellular Biology of Wound Repair. New York: Plenum Press, 1996:427–474.
12. Pannell R, Black J, Gurewich V. The complementary modes of action of tissue plasminogen activator and pro-urokinase by their synergistic effect on clot lysis may be explained. J Clin Invest 1988;81:853–859.
13. Padro T, van den Hoogen CM, Emeis JJ. Distribution of tissue-type plasminogen activator (activity and antigen) in rat tissues. Blood Coagul Fibrinolysis 1990;1:601–608.
14. Risberg B, Eriksson E, Björk S, Hansson GK. Immunohistochemical localization of plasminogen activators in human saphenous veins. Thromb Res 1986;37:301–308.
15. van Hinsbergh VWM, Kooistra T, Scheffer MA, van Bockel JH, van Muijen GNP. Characterization and fibrinolytic properties of human omental tissue mesothelial cells. Comparison with endothelial cells. Blood 1990;75:1490–1497.
16. Wodzinski MA, Bardhan KD, Reilly JT, Preston FE. Reduced tissue type plasminogen activator activity of the gastroduodenal mucosa in peptic ulcer disease. Gut 1993;34: 1310–1314.
17. Thompson JN, Paterson Brown S, Harbourne T, Whawell SA, Kalodiki E, Dudley HAF. Reduced human peritoneal plasminogen activating activity: possible mechanism of adhesion formation. Br J Surg 1989;76:382–384.
18. Vipond MN, Whawell SA, Thompson JN, Dudley HA. Peritoneal fibrinolytic activity and intra-abdominal adhesions. Lancet 1990;335:1120–1122.
19. Whawell SA, Wang Y, Fleming KA, Thompson EM, Thompson JN. Localization of plasminogen activator inhibitor-1 production in inflamed appendix by in situ mRNA hybridization. J Pathol 1993;169:67–71.
20. Whawell SA, Vipond MN, Scott-Coombes D, Thompson JN. Plasminogen activator inhibitor 2 reduces peritoneal fibrinolytic activity in inflammation. Br J Surg 1993;80: 107–109.

21. Nkere UU, Whawell SA, Thompson EM, Thompson JN, Taylor KM. Changes in pericardial morphology and fibrinolytic activity during cardiopulmonary bypass. J Thorac Cardiovasc Surg 1993;106:339–345.
22. Holmdahl L, Eriksson E, Risberg B. Fibrinolysis in human peritoneum during operation. Surgery (St. Louis) 1996; 119:701–705.
23. Holmdahl L, Falkenberg M, Ivarsson ML, Risberg B. Plasminogen activator and inhibitors in peritoneal tissue. APMIS 1997;105:25–30.
24. Holmdahl L, Eriksson E, Risberg B. Measurement of fibrinolytic components in human tissue. Scand J Clin Lab Invest 1997;57:445–452.
25. Holmdahl L, Eriksson E, Eriksson Bl, Risberg B. Depression of peritoneal fibrinolysis during surgery is a local response to trauma. Surgery (St. Louis) 1998;123:539–544.
26. Ivarsson M-L, Holmdahl L, Eriksson E, Söderberg R, Risberg B. Expression and kinetics of fibrinolytic components in plasma and peritoneum during abdominal surgery. Fibrinolysis 1998;12:61–67.
27. Rånby M. Studies on the kinetics of plasminogen activation by tissue plasminogen activator. Biochim Biophys Acta 1982;704:461–469.
28. Verheijen JH, Chang GTG, Kluft C. Evidence for the occurrence of a fast-acting inhibitor for tissue-type plasminogen activator in human plasma. Thromb Haemostasis 1984;51:392–395.
29. Juhan-Vague I, Moerman B, DeCock F, Aillaud MF, Collen D. Plasma levels of a specific inhibitor of tissue-type plasminogen activator (and urokinase) in normal and pathological conditions. Thromb Res 1984;33:523–530.
30. Drapier JC, Tenu JP, Lemaire G, Petlt JF. Regulation of plasminogen activator secretion in mouse peritoneal macrophages. Biochimie (Paris), 1979;61:463–471.
31. Freyria AM, Paul J, Belleville J, Broyer P, Eloy R. Rat peritoneal macrophage procoagulant and fibrinolytic activities. An expression of the local inflammatory response. Comp Biochem Physiol A 1991;99:517–524.
32. Grulich-Henn J, Preissner KT, Muller-Berghaus G. Heparin stimulates fibrinolysis in mesothelial cells by selective induction of tissue-plasminogen activator but not plasminogen activator inhibitor-1 synthesis. Thromb Haemostasis 1990;64:420–425.
33. Idell S, Zwieb C, Kumar A, Koenig KB, Johnson AR. Pathways of fibrin turnover of human pleural mesothelial cells in vitro. Am J Respir Cell Mol Biol 1992;7:414–426.
34. Ivarsson M-L, Holmdahl L, Falk P, Mölne J, Risberg B. Characterization and fibrinolytical properties of mesothelial cells isolated from peritoneal lavage. Scand J Clin Lab Invest 1998;58:195–204.
35. Rånby M, Bergsdorf N, Nilsson T. Enzymatic properties of the one- and two-chain form of tissue plasminogen activator. Thromb Res 1982;27:175–183.
36. Grøndahl-Hansen J, Christensen IJ, Rosenquist C, et al. High levels of urokinase-type plasminogen activator and its inhibitor PAI-1 in cytosolic extracts of breast carcinomas are associated with poor prognosis. Cancer Res 1993; 53:2513–2521.
37. Nykjaer A, Petersen CM, Møller B, Andreasen PA, Gliemann J. Identification and characterization of urokinase receptors in natural killer cells and T-cell-derived lymphokine activated killer cells. FEBS Lett 1992;300:13–17.
38. Vassalli JD, Wohlwend A, Belin D. Urokinase-catalyzed plasminogen activation at the monocyte/macrophage cell surface: a localized and regulated proteolytic system. Curr Top Microbiol Immunol 1992;181:65–86.
39. Casslen B, Gustavsson B, Åstedt B. Cell membrane receptors for urokinase plasminogen activator are increased in malignant ovarian tumours. Eur J Cancer 1991;27: 1445–1448.
40. Vassalli JD, Dayer JM, Wohlwend A, Belin D. Concomitant secretion of prourokinase and of a plasminogen activator-specific inhibitor by cultured human monocytes-macrophages. J Exp Med 1984;159:1653–1668.
41. Lu HR, Wu Z, Pauwels P, Lijnen HR, Collen D. Comparative thrombolytic properties of tissue-type plasminogen activator (t-PA), single-chain urokinase-type plasminogen activator (u-PA) and K1K2Pu (a t-PA/u-PA chimera) in a combined arterial and venous thrombosis model in the dog. J Am Coll Cardiol 1992;19:1350–1359.
42. Collen D, Lijnen RH. Fibrin-specific fibrinolysis. Ann NY Acad Sci 1992;667:259–271.
43. Yamamoto K, Loskutoff DJ. Fibrin deposition in tissues from endotoxin-treated mice correlates with decreases in the expression of urokinase-type but not tissue-type plasminogen activator. J Clin Invest 1996;97:2440–2451.
44. Møller LB. Structure and function of the urokinase receptor. Blood Coagul Fibrinolysis 1993;4:293–303.
45. Blasi F. Urokinase and urokinase receptor: a paracrine/autocrine system regulating cell migration and invasiveness. Bioessays 1993;15:105–111.
46. Duffy MJ. Urokinase-type plasminogen activator and malignancy. Fibrinolysis 1993;7:295–302.
47. van Hinsbergh VWM, Kooistra T, van den Berg EA. Tumor necrosis factor increases the production of plasminogen activator inhibitor in human endothelial cells in vitro and in rats in vivo. Blood 1988;72:1467–1473.
48. Emeis JJ, Kooistra T. Interleukin-1 and lipopolysaccarides induce an inhibitor of tissue-type plasminogen activator in vivo and in cultured endothelial cells. J Exp Med 1986; 163:1260–1266.
49. Nordt TK, Klassen KJ, Schneider DJ, Sobel BE. Augmentation of synthesis of plasminogen activator inhibitor type-1 in arterial endothelial cells by glucose and its implications for local fibrinolysis. Arterioscler Thromb 1993;13: 1822–1828.
50. Wohlwend A, Belin D, Vassalli J-D. Plasminogen activator-specific inhibitors in mouse machrophages: in vivo and vitro modulation of their synthesis and secretion. J Immunol 1987;139:1278–1284.
51. Kuraoka S, Campeau JD, Rodgers KE, Nakamura RM, diZerega GS. Effects of interleukin-1 (IL-1) on postsurgical macrophage secretion of protease and protease inhibitor activities. J Surg Res 1992;52:71–78.
52. Idell S, Zwieb C, Boggaram J, Holiday D, Johnson AR, Raghu G. Mechanisms of fibrin formation and lysis by human lung fibroblasts: influence of TGF-beta and TNF-alpha. Am J Physiol 1992;263:L487–L494.
53. Carmassi F, De Negri F, Morale M, Puccetti R, Song KY, Chung SI. Assessment of coagulation and fibrinolysis in

synovial fluid of rheumatoid arthritis patients. Fibrinolysis 1994;8:162–171.
54. Casslen B, Urano S, Ny T. Progesterone regulation of plasminogen activator inhibitor 1 (PAI-1) antigen and mRNA levels in human endometrial stromal cells. Thromb Res 1992;66:75–87.
55. Erickson LA, Ginsberg MH, Loskutoff DJ. Detection and partial characterization of an inhibitor of plasminogen activator in human platelets. J Clin Invest 1984;74: 1465–1472.
56. Schwartz BS, Monroe MC, Bradshaw JD. Endotoxin-induced production of plasminogen activator inhibitor by human monocytes is autonomous and can be inhibited by lipid X. Blood 1989;73:2188–2195.
57. Eriksson E, Risberg B. Tissue plasminogen activator and its inhibitor following major surgery in relation to ventilatory pattern. Acta Chir Scand 1988;154:57–60.
58. Kluft C, De Bart ACW, Barthels M. Short term extreme increases in plasminogen activator inhibitor (PAI-1) in plasma of polytrauma patients. Fibrinolysis 1988;2: 221–226.
59. Eriksson BI, Eriksson E, Gyzander E, Teger-Nilsson A-C, Risberg B. Thrombosis after hip replacement. Relationship to the fibrinolytic system. Acta Orthop Scand 1989; 60:159–163.
60. Engebretsen LF, Keirulf P, Brandtzaeg P. Extreme plasminogen activatior inhibitor and endotoxin values in patients with meningococcal disease. Thromb Res 1986;42: 713–716.
61. Wilson HM, Reid FJ, Brown PA, Power DA, Haites NE, Booth NA. Effect of transforming growth factor-beta 1 on plasminogen activators and plasminogen activator inhibitor-1 in renal glomerular cells. Exp Nephrol 1993;1: 343–350.
62. Gerwin BI, Keski Oja J, Seddon M, Lechner JF, Harris CC. TGF-beta 1 modulation of urokinase and PAI-1 expression in human bronchial epithelial cells. Am J Physiol 1990; 259:L262–L269.
63. Wiman B, Almquist Å, Sigurdardottir O, Lindahl T. Plasminogen activator inhibitor 1 (PAI) is bound to vitronectin in plasma. FEBS Lett 1988;242:125–128.
64. Podor TJ, Loskutoff DJ. Immunoelectron microscopic localization of type 1 plasminogen activator inhibitor in the extracellular matrix of transforming growth factor-β activated endothelial cells. Ann NY Acad Sci 1992;667:46–49.
65. Sprengers ED, Kluft C. Plasminogen activator inhibitors. Blood 1987;69:381–387.
66. Sancho E, Tonge DW, Hockney RC, Booth NA. Purification and characterization of active and stable recombinant plasminogen-activator inhibitor accumulated at high levels in *Escherichia coli*. Eur J Biochem 1994;224:125–134.
67. Kawano T, Morimoto K, Uemura Y. Urokinase inhibitor in human placenta. Nature (Lond) 1968;217:253–254.
68. Åstedt B, Lecander I, Ny T. The placental type plasminogen activator inhibitor PAI-2. Fibrinolysis 1987;1:203–208.
69. Marshall BC, Xu QP, Rao NV, Brown BR, Hoidal JR. Pulmonary epithelial cell urokinase-type plasminogen activator. Induction by interleukin-1 beta and tumor necrosis factor-alpha. J Biol Chem 1992;267:11462–11469.
70. Andreasen PA, Georg B, Lund LR, Riccio A, Stacey SN. Plasminogen activator inhibitors: hormonally regulated serpins. Mol Cell Endocrinol 1990;68:1–19.
71. Heeb MJ, Espana F, Geiger M, Collen D, Stump DC, Griffin JH. Immunological identity to heparin-dependent plasma and urinary protein C inhibitor and plasminogen activator inhibitor-3. J Biol Chem 1987;262:15813–15816.
72. Ecke S, Geiger M, Resch I, et al. Inhibition of tissue kallikrein by protein C inhibitor. Evidence for identity of protein C inhibitor with the kallikrein binding protein. J Biol Chem 1992;267:7048–7052.
73. Plow EF, Felez J, Miles LA. Cellular regulation of fibrinolysis. Thromb Haemostasis 1991;66:32–36.
74. Weisel JW, Cederholm-Williams SA. Fibrinogen and fibrin. In: Domb AJ, Kost J, Wiseman DM, eds. Handbook of Biodegradable Polymers. Amsterdam: Harwood, 1997:347–365.
75. Harris ES, Morgan RF, Rodeheaver GT. Analysis of the kinetics of peritoneal adhesion formation in the rat and evaluation of potential antiadhesive agents. Surgery (St. Louis) 1995;17:663–669.
76. Falk E. Dynamics in thrombus formation. Ann NY Acad Sci 1992;667:204–223.
77. Muzaffar TZ, Youngson GG, Bryce WAJ, Dhall DP. Studies on fibrin formation and effects of dextran. Thromb Haemostasis 1972;28:244–256.
78. Ellis H. The aetiology of postoperative abdominal adhesions: an experimental study. Br J Surg 1962;50:10–16.
79. James DCO, Ellis H, Hugh TB. The effect of streptokinase on experimental intraperitoneal adhesion formation. J Pathol Bacteriol 1965;90:279–287.
80. Gervin AS, Puckett CL, Silver D. Serosal hypofibrinolysis. Am J Surg 1973;125:80–88.
81. Buckman RF, Woods M, Sargent L, Gervin AS. A unifying pathogenetic mechanism in the etiology of intraperitoneal adhesions. J Surg Res 1976;20:1–5.
82. Raftery AT. Effect of peritoneal trauma on peritoneal fibrinolytic activity and intraperitoneal adhesion formation. Eur Surg Res 1981;13:397–401.
83. Raftery AT. Regeneration of parietal and visceral peritoneum: an electron microscopical study. J Anat 1973;115: 375–392.
84. Myhre-Jensen O, Bergman Larsen S, Astrup T. Fibrinolytic activity in serosal and synovial membranes. Arch Pathol Lab Med 1969;88:623–630.
85. Porter JM, Ball AP, Silver D. Mesothelial fibrinolysis. J Thorac Cardiovasc Surg 1971;62:725–730.
86. Scott-Coombes DM, Whawell SA, Vipond MN, Thompson JN. The human intraperitoneal fibrinolytic response to elective surgery. Br J Surg 1995;82:414–417.
87. Raftery AT. Regeneration of peritoneum: a fibrinolytic study. J Anat 1979;129:659–664.
88. Merio G, Fausone G, Barbero C, Castagna B. Fibrinolytic activity of the human peritoneum. Eur Surg Res 1980;12: 433–438.
89. Pugatch EMJ, Poole JCF. Inhibitor of fibrinolysis from mesothelium. Nature (Lond) 1969;221:269–270.
90. Hau T, Payne WD, Simmons RL. Fibrinolytic activity of the peritoneum during experimental peritonitis. Surg Gynecol Obstet 1979;148:415–418.

91. Lundin C, Sullins KE, White NA, Clem MF, Debowes RM, Pfeiffer CA. Induction of peritoneal adhesions with small intestinal ischaemia and distention in the foal. Equine Vet J 1989;21:451–458.
92. Fedor E, Mikó I, Nagy T. The role of ischaemia in the formation of postoperative intra-abdominal adhesions. Acta Chir Hung 1983;145:3–8.
93. Nishimura K, Nakamura RM, diZerega GS. Ibuprofen inhibition of postsurgical adhesion formation: a time and dose response biochemical evaluation in rabbits. J Surg Res 1984;36:115–124.
94. Nishimura K, Nakamura RM, diZerega GS. Biochemical evaluation of postsurgical wound repair: prevention of intraperitoneal adhesion formation with ibuprofen. J Surg Res 1983;34:219–226.
95. Rodgers K, Girgis W, diZerega GS, Bracken K, Richer L. Inhibition of postsurgical adhesions by liposomes containing nonsteroidal antiinflammatory drugs. Int J Fertil 1990;35:315–320.
96. Rodgers K, Girgis W, diZerega GS, Johns DB. Intraperitoneal tolmetin prevents postsurgical adhesion formation in rabbits. Int J Fertil 1990;35:40–45.
97. Abe H, Rodgers KE, Campeau JD, Girgis W, Ellefson D, diZerega GS. The effect of intraperitoneal administration of sodium tolmetin-hyaluronic acid on the postsurgical cell infiltration in vivo. J Surg Res 1990;49:322–327.
98. Hill West JL, Chowdhury SM, Sawhney AS, Pathak CP, Dunn RC, Hubbell JA. Prevention of postoperative adhesions in the rat by in situ photopolymerization of bioresorbable hydrogel barriers. Obstet Gynecol 1994;83:59–64.
99. Hill West JL, Dunn RC, Hubbell JA. Local release of fibrinolytic agents for adhesion prevention. J Surg Res 1995; 59:759–763.
100. Vipond MN, Whawell SA, Thompson JN, Dudley HAF. Effect of experimental peritonitis and ischemia on peritoneal fibrinolytic activity. Eur J Surg 1994;160:471–477.
101. Scott-Coombes DM, Whawell SA, Thompson JN. The operative peritoneal fibrinolytic response to abdominal operation. Eur J Surg 1995;161:395–399.
102. Kluft C. Fibrinolytic shut-down after surgery. In: Sawaya R, ed. Fibrinolysis and the Central Nervous System, Philadelphia: Hanley & Belfus, 1990:127–140.
103. D'Angelo A, Kluft C, Verheijen JH, Rijken DC, Mozzi E. Fibrinolytic shutdown after surgery: impairment of the balance between tissue type plasminogen activator and its specific inhibitor. Eur J Clin Invest 1985;15:308–312.
104. Holmdahl L, Eriksson E, Rippe B, Risberg B. Kinetics of transperitoneal tissue-type plasminogen (t-PA) absorption. Fibrinolysis 1996;10:1–7.
105. Parmer RJ, Mahata M, Mahata S, Sebald MT, O'Connor DT, Miles LA. Tissue plasminogen activator (t-PA) is targeted to the regulated secretory pathway. J Biol Chem 1997;272:1976–1982.
106. Emeis JJ, van den Hoogen CM, Diglio CA. Synthesis, storage and regulated secretion of tissue-type plasminogen activator by cultured rat heart endothelial cells. Fibrinolysis 1998;12:9–16.
107. Sitter T, Gödde M, Spannagl M, Fricke H, Kooistra T. Intraperitoneal coagulation and fibrinolysis during inflammation: *in vivo* and *in vitro* observations. Fibrinolysis 1996;10(suppl 2):99–104.
108. Tietze L, Elbrecht A, Schauerte C, et al. Modulation of pro- and antifibrinolytic properties of human peritoneal mesothelial cells by transforming growth factor $\beta1$ (TGF-$\beta1$), tumor necrosis factor α (TNF-α) and interleukin 1β (IL-1β). Thromb Haemostasis 1998;79:362–370.
109. Roberts AB, Spom MB. Transforming growth factor-β. In: Clark RAF, ed. The Molecular and Cellular Biology of Wound Repair. New York: Plenum Press, 1996: 275–308.
110. Whawell SA, Thompson JN. Cytokine-induced release of plasminogen activator inhibitor-1 by human mesothelial cells. Eur J Surg 1995;161:315–317.
111. Lundgren CH, Sawa H, Sobel BE, Fujii S. Modulation of expression of monocyte/macrophage plasminogen activator activity and its implications for attenuation of vasculopathy. Circulation 1994;90:1927–1934.
112. Weibel M, Majno AG. Peritoneal adhesions and their relation to abdominal surgery. A postmortem study. Am J Surg 1973;126:345–353.
113. Luijendijk RW, de Lange DCD, Wauters CCAP, et al. Foreign material in postoperative adhesions. Ann Surg 1996;223:242–248.
114. Ivarsson M-L, Bergström M, Eriksson E, Risberg B, Holmdahl L. Tissue markers as predictors of post-surgical adhesions. Br J Surg 1998;85:1549–1554.
115. Diamond MP, Daniell JF, Feste J, et al. Adhesion reformation and de novo adhesion formation after reproductive pelvic surgery. Fertil Steril 1987;47:864–866.
116. Menzies D, Ellis H. Intestinal obstruction from adhesions—how big is the problem? Ann R Coll Surg Engl 1990;72:60–63.
117. Sancho E, Declerck PJ, Price NC, Kelly SM, Booth NA. Conformational studies on plasminogen activator inhibitor (PAI-1) in active, latent, substrate, and cleaved forms. Biochemistry 1995;34:1064–1069.
118. Aalto M, Kulonen E, Penttinen R, Renvall S. Collagen synthesis in cultured mesothelial cells. Acta Chir Scand 1981;147:1–6.
119. Arici A, Tazuke SI, Attar E, Kliman HJ, Olive DL. Interleukin-8 concentration in peritoneal fluid of patients with endometriosis and modulation of interleukin-8 expression in human mesothelial cells. Mol Hum Reprod 1996; 2:40–45.
120. Baer AN, Green FA. Cyclooxygenase activity of cultured human mesothelial cells. Prostaglandins 1993;46:37–49.
121. Beavis J, Harwood JL, Coles GA, Williams JD. Synthesis of phospholipids by human peritoneal mesothelial cells. Perit Dial Int 1994;14:348–355.
122. Bermudez E, Everitt J, Walker C. Expression of growth factor and growth factor receptor RNA in rat pleural mesothelial cells in culture. Exp Cell Res 1990;190:91–98.
123. Betjes MGH, Tuk CW, Struijk DG, et al. Interleukin-8 production by human peritoneal mesothelial cells in response to tumor necrosis factor-α, interleukin-1, and medium conditioned by macrophages cocultured with *Staphylococcus epidermidis*. J Infect Dis 1992;168: 1202–1210.

124. Bittinger F, Klein CL, Skarke C, et al. PECAM-1 expression in human mesothelial cells: an in vitro study. Pathobiology 1996;64:320–327.
125. Bottles KD, Laszik Z, Morrissey JH, Kinasewitz GT. Tissue factor expression in mesothelial cells: induction both in vivo and in vitro. Am J Respir Cell Mol Biol 1997;17:164–172.
126. Breborowicz A, Korybalska K, Grzybowski A, Wieczorowska Tobis K, Martis L, Oreopoulos DG. Synthesis of hyaluronic acid by human peritoneal mesothelial cells: effect of cytokines and dialysate. Perit Dial Int 1996;16:374–378.
127. Bult H, Coene M-C, Rampart M, Herman AG. Complement derived factors and prostacyclin formation by rabbit isolated peritoneum and cultured mesothelial cells. Agents Actions Suppl 1984;14:237–247.
128. Cannistra SA, Ottensmeier C, Tidy J, DeFranzo B. Vascular cell adhesion molecule-1 expressed by peritoneal mesothelium partly mediates the binding of activated human T lymphocytes. Exp Hematol 1994;22:996–1002.
129. Cicila GT, O'Connel TM, Hahn WC, Reinwald JG. Cloned cDNA sequence for the human mesothelial protein 'mesosecrin' discloses its identity as a plasminogen activator inhibitor (PAI-1) and a recent evolutionary change in transcript processing J Cell Sci 1989;94:1–10.
130. Coene MC, Solheid C, Clates M, Herman AG. Prostaglandin production by cultured mesothelial cells. Arch Int Pharmacodyn 1981;249:316–318.
131. Coene M-C, van Hove C, Claeys M, Herman A. Arachidonic acid metabolism by cultured mesothelial cells. Different transformations of exogenously added and endogenously released substrate. Biochim Biophys Acta 1982;710:437–445.
132. Davies M, Stylianou E, Yung S, Thomas GJ, Coles GA, Williams JD. Proteoglycans of CAPD-dialysate fluid and mesothelium. Contrib Nephrol 1990;85:134–141.
133. Dobbie JW, Pavlina T, Lloyd J, Johnson RC. Phosphatidylcholine synthesis by peritoneal mesothelium: its implication for peritoneal dialysis. Am J Kidney Dis 1988;12:31–36.
134. Douvdevani A, Rapoport J, Konforty A, Argov S, Ovnat A, Chaimovitz C. Human peritoneal mesothelial cells synthesize IL-1 alpha and beta. Kidney Int 1994;46:993–1001.
135. Ferriola PC, Stewart W. Fibronectin expression and organization in mesothelial and mesothelioma cells. Am J Physiol 1996;271:L804–L812.
136. Griffith DE, Miller EJ, Gray LD, Idell S, Johnson AR. Interleukin-1-mediated release of interleukin-8 by asbestos-stimulated human pleural mesothelial cells. Am J Respir Cell Mol Biol 1994;10:245–252.
137. Harvey W, Amlot PL. Collagen production by human mesothelial cells in vitro. J Pathol 1983;139:337–347.
138. Hjelle JT, Golinska BT, Waters DC, et al. Lectin staining of peritoneal mesothelial cells in vitro. Perit Dial Int 1991;11:307–316.
139. Hjelle JT, Ho AK, Dobbie JW, Steidley KR, Duffield R. Evidence of muscarinic acetylcholine receptors and GTP-binding proteins in peritoneal mesothelial cells in vitro. Adv Perit Dial 1993;9:303–306.
140. Honda A, Noguchi N, Takehara H, Ohashi Y, Asuwa N, Mori Y. Cooperative enhancement of hyaluronic acid synthesis by combined use of IGF-1 and EGF, and inhibition by tyrosine kinase inhibitor genistein, in cultured mesothelial cells from rabbit pericardial cavity. J Cell Sci 1991;98:91–98.
141. Honda A, Sekiguchly, Mori Y. Prostaglandin E2 stimulates cyclic AMP-mediated hyaluronan synthesis in rabbit pericardial mesothelial cells. Biochem J 1993;292:497–502.
142. Jonjic N, Peri G, Bernasconi S, et al. Expression of adhesion molecules and chemotactic cytokines in cultured human mesothelial cells. J Exp Med 1992;176:1165–1174.
143. Kawata Y, Mimuro J, Kaneko M, Shimada K, Sakata Y. Expression of plasminogen activator inhibitor 2 in the adult and embryonic mouse tissues. Thromb Haemostasis 1996;76:569–576.
144. Korybalska K, Breborowicz A, Martis L, Oreopoulos DG. In vitro detection of hydrogen peroxide in mesothelial cells. Adv Perit Dial 1996;12:7–10.
145. Kumar A, Koenig KB, Johnson AR, Idell S. Expression and assembly of procoagulant complexes by human pleural mesothelial cells. Thromb Haemostasis 1994;71:587–592.
146. Lanfrancone L, Boraschi D, Ghiara P, et al. Human peritoneal mesothelial cells produce many cytokines (granulocyte colony-stimulating factor [CSF], granulocyte-monocyte-CSF, macrophage-CSF, interleukin-1 [IL-1], and IL-6) and are activated and stimulated to grow by IL-1. Blood 1992;80:2835–2842.
147. Marshall BC, Santana A, Xu QP, et al. Metalloproteinases and tissue inhibitor of metalloproteinases in mesothelial cells. Cellular differentiation influences expression. J Clin Invest 1993;91:1792–1799.
148. Morganti M, Budianto D, Amo Takiy B, et al. Detection of minimal but significant amount of von Willebrand factor in human omentum mesothelial cell cultures. Biomed Pharmacother 1996;50:369–372.
149. Owens MW, Grisham MB. Nitric oxide synthesis by rat pleural mesothelial cells: induction by cytokines and lipopolysaccaride. Am J Physiol 1993;265:110–116.
150. Raftery AT. An enzyme histochemical study of mesothelial cells in rodents. J Anat 1973;115:365–373.
151. Rougier JP, Moullier P, Piedagnel R, Ronco PM. Hyperosmolality suppresses but TGF beta 1 increases MMP9 in human peritoneal mesothelial cells. Kidney Int 1997;51:337–347.
152. Rougier JP, Guia S, Hagege, Nguyen G, Ronco PM. PAI-1 secretion and matrix deposition in human peritoneal mesothelial cell cultures: transcriptional regulation by TGF-beta 1. Kidney Int 1998;54:87–98.
153. Shanthaveerappa TR, Bourne GH. Histochemical studies on the localization of oxidative and dephosphorylating enzymes and esterases in the peritoneal mesothelial cells. Histochemistry 1965;5:331–338.
154. Shostak A, Pivnik E, Gotloib L. Cultured rat mesothelial cells generate hydrogen peroxide: a new player in peritoneal defense? J Am Soc Nephrol 1996;7:2371–2378.
155. Sitter T, Toet K, Fricke H, Schiffl H, Held E, Kooistra T. Modulation of procoagulant and fibrinolytic system com-

ponents of mesothelial cells by inflammatory mediators. Am J Physiol 1996;271:R1256–R1263.
156. Suassuna JH, Das Neves FC, Hartley RB, Ogg CS, Cameron JS. Immunohistochemical studies of the peritoneal membrane and infiltrating cells in normal subjects and in patients on CAPD. Kidney Int 1994;46:443–454.
157. Topley N, Jörres A, Luttman W, et al. Human peritoneal mesothelial cells synthesize interleukin-6: induction by Il-1β and TNF-α. Kidney Int 1993;43:226–233.
158. Topley N, Jörres A, Luttman W, et al. Human peritoneal mesothelial cells synthesize interleukin-8: synergistic induction by interleukin-1β and tumor necrosis factor-α. Am J Pathol 1993;142:1876–1886.
159. Topley N, Petersen MM, Mackenzie R, et al. Human peritoneal mesothelial cell prostaglandin synthesis: induction of cyclooxygenase mRNA by peritoneal macrophage-derived cytokines. Kidney Int 1994;46:900–909.
160. Verhagen HJ, Heijnen Snyder GJ, Vink T, et al. Tissue factor expression on mesothelial cells is induced during in vitro culture—manipulation of culture conditions creates perspectives for mesothelial cells as a source for cell seeding procedures on vascular grafts. Thromb Haemostasis 1995;74:1096–1102.
161. Visser CE, Brouwer Steenbergen JJ, Betjes MG, Koomen GC, Beelen RH, Krediet RT. Cancer antigen 125: a bulk marker for the mesothelial mass in stable peritoneal dialysis patients. Nephrol Dial Transplant 1995;10:64–69.
162. Whawell SA, Scott-Coombes DM, Vipond MN, Terbutt SJ, Thompson JN. Tumor necrosis factor-mediated release of plasminogen activator inhibitor 1 by human mesothelial cells. Br J Surg 1994;81:214–216.
163. Witowski J, Jorres A, Coles GA, Williams JD, Topley N. Superinduction of IL-6 synthesis in human peritoneal mesothelial cells is related to the induction and stabilization of IL-6 mRNA. Kidney Int 1996;50:1212–1223.
164. Witowski J, Breborowicz A, Topley N, Martis L, Knapowski J, Oreopoulos DG. Insulin stimulates the activity of Na+/K(+)-ATPase in human peritoneal mesothelial cells. Perit Dial Int 1997;17:186–193.
165. Yung S, Coles GA, Williams JD, Davies M. The source and possible significance of hyaluronan in the peritoneal cavity. Kidney Int 1994;46:527–533.
166. Yung S, Thomas GJ, Stylianou E, Williams JD, Coles GA, Davies M. Source of peritoneal proteoglycans. Human peritoneal mesothelial cells synthesize and secrete mainly small dermatan sulfate proteoglycans. Am J Pathol 1995; 146:520–529.
167. Yung S, Coles GA, Davies M. IL-1 beta, a major stimulator of hyaluronan synthesis in vitro of human peritoneal mesothelial cells: relevance to peritonitis in CAPD. Kidney Int 1996;50:1337–1343.
168. Zeillemaker AM, Verbrugh HA, Hoynck van Papendrecht AA, Leguit P. CA 125 secretion by peritoneal mesothelial cells. J Clin Pathol 1994;47:263–265.
169. Zeillemaker AM, Mul FP, Hoynck van Papendrecht AA, et al. Polarized secretion of interleukin-8 by human mesothelial cells: a role in neutrophil migration. Immunology 1995;84:227–232.

9

Peritoneal Fibrinolysis and Adhesion Formation

Jeremy Thompson

CONTENTS

The aim of this chapter is to examine our current knowledge of peritoneal fibrinolysis. The fibrinolytic activity of the normal peritoneum and the changes that occur following peritoneal injury are described. These changes are believed to be of pivotal importance in the pathogenesis of intraperitoneal adhesion formation. Many biologic systems are involved in the response of the peritoneum to injury in addition to fibrinolysis, for example, the coagulation system and acute inflammatory mechanisms. Some of these systems are discussed elsewhere in this volume, including the processes underlying peritoneal tissue repair (Chapters 1 and 4), the cytokine response to peritoneal injury (Chapter 5), and the action of growth factors in peritoneal wound repair (Chapter 3).

The Pathology of Adhesion Formation

Adhesions are deposits of fibrous tissue that occur in many sites including the peritoneal, pericardial, and pleural cavities. Although they may occasionally be congenital in origin, adhesions are usually the result of injury to the lining membrane of such cavities. John Hunter was probably one of the first to study the pathogenesis of adhesion formation when he noted the early development of a fibrinous peritoneal deposit following inflammation.[1] This was later identified as fibrin following the development of specific histologic staining tech-

TABLE 9.1. Causes of intraperitoneal adhesions

Operative injury
Bacterial peritonitis
Radiotherapy
Visceral ischemia
Foreign bodies reactions, e.g., starch, talc
Chemical peritonitis

niques.[2,3] At the beginning of the twentieth century, Hertzler[4] clearly described the pathologic progression from injury to fibrinous exudate followed by gradual conversion into fibrous tissue by 3 or 4 days. These and later studies have confirmed the pathophysiologic progression from peritoneal injury to tissue inflammation with its associated inflammatory exudate leading to deposition of fibrin and the formation of fibrinous adhesions. These fibrinous adhesions then become organized, and the resultant fibroblast invasion leads to collagen deposition. Collagen maturation then occurs with the formation of permanent fibrous adhesions.

A large number of experimental models of adhesion formation have been reported using different mechanisms of peritoneal injury; these have included tissue ischemia, mechanical injury, bacterial peritonitis, and chemical peritoneal injury.[5,6] In modern clinical practice, iatrogenic operative injury to the peritoneum and infective peritonitis are the common causes of intraperitoneal adhesion formation. Indeed, up to 90% of patients develop intraabdominal adhesions following laparotomy.[7,8] There is however a wide range of recognized causes of intraperitoneal adhesion formation (Table 9.1). Intraperitoneal adhesions are a major cause of morbidity, being the most common cause of small-bowel obstruction,[9–11] and a common cause of both primary and secondary female infertility and pelvic pain.[12,13]

For many years it has been recognized that peritoneal injury does not inevitably lead to the formation of permanent fibrous adhesions. Boys was one of the first to describe the clearance of fibrin from the peritoneum,[14] an observation subsequently confirmed by Jackson who observed that the majority of experimental fibrinous adhesions were absorbed by 48 to 96 hours after injury.[15] Thus, it has long been recognized that lysis of intraperitoneal fibrinous deposits may occur and that this process is important in the prevention of permanent adhesion formation (Fig. 9.1).

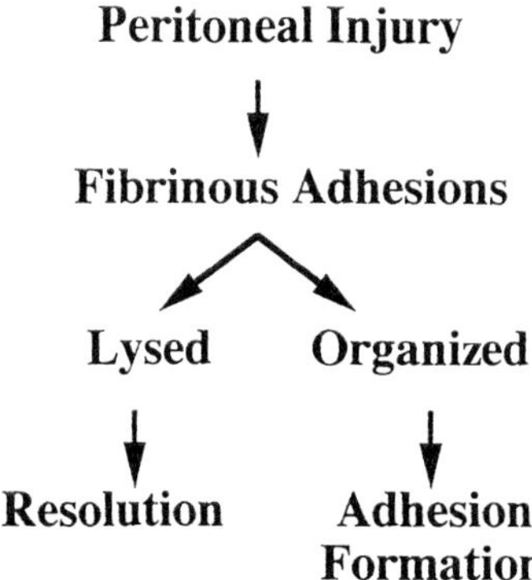

FIG. 9.1. The pathway to adhesion formation.

The Fibrinolytic System

The first description of fibrinolysis in tissues arose from the pioneering tissue culture experiments of Fleischer and Loeb.[16] Three lines of investigation—the fibrinolytic activity of cultures of hemolytic streptococci, the proteolytic activity of blood, and the spontaneous lysis of clotted blood[17–19]—led to the gradual identification of individual fibrinolytic system mediators.[20–22] Our current concept of the fibrinolytic system is shown in Fig. 9.2. There is a complicated interplay between activators and inhibitors of this system, and the important mediators vary considerably at different biologic sites.

Plasminogen and Plasmin

The final common pathway of the fibrinolytic system is the formation of plasmin, which is a fully active serine protease formed by the action of plasminogen activators on its zymogen precursor, plasminogen. Activation converts inactive single-chain plasminogen into an active two-chain disulfide-linked protease, the main role of which is the degradation of fibrin. Plasmin is also active on other susceptible circulating proteins including fibrinogen, clotting factors V and VIII, and platelet membrane receptors.[23,24] Plasmin is weakly inhibited by alpha-2-antiplasmin, which acts by the formation of an inactive one-to-one stoichiometric complex.[23,25]

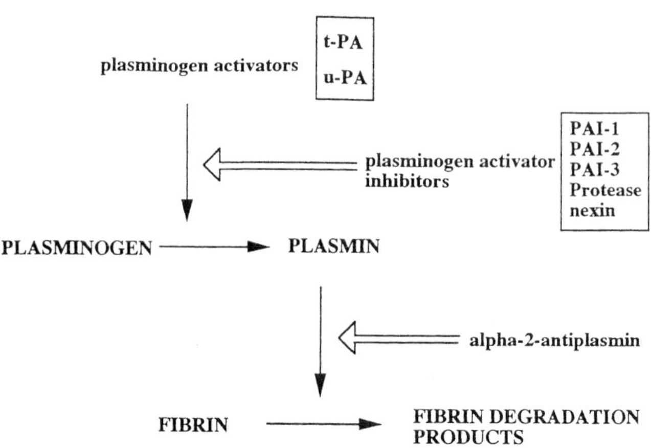

FIG. 9.2. Schematic representation of the fibrinolytic system. tPA, tissue plasminogen activator; uPA, urokinase; PAI, plasminogen activator inhibitor.

Tissue Plasminogen Activator

Human tissue plasminogen activator (tPA) was first isolated from uterine tissue.[26] It exists in both single- and double-chain forms, the two-chain structure being formed by proteolytic cleavage of the single-chain molecule.[27] Tissue plasminogen activator is present in many human tissues and body fluids, including the thyroid, kidney, heart, uterus, prostate, blood, semen, saliva, and tears.[28]

Urokinase

Urokinase (uPA) was first isolated from human urine[29] but has since been isolated from a number of tissues including the kidney, lung, placenta, bladder, epidermal cells, fibroblasts, and monocyte-macrophages.[23,30] Urokinase is synthesized in a single-chain form that has very limited capacity to activate plasminogen.[24] Limited cleavage by plasmin itself converts the single-chain urokinase into a two-chain disulfide form that activates plasminogen approximately 1000 times faster than its single-chain precursor.[23]

Plasminogen Activator Inhibitors

Plasminogen activator inhibitor-1 (PAI-1) is a glycoprotein first isolated from cultured human endothelial and rat hepatoma cells.[31–33] PAI-1 is a member of the serpin superfamily and has been detected in the alpha granules of human platelets, in human plasma and smooth muscle cells.[32,34,35] PAI-1 is a powerful inhibitor of both tissue plasminogen activator and urokinase.[31,36]

Plasminogen activator inhibitor-2 (PAI-2) was first isolated from human placenta[37] and is also a member of the serpin superfamily.[38] PAI-2 has been localized to the trophoblastic epithelium of the placenta,[39] amniotic fluid,[40] plasma of pregnant women,[41] and leukocytes, principally of the mononuclear type.[42–44] PAI-2 avidly inhibits urokinase and inhibits tissue plasminogen activator with a marginally slower reaction rate.[42,45] PAI-2 reacts with both plasminogen activators at a slower rate than PAI-1.[42]

Protease nexin has been found in human fibroblasts and possesses a broad spectrum of activity inhibiting uPA, tPA, thrombin, trypsin, plasmin, and factor Xa.[46,47] Plasminogen activator inhibitor-3 (PAI-3), which was originally identified from human urine,[48] and acts by inhibiting two-chain urokinase.[49]

Regulation of Fibrinolysis

Fibrinolytic activity is regulated both at the cellular level and by complex interactions between individual fibrinolytic system mediators. The rate of cellular synthesis and release of individual fibrinolytic components can be influenced by a variety of hormonal, physiologic, and neural stimuli.[25] Tissue plasminogen activator release from endothelial or granulosa cell lines in culture can be stimulated by thrombin, histamine, butyrate, follicle-stimulating hormone, and gonadotrophin-releasing hormone.[50–54] A variety of other stimuli, including venostasis, exercise, infusions of vasoactive drugs including vasopressin analog, and anabolic steroids,[55–58] are known to increase plasma concentrations of tissue plasminogen activator.

Plasminogen activator inhibitor-1 production synthesis or release has been stimulated in endothelial cell culture by dexamethasone, thrombin, endotoxin, interleukin-1, and tissue necrosis factor.[59–62] PAI-1 appears to be an acute-phase reactant protein.[63,64] Plasminogen activator inhibitor-2 synthesis or release has also been stimulated in vitro by endotoxin and tumor necrosis factor (TNF).[65,66]

At the local level, fibrinolysis is regulated in part by the fibrin enhancement of plasminogen activation and in part by the rapid inactivation of both plasmin and tissue plasminogen activator by their specific inhibitors. Plasminogen is preferentially activated by tissue plasminogen activator upon the surface of fibrin, tPA binding to a fibrin at a specific receptor,[67] which leads to the exposure of a strong plasminogen-binding site on the surface of the fibrin molecule.[68,69] In this way plasminogen activation is markedly potentiated (up to 1000 fold) in the presence of fibrin, and the fibrin-bound plasmin is protected against inhibition by alpha-2-antiplasmin.[69] Following lysis of fibrin, both plasmin and tPA are released and then rapidly bound by their respective inhibitors, effectively confining the activation of plasmin to the surface of fibrin.

Peritoneal Fibrinolysis

Early Studies

Although Boys[14] and Jackson.[15] both recognized that fibrinous adhesions may resolve rather than progress to fibrous adhesions, it was probably Benzer[70] who first recognized that the peritoneum itself possessed fibrinolytic activity. Myhre-Jensen et al. confirmed this finding in a variety of animal models and also demonstrated the existence of interspecies variation.[71] At about the same time, plasminogen-activating activity was first described in human mesothelium.[72] Whitaker and coworkers first demonstrated fibrinolytic activity in a cell-free preparation of peritoneal fluid from the rat using the fibrin plate technique.[73] Pattinson and colleagues[74] demonstrated the presence of both plasminogen and plasmin–antiplasmin complexes together with a high concentration of fibrinogen degredation products in peritoneal fluid obtained from women undergoing investigation for infertility. More recent studies have demonstrated the presence of plasminogen-activating activity in the pelvic fluid of both women and rabbits.[75,76]

Localization of Peritoneal Plasminogen-Activating Activity

A number of techniques have been used in an attempt to localize peritoneal plasminogen-activating activity. Porter and colleagues used the fibrin slide technique, which demonstrated activity in human peritoneal tissue related to submesothelial blood vessels and subsequently along the mesothelial border.[77] Using Hautchen preparations of rat peritoneum, Raftery localized plasminogen-activating activity to the mesothelium.[78–80] These findings were subsequently confirmed by other workers.[73,81,82] Biopsied material from human peritoneum obtained at the time of operation has been shown to possess plasminogen-activating activity.[83,84] Although there is considerable variation in plasminogen-activating activity between biopsies from different patients, similar levels of plasminogen-activating activity have been found in both visceral and parietal biopsies taken from a number of abdominal sites.[83]

Characterization of Peritoneal Fibrinolytic Mediators

Moore and colleagues first proposed that tissue plasminogen activator (tPA) was the primary mediator of plasminogen-activating activity in the peritoneal cavity.[85] Mayer and coworkers demonstrated that human peritoneal tissue plasminogen-activating activity was markedly suppressed by the addition of an antiserum raised against human tissue plasminogen activator.[86] Vipond and colleagues confirmed the inhibition of human peritoneal plasminogen-activating activity by anti-tPA antibody, whereas antiurokinase antibody had minimal effect.[87] In addition, they quantified the concentration of tPA within peritoneal tissue and showed that this correlated well with overall plasminogen-activating activity. These and subsequent studies have confirmed that tPA is the principal physiologic plasminogen activator in human peritoneal tissue.[87,88]

The presence of an inhibitor of fibrinolysis was first described by Pugatch and Poole,[89] who postulated that the presence of an inhibitor might explain the marked interspecies variation in plasminogen-activating activity previously demonstrated.[71] Buckman and colleagues noted a reduction in plasminogen-activating activity of the peritoneum surrounding an experimental free peritoneal graft.[90] van Hinsburgh and coworkers reported that human omental mesothelial cells in culture could produce plasminogen activator inhibitor-1 and -2 in addition to tissue plasminogen activator.[65] Plasminogen activator inhibitors have been either not detectable or found to be present in very low concentrations in normal human peritoneal tissue.[87,91,92]

Effect of Peritoneal Injury or Inflammation on Fibrinolytic Activity

A number of workers have suggested that loss of peritoneal fibrinolytic activity might be important in the development of permanent fibrous adhesions.[71,72,93] Porter and colleagues demonstrated that both mechanical abrasion and chemical injury reduce peritoneal plasminogen-activating activity in dogs.[72] Since then, a number of studies have confirmed this finding both in experimental models and in man; some of these are listed in Table 9.2.[6,72,83,94–98] Different mechanisms of peritoneal injury all appear to lead to a reduction in peritoneal plasminogen-activating activity, which is regarded as central to the pathogenesis of adhesion formation. Marked reduction in plasminogen-activating activity has been seen experimentally in rats when a free peritoneal graft has been studied,[90,98] whereas raw, un-

TABLE 9.2. Studies of peritoneal plasminogen-activating activity following injury

Study	Species	Type of injury	Magnitude of reduction in peritoneal plasminogen-activating activity
Porter et al. 1969[72]	Dog	i. Mechanical ii. Chemical	i. 25% ii. 45%–100%
Gervin et al. 1973[94]	Dog	Mechanical abrasion	20%–100%
Ryan et al. 1973[95]	Rat	Drying	100%
Buckman et al. 1976[96]	Rat	i. Mechanical abrasion ii. Ischemia	i. 40% ii. 60%
Hau et al. 1979[97]	Dog	Peritonitis (ischemic loop of small bowel)	100%
Raftery 1981[80]	Rat	i. Diathermy ii. Ischemia	i. 100% ii. 90%
Thompson et al. 1989[83]	Human	Appendicitis	69%
Vipond et al. 1994[6]	Rat	i. Ischemia ii. Chemical injury iii. Bacterial peritonitis	60%–100%

covered peritoneal defects (at least in this experimental model) contained significantly more fibrinolytic activity. These experimental results are consistent with Ellis' view[99] that peritoneal defects should not be closed under tension. Although it is difficult to directly relate reduction in peritoneal plasminogen-activating activity to subsequent fibrous adhesion formation, a number of experimental studies have demonstrated good correlation between the reduction in peritoneal fibrinolytic activity produced by a particular injury and the degree of adhesion formation associated with the same experimental injury.[6,90,94,96,98]

A number of studies have examined the time course of the reduced plasminogen-activating activity associated with peritoneal injury. Studies of sequential biopsies taken during prolonged open operation have demonstrated reductions in plasminogen-activating activity of the peritoneal tissue during surgery, which appears to be largely related to reduced concentrations of tissue plasminogen activator rather than the presence of detectable plasminogen activator inhibitors.[84,100] Experimental studies have demonstrated a reduction in plasminogen-activating activity for up to 24 hours after peritoneal injury, but following this period a rebound increase in peritoneal fibrinolytic activity has been observed by a number of investigators.[6,79,90,95,97] Studies of postoperative peritoneal drain fluid have shown a progressive reduction in plasminogen-activating activity, in the first few hours following operation, to undetectable levels of activity, followed by complete loss of fibrinolytic activity up to 72 hours after operation.[101] In clinical practice, the duration of reduced peritoneal plasminogen-activating activity will depend on the nature and degree of peritoneal injury and whether the injury is ongoing, such as seen in patients with bacterial peritonitis or foreign-body deposition, or limited, for example, operative injury. Experimental studies suggest that a period of 4 to 5 days is required before fibrinous adhesions undergo irreversible organization, and there are sound reasons for believing that the time course in patients is similar.

Mechanism of Reduced Peritoneal Plasminogen-Activating Activity Following Injury

Some workers initially attributed the reduction in fibrinolytic activity to the loss of mesothelial cells from the peritoneal surface, but subsequent studies have shown that the production and release of plasminogen activator inhibitors is the major factor in the loss of peritoneal fibrinolytic activity. An improved understanding of the fibrinolytic system and development of specific mediator assays allowed a number of groups to demonstrate that the reduced plasminogen-activating activity seen in peritonitis and following peritoneal injury is related to the production and release of plasminogen activator inhibitors.[84,87,91] Both plasminogen activator inhibitor-1 and -2 have been found in high concentrations in biopsies taken from inflamed human peritoneum, and these inhibitors reduce and subsequently abolish all peritoneal fibrinolytic activity. The same phenomenon can be observed in postoperative peritoneal fluid[101] where the changes in plasminogen-activating activity and PAI-1 and PAI-2 concentrations are shown (Figs. 9.3 through 9.5). Antigenic assays of extracts of inflamed peritoneal tissue

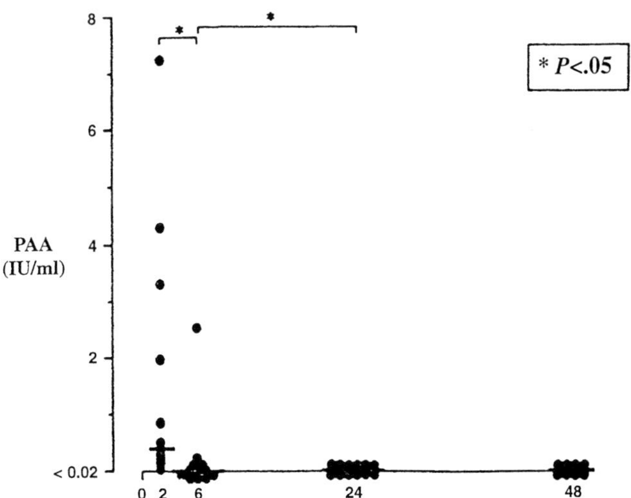

FIG. 9.3. Postoperative peritoneal fluid plasminogen-activating activity (PAA).

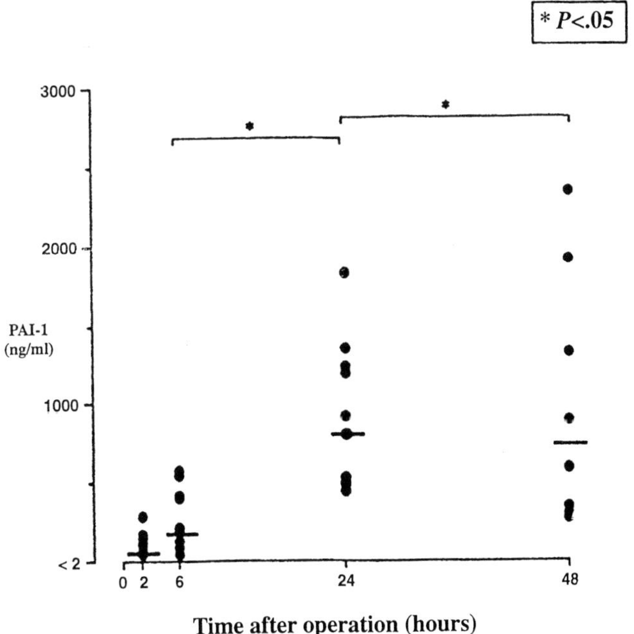

FIG. 9.4. Postoperative peritoneal fluid plasminogen activator inhibitor-1 (PAI-1) concentrations.

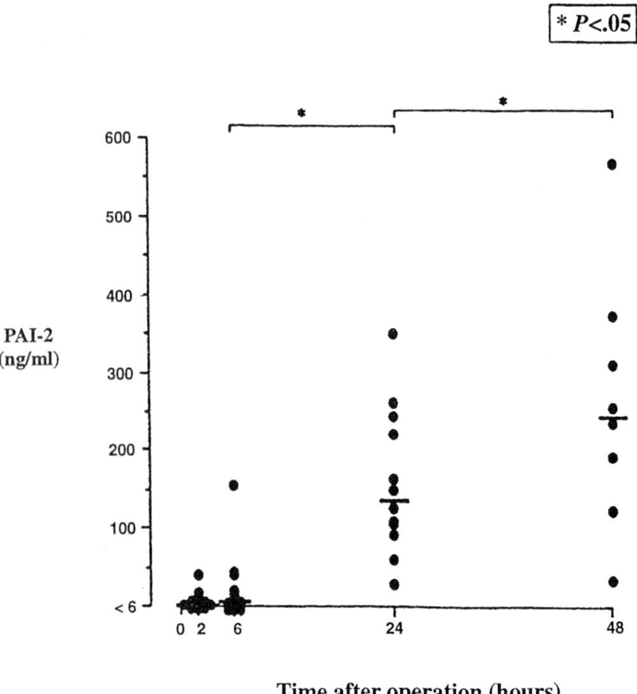

FIG. 9.5. Postoperative peritoneal fluid plasminogen activator inhibitor-2 (PAI-2) concentrations.

show detectable levels of tissue plasminogen activator but low or undetectable plasminogen-activating activity, because tPA activity has been completely abolished by plasminogen activator inhibitors.[84,87,91]

Localization of Plasminogen Activator Inhibitor Production

Both immunohistochemistry and messenger RNA in situ hybridization techniques have been used to localize the cellular site of both plasminogen activators and inhibitors in peritoneal tissue.[92,102,103] Whawell and coworkers have localized plasminogen activator inhibitor-1 production to the mesothelium and the endothelial cells lining submesothelial blood vessels in inflamed human peritoneum using mRNA in situ hybridization.[102] Using a similar technique, they also localized plasminogen activator inhibitor-2 to the mesothelium and to monocytes within the submesothelial tissues.[103] Examples of the studies are shown in Figs. 9.6 and 9.7. Holmdahl and colleagues have used immunohistochemistry to localize tissue plasminogen activator to normal human mesothelium and subserosal capillary walls, this localization being lost in inflamed tissue.[92] Plasminogen activator inhibitor-1 immunoreactivity was detectable in normal mesothelium but substantially increased in inflammation, when it was also seen throughout the submesothelial tissue and localized to macrophage cells. These morphologic observations are supported by the finding that cultures of human omental mesothelial cells and a human mesothelial cell line produce both tissue plasminogen activator and plasminogen activator inhibitors.[65,104,105]

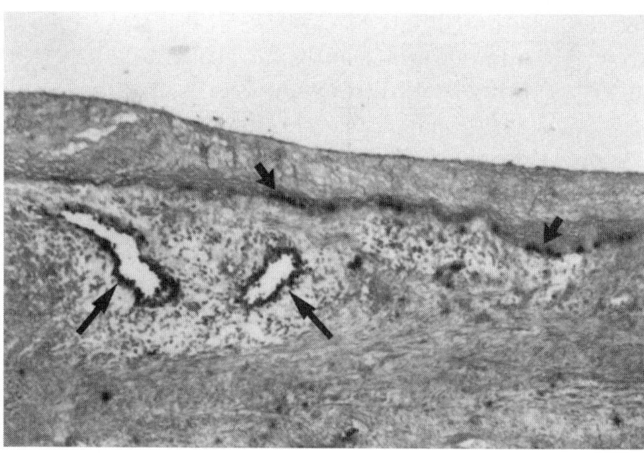

FIG. 9.6. Plasminogen activator inhibitor-1 production localized to mesothelial (*small arrows*) and submesothelial endothelial (*large arrows*) cells in inflamed human peritoneum using mRNA in situ hybridization. *Please see insert for color reproduction of this figure.*

Role of Proinflammatory Cytokines in the Peritoneal Production of Plasminogen Activator Inhibitors

The association between inflamed peritoneum and the production of plasminogen activator inhibitor-1 and -2 with resultant loss in fibrinolytic activity suggests that the inflammatory process results in stimulation of PAI-1 and PAI-2 production. The role of cytokines in peritoneal inflammation is discussed in Chapter 5. High levels of proinflammatory cytokines are found in inflamed peritoneal tissue,[106,107] and the concentration seen in perito-

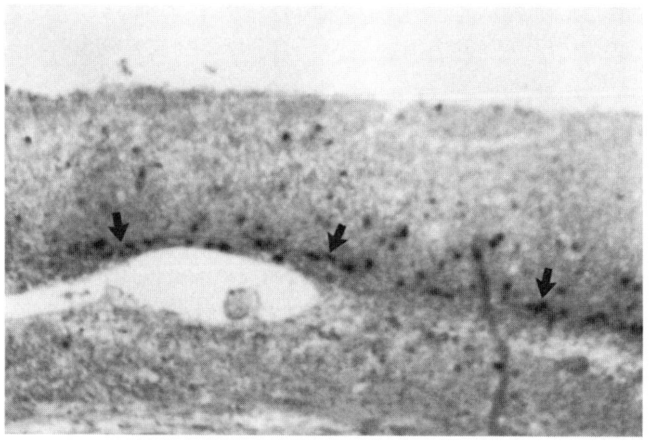

FIG. 9.7. Plasminogen activator inhibitor-2 production localized to mesothelial cells (*arrowed*) on the surface of an inflamed appendix using mRNA in situ hybridization. *Please see insert for color reproduction of this figure.*

neal tissue are several hundredfold higher than those in the plasma, as would be expected because of the predominantly paracrine nature of their activity.[106] Studies of mesothelial cells derived either from human omentum or from a human mesothelial cell line have demonstrated that the inflammatory cytokines tumor necrosis factor-alpha (TNF-α), interleukin-1, interleukin-6, and transforming growth factor-beta (TGF-β), together with lipopolysaccharide (endotoxin), all resulted in increased plasminogen activator inhibitor-1 release.[104,105,108,109] Whawell and colleagues[104] showed that the proinflammatory cytokines TNF-α, interleukin-1, and interleukin-6 both individually and synergistically stimulated mesothelial cell PAI-1 production in vitro. Studies of postoperative peritoneal fluid have shown that the time course of peritoneal cytokine production is in keeping with their de novo stimulation of plasminogen activator inhibitor production and release (Fig. 9.8). These observations strongly support the hypothesis that proinflammatory cytokines directly stimulate mesothelial cells to synthesize and release plasminogen activator inhibitors.

Adhesion Prevention Using Fibrinolytic Enhancement

The observation that decreased peritoneal fibrinolytic activity may well be of prime importance in the development of permanent fibrous adhesions stimulated a number of workers to attempt adhesion prevention by fibrinolytic enhancements. Early studies used either streptokinase or plasmin, with conflicting experimental results.[110–115] Rivkind and colleagues were unable to demonstrate any benefit from urokinase in a rat model of adhesion formation.[116] The availability of recombinant tissue plasminogen activator resulted in a number of experimental studies of its effect on adhesion formation. These models either have used intraperitoneal perfusion of tPA[117,118] or have incorporated tPA into a gel with resultant delayed release and absorption.[119–121] These approaches have been used because tPA is rapidly absorbed from the peritoneal cavity, and a prolonged enhancement of fibrinolysis over a period of several days is likely to be required for effective adhesion prevention. Most of these studies have shown significant reductions in experimental adhesion formation, without significant intraperitoneal hemorrhage or obvious impairment of wound healing.[117–121] Despite these encouraging experimental studies, very little information on the use of tPA in patients to prevent adhesion formation is currently available.

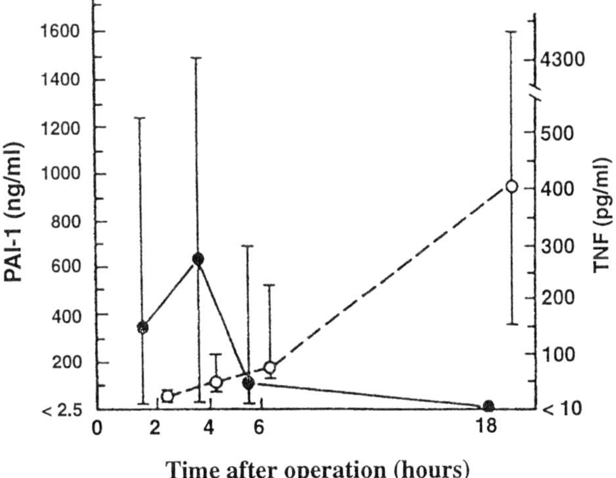

FIG. 9.8. Time course of postoperative peritoneal fluid tumor necrosis factor-α (TNF, *solid circles*) and plasminogen activator inhibitor-1 (PAI-1, *open circles*) concentrations.

Summary

The peritoneum possesses plasminogen-activating activity that acts to prevent the deposition of fibrin within the peritoneal cavity. Peritoneal inflammation leads to loss of this activity and allows the deposition of fibrin to occur within the inflammatory peritoneal exudate. This fibrin deposition results in fibrinous adhesions between viscera and to the parietal peritoneum. Prolonged depression of peritoneal fibrinolysis permits organization of these fibrinous adhesions into permanent fibrous structures. In this way, the fibrinolytic activity of the peritoneum is of pivotal importance in the development of fibrous adhesions.

The plasminogen-activating activity of human peritoneum is largely mediated through tissue plasminogen activator. Peritoneal inflammation results in the production and release of plasminogen activator inhibitors, the synthesis and release of which appear to be stimulated by proinflammatory cytokines. Modification of this pathophysiologic sequence either by reduction of inflammation or by enhancement of peritoneal fibrinolytic activity may provide a sound basis for future attempts at adhesion prevention.

References

1. Palmer JF. The surgical works of John Hunter, Vol. 3. London: Longman Rees Orme Brown Green and Longman, 1835.
2. Warbasse JP. Graser on the adhesions of serous membranes. Ann Surg 1895;22:811–816.
3. Baillie M. The Morbid Anatomy of Some of the Most Important Parts of the Human Body, 5th Ed. London: G&W Nicol, 1818:133–136.
4. Hertzler AE. The development of fibrous tissue in peritoneal adhesions. Anat Rec 1915;9:83.
5. Ellis H. The causes and prevention of intestinal adhesions. Br J Surg 1982;69:241–243.

6. Vipond MN, Whawell SA, Thompson JN, et al. Effect of experimental peritonitis and ischaemia on peritoneal fibrinolytic activity. Eur J Surg 1994; 160:471–477.
7. Menzies D, Ellis H. Intestinal obstruction from adhesions—how big is the problem? Ann R Coll Surg Engl 1990;72:60–63.
8. Thompson JN, Whawell SA. The pathogenesis and prevention of adhesion formation. Br J Surg 1995;82:3–5.
9. Bevan PG. Adhesive obstruction. Ann R Coll Surg Engl 1984;66:164–169.
10. McEntee G, Pender D, Mulvin D, et al. Current spectrum of intestinal obstruction. Br J Surg 1987;74:976–980.
11. Füzün M, Kaymak E, Harmancioglu Ô, et al. Principal causes of mechanical bowel obstruction in surgically treated adults in Western Turkey. Br J Surg 1991;78: 202–203.
12. Hull MGR, Glazener CMA, Kelly NJ, et al. Population study of causes, treatment and outcome of infertility. Br Med J 1985;291:1693–1697.
13. Bronson RA, Wallach EE. Lysis of periadnexal adhesions for correction of infertility. Fertil Steril 1977;278:613–619.
14. Boys F. The prophylaxis of peritoneal adhesions. Surgery (St. Louis) 1942;11:118–168.
15. Jackson BB. Observations on intraperitoneal adhesions: an experimental study. Surgery (St. Louis) 1958;44:507–514.
16. Fleischer MS, Loeb L. On tissue fibrinolysins. J Biol Chem 1915;21:477–501.
17. Tillett WS, Garner RL. The fibrinolytic activity of hemolytic streptococci. J Exp Med 1933;58:485–502.
18. Tagnon HJ. The significance of fibrinolysis in mechanism of coagulation of blood. J Lab Clin Med 1942;27: 1119–1131.
19. Mole RH. Fibrinolysis and the fluidity of blood post mortem. J Pathol Bacteriol 1948;60:413–427.
20. Fischer A. Mechanism of the proteolytic activity of malignant tissue cells. Nature (Lond) 1946;157:442.
21. Sherry S. The fibrinolytic system and its pharmacologic activation for thrombolysis. Cardiol Clin 1987;5:1–11.
22. Astrup T. The tissue plasminogen activator—an historical account. In: Kluft C, ed. Tissue-Type Plasminogen Activator (t-PA): Physiological and Clinical Aspects, Vol. 1. Florida: CRC Press, 1988:4–18.
23. Hekman CM, Loskutoff DJ. Fibrinolytic pathways and the endothelium. Semin Thromb Hemostasis 1987;13:514–527.
24. Runge MS, Quertermous T, Haber E. Plasminogen activators: the old and the new. Circulation 1989;79:217–224.
25. Ranby M, Brändström A. Biological control of tissue plasminogen activator mediated fibrinolysis. Enzyme (Basel) 1998;40:130–143.
26. Rijken DC, Wijngaards G, Jong MZ-D, et al. Purification and partial characterisation of plasminogen activator from human uterine tissue. Biochim Biophys Acta 1979;580: 140–153.
27. Pennica D, Holmes WE, Kohr WJ, et al. Cloning and expression of human tissue-type plasminogen activator cDNA in *E. coli*. Nature (Lond) 1983;301:214–220.
28. Rijken DC, Collen D. Purification and characterisation of the plasminogen activator secreted by human melanoma cells in culture. J Biol Chem 1981;256:7035–7041.
29. Williams JRB. The fibrinolytic activity of urine. Br J Exp Biol 1951;32:530–537.
30. Saksela O, Hovi T, Vaheri A. Urokinase-type plasminogen activator and its inhibitor secreted by cultured human monocyte-macrophages. J Cell Physiol 1985;122:125–132.
31. van Mourik JA, Lawrence DA, Loskutoff DJ. Purification of an inhibitor of plasminogen activator (antiactivator) synthesised by endothelial cells. J Biol Chem 1984;259: 14914–14921.
32. Erickson LA, Ginsberg MH, Loskutoff DJ. Detection and partial characterisation of an inhibitor of plasminogen activator in human platelets. J Clin Invest 1984;74: 1465–1472.
33. Coleman PL, Barouski PA, Gelehrter TD. The dexamethasone-induced inhibitor of fibrinolytic activity in hepatoma cells. J Biol Chem 1982;257:4260–4264.
34. Chmielewska J, Rånby M, Wiman B. Evidence for a rapid inhibitor to tissue plasminogen activator in plasma. Thomb Res 1983;31:427–436.
35. Laug WE. Human vascular smooth muscle cells (HVSMC) produce plasminogen activator inhibitor-1 (PAI-1) and protease Nexin (PN). Thromb Haemostasis 1987;58:14.
36. Kuithof EKO, Tran-Thang C, Ransijn A, et al. Demonstration of a fast-acting inhibitor of plasminogen activators in human plasma. Blood 1984;64:907–913.
37. Kawano T, Morimoto K, Uemura Y. Urokinase inhibitor in human placenta. Nature (Lond) 1968;217:253–254.
38. Webb AC, Collins KL, Synder SE, et al. Human monocyte ARG-serpin cDNA: sequence, chromosomal assignment, and homology to plasminogen activator-inhibitor. J Exp Med 1987;166:77–94.
39. Åstedt B, Hägerstrand I, Lecander I. Cellular localisation in placenta of placental type plasminogen activator inhibitor. Thromb Haemostasis 1986;56:63–65.
40. Kjaeldgaard A, Pscera H, Larsson B, et al. Plasminogen activators and inhibitors in amniotic fluid. Fibrinolysis 1989;3:203–206.
41. Lecander I, Åstedt B. Isolation of a new specific plasminogen activator inhibitor from pregnancy plasma. Br J Haematol 1986;62:221–228.
42. Kopitar M, Rozman B, Babnik J, et al. Human leukocyte urokinase inhibitor—purification, characterisation and comparative studies against different plasminogen activators. Thromb Haemostasis 1985;54:750–755.
43. Golder JP, Stephens RW. Minactivin: a human monocyte product which specifically inactivates urokinase-type plasminogen activators. Eur J Biochem 1983;136:517–522.
44. Schwartz BS, Monroe MC, Bradshaw JD. Endotoxin-induced production of plasminogen activator inhibitor by human monocytes is autonomous and can be inhibited by lipid X. Blood 1989;73:2188–2195.
45. Kruithof EKO, Tran-Thang C, Bachmann F. The fast-acting inhibitor of tissue-type plasminogen activator in plasma is also the primary plasma inhibitor of urokinase. Thromb Haemostasis 1986;55:65–69.
46. Baker JB, Low DA, Simmer RL, et al. Protease Nexin: a cellular component that links thrombin and plasminogen activator and mediates their binding to cells. Cell 1980; 21:37–45.
47. Scott RW, Baker JB. Purification of human protease Nexin. J Biol Chem 1983;258:10439–10444.
48. Stump DC, Thienpont M, Collen D. Urokinase-related proteins in human urine. J Biol Chem 1986;261:1267–1273.
49. Stump DC, Theinpont M, Collen D. Purification and characterisation of a novel inhibitor of urokinase from human urine. J Biol Chem 1986;261:12759–12766.
50. Gelehrter TD, Sznycer-Laszuk R. Thrombin induction of plasminogen activator-inhibitor in cultured human endothelial cells. J Clin Invest 1986;77:165–169.

51. Hanss M, Collen D. Secretion of tissue-type plasminogen activator and plasminogen activator inhibitor by cultured human endothelial cells: modulation by thrombin, endotoxin, and histamine. J Lab Clin Med 1987;109:97–104.
52. Kooistra T, Van Den Berg J, Töns A, et al. Butyrate stimulates tissue-type plasminogen activator synthesis in cultured human endothelial cells. Biochem J 1987;247: 605–612.
53. O'Connell ML, Canipari R, Strickland S. Hormonal regulation of tissue plasminogen activator secretion and mRNA levels in rat granulosa cells. J Biol Chem 1987; 262: 2339–2344.
54. Ny T, Liu Y-X, Ohlsson M, et al. Regulation of tissue-type plasminogen activator activity and messenger RNA levels by gonadotrophin-releasing hormone in cultured rat granulosa cells and cumulus-oocyte complexes. J Biol Chem 1987;262:11790–11793.
55. Nicoloso G, Hauert J, Kruithof EKO, et al. Fibrinolysis in normal subjects—comparison between plasminogen activator inhibitor and other components of the fibrinolytic system. Thomb Haemostasis 1988;59:299–303.
56. Bachmann F, Egbert IR, Kruithof EKO. Tissue plasminogen activator: chemical and physiological aspects. Semin Thromb Hemostasis 1984;10:6–17.
57. Gader AMA, da Costa J, Cash JD. A new vasopressin analogue and fibrinolysis. Lancet 1973;ii:1417–1418.
58. Kluft C, Preston FE, Malia RG, et al. Stanozolol-induced changes in fibrinolysis and coagulation in healthy adults. Thromb Haemostasis 1984;51:157–164.
59. Loskutoff DJ, Roegner K, Erickson LA, et al. The dexamethasone-induced inhibitor of plasminogen activator in hepatoma cells is antigenetically related to an inhibitor produced by bovine aortic endothelial cells. Thromb Haemostasis 1986;55:8–11.
60. Colucci M, Paramo JA, Collen D. Generation in plasma of a fast-acting inhibitor of plasminogen activator in response to endotoxin stimulation. J Clin Invest 1985;75:818–824.
61. Nachman RL, Hajjar KA, Silverstein RL, et al. Interleukin-1 induces endothelial cell synthesis of plasminogen activator inhibitor. J Exp Med 1986;163:1595–1600.
62. van Hinsburgh VWM, Kooistra T, Fiers W, et al. Tumour necrosis factor increases the production of plasminogen activator inhibitor in human endothelial cells in vitro and in rats in vivo. Thromb Haemostasis 1987;58:15.
63. de Boer JP, Abbink JJ, Brouwer MC, et al. PAI-1 synthesis in the human hepatoma cell line Hep G2 is increased by cytokines—evidence that the liver contributes to acute phase behaviour of PAI-1. Thromb Haemostasis 1991;65: 181–185.
64. Olofsson BO, Dahlén G, Nilsson TK. Evidence for increased levels of plasminogen activator inhibitor and tissue plasminogen activator in plasma of patients with angiographically verified coronary artery disease. Eur Heart J 1989;10:77–82.
65. van Hinsburgh VWM, Kooistra T, Scheffer MA, et al. Characterisation and fibrinolytic properties of human omental tissue mesothelial cells. Comparison with endothelial cells. Blood 1990;75:1490–1497.
66. Pytel BA, Peppel K, Baglioni C. Plasminogen activator inhibitor type-2 is a major protein induced in human fibroblasts and SK-MEL-109 melanoma cells by tumour necrosis factor. J Cell Physiol 1990;144:416–422.
67. Ichinose A, Takio K, Fujikawa K. Localisation of the binding site of tissue-type plasminogen activator to fibrin. J Clin Invest 1986;78:163–169.
68. Norrman B, Wallen P, Ranby M. Fibrinolysis mediated by tissue plasminogen activator; disclosure of a kinetic transition. Eur J Biochem 1985;149:193–200.
69. Collen D, Lijnen HR, Todd PA, et al. Tissue-type plasminogen activator: a review of its pharmacology and therapeutic uses as a thrombolytic agent. Drugs 1989;38:346–388.
70. Benzer Von H, Blümel G, Piza F. Ueber zusammenhänge zwischen fibrinolyse und intraperitonealen adhäsionen. Weiner Klin Wochenschr 1963;75:881–883.
71. Myhre-Jensen O, Larsen SB, Astrup T. Fibrinolytic activity in serosal and synovial membranes. Arch Pathol 1969; 88:623–630.
72. Porter JM, McGregor GH, Mullen DC, et al. Fibrinolytic activity of mesothelial surfaces. Surg Forum 1969;20:80–82.
73. Whitaker D, Papadimitriou JM, Walters MN-I. The mesothelium: its fibrinolytic properties. J Pathol 1981;136: 291–299.
74. Pattinson HA, Konickx PR, Brosens IA. Clotting and fibrinolytic activities in peritoneal fluid. Br J Obstet Gynaecol 1981;88:160–166.
75. Batzofin JH, Holmes SD, Gibbons WE, et al. Peritoneal fluid plasminogen activator activity in endometriosis and pelvic adhesive disease. Fertil Steril 1985;44:277–279.
76. Bouckaert PXJM, Land JA, Brommer EJP, et al. The impact of peritoneal trauma on intra-abdominal fibrinolytic activity, adhesion formation and early embryonic development in a rabbit longitudinal model. Hum Reprod 1990; 5:237–241.
77. Porter JM, Ball AP, Silver D. Mesothelial fibrinolysis. J Thorac Cardiovasc Surg 1971;62:725–730.
78. Raftery AT. Method for measuring fibrinolytic activity in a single layer of cells. Br J Surg 1977;64:825–826.
79. Raftery AT. Regeneration of peritoneum: a fibrinolytic study. J Anat 1979;129:659–664.
80. Raftery AT. Method for measuring fibrinolytic activity in a single layer of cells. J Clin Pathol 1981;34:625–629.
81. Merlo M, Fausone G, Barbero C, et al. Fibrinolytic activity of human peritoneum. Eur Surg Res 1980;12:433–438.
82. Carlin G, Santerre RF, Bang NU. Functional properties of human mesothelial cells in culture. Thromb Haemostasis 1983;50:145.
83. Thompson JN, Paterson-Brown S, Harbourne T, et al. Reduced human peritoneal plasminogen activating activity: a possible mechanism of adhesion formation. Br J Surg 1989;76:382–384.
84. Holmdahl L, Risberg B, Beck DE, et al. Adhesions: pathogenesis and prevention—panel discussion and summary. Eur J Surg 1997;577(suppl):56–62.
85. Moore KL, Bang NU, Broadie TA, et al. Peritoneal fibrinolysis: evidence for the efficiency of tissue-type plasminogen activator. J Lab Clin Med 1983;101:921–929.
86. Mayer M, Yedgar S, Hurwitz A, et al. Effect of viscous macromolecules on peritoneal plasminogen activator activity: a potential mechanism for their ability to reduce postoperative adhesion formation. Am J Obstet Gynaecol 1988;159:957–963.
87. Vipond MN, Whawell SA, Thompson JN, et al. Peritoneal fibrinolytic activity and intraabdominal adhesions. Lancet 1991;i:1120–1122.

88. Holmdahl L, Eriksson E, Al-Jabreen M, et al. Fibrinolysis in human peritoneum during operation. Goteborg, Sweden: Department of Surgery, University of Goteborg, 1996;119(6):701–705.
89. Pugatch EMJ, Poole JCF. Inhibitor of fibrinolysis from mesothelium. Nature (Lond) 1969;221:269–270.
90. Buckman RF, Buckman PD, Hufnagel HV, et al. A physiologic basis for the adhesion-free healing of deperitonealised surfaces. J Surg Res 1976;21:67–76.
91. Whawell SA, Vipond MN, Scott-Coombes DM, et al. Plasminogen activator inhibitor-2 inhibits peritoneal fibrinolytic activity in inflammation. Br J Surg 1993;80: 107–109.
92. Holmdahl L, Falkenberg M, Ivarsson ML, et al. Plasminogen activators and inhibitors in peritoneal tissue. APMIS 1997;105:25–30.
93. Raftery AT. Serosae. In: Bucknell TE, Ellis H, eds. Wound Healing for Surgeons. London: Ballière-Tindall, 1984: 143–160.
94. Gervin AS, Puckett CL, Silver D. Serosal hypofibrinolysis: a cause of postoperative adhesions. Am J Surg 1973;125: 80–87.
95. Ryan GB, Grobéty J, Majno G. Mesothelial injury and recovery. Am J Pathol 1973;71:93–112.
96. Buckman RF, Woods M, Sargent L, et al. A unifying pathogenic mechanism in the etiology of intraperitoneal adhesions. J Surg Res 1976;20:1–5.
97. Hau T, Payne WD, Simmons RL. Fibrinolytic activity of the peritoneum during experimental peritonitis. Surg Gynaecol Obstet 1979;148:415–418.
98. Raftery AT. The effect of peritoneal trauma on peritoneal fibrinolytic activity and intraperitoneal adhesion formation. Eur Surg Res 1981;13:397–401.
99. Ellis H. The aetiology of post-operative abdominal adhesions: an experimental study. Br J Surg 1962;50:10–16.
100. Scott-Coombes DN, Whawell SA, Thompson JN. The operative peritoneal fibrinolytic response to abdominal operation. Eur J Surg 1995;161:395–399.
101. Scott-Coombes DN, Whawell SA, Vipond MN, et al. The human intraperitoneal fibrinolytic response to elective surgery. Br J Surg 1995;82:414–417.
102. Whawell SA, Wang Y, Fleming KA, et al. Localisation of plasminogen activator inhibitor-1 production in inflamed appendix by in situ mRNA hybridisation. J Pathol 1993; 169:67–71.
103. Whawell SA, Thompson EM, Fleming KA, et al. Plasminogen activator inhibitor-2 expression in inflamed appendix. Histopathology (Oxf) 1995;27:75–78.
104. Whawell SA, Scott-Coombes DN, Vipond MN, et al. Tumour necrosis factor mediated release of plasminogen activator inhibitor-1 by human peritoneal mesothelial cells. Br J Surg 1994;81:214–216.
105. Ivarsson ML, Holmdahl L, Falk P, et al. Characterisation and fibrinolytic properties of mesothelial cells isolated from peritoneal lavage. Scand J Clin Lab Invest 1998;58: 195–203.
106. Badia JM, Scott-Coombes DN, Whawell SA, et al. Peritoneal and systemic cytokine response to laparotomy. Br J Surg 1996;83:347–348.
107. Appleton SG, Thompson JN. Cytokines and postoperative abdominal adhesions. In: Schein M, Wise L, eds. Cytokines and the Abdominal Surgeon. Texas: Landes, 1998:53–62.
108. van Hinsburgh VWM, Bauer KA, Kooistra T, et al. Progress of fibrinolysis during tumour necrosis factor infusions in humans. Concomitant increase in tissue-type plasminogen activator, plasminogen activator inhibitor type-1, and fibrin(ogen) degradation products. Blood 1990;76:2284–2289.
109. Tietz EL, Handt S, Ellbrecht A, et al. Decreased fibrinolytic activity of human mesothelial cells in vitro following stimulation with transforming growth factor-β1, interleukin-1 β, and tumour necrosis factor-alpha. In: Treutner K-H, Schumpelick V, eds. Peritoneal Adhesions. Berlin: Springer, 1997:146–159.
110. Wright LT, Smith DH, Rothman M, et al. Prevention of postoperative adhesions in rabbits with streptococcal metabolites. Proc Soc Exp Biol Med 1950;75:602–604.
111. Sherry S, Callaway DW, Freiberg R. Prevention of postoperative adhesions in the dog by intravenous injections of plasminogen activators. Proc Soc Exp Biol Med 1955; 90:1–4.
112. James DCO, Ellis H, Hugh TB. The effect of streptokinase on experimental adhesion formation. J Pathol Bacteriol 1965;90:279–287.
113. Luttwak EM, Behar AJ, Saltz NJ. Effect of fibrinolytic agents and corticosteroid hormones on peritoneal adhesions. Arch Surg 1956;75:96–101.
114. Jewett TC, Ambrus JL, Ambrus CM, et al. Effect of fibrinolytic enzymes on experimentally induced peritoneal adhesions. Surgery (St. Louis) 1965;57:280–284.
115. Bryant LR. An evaluation of the effect of fibrinolysin on intraperitoneal adhesion formation. Am J Surg 1963; 106:892–897.
116. Rivkind AI, Lieberman N, Durst AL. Urokinase does not prevent adhesion formation in rats. Eur Surg Res 1985; 17:254–258.
117. Orita H, Fukasawa M, Gergis W, et al. Inhibition of postsurgical adhesions in a standardised rabbit model: intraperitoneal treatment with tissue plasminogen activator. Int J Infertil 1991;36:172–177.
118. Dunn RC, Buttram VC. Tissue-type plasminogen activator as an adjuvant for postsurgical adhesions. Prog Clin Biol Res 1990;358:113–118.
119. Menzies D, Ellis H. Intra-abdominal adhesions and their prevention by topical tissue plasminogen activator. J R Soc Med 1989;82:534–535.
120. Doody KJ, Dunn RC, Buttram V. Recombinant tissue plasminogen activator reduces adhesion formation in a rabbit uterine horn model. Fertil Steril 1989;51:509–512.
121. Vipond MN, Whawell SA, Scott-Coombes DM, et al. Experimental adhesion prophylaxis with recombinant tissue plasminogen activator. Ann R Coll Surg Engl 1994;76: 412–415.

Section 3
Surgical Technique

10

Laparoscopic Myomectomy

Jean-Bernard Dubuisson, Arnaud Fauconnier, and Charles Chapron

CONTENTS

The technique of laparoscopic myomectomy (LM) appeared only recently, with the first cases being described for subserous myomas in the 1980s.[1,2] Since the beginning of the 1990s, several teams have reported their experience with LM for interstitial myomas.[3–6] Although there has been some hesitation on the part of many surgeons, LM has gradually come into more widespread use. The large number of studies addressing the subject show that the technique has reached maturity.[4–24] LM has been the subject of several prospective randomized studies.[14,25,26] One of these studies compared the LM technique with laparotomy.

In our center we have acquired considerable experience with this technique, as we carried out 373 LM between March 1989 and July 1998. The purpose of this chapter, therefore, is to focus on the operative technique and describe the advantages, limitations, and risks involved.

Procedures for Myomectomy Using Laparoscopy

Four different myomectomy procedures using laparoscopy can be described: intraperitoneal myomectomy, laparoscopy-assisted myomectomy (LAM), laparoconversion, and diagnostic laparoscopy.

Intraperitoneal myomectomy

All phases of the myomectomy are carried out by laparoscopy (hysterotomy, enucleation, and suture of the hysterotomy).

Laparoscopic-Assisted Myomectomy

In 1994, Nezhat et al.[27] defined a myomectomy procedure that is midway between laparotomy and laparoscopy: LAM. In the initial description by this author, laparoscopy was used solely to treat any associated lesions (adhesions) and to facilitate the exposure of the myoma(s). Enucleation, extraction, and suture of the hysterotomy were carried out by minilaparotomy. Our method of myomectomy assisted by laparoscopy (partial LAM) is a little different, consisting of carrying out only the hysterotomy suture and the extraction of the myoma through the minilaparotomy, with hysterotomy and enucleation of all the myomas achieved totally by laparoscopy.

Laparo-Conversion

In the category of laparo-conversion, we include all operations in which recourse to laparotomy is required when the initial phase of myomectomy had been started by laparoscopy. Conversion may be needed because of technical difficulties (difficulties in dissecting the myoma or in achieving hemostasis), or complications connected with the myomectomy (hemorrhage) or not connected (anesthesia complication; hypercapnia, for example).

Diagnostic Laparoscopy

We include under diagnostic laparoscopy all myomectomies that use laparoscopy to assess the characteristics of the myomas and to decide whether laparoscopic myomectomy is feasible, but for which none of the operative steps for the actual myomectomy is carried out by laparoscopy. We also include under this name all procedures carried out by laparoscopy and aimed at allowing satisfactory exploration of the pelvis and myomas (adhesiolysis).

By "laparoscopic myomectomy," we mean all myomectomy procedures for which at least the first step for myomectomy was started by laparoscopy. The term thus covers all laparo-conversions, intraperitoneal myomectomies, and LAM. In our work almost all LM are in fact intraperitoneal myomectomies. Alternatives have been proposed for LM, such as the use of pneumosuspension[28] and myolysis techniques.[29–31]

Operative Technique

Principles

The LM technique we use in our institution[32] comprises four main phases, schematically speaking hysterotomy and revelation of the myoma, enucleation, suture of the myomectomy site, and extraction of the myoma. The main difficulties with the operation, as with myomectomy by laparotomy, are the risk of intraoperative hemorrhage and the prevention of postoperative adhesions. Use of the laparoscopic route for the myomectomy also raises certain particular problems connected with this approach; a bloodless enucleation of the myomas is absolutely needed, and a perfect suture must be done to obtain a good-quality scar.

The use of the LM technique, therefore, is based on several basic principles:

1. The principles of microsurgery must be applied to LM: avoidance of intraperitoneal contamination, use of fine and atraumatic instruments, and gentle and atraumatic manipulation of the uterus without grasping the pelvic organs (except the myoma itself). These precautions make it possible to keep postoperative adhesions to a minimum.
2. With LM each myoma must be excised via its own hysterotomy; it is not possible to apply the same technique as with myomectomy by laparotomy,[33,34] that is, removing all the myomas present on the uterus via a longitudinal hysterotomy.
3. A distinct cleavage plane separates the myoma from the adjacent myometrium. This cleavage plane is bounded by a pseudocapsule made up of compressed muscular fibers and diverted uterine vessels.[35] Vascularization of the myoma is plurifocal through the cleavage plane by means of a mulltitude of small nourishing vessels, and there is no true vascular pedicle.[36] Dissection must take place in every case along this cleavage plane for two reasons: on the one hand, preservation of healthy adjacent myometrium is one of the conditions for obtaining a good-quality uterine scar, and on the other, this also helps avoid damaging the perimyomatous vessels, which are often distended because of compression by the myoma.[37] The large veins may be the origin of considerable hemorrhage. Another advantage with the laparoscopic approach is that the small nourishing vessels can be viewed clearly, thus permitting elective coagulation.
4. Electrocoagulation must be used as sparingly as possible to achieve hemostasis of the edges after myomectomy. Certain cases of uterine rupture during pregnancy reported after LM[4,38,39] suggest that the use of electrocoagulation may induce necrosis of the myometrium, resulting in a postoperative fistula. Furthermore, electrocoagulation is responsible for delayed healing,[40] which could also adversely affect the solidity of the myomectomy scar.
5. Suture of the hysterotomy must always respect a certain number of principles. Indeed, any technical deficiency when carrying it out may result in uterine rupture during a subsequent pregnancy.[39] Apart from pedunculated myomas or certain sessile subserous myomas with a narrow implantation base, the myomectomy sites must always be sutured. In the experience of certain teams at the beginning, when no su-

ture was carried out the resulting scars were fine or dehiscent.[4,41] The suture must always take up the full depth of the edges of the hysterotomy and result in total contact over the whole of the myomectomy site so as to avoid secondary constitution of a hematoma deep inside the myometrium. This kind of hematoma can cause weakness in the scar tissues and the constitution of a secondary fistula.[17,41] The uterine suture does not necessarily have to use several planes, despite the recommendation of certain authors.[42,43] Suture of the uterine serosa is unnecessary and could increase the risk of postoperative adhesions.[40,44,45] Sometimes it is necessary to make a suture in two or three planes if the uterine cavity has been broached or if the myomectomy site is very deep. It is possible to make this type of suture in several planes by laparoscopy.[17,19,46] However, if this approach proves difficult there should be no hesitation in using a minilaparotomy to complete the procedure successfully.

Instrumentation

In addition to the standard instrumentation for any operative laparoscopy, certain specific instruments are useful when carrying out LM. Short curved monopolar scissors enable incision of the myometrium and section of the tracti between the myoma and myometrium. Other instruments are useful when making the intra- or extracorporeal sutures needle holders, atraumatic forceps with no slot nor claws, and a suture pusher. A strong grasping forceps specifically for myomas (Museux forceps type) means that efficient traction can be exerted on the myoma.

Ideally, an electric morcellation device such at the Steiner morcellator[47] allows myomas larger than 4 cm to be extracted by the suprapubic port. In our experience this device proved easy to use after a certain learning phase and has enabled us to reduce the duration of our operations considerably. The relatively high cost of this device is compensated by shorter operation times.[48]

Positioning

The patient lies in the following position: thighs spread with abduction providing access to the vagina and buttocks protruding generously over the edge of the table to allow manipulation of the uterus with an intrauterine cannula. The main surgeon stands to the patient's left, with the first assistant opposite and the second assistant between the patient's legs. Injection of undiluted methylene blue into the uterine cavity at the beginning of the operation makes it possible to see when dissection of intramural myomas is coming close to the endometrium and to know when the uterine cavity is broached during the procedure. The uterus is then cannulated, enabling it to be manipulated during the operation.

Two 5-mm lateral trocars and one 10- to 12-mm midline trocar are inserted in the suprapubic position. The position of the trocars should be adapted whenever possible to the size and location of the myomas. Generally speaking, the two lateral trocars should be placed relatively high and outside the epigastric vessels so that good accessibility is provided for myomas in various locations and to ensure that the surgeon has sufficient scope for movement when carrying out the sutures.

Incision of the Myometrium and Myoma Exposure

The hysterotomy is direct, lined up with the myoma (Fig. 10.1). We place no importance on the direction in our practice, and it may be either sagittal, oblique, or transversal. We tend to use sagittal hysterotomies because they are easier to suture. The myometrium is incised using low-voltage monopolar current in section mode to safeguard the myometrium as much as possible. Hemostasis of the intramyometrial vessels is carried out progressively (and preventively, if possible) using monopolar or bipolar current. Identification of the avascular plane surrounding the myoma is helped by the magnifying effect of the laparoscopic images. The myoma is easy to recognize by its smooth appearance and pearly-white color, which contrasts with the adjacent myometrium. In addition the myoma is firm to the touch, in contrast to the myometrium, and this can be felt via the laparoscopic instruments.

Enucleation

Dissection of the myoma should run inside the avascular plane, leaving the pseudocapsule around the outside and the uterine vessels pushed back (Fig. 10.2). Dissection is easier if the following maneuver is used: the my-

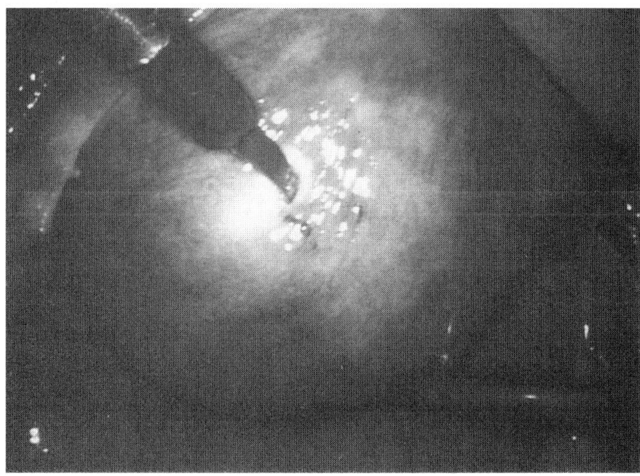

FIG. 10.1. Posterior intramural myoma: incision of the serosa using monopolar scissors.

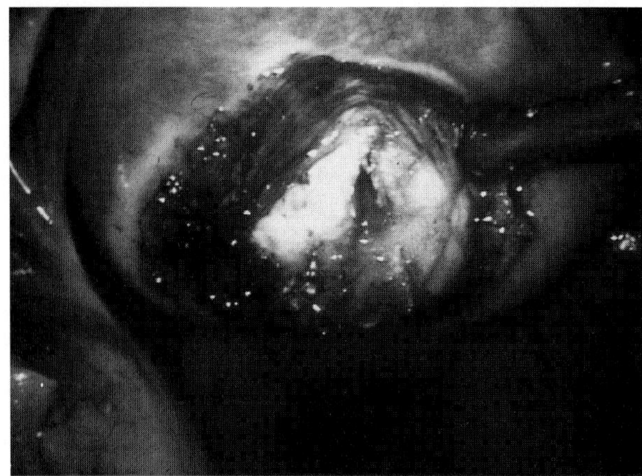

FIG. 10.2. Atraumatic enucleation of the myoma.

oma is grasped with a strong grasping forceps (Museux type) and pulled hard toward the anterior abdominal wall or upward at the same time, the surgeon or his assistant exerts traction in the opposite direction using the endouterine cannula and by pushing on the edges of the hysterotomy with an instrument. This dissection proceeds from the superficial areas inward, and always under visual control to identify the fine tissue bands adhering to the myoma. The tip of a blunt instrument is used (curved scissors or bipolar forceps) to press against the myoma. The bands adhering to the myoma are coagulated (as close as possible to the myoma), then sectioned.

Some authors recommend the use of "atraumatic" dissection instruments (harmonic scalpel, ultrasonically activated laparosonic coagulating shears, aquadissector, laser) (Fig. 10.3).[21,49,50] The use of such instruments is supposed to preserve the adjacent myometrium even better. The ultrasonically activated laparosonic coagulating shears is reputed to make dissection of the myoma easier than with standard instruments.[17] We have no experience with this instrument in our institution. The bed of the myomectomy is most often free from hemorrhage at the end of dissection if care has been taken to follow the avascular cleavage plane, and thus there is no need to take further steps for hemostasis.

Hysterotomy Suture

We use fine resorbable suture, diameter 00-gauge, mounted on a curved needle with atraumatic tip (Vicryl, Polyglactine 910;Ethicon, Neuilly, France). The suture is usually carried out in a single plane (Fig. 10.4). We use single, separate knots, tied in or outside the body. These stitches go through the whole thickness of the edges of the hysterotomy and through the uterine serosa. They are placed sufficiently close for the edges to be approximated completely yet far enough apart to avoid making the myometrium too fragile (Fig. 10.5).

When the myomectomy is located deeply, or the uterine cavity has been opened, we suture along a deep plane with a few single stitches deep in the myometrium, and along a superficial plane taking in the serosa and the superficial part of the myometrium. The superficial plane can be handled using a running suture or with individual stitches. When suturing the deep plane, it can sometimes be difficult to take the needle through the thickness of the defect. In this case it can be an advantage to use Vicryl 1 with a curved needle or a U-shaped transfixing stitch, the "belt stitch,"[41] running through the uterine serosa and taking in the whole thickness of the edges of the myomectomy. One or two of these stitches are sufficient to ensure that all the deep part of the hysterotomy is brought into contact. When the uterine suture proves difficult to carry out, it is essential to know when to stop and use a minilaparotomy for the suture.

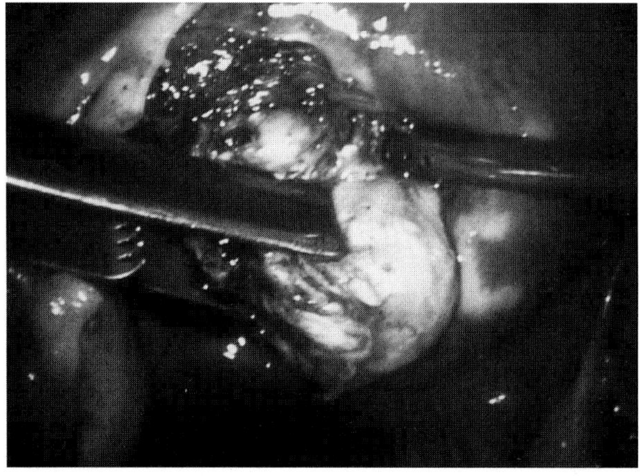

FIG. 10.3. The dissection is facilitated by traction using a grip forceps.

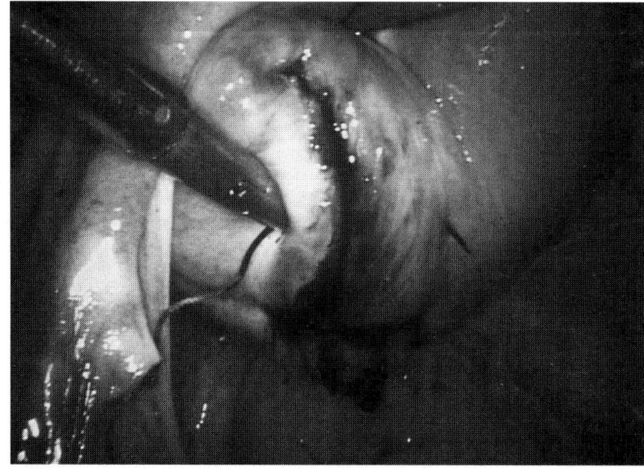

FIG. 10.4 The uterine suture is performed atraumatically using vicryl 2/0 sutures.

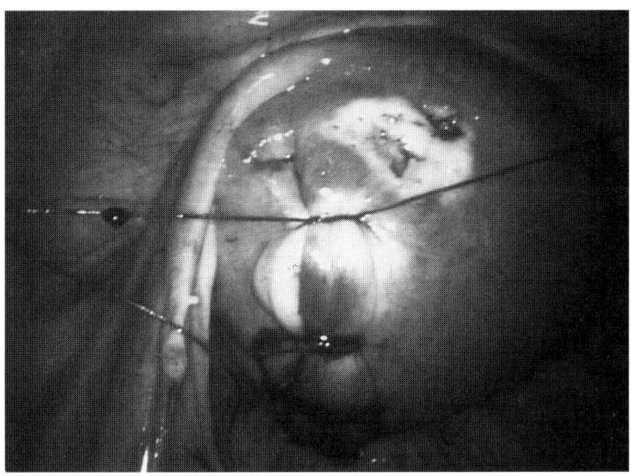

Fig. 10.5. Final result of myomectomy.

Extraction of the Myoma

There are various methods possible for extraction: direct extraction, standard intraabdominal morcellation, electric morcellation, extraction via posterior colpotomy (Fig. 10.6), and extraction via minilaparotomy. Direct suprapubic extraction is appropriate only for myomas measuring less than 3 cm. Extraction takes place through the midline suprapubic incision, which may be enlarged if needed. It is important when using ports larger than 10 mm to close the abdominal wall correctly to avoid incisional hernias.[51] Standard morcellation is carried out either with the scissors or with scapels and is appropriate for small myomas (less than 4 or 5 mm in diameter). Electric morcellation uses the Steiner morcellator.[47] This device has proved easy to use and without danger, but the position of the blade in the device must be under perfect control at all times to avoid any risk of damaging any neighboring organs. Posterior colpotomy also allows large myomas to be extracted.[15] Some authors have suggested that postoperative adhesions involving the colpotomy scar are possible,[6,17] but we ourselves have not found any increase in this risk in our study on adhesions after LM.[44] Since the advent of the electric morcellator, we almost never use a posterior colpotomy to extract myomas.

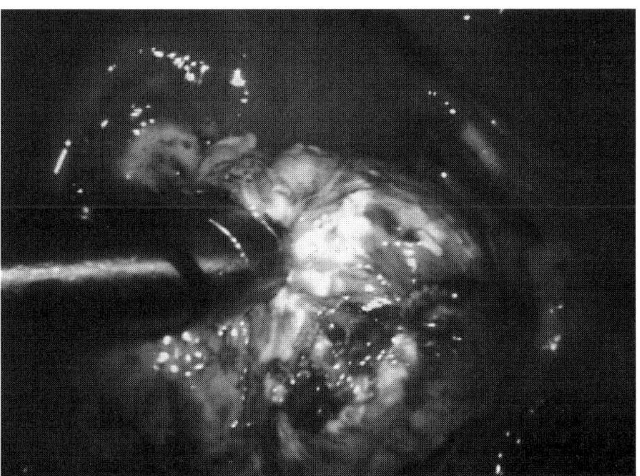

Fig. 10.6. Morcellation of the myoma using an electric morcellator.

Results of Laparoscopic Myomectomy

Advantages

It is now accepted that the technique is both feasible and reproducible, as can be seen from the many teams who now use LM and have reported their experience.[4–14,16,17,20–24] Analysis of these series of LM together with the experience gained in our own institution[52] enables us to state that this technique does not involve a higher risk of perioperative or immediate postoperative complications as compared with myomectomy via laparotomy. Furthermore, two controlled studies suggest that the risk of peroperative hemorrhage and the risk of postoperative complications are reduced.[9,53]

From the cosmetic point of view, the absence of a scar is very much appreciated by our patients. As for the functional point of view, the fact that the patients are more comfortable has been proved by a clinical trial: by using LM there is less postoperative pain and the hospital stay is shorter.[14] LM could in particular reduce the risk of adhesions after myomectomy. In our study on second look after LM, we observed in the 45 patients who underwent the check that there was a 36% rate of adhesions; if only adhesions involving the adnexa were taken into account, the rate was 24%.[44] These rates are low in comparison with those observed at second look after myomectomy via laparotomy, which reach nearly 90% with nearly two-thirds of the cases showing involvement of the adnexa.[54–57] Two controlled studies also suggest a lower risk of adhesions after LM.[7,53] This reduction in postoperative adhesions presents a particular advantage when the myomectomy is carried out in a context of infertility because it could help improve the fertility of the patients operated.

The results of LM relative to fertility have been assessed.[58] In our series of 91 infertile patients, we observed a cumulative conception rate of 44% at 2 years. This rate was 70% when no other factor was found for infertility other than the myoma. These results are comparable to those of the series of myomectomy via laparotomy, which in our opinion justifies preferential use of the laparoscopic approach whenever the myomas are medium-sized and few in number. However there has been no randomized clinical trial to validate this proposal.

Limits and Risks

Laparoscopic myomectomy, in particular in the case of interstitial myomas, is nevertheless a difficult technique that requires surgeons highly experienced in laparoscopic surgery.[32,52] Moreover, it takes time, and the operations do seem to last longer than with laparotomy.[53]

We consider that the maximum size of myomas operated by LM should not exceed 8 cm and that no more than three myomas should be removed in total.[59] In practice we do sometimes go beyond these limits, and some teams have also reported carrying out LM for far larger myomas, up to 16 cm.[23] However, in using LM for large myomas we run up against difficulties in obtaining cleavage of the myomas for several reasons: the growth of certain myomas results in reorganization of the myomatous tissues and neighboring myometrium, making the attachments of the myomas more dense and difficult to cleave; the depth of the site of the myoma hampers access for the instruments and visibility of the tissues to be dissected; the larger myomas have a more highly developed vascularization, which results in an increased risk of perioperative hemorrhage; and finally, the time required for electric morcellation increases considerably with the size of the myoma. When we first started, we planned to use gonadotropin-releasing hormone (GnRH) analogs preoperatively to reduce the size of the myomas to be operated. This approach proved to be inefficient because the tissue reorganization induced by the analogs caused the cleavage plane around the myoma to become less distinct.

To date, five cases of uterine rupture during pregnancy have been reported after LM, in particular one in our institution.[16,38,39,60,61] These accidents raise the question of the quality of the scars after LM, and some authors[27,62] consider that the laparoscopic route is not satisfactory to make solid sutures of the myometrium in the case of a deep defect.

We have several arguments to counter these criticisms:

1. Although experience with pregnancies after myomectomy via laparotomy shows that uterine rupture is rare (no case in the largest series published),[63,64] observations of uterine rupture after laparotomy are nevertheless regularly reported in the literature.[65–68] Cases of rupture have also been reported after hysteroscopy.[69]
2. At present there is no knowledge concerning the real incidence of rupture after LM, because only the cases themselves are reported. The incidence is probably low; in our population, for example, we observed a single case of rupture for 92 pregnancies after LM (unpublished data).
3. There may be a publication bias connected with the newness of the technique for LM that could explain the number of cases reported in the literature during a short period. In contrasting myomectomy via laparotomy, observations of uterine rupture are only reported when the particular circumstances under which they occur make them interesting enough to publish.
4. It took a long time to arrive at a good suture technique by laparoscopy, and at the beginning certain teams (including ours) did not immediately apply certain principles that have since become clear for making the uterine sutures. Some authors did not systematically suture the myomectomy sites[4] at the beginning of their experience. In addition, our observation[39] suggests that electrocautery plays a part in the secondary development of parietal necrosis, resulting in a fistula.

At the present time, although suturing by the intraperitoneal route remains a technically difficult technique requiring surgeons skilled in laparoscopic surgery, we agree with other teams[17,41] in considering that provided the technique is meticulous, the uterine suture can be carried out satisfactorily by the purely laparoscopic route. Nevertheless we remain vigilant, which is one of the reasons why, when there is a desire for pregnancy, we propose systematically to take a second look by laparoscopy, which enables the appearance of the uterine scars after LM to be assessed.

Conclusions

LM enables subserous and interstitial myomas to be treated surgically using minimally invasive techniques. Analysis of the ratio of advantages to risk for this operation as compared with the use of laparotomy for myomectomy pleads in favor of its use for medium-sized myomas (<8 cm) when few in number. LM appears to present particular advantages when operating in a context of infertility because it may reduce the risk of postoperative adhesions. If good quality healing is to be attained, the surgeons must be experienced in laparoscopic surgery techniques, and the principles for making uterine sutures defined for myomectomy via laparotomy must be applied.

References

1. Semm K, Mettler L. Technical progress in pelvic surgery via operative laparoscopy. Am J Obstet Gynecol 1980; 138(2):121–127.
2. Kolmorgen K. [Ovariectomy by laparoscopy.] Zentralbl Gynaekol 1989;111(9):613–617.
3. Dubuisson JB, Lecuru F, Foulot H, Mandelbrot L, Aubriot FX, Mouly M. Myomectomy by laparoscopy: a preliminary report of 43 cases. Fertil Steril 1991;56(5):827–830.
4. Nezhat C, Nezhat F, Silfen SL, Schaffer N, Evans D. Laparoscopic myomectomy. Int J Fertil 1991;36(5):275–280.

5. Daniell JF, Gurley LD. Laparoscopic treatment of clinically signifiant symptomatic uterine fibroids. J Gynecol Surg 1991;7:37–39.
6. Hasson HM, Rotman C, Rana N, Sistos F, Dmowski WP. Laparoscopic myomectomy Obstet Gynecol 1992;80(5): 884–888.
7. Bulletti C, Polli V, Negrini V, Giacomucci E, Flamigni C. Adhesion formation after laparoscopic myomectomy. J Am Assoc Gynecol Laparosc 1996;3(4):533–536.
8. Andrei B. Myomectomy by pelvicoscopy. Int Surg 1996;81 (3):271–275.
9. Carter JE, McCarus S, Baginiski L, Bailey TS. Laparoscopic outpatient treatment of large myomas. J Am Assoc Gynecol Laparosc 1996;3(suppl 4):S6.
10. Cittadini E. Laparoscopic myomectomy: the Italian experience. J Am Assoc Gynecol Laparosc 1998;5(1):7–9.
11. Daraï E, Deval B, Darles C, Benifla JL, Guglielmina JN, Madelenat P. Myomectomie: coelioscopie ou laparotomie. Contracept Fertil Sex 1996;24(10):751–756.
12. Dubuisson JB, Chapron C. Laparoscopic myomectomy. Operative procedure and results. Ann NY Acad Sci 1994; 734:450–454.
13. Kolmorgen K. [Laparoscopic myomectomy.] Zentralbl Gynaekol 1995;117(12):659–662.
14. Mais V, Ajossa S, Guerriero S, Mascia M, Solla E, Melis GB. Laparoscopic versus abdominal myomectomy: a prospective, randomized trial to evaluate benefits in early outcome. Am J Obstet Gynecol 1996;174(2):654–658.
15. Mangeshikar PR. New instrumentation and technique for laparoscopic myomectomy. J Am Assoc Gynecol Laparosc 1995;2(suppl 4):S29.
16. Mecke H, Wallas F, Brocker A, Gertz HP. [Pelviscopic myoma enucleation: technique, limits, complications.] Geburtsh Frauenheilkd 1995;55(7):374–379.
17. Miller CE, Johnston M, Rundell M. Laparoscopic myomectomy in the infertile woman. J Am Assoc Gynecol Laparosc 1996;3(4):525–532.
18. Montevecchi L, Bagnini C, Campo S, et al. Laparoscopic myomectomy. J Am Assoc Gynecol Laparosc 1995;2(suppl 4):S34.
19. Ostrzenski A. A new laparoscopic myomectomy technique for intramural fibroids penetrating the uterine cavity. Eur J Obstet Gynecol Reprod Biol 1997;74(2):189–193.
20. Parker WH, Rodi IA. Patient selection for laparoscopic myomectomy. J Am Assoc Gynecol Laparosc 1994;2(1): 23–26.
21. Reich H. Laparoscopic myomectomy. Obstet Gynecol Clin North Am 1995;22(4):757–780.
22. Seinera P, Arisio R, Decko A, Farina C, Crana F. Laparoscopic myomectomy indications, surgical technique and complications. Hum Reprod (Oxf) 1997;12(9):1927–1930.
23. Stringer NH. Laparoscopic myomectomy in African-American women. J Am Assoc Gynecol Laparosc 1996; 3(3):375–381.
24. Wood EC, Maher P. New strategies for endoscopic myomectomy. J Am Assoc Gynecol Laparosc 1995;2(suppl 4): S60–S61.
25. Mais V, Ajossa S, Piras B, Guerriero S, Marongiu D, Melis GB. Prevention of denovo adhesion formation after laparoscopic myomectomy: a randomized trial to evaluate the effectiveness of an oxidized regenerated cellulose absorbable barrier. Hum Reprod 1995;10(12):3133–3135.
26. Zullo F, Pellicano M, De Stefano R, Zupi E, Mastrantonio P. A prospective randomized study to evaluate leuprolide acetate treatment before laparoscopic myomectomy efficacy and ultrasonographic predictors. Am J Obstet Gynecol 1998;178(1 Pt 1):108–112.
27. Nezhat C, Nezhat F, Bess O, Nezhat CH, Mashiach R. Laparoscopically assisted myomectomy: a report of a new technique in 57 cases. Int J Fertil Menopausal Stud 1994; 39(1):39–44.
28. Chang FH, Soon YK, Lee CL, Lai YM, Wang HS. Laparoscopic removal of a large leiomyoma using airlift gasless laparoscopy. J Am Assoc Gynecol Laparosc 1996;3(suppl 4):S7.
29. Olive DL, Rutherford T, Zreik T, Palter S. Cryomyolysis in the conservative treatment of uterine fibroids. J Am Assoc Gynecol Laparosc 1996;3(Suppl 4):S36.
30. Nisolle M, Smets M, Malvaux V, Donnez J. Laparoscopic myolysis with the Nd-Yag laser. J Gynecol Surg 1993;9: 95–98.
31. Goldfarb H. Laparoscopic coagulation of myomas (myolysis). Obstet Gynecol Clin North Am 1995;22:807–819.
32. Dubuisson JB, Chapron C, Fauconnier A, Kreiker G. Laparoscopic myomectomy and myolysis. Curr Opin Obstet Gynecol 1997;9(4):233–238.
33. Bonney V. The technique and results of myomectomy. Lancet 1931;220:171–173.
34. Buttram VC, Reiter R. Uterine leiomyomata: etiology, symptomatology and management. Fertil Steri 1981; 36: 433–445.
35. Vollenhoven BJ, Lawrence AS, Hely DL. Uterine fibroids: a clinical review. Br J Obstet Gynaecol 1990;97:285–298.
36. Acien P, Quereda F. Abdominal myomectomy: results of a simple operative technique. Fertil Steril 1996;65(1):41–51.
37. Farrer-Brown G, Beilby J, Tarbit MH. Venous changes in the endometrium of myomatous uteri. Obstet Gynecol 1971;38:743.
38. Harris WJ. Uterine dehiscence following laparoscopic myomectomy Obstet Gynecol 1992;80(3 Pt 2):545–546.
39. Dubuisson JB, Chavet X, Chapron C, Gregorakis SS, Morice P. Uterine rupture during pregnancy after laparoscopic myomectomy. Hum Reprod (Oxf) 1995;10(6): 1475–1477.
40. Elkins TE, Stoval TG, Warren J, et al. A histologic evaluation of peritoneal injury and repair. Obstet Gynecol 1987; 70:225–228.
41. Hasson H. Laparoscopic myomectomy. Infertil Reprod Med Clin North Am 1996;7(1):143–159.
42. Davids AM. Myomectomy in the relief of infertility and sterility and in pregnancy. Surg Clin North Am 1957;37: 563.
43. Verkauf BS. Myomectomy for fertility enhancement and preservation. Fertil Steril 1992;58(1):1–15.
44. Dubuisson JB, Fauconnier A, Chapron C, Kreiker G, Norgaard C. Second-look after laparoscopic myomectomy. Hum Reprod (Oxf) 1998;13(8):2102–2106.
45. Mac Donald M, Elkins TE, Wortham GF, et al. Adhesion formation and prevention after peritoneal injury and repair in the rabbit. J Reprod Med 1988;33:436–439.

46. Dubuisson JB, Chapron C, Chavet X, Morice P, Foulot H, Aubriot FX. Traitement coeliochirurgical des volumineux fibromes utérins. Technique opératoire et résultats. J Gynecol Obstet Biol Reprod 1995;24(7):705–710.
47. Steiner R, Wight E, Tadir Y, Haller U. Electrical device for removal of tissue from the abdominal cavity. Obstet Gynecol 1993;81:471–474.
48. Carter JE, McCarus SD. Laparoscopic myomectomy. Time and cost analysis of power vs. manual morcellation. J Reprod Med 1997;42(7):383–388.
49. Stringer NH, Strassner HT. Pregnancy in five patients after laparoscopic myomectomy with the harmonic scalpel. J Gynecol Surg 1996;12:129–133.
50. Starks GC. CO_2 laser myomectomy in an infertile population. J Reprod Med 1988;33(2):184–186.
51. Boike GM, Miller CE, Spirtos NM, et al. Incisional bowel herniations after operative laparoscopy: a series of nineteen cases and review of the literature. Am J Obstet Gynecol 1995;172(6):1726–1731 (discussion, 1731–1733).
52. Dubuisson JB, Chapron C, Lévy L. Difficulties and complications of laparoscopic myomectomy. J Gynecol Surg 1996; 12:159–165.
53. Stringer NH, Walker JC, Meyer PM. Comparison of 49 laparoscopic myomectomies with 49 open myomectomies. J Am Assoc Gynecol Laparosc 1997;4(4):457–464.
54. Myectomy Adhesion Multicenter Study Group (M.A.M.S.G.). An expanded polytetrafluoroethylene barrier (Gore-Tex Surgical Membrane) reduces post-myomectomy adhesion formation. The Myomectomy Adhesion Multicenter Study Group. Fertil Steril 1995;63(3):491–493.
55. Tulandi T, Murray C, Guralnick M. Adhesion formation and reproductive outcome after myomectomy and second-look laparoscopy. Obstet Gynecol 1993;82:213–215.
56. Ugur M, Turan C, Mungan T, Aydogdu T, Sahin Y, Gokmen O. Laparoscopy for adhesion prevention following myomectomy. Int J Gynaecol Obstet 1996;53(2):145–149.
57. Diamond MP. Reduction of adhesions after uterine myomectomy by Seprafilm membrane (HAL-F): a blinded, prospective, randomized, multicenter clinical study. Seprafilm Adhesion Study Group. Fertil Steril 1996;66(6): 904–910.
58. Dubuisson J, Fauconnier A, Chapron C, Kreiker G, Nørgaard C. Reproductive outcome after laparoscopic myomectomy in infertile patients. J Reprod Med. (in press).
59. Dubuisson JB, Chapron C. Laparoscopic myomectomy today. A good technique when correctly indicated. Hum Reprod (Oxf) 1996;11(5):934–935.
60. Friedmann W, Maier RF, Luttkus A, Schafer AP, Dudenhausen JW. Uterine rupture after laparoscopic myomectomy. Acta Obstet Gynecol Scand 1996;75(7):683–684.
61. Pelosi M, Pelosi MA. Spontaneous uterine rupture at thirty-three weeks subsequent to previous superficial laparoscopic myomectomy. Am J Obstet Gynecol 1997;177(6): 1547–1549.
62. Tulandi T, Youssef H. Laparoscopy assisted myomectomy of large uterine myomas. Gynaecol Endosc 1997;6: 105–108.
63. Davids A. Myomectomy: surgical technique and results in series of 1150 cases. Am J Obstet Gynecol 1952;63: 592–604.
64. Brown AB, Chamberlain R, Te Linde RW. Myomectomy. Am J Obstet Gynecol 1956;71:759–763.
65. Garnet J. Uterine rupture during pregnancy. Obstet Gynecol 1964;23:898.
66. Georgakopoulos P, Bersis G. Sigmoido-uterine rupture in pregnancy after multiple myomectomy. Int Surg 1981;66: 367–368.
67. Golan D, Aharoni A, Gonon R, Boss Y, Sharf M. Early spontaneous rupture of the post myomectomy gravid uterus. Int J Gynaecol Obstet 1990;31:167–170.
68. Palerme G, Friedman E. Rupture of the gravid uterus in the third trimester. Am J Obstet Gynecol 1966;94(4): 571–576.
69. Yaron Y, Shenhav M, Jaffa A, Lessing J, Peyser M. Uterine rupture at 33 weeks gestation subsequent to hysteroscopic perforation. Am J Obstet Gynecol 1994;170:786–787.

11

Foreign Materials

Kristina Falk and Lena Holmdahl

CONTENTS

During the twentieth century there has been an unprecedented progression in medical care. In this process, the abdominal cavity has been increasingly explored and utilized for a variety of purposes. Exploitation of the peritoneal cavity has by no means been limited to abdominopelvic surgery, but includes chemotherapy, drug delivery, nutrition, peritoneal dialysis, and transplantation of various tissues. As an unanticipated consequence, many of these attempts have resulted in adhesion formation or intraperitoneal fibrosis, limiting further access. Interestingly, drugs administered elsewhere may still affect the peritoneum and induce fibrosis,[1,2] indicating that the peritoneum can react through indirect mechanisms to certain agents. Observations like this might provide clues as to how peritoneal fibrosis is induced. This chapter, however, focuses on intraabdominal deposition of foreign materials, defined as those having an exogenous component, and the ensuing peritoneal reaction. Because of the lack of noninvasive methods of assessing the intraabdominal response to a specific agent and the clinical and ethical restrictions to reentering the peritoneal cavity for evaluation, much of the existing knowledge in this area originates from animal experiments. Nonetheless, whenever possible information originating from observations in humans has been included.

The peritoneum is an active organ likely to have several functions, some of which are presently understood. There may be others yet to be realized. It serves to minimize friction and thus facilitate free movement of ab-

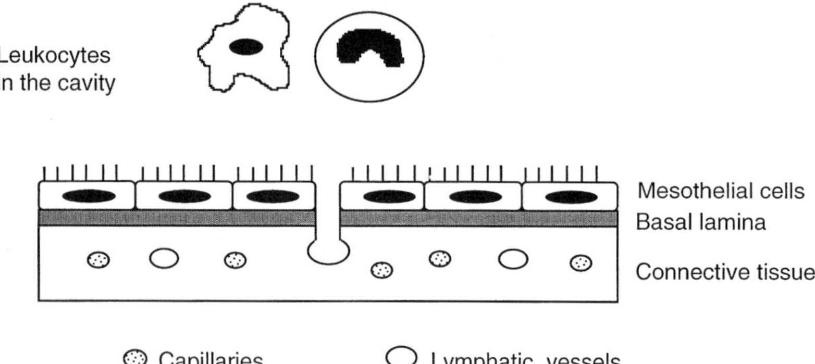

FIG. 11.1. Schematic illustration of the peritoneal environment. The peritoneum consists of a loose connective tissue, a basal lamina, and a single layer of mesothelial cells. The monolayer of mesothelial cells is covered by numerous microvilli. The peritoneum is richly supplied with blood and lymphatic vessels located in the submesothelial connective tissue. Occasionally, large lymphatic lacunae open up to the cavity, large enough to accommodate even cells.

dominal organs, and to resist or localize infections. Fluid is both filtered into and absorbed from the peritoneal cavity through the peritoneum. Smaller solutes and water are mainly transported to systemic circulation via uptake in peritoneal microvasculature, whereas larger molecules (>30 kDa) reach the systemic circulation via the lymphatics, either by tissue diffusion or through the peritoneal lymphatic lacunae.[3,4] Numerous large lymphatic lacunae, which are especially abundant in the subdiaphragmatic area, drain fluid, substances, particles, and entire cells from the abdominal cavity to the systemic circulation via the right thoracic duct.[5–8] This diaphragmatic lymphatic drainage system has been suggested to play an important role in the absorption of materials from the peritoneal cavity.[9] This concept implies that *anything* put in the peritoneal cavity can reach the systemic circulation, either intact, fragmented, in a partially degraded state, or as degradation products. Furthermore, the peritoneal response to a given material could be propagated systemically.

There are several cell types present in the peritoneal cavity. Mesothelial cells line the cavity, and within the cavity is a mixed population of free-floating cells including monocytes, B- and T lymphocytes, granulocytes, and mesothelial cells.[10] To investigate the peritoneal environment postsurgically, either cells have been harvested from peritoneal exudate (mainly macrophages), or tissue repair cells obtained from the injured peritoneal surface after abrasion (mainly fibroblasts)[11–13] have been used. Thus, the peritoneal environment represents a heterogeneous cell population with an even more complex composition postsurgically when the various cells are likely to be activated and capable of reacting to various substances entering the cavity. The peritoneal environment is schematically illustrated in Fig. 11.1.

Materials Used in Surgery

Sutures and Ligatures

Sutures and ligatures are widely used in abdominopelvic surgery to create anastomoses, to appose tissues, to tie off vessels, and to reapproximate peritoneum. Sutures, which are discussed in another chapter in this volume, are not treated extensively here. However, in the context of foreign materials it is worthwhile to mention, for example, that the suture material seems to be important because different suture materials apparently have different impacts on peritoneal tissue repair and adhesion formation. This effect was more prominent than the knot configuration or suture gauge,[14] both of which reflect the amount of suture material used. The type of suture material composing the suture thus may be more important than the amount of material in determining peritoneal reaction. Interestingly, in the study of Bakkum et al., no convincing correlation occurred between the degree of inflammatory response and adhesion formation.[14]

Typically, when new suture materials are evaluated, the mechanical properties over time and the "biocompatibility," often described in terms of inflammatory reaction, are considered. Adhesion-inducing properties are rarely investigated. Neglecting to do this should raise serious concerns because of the discrepancies just described in adhesion-inducing properties of sutures and between inflammation and adhesion formation, in addition to a recent observation that suture granulomas were found in 25% of patients at reoperation.[15] Therefore, it seems to be of utmost importance to investigate effects of suture materials on peritoneal repair processes, at least for suture materials intended for intraabdominal use. Failure to do this might result in adverse events and increased adhesion formation, elements that are incompatible with high-quality medical care.

Another observation is the consequences of peritoneal reapproximation, widely practiced among surgeons and gynecologists to restore tissue continuity after surgical excision because it is believed to decrease adhesion formation. Even though to some extent possibly influenced by the suture itself,[16] there are numerous experimental reports concluding that reapproximation of the peritoneum is superfluous or induces adhesions, or both. The compelling arguments against peritoneal closure can be subdivided into (1) the peritoneum regenerates rapidly without reapproximation in animals[17–29] and humans;[30–32] (2) suturing the peritoneum stimulates adhesion formation;[24,25,33–46] (3) nonclosure has not been observed to be harmful, and has even reduced postoperative complications;[47–60] and (4) the reduced surgical intervention and operating time resulting from nonclosure[50,52,54,56,59] is beneficial to the patient and reduces costs. Thus, abandoning peritoneal reapproximation would achieve several important objectives: (1) the total amount of foreign material present in the abdominal cavity would be reduced; (2) adhesion formation may be minimized; (3) postoperative complications would be reduced; and (4) last, but not least, costs would be reduced.

Perioperative Contamination

Of the great diversity of materials present in operating rooms, two main types can be identified: those intended for implantation and those that are accidentally deposited in the body. Those intentionally used are considered under headings reflecting their purpose or potential action(s), whereas foreign materials unintentionally left behind are presented here. These materials include glove powder, fabric, lint, and other particles, many of which become airborne in the operating room.

Swabs and Sponges

Sponges and swabs have a potential to shed particles. Experiments in rats demonstrated that small particles of lint, from gauze sponges induced adhesions and granulomas. Furthermore, it was shown that moist sponges shed fewer particles than dry ones,[61] thereby suggesting that wet swabs are less adhesiogenic. Indeed, experimentally it can be demonstrated that dry gauze swabs, when used rather vigorously in the peritoneal cavity of rats, were associated with more adhesions than the similar use of wet gauze swabs.[38]

Besides the shedding of particles, gauze swabs have an abrasive effect on the serosal surface that may be even more important. A study using rats demonstrated that adhesion formation was significantly more frequent with a cotton abdominal swab than with a nonwoven counterpart, explained by the finding that nonwoven material was significantly less traumatizing to the serosa than were conventional cotton swabs.[62] The issue was further explored in a rat model where the adhesiogenic potential of two commercially available brands of surgical packs was tested. Both brands were shown to cause a significant increase in the incidence of postoperative peritoneal adhesions, regardless of whether the packs were used wet or dry. The conclusion was that the foreign debris from surgical sponges after intraabdominal use was not the main cause of peritoneal adhesions. Instead, the abrasive effect of the sponge was considered to produce mesothelial trauma, sufficient to initiate adhesion formation.[63,64] This notion has recently been confirmed by an observation in rats showing that standard surgical gauze traumatized the peritoneum and promoted adhesion formation whereas a less abrasive nonsurgical textile did not.[65]

It is well known clinically that an abdominal operation might greatly enhance the growth and spread of intraabdominal tumors. Recently, it was found that there was a significant correlation between the amount of peritoneal trauma and the degree of tumor take at damaged peritoneal surfaces. Moreover, the tumor take could be reduced by using a nonabrasive gauze.[66] Thus, it is possible that by reducing peritoneal trauma through the use of less abrasive, nonshedding gauze both the likelihood of adhesions and the peritoneal dissemination of intraabdominal tumors may be reduced. Thus, there seem to be possibilities to reduce peritoneal trauma by using a less abrasive gauze, preferably one that does not shed, thereby reducing not only the likelihood of adhesion formation but also the spread of cancer.

Fibers

Foreign materials from surgical gowns, dressings, masks, and sponges (fabric, fibers, fluff, lint) may be introduced into the abdomen either through direct contact or indirectly by being aerosolized. These materials may also interfere with peritoneal tissue repair and cause adhesions and granulomas.[67,68] A recent study indicated that foreign microbodies were present in more than 90% of all reoperated patients in which adhesions were analyzed for evidence of external contamination. Many of these foreign microbodies contained remnants of fabric.[69,70] Although it remains debatable if these foreign materials caused the adhesions, or were simply trapped in the fibrinous mesh caused by the surgical injury, it seems reasonable to assume that they affect the peritoneal repair process by intensifying and sustaining the inflammatory reaction. The result would be a shift in the delicate balance between fibrin deposition and degradation toward an accumulation of fibrin, leading to adhesion development. In the context of fibers, it is noteworthy that certain fibers may actually act as carcinogens.[71]

Glove Powder

Preceded by some experimentation with other types of dusting powder, talc became the first donning agent to be used on a larger scale. It was observed early on that talc introduced into the abdomen triggered foreign-body reactions leading to peritoneal adhesions, granulomas, fistula formation, and impaired wound healing.[72–83] Although considered to be inert in the initial study in 1947 by Lee and Lehman,[84] the glove powder (primarily cornstarch that has been treated with epichlorhydrine and mixed with 2.3% magnesium oxide as a desiccating agent) was soon to be reappraised. Absorption experiments with starch powder in dogs and rabbits revealed that the starch often, but not always, disappeared and that adhesions could develop.[85] In dogs, starch was demonstrated to cause inflammatory reactions and adhesions. The authors concluded that glove powder was potentially harmful and had to be washed off.[86] This precaution has had a variable penetration clinically.[87]

Later, glove powder was demonstrated to cause or augment adhesion formation in rats and rabbits.[88–93] The effect of glove powder was shown to be dose dependent[94] and was potentiated by a simultaneous serosal injury.[95,96] Experimental animals that underwent a standardized abdominal operation with powdered surgical gloves developed significantly more adhesions than those operated with powder-free gloves,[97] indicating that the amount of powder on the exterior surface of a powdered glove was sufficient to affect peritoneal tissue repair (Fig. 11.2). Histopathologic studies of human adhesion tissue have revealed that adhesions contain starch particles and other foreign materials, similar to the findings in animals.[15,95,97,98]

In addition to the adhesiogenic potential, glove powder may cause granulomas in animals and humans.[94,99–133] These granulomas can become very large, and in some cases have been misdiagnosed as malignant tumors or peritoneal carcinomatosis.[134] Although of scientific interest, the mechanism leading to granuloma formation is not fully understood. Because of reports that food starch caused granulomatous peritonitis after ingestion and entering into the peritoneal cavity through gastrointestinal perforations,[127,135] it seems likely that the starch itself induces the granuloma development. Starch glove powder not only affects tissues in the peritoneal cavity but also has been reported to cause adverse events in the urogenital tract, pleura, and central nervous system, as comprehensively reviewed by Ellis.[136] In addition, deleterious effects of glove powder have been observed in joints[137] and in the ear–nose–throat region.[103,138] Inflammatory and granulomatous reactions in the myo- or pericardium have also been reported[139–141] and reproduced experimentally.[142]

Starch Peritonitis

There are numerous reports of glove powder peritonitis in the literature,[102,106,109–112,114,115,117,118,120,128,133,143–152] and some other reports have been reviewed by Klink and Boynton.[153] These authors also described the starch peritonitis syndrome.[153] Typically, the patient returns 3 to 4 weeks after an uneventful procedure. The dominating symptoms are abdominal pain and distension. Fever, typically low grade, could be present. The white blood cell response is inconsistent, but eosinophilia is often present. The severity of the syndrome is variable, ranging from mild to a life-threatening condition, and deaths have been reported. Most patients eventually are treated surgically. When the abdomen is opened, there is a substantial amount of fluid, with miliary seedlings and nodules on the visceral and parietal peritoneum. Treatment with corticosteroids has been reported to be successful. Because of the dramatic effect of steroids and the frequent eosinophilia, several authors proposed that the

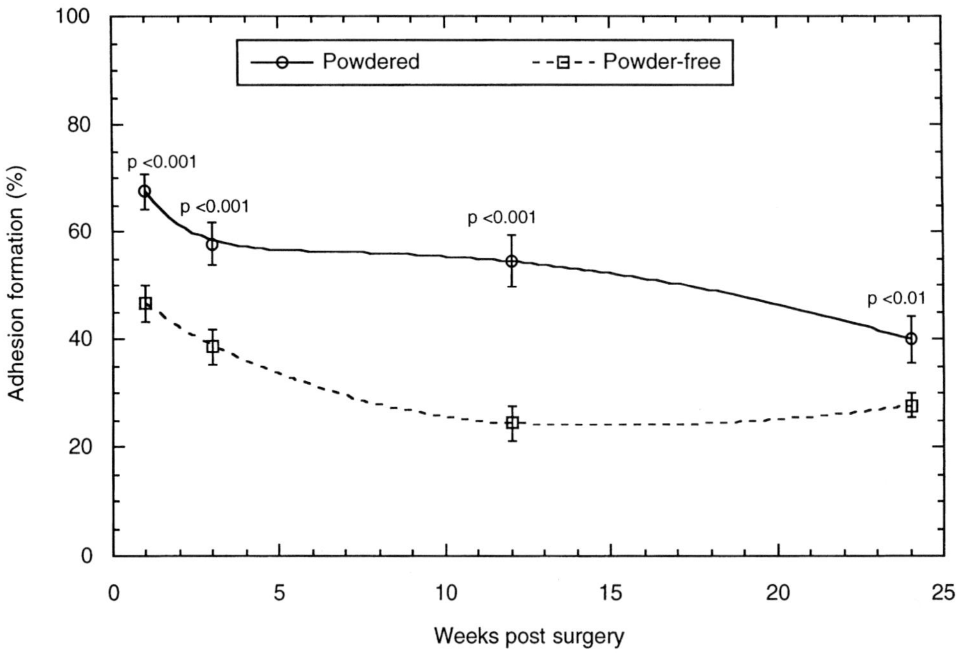

FIG. 11.2. Adhesion formation in an experimental rat model. The rats underwent a standardized operation in which the surgeon randomly operated with powdered or powder-free gloves. (Redrawn from Holmdahl et al.[97])

syndrome was a delayed hypersensitivity to the glove powder. Using other approaches, immunologic mechanisms were clearly demonstrated to be involved.[154–156]

Glove Powder Action in the Peritoneal Cavity

From experimental animal studies it was known that glove powder could affect the peritoneal repair processes and stimulate adhesion formation, but the mechanism(s) of action were not known. Based on findings related to the starch peritonitis syndrome, it was known that glove starch powder could elicit biologic responses involving the immune system. Additionally, it was accidentally discovered that glove powder was cytotoxic to cultured endothelial cells,[157] indicating another mode of action.

As mentioned earlier, there are several cell types present in the peritoneal cavity, among which monocytes/macrophages and mesothelial cells dominate. An important contribution to the understanding of how glove powder affected the peritoneal cavity was reported by Renz and coworkers.[158] They found in separate experiments that rat peritoneal macrophages and human monocytes that were incubated in vitro with glove starch particles obtained from three commonly used types of surgical gloves released large amounts of tumor necrosis factor-alpha (TNF-α), interleukin-1 (IL-1), prostaglandin E_2, thromboxane B_2, and hydrogen peroxide. Moreover, release of these inflammatory mediators was associated with progressive cell death of macrophages.

TNF-α Production

The mesothelium has been suggested to be the main defense against the development of adhesions by being the provider of tissue-type plasminogen activator (tPA),[159] the prevailing activator of fibrinolysis in the peritoneal cavity.[160] Release of these proinflammatory mediators in the peritoneal cavity undoubtedly affects the mesothelium. Indeed, TNF-α was found to decrease the release of tPA by cultured human peritoneal mesothelial cells[161] as well as by omentally derived mesothelial cells.[162–165] Furthermore, the release of the major inhibitor of fibrinolysis, plasminogen activator inhibitor type-1 (PAI-1), was increased in both types of mesothelial cells after exposure to TNF-α.[161–167] The combination of decreased tPA and increased PAI-1 expression leads to a powerful reduction of fibrinolytic capacity that favors the development of adhesions. Il-1, also secreted by macrophages exposed to glove starch powder, has been demonstrated to have similar effects.[163–166] Moreover, these proinflammatory mediators stimulate mesothelial cells to produce interleukin-8, which stimulates the recruitment of granulocytes into the peritoneal cavity,[168,169] and the release of interleukin-6,[170] IL-1α, and IL-1β.[171]

Prostaglandins and Hydrogen Peroxide

Mesothelial cells produce prostaglandins and other arachidonic acid metabolites.[172–178] Prostaglandin E_2 stimulates the synthesis of hyaluronic acid in rabbit pericardial mesothelial cells.[179] However, the biologic consequences of this is not fully understood. Glove-powder-exposed macrophages also produced hydrogen peroxide, a reactive oxygen species. This reaction might cause increased damage to the peritoneum because human mesothelial cells seem to be more susceptible to oxidative damage than other cell types investigated.[180]

Endotoxin

Surgical gloves may act as vehicles for foreign materials and other contaminants. Asplund-Peiró and coworkers

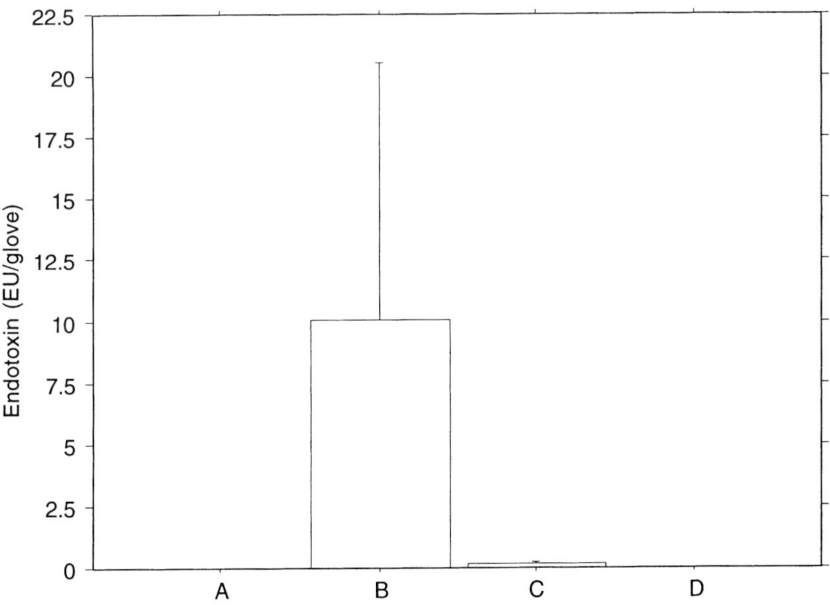

FIG. 11.3. Endotoxin concentration in washings from the outer surface of four different brands (*A–D*) of powder-free surgical gloves. Values are expressed as means; error bars indicate 1 SD. (Redrawn from Holmdahl and Chegini.[182])

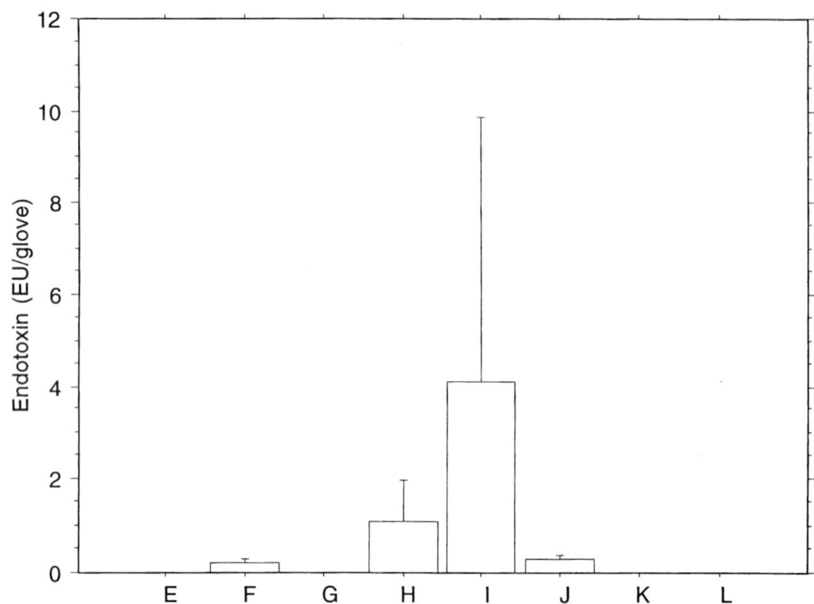

FIG. 11.4. Endotoxin concentration in washings from the outer surface of eight different brands (*E–L*) of powdered surgical gloves. Values are expressed as means; error bars indicate 1 SD. (Redrawn from Holmdahl and Chegini.[182])

observed that some commercially available gloves were heavily contaminated with endotoxin, in amounts sufficient to cause febrile reactions.[181] Endotoxin was detectable in powder samples obtained from manufacturers, but the levels corresponded to only a minor fraction of the amount of endotoxin found on the exterior surface of a glove. Recently, when a variety of surgical gloves were investigated for possible contamination on the exterior surface, endotoxin was present on several, including a powder-free glove (Figs. 11.3 and 11.4). This study demonstrated that powder can be one source but is not the sole source of endotoxin, however detectable in powder (Fig. 11.5).[182] The presence of endotoxin on some gloves and in powder might in part explain the adhesion-instigating effect of glove powder because mesothelial cells from various sources exposed to endotoxin have a reduced fibrinolytic capacity; this reduction is considered to be a crucial factor in the early formation of adhesions.[161–163]

Particulate Matter

The amount of particulate contamination present on a surgical glove varied greatly among the different brands of gloves (Fig. 11.6 and, Fig. 11.7). Although particulate contamination was considerably less on powder-free gloves, only one brand of the powder-free gloves was actually free from particulates (Fig. 11.6). Thus, "powder-free" does not mean "particulate-free." The effects of the particulate contamination in the peritoneal cavity remain to be elucidated. Photomicrographs of the recovered particles are displayed in Fig. 11.8.

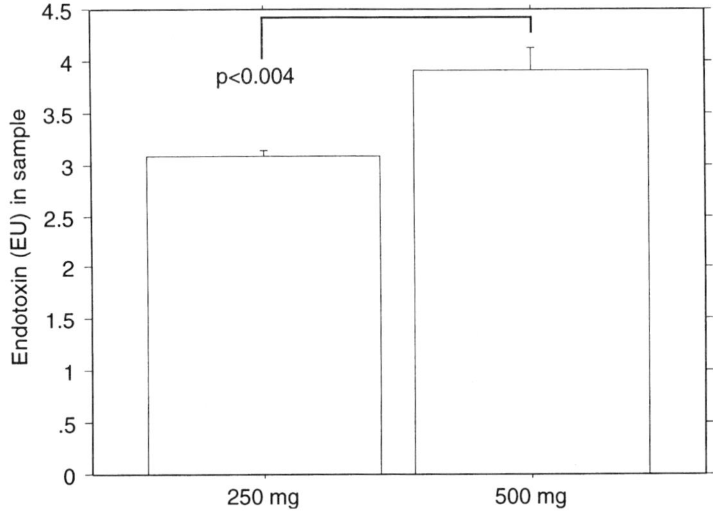

FIG. 11.5. Concentration of endotoxin in sterile glove powder commonly used as a donning agent. The powder contained detectable amounts of endotoxin, increasing with increasing amounts of powder. Values are expressed as means; error bars indicate 1 SD. (Redrawn from Holmdahl and Chegini.[182])

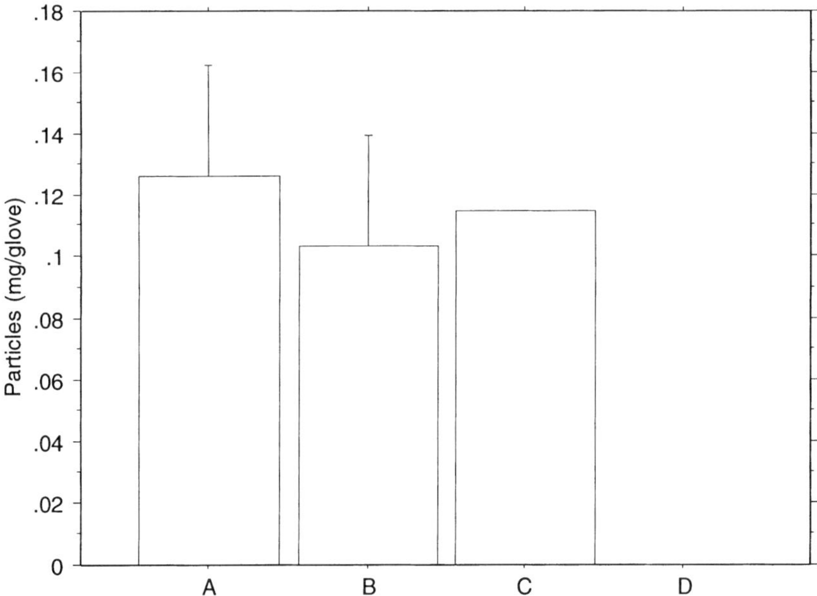

FIG. 11.6. The amount of particulate matter on the outer surface of powder-free surgical gloves. Only one of the four investigated brands (*A–D*) did not carry any particulate contamination. Values are expressed as means; error bars indicate 1 SD. (Redrawn from Holmdahl and Chegini.[182])

Glove Powder Has Deleterious Effects on Wound Healing

Glove powder can contaminate wounds directly or indirectly by being aerosolized. It has been demonstrated that starch powder significantly decreased the ultimate strength, resilience, and toughness of abdominal incisional wounds in immunocompetent animals. Healing in the presence of powder was not affected in T-cell-depleted rats.[183] Thus, starch powder seems to affect integral parts of the immune system involved in healing.

Latex Allergy

The prevalence of latex allergy among medical personnel has increased steadily over the past few years. It is now thought to be between 5% and 15%,[184,185] and is expected to increase even more with extended exposure to latex allergens. Most alarming is the increasing prevalence of type I allergic reactions, associated with systemic manifestations and anaphylaxis, among medical staff and patients.[185–187] There is no doubt that repeated exposure to latex antigens (e.g., in gloves, catheters, balloons, condoms, and a variety of household products) can provoke latex allergy. For surgical patients, the risk increases with increasing number of surgical interventions.[188,189] Exposure is not limited to direct contact with the latex, but also includes exposure to glove powder, which has been found to act as a vehicle for latex allergens.[190–192] Fortunately, the problem of latex sensitiza-

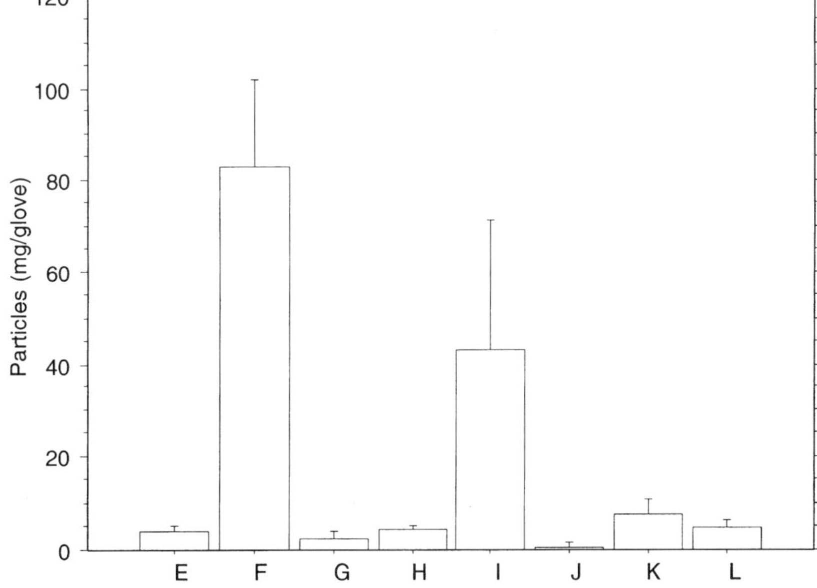

FIG. 11.7. The amount of particulate matter on the outer surface of powdered surgical gloves. The amount of particles retrieved from glove washings differed substantially. Most gloves carried less than 10 mg of particulate debris, but two of the eight investigated brands (*E–L*) carried large amounts of particulate matter. Values are expressed as means; error bars indicate 1 SD. (Redrawn from Holmdahl and Chegini.[182])

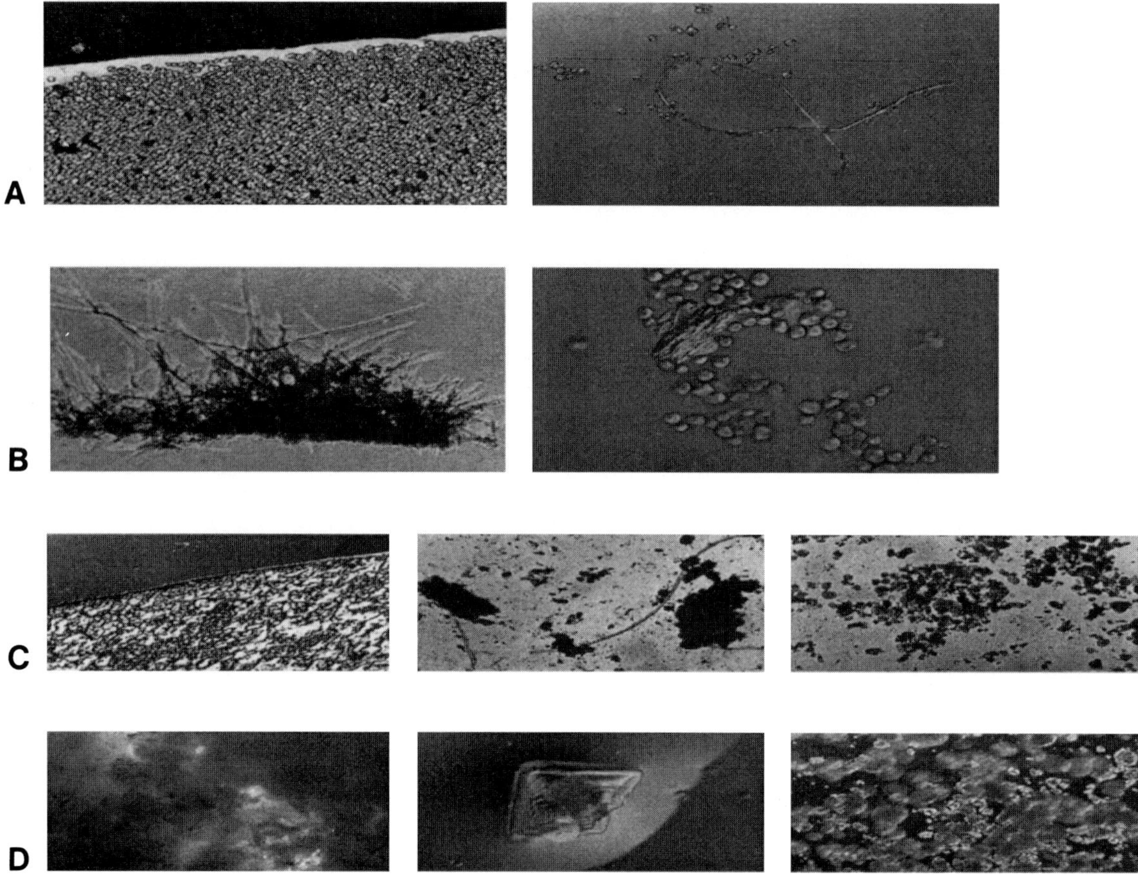

FIG. 11.8. Photomicrographs showing examples of particulate matter pelleted from glove washings. Rows *A* and *B* depict particulate matter from powdered gloves and rows *C* and *D* that from powder-free gloves. Photomicrographs are from experiments reported in Holmdahl and Chegini.[182]

tion and allergic reactions seems to be manageable with strict prophylaxis,[193] including the use of nonlatex gloves or powder-free gloves that contain very low levels of natural rubber latex proteins.

Gastrointestinal Contents

Although contained within the body, gastrointestinal contents typically cause an aggressive peritoneal reaction when introduced into the peritoneal cavity, such as by rupture or during surgical procedures. It is well known that gastric juice and feces cause intense and often life-threatening conditions. Bile can produce peritonitis, with a purulent exudate and destruction of subperitoneal muscle,[96] as well as greatly exacerbate peritoneal inflammation associated with the presence of *E. coli* bacteria.[194] The introduction of laparoscopic cholecystectomy has put focus on the retention of gallstones in the peritoneal cavity. Although controversial, retained gallstones have been found to induce adhesions.[195,196] The combination of bile and gallstones in the peritoneal cavity seems to be especially ominous, resulting in an increased risk of intraabdominal adhesion and abscess formation.[197,198]

Medical Devices

Adhesion Control

Adjunct therapies for adhesion control are covered in other chapters. However, in the context of foreign materials it should be pointed out that devices for adhesion control may contain compounds capable of eliciting adverse reactions in the peritoneal cavity.[199,200] The presence of blood can reduce the efficacy of such materials and reportedly increase adhesion formation, for example, oxidized regenerated cellulose (Interceed).[201–203] Furthermore, it should be observed that being "endogenous" does not preclude a material from having harmful effects in the peritoneal cavity; the peritoneal environment may not be the place where the material typically is found. Excess intraperitoneal amounts of a material may saturate defense systems, or activate the mesothelium and the resident population of leukocytes, and thus trigger an inflammatory reaction.

Hemostatic Agents

To some extent, oxidized regenerated cellulose (Surgicel) has been investigated experimentally for its effect on peritoneal tissue repair. It does not seem to increase adhesion formation, but its efficacy in reducing adhesion development is questionable.[199,204,205] Fibrin glue, often used as a hemostatic agent, can affect peritoneal repair processes. In experimental studies it has been reported to reduce adhesion formation.[206,207] However, the efficacy seems not to be consistent, and several reports indicated that fibrin glue was ineffective,[208–210] or that it increased adhesion formation[211] or may adversely affect intestinal healing.[212,213] Other major concerns have been the possibility of viral transmission and antibody formation against fibrin glue components.[214]

Translocation of Foreign Materials

Foreign bodies have been reported to be introduced into the peritoneal cavity via the female genital tract. In 1963, Saxen et al. reported a case of starch peritonitis without previous surgery that was caused by condom emulsion.[215] Another case in which an ovarian starch granuloma was presumably caused by prolonged use of a powder suspension in water by the patient as a douche has been reported.[123]

Intrauterine contraceptive devices occasionally also find their way into the peritoneal cavity, usually through a uterine perforation.[216–218] A large proportion of perforations occur at insertion.[219] Cases of translocation via the fallopian tubes have also been reported.[220] Copper devices have been shown to elicit a much stronger peritoneal reaction than other devices,[218,314,315] with tissue necrosis, granulation tissue, a severe infiltration of polymorphonuclear leukocytes, and the entire device covered by dense adhesions.[218,314,315] Prevo et al. showed that intrauterine progesterone contraceptive devices produced a minimal peritoneal response, similar to that of a plastic "nonmedicated" contraceptive.[314] This response was attributed to the fact that progesterone in high local concentration exerts a significant antiinflammatory activity.[221] The urgency with which an intraperitoneally translocated contraceptive device should be removed depends therefore on the type of device used. Copper devices should be removed as soon as possible after diagnosis to reduce their tissue-damaging effects.[222]

Not only exogenous materials deposited in the uterus may cause peritoneal inflammation. Peritoneal foreign-body granulomas caused by keratin from uterine adenocarcinomas with squamous metaplasia have been reported.[223–225] The presence of peritoneal keratin granulomas therefore should alert the pathologist that a neoplastic disease may be the cause and that it may not be a benign cystic teratoma of the ovary but a transtubal spread from the uterus.

The Peritoneum As an Exchange Area

Tissue Implantation and Microencapsulation

Microencapsulation of implantable tissues, such as the islets of Langerhans, has been studied for many years. The protective capsules aim to avoid rejection from the host's immune system without immunosuppressive therapy by preventing access of antibodies and immunocompetent cells to the tissue. Simultaneously, the capsules must allow access for nutrients and diffusion of glucose and insulin to and from the islets. The peritoneal cavity has been considered a practical implantation site for this tissue.[226] Biocompatibility of the encapsulated tissue is of importance to the survival of the graft, because a foreign-body reaction leading to fibrosis around the capsule will lead to graft failure through impaired diffusion of nutrients and oxygen to the cells. The tissue reaction strongly depends on the surface characteristics of the implants.

As pointed out by Sawhney et al., an ideal microencapsulating device should be "non-cytotoxic, have suitable permeability characteristics, and be mechanically stable and non-biodegradable, as well as biocompatible."[227] Many of the encapsulating materials studied have contained alginate and poly-L-lysine.[227–232] The advantage of alginates (originating from seaweeds) for cell entrapment is that the immobilization is performed under very mild conditions so that there is little cell loss.[233] Polyurethane[234] and agarose[235] are other examples of materials used for immunoisolation of endocrine tissue transplants.

Cell adhesion to synthetic surfaces is partly mediated by interaction between cell-surface receptors and adhesion proteins adsorbed to the surface of the implant. Fibrosis on implanted microcapsules is probably the result of the adhesion and activation of resident macrophages, and of the secretion of interleukins and cytokines, which attract nonresident macrophages, neutrophils, and lymphocytes.[236] Different approaches have been used to try to diminish the tissue reaction and the formation of a fibrous capsule around the cell transplant devices. The group of Christenson showed that the intensity of the tissue reaction to inraperitoneally implanted capsules can be reduced by dexamethasone given orally.[237] Local release of even smaller amounts of dexamethasone in a polymeric drug delivery capsule, given intraperitoneally, was even more successful in reducing the formation of a fibrous capsule around the implant.[238] The effect could be explained by decreased production of macrophage-derived factors and inhibited mast cell degranulation. By covering alginate-poly-L-lysine microcapsules with a polyethylene glycol-based hydrogel, Sawhney et al. could reduce the fibrotic and inflammatory response by reducing protein adsorption and complement binding.[227]

Polyethylene glycol, a nonionic polymer, can also prevent proteoglycan-mediated cell adhesion to charged surfaces. Soon-Shiong et al. managed to improve the mechanical integrity and chemical stability of alginate-based encapsulated islets by controlling the kinetics of their formation and by using alginate high in glucuronic acid.[316] Phase I–II human clinical trials have demonstrated insulin secretion from the encapsulated islets for more than 20 months. The concept of microencapsulated cells has proven effective in many animal experiments and seems to have become an important therapeutic alternative. However, the long-term effects on the peritoneal cavity remains to be elucidated.

Pumps

If transplantation of microencapsulated islets of Langerhans is still an experimental treatment of diabetes mellitus, continuous peritoneal insulin infusion (CPII) is definitely in clinical practice. Both external portable pumps and implantable devices are available on the market. Insulin can then be infused intravenously or intraperitoneally. An advantage of the peritoneal route is that it represents a more physiologic delivery route by absorption of insulin through the portal circulation, resulting in improved bioavailability and lower peripheral insulinemia, as compared to the intravenous route.[239] Catheter obstruction, catheter migrations, and breaks or infections are complications that can occur from CPII. Infections are less common with the implantable systems. Complications include the formation of a fibrin clot at the catheter tip or the development of omental encapsulations around the peritoneal part of the catheter.[240] Tissue encapsulation seems to be an immunoinflammatory reaction involving catheter components and/or insulin, with amyloid deposits reacting to antiinsulin antibodies in some cases.[240]

Peritoneal Dialysis

Much could be learned about peritoneal responses to foreign materials from experiences with peritoneal dialysis. The extensive use of the peritoneum as an exchange area often results in the development of adhesions, which limit further use of the peritoneal cavity and make abdominal surgery cumbersome. In recent years a growing body of information on the biocompatibility and peritoneal reactions to peritoneal dialysis has accumulated. Di Paolo et al. defined biocompatibility in this context as being the capacity to leave the anatomic and physiologic characteristics of the peritoneum unchanged in time.[241] Factors influencing these characteristics are the peritoneal catheter, the solution bags, and most importantly the dialysis solutions themselves. The conventional dialysis solutions contain high concentrations of glucose to create an osmolality sufficient to achieve water ultrafiltration over the peritoneal membrane. Many recent research efforts have been focused on trying to clarify the effects of the different constituents of the dialysis solutions on the peritoneum and on trying to find more physiologic alternatives.

The peritoneal membrane plays an important role in the control of the inflammatory reaction through secretion of prostaglandins and pro- and immunomodulatory cytokines and chemokines recruiting leukocytes during infection.[174] During peritoneal dialysis, macrophages and lymphocytes seem to be in a state of chronic activation, with enhanced expression of surface antigens such as HLA-DR, IL-2 receptor (CD25), and transferrin receptor (CD71),[242–244] which hypothetically could result in the chronic production of fibrogenic cytokines and oxidative free radicals. In the past, lactate has been used to buffer the pH of the solutions to 5.2–5.5.[245] Leukocyte function has been shown to be suppressed by low pH and lactate, as demonstrated by decreased phagocytosis, bactericidal activity, respiratory burst, leukotriene synthesis, and production of IL-6 and TNF-α.[246] IL-6 is believed to induce B-cell differentiation and immunoglobulin synthesis. These effects could render continuous ambulatory peritoneal dialysis patients more susceptible to peritonitis and fibrosis and failure to achieve sufficient ultrafiltration. In addition, the IgG and complement normally residing in the peritoneal fluid is greatly diluted by the dialysis solution, resulting in a significant decrease in opsonic activity.

Mesothelial cells are known to sometimes become very large in cell cultures. This is not a specific reaction for mesothelial cells, but is known to occur in many different cell lines. Gotloib et al. recently observed very large mesothelial cells in rats undergoing peritoneal dialysis, indicating that these cells may also increase in size in vivo during peritoneal dialysis.[247] Di Paolo et al. showed that peritoneal dialysis in rabbits caused a large increase in the size of mesothelial cells and that the increase seemed to be correlated with increasing osmotic pressure. It has also been reported that giant mesothelial cells with atypical morphology occur in dialysis liquid from patients with peritonitis, a condition in which mesothelial cells are detached from the basal lamina in large numbers. Similar cells were observed in rats undergoing peritoneal dialysis without peritonitis, using a peritoneal imprint technique capable of separating the mesothelial cells from the basal lamina.[247] These morphologic changes are likely to be caused by the increased mesothelial turnover in peritoneal dialysis.[248] and perhaps the chemical and physical stress applied to the peritoneum. The functional characteristics of the mesothelium are also changed by exposure to large amounts of peritoneal dialysis solutions, including a decrease in fibrinolytic potential, lubricating capacity (through decreased phospholipid production), secretory properties, and impaired leukocyte- and macrophage-mediated response to infection.[249] These observations are likely, at least in part, to explain the tendency for peritoneal dialysis to induce adhesions.

Substitution of lactate with bicarbonate as the buffering substance improves macrophage phagocytic function.[245,250] Pyrovate-based solutions also cause less injury to mesothelial cells, as compared to lactate-based solutions.[251] The macrophage phagocytic function and oxidative metabolism seemed to improve when the hyperosmolar glucose-based solution was replaced by an isoosmolar glucose-polymer solution.[252] A filter-sterilized fluid induced less changes in leukocyte function than the heat-sterilized fluid.[253] These findings are likely to be relevant when compounding irrigation fluids for intraperitoneal use.

The peritoneal catheter may cause problems such as exit site infection and peritonitis. Bacterial adhesion to biomaterials and intraluminal contamination and colonization may be a cause of peritonitis. The most commonly used catheters are made of silicone rubber or Silastic. Silver-coated silicone catheters prevent bacterial colonization through the bactericidal activities of silver, but the long-term effects of silver are not fully known.[254] The search for new biomaterials to prevent bacterial attachment continues, and such observations are likely to be applicable when developing drains for intraperitoneal use.

The bags containing dialysis solutions have been proposed as a source of toxic substances such as phthalates, a plasticizer, and particles of plastics. Residues of plastics have in fact been identified in peritoneal biopsies from dialysis patients.[241] Phthalate-free bags have been tried and found to have reduced toxicity toward the mesothelial cells in vitro and less stimulating effect on the peritoneal fibroblasts.[255] These observations should be considered when designing containers for irrigation fluids. In conclusion, peritoneal dialysis remains an important instigator of intraabdominal adhesions complicating peritoneal surgery, and important lessons could be learned from research in this area.

Experiences from Peritoneal Implant Studies in Animals

When a device is implanted in the body, the first event that takes place is an adsorption of proteins such as fibronectin, immunoglobulins, and complement factors to the surface of the implant. This process is determined by the nature of the proteins, the composition of the biologic fluid where it takes place, and the surface characteristics of the implant. The adsorbed proteins then might activate polymorphonuclear leukocytes and macrophages and initiate an inflammatory response.

It has been shown that when leukocytes encounter a noningestible material, they are activated to produce reactive oxygen species and release their granules, thereby inducing a local inflammatory reaction.[256] This process is known as frustrated phagocytosis. Henson showed that larger particles induced greater amounts of enzyme release.[257] This result suggests that the inflammatory response in the peritoneal cavity is dependent on the size of the implant and that a material in powder or particulate form, suitable for phagocytosis, may provoke a different response than the same material in a nonphagocytosable form, that is, a film.

Early in the response to an implant, polymorphonuclear leukocytes (PMNs) are the most prevalent cells, but eventually macrophages become the predominant cell type, resulting in chronic inflammatory response. Later, neovascularization, foreign-body giant cells, and fibroblasts enter the scene, leading to fibrosis around the foreign material. As indicated earlier, the amount of foreign-body reaction depends on the characteristics of the surface of the implant.

Biomaterial-Related Infections

Biomaterial-associated infection is a major problem in the usage of biomedical devices. Infections may arise from contamination at implantation or from bacterial migration along transcutaneous tracts. Infections in association with intraabdominal devices, however, are often caused by enteric bacteria, in the absence of intestinal perforation.[258] Mora et al. demonstrated that enteric bacteria can translocate to sterile intraperitoneal implants. The translocation was believed to involve phagocytosis of bacteria within the bowel wall and chemotactic attraction to nearby sites of inflammation. Guo et al. studied the effect of different intraperitoneal biomaterials on reticuloendothelial system (RES) and bacterial translocation. They showed an impaired RES function in the gut-associated lymphoid tissues that was believed to predispose to the bacterial translocation which was observed concomitantly.[259] They also showed that splenectomy reduced the rate of enteric bacterial translocation induced by intraperitoneal biomaterial implantation in the rat, which was partly attributed to a decrease in the production of bioactive mediators, thereby protecting the mucosal barrier from products from the host–biomaterial interface.[260]

The biomaterial surface provides a substrate to which bacteria can adhere and create what are known as protected environments in the form of biofilms.[261] Many bacterial strains have the ability to produce expolysaccharides, or glycocalyx, that help them to attach to the surface,[262] where they can surround themselves with additional glycocalyx and replicate within the biofilm to form microcolonies. The microcolonies then act as a nucleus for attracting other bacteria. Bacteria in biofilms are resistant to host defense mechanisms and antibiotic therapy, which is why treatment of these infections often requires removal of the implant. At the same time, the host defense mechanisms are altered. The process of frustrated phagocytosis causes a decreased leukocyte killing activity, with loss of ability to release hydrogen peroxide and superoxide anion, combined with an enhanced degranulation. Release of granule contents results in membrane damage and an exhaustion of PMN function,[263] which may partly explain why *Candida* yeasts frequently are isolated from patients with continuous ambulatory peritoneal dialysis (CAPD) peritonitis or other biomaterial-related infections.[264] Rozalska et al. showed that the surface of an implant of heparinized polyethylene was quickly covered by fibronectin and that staphylococci equipped with fibronectin-binding proteins could form a biofilm on the biomaterial surface.[256] In this way, the bacteria could avoid eradication by humoral defense mechanisms and staphylococci could be demonstrated long after eradication of the bacteria from the peritoneal cavity, spleen, liver, and kidney. Coating the material with recombinant granulocyte-macrophage colony-stimulating factor (rGM-CSF) improved the elimination of staphylococci from mouse peritoneum, and the number of bacteria in the biofilms covering the implants was significantly lower.[265]

Not all biomaterials seem to have the same impairing effect on leukocyte bactericidal activity. The use of a polyglycolic acid (PGA) mesh as an intestinal sling to elevate the small bowel from the true pelvis during postoperative radiation has been associated with an unusual lack of pelvic infections as observed by Devereaux et al. They also demonstrated that a PGA mesh surgically implanted in the peritoneal cavity of rats stimulated the respiratory burst by peritoneal cells, which may partly be responsible for the lack of infections seen with the use of this material.[317]

Peritoneal Cavity and Biocompatibility Studies

The mouse peritoneal cavity has been used extensively as a model compartment for screening for biocompatibility of a vast array of biomaterials,[266–269] not only for biomaterials intended for use in the abdominal cavity but for screening of all types of materials, including bone cements,[270] prosthetic anterior cruciate ligaments,[271] and vascular prosthesis.[272–274] The peritoneal cavity contains an easily quantifiable cell population consisting of the cells normally involved in the inflammatory reaction including macrophages, lymphocytes, mast cells, eosinophils, and polymorphonuclear leukocytes. The cell population is easily retrievable for analysis by peritoneal lavage.

Attempts to Increase Biocompatibility

A common definition of biocompatibility is "the ability of a material to perform with an appropriate host response in a specific application." Ratner has proposed a new definition: "the exploitation by materials of the proteins and cells of the body to meet a specific performance goal."[275] The intention was to stress the central role of the interfacial proteins and cellular recognition processes in biocompatibility and to emphasize the need of an active role of the biomaterial. Instead of the nonspecific reactions mostly seen with today's biomaterials, a future role for bioengineered surfaces eliciting precise reactions with proteins and cells, according to what is needed, is suggested. Even if such bioengineered materials are not a reality today, many attempts to improve biocompatibility have been made, slowly approaching that vision.

Drug Delivery

Intraperitoneal administration of cytostatic agents has been extensively studied in connection with ovarian cancer[276,277] because ovarian cancer often remains confined to the peritoneal cavity until late in its course. It is therefore an attractive concept to deliver the cytotoxic agents locally in the peritoneal cavity to achieve a high concentration in the tumor and reduced systemic side effects, compared to traditional administration routes.

The ideal cytostatic drug in intraperitoneal therapy was described by Tranberg et al. as having the following properties: a peritoneal clearance that is slow relative to clearance from blood, ability to diffuse into the tumor, producing no or acceptable chemical peritonitis (pain) in therapeutic concentrations, and a steep dose–response relationship in the concentration range to be used.[278] Chemical peritonitis and abdominal pain are limiting for many drugs. Some drugs administered intraperitoneally have a documented sclerotic effect on the peritoneum,[279] causing intraabdominal adhesions.[280] For carboplatinum, adhesion development is related to the dose of the drug.[281] Some agents given intraperitoneally (^{32}P and mitoxantrone) are reported to cause adhesion formation or fibrosis leading to small-bowel obstruction.[282,283]

Other major complications are infectious peritonitis and adhesion formation.[278] Adhesions or tumor masses may limit distribution by creating pockets with high concentrations of the drug. Most information regarding peritoneal access and its complications come from the field of peritoneal dialysis. Several characteristics of intraperitoneal chemotherapy differ from those of peritoneal dialysis: higher incidence of previous laparotomy, presence of known pathology in the peritoneal cavity, fewer intraperitoneal accessions for treatment, and the unknown effect of cytotoxic agents on normal functions or peritoneal cells.[284] Although of potential benefit as adjuvant therapy in gastrointestinal or gynecologic cancer, intraperitoneal administration of cytostatic drugs can cause serious complications in the peritoneal cavity. Available drugs may be rendered more suitable for intraperitoneal use by coadministration of agents with lower peritoneal clearance to increase tumor penetration, reduce chemical peritonitis, and combat toxic levels in the systemic circulation. Examples of drug delivery devices investigated are a carrier solution, Icodextrin 20, allowing prolonged intraperitoneal infusion,[285] poly (glycolide-co-lactide) microspheres with a slow release over 3 weeks,[286,287] liposomes, and immunoliposomes with monoclonal antibodies.[288]

Nutritional supplementation by way of the peritoneal cavity has been attempted.[289-296] Although this was not extensively investigated, episodes of peritonitis were reported and there were morphologic changes in the mesothelium.[297,298]

Abdominal Wall Substitutes

Synthetic materials to repair defects of the abdominal wall have been used for many years. Among the most commonly used materials are polypropylene (Marlex, Prolene, Trelex) and expanded polytetrafluoroethylene (ePTFE) in different compositions. Many studies have been performed to compare the efficacy of these two materials. Their different properties clearly demonstrate some central principles crucial to the performance of an abdominal wall substitute.

Polypropylene meshes are macroporous materials (1-mm pores in Marlex and 2-mm pores in Prolene). As wound healing progresses, the polypropylene mesh is completely incorporated in fibrocollagenous tissue. Ingrowth of fibrocollagenous tissue is mainly determined by the pore size. The ePTFE patch (Gore-Tex Soft-Tissue Patch; W.L. Gore) has a pore size of approximately 20 μm, which is too small to allow ingrowth of fibroblasts. Consequently there is very little ingrowth of fibrocollagenous tissue to these prostheses,[299,300] which results in an increased risk of reherniation at the fascia and patch interface from insufficient anchorage of the patch to the surrounding tissue.[301]

An unwanted side effect of abdominal wall substitutes is adhesion formation to the implant, particularly when applied intraperitoneally. Besides a potential risk of adhesions, in this context adhesion formation might be the first stage of biomaterial-related fistula formation. The use of the ePTFE patch was associated with significantly less frequent and severe adhesions than the polypropylene mesh and induced a less prominent foreign-body reaction.[299] The polypropylene mesh has also been shown to become distorted by contracture of the scar tissue, causing mechanical irritation that can cause mesh erosion into the skin or intestine.[302,303]

In addition to studying the tissue integration and adhesion-promoting or -preventing effect, it is of utmost importance to determine the biomaterial behavior in the presence of infection. These defects are often the result of (semi)open treatment of generalized peritonitis. Although the use of foreign materials is typically avoided in the presence of an infection, there might be occations when this is needed. If so, Bleichrodt et al. showed that ePTFE patches are unsuitable for reconstruction of contaminated abdominal wall defects after observing the disintegration of the patch, and they were forced to remove the patch in two patients for ongoing sepsis.[304]

Because neither the macroporous polypropylene meshes nor the microporous ePTFE patches were shown to be ideal as an abdominal wall substitute, the hypothesis was that a nonporous layer facing the peritoneal cavity on a porous layer facing the subcutaneous tissue would lead to tissue integration and increased tensile strength at the same time as adhesions and fistulae formation could be reduced. An ePTFE prosthesis with the peritoneal face consisting of a nonporous PTFE and the other face with a chosen porosity (Dual Mesh) was tried out.[305-307] Compared to a polypropylene mesh, Dual Mesh was associated with less adhesion formation but less resistance to traction.[307] There have also been attempts to combine polypropylene with different nonporous layers, such as Silastic sheeting and polypropylene sheeting on the intestinal side.[308] Indeed, the composite materials gave less adhesion formation than the pure polypropylene mesh, as did a combination of polypropylene and polyurethane used in both infected and uninfected conditions,[309] as well as a composite mesh of polypropylene and a nonporous layer of ePTFE.[310] Another ePTFE mesh examined is the Mycro Mesh, which combines the features of both macro- and microporous ePTFE. Mycro Mesh consists of a laminar base similar to the Soft-Tissue Patch with 2-mm perforations. The Mycro Mesh prosthesis induced little adhesion formation, and, in the perforations, bridges of tissue linked the peritoneal and the subcutaneous sides, thereby providing improved tissue integration.[133]

The development of biocompatible and low-adhesiogenic materials for abdominal wall substitutes is ongoing, and a novel synthetic material is reported to have less adhesiogenic potential than others.[311] The development of adjunct therapies might also prove useful, without compromising abdominal wall tissue integration. Successful attempts has been made with Seprafilm, an adhesion prevention barrier, with no adverse effects on wound healing at least in animals.[312]

In spite of the improvements achieved in the area of biocompatibility of abdominal wall substitutes, the only way to definitely prevent adhesion formation still is to leave the peritoneum intact, as demonstrated by Bellon et al., who showed that the formation of adhesions was almost inhibited when the parietal peritoneum was left unbreached.[313]

References

1. Myllärniemi H, Leppäniemi A. Peritoneal fibrosis due to practolol. Acta Chir Scand 1981;147:137–142.
2. Agarwal DK, Barthwal SP, Agarwal R, Tandon S, Agarwal RL. Peritoneal fibrosis—an expression of atenolol toxicity. J Assoc Physicians India 1994;42:152.
3. Flessner MF, Dedrick RL, Schultz JS. Exchange of macromolecules between peritoneal cavity and plasma. Am J Physiol 1985;240:H15–H25.
4. Flessner MF, Fenstermacher JD, Dedrick RL, Blasberg RG. A distributed model of peritoneal-plasma transport: tissue concentration gradients. Am J Physiol 1985;248:425–435.
5. Bettendorf U. Lymph flow mechanism of the subperitoneal diaphragmatic lymphatics. Lymphology 1978;11: 111–116.
6. Flessner MF, Parker RJ, Sieber SM. Peritoneal lymphatic uptake of fibrinogen and erythrocytes in the rat. Am J Physiol 1983;244:H89–H96.
7. Abu Hijleh MF, Habbal OA, Moqattash ST. The role of the diaphragm in lymphatic absorption from the peritoneal cavity. J Anat 1995;186:453–467.
8. Shinohara H. Lymphatic system of the mouse diaphragm: morphology and function of the lymphatic sieve. Anat Rec 1997;249:6–15.
9. Li J, Zhao Z, Zhou J, Yu S. A study of the three-dimensional organization of the human diaphragmatic lymphatic lacunae and lymphatic drainage units. Anat Anz 1996;178:537–544.
10. Kubicka U, Olszewski WL, Maldyk J, Wierzbicki Z, Orkiszewska A. Normal human immune peritoneal cells: phenotypic characteristics. Immunobiology 1989;180:80–92.
11. Fukasawa M, Bryant SM, Orita H, Campeau JD, diZerega GS. Modulation of proline and glucosamine incorporation into tissue repair cells by peritoneal macrophages. J Surg Res 1989;46:166–171.
12. Fukasawa M, Campeau JD, Yanagihara DL, Rodgers KE, diZerega GS. Mitogenic and protein synthetic activity of tissue repair cells: control by the postsurgical macrophage. J Invest Surg 1989;2:169–180.
13. Fukasawa M, Yanagihara DL, Rodgers KE, diZerega GS. The mitogenic activity of peritoneal tissue repair cells: control by growth factors. J Surg Res 1989;47:45–51.
14. Bakkum EA, Dalmeijer RA, Verdel MJ, Hermans J, van Blitterswijk CA, Trimbos JB. Quantitative analysis of the inflammatory reaction surrounding sutures commonly used in operative procedures and the relation to postsurgical adhesion formation. Biomaterials 1995;16:1283–1289.
15. Luijendijk RW, de Lange DCD, Wauters CCAP, et al. Foreign material in postoperative adhesions. Ann Surg 1996; 223:242–248.
16. Hurd WW, Himebaugh KS, Cofer KF, Gauvin J, Elkins TE. Etiology of closure-related adhesion formation after wedge resection of the rabbit ovary. J Reprod Med 1993; 38:465–468.
17. Ellis H. The aetiology of postoperative abdominal adhesions: an experimental study. Br J Surg 1962;50:10–16.
18. Ellis H, Harrison W, Hugh TB. The healing of peritoneum under normal and pathological conditions. Br J Surg 1965;52:471–476.
19. Hubbard TB, Khan MZ, Carag WR, Albites VE, Hricko GM. The pathology of peritoneal repair: its relation to the formation of adhesions. Ann Surg 1966;165:908–916.
20. Eskeland G. Regeneration of parietal peritoneum in rats. A light microscopical study. Acta Pathol Microbiol Scand 1966;68:355–378.
21. Swanwick RA, Milne FJ. The non-suturing of parietal peritoneum in abdominal surgery of the horse. Vet Rec 1973; 93:328–335.
22. Raftery AT. Regeneration of parietal and visceral peritoneum. A light microscopical study. Br J Surg 1973;60: 293–299.
23. Raftery AT. Regeneration of parietal and visceral peritoneum: an electron microscopical study. J Anat 1973;115: 375–392.
24. McDonald MN, Elkins TE, Worthman GF, Stowall TG. Adhesion formation and prevention after peritoneal injury and repair in the rabbit. J Reprod Med 1988;33:436–439.
25. Holmdahl L, Al-Jabreen M, Risberg B. Experimental models for quantitative studies on adhesion formation in rats and rabbits. Eur Surg Res 1994;26:248–256.
26. Ryan GB, Grobéty J, Majno G. Mesothelial injury and recovery. Am J Pathol 1973;71:93–102.
27. Watters WB, Buck RC. Scanning electron microscopy of mesothelial regeneration in the rat. Lab Invest 1972;26: 604–609.
28. Raftery AT. Regeneration of peritoneum: a fibrinolytic study. J Anat 1979;129:659–664.
29. Elkins TE, Stovall TG, Warren J, Ling FW, Meyer NL. A histologic evaluation of peritoneal injury and repair: implications for adhesion formation. Obstet Gynecol 1987;70: 225–228.
30. Robbins GF, Brunschwig A, Foote FW. Deperitonealization: clinical and experimental observations. Ann Surg 1949;130:466–479.
31. Trimpi HD, Bacon HE. Clinical and experimental study of denuded surfaces in extensive surgery of the colon and rectum. Am J Surg 1952;74:596–603.

32. Williams DC. The peritoneum. A plea for a change in attitude towards this membrane. Br J Surg 1955;42:401–405.
33. Bakkum EA, van Blitterswijk C, Dalmeijer RA, Trimbos JB. A semiquantitative rat model for intraperitoneal postoperative adhesion formation. Gynecol Obstet Invest 1994; 37:99–105.
34. diZerega GS. Contemporary adhesion prevention. Fertil Steril 1994;61:219–235.
35. Duffy DM, diZerega GS. Is peritoneal closure necessary? Obstet Gynecol Surv 1994;49:817–822.
36. Kyzer S, Bayer I, Turani H, Chaimoff C. The influence of peritoneal closure on formation of intraperitoneal adhesions: an experimental study. Int J Tissue React 1986;8: 355–359.
37. O'Leary DP, Coakley JB. The influence of suturing and sepsis on the development of postoperative peritoneal adhesions. Ann R Coll Surg Engl 1992;74:134–137.
38. Conolly WB, Stephens FO. Factors influencing the incidence of intraperitoneal adhesions: an experimental study. Surgery (St. Louis) 1968;63:976–979.
39. Storey BG, Lawrenson KB, Chant S, Stephens FO. Factors influencing the incidence of postoperative abdominal adhesions: an experimental study. Aust N Z J Surg 1971; 40:388–390.
40. Lindenberg S, Lauritsen JG. Prevention of peritoneal adhesion formation by fibrin sealant. An experimental study in rats. Ann Chir Gynaecol 1984;73:11–13.
41. McGaw T, Elkins TE, DeLancey JO, McNeeley SG, Warren J. Assessment of intraperitoneal adhesion formation in a rat model: can a procoagulant substance prevent adhesions? Obstet Gynecol 1988;71:774–778.
42. Nezhat C, Nezhat F, Silfen SL, Schaffer N, Evans D. Laparoscopic myomectomy. Int J Fertil 1991;36:275–280.
43. Meyer WR, Grainger DA, DeCherney AH, Lachs MS, Diamond MP. Ovarian surgery on the rabbit. Effect of cortex closure on adhesion formation and ovarian function. J Reprod Med 1991;36:639–643.
44. Ansari AG. Adhesion formation to incisional abdominal wound in response to polyamide "6" and polyglactin "910" sutures. J Pak Med Assoc 1992;42:184–185.
45. Durstein-Decker C, Brick WG, Gadacz TR, Crist DW, Ivey RK, Windom KW. Comparison of adhesion formation in transperitoneal laparoscopic herniorrhaphy techniques. Am Surg 1994;60:157–159.
46. Holmdahl L, Al-Jabreen M, Risberg B. The role of fibrinolysis in the formation of postoperative adhesions. Wound Repair Regen 1994;7:171–176.
47. Mok SD, Li AK. Is reperitonealization of the gallbladder bed a ritual or necessity? Am J Surg 1989;157:312–314.
48. Gilbert JM, Ellis H, Foweraker S. Peritoneal closure after lateral paramedian incision. Br J Surg 1987;74:113–115.
49. Ellis H, Heddle R. Does the peritoneum need to be closed at laparotomy? Br J Surg 1977;64:733–736.
50. Hull DB, Varner MW. A randomized study of closure of the peritoneum at Cesarean delivery. Obstet Gynecol 1991;77:818–821.
51. Tulandi T, Hum HS, Gelfand M. Closure of laparotomy incisions with or without peritoneal suturing and second look laparoscopy. Am J Obstet Gynecol 1987;158:536–537.
52. Pietranoni M, Parsons MT, O'Brien WF, Collins E, Knuppel RA, Spellacy WN. Peritoneal closure or non-closure at Cesarean. Obstet Gynecol 1991;77:293–296.
53. Than GN, Arany AA, Schunk E, Vizer M, Krommer KF. Closure or non-closure of visceral peritoneums after abdominal hysterectomies and Wertheim-Meigs radical abdominal hysterectomies. Acta Chir Hung 1994;34:79–86.
54. Irion O, Luzuy F, Beguin F. Nonclosure of the visceral and parietal peritoneum at caesarean section: a randomised controlled trial. Br J Obstet Gynaecol 1996;103:690–694.
55. Lipscomb GH, Ling FW, Stovall TG, Summit RL Jr. Peritoneal closure at vaginal hysterectomy: a reassessment. Obstet Gynecol 1996;87:40–43.
56. Nagele F, Karas H, Spitzer D, et al. Closure or nonclosure of the visceral peritoneum at cesarean delivery. Am J Obstet Gynecol 1996;174:1366–1370.
57. Hugh TB, Nankivell C, Meagher AP, Li B. Is closure of the peritoneal layer necessary in the repair of midline surgical abdominal wounds? World J Surg 1990;14:231–234.
58. Fasth S, Hultén L, öjerskog B. Omission of pelvic peritoneal closure after abdominoperineal rectal excision. Ann Chir Gynaecol 1977;66:181–183.
59. Kadanali S, Erten O, Kucukozkan T. Pelvic and periaortic pertioneal closure or non-closure at lymphadenectomy in ovarian cancer: effects on morbidity and adhesion formation. Eur J Surg Oncol 1996;22:282–285.
60. Franchi M, Ghezzi F, Zanaboni F, Scarabelli C, Beretta P, Donadello N. Nonclosure of peritoneum at radical abdominal hysterectomy and pelvic node dissection: a randomized study. Obstet Gynecol 1997;90:622–627.
61. Sturdy JH, Baird RM, Gerein AN. Surgical sponges: a cause of granuloma and adhesion formation. Ann Surg 1967;165:128–134.
62. Swolin K, Bendz A, Larsson B, et al. Traumatization of the abdominal serosa. A comparison between non-woven and cotton abdominal swabs. Acta Chir Scand 1973;140: 203–204.
63. Down RHL, Whitehead R, Watts JM. Do surgical packs cause peritoneal adhesions? Aust N Z J Surg 1979;49: 379–382.
64. Down RHL, Whitehead R, Watts JM. Why do surgical packs cause peritoneal adhesions? Aust N Z J Surg 1980;50: 83–85.
65. van den Tol MP, van Stijn I, Bonthuis F, Marquet RL, Jeekel J. Reduction of intraperitoneal adhesion formation by use of non-abrasive gauze. Br J Surg 1997;84:1410–1415.
66. van den Tol PM, van Rossen EE, van Eijck CH, Bonthuis F, Marquet RL, Jeekel H. Reduction of peritoneal trauma by using nonsurgical gauze leads to less implantation metastasis of spilled tumor cells. Ann Surg 1998;227:242–248.
67. Godleski JJ, Gabriel KL. Peritoneal responses to implanted fabrics used in operating rooms. Surgery (St. Louis) 1981; 90:828–834.
68. Weibel M, Majno AG. Peritoneal adhesions and their relation to abdominal surgery. A postmortem study. Am J Surg 1973;126:345-353.
69. Duron JJ, Olivier L, Khosrovani C, Gineste D, Jost JL, Keilani K. Natural history of postoperative intraperitoneal adhesions. Surely, a question of the day. J Chir (Paris) 1993;130:385–390.

70. Duron JJ, Ellian N, Olivier O. Post-operative peritoneal adhesions and foreign bodies. Eur J Surg 1997;579(suppl): 15–16.
71. Unfried K, Roller M, Pott F, Friemann J, Dehnen W. Fiber-specific molecular features of tumors induced in rat peritoneum. Environ Health Perspect 1997;105(suppl 5):1103–1108.
72. Antopol W. Lycopodium granuloma, its clinical and pathologic significance together with a note on granuloma produced by talc. Arch Pathol 1933;16:326–331.
73. Owen M. Peritoneal response to glove powder containing talcum. Texas State J Med 1936;32:482–485.
74. Fienberg R. Talcum powder granuloma. Arch Pathol Lab Med 1937;24:36–42.
75. Eiseman B, Seelig MG, Womack NA. Talcum powder granuloma: a frequent and serious postoperative complication. Ann Surg 1949;126:820–832.
76. Lichtman A, McDonald J, Dixon C, Mann F. Talcum granulomas. Surg Gynecol Obstet 1946;83:531–546.
77. German WM. Dusting powder granulomas following surgery. Surg Gynecol Obstet 1943;76:501–507.
78. McCormick EJ, Ramsey TL. Postoperative peritoneal granulomatous inflammation caused by magnesium silicate. JAMA 1941;116:817.
79. Mackey A, Gibson JB. Siliceous granuloma due to talc. Br Med J 1943;1:1077.
80. Roberts GBS. Granuloma of the fallopian tube due to surgical glove talc. Br J Surg 1947;34:417–423.
81. Chamlin M. Effect of talc in ocular surgery. Arch Ophthalmol 1945;34:369–371.
82. Gruenfeld GE. Granulomas of large size caused by implantation of talcum (talcum sarcoids). Arch Surg 1949;59: 917–924.
83. Saxen A, Tuovinen PJ. Experimental and clinical observations on granulomas caused by talc and some other substances. Acta Chir Scand 1947;96:131–151.
84. Lee CM, Lehman EP. Experiments with non-irritating glove powder. Surg Gynecol Obstet 1947;84:689–695.
85. Postlethwait RW, Howard HL, Schanher P. Comparison of tissue reaction to talc and modified starch glove powder. Surgery (St. Louis) 1949;25:22–29.
86. Lee CM, Collins WT, Largen TLA. A reappraisal of absorbable glove powder. Surg Gynecol Obstet 1952;95: 725–737.
87. Holmdahl L, Risberg B. Adhesion prevention and complications in general surgery. Eur J Surg 1997;163:169–174.
88. Mazuji MK, Fadhli HA. Peritoneal adhesions; prevention with povidone and dextran 75. Arch Surg 1965;91: 872–874.
89. Myllärniemi H, Frilander M, Turunen M, Saxen L. The effect of glove powders and their constituents on adhesion and granuloma formation in the abdominal cavity of the rabbit. Acta Chir Scand 1966;131:312–318.
90. McEntee GP, Stuart RC, Byrne PJ, Leen E, Hennessy TP. Experimental study of starch-induced intraperitoneal adhesions. Br J Surg 1990;77:1113–1114.
91. Kamffer WJ, Jooste EV, Nel JT, de Wet JI. Surgical glove powder and intraperitoneal adhesion formation. An appeal for the use of powder-free surgical gloves. S Afr Med J 1992;81:158–159.
92. Reikeras O, Nordstrand K. Use of dextran to prevent intraperitoneal adhesions caused by maize starch powder. Eur Surg Res 1985;17:251–253.
93. Pelling D, Evans JG. Long-term peritoneal tissue response in rats to mould-release agents and lubricant powder used on surgeons gloves. Food Chem Toxicol 1986;24:425–430.
94. Nordstrand K, Melhus O, Eide TJ, Larsen T, Giercksky KE. Intraabdominal granuloma reaction in rats after introduction of maize-starch powder. Acta Pathol Microbiol Immunol Scand 1987;95:93–98.
95. Jagelmann DG, Ellis H. Starch and intraperitoneal adhesion formation. Br J Surg 1973;60:111–114.
96. Walker EM. Effects of blood, bile and starch in the peritoneal cavity of the rat. J Anat 1978;126:495–507.
97. Holmdahl L, Al-Jabreen M, Xia G, Risberg B. The impact of starch-powdered gloves on the formation of adhesions in rats. Eur J Surg 1994;160:257–261.
98. Cooke SA, Hamilton DG. The significance of starch powder contamination in the aetiology of peritoneal adhesions. Br J Surg 1977;64:410–412.
99. Sneierson H, Woo ZP. Starch powder granuloma. A report of two cases. Ann Surg 1955;142:1045–1050.
100. McAdams GB, Conn H. Granulomata caused by absorbable starch glove powder. Surgery (St. Louis) 1956; 39:329–336.
101. Paine CG, Smith P. Starch granulomata. J Clin Pathol 1957;10:51–55.
102. Myers RN, Deaver JM, Brown CE. Granulomatous peritonitis due to starch glove powder. Ann Surg 1960;151: 106–112.
103. Ising U. Foreign-body granuloma resulting from the use of starch glove powder at surgery. Acta Chir Scand 1960; 120:95–99.
104. Saxen L, Saxen E. Starch granulomas as a problem in surgical pathology. Acta Pathol Microbiol Scand 1965;64: 55–70.
105. Epstein WL. Granulomatous hypersensitivity. Prog Allergy 1967;11:36–88.
106. Taft DA, Lasersohn JT, Hill LD. Glove starch granulomatous peritonitis. Am J Surg 1970;120:231–236.
107. Cox KR. Starch Granuloma (pseudo-malignant seedlings). Br J Surg 1970;57:650–653.
108. Swingler GR. Starch granulomatosis of the peritoneum. Br Med J 1971;4:116.
109. Sobel HJ, Schiffman RJ, Schwarz R, Albert WS. Granulomas and peritonitis due to starch glove powder. Arch Pathol 1971;91:559–568.
110. Hornung JR, Kremen AJ. Granulomatous peritonitis induced by cornstarch powder. Minn Med 1972;55:427–429.
111. Coder DM, Olander GA. Granulomatous peritonitis caused by starch glove powder. Arch Surg 1972;105:83–86.
112. Humphreys SR, Cameron AJ, Harrison EG Jr. Acute granulomatous peritonitis due to starch glove powder. Gastroenterology 1972;63:1062–1065.
113. Davies JD, Neely J. The histopathology of peritoneal starch granulomas. J Pathol 1972;107:265–278.
114. Soderberg CJ, Lou TY, Randall HT. Glove starch granulomatous peritonitis. Am J Surg 1973;125:455–460.
115. Kirshen EJ, Naftolin F, Benirschke K. Starch glove powders and granulomatous peritonitis. Am J Obstet Gynecol 1974;15:799–804.
116. Cutright DE, Becker PD, Bunge JL. Granulomas caused by starch powder from surgeons' gloves. Oral Surg Oral Med Oral Pathol 1974;37:699–704.

117. Sugarbaker PH, McReynolds RA, Brooks JR. Glove starch granulomatous disease. An unsolved surgical problem. Am J Surg 1974;128:3–7.
118. Ehrlich CE, Wharton JT, Gallager HS. Starch granulomatous peritonitis. South Med J 1974;67:443–446.
119. Vellar ID. The starch granuloma syndrome. Med J Aust 1975;1:60–62.
120. Neely J. Starch granuloma peritonitis. Nurs Mirror Midwives J 1975;140:62–63.
121. Cade D, Ellis H. The peritoneal reaction to starch and its modification by prednisone. Eur Surg Res 1976;8: 471–479.
122. Stiegler FS. Starch granulomatosis. A preventable iatrogenic disease. Minn Med 1977;60:795–796.
123. Hidvegi D, Hidvegi I, Barret J. Douche-induced pelvic peritoneal starch granuloma. Obstet Gynecol Suppl 1978; 52:15–18.
124. Yaffe H, Beyth Y, Reinhartz T, Levij I. Foreign body granulomas in peritubal and periovarian adhesions: a possible cause for unsuccessful reconstructive surgery in infertility. Fertil Steril 1980;33:277–279.
125. Chenowenth CV. Retroperitoneal fibrosis due to starch granuloma. Urology 1981;17:157–159.
126. Wilson DF, Garach V. Surgical glove starch granuloma. Oral Surg Oral Med Oral Pathol 1981;51:342–345.
127. Davies JD, Ansell ID. Food-starch granulomatous peritonitis. J Clin Pathol 1983;36:435–438.
128. Michowitz M, Stavorovsky M, Ilie B. Granulomatous peritonitis caused by glove starch. Postgrad Med J 1983;59: 593–595.
129. Sheikh KM, Duggal K, Relfson M, Gignac S, Rowden G. An experimental histopathologic study of surgical glove powders. Arch Surg 1984;119:215–219.
130. Nordstrand K, Giercksky KE, Melhus O, Eide TJ, Flægstad T. Corn starch glove powder. A life-threatening peritoneal reaction. Tidsskr Nor Lægeforen 1986;106:494–495.
131. Carrington AC. Starch granuloma: the problems caused by surgical glove powder. Natnews 1987;24:9–10.
132. Ohtsuki Y, Sonobe H, Takahashi K, et al. Postoperative starch granuloma revealed as femoral herniation. A case report. Acta Pathol Jpn 1988;38:1235–1240.
133. Howard PM, Maxwell JG. Corn starch granulomatous peritonitis. Rocky Mt Med J 1965;62:46–48.
134. Giercksky K-E, Qvist H, Giercksky TC, Warloe T, Nesland JM. Multiple glove powder granulomas masquerading as peritoneal carcinomatosis. J Am Coll Surg 1994;179: 299–304.
135. Veress B, Alafuzoff I, Juliusson G. Granulomatous peritonitis and appendicitis of food starch origin. Gut 1991; 32:718–720.
136. Ellis H. The hazards of surgical glove dusting powders. Surg Gynecol Obstet 1990;171:521–527.
137. Singh I, Chow WL, Chablani LV. Synovial reaction to glove powder. Clin Orthop 1974;99:285–292.
138. Rock EH. Surgeon's glove powder (starch) middle ear granuloma. Arch: Otolaryngol 1967;86:8–17.
139. Brynjolfson G, Eshaghy B, Talano JV, Gunnar R. Granulomatous myocarditis secondary to cornstarch. Am Heart J 1977;94:353–358.
140. McKee PH, McKeovn EF. Starch granulomata of the endocardium. J Pathol 1978;126:103–105.
141. Osborne MP, Paneth M, Hinson KFW. Starch granules in the pericardium as a cause of the postcardiotomy syndrome. Thorax 1974;199:199–203.
142. Reikerås O, Nordstrand K, Sörlie D. Use of dextran to prevent pericardial adhesions caused by maize starch powder. Eur Surg Res 1987;19:62–64.
143. Berkson PM, Grinvalsky HT. Starch glove powder peritonitis. NY State J Med 1971;71:2874–2876.
144. Dutra FR, Jensen CD. Peritonitis from starch glove powder. Calif Med 1972;117:8–12.
145. Goodrich EJ, Prine JR, Wilson JS. Iodized starch granules as a cause of starch peritonitis. Surg Forum 1974;25: 372–374.
146. Kaufman M, Gloor F, Maurer W, Miller G. Peritonitis fibroplastica incapsulata with superadded post-operative starch powder peritonitis. Scand J Gastroenterol 1975; 10:801–804.
147. Malmfors G. 2 cases of peritonitis caused by starch from surgical gloves. Lakartidningen 1972;69:6014–6015.
148. Norgren L. Excessive foreign-body reaction following abdominal surgery. A case report. Acta Chir Scand 1978; 144:121–122.
149. Vandamme JP. Glove starch peritonitis. Acta Chir Belg 1974;73:333–340.
150. Warshaw AL. Diagnosis of starch peritonitis by paracentesis. Lancet 1972;2:1054–1056.
151. Warshaw AL. Management of starch peritonitis without the unnecessary second operation. Surgery (St. Louis) 1973;73:681–685.
152. Hugh TB, Scoppa J, Tsang J. Starch peritonitis—a hazard of surgical glove powder. Med J Aust 1975;1:63–64.
153. Klink B, Boynton CJ. Starch peritonitis. A case report and clinicopathologic review. Am Surg 1990;56:672–674.
154. Holgate ST, Wheeler JH, Bliss BP. Starch peritonitis: an immunological study. Ann R Coll Surg Engl 1973;52: 182–188.
155. Grant JB, Davies JD, Jones JV. Allergic starch peritonitis in the guinea-pig. Br J Surg 1976;63:867–869.
156. Grant JB, Davies JD, Jones JV, Espiner HJ, Eltringham WK. The immunogenicity of starch glove powder and talc. Br J Surg 1976;63:864–866.
157. Sharefkin JB, Fairchild KD, Albus RA, Cruess DF, Rich NM. The cytotoxic effect of surgical glove powder particles on adult human vascular endothelial cell cultures: implications for clinical uses of tissue culture techniques. J Surg Res 1986;41:463–472.
158. Renz H, Schmidt A, Hofman P, Amann S, Gemsa D. Tumor necrosis factor-alpha, interleukin 1, eicosanoid, and hydrogen peroxide release from macrophages exposed to glove starch particles. Clin Immunol Immunopathol 1993;68:21–28.
159. Holmdahl L, Falkenberg M, Ivarsson ML, Risberg B. Plasminogen activator and inhibitors in peritoneal tissue. APMIS 1997;105:25–30.
160. Holmdahl L, Eriksson E, Risberg B. Fibrinolysis in human peritoneum during operation. Surgery (St. Louis) 1996; 119:701–705.
161. Ivarsson M-L, Holmdahl L, Falk P, Mölne J, Risberg B. Characterization and fibrinolytical properties of mesothelial cells isolated from peritoneal lavage. Scand J Clin Lab Invest 1998;58:195–204.

162. van Hinsbergh VWM, Kooistra T, Scheffer MA, van Bockel JH, van Muijen GNP. Characterization and fibrinolytic properties of human omental tissue mesothelial cells. Comparison with endothelial cells. Blood 1990;75: 1490–1497.
163. Sitter T, Gödde M, Spannagl M, Fricke H, Kooistra T. Intraperitoneal coagulation and fibrinolysis during inflammation: *in vivo* and *in vitro* observations. Fibrinolysis 1996;10(suppl 2):99–104.
164. Sitter T, Toet K, Fricke H, Schiffl H, Held E, Kooistra T. Modulation of procoagulant and fibrinolytic system components of mesothelial cells by inflammatory mediators. Am J Physiol 1996;271:R1256–R1263.
165. Tietze L, Elbrecht A, Schauerte C, et al. Modulation of pro- and antifibrinolytic properties of human peritoneal mesothelial cells by transforming growth factor β1 (TGF-β1), tumor necrosis factor-α (TNF-α) and interleukin 1β (IL-1β). Thromb Haemostasis 1998;79:362–370.
166. Whawell SA, Thompson JN. Cytokine-induced release of plasminogen activator inhibitor-1 by human mesothelial cells. Eur J Surg 1995;161:315–317.
167. Whawell SA, Scott-Coombes DM, Vipond MN, Terbutt SJ, Thompson JN. Tumor necrosis factor-mediated release of plasminogen activator inhibitor 1 by human mesothelial cells. Br J Surg 1994;81:214–216.
168. Betjes MG, Tuk CW, Struijk DG, et al. Interleukin-8 production by human peritoneal mesothelial cells in response to tumor necrosis factor-α, interleukin-1, and medium conditioned by macrophages cocultured with *Staphylococcus epidermidis*. J Infect Dis 1993;168:1202–1210.
169. Topley N, Jorres A, Luttman W, et al. Human peritoneal mesothelial cells synthesize interleukin-8: synergistic induction by interleukin-1β and tumor necrosis factor-α. Am J Pathol 1993;142:1876–1886.
170. Topley N, Jorres A, Luttman W, et al. Human peritoneal mesothelial cells synthesize interleukin-6: induction by Il-1β and TNF-α. Kidney Int 1993;43:226–233.
171. Douvdevani A, Rapoport J, Konforty A, Argov S, Ovnat A, Chaimovitz C. Human peritoneal mesothelial cells synthesize IL-1 alpha and beta. Kidney Int. 1994;46: 993–1001.
172. Coene MC, Solheid C, Clates M, Herman AG. Prostaglandin production by cultured mesothelial cells. Arch Int Pharmacodyn 1981;249:316–318.
173. Coene M-C, van Hove C, Claeys M, Herman A. Arachidonic acid metabolism by cultured mesothelial cells. Different transformations of exogenously added and endogenously released substrate. Biochim Biophys Acta 1982;710:437–445.
174. Topley N, Petersen MM, Mackenzie R, et al. Human peritoneal mesothelial cell prostaglandin synthesis: induction of cyclooxygenase mRNA by peritoneal macrophage-derived cytokines. Kidney Int 1994;46:900–909.
175. Baer AN, Green FA. Cyclooxygenase activity of cultured human mesothelial cells. Prostaglandins 1993;46:37–49.
176. Chegini N, Rossi M, Holmdahl L. Cellular distribution of 5-lipooxygenase and receptors for leukotrienes in peritoneal wound healing. Wound Repair Regen 1997;5: 235–242.
177. Di Paolo N, Sacchi G. Anatomy and physiology of the peritoneal membrane. In: Scarpioni LL, Ballocchi S, eds. Evolution and Trends in Peritoneal Dialysis, Vol. 84. Basel: Karger, 1990:10–26.
178. Stylianou E, Jenner LA, Davies M, Coles GA, Williams JD. Isolation, culture and characterization of human peritoneal mesothelial cells. Kidney Int 1990;37:1563–1570.
179. Honda A, Sekiguchi Y, Mori Y. Prostaglandin E_2 stimulates cyclic AMP-mediated hyaluronan synthesis in rabbit pericardial mesothelial cells. Biochem J 1993;292: 497–502.
180. Chen JY, Yang AH, Lin YP, Lin JK, Yang WC, Huang TP. Absence of modulating effects of cytokines on antioxidant enzymes in peritoneal mesothelial cells. Perit Dial Int 1997;17:455–466.
181. Asplund-Peiró S, Kulander L, Eriksson Ö. Quantitative determination of endotoxins on surgical gloves. J Hosp Infect 1990;16:167–172.
182. Holmdahl L, Chegini N. Endotoxin and particulate matter on surgical gloves. J Long-Term Effic Med Impl 1997;7:225–234.
183. Corless DJ, Holland J, Wastell C. Effect of starch-containing glove powder on wound healing in the rat. Br J Surg 1995;82:368–370.
184. Charous B, Hamilton R, Yunginger J. Occupational latex exposure: characteristics of contact and systemic reactions in 47 workers. J Allergy Clin Immunol 1994;94: 12–18.
185. Heese A, Peters K-P, Koch HU. Type I allergies to latex and the aeroallergic problem. Eur J Surg 1997;579 (suppl):19–22.
186. Meric F, Teitelbaum DH, Geiger JD, Harmon CM, Groner JI. Latex sensitization in general pediatric surgical patients: a call for increased screening of patients. J Pediatr Surg 1998;33:1108–1111.
187. Kelly KJ, Pearson ML, Kurup VP, et al. A cluster of anaphylactic reactions in children with spina bifida during general anesthesia: epidemiologic features, risk factors, and latex hypersensitivity. J Allergy Clin Immunol 1994; 94:53–61.
188. Bode CP, Fullers U, Roseler S, Wawer A, Bachert C, Wahn V. Risk factors for latex hypersensitivity in childhood. Pediatr Allergy Immunol 1996;7:157–163.
189. Chen Z, Cremer R, Baur X. Latex allergy correlates with operation. Allergy (Cph) 1997;52:873.
190. Baur X, Jäger D. Airborne antigens from latex gloves. Lancet 1990;335:912.
191. Turjanmaa K, Reunala T, Alenius H, Brummer-Korvenkontio H, Palosuo T. Allergens in latex surgical gloves and glove powder. Lancet 1990;336:1588.
192. Beezhold D, Beck WC. Surgical glove powder bind latex antigens. Arch Surg 1992;127:1354–1357.
193. Cremer R, Hoppe A, Kleine-Diepenbruck U, Blaker F. Longitudinal study on latex sensitization in children with spina bifida. Pediatr Allergy Immunol 1998;9:40–43.
194. Andersson R, Willen R, Massa G, Tranberg KG, Carlen B, Bengmark S. Effect of bile on peritoneal morphology in *Escherichia coli* peritonitis. Scand J Gastroenterol 1990; 25:405–411.

195. Cline RW, Poulos E, Clifford EJ. An assessment of potential complications caused by intraperitoneal gallstones. Am Surg 1994;60:303–305.
196. Yerdel MA, Alacayir I, Malkoc U, et al. The fate of intraperitoneally retained gallstones with different morphologic and microbiologic characteristics: an experimental study. J Laparoendosc Adv Surg Tech A 1997;7:87–94.
197. Johnston S, O'Malley K, McEntee G, Grace P, Smyth E, Bouchier Hayes D. The need to retrieve the dropped stone during laparoscopic cholecystectomy. Am J Surg 1994;167:608–610.
198. Agalar F, Sayek I, Agalar C, Cakmakci M, Hayran M, Kavuklu B. Factors that may increase morbidity in a model of intra-abdominal contamination caused by gallstones lost in the peritoneal cavity. Eur J Surg 1997;163: 909–914.
199. Larsson B, Nisell H, Granberg L. Surgicel—an absorbable hemostatic material—in prevention of peritoneal adhesion in rats. Acta Chir Scand 1978;144:375–378.
200. Kershisnik MM, Ro JY, Cannon GH, Ordonez NG, Ayala AG, Silva EG. Histiocytic reaction in pelvic peritoneum associated with oxidized regenerated cellulose. Am J Clin Pathol 1995;103:27–31.
201. Nishimura K, Bieniarz A, Nakamura RM, diZerega GS. Evaluation of oxidized regenerated cellulose for prevention of postoperative intraperitoneal adhesions. Jpn J Surg 1983;13:159–163.
202. Larsson B. Efficacy of Interceed in adhesion prevention in gynecologic surgery: a review of 13 clinical studies. J Reprod Med 1996;41:27–34.
203. diZerega GS. Use of adhesion prevention barriers in ovarian surgery, tubalplasty, ectopic pregnancy, endometriosis, adhesiolysis, and myomectomy. Curr Opin Obstet Gynecol 1996;8:230–237.
204. Schröder M, Willumsen H, Hansen JP, Hansen OH. Peritoneal adhesion formation after the use of oxidized cellulose (Surgicel) and gelatin sponge (Spongostan) in rats. Acta Chir Scand 1982;148:595–596.
205. Raftery AT. Absorbable haemostatic materials and intraperitoneal adhesion formation. Br J Surg 1980;67: 57–58.
206. de Virgilo C, Dubrow T, Sheppard BB, et al. Fibrin glue inhibits intraabdominal adhesion formation. Arch Surg 1990;125:1378–1381.
207. Sheppard BB, de Virgilio C, Bleiweis M, Milliken JC, Robertson JM. Inhibition of intra-abdominal adhesions: fibrin glue in a long term model. Am Surg 1993;59: 786–790.
208. Bilgin T, Cengiz C, Demir U. Postoperative adhesion formation following ovarian reconstruction with fibrin glue in the rabbit. Gynecol Obstet Invest 1995;39:186–187.
209. van der Ham AC, Kort WJ, Weijma IM, van den Ingh HF, Jeekel H. Healing of ischemic colonic anastomosis: fibrin sealant does not improve wound healing. Dis Colon Rectum 1992;35:884–891.
210. Evrard VA, De Bellis A, Boeckx W, Brosens IA. Peritoneal healing after fibrin glue application: a comparative study in a rat model. Hum Reprod (Oxf) 1996;11:1877–1880.
211. Gauwerky JFH, Mann J, Bastert G. The effect of fibrin glue and peritoneal grafts in the prevention of intraperitoneal adhesions. Arch Gynecol Obstet 1990;247: 161–166.
212. Byrne DJ, Hardy J, Wood RA, McIntosh R, Hopwood D, Cuschieri A. Adverse influence of fibrin sealant on the healing of high-risk sutured colonic anastomoses. J R Coll Surg Edinb 1992;37:394–398.
213. van der Ham AC, Kort WJ, Weijma IM, van den Ingh HF, Jeekel J. Effect of fibrin sealant on the healing colonic anastomosis in the rat. Br J Surg 1991;78:49–53.
214. Seifert J, Klause N, Stobbe J, Egbers HJ. Antibodies formed against fibrin glue components and their circulatory relevance. J Invest Surg 1994;7:167–171.
215. Saxen L, Kassinen A, Saxen E. Peritoneal foreign body reaction caused by condom emulsion. Lancet 1963;1:1295–1296.
216. Esposito JM, Zarou DM, Zarou GS. Localized inflammation secondary to intraperitoneal IUCD. J Reprod Med 1972;8:147–150.
217. MacKay DH, Mowat J. Translocation of intrauterine contraceptive devices Lancet 1974;1:652–653.
218. Avni A, David MP, Pauzner D. The peritoneal reaction to the translocated copper intrauterine device in women and female rats. Fertil Steril 1983;39:193–196.
219. Dhall K, Dhall GI, Gupta BB. Uterine perforation with the Lippes loop. Detection by hysterography. Obstet Gynecol 1969;34:266–270.
220. Nohr M. Tubal migration of the Nova-T intrauterine device to the peritoneal cavity. Ugeskr Laeg 1984;146: 1048–1049.
221. Siiteri PK, Febres F, Clemens LE, Chang RJ, Gondos B, Stites D. Progesterone and maintenance of pregnancy: is progesterone nature's immunosuppressant? Ann N Y Acad Sci 1977;286:384–397.
222. Adoni A, Ben Chetrit A. The management of intrauterine devices following uterine perforation. Contraception 1991;43:77–81.
223. Chen KT, Kostich ND, Rosai J. Peritoneal foreign body granulomas to keratin in uterine adenocanthoma. Arch Pathol Lab Med 1978;102:174–177.
224. Williams WD, Amazon K, Rywlin AM. Peritoneal keratin globules in uterine adenosquamous carcinoma. South Med J 1984;77:1316–1318.
225. Wotherspoon AC, Benjamin E, Boutwood AA. Peritoneal keratin granulomas from transtubal spread of endometrial carcinoma with squamous metaplasia (adenoacanthoma). Br J Obstet Gynaecol 1989;96:236–240.
226. Gin H, Dupuy B, Bonnemaison-Bourignon D, et al. Biocompatibility of polyacrylamide microcapsules implanted in peritoneal cavity or spleen of the rat. Effect on various inflammatory reactions in vitro. Biomater Artif Cells Artif Organs 1990;18:25–42.
227. Sawhney AS, Hubbell JA. Poly(ethylene oxide)-graft-poly(L-lysine) copolymers to enhance the biocompatibility of poly(L-lysine)-alginate microcapsule membranes. Biomaterials 1992;13:863–870.
228. De Vos P, De Haan B, Van Schilfgaarde R. Effect of the alginate composition on the biocompatibility of alginate–polylysine microcapsules. Biomaterials 1997;18: 273–278.
229. De Vos P, De Haan BJ, Wolters GH, Strubbe JH, Van Schilfgaarde R. Improved biocompatibility but limited

graft survival after purification of alginate for microencapsulation of pancreatic islets. Diabetologia 1997;40:262–270.
230. Pasquier C, Marty N, Dournes JL, Chabanon G, Pipy B. Implication of neutral polysaccharides associated to alginate in inhibition of murine macrophage response to *Pseudomonas aeruginosa*. FEMS Microbiol Lett 1997;147: 195–202.
231. Petruzzo P, Cappai A, Ruiu G, Dessy E, Rescigno A, Brotzu G. Development of biocompatible barium alginate microcapsules. Transplant Proc 1997;29:2129–2130.
232. Wong H, Chang TM. The microencapsulation of cells within alginate poly-L-lysine microcapsules prepared with the standard single step drop technique: histologically identified membrane imperfections and the associated graft rejection. Biomater Artif Cells Immobilization Biotechnol 1991;19:675–686.
233. Kost J, Goldbart R. Natural and modified polysaccharides. In: Domb AJ, Kost J, Wiseman DM, eds. Handbook of Biodegradable Polymers. Amsterdam: Harwood, 1997: 275–289.
234. Zondervan GJ, Hoppen HJ, Pennings AJ, Fritschy W, Wolters G, van Schilfgaarde R. Design of a polyurethane membrane for the encapsulation of islets of Langerhans. Biomaterials 1992;13:136–144.
235. Iwata H, Takagi T, Amemiya H, et al. Agarose for a bioartificial pancreas. J Biomed Mater Res 1992;26:967–977.
236. Sawhney AS, Pathak CP, Hubbell JA. Interfacial photopolymerization of poly(ethylene glycol)-based hydrogels upon alginate-poly(L-lysine) microcapsules for enhanced biocompatibility. Biomaterials 1993;14: 1008–1016.
237. Christenson L, Aebischer P, McMillan P, Galletti PM. Tissue reaction to intraperitoneal polymer implants: species difference and effects of corticoid and doxorubicin. J Biomed Mater Res 1989;23:705–718.
238. Christenson L, Wahlberg L, Aebischer P. Mast cells and tissue reaction to intraperitoneally implanted polymer capsules. J Biomed Mater Res 1991;25:1119–1131.
239. Nelson JA, Stephen R, Landau ST, Wilson DE, Tyler FH. Intraperitoneal insulin administration produces a positive portal-systemic blood insulin gradient in unanesthetized, unrestrained swine. Metabolism 1982;31:969–972.
240. Renard E, Baldet P, Picot MC, et al. Catheter complications associated with implantable systems for peritoneal insulin delivery. An analysis of frequency, predisposing factors, and obstructing materials. Diabetes Care 1995; 18:300–306.
241. Di Paolo N, Garosi G, Monaci G, Brardi S. Biocompatibility of peritoneal dialysis treatment. Nephrol Dial Transplant 1997;12(suppl 1):78–83.
242. Lewis SL, Norris PJ, Holmes CJ. Phenotypic characterization of monocytes and macrophages from CAPD patients. Trans Am Soc Artif Intern Organs 1990;XXXVI: M575–M577.
243. Davies SJ, Suassuna J, Ogg CS, Cameron JS. Activation of immunocompetent cells in the peritoneum of patients treated with CAPD. Kidney Int 1989;36:661–668.
244. Moughal NA, McGregor SJ, Brock JH, Briggs JD, Junor BJ. Expression of transferrin receptors by monocytes and peritoneal macrophages from renal failure patients treated by continuous ambulatory peritoneal dialysis (CAPD). Eur J Clin Invest 1991;21:592–596.
245. Jorres A, Gahl GM, Ludat K, Frei U, Passlick-Deetjen J. In vitro biocompatibility evaluation of a novel bicarbonate-buffered amino-acid solution for peritoneal dialysis. Nephrol Dial Transplant 1997;12:543–549.
246. Jorres A, Jorres D, Gahl GM, et al. Leukotriene B4 and tumor necrosis factor from leukocytes: effect of peritoneal dialysate. Nephron 1991;58:276–282.
247. Gotloib L, Wajsbrot V, Shostak A, Kushnier R. Experimental approach to peritoneal morphology. Perit Dial Int 1994;14(suppl 3):S6–S11.
248. Dobbie JW, Anderson JD, Hind C. Long-term effects of peritoneal dialysis on peritoneal morphology. Perit Dial Int 1994;14:S16–S20.
249. Dobbie JW. Morphology of the peritoneum in CAPD. Blood Purif 1989;7:74–85.
250. Topley N. In vitro biocompatibility of bicarbonate-based peritoneal dialysis solutions. Perit Dial Int 1997;17:42–47.
251. Brunkhorst R, Mahiout A. Pyruvate neutralizes peritoneal dialysiate cytotoxicity: maintained integrity and proliferation of cultured human mesothelial cells. Kidney Int 1995;48:177–181.
252. de Fijter CW, Verbrugh HA, Oe LP, et al. Biocompatibility of a glucose-polymer-containing peritoneal dialysis fluid. Am J Kidney Dis 1993;21:411–418.
253. Cendoroglo M, Sundaram S, Jaber BL, Pereira BJ. Effect of glucose concentration, osmolality, and sterilization process of peritoneal dialysis fluids on cytokine production by peripheral blood mononuclear cells, and polymorphonuclear cell functions in vitro. Am J Kidney Dis 1998;31:273–282.
254. Dasgupta MK. Silver-coated catheters in peritoneal dialysis. Perit Dial Int 1997;17(Suppl 2):S142–S145.
255. Carozzi S, Nasini MG, Schelotto C, Caviglia PM, Santoni O, Pietrucci A. A biocompatibility study on peritoneal dialysis solution bags for CAPD. Adv Perit Dial 1993;9: 138–142.
256. Rozalska B, Burow A, Ljungh A, Rudnicka W. The influence of long-lasting implantation on the function of phagocytes towards staphylococci. Acta Microbiol Pol 1995;44:243–254.
257. Henson PM. The immunologic release of constituents from neutrophil leukocytes: I. The role of antibody and complement on nonphagocytosable surfaces or phagocytosable particles. J Immunol 1971;107:1535–1546.
258. Mora EM, Cardona MA, Simmons RL. Enteric bacteria and ingested inert particles translocate to intraperitoneal prosthetic materials. Arch Surg 1991;126:157–163.
259. Guo W, Andersson R, Wang X, Bengmark S. Effect of intraperitoneal prosthetic materials on reticuloendothelial function in the rat. J Surg Res 1993;55:80–86.
260. Guo W, Andersson R, Willen R, et al. Bacterial translocation after intraperitoneal implantation of rubber fragments in the splenectomized rat. J Surg Res 1994;57:408–415.
261. Khardori N, Yassien M. Biofilms in device-related infections. J Ind Microbiol 1995;15:141–147.
262. Costerton JW, Irvin RT, Cheng KJ. The bacterial glycocalyx in nature and disease. Annu Rev Microbiol 1981;35: 299–324.
263. Klock JC, Bainton DF. Degranulation and abnormal bactericidal function of granulocytes procured by reversible adhesion to nylon wool. Blood 1976;48:149–161.

264. Rozalska B, Ljungh A, Burow A, Rudnicka W. Biomaterial-associated infection with *Candida albicans* in mice. Microbiol Immunol 1995;39:443–450.
265. Rozalska B, Ljungh A, Paziak-Domanska B, Rudnicka W. Effects of granulocyte-macrophage colony stimulating factor (GM-CSF) on biomaterial-associated staphylococcal infection in mice. Microbiol Immunol 1996;40: 931–939.
266. Wortman RS, Merritt K, Brown SA. The use of the mouse peritoneal cavity for screening for biocompatibility of polymers. Biomater Med Devices Artif Organs 1983;11: 103–114.
267. Keller JC, Marshall GW, Kaminski EJ. An in vivo method for the biological evaluation of metal implants. J Biomed Mater Res 1984;18:829–844.
268. Freyria AM, Chignier E, Guidollet J, Louisot P. Peritoneal macrophage response: an in vivo model for the study of synthetic materials. Biomaterials 1991;12:111–118.
269. van der Meulen J, Verhoeven MC, Koerten HK. Mouse peritoneal cavity; a model compartment for degradation studies. Eur J Morphol 1993;31:9–12.
270. Thomson LA, Law FC, James KH, Matthew CA, Rushton N. Biocompatibility of particulate polymethylmethacrylate bone cements: a comparative study in vitro and in vivo. Biomaterials 1992;13:811–818.
271. Marois Y, Roy R, Vidovszky T, et al. Histopathological and immunological investigations of synthetic fibres and structures used in three prosthetic anterior cruciate ligaments: in vivo study in the rat. Biomaterials 1993;14: 255–262.
272. Marois Y, Roy R, Marois M, et al. T lymphocyte modification with the UTA microporous polyurethane vascular prosthesis: in vivo studies in rats. Clin Invest Med 1992; 15:141–149.
273. Bakker WW, van der Lei B, Nieuwenhuis P, Robinson P, Bartels HL. Reduced thrombogenicity of artificial materials by coating with ADPase. Biomaterials 1991;12: 603–606.
274. Marois Y, Chakfe N, Guidoin R, et al. An albumin-coated polyester arterial graft: in vivo assessment of biocompatibility and healing characteristics. Biomaterials 1996;17: 3–14.
275. Ratner BD. New ideas in biomaterials science—a path to engineered biomaterials. J Biomed Mater Res 1993;27: 837–850.
276. Walton LA. Intraperitoneal chemotherapy in gynecologic malignancies. In: G Deppe, ed. Chemotherapy of Gynecologic Cancer. New York: Liss, 1984:321–330.
277. Topuz E, Aydiner A, Saip P, Bengisu E, Berkman S, Disci R. Intraperitoneal cisplatin-mitoxantrone in ovarian cancer patients with minimal residual disease. Eur J Gynaecol Oncol 1997;18:71–74.
278. Tranberg K-G, Andersson K-E, Bengmark S. Peritoneum and peritoneal cytostatic treatment. In: Bengmark S, ed. The Peritoneum and Peritoneal Access. London: Butterworth, 1989:168–178.
279. Atiq OT, Kelsen DP, Shiu MH, et al. Phase II trial of postoperative adjuvant intraperitoneal cisplatin and fluorouracil and systemic fluorouracil chemotherapy in patients with resected gastric cancer. J Clin Oncol 1993;11: 425–433.
280. Jacquet P, Sugarbaker PH. Effects of postoperative intraperitoneal chemotherapy on peritoneal wound healing and adhesion formation. Cancer Treat Res 1996;82: 327–335.
281. Hopkins MP, Shellhaas C, Clark T, Stakleff KS, Jenison EL. The effect of immediate intraperitoneal carboplatinum on wound healing. Gynecol Oncol 1993;51:210–213.
282. Vlasveld LT, Taal BG, Kroon BB, Gallee MP, Rodenhuis S. Intestinal obstruction due to diffuse peritoneal fibrosis at 2 years after the successful treatment of malignant peritoneal mesothelioma with intraperitoneal mitoxantrone. Cancer Chemother Pharmacol 1992;29:405–408.
283. Tharp M, Hornback NB. Complications associated with intraperitoneal 32P. Gynecol Oncol 1994;53:170–175.
284. Piccart MJ, Speyer JL, Markman M, et al. Intraperitoneal chemotherapy: technical experience at five institutions. Semin Oncol 1985;12:90–96.
285. Kerr DJ, Young AM, Neoptolemos JP, et al. Prolonged intraperitoneal infusion of 5-fluorouracil using a novel carrier solution. Br J Cancer 1996;74:2032–2035.
286. Hagiwara A, Takahashi T, Sawai K, et al. Pharmacological effects of 5-fluorouracil microspheres on peritoneal carcinomatosis in animals. Br J Cancer 1996;74:1392–1396.
287. Hagiwara A, Sakakura C, Shirasu M, et al. Therapeutic effects of 5-fluorouracil microspheres on peritoneal carcinomatosis induced by Colon 26 or B-16 melanoma in mice. Anticancer Drugs 1998;9:287–289.
288. Crosasso P, Brusa P, Dosio F, et al. Antitumoral activity of liposomes and immunoliposomes containing 5-fluorouridine prodrugs. Pharm Sci 1997;86:832–839.
289. Stone MM, Mulvihill SJ, Lewin KJ, Fonkalsrud EW. Long-term total intraperitoneal nutrition in a rabbit model. J Pediatr Surg 1986;21:267–270.
290. Stabile BE, Calabria R. Intraperitoneal nutritional support: initial results in a canine model. J Surg Res 1987; 42:362–368.
291. Stabile BE, Borzatta M. Transperitoneal absorption of glucose and amino acids for nutritional support. Arch Surg 1987;122:344–348.
292. Albert A, Takamatsu H, Fonkalsrud EW. Absorption of glucose solutions from the peritoneal cavity in rabbits. Arch Surg 1984;119:1247–1251.
293. Adkins ES, Salman FT, Fonkalsrud EW. Triglyceride absorption in transperitoneal alimentation. Am J Surg 1990;159:237–240.
294. Klein MD, Coran AG, Drongowski RA, Wesley JR. The quantitative transperitoneal absorption of a fat emulsion: implications for intraperitoneal nutrition. J Pediatr Surg 1983;18:724–731.
295. Mahedero G, Moran JM, Salas J, Blanco M. Absorption of Intralipid and interferences from nutrients infused into the peritoneal cavity of the rat. Am J Surg 1992;164: 45–50.
296. Moran J, Cruz G, Nogue-Rales F, Requena F, Vinagre L, Garcia-Sancho L. Transperitoneal absorption of intralipid in rats: total serum fatty acids and triglyceride after absorption. J Parenter Enteral Nutr (JPEN) 1986;10: 604–608.
297. Garcia-Gamito FJ, Moran JM, Mahedero G, Pimentel JJ, Martinez MC, Vinagre LM. Long term peritoneal nutrition in dogs, both normal and after intestinal resection. Int Surg 1991;76:235–240.

298. Moran JM, Garcia-Gamito FJ, Mahedero G, et al. Peritoneal nutrition in dogs after intestinal resection: comparative study. Nutrition 1989;5:315–320.
299. Bellon JM, Bujan J, Contreras L, Hernando A. Integration of biomaterials implanted into abdominal wall: process of scar formation and macrophage response. Biomaterials 1995;16:381–387.
300. Simmermacher RK, Schakenraad JM, Bleichrodt RP. Reherniation after repair of the abdominal wall with expanded polytetrafluoroethylene. J Am Coll Surg 1994; 178:613–616.
301. van der Lei B, Bleichrodt RP, Simmermacher RRJ. Expanded polytetrafluoroethylene patch for the repair of large abdominal wall defects. Br J Surg 1989;76:803–805.
302. Voyles CR, Richardson JD, Bland KI, Tobin GR, Flint LM, Polk HC Jr. Emergency abdominal wall reconstruction with polypropylene mesh. Short term benefits versus long term complications. Ann Surg 1981;194:219–223.
303. Elliott MP, Juler GL. Comparison of Marlex mesh and microporous teflon sheets when used for hernia repair in the experimental animal. Am J Surg 1979;137:342–344.
304. Bleichrodt RP, Simmermacher RK, van der Lei B, Schakenraad JM. Expanded polytetrafluoroethylene patch versus polypropylene mesh for the repair of contaminated defects of the abdominal wall. Surg Gynecol Obstet 1993;176:18–24.
305. Bellon JM, Contreras LA, Bujan J, Carrea San Martin A. Experimental assay of a Dual Mesh polytetrafluoroethylene prosthesis (non-porous on one side) in the repair of abdominal wall defects. Biomaterials 1996;17:2367–2372.
306. Christoforoni PM, Kim YB, Preys Z, Lay RY, Montz FJ. Adhesion formation after incisional hernia repair: a randomized porcine trial. Am Surg 1996;62:935–938.
307. Bellon JM, Contreras LA, Bujan J, Carrera-San Martin A. The use of biomaterials in the repair of abdominal wall defects: a comparative study between polypropylene meshes (Marlex) and a new polytetrafluoroethylene prosthesis (Dual Mesh). J Biomater Appl 1997;12:121–135.
308. Amid PK, Shulman AG, Lichtenstein IL, Sostrin S, Young J, Hakakha M. Experimental evaluation of a new composite mesh with the selective property of incorporation to the abdominal wall without adhering to the intestines. J Biomed Mater Res 1994;28:373–375.
309. Aliabadi-Wahle S, Choe EU, Jacob-LaBarre J, Flint LM, Ferrara JJ. Evaluation of a novel synthetic material for closure of large abdominal wall defects. Surgery (St. Louis) 1996;119:141–145.
310. Bellon JM, Bujan J, Contreras LA, Jurado F. Use of nonporous polytetrafluoroethylene prosthesis in combination with polypropylene prosthetic abdominal wall implants in prevention of peritoneal adhesions. J Biomed Mater Res 1997;38:197–202.
311. Cnota MA, Aliabadi Wahle S, Choe EU, Jacob JT, Flint LM, Ferrara JJ. Development of a novel synthetic material to close abdominal wall defects. Am Surg 1998;64: 415–418.
312. Alponat A, Lakshminarasappa SR, Yavuz N, Goh PM. Prevention of adhesions by Seprafilm, an absorbable adhesion barrier: an incisional hernia model in rats. Am Surg 1997;63:818–819.
313. Bellon JM, Contreras LA, Bujan J, Palomares D, Carrera-San Martin A. Tissue response to polypropylene meshes used in the repair of abdominal wall defects. Biomaterials 1998;19:669–675.
314. Prevo M, Langston JB, Pharriss BB, Reno FE, Sheldon JJ. Local effects of intrauterine contraceptives placed within the peritoneal cavities of rabbits. J Reprod Med 1980; 24:32–38.
315. Shahani S, Gadgil BA, Devi PK. Tissue reaction to extrauterine copper TCu 200 & TCu 380: An experimental study. Indian J Exp Biol 1975;13:560–561.
316. Soon-Shiong P, Heintz R, Merideth N, Yao Qiang X, Yao Z, Zheng T, Murphy M, Moloney M, Schmehl M, Harris M, Mendez R, Sandford P. Insulin independence in a Type I diabetic patient after encapsulated islet transplantation. Lancet 1994;343(8903):950–951.
317. Devereaux DF, O'Connell SM, Liesch JB, Weinstein M, Robertson FM. Induction of leukocyte activation by mesches surgically implanted in the peritoneal cavity. The American Journal of Surgery 1990;16:243–246.

12

The Peritoneum and Laparoscopy

Douglas E. Ott

CONTENTS

The Peritoneum and Laparoscopy

Gas used to create a laparoscopic pneumoperitoneum is unsterile, cold, and bone dry. The peritoneal cavity is sterile, warm, and wet. The difference between the normal condition of the abdomen and a pneumoperitoneum is the basis of understanding the preventable deleterious effects and hazards posed by the distending gas and its effects on the peritoneal cavity. The currently used laparoscopic gas is unsterile, cold, and dry ("raw" gas). These characteristics expose the peritoneum to rapid temperature changes, rapid evaporation, tissue desiccation and initiate inflammatory activity. Maintaining a normal physiologic homeostatic condition within the peritoneal cavity during laparoscopy is necessary to reduce any damage and the consequences associated with "raw gas" pneumoperitoneum. The stark differences between the normal condition of the abdomen and that created by a pneumoperitoneum are physically apparent, well defined, clinically discernible, and correctable.

Current laparoscopic gas insufflation converts the peritoneal environment from sterile to unsterile, from warm to cold, and from moist to dry. Preserving the normal peritoneal environment is necessary to maintain normal intraabdominal homeostatis and reduce the risks of raw gas. Preconditioning the insufflation gas by filtering, heating, and hydrating changes the gas from one that creates a hostile environment which has negative consequences and alters homeostasis to one that preserves homeostasis. Maintaining the normal intraabdominal physiologic condition minimizes tissue damage and increases patient safety. Modifying the gas to the normal physiologic state before it enters the peritoneal cavity is preferred as a preventative precaution rather than trying to "cure" the problems caused by raw gas after they occur. the benefits from preconditioning laparoscopic gas to a normal physiologic state are preservation of the sterile, warm, moist peritoneal environment. The changes that occur because of raw gas insufflation are well recognized. Correcting these problems is an improvement over the damaging effects to the peritoneum with current gas conditions, improves surgical outcomes, and established a new standard of care during laparoscopy.

Surgical principles require attention to detail, keeping peritoneal tissue surfaces moist, reducing foreign-body contamination, maintaining normal physiologic conditions, gentle tissue handling, meticulous hemostasis, and magnification when appropriate to maximize surgical benefits and reduce peritoneal damage and adhesion formation.[1,2] These principles also apply to laparoscopic surgery. Changes attributed to the raw gas used during insufflation to create a pneumoperitoneum include local tissue and core hypothermia, unrecognized peritoneal damage, postoperative pain, altered immune response, anoxia, damaging effects to the peritoneum and surgical outcome, and prolonged recovery room stay.[3–9]

Changing the quality of the gas from the raw state to the normal condition by filtering, heating, and hydrating reduces these iatrogenic consequences and maintains a more normal physiologic intraabdominal state. Creating and maintaining a normal sterile, warm, moist intraabdominal environment throughout laparoscopy is a necessary and attainable improvement to preserve peritoneal integrity.

Standards for Insufflation Gases

The standards for the gases used during laparoscopy are defined in the United States Phamacopeia (USP) and National Formulary (Table 12.1). These characteristics relate to gas purity and require that the gas have less than 200 parts per million (ppm) of water vapor (0.0002%; "bone dry")[3,10–12] The nonsterile and dry condition of the gas makes it "raw" and harsh compared to the normal intraabdominal environment. To maintain the normal intraabdominal condition, it is important that the gas used to create the pneumoperitoneum be contaminant free, sterile, warm, and wet, which does not occur when raw gas is used. The gas delivery system further compounds the problem by throttling the gas through insufflators at high flow rates that reach 45 miles per hour through narrow or partially occluded delivery ports, causing a "jet stream" and "wind chill" effect on peritoneal surfaces.

Laparoscopic insufflators and the gas cylinders are contaminated with inorganic and organic debris. This foreign material is forced with the gas stream into the sterile peritoneal cavity during insufflation.[3,12] Removal of this foreign material from the gas stream by using a 0.2- to 0.3-µm filter was introduced in 1989.[3] This filtration results in a sufficient level of sterility without affecting insufflation flow rates.

Hypothermia

The current physical state of raw gas contributes to laparoscopic hypothermia.[7] The temperature of the gas as it enters the abdomen is 21°C. Using raw gas causes a minimal loss of 0.3°C per hour for each 60 L of gas consumed.[3] Attempts to prevent laparoscopic gas-induced hypothermia by only heating the gas has little to no effect because the gas remains bone dry and evaporative losses continue with gas insufflation.[8] Heating the gas alone without adding water also does not adequately prevent laparoscopic hypothermia.[4,5] Further, the gas warmed within an insufflator loses more than 80% of its heat before it enters the abdomen. These findings demonstrate that there is more to a proper pneumoperitoneum than just warming the gas; it is necessary to precondition the gas by heating and hydrating with water vapor to have the maximal intraoperative thermal stability. The steady state of high water vapor content in the abdomen from the peritoneal fluid-covered tissue surfaces is severely altered by insufflation of the standard raw dry gas.

TABLE 12.1. Impurity limits for laparoscopic carbon dioxide. The carbon dioxide must contain 200 ppm (0.0002%) or less water vapor, creating a hostile environment for the peritoneum.

CO_2 must be 99% pure	
Carbon monoxide	10.0 ppm
Hydrogen disulfide	1.0 ppm
Nitric oxide	2.5 ppm
Ammonia	25.0 ppm
Sulfur dioxide	5.0 ppm
Water	200.0 ppm
Odor	none

Insufflation with raw CO_2 in experimental studies showed a significant decrease in core temperature;[4] this demonstrated that with warmed gas alone there is more heat expenditure to humidify the dry gas than is used to raise the ambient temperature of the gas to a physiologic temperature. The latent heat to evaporate water is significant and during laparoscopic conditions causes significant heat loss. Comparing cold dry gas to warmed humidified gas shows that the regression lines for cold and warmed gas are indistinguishable and that the temperature loss is caused by the latent heat of vaporization of peritoneal fluid from peritoneal surfaces. The calculated loss is 1.2°C per hour. The clinical hypothermic impact can be profound on prolonged cases. The difference in operative temperature loss using cold dry gas versus warmed humidified gas clinically ranges from 0.6 to 1.2°C per hour.[3–5] With heated hydrated gas there is a significant improvement in heat preservation, with losses of only 0.1° per hour. Therefore, eliminating water loss is the most important factor in preventing laparoscopic hypothermia. Warm wet gas maintains the appropriate environment for tissue surfaces and nullifies the effects of jet cooling and wind chill caused by gas delivery through restricted entry ports.[13,14]

Operative hypothermia requires monitoring, care, and time to correct. Postoperative hypothermia has both metabolic and economic costs,[15] including increased time in the recovery area, use of alternative warming methods, and increased need for analgesic medicines. Clinical hypothermia is defined as a core temperature less than 36°C (96.8°F).[16] The changes resulting from mild and moderate hypothermia (32–35°C) are significant (Table 12.2) Surgery stresses normal body temperature and modified the normal regulatory mechanisms, resulting in an alteration in the balance of heat production and heat loss. The result is a shift of temperature outside the normal physiologic range. The thermoregulatory system attempts to maintain the core temperature in a 0.2°C range to counteract the negative effects of hy-

TABLE 12.2. Definition of clinical ranges of hypothermia.

Temperature (°C)	Degree of hypothermia
35–36	Mild
32–35	Moderate
Less than 32	Severe

pothermia during surgery. Even mild operative hypothermia directly impairs immune function and vasoconstriction (by decreasing partial pressure of oxygen in tissues), induces hypokalemia, impairs myocardial function, depresses respiration, influences nitrogen balance,[17] depletes clotting factors, induces thrombocytopenia,[18] decreases collagen synthesis,[19] impairs chemotaxis and phagocytosis of neutrophils, and decreases the production of antibodies. Mild hypothermia alters drug metabolism and pharmacokinetics and significantly prolongs recovery room time.[20,21] Mild hypothermia is associated with postoperative shivering, substantial adrenergic activation,[22] and patient discomfort.[23] A 1.5°C decrease in core temperature causes a threefold increase in ventricular tachycardia,[24] increases postoperative ventilation and oxygen consumption, and changes peripheral vascular tone. These changes are all seen at laparoscopy because of hypothermia resulting from cold dry gas and are prevented or corrected by using heated hydrated gas.

The normal thermal steady state is one in which heat loss is equal to metabolic heat production. This distribution is not uniform during surgery. Thermoregulatory mechanisms try to keep the core temperature nearly constant, while the periphery is simultaneously at a lower temperature because of tonic vasoconstriction.[25] The evaporative cooling effects caused by the dry laparoscopic gas and gas flow alter the normal intraabdominal conditions and decrease the heat available for redistribution, upsetting the body's normal balance of heat retention and heat loss. The heat normally sequestered in the abdomen is lost because of evaporation of water from peritoneal surfaces and the resultant chilling effect.

Gas that now contains heat and water evaporated from tissue surfaces is removed and replaced with cold dry gas that further contributes to thermal instability. Postoperatively, the normal core heat sink is unavailable for thermoregulation and redistribution and leads to a cool periphery and a cool core, further compounding the hypothermic effect. Using laparoscopic gas containing water vapor allows maintenance of the normal heat sink and reduces or prevents laparoscopic-induced hypothermia. Rewarming the core using a surface convection warming device is an inefficient method to maintain global euthermia for laparoscopic-induced hypothermia and offers no protection to the peritoneum from the effects of desiccation. Directly reducing intraabdominal thermal losses by heating and hydrating the gas is more efficient and maintains the integrity of the peritoneum.

The results of tests that model the effects of evaporative jet cooling from peritoneal tissues surfaces at laparoscopy demonstrate the comparison between dry and wet gas.[13] The fluid dynamics of the gas delivered through constricted laparoscopic entry ports on the wet peritoneal tissue surfaces lead to surface evaporation and severe tissue temperature changes. Peritoneal damage occurs not only at the sight of surgical injury that is the area of surgical focus but also in areas where gas flow is directed, as occurs through entry needles and ports at any time the abdomen is initiating or maintaining a pneumoperitoneum. This directed gas flow is a jet stream and causes rapid, dramatic lowering of tissue temperature and surface desiccation.

Figure 12.1 shows the temperature effect using different flow rates through different-sized ports. The surface temperature drop that occurs is relatively independent of the type or size of gas port through which the gas is delivered. A 5-L flow rate of raw gas causes a surface temperature drop of 20°C within 5 seconds for tissue areas up to 2 cm^2 (Figure 12.2). Using preheated humidified gas causes no local surface cooling. Thermal losses caused by directed raw gas flow can cause local tissue abnormalities and contribute to postoperative ileus.

Peritoneal Drying

Histologic evaluation of peritoneum exposure to directed gas flows from laparoscopic surgical conditions shows that using the current raw dry gas causes cells to be lost from the peritoneal surface with disruption of attachments at the periphery. These denuded sites extend to 2 cm in diameter depending on gas flow rate, gas entry distance from the tissue surface, and diameter of the gas stream. Dry gases cause immediate (in less than 2 seconds) surface drying with 0.5 L/min flow rate through a Verres needle at any distance from 1 to 5 cm. Even with a 1 L/min flow rate through a 10-mm empty port, peritoneum is lost up to a 2 cm in diameter in less than 10 seconds at a 5-cm distance. When moist (95% water vapor) gas is used, no peritoneum is lost, even with high flow rates at close gas tissue approximations through restricted ports.

Latent heat of vaporization causes heat loss and tissue damage. The rapid evaporation of surface fluids causes significant heat loss, decreased tissue temperatures, tissue desiccation, and damage and loss of peritoneal cells with exposure to underlying connective tissue. The degree of cooling, tissue temperature, and amount of cellular damage are directly related to the amount of gas used, flow rate, and size of the gas delivery orifice. Even with large gas entry ports the stark difference between moist tissue surfaces and the dry gas over exposed peritoneal surface causes significant evaporative losses and

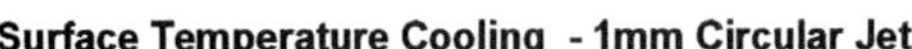

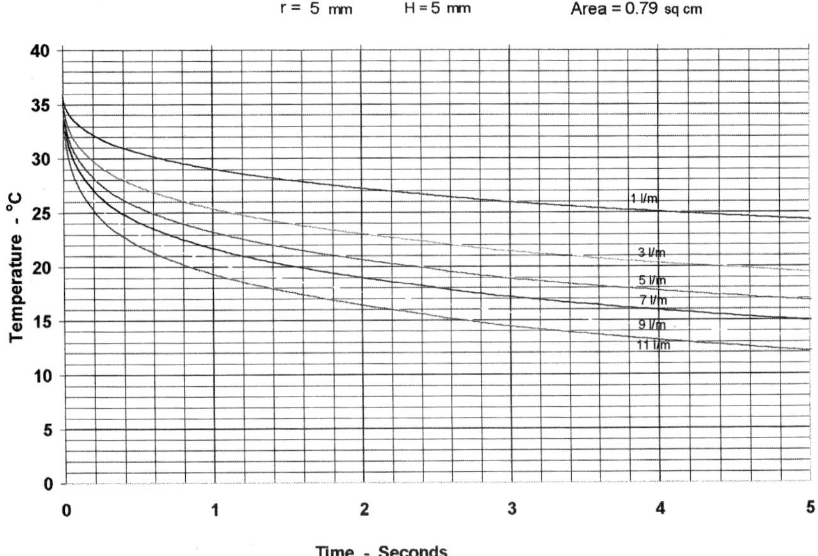

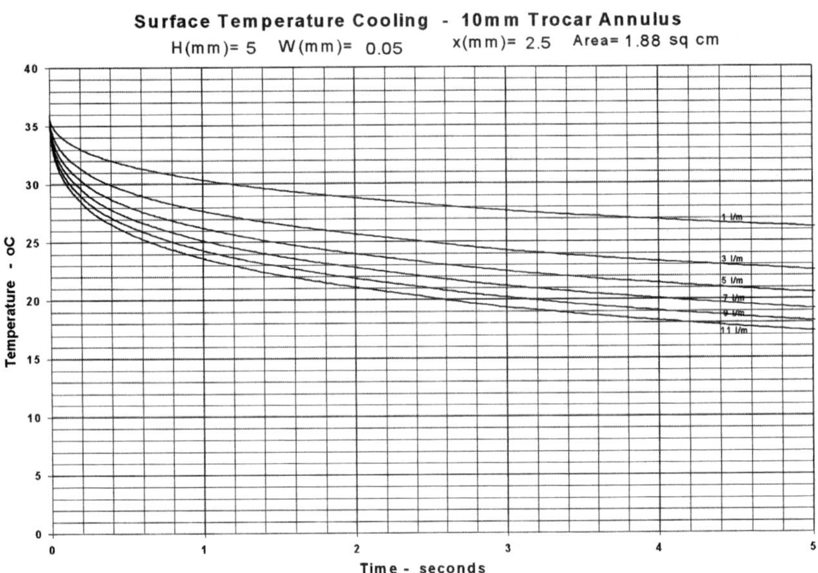

FIG. 12.1. Surface temperature cooling effects for a 1-mm circular and a 0.05-mm annular slot at a 5-mm distance from the tissue surface at various flow rates. A drop to 14°C within 4 seconds is found for a 2-cm^2 diameter.

tissue drying. The distance of the directed gas stream from tissue, the effective diameter of the gas delivery site, and volume of gas delivered to the abdomen determine the amount of evaporative effects. The longer the procedure or the larger the volume of gas used, the greater the consequences. The constant evaporative effect caused by the attempt to equilibrate water vapor in the closed abdomen stresses the peritoneal cells, causing cell shrinkage, breakage, and desmosome detachment in addition to loss of peritoneal continuity and integrity, resulting in profuse prostaglandin release. This effect reduces the number of areas for coaptation and possibly de novo adhesion formation.

The adverse effects of peritoneal drying at laparotomy are well known. Peritoneal drying induced during laparoscopy is no less important but has received little attention. Peritoneal exposure to raw gas causes significant tissue drying and damage, hypothermia, prostaglandin release that alters intraabdominal physiologic homeostasis, and many be a factor in de novo adhesion formation. The peritoneal fluid and its water content keep tissue surfaces moist, maintain tissue integrity and cellular hydrostatic pressure, and preserve peritoneal homeostasis. The integrity of the peritoneum and peritoneal fluid is important to provide an uninterrupted, smooth, nonadhering lubricated surface that minimizes the friction of visceral movements, maintains normal physiologic moist tissue conditions, and reduces the potential of adhesion formation. Peritoneal fluid viscosity is altered by evaporation caused by the dry gas. The normal proteinaceous peritoneal fluid transudate forms a reactive coagulum and with precipitates, which increases drag and friction impeding the normal peritoneum over peritoneum movement. The result is increased contact time for

FIG. 12.2. **A.** Temperature transients for tissue at various flow rates caused by a 1-mm circular gas jet and a 0.05-mm annular clot 10-mm length. **B.** Elimination of tissue temperature loss at laparoscopy by heating and hydrating the gas.

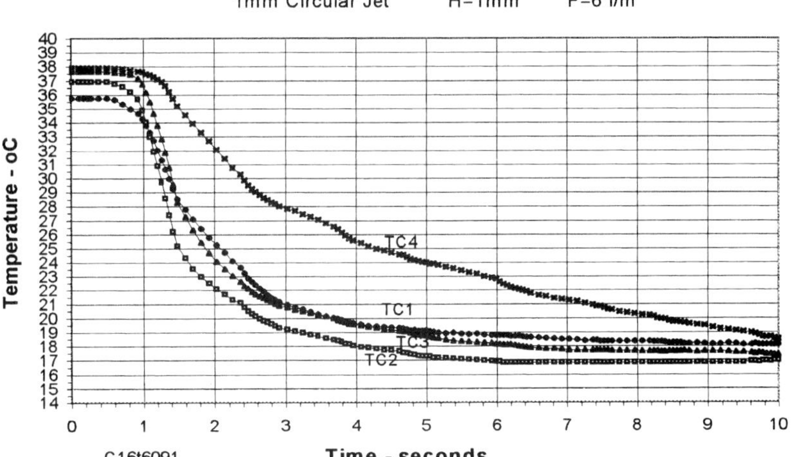

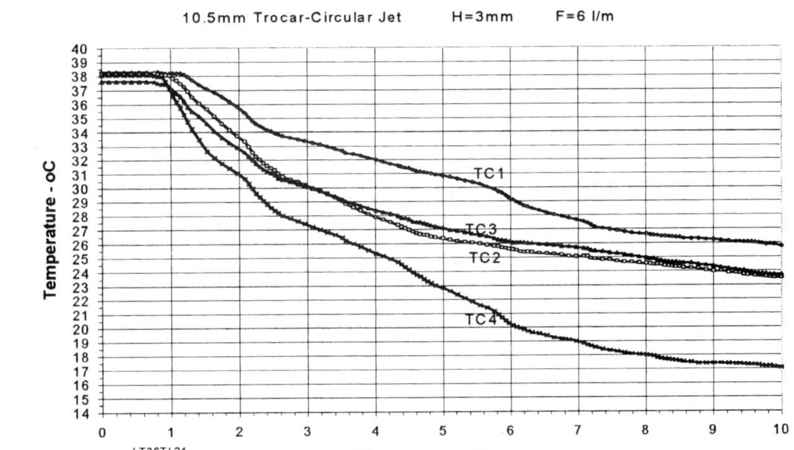

A

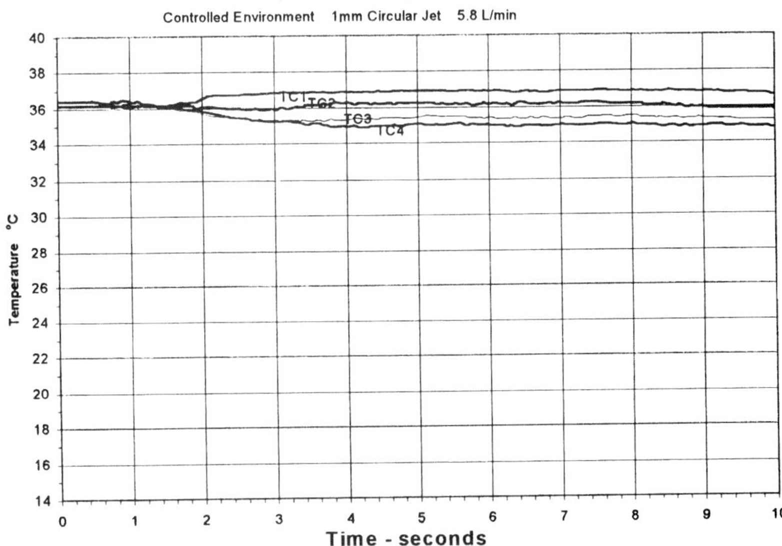

B

chemical reactions, exchange of vasoactive and chemotactic factors, and increased macrophage activity. Macrophage movement is impaired by the increase in viscosity of peritoneal fluid and altered peritoneal physiologic dynamics. There is also delay in normal peritoneal fluid transudate formation and macrophage replenishment while the process of adhesion formation or fibrinolytic activity is taking place.

Evidence shows that two of the major components and prerequisites of adhesion formation are tissue drying and peritoneal damage. Both these predisposing conditions occur during insufflation of raw gas into the abdomen during laparoscopy and do not occur when the gas contains a sufficient quantity of water vapor. Immediately after drying, normal peritoneal architecture is severely disrupted at laparotomy;[26] this also occurs at laparoscopy and is directly attributable to peritoneal exposure to raw gas dryness. The evaporative effects cause loss of peritoneal cells, tissue drying, loss of integrity, cellular compromise, and exposure of the underlying loose areolar peritoneal matrix, setting in motion release of chemically active substances that contribute to pain, the inflammatory process, and adhesion formation. Tissue desiccation, damaged peritoneum, and release of chemically active kinins and prostaglandins increase the susceptibility to adhesion formation when apposing defects are present and probably contribute to de novo adhesion formation. Preconditioning the gas to the normal moist condition reproduces the intraabdominal environment, maintains and sustains the normal environment, and reduces the hazards and risks attributable to the raw gas.

Hydrating the gas from the bone-dry condition to 95% relative humidity maintains the normal peritoneum–peritoneal fluid relationship and the normal moist tissue–gas vapor pressure relationship that are critical for peritoneal cell integrity. A proper amount of water vapor also maintains the normal cellular hydrostatic pressure and proper peritoneal fluid viscosity on tissue surfaces. Changes in peritoneal fluid viscosity and in the concentration of its components can affect tissue healing.

Perspective

Total laparoscopic gas consumption is influenced by creation of the initial pneumoperitoneum, incision leaks around trocar sites, instrument exchanges through trocars, smoke and fluid evacuation, and maintenance of abdominal distension. The gas instillation process repetitively and progressively dries the tissue surfaces by the intermittent throttling of dry gas instillation, causing rapid surface evaporation from the peritoneal fluid covering the abdominal surfaces and then from the cells themselves. The severity of the drying effect is directly related to water content of the gas, total amount of gas consumed, length of the procedure, gas flow rate, effective diameter of the gas entrance port, distance of the delivery port from the tissue surface, amount and direction of irrigation, and frequency of gas evacuation.

Clinical studies show dramatic and statistically significant improvements in reduction of hypothermia, decreased need for postoperative analgesia, shortened time to return to full function, and economic benefits from heating and hydrating laparoscopic gas compared to cold dry raw gas. These prospective, randomized, controlled studies compared outcome parameters assessing single and combined variables. Preconditioned laparoscopic gas is well tolerated with no adverse effects. The safety profile of the preconditioned gas has significant benefits compared to currently used raw gas. The improvements gained by preconditioning the gas are efficacious, maintain the integrity of the normal intraabdominal condition, and reduce peritoneal desiccation and damage allowing the patient to return to normal function quickly and with decrease postoperative pain.[9,14] A significant difference in postoperative pain was found between raw and heated hydrated gas. Pain intensity was directly related to gas volume used and length of surgery in both groups, but was significantly reduced in the heated hydrated group at all time parameters compared to the standard raw gas group regardless of volume of gas consumed or length of surgery.[8,9,27]

The conclusions of these studies are that warmed hydrated gas protects the physical and chemical integrity of the peritoneum, leads to significant reduction of pain, reduces postoperative pain, and reduces postoperative recovery time.[8,9] Temperature-sensitive transmitters may be affected by acute local thermal changes and account for loss of the integrity of temperature regulation and pain sensation. It is suspected that the decrease in peritoneal damage using the hydrated gas decreases prostaglandin release and is probably the reason there is less pain.

Conclusion

Laparoscopic gas insufflation affects the peritoneum. To minimize the harmful effects of the raw unconditioned gas, filtered, heated, and hydrated gas must be used for laparoscopy. The damaging effects and consequences of the currently used raw bone-dry gas are preventable and confirmed by clinical studies. The comparison of unconditioned gas versus heated hydrated gas shows that maintaining normal peritoneal homeostasis is important. Insufflating cold dry gas into the contaminant-free, warm, moist peritoneal cavity is undesirable, unnatural, and detrimental to tissue, surgical outcome, and economic consequences. Insufflation of heated gas containing water vapor during laparoscopy maintains the normal intraabdominal condition and allows maximal peritoneal preservation. Changing the physical nature of the gas by filtering, heating, and hydrating improves gas safety profile, prevents peritoneal damage, improves surgical outcome, and preserves peritoneal integrity compared to the raw gas currently used. Preventing deleterious iatrogenic peritoneal effects before they occur by preconditioning the gas with heat and water vapor is advocated,[4,5] and is a practical technologic cost effective reality.[14,28]

References

1. Diamond MP. Adhesion prevention. In: Gershenson DM, DeCherney AH, Curry SL, eds. Operative Gynecology. Philadelphia: Saunders, 1993:147–158.
2. diZerega GS. The peritoneum and its response to surgical injury. In: diZerga GS, Malinak LR, Diamond MP, Linsky CB, eds. Treatment of Post Surgical Adhesions. New York: Wiley-Liss, 1990.
3. Ott DE. Contamination via gynecologic endoscopy insufflation. J Gynecol Surg. 1989;5:205–208.
4. Bessell JR, Karatassas A. Patterson JR, Jamieson GG, Maddern GJ. Hypothermia induced by laparoscopic insufflation. Surg Endosc 1995;9:791–796.
5. Bessell JR, Maddern GJ. Influence of gas temperature during laparoscopic procedures. In: Rosenthal RJ, Friedman RL, Phillips EH, eds. The Pathophysiology of Pneumoperitoneum. Berlin: Springer, 1998.
6. Ott DE. Correction of laparoscopic insufflation hypothermia. J Laparoendosc Surg 1991:1:183–186.
7. Ott DE. Laparoscopic hypothermia. J. Laparoendosc Surg 1991;1:127–131.
8. Korell M, Schmaus F, Strowitzki T, Schneeweiss SG, Hepp H. Pain intensity following laparoscopy. Surg Laparosc Endosc 1996;6:375–379.
9. Mouton WG, Bessell JR, Millard SH, Maddern GL. A randomized controlled trial assessing the benefit of humidified insufflation gas during laparoscopic surgery. Abstract, World Congress Endoscopy, Rome. Endosc Surg (in press).
10. United States Pharmacopeia and National Formulary and Supplements, Vol. XXI-NF. Washington, DC: U.S. Government Printing Office, 1984.
11. Ott DE. Microbial colonization of laparoscopic gas delivery systems: a quantitative analysis. Journal of the Society of Laparoendoscopic Surgeons 1997;1:325–329.
12. Couper GW, Ewen SW, Krukowski ZH. Risk of contamination from laparoscopic carbon dioxide insufflators. J R Coll Surg Edinb 1997;42:231–232.
13. Gray RI, Henderson AC, Ott DE. Severe local hypothermia from laparoscopic gas: evaporative jet cooling. Ann Biomed Eng 1997;25(suppl 1):Abstr 28.
14. Ott DE, Reich H, Liu CY. Reduction of laparoscopic induced hypothermia, post-operative pain and recovery room length of stay by pre-conditioning gas with the Insuflow* device: a prospective randomized controlled multicenter study. Journal of the Society of Laproendoscopic Surgeons 1998;2:321–329.
15. Conahan TJ. Heating reduces recovery time (cost) in outpatients. Anesthesiology 1982;67:128–130.
16. Morris RH, Kumar A. The effect of warming blankets on maintenance of body temperature of the anesthetized, paralyzed adult patient. Anesthesiology 1970;36:408–411.
17. Carli F. Emery PW, Freemantle CAJ. Effect of perioperative normothermia on postoperative protein metabolism. Br J. Anaesth 1989;63:276–282.
18. Michelson AD, MacGregor H, Barnard MR, Kestin AS, Roher MJ, Valeri CR. Reversible inhibition of human platelet activation by hypothermia in vivo and in vitro. Throm Haemostasis 1994;71:633–640.
19. Kurz A. Sessler DI, Lenhardt R. Perioperative normothermia to reduce the incidence of surgical-wound infection and shorten hospitalization. N Engl J Med 1996;334: 1209–1215.
20. Lenhardt R. Kurz A, Sessler DI, Marker E, Narzt E, Lackner F. Intraoperative hypothermia prolongs duration of postoperative recovery. Anesthesiology 1995;83(Suppl A): 1114(abstract).
21. Lenhardt R. Marker E, Goll V, et al. Mild intraoperative hypothermia prolongs postanesthetic recovery. Anesthesiology 1997;87:1318–1323.
22. Frank SM, Higgins MS, Breslow NJ, et al. The catecholamine, cortisol and hemodynamic responses to mild perioperative hypothermia: a randomized clinical trial. Anesthesiology 1995;82:83–93.
23. Kurz A, Sessler DI, Nartz E, et al. Postoperative hemodynamic and thermoregulatory consequences of intraoperative core hypothermia. J Clin Anesthiol 1995; 7359–7366.
24. Frank SM, Fleisher LA, Breslow NJ, et al. Perioperative maintenance of normothermia reduces the incidence of morbid cardiac events; a randomized clinical trial. JAMA 1997;227:1127–1134.
25. Sessler DI. Perianesthetic thermoregulation and heat balance in humans. FASEB J 1993;7:638–644.
26. Ryan GB, Groberty J, Majno G. Mesothelial injury and repair. Am J Pathol 1973;71:93–112.
27. Semm K. Arp WD, Trappe M, Kube D. Pain reduction after pelvilaparoscopic interventions by insufflation of CO_2 gas at body temperature. Geburtsh Frauenheilkd 1994; 4:300–304.
28. Gray RI, Ott DE, Henderson SA, Cochran EA, Roth EA. Severe local hypothermia from laparoscopic gas evaporative jet cooling: a possible mechanism to explain widespread clinical observations. J Soc Laparoendoscopic Surg (in press).

13

Adhesions: Laparoscopy Versus Laparotomy

Jean-Luc Pouly and Sonteara Seak-San

CONTENTS

It has long been agreed that laparoscopic procedures induce fewer adhesions than laparotomy, but this often-heard and well-accepted affirmation is not as simple and definite as it seemed at first glance. The problem stems from the considerable lack of human data about this precise subject.

First, to avoid any confusion in terms, we employ and define here three types of situations often encountered:

Adhesion formation is the occurrence of adhesion at an operated site that did not involve any adhesion before the surgical procedure.
Adhesion reformation is the recurrence of adhesion at an operated site; it is treated by adhesiolysis by laparotomy or laparoscopy.
De novo adhesion formation is the occurrence of adhesion at a nonoperated site that had no adhesion before the surgical procedure.

In this chapter, we review animal experimental data and the available human data, and then discuss different points of view that may explain the difference between laparoscopy and laparotomy.

Animal Data

Luciano et al.[1] tested the hypothesis that intraperitoneal adhesion formation and reduction after laser surgery were the same whether the surgery is performed by laparoscopy or laparotomy. Twenty rabbits were randomly assigned to either laparoscopy or laparotomy and subjected to standardized laser incisions over one uterine horn and over the peritoneal surface of either lower quadrant. Three weeks later, 5 animals from each group underwent laparoscopy and the other 5 were submitted to laparotomy to score the extent of postoperative adhesions formed and to carry out laser adhesiolysis. The same power density was delivered to tissues in both procedures. Three weeks after the second operative intervention, the animals were killed and the intraperitoneal adhesions blindly scored. After the initial procedure, adhesions were absent in the laparoscopy group, but in the laparotomy group, adhesions were frequently present, not only at the operative sites of the peritoneal surfaces and uterine horn but also on the bowel, bladder, and opposite uterine horn where no apparent injury had been inflicted ($p < 0.005$). Three weeks after adhesiolysis, a significant reduction was observed in the mean adhesion scores in the laparoscopy group but not in the laparotomy group. The first part of this study suggested that laparoscopy avoids both adhesion formation and de novo adhesion formation, and the second part suggested that laparoscopy reduces the risk of adhesion reformation.

Marana et al.[2] also studied this problem in a rabbit model. The purpose was to compare postoperative adhesion formation and reproductive outcome after the same ovarian surgical procedure performed by laparoscopy or laparotomy by means of microsurgical techniques. For the study, 28 female rabbits were randomly assigned to laparotomy or laparoscopy for the same standardized surgical procedure: both ovaries were grasped with a traumatic forceps and longitudinally incised on the antimesenteric side from the cortex to the hilum with a microelectrode delivering a tissue power density of 66,666.00 W/cm^2. The rabbits were then mated, and 2 weeks later a second-look laparotomy was performed by a blinded observer for the evaluation of postoperative adhesions, number of corpora lutea in each ovary, number of embryos in the ipsilateral uterine horn, and nidation index for each side. At second look, no statistically significant differences were found in postoperative adhesion formation, number of corpora lutea, number of embryos, or nidation index between the laparoscopy and the laparotomy groups. The conclusion of this study is totally different from the previous one: laparoscopy or laparotomy for ovarian conservative surgery do not appear significantly different in adhesion formation and de novo adhesion formation. There were, however, three crucial differences compared to the previous study. The comparison was between laparoscopy and microsurgery by laparotomy, and of electrosurgery versus laser surgery; also, the operated area was the ovary instead of the uterine horn or the peritoneum.

Filmar et al.[3] compared the occurrence of adhesions after a standard uterine injury inflicted by laparoscopy or laparotomy during which microsurgical principles were observed. The cross-sectional areas of adhesions involving the uterus were assessed, and the 31 rats operated upon laparoscopically were compared with the 30 rats subjected to a laparotomy. The mean area of uterine adhesions formed was 4.29 mm^2 in the laparotomy group and 8.88 mm^2 in the laparoscopy group. The difference was not statistically significant. Again, these results imply that a standard electrical tissue injury to uterine tissue, whether conducted by laparoscopy or via laparotomy, carries the same potential to induce adhesion formation (de novo).

The comparison in these three studies suggests that the differences in the Luciano study at least partially result from laser use. The study by Schemmel et al.,[4] however, adds to the confusion. They used a rabbit model to perform ovarian wedge resection and removal of the distal uterine horn by laparotomy using three different surgical technologies: ultrasonic scalpel, CO_2 laser, and electrosurgery. When hemostatic properties, coagulation necrosis, and adhesion formation were assessed, no differences among the different systems used were found.

Chen et al.[5] and Fowler et al.[6] in two successive studies tried to determine whether there was a difference in adhesion formation after pelvic and paraaortic lymphadenectomy with transperitoneal laparoscopy, compared with both extraperitoneal laparotomy and transperitoneal laparotomy, in a porcine model. Ninety female hogs underwent pelvic and paraaortic lymphadenectomy: 40 with transperitoneal laparoscopy, 40 with extraperitoneal laparotomy, and 10 with transperitoneal laparotomy. Three weeks after the initial surgery, a laparotomy was performed to assess adhesion formation. The transperitoneal laparotomy group had significantly higher adhesion formation, with a 100% (10 of 10) adhesion rate. In the transperitoneal laparoscopy group, 12 of 40 hogs (30%) developed adhesions versus 8 of 38 (21%) in the extraperitoneal laparotomy group (p = not significant). Also, no differences were found in the transperitoneal laparoscopy and extraperitoneal laparotomy groups when comparing adhesion thickness or the total surface area of adhesions, but more anterior abdominal wall adhesions were noted in the extraperitoneal laparotomy group (5 of 38) than in the transperitoneal laparoscopy group (0 of 40; $p = 0.02$). These studies confirm that the crucial point during a laparotomy is the opening of the peritoneal cavity. The difference in adhesion location that was found between laparoscopy and extraperitoneal laparotomy, however, is more difficult to explain. One can imagine that extraperitoneal laparotomy induces more trauma, more dryness, and more devascularization, which ultimately cause adhesions to the anterior abdominal wall of the peritoneum, which is less injured during a laparoscopy.

The conclusions drawn from the animal model experiments remain unclear after this analysis, but no one study was in favor of laparotomy compared to laparoscopy. The subjective impression is that the potential benefits of laparoscopy are mainly a very low rate of de novo adhesion formation.

Human Data

To our knowledge, no prospective randomized studies are available in human except that by Lundorff et al.[7] Among 105 patients with ectopic tubal pregnancy who were randomized to surgery by laparoscopy or laparotomy, 73 patients with a strong desire for pregnancy underwent a second-look laparoscopy to evaluate adhesion formation and tubal status. Adhesion status at the ipsilateral and contralateral side at primary surgery was compared with status at second-look laparoscopy. Adhesions were found in 58% of patients who were adhesion free at the initial laparoscopy after second-look laparoscopy and in 79% after laparotomy. Among the patients who were found to have adhesions during the first procedure, the adhesion status was slightly impaired after laparoscopy, and adhesions developed dramatically after laparotomy, on the ipsilateral tube as well as on the contralateral side. All these differences were statistically significant. The group of patients submitted to adhesiolysis during the first procedure was too small to provide any significant data. From this study one can conclude that laparoscopic surgery induces less de novo adhesion formation and accompanies a reduction in the risk of adhesion formation.

Although the other human studies are less clear, they provide some additional data. Bulletti et al.,[8] in a case-control study, have compared adhesion formation after myomectomy performed by laparoscopy or by open surgery in 28 patients. All were submitted to a second-look laparoscopy. In comparison with laparotomy, laparoscopy resulted in adhesion formation in significantly fewer patients, and in significantly lower scores when adhesions were detected. This study demonstrated that adhesion formation is reduced with laparoscopy, as well as do novo adhesion formation, which was rare.

Levrant et al.[9] determined the frequency of postoperative adhesions to the anterior abdominal wall in a prospective cohort study of 215 women, 124 with prior abdominal surgery (45 laparoscopy, 29 midline vertical incision, 39 suprapubic transverse incision) and 91 with no prior surgery. No anterior abdominal wall adhesions occurred in 91 patients with no previous surgery or in 45 patients with previous laparoscopy (12 had more than 1 laparoscopy; $p < 0.001$ vs. laparotomy). Of 29 patients with a midline vertical incision, 17 (59%) had anterior wall adhesions ($p < 0.05$ vs. suprapubic transverse incision) and 11 (28%) of 39 with a suprapubic transverse incision also had anterior wall adhesions ($p < 0.001$ vs. no surgery or laparoscopy); 96% of adhesions involved omentum and 29% included bowel. This study clearly demonstrated that omentum or bowel abdominal wall adhesions are very infrequent after laparoscopy by comparison with laparotomy. It also appears that the kind of abdominal wall incision leads to differences in adhesion frequency.

The final interpretation of this study is unclear on one crucial point, however: should these adherences be considered as de novo adhesion formation or as adhesion formation? Moreover, no data were available regarding peritoneal closure during the first operation. This point was not trivial, according to McNally and Curtain,[10] who studied postoperative adhesion formation in a series of 100 patients who had previous cesarean section with or without peritoneum closure. Adhesions were present in 28% of the closed peritoneum group versus 14% in the open peritoneum group cases. Supporting these data, it is possible that some of the differences found in the Levrant study[9] result from suturing the peritoneum rather than the basic difference between laparotomy and laparoscopy.

Some indirect conclusions may be drawn. For instance, Diamond et al.[11] noted adhesions in at least one new location at second-look laparoscopy after microsurgical procedures by laparotomy, among 82 of 161 women (51%). Among 121 women with adhesions at the initial operative procedure, the rate and type of recurrence assessed on the ovaries, fimbriae, and other sites were independent of the initial adhesion type. Additionally, neither the rate nor the type of adhesion recurrence observed at the time of second-look laparotomy was determined by the variable amount of time between the initial and the second-look operative procedures. They concluded that reproductive pelvic surgical procedures are frequently complicated not only by adhesion reformation but by de novo adhesion formation as well.

In a second paper, Diamond et al.[12] reported adhesion reformation and de novo formation after laparoscopic infertility surgery among 68 patients. The frequency and severity of adhesion reformation and de novo adhesion formation after operative laparoscopy were assessed during an early second-look procedure after an initial operative laparoscopy; in all 68 subjects the operative laparoscopic procedure included adhesiolysis. The second operative procedure was performed within 90 days. The total mean adhesion score decreased from 11.4 ± 0.7 at the initial operative procedure to 5.5 ± 0.4 at the second-look procedure, with a decrease of 52% in adhesion rate. At the time of the second-look procedure, 66 of 68 women (97.1%) had pelvic adhesions. Adhesion reformation occurred in 66 of 68 women and at 230 of 351 sites (66%) at which adhesions were lysed. Despite this high incidence of adhesion reformation, de novo adhesion formation after operative laparoscopy occurred in only 8 of 68 women (12%) and at 11 of 47 available sites in these 8 women. The main conclusion is that adhesion reformation is quite as frequent after operative laparoscopy as after microsurgery by laparotomy, but that de novo adhesion formation appears to occur much less frequently after laparoscopic surgery.

Roushdy et al.[13] evaluated the rate of de novo adhesion formation, adhesion formation, and reformation after different laparoscopic procedures such as ovarian cystectomy, ovarian drilling, salpingostomy for ectopic pregnancy, endometriosis, myomectomy, and adhesiolysis. Eighteen patients had no initial adhesions and at second-look laparoscopy, the adhesion score was 1.6 ± 2.2; the other 29 patients had an initial score of 3.2 ± 0.7.

The higher the initial adhesion score found at the primary procedure, the more likely the adhesion recurrence. Of 29 patients who underwent adhesiolysis, 26 either improved or became totally free of adhesions. Thick and extensive adhesions are less likely to give a favorable result after adhesiolysis. The conclusion is that by laparoscopic surgery, de novo adhesion formation is infrequent, that adhesion formation is not important, but that adhesion reformation is frequent and depends on the initial extent.

Jansen[14] published an interesting but very complex paper. He performed a second-look laparoscopy 12 days after 256 consecutive operations for infertility to make an early diagnosis and treatment of postoperative adhesions. He noted that, despite scrupulous microsurgical techniques, complete absence of adnexal adherences was present in only 31 of 73 (42.5%) patients without initial adhesions and in 15 of 183 (8.2%) patients who had previous adhesions lysed. New or reformed adhesions usually were easily separable, often without bleeding, and often with much apparent improvement in fimbrio-ovarian anatomy. Unfortunately, no quantification of the adhesion was made in this first part of the study. In a second part, 38 of the patients were submitted to a third-look laparoscopy and adhesions were then quantified using a modified 1979 American Fertility Society (AFS) endometriosis scoring system. Adhesions were worse as the result of the laparoscopic procedure in 0 patients, unchanged in 5 patients, and improved in 33 patients; overall, there was a significant reduction in median adhesion scores from 8 at laparoscopy (95% confidence limits of median, 6–10) to 2 at final observation (95% limits, 0–4; $p < 0.001$). This study suggests that adhesion formation occurs in half or more patients treated by microsurgical technique and laparotomy and that adhesion reformation occurs in 90% of cases. In opposition, it seems that laparoscopic surgery does not induce a very large amount of adhesion reformation and that de novo adhesion formation is extremely infrequent. It is evident however that these conclusions are putative according to the nonexperimental, nonprospective, and noncomparative nature of this study.

Nezhat et al.[15] studied the postoperative adhesion in two groups of patients submitted to an initial videolaseroscopy for the treatment of endometriosis-associated infertility. The first group consisted of 135 patients who underwent second-look laparoscopy for persistent infertility or recurrence of pelvic pain. The second group consisted of 22 patients who achieved pregnancy after initial surgery and underwent second-look laparoscopy for evaluation of ectopic pregnancy or in association with uterine evacuation for first-trimester spontaneous abortion. In both groups of patients, they found a significant reduction in adhesion scores involving the ovaries, tubes, posterior cul-de-sac, anterior cul-de-sac, and omentum/bowel. He concluded that videolaseroscopy is effective in reducing adhesion formation (by comparison with his experience in microsurgery), is associated with a low frequency of adhesion reformation, and appears to completely avert de novo adhesion formation. Moreover, the comparison between the two groups clearly demonstrated that adhesions were more frequent in the first group than in the second one and that adhesion formation or reformation is one of the main causes of failure in infertility surgery for endometriosis.

From all these human studies, no definitive conclusion can be drawn, but all suggest that de novo adhesion formation is rare after laparoscopy as compared with laparotomy. For adhesion formation, some improvements seem to exist. In contrast, adhesion reformation does not appear to be significantly reduced by laparoscopic surgery.

Clinical Perspective

Before going any further at this level of our analysis, we have to concern ourselves with some remaining controversies. The most important question is to really appreciate the main differences in tissue effects between laparoscopy and laparotomy. Laparoscopy avoids physical and chemical contact between peritoneum and serosa with atmospheric gases; it avoids peritoneal dryness and is not accompanied by setting surgical tissue into the pelvic cavity to move the viscera away from the surgical field, which unfortunately creates a microtrauma. Moreover, the laparoscopic surgical technique is by itself completely different from laparotomy, and we wonder if this makes any difference. Finally, different anatomic and surgical sites are involved in adhesion formation.

Chemical and Physical Differences Between Laparoscopy and Laparotomy

Portz et al.[16] demonstrated, in a laparotomy rabbit model, that the combined instillation of superoxide dismutase and catalase significantly reduced the formation of intraperitoneal adhesions at endometriosis sites. These two drugs have the potential to block the toxic effects of superoxide anion (O_2) and hydrogen peroxide (H_2O_2), which are associated with the production of endometriosis and inflammation.

Taskin et al.[17] investigated the effects of peritoneal exposure to carbon dioxide (CO_2) on peritoneal microcirculation and free radical scavenger (FRS) metabolism, and its precise role in potential adhesion formation after operative laparoscopy, by comparing excised peritoneal flap at the beginning and at the end of a laparoscopic procedure in different patients. He concluded that CO_2 exposure had adverse effects on peritoneal microcirculation and cell-protective systems, which are some of the proposed mechanisms in adhesion formation. As FRS are mainly released by the macrophages, he suggest that avoiding long CO_2 exposure and copiously irrigating the abdominal cavity (to remove the free-floating peritoneal macrophages) throughout surgery may diminish these effects. the potential role of the peritoneal FRS system on postoperative adhesion formation and its relation to estrogen status mandates further studies.

The possible involvement of inflammatory mediators such as nitric oxide (NO), and reports of protective effects of antioxidants, led Galili et al.[18] to test the effectiveness of methylene blue and NO synthesis inhibitor in reducing adhesion formation in rats. Adhesion development was obtained by scraping the anterior uterine hem wall, followed by intraperitoneal administration of saline, methylene blue, or Na-*t*-BOC-ω-nitro-L-arginine. Additional rats received identical treatment, but without the serosal damage. Two weeks later, adhesions were found in less than 5% of the rats with sham surgery, regardless of treatment. In the experimental group, more than 95% of the rats treated with saline or NO synthetase inhibitor had severe adhesions, in contrast to 5% of the methylene blue-treated rats. Severity of adhesion was less in the methylene blue group ($p < 0.001$). They concluded that methylene blue was very effective in preventing formation of peritoneal adhesions and that its activity is probably through inhibition of free radical generation and not of nitric oxide action.

These three studies suggest that there is a strong relation between the presence of free oxygen radicals in the peritoneal cavity and the occurrence of adhesions. Of course these radicals are mainly liberated by macrophages in reaction to an inflammatory process, but whether the contact of CO_2 versus air make a difference in this metabolism remains unknown. We were unable to find any publication on this point. Dryness of the peritoneum is certainly a crucial point in inducing macrophage reaction, but variation in local pH can be another concern, one that should be tested because it is possible that potential reduction of de novo adhesion formation or adhesion formation could also be achieved by using humid and inert gas during laparoscopy rather than dry CO_2, as is often used at present.

Ambulation

Another curious idea was checked by Das et al.,[19] who performed a study to assess the effects of unrestrained ambulation and of passive motion and delayed ambulation on the occurrence of adhesions after controlled uterine injuries, produced by conventional surgical techniques, in rats. Animals were divided into four groups; some were allowed to ambulate without restriction following recovery from the anesthetic, some were maintained without motion for 12 to 24 hours, and others were submitted to passive motion. The rats allowed to ambulate developed fewer adhesions. Das et al. suggested that either passive motion or delayed ambulation may be associated with increased postoperative uterine adhesion formation. This result provides another possible explanation for the unconfirmed clinical observation of decreased postoperative adhesions formation following laparoscopic surgery as compared with laparotomy.

Surgical Technologies

It is evident that the operative technology generally used during a laparotomy or a laparoscopy largely differs. Sutures are commonly used in laparotomy and rarely in laparoscopy. Electrosurgery is used in both, but usually monopolar energy is used during a laparotomy and bipolar during a laparoscopy. Lasers are mainly used by laparoscopy and, moreover, there are major differences among the lasers (Nd:Yag, holmium, CO_2, KTP, or argon lasers). On the other hand, the size of the instruments is quite different. Laparoscopic tools are much smaller than those used during laparotomy but are larger than those for microsurgery. In response to that opinion, microsurgical endoscopic instrumentation has been developed. Should these differences in operative techniques explain totally or partially the differences found in the adhesion process between laparotomy and laparoscopy? That is the topic of the next section.

Electrosurgery, Laser, and the Ultrasonic Scalpel

Some animal experiments have been published. Schemmel et al.[4] used a rabbit model to perform an ovarian wedge resection and removal of the distal uterine horn to test an ultrasonic scalpel, CO_2 laser, and electrosurgery. Observations of hemostatic properties, coagulation necrosis, and adhesion formation indicated no differences among the different surgical tools in adhesion formation or de novo adhesion formation.

De Leon et al.[20] also found that using laser surgery did not offer a significant reduction in postoperative adhesion formation in comparison with standard microsurgery technique when performing ovarian wedge resection in rats. Marana et al.,[21] in a first publication, reported studies in rabbits in which, at random, one ovary was longitudinally bivalved with a scalpel and then reconstructed by microsurgery. The contralateral ovary was similarly cut, but with a CO_2 laser set at a superpulsed mode. Four weeks after surgery, no difference in adhesion formation was found following this ovarian surgery by microsurgery or CO_2 laser. Bhatta et al.[22]

studied the role of bleeding, acute thermal damage, and charring in adhesion formation by submitting 96 rabbit ovaries to an ovarian wedge resection using different lasers, electrosurgery, and scalpel. Bleeding and charring correlated with adhesion formation, but the histologic depth of thermal damage did not. The adhesion scores were 11.6 ± 8.0 with pulsed Er:YAG laser; 11.9 ± 7.5 with scalpel; 8.3 ± 9.3 with electrocautery; 6.7 ± 8.8 with a continuous wave (c.w.) Nd:YAG laser; 5.3 ± 4.8 with c.w. CO_2 laser; 3.1 ± 2.7 with pulsed CO_2 laser; 1.7 ± 1.8 with pulsed Ho:YAG laser; and 0.8 ± 1.5 in the control (no resection) group. The main conclusion of this study is that different surgical tools can lead to very different results in adhesion formation.

It is difficult to draw any clear conclusion from these four studies. All were done by laparotomy; three of four studies concluded there was no difference, but the most precise study found a large difference. This last publication underlines the fact that rather than the technology itself, the bleeding and charring are the crucial points in adhesion formation. That result can certainly explain why using the same technology, in the same conditions but in different hands, can lead to different adhesion formation levels.

Marana et al.[23] performed a second study in which each ovary was longitudinally bivalved with a scalpel, but only one ovary was reconstruction microsurgically (with sutures), whereas the contralateral ovary was left open. No significant differences were found between the microsurgically sutured and the nonsutured ovaries for adhesion formation.

Lin and Chou[24] performed a study in pigs to evaluate adhesion formation from created peritoneal defects following laparoscopic surgery. A second-look laparotomy was performed 3 to 6 weeks later. In the group with peritoneal defects left open, 22% (2/9) of the pigs had grade I adhesions. In the group with peritoneal defects repaired with staples, 11% (1/9) of the pigs had grade I adhesions. However, no significant difference in adhesions was noted between these two groups ($p > 0.05$). They concluded that repairing the large peritoneal defect remaining from laparoscopic surgery is not necessary to reduce postoperative pelvic adhesions.

Peritoneal Closure

We should also include here the report by McNally and Curtain,[10] who studied postoperative adhesion formation in a series of 100 patients who had previous Cesarean with or without closure of the peritoneum. Adhesions were present in 28% of the closed group cases versus 14% in the open group cases. Finally, it seems that closing or suturing peritoneal or ovarian raw areas has no advantage when it is done according to microsurgical techniques and probably induces more adhesion formation when it is done in a classical manner.

Organs and Adhesions

Does the rate of adhesion formation differ from one site to another? The data from Levrant et al.,[9] who found a 59% adhesion rate to the anterior abdominal wall after a midline vertical incision versus 28% after a suprapubic transverse incision, suggest that the areas in the peritoneal cavity are not equivalent for adhesions formation or reformation. We review this problem here; the point is important in our chapter because the type of surgery is often different. Generally, laparoscopy is devoted more to reconstructive infertility surgery and laparotomy to surgery involving resection of organs; however, we must also keep in mind that any surgical procedure acts on an organ and on a disease. Saravelos and Li[25] studied postoperative adhesion formation after laparoscopic electrosurgical treatment for polycystic ovarian syndrome in a prospective, randomized, controlled clinical study. The main aim of the study was to check the efficiency of Interceed. At the second-look laparoscopy, periadnexal adhesions of significant extent and severity developed in 57% of the women and 38% of the adnexa without difference according to the use of Interceed.

Naether and Fischer[26] studied adhesion formation after laparoscopic electrocoagulation of the ovarian surface in polycystic ovary patients in 62 cases. They concluded that the incidence of adhesion formation caused by laparoscopic electrocoagulation of the ovarian surface is low, and is much lower than after ovarian wedge resection (by laparotomy), and that this could be reduced by abdominal lavage and artificial ascites.

Uterus

Murray and Tulandi[27] found that myomectomy by laparotomy is associated frequently with de novo adhesion formation on the adnexa in 80% of the cases, but this frequency differed according to the incision location on the uterus. It was more frequent after posterior incision (93.7%) than after fundic or anterior incision (55.5%). Moreover, the extent and the severity of adhesion were also related to the type of incision. This is an interesting consideration because uterine incisions by laparotomy are more likely to be anterior, and in contrast, by laparoscopy the location of the uterus incision is generally fundic or posterior. Other than the study of Bulletti et al.,[8] the reports are not clear, but it seems that the main advantage of laparoscopic myomectomy is to decrease the risk of de novo adhesion formation and adhesion formation.

Cul-de-sac

Mais et al.[28] studied postoperative adhesion formation in 32 premenopausal nonpregnant women with severe endometriosis and complete posterior cul-de-sac obliteration who submitted to laparoscopic surgery. The main purpose of the study was to assess the efficacy of Interceed. In the control group, only 12.5% of the patients were free to adhesions versus 75% in the Interceed group. Nezhat et al.[29] noted adhesion formation in the cul-de-sac among 21 patients operated by laparoscopy for various procedures (myomectomy, dermoid cystectomy, serious cystadenoma removal, salpingo-oophorectomy for severe endometriosis) who had submitted to a laparoscopic posterior colpotomy.

These publications suggest that de novo adhesion formation is rare in this area after laparoscopy, but that adhesion formation or reformation frequently occurs. For formation after laparotomy, no precise data are available, but in our past experience of infertility surgery by laparotomy de novo adhesion formation was a current complication. Adhesion formation and reformation were also very frequent. Thus, we again come to the conclusion that the main advantage of laparoscopic surgery is to prevent the occurrence of de novo adhesion.

Adjuvants

Ortega-Moreno and Caballero-Gomez[30] tested the efficacy of Interceed in rat model in which 48 uterine horns were kept in uniform contact with the intestinal serosa layer by means of two 8/0 nylon stitches. Twelve rats were also submitted only to a 1-cm cut of the serosal layer, 12 were surround with only three layers of Interceed, 12 were incised and wrapped with Interceed, and 12 were left intact. Results in adhesion formation were similar in the two groups where the uterine horn was cut without respect to Interceed placement. Less adhesion were noted when no uterine incision was done and mainly when no Interceed was used. This result again demonstrates that the type of surgery and the way the tissue is handled are important points in adhesion formation.

Keckstein et al.[31] studied adhesion formation on the ovary after laparoscopic ovarian cystectomy in 25 patients requiring laparoscopic bilateral ovarian cystectomy. the main aim of the studies was to evaluate the efficacy of Interceed. Only 35% (6/17) of the controlled ovaries were free of adhesions, but no ovary was involved in vascular or dense adhesion. This rate was increased by the use of Interceed. On the other hand, this study demonstrated that there was no difference in postoperative adhesions in cases of endometriomas versus serous or mucinous cysts. Moreover, they demonstrated that suturing the ovaries leads to an increased frequency and extension of adhesions.

During the same period, Greenblatt and Casper[32] performed a prospective, randomized, blinded, clinical study of laparoscopic ovarian cautery with application of Interceed to one ovary, followed by short-interval second-look laparoscopy, scoring of adhesions, and clinical follow-up. Periovarian adhesions of varying severity developed in all women after laparoscopic ovarian cautery. Interceed showed no protective effect. Such a major differences between these two studies and their conclusions is difficult to understand.

Takeuchi et al.[33] evaluated the formation of adhesions after laparoscopic excision of endometriomas in 25 patients submitted to laparoscopic resection of endometriomas. The main aim of this study was to check the effects of fibrin glue in adhesion prevention. This method was demonstrated to be efficient, but this study also demonstrated that endometriomas of 5 cm or more in diameter and for those with a preoperative adhesion score of 8 or higher are more frequently associated with major postoperative adhesions.

From these five publications, it is again difficult to draw a clear and comprehensive conclusion. Adhesion formation on a "nearly normal ovary" (PCO) is frequent but the different publications provide such different results when using the same technology that the way that electrocautery is used is probably the cause of the difference. On pathologic ovaries, adhesion formation occurred in two-thirds of the cases but the type of pathology does not seem to have an effect on this rate. In contrast, adhesion reformation is common after laparotomy (74%)[34] and after laparoscopy (80%)[35] but its severity depends on the severity of the initial adhesion and on the presence of endometriosis adnexa.

A putative comparison can be made in comparing two series of early second-look laparoscopies, one after microsurgery by laparotomy[34] and one after laparoscopic tuboplasty.[35] Precise data were available for laparotomy from the Nordic Adhesion Prevention Study Group[34] in the study about Interceed. It was found that adhesion reformation after microsurgery was present on 74% of the ovaries, 76% of the tubes, and only 62% of the fimbria in the control group ($p < 0.05$). It was also demonstrated that recurrence implied less severe adhesion, at least during an early second-look laparoscopy (4–10 weeks). The operative laparoscopy study group[35] published data after laparoscopic infertility surgery showing that adhesion reformation occurred at 80.3% of the ovaries and 67% of the tubes. This study also confirmed that adhesion reformation depends on the type of the initial adhesion. The adhesion reformation rate was 45% after filmy adhesion lysis, 60.9% after dense or vascular adhesion lysis, and 79.3% after cohesive adhesion. A ratio of 12% de novo adhesion formation was reported. From this comparison, it appears that laparoscopy does not decrease the risk of adhesion reformation and that its risk to induce de novo adhesion exists even if it is limited. According to Lundorff et al.,[7] however, laparoscopy seems to reduce the risk of adhesion formation.

Estrogens and Adhesion Formation

In the era of microsurgery, it was admitted that the patients should be operated on in the early postmenstrual period. The main argument was to avoid bleeding from the corpus luteum or mature follicule. With laparoscopic procedures, this point is less frequently taken into account, but several reports have pointed out the deleterious role of estrogen in the genesis of adhesions.

Wiczyk et al.[36] evaluated female pelvic adhesion tissue for the presence of estrogen receptor (ER), progesterone receptor (PR), basic fibroblastic growth factor (basic FGF), and vascular endothelial growth factor (VEGF). Nineteen of 19 specimens were positive for PR; 16 of 19 specimens were positive for ER, which was present in a variety of the different cell types constituting adhesion; and VEGF and basic FGF were detected in endothelial cells of blood vessels supplying this tissue as well as in mesothelial cells. Adhesion tissue contained ER, PR, and growth factors that may be important in the genesis of the permanent fibrovascular bands between pelvic organs. This report supports the possibility of hormonal manipulation of these tissues to negatively influence postoperative pelvic adhesion formation.

Grow et al.[37] studied the occurrence of postoperative adhesions after uterine surgery in a randomized, prospective study in nonhuman primates according to different treatments that influence the E_2 (estradiol) and progesterone levels. GnRH-a and mifepristone were compared to a control group. Significantly fewer utero-omental adhesions were found with these drugs, suggesting that E_2 has a dramatic effect on the formation of pelvic adhesions after myometrial surgery.

Conclusions

The common concept that laparoscopic surgery is associated with fewer adhesions is not supported by hard human data. Even animal data are not so convincing. There are many difficulties with this literature review and analysis because of the lack of conclusive animal and human data. The most common evaluation procedure used was a second-look laparoscopy. At early second-look laparoscopy, Trimbos-Kemper et al.[38] found de novo adhesions in 50% of the cases after tubal microsurgery, but this permits secondary adhesiolysis, which was proven efficient by a late third-look laparoscopy. One can be doubtful about the reliability of this procedure to evaluate adhesions genesis, however, as the adhesion situation seems to differ with time. DeCherney and Mezer[39] compared early (4–10 weeks) and late (1 year) second-look laparoscopic findings in two groups of patients, finding the overall adhesion frequency was similar (25% versus 24%) but that the severity was totally different. In the early control group, 60% of the patients were classified as grade I, 10% as a grade II, and 5% at grade III. In the late control group, only 12% were classified in grade I, 41% in grade II, and 22% in grade III. This point coupled with the difficulty (or the impossibility) of proposing a reliable classification can certainly explain some of the major divergences that we have reported.

The final conclusions of this review are the following:

- There are major data showing that laparoscopic surgery decreases the risk of de novo adhesion formation.
- Some evidence indicates that laparoscopic surgery decreases adhesion formation mainly for uterine surgery, but this has not been proven for other ovarian and adnexal surgery, at least in comparison with microsurgery.
- There is no evidence that laparoscopic surgery decreases the incidence of adhesion reformation, but there is some question that its severity is decreased.
- The type of surgical technology does not seem to affect adhesion formation or reformation if correctly used.
- Suturing the peritoneum by laparoscopy is unnecessary or even deleterious.
- The best way to decrease the incidence and severity of adhesion formation or reformation is to use microsurgical principles by laparoscopy or by laparotomy. These techniques include a perfect hemostasis, frequent peritoneal washing, and gentle handling of the tissue to avoid large coagulation and charring.
- Laparoscopic surgery cannot be considered as nonadhesiogenic, and adhesion prevention by barrier methods (Intergel, Interceed, Goretex) or other chemicals substances (corticosteroids, pretreatment with GnRH analogs is mandatory in this type of surgery.
- Prospective studies should be undertaken to analyze the deleterious effect of free oxygen radicals in adhesion formation by modifying some physicochemical principles of laparoscopy.

References

1. Luciano AA, Maier DB, Koch EI, et al. A comparative study of postoperative adhesion following laser surgery by laparoscopy versus laparotomy in a rabbit model. Obstet Gynecol 1989:74:220–224.
2. Marana R, Luciano AA, Muzii I. Laparoscopy versus laparotomy for ovarian conservative surgery: a randomized trial in the rabbit model. Am J Obstet Gynecol 1994;171: 861–864.
3. Filmar F, Gomel V, Macomb P. Operative laparoscopy versus open abdominal surgery: a comparative study on postoperative adhesion formation on the rat model. Fertil Steril 1987;48:486–489.
4. Schemmel M, Haefner HK, Selvaggi SM, Warren JS, Termin CS, Hurd WW. Comparison of the ultrasonic scalpel to CO_2 laser and electrosurgery in terms of tissue injury

and adhesion formation in a rabbit model. Fertil Steril 1997;67/2:382–386.

5. Chen MD, Teigen TA, Reynolds HT, et al. Laparoscopy versus laparotomy: an evaluation of adhesion formation after pelvic and para-aortic lymphadenectomy in a porcine model. Am J Obstet Gynecol 1998;178:499–503.
6. Fowler JM, Hartenbach EM, Reynolds HT, et al. Pelvic adhesion formation after pelvic lymphadenectomy: comparison between transperitoneal laparoscopy and extraperitoneal laparotomy in a porcine model. Gynecol Oncol 1994;55:25–28.
7. Lundorff P, Hahlin M, Kallfelt B, Thorburn J, Lindblom B. Adhesion formation after laparoscopic surgery in tubal pregnancy: a randomized trial versus laparotomy. Fertil Steril 1991;55/5:911–915.
8. Bulletti C, Polli V, Negrini V, Giacomucci E, Flamigni C. Adhesion formation after laparoscopic myomectomy. J Am Assoc Gynecol Laparosc 1996;3/4:533–536.
9. Levrant SG, Bieber EJ, Barnes RB. Anterior abdominal wall adhesions after laparotomy or laparoscopy. J Am Assoc Gynecol Laparosc 1997;4/3:353–356.
10. McNally OM, Curtain AC. Does closure of the peritoneum during caesarian section influence postoperative morbidity and subsequent bladder adhesion formation? J Obstet Gynecol 1997;17/3:239–241.
11. Diamond MP, Daniell JF, Feste J. Adhesion reformation and de novo adhesion formation following reproductive pelvic surgery. Fertil Steril 1987;47:864.
12. Diamond MP, Daniell JF, Johns DA. Adhesion formation and reformation after operative laparoscopy: assessment at early second-look procedures. Fertil Steril 1991;55: 500–504.
13. Roushdy M, Farag O, Kinawy G. Adhesion formation after laparoscopic surgery. Middle East Fertil Soc J 1996;1/3: 211–216.
14. Jensen RPS. Early laparoscopy after pelvic operations to prevent adhesions: safety and efficacy. Fertil Steril 1988; 49/1:26–31.
15. Nezhat CR, Nezhat FR, Metzer DA, Luciano AA. Adhesion reformation after reproductive surgery by videolaseroscopy. Fertil Steril 1990;53/6:1008–1011.
16. Portz DM, Elkins TE, White R, Warren J, Adadevoh S, Randolph J. Oxygen free radicals and pelvic adhesion formation: blocking oxygen free radical toxicity to prevent adhesion formation in an endometriosis model. Int J Fertil 1991;36/1:39–42.
17. Taskin O, Buhur A, Birincioglu M, Burak F, Atmaca R, Yilmaz I, Wheeler JM. The effects of duration of CO_2 insufflation and irrigation on peritoneal microcirculation assessed by free radical scavengers and total glutathion levels during operative laparoscopy. J Am Assoc Gynecol Laparosc 1998;5/2:129–133.
18. Galili Y, Ben-Abraham R, Rabau M, Klausner J, Kluger Y. Reduction of surgery-induced peritoneal adhesions by methylene blue. Am J Surg 1998;175/1:30–32.
19. Das K, Penney LL, Critser JK. Effects of passive motion and early vs. delayed ambulation on adhesion formation in rat uterine surgery Int J Fertil 1990;35/4:245–248.
20. De Leon FD, Edwards M, Heine MW. A comparison of microsurgery and laser surgery for ovarian wedge resections. Int J. Fertil 1990;35/3:177–179.
21. Marana R, Luciano AA, Marendino VE, et al. Reproductive outcome after ovarian surgery: microsurgery versus CO_2 laser. J Gynecol Surg 1991;7/3:159–162.
22. Bhatta N, Isaacson K, Flotte T, Schiff I, Anderson RR. Injury and adhesion formation following ovarian wedge resection with different thermal surgical modalities. Lasers Surg Med 1993;13/3:344–352.
23. Marana R, Luciano AA, Muzii L, et al. Reproductive outcome after ovarian surgery: suturing versus nonsuturing of the ovarian cortex. J Gynecol Surg 1991;7/3:155–158.
24. Lin Y-S, Chou C-Y. Evaluation of pelvic adhesions from peritoneal defects following laparoscopic surgery: an animal study. J Gynecol Surg 1996;12/2:95–98.
25. Saravelos H, Li T-C. Post-operative adhesions after laparoscopic electrosurgical treatment for polycystic ovarian syndrome with the application of Interceed to one ovary: a prospective randomized controlled study. Hum Reprod (Oxf) 1996;11/5:992–997.
26. Naether OGJ, Fischer R. Adhesion formation after laparoscopic electrocoagulation of the ovarian surface in polycystic ovary patients. Adhesion formation was detected in 19.3%. Fertil Steril 1993;60/1:95–98.
27. Murray C, Tulandi T. Prevention of postmyomectomy adhesions. Infertil Reprod Med Clin North Am 1996;7/1: 169–177.
28. Mais V, Ajossa S, Marongiu D, Peiretti RF, Guerriero S, Melis GB. Reduction of adhesion reformation after laparoscopic endometriosis surgery: a randomized trial with an oxidized regenerated cellulose absorbable barrier. Obstet Gynecol. 1995;86/4:512–515.
29. Nezhat F, Brill AI, Nezhat CH, Nezhat C. Adhesion formation after endoscopic posterior colpotomy. J Reprod Med Obstet Gynecol 1993;38/7:534–536.
30. Ortega-Moreno J, Caballero-Gomez JM. Postoperative adhesion after uterine horn surgery in the rat, with the use of TC7. Eur J Obstet Gynecol Reprod Biol 1993;48/1:51–59.
31. Keckstein J, Ulrich U, Sasse V, Roth A, Karageorgieva E. Reduction of postoperative adhesion formation after laparoscopic ovarian cystectomy. Hum Reprod (Oxf) 1996; 11/3:579–582.
32. Greenblatt EM, Casper RF. Adhesion formation after laparoscopic ovarian cautery for polycystic ovarian syndrome: lack of correlation with pregnancy rate. Fertil Steril 1993; 60/5:766–770.
33. Takeuchi H, Awaji M, Hashimoto M, Nakano Y, Mitsuhashi N, Kuwabara Y. Reduction of adhesions with fibrin glue after laparoscopic excision of large ovarian endometriomas. J Am Assoc Gynecol Laparosc 1996;3/4:575–579.
34. Nordic Adhesion Prevention Study Group. The efficacy of Interceed for prevention of reformation of postoperative adhesions on ovaries, fallopian tubes, and fimbriae in microsurgical operations for fertility: a multicenter study. Fertil Steril 1995;63/4:709–714.
35. Operative Laparoscopy Study Group. Postoperative adhesion development after operative laparoscopy evaluation at early second-look procedures. Fertil Steril 1991;55: 700–704.
36. Wiczyk HP, Grow DR, Adams LA, O'Shea DL, Reece MT. Pelvic adhesions contain sex steroid receptors and produce angiogenesis growth factors. Fertil Steril 1998; 69/3:511–516.

37. Grow DR, Coddington CC, Hsiu J-G, Mikich Y, Hodgen GD. Role of hypoestrogenism or sex steroid antagonism in adhesion formation after myometrial surgery in primates. Fertil Steril 1996;66/1:140–147.
38. Trimbos-Kemper TCM, Trimbos JB, Van Hall EV. Adhesion formation after tubal surgery: results of the eight-day laparoscopy in 188 patients. Fertil Steril 1985;43:395–400.
39. De Cherney AH, Mezer HC. The nature of posttuboplasty pelvic adhesions as determined by early and late laparoscopy. Fertil Steril 1984;41/4:643–646.

14

Reducing Adhesion Formation in Gynecologic Procedures Using Laparoscopic Surgery

Salli Tazuke and Camran Nezhat

CONTENTS

Abdominal adhesions are estimated to occur in as high as 90% of patients who have undergone major gynecologic surgery[1] and represent one of the most common causes of intestinal obstruction.[2] Complications that often accompany adhesions include chronic pelvic pain and infertility, both of which frequently require additional surgery. In 1994, 1% of all U.S. hospital admissions involved adhesiolysis treatment, resulting in $1.33 billion of health care expenditure.[3] To reduce the need for adhesion-related treatment of patients who have had gynecologic surgery, surgeons should optimize surgical techniques and apply adjuvants to reduce postoperative adhesion formation. This chapter reviews the operative techniques and adjuvants currently available for the prevention and management of pelvic adhesions.

Peritoneal Surgery and Adhesion Formation

Adhesion formation is a physiologic consequence of peritoneal tissue repair. After the initial injury, mesothelial cells secrete fibrinous exudate to cover the defect. This fibrinous exudate, if left alone, will induce fibroblast migration and proliferation in the area, collagen deposition, and ultimately fibrous adhesion formation and neovascularization. In the initial 72 to 96 hours, fibrinolytic activity by the peritoneum suppresses the accumulation of fibrinous exudate, permitting mesothelial cell migration and repair of the damaged area within 5 days of initial trauma.

As demonstrated more than a century ago in animal models, uncomplicated peritoneal injuries can heal without adhesions.[4–6] Although some patients are more prone to adhesion formation, careful surgical techniques can minimize factors that promote adhesion development. Most notable are surgical techniques that will suppress the fibrinolytic activity of the peritoneum during the initial 72 to 96 hours. Surgical techniques that lead to tissue ischemia, infection, or peritoneal or adnexal trauma are known to be associated with increased adhesion formation via the suppression of fibrinolytic activity needed during the initial 72 to 96 hours. Other detrimental surgical practices include traction of the peritoneum, drying of serosal surface, excessive suturing, retention of blood clots, and use of omental patches. Such clinical practices can lead to excessive fibroblast activity in the peritoneal cavity, resulting in postoperative adhesion formation.[6]

For many different gynecologic procedures, laparoscopy rather than the laparotomy approach is associated with decreased postoperative adhesion formation.[7–11] Operative laparoscopy is preferable because it permits gentle handling of tissue, use of microsurgical instruments, precise treatment of the diseased area, meticulous hemostasis, constant irrigation, and nonexposure to talc powder intraabdominally, all of which minimize adhesion formation. It is important to emphasize, however, that a laparoscopic approach is not a panacea to adhesion prevention.

Data from animal[12–14] and clinical studies[15–19] suggest that once adhesions have formed and present a clinical problem, laparoscopic surgery is more effective for adhesiolysis because it causes fewer de novo adhesions than a laparotomy and reduces impairment of tubo-ovarian function.[7]

Laparoscopy in Patients with Prior Surgery

In patients with a history of previous laparotomy or advanced endometriosis, the intraabdominal anatomy may be distorted. Many of the injuries during laparoscopy in such patients occur during the blind insertion of the primary trocar and can be very dangerous. Inflexible adhesive bridging between the intestine and abdominal wall can nullify any protection from trocar injury usually afforded by elevating the abdominal wall, creating a pneumoperitoneum, Trendelenburg positioning, and bowel motility. Review of prior operative notes can help identify those particularly at risk for initial trocar injury.

An analysis of 360 women with prior intraabdominal operations led to the following observations:[20]

1. Patients with prior midline incisions have more adhesions than those with prior Pfannenstiel.
2. Patients with multiple prior incisions do not have more adhesions than those with a single prior incision.
3. Patients with prior midline or Pfannenstiel incisions for gynecologic surgery have more adhesions than those having undergone obstetric surgery.
4. Patients with prior midline incisions for obstetric surgery do not have more adhesions than those with a prior Pfannenstiel incision for obstetric surgery.
5. Incidence of subumbilical bowel adhesions and subsequent bowel injury is related more closely to the indication for previous laparotomy than the type or number of previous laparotomies. Severe adhesions are associated with previous adhesions, generalized peritonitis, bowel resection after bowel obstruction, oncologic procedures with omentectomy, previous radiation, and intraperitoneal chemotherapy.

Before the operation, every patient should be assessed for abdominal wall bowel adhesion risks. For those at risk, preoperative bowel preparation is important. In patients with a history of laparotomies, open or closed techniques to trocar insertions are used. If the closed technique is used, a disposable trocar with a bullet shield is preferable. Either direct trocar insertion or establishment of a pneumoperitoneum by Veress needle can be used depending on the surgeon's preference and experience. Trocar entry should be controlled and at a vertical, not obligue, angle. If a Veress needle is used, the subumbilical area may be searched for bowel adhesions before trocar insertion.

In patients who may have a high likelihood of bowel adhesion to the anterior abdominal wall, a pneumoperitoneum may also be created by placing the Veress needle in the left-upper quadrant of the abdomen, in the midclavicular line, after aspirating with a syringe to rule out bowel entry. The only exception to this access is in patients who have a history of splenectomy. The abdomen is insufflated after ruling out bowel entry, and then the area is explored using a 20-gauge needle to inject saline. If no fluid is aspirated, a 5-mm trocar and laparoscope are inserted to visualize the peritoneal cavity. Once a safe entry is confirmed, secondary trocars may be placed under direct observation. However, even under direct visualization, placement of an ancillary trocar may deviate from the intended track of insertion and result in bowel injury. The insertion track may also be simulated first with a 21-gauge spinal needle to confirm the angle and safety of the path chosen. While leaving the needle in place, the trocar can be introduced immediately adjacent to the needle.[20]

An alternative method was proposed by DeCherney, who used a 2- to 3-mm-diameter needle laparoscope to visualize the area immediately subperitoneal to the umbilicus. A Veress needle is then inserted under visualization before insufflation of the cavity. The periumbilical area can also be explored using an 18-gauge needle attached to a syringe after establishment of pneumoperitoneum.[21]

Adhesiolysis

To perform adhesiolysis adequately, two to three ancillary trocars are placed in the lower, lateral suprapubic area at the level of the iliac crests. An atraumatic grasper can be inserted by the assistant to hold the adhesion or involved organs. The adhesion can be gently retracted to identify its extent and vascularity. The surgeon can approach the adhesions close to the affected organs, preferably at both ends and removed from the abdominal cavity.

If the adhesion is avascular, microscissors or lasers can be used to resect the adhesions (Figs. 14.1–14.4). Adhesions containing vasculature can be coagulated then incised with a microelectrode (15–20 W cutting mode) or CO_2 laser, superpulse (40 W), ultrapulse (20–80 W and 25–200 millijoules), or fiber laser (15–25 W). Microscissors or laser can be used to resect the adhesions.

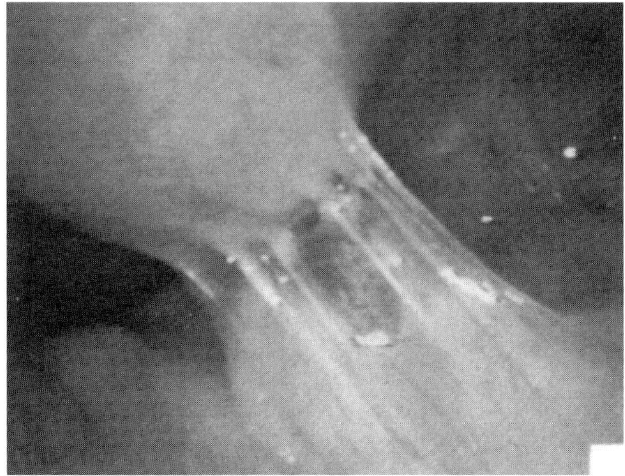

Fig. 14.1. Avascular adhesions between the uterus and omentum are gently stretched before dissection with scissors. (From Nezhat CR, Nezhat FR, Luciano AA, et al.[20] by permission of Operative Gynecologic Laparoscopy: Principles and Techniques.)

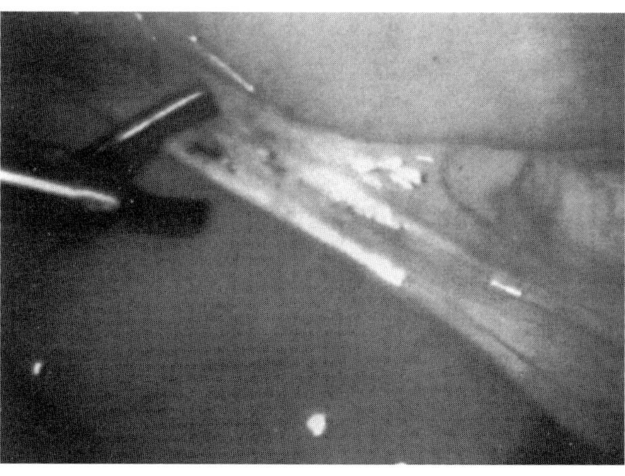

Fig. 14.3. Thick, vascular adhesions are coagulated before dissection with a bipolar cautery. (From Nezhat CR, Nezhat FR, Luciano AA, et al.[20] by permission of Operative Gynecologic Laparoscopy: Principles and Techniques.)

If adhesions are extensive, a strategy allowing for progressive exposure of the abdominal and pelvic structures should be utilized. Typically, this means that the bowel adhesions are severed first, followed by periovarian and peritubal adhesions. Once the intestines are freed, they can be placed cephalad, away from the operative field. With dense adhesions between different organs, the plane of dissection may be sometimes difficult to identify. A pressurized suction irrigator probe can hydrodissect and create tissue planes before resection (Fig. 14.5). The advantages of hydrodissection include the use of fluid as a backstop for the laser and the ability to prevent desiccation of the serosal surface.

Adnexal trauma increases the likelihood of subsequent pelvic adhesions. Therefore, whenever possible, either the adhesion or the ovarian ligaments should be grasped instead of the ovarian cortex. Filmy adhesions on the ovary that are difficult to identify can be visualized when the adnexa is floated in lactated Ringer's fluid. These adhesions can be grasped with forceps and resected, preferably with microscissors or an ultrapulse laser at the base of its attachment to the ovary. In gen-

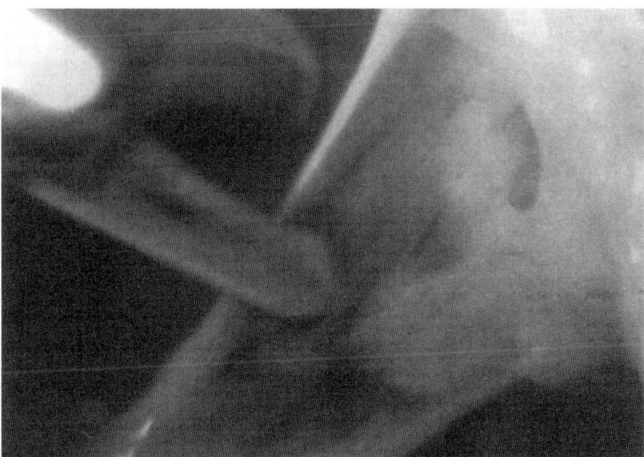

Fig. 14.2. Avascular adhesions are dissected with scissors. (From Nezhat CR, Nezhat FR, Luciano AA, et al.[20] by permission of Operative Gynecologic Laparoscopy: Principles and Techniques.)

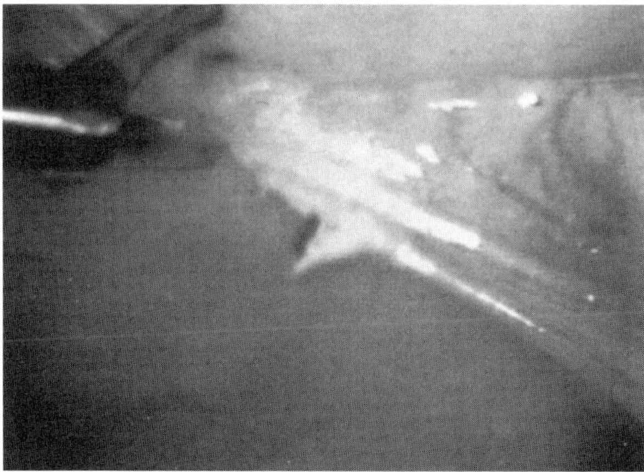

Fig. 14.4. A coagulated vascular adhesion is lysed with scissors after cauterization. (From Nezhat CR, Nezhat FR, Luciano AA, et al.[20] by permission of Operative Gynecologic Laparoscopy: Principles and Techniques.)

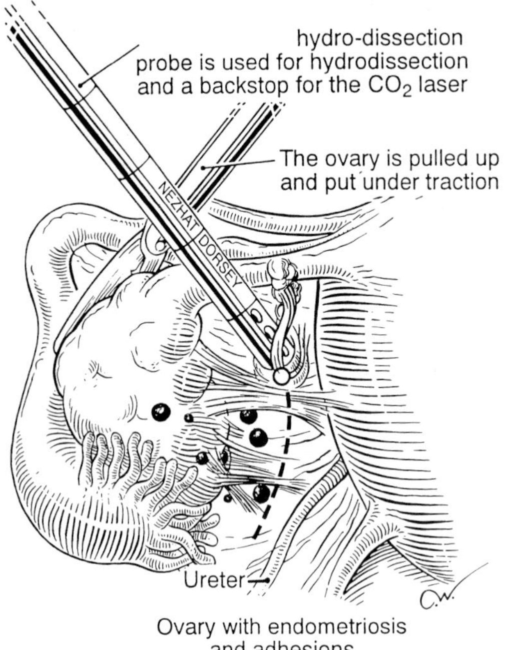

FIG. 14.5. Adhesiolysis between the ovary, uterus, and the pelvic sidewall using the CO_2 laser. The ovary is gently grasped and placed under traction with an atraumatic grasper. The suction irrigator is used for a backstop, and the adhesions are lysed using the CO_2 laser. (From Nezhat CR, Nezhat FR, Luciano AA, et al.[20] by permission of Operative Gynecologic Laparoscopy: Principles and Techniques.)

eral, the laser beams other than the ultrapulse are at least 1 mm in diameter and are too wide for the narrow bands of adhesions. Electrosurgery and fiber lasers (Nd: YAG, KTP, or argon) induce thermal damage to the immediately surrounding tissue, which will increase the risk of adhesion recurrence.

Laparoscopic surgery and microsurgical techniques can reduce but not eliminate adhesion formation. To further reduce the risk of adhesion formation, various adjuvants have been developed and utilized.

Hydroflotation: Adhesion Prevention Adjuvant Barriers

Instillation of crystalloids in the peritoneal cavity of the end of surgical procedures to prevent adhesion formation is a common practice among surgeons and gynecologists. Theoretically speaking, however, crystalloids cannot be expected to effectively prevent adhesion formation because these are rapidly absorbed within 24 hours, far short of the 5-day window during which mesothelial cells reepitheliaze the peritoneum. Several clinical studies confirm the shortcomings of crystalloid instillation in adhesion prevention during laparoscopic procedures. Laparoscopic electrocoagulation or laser vaporization of ovarian surface for treatment of polycystic ovarian disease is complicated frequently by postoperative adhesion formation. Instillation of 150 mL of lactated Ringer's solution did not improve the incidence of adhesion formation by second-look laparoscopy.[22] Similarly, no benefit was reported with 500 mL of lactated Ringer's solution at the end of laparoscopic removal of ovarian endometrioma.[23]

Hyskon is a high molecular weight dextran-70 suspended in 10% dextrose solution (Pharmacia, Uppsala, Sweden) that has an osmotic effect, drawing fluid into the peritoneal cavity. The hydroflotation of peritoneal organs and fluid barrier between the raw surgical surfaces and structures are thought to reduce adhesion formation. Clinical studies in the 1980s however demonstrated inconsistent results,[24] and complications such as coagulopathy, fluid overload, infection, and allergic reactions have rendered this adjuvant unfavorable.[25–28] Several materials have been developed as mechanical barriers to cover the areas denuded from the surgical procedures (Table 14.1).

Interceed T7 (Johnson & Johnson Patient Care, Somerville, NJ, USA) is composed of oxidized regenerated cellulose, which becomes gelatinous within 8 hours of application in the intraperitoneal cavity and is slowly absorbed over 28 days. In two multicenter trials, Inter-

TABLE 14.1. Adhesion prevention adjuvants.

Adjuvants	Mechanism
Crystalloid	Fluid barrier. Rapidly absorbed, and clinical efficacy limited
Dextran 70 (Hyskon)	Osmotically draws fluid into the peritoneal cavity, resulting in hydroflotation of organs
Interceed TC7	Oxidized regenerated cellulose that separates opposing surfaces. A procoagulant, which may increase adhesion formation in the presence of blood
ePTFE (Gore-Tex)	Nonreactive, nonresorbable mechanical barrier separating opposing surfaces. Requires suturing, and is a permanent material unless removed
Seprafilm (HAL-F)	Hyaluronic acid coupled with carboxymethyl cellulose. Nonreactive, nonimmunogenic, and has good efficacy even in the presence of some blood. Cannot be applied through the laparoscope
Fibrin glue	Polymerizes to solid film after application and produces mechanical barrier
Poloxamer 407	Polymer of propylene oxide, ethylene oxide. Animal studies only
Repel	Polyethylene glycol 6000 and polylactic acid block copolymers. Animal studies only

ceed was placed on one of the two pelvic sidewalls, which had been treated for comparable disease, at the conclusion of the operation. At second-look laparoscopy, approximately twice as many Interceed-treated sidewalls were free of adhesions as untreated sidewalls.[29,30] These observations were confirmed by four other studies, where one of the two ovaries were wrapped with Interceed and compared to the unwrapped similarly operated ovary. Again, approximately twice as many ovaries without the Interceed developed adhesions at second-look laparoscopy.[31–33]

Despite the favorable initial reports, subsequent studies have not shown consistent efficacy, likely because of the limitation of Interceed strictly to surfaces completely free of blood. The oxidized regenerated cellulose is a procoagulant that can actually induce fibrin deposition if hemostasis is not complete. Furthermore, the material is acidic and can cause necrosis of cells. Degradation of Interceed requires an inflammatory response, and hence the intraperitoneal leukocyte population can also counter the beneficiary effect of Interceed by promoting adhesion formation.

Another barrier material with extensive clinical data is expanded polytetrafluoroethylene (ePTFE; Gore-Tex Surgical Membrane, W.L. Gore & Associates, Flagstaff, AZ, USA). PTFE has been utilized extensively as a pericardium or peritoneal substitute with excellent outcome. The material is nonreactive and has been reported to produce similar reduction in adhesion formation as Interceed when placed on pelvic sidewalls after adhesionlysis.[34] However, the material is hydrophobic and does not adhere well to organs without suturing, which requires advanced laparoscopic dexterity. Furthermore, because it is nonresorbable in nature, concern remains regarding the permanent presence of a foreign material in the abdominal cavity.

A newer compound for barrier material, utilized in open procedures, is composed of hyaluronic acid, a component of nascent extracellular matrix, coupled with carboxymethylcellulose. Seprafilm (Genzyme Corp., Cambridge, MA, USA) is a bioresorbable membrane that is nontoxic, nonimmunogenic, and biocompatible. The film adheres to moist surfaces well, gelatinizes rapidly, and remains at the site for as long as 28 days. Unlike Interceed, Seprafilm is not a procoagulant and can reduce adhesion formation regardless of incomplete hemostasis. A recent clinical trial demonstrated Seprafilm to be effective in reducing adhesion formation after abdominal myomectomy.[35,36] Unfortunately, the material cannot be applied laparoscopically. Furthermore, there have been case reports of postoperative pulmonary embolism and intraperitoneal abscesses occurring at a higher frequency in patients receiving Seprafilm than those in the control group, who did not receive Seprafilm.[37] Although the precise mechanism is unknown, it is postulated that relative differences in dissolution of the material may lead to fragmentation of the film resulting in thrombosis formation. A similar compound to Seprafilm in a gel form (Sepra-gel) has been reported to be as efficacious in several animal models and awaits clinical trials.[37,38]

Fibrin Glue

Fibrin glue or fibrin sealant is a two component substance that becomes a highly polymerized solid film shortly after mixing. As a hydrogel, this can be applied easily during laparoscopy. However, in both animal and human studies, its efficacy has not been consistent, nor is there evidence that fibrin glue is superior to other antiadhesion substances. Fibrin glue is made from the pooled plasma of several donors. Although viruses and other infectious agents are likely inactivated during the processing of fibrin glue, concern remains regarding the potential for disease transmission.[39–42]

Second-Look Laparoscopy

Finally, despite use of good surgical technique and adjuvants, postsurgical adhesions are currently not yet preventable. Second-look laparoscopy has been utilized to not only evaluate but also to lyse early adhesions. The optimal time for second-look laparoscopy to lyse early adhesions is between 2 and 6 weeks after the initial surgery. De novo adhesions from the original surgery are gelatinous and can be lysed with gentle blunt dissection. Such early second-look laparoscopy and treatment of adhesions have been associated with an increased pregnancy rate compared to those performed 1 year after the initial surgery.[43–45] This approach is unfortunately not undertaken in the United States because of the lack of insurance coverage for second-look laparoscopy.

Summary

In conclusion, the clinical consequences of postsurgical adhesions and their complications are significant. In recent years, the pathophysiology of adhesions formation has been increasingly characterized and has led to the identification of adhesion-promoting factors and techniques, as well as the development of a number of adhesion prevention adjuvants and barriers. Many studies have demonstrated that laparoscopic surgery is associated with decreased adhesion formation when compared to a laparotomy for similar procedures. Operative laparoscopy is also superior to a laparotomy for the treatment of postoperative adhesions. However, laparoscopy is not a panacea to adhesion formation, and good surgical techniques and basic principles of microsurgery should be followed to minimize adhesion formation. Although several adjuvants have been developed, there are currently no perfect adhesion prevention adjuvants. It is hoped that continued investigation and development of adhesion prevention adjuvants will soon allow peritoneal healing without associated adhesions.

References

1. Stricker B, Blanco J, Fox HE. The gynecologic contribution to intestinal obstruction in females. J Am Coll Surg 1994;178:617–620.
2. Monk BJ, Berman ML, Montz FJ. Adhesions after extensive gynecologic surgery: clinical significance, etiology, and prevention. Am J Obstet Gynecol 1994;170: 1396–1403.
3. Ray NF, Denton WG, Thamer M, et al. Abdominal adhesiolysis: inpatient care and expenditure in the United States in 1994. J Am Coll Surg 1998;186:1–9.
4. Von Dembowski T. Uber die urasachen der peritonealein adhaseonen nach cirurgischen mit Rucksicht auf die Frage des Ileus nach Laparotomien. Arch Klin Chir 1888; 37:745.
5. Franz K. Uber die Bedeutung der Branchorfe in der Bauchhohle. Z Geburtshilfe Gynaekol 1902;47:64–75.
6. Ellis H. The cause and prevention of postoperative intraperitoneal adhesions. Surg Gynecol Obstet 1971;133: 497–511.
7. Lundorff P, Hahlin M, Kallfelt B, et al. Adhesion formation after laparoscopic surgery in tubal pregnancy: a randomized trial versus laparotomy. Fertil Steril 1991;55: 911–915.
8. Nezhat CR, Nezhat FR, Metzger DA, et al. Adhesion reformation after reproductive surgery by videolaserlaparoscopy. Fertil Steril 1990;53:1008–1011.
9. Operative Laparoscopy Study Group. Postoperative adhesion development after operative laparoscopy: evaluation at early second-look laparoscopy. Fertil Steril 1991;55: 700–704.
10. Bulletti C, Polli V, Negrini E, et al. Adhesion formation after laparoscopic myomectomy. J Am Assoc Gynecol Laparosc 1996;4:533–536.
11. Mais V, Ajossa S, Mascia M, et al. Laparoscopy versus abdominal myomectomy: a prospective randomized trial to evaluate benefits in early outcome. Am J Obstet Gynecol 1996;174:654–658.
12. Filmar S, Gomel V, McComb P. Operative laparoscopy versus open abdominal surgery: a comparative study on postoperative adhesion formation in the rat model. Fertil Steril 1987;48:486–490.
13. Luciano AA, Maier DB, Nulsen ZC, et al. A comparative study of postoperative adhesion formation following laser surgery by laparoscopy versus laparotomy in the rabbit model Obstet Gynecol 1989;74:220–224.
14. Maier DB, Nulsen J, Klock A, et al. Laser laparoscopy vs. laparotomy in lysis of dense and incidental pelvic adhesions. J Reprod Med 1992;37:965–968.
15. Diamond MP, Daniell SF, Feste J, et al. Adhesion reformation and de novo formation after reproductive pelvic surgery. Fertil Steril 1987;47:864–866.
16. Luciano AA, Moufauino-Oliva M. Comparison of postoperative adhesion formation—laparoscopy versus laparotomy. Infertil Reprod Med Clin North Am 1994;5:437–457.
17. Marana R, Luciano AA, Morendino VE, et al. Reproductive outcome after ovarian surgery: microsurgery versus CO_2 laser. J Gynecol Surg 1991;7:159–162.
18. Mueller MD, Tschudi J, Herrman U, et al. An evaluation of laparoscopic adhesiolysis in patients with chronic abdominal pain. Surg Endosc 1995;9:802–804.
19. Trimbos-Kemper TCM, Trimbos JB, van Hall EV. Adhesion formation after tubal surgery: results of the 8 day laparoscopy in 188 patients. Fertil Steril 1985;43:395–400.
20. Nezhat CR, Nezhat FR, Luciano AA, et al. Laparoscopy. In: Nezhat CR, Nezhat FR, Luciano AA, Siegler Am, Metzger DA, Nezhat CH, eds. Operative Gynecologic Laparoscopy: Principles and Techniques. New York: McGraw-Hill, 1995: 79–96.
21. DeCherney AH. Laparoscopy with unexpected viscous penetration. In: Nichols DH, DeLancey JOL, eds. Clinical Problems, Injuries and Complication of Gynecologic Surgery. Baltimore: Williams & Wilkins, 1988:62–63.
22. Gurgan T, Kinisci H, Yarali H, et al. Evaluation of adhesion formation after laparoscopic treatment of polycystic ovarian disease. Fertil Steril 1991;56:1176–1178.
23. Gurgan T, Urman B, Yarali H. Adhesion formation and reformation after laparoscopic removal of ovarian endometriomas. J Am Assoc Gynecol Laparosc 1996;3: 389–392.
24. diZerega GS. Contemporary adhesion formation. Fertil Steril 1994;61:219–235.
25. Luciano AA, Hauser KS, Benda J. Evaluation of commonly used adjuvants in the prevention of postoperative adhesions. Am J Obstet Gynecol 1983;146:88–92.
26. Rosenberg SM, Board JA. High molecular weight dextran in human fertility surgery. Am J Obstet Gynecol 1984; 148:380–385.
27. diZerega GS, Hodger GD. Reduction of postoperative pelvic adhesions with intraperitoneal 32% dextran 70: a prospective randomized clinical trial. Fertil Steril 1983; 40:612–619.
28. Borten M, Seibert CP, Taymor ML. Recurrent anaphylactic reaction to intraperitoneal dextran 70 used for prevention of postsurgical adhesions. Obstet Gynecol 1983;61: 755–757.
29. Azziz R, INTERCEED Barrier Study Group. Microsurgery alone or with INTERCEED Absorbable Adhesion Barrier for pelvic sidewall adhesion reformation. Surg Gynecol Obstet 1993;177:135–139.
30. Sekiba K, Obstetrics and Gynecology Adhesion Prevention Committee. Use of Interceed (TC7) absorbable adhesion barrier to reduce postoperative adhesion reformation in infertility and endometriosis surgery. Obstet Gynecol 1992;79:518–522.
31. Franklin RR. Reduction of ovarian adhesions by the use of Interceed. Ovarian Adhesion Study Group. Obstet Gynecol 1995;86:335–340.
32. Keckstein J, Ulrich U, Sasse V, et al. Reduction of postoperative adhesion formation after laparoscopic ovarian cystectomy. Hum Reprod (Oxf) 1996;11:579–582.

33. Larsson B, Berg AA, Bryman I, et al. The efficacy of Interceed Absorbable Adhesion Barrier (TC7) for prevention of reformation postoperative adhesions on ovaries, fallopian tubes, and fimbriae in microsurgical operation for fertility. Fertil Steril 1995;63:709–714.
34. Haney AF, Hesla J, Hurst BS, et al. Expanded polytetrafluoroethylene (Gore-Tex Surgical Membrane) is superior to oxidized regenerated cellulose (Interceed TC7) in preventing adhesions. Fertil Steril 1995;63:1021–1026.
35. Diamond MP, Seprafilm Adhesions Study Group. Reduction of adhesions after uterine myomectomy by Seprafilm membrane (HAL-F): a blinded, prospective, randomized; multicenter clinical study. Fertil Steril 1996;66:904–910.
36. DeCherney AH, diZerega GS. Clinical problem of intraperitoneal postsurgical adhesion formation following general surgery and the use of adhesion prevention barriers. Surg Clin North Am 1997;77:671–688.
37. Becker JM, Dayton MT, Fazio VW, et al. Prevention of postoperative abdominal adhesions by a sodium hyaluronate-based bioresorbable membrane: A prospective, randomized, double-blind multicenter study. J Am Coll Surg 1996;183:297–306.
38. DeIaco PA, Stefanetti M, Pressato D, et al. A novel hyaluronan-based gel in laparoscopic adhesion prevention: preclinical evaluation in an animal model. Fertil Steril 1998; 69:318–323.
39. Cabarello J, Tulandi T. Effects of Ringer's lactate and fibrin glue on postsurgical adhesions. J Reprod Med 1992; 37:141–143.
40. Evrard VAC, De Bellis A, Boeckx W, et al. Peritoneal healing after fibrin glue application: a comparative study in a rat model. Hum Reprod (Oxf) 1996;11:1877–1880.
41. Vandendael A, Struwig D, Nel JT, et al. Efficacy of fibrin sealant in prevention of adhesion formation on ovarian surgical wounds in a rabbit mode. Gynaecol Endosc 1996; 5:169–172.
42. Takeuchi H, Awaji M, Hashimoto M, et al. Reduction of adhesions with fibrin glue after laparoscopic excision of large ovarian endometriomas. J Am Assoc Gynecol Laparosc 1996;4:575–579.
43. Ugur M, Turan C, Mungan T, et al. Laparoscopy for adhesion formation following myomectomy. Int J Gynecol Obstet 1996;53:145–149.
44. Raiga J, Canis M, Le Boudec G, et al. Laparoscopic management of adnexal abscesses: consequences for fertility. Fertil Steril 1996;66:712–717.
45. Savarelos HG, Li TC, Cooke ID. An analysis of the outcome of microsurgical and laparoscopic adhesiolysis for infertility. Hum Reprod (Oxf) 1995;10:2887–2894.

15

Role of Sutures and Suturing in the Formation of Postoperative Adhesions

Daniel P. O'Leary

CONTENTS

Adhesions and Surgery

Peritoneal adhesions mostly follow abdominal operations.[1,2] Menzies et al. observed that 93% of patients who had previously undergone a laparotomy had adhesions, compared with 10.4% of those with no history of abdominal surgery.[2] In an earlier study, among 1,477 patients requiring operation for adhesion obstruction of the small intestine, 86% had previously undergone an abdominal operation, mostly an appendicectomy or gynecological surgery.[3]

Factors that contribute to the formation of postoperative peritoneal adhesions include abrasive surgical trauma,[4] the presence of blood clot or foreign materials in the peritoneal cavity,[5,6] peritoneal ischaemia,[7] and infection.[8] Some of these factors appear to act synergistically.[5,8]

Peritoneal Suturing and Adhesions

Suturing peritoneum introduces a foreign material and implies a degree of trauma and potential for peritoneal ischaemia, factors known to promote adhesion formation. This chapter reviews the evidence concerning the need to suture peritoneum and the potential for inducing adhesions by doing so under four headings:

Healing of peritoneal defects: sutured and unsutured
Suturing the parietal peritoneum during abdominal wound closure
Incorporation of visceral peritoneum in suture lines
Use of prosthetic materials in hernia repair

Healing of Peritoneal Defects: Sutured and Unsutured

Historical Perspective

Surgical interventions often cause defects in the parietal peritoneum or deperitonealization of viscera, for example, after abdominoperineal resection of the rectum or pelvic exenteration. Traditionally, it has been assumed that peritoneal defects, like unsutured skin defects, heal from the edges inward with fibrotic scarring and that this results in adhesions.[9] Defects in parietal peritoneum have been sutured closed in the hope that this would reduce the likelihood of adhesions and the potential for small intestine obstruction caused by herniation through peritoneal defects or adhesion to the exposed raw surfaces.[9] Indeed, Smith estimated that 2% of postoperative deaths could be prevented by suturing peritoneal defects.[9] Several surgical texts perpetuate this approach by advising closure of peritoneal defects, such as after abdominoperineal resection.[10–12]

Current Concepts of Peritoneal Healing

In fact, healing of peritoneal defects is quite unlike healing of skin defects. More than a century ago von Dembowski reported that experimentally created parietal peritoneal defects that were left unsutured healed to form a smooth serosal layer without adhesions.[13] This report has been confirmed by numerous researchers[7,14–18] (Table 15.1). Similar observations have been made concerning defects in visceral peritoneum.[15,19–21] Although adhesions may form in relation to peritoneal defects (possibly because of injury to a second contiguous, peritoneal surface),[22] the predominant tendency is for peritoneal defects to regenerate a smooth serosa. Large defects heal as rapidly as small ones,[16,17,23,24] suggesting that healing is not dependent on ingrowth from the peritoneal edges. The new mesothelium appears to be formed from primitive mesenchymal cells from the deeper layers or from the peritoneal cavity.[17,24–26] In the case of parietal peritoneal defects the new mesothelium is macroscopically indistinguishable from the surrounding serosa by 7 days.[7,17]

Suturing Peritoneal Defects

In contrast to the healing of unsutured peritoneal defects, Thomas and Rhoads[19] and Singleton et al.[15] showed that suturing visceral peritoneal defects increased the incidence of adhesions. Hubbard et al. found that unsutured visceral peritoneal defects created in small intestinal serosa healed with a 30% incidence of adhesions, compared with 82% and 90% ($p < 0.001$) when sutured with silk or chromic catgut, respectively.[17]

Later, in an elegant series of experiments, Ellis created defects measuring from 1 × 1 cm to 2 × 3 cm in the parietal peritoneum of dogs.[7] Fifty-eight defects were left unsutured, among which 53 healed without adhesions within 1 week, only 5 (8.6%) forming adhesions. In contrast, among 19 similar defects sutured with fine silk, 16 (84.2%; $p < 0.01$) formed adhesions (Table 15.1).

TABLE 15.1. Healing of experimental defects in parietal peritoneum: sutured versus unsutured.

Reference	Peritoneum sutured adhesions/*n*	Peritoneum open adhesions/*n*	*p*
Singleton (1952)[15]	—	1/10	
Williams (1955)[16]	—	1/8	
Hubbard (1967)[17]	59/60	29/60	<0.01
Ellis (1962)[7]	16/19	5/58	<0.01
Raftery (1981)[18]	—	1/20	

Lengths of silk sutured loosely in the peritoneal layer did not promote adhesions, suggesting that adhesion formation resulted from suturing under tension rather than as a reaction to the suture material. Ellis proposed that the adhesions were a response to ischemia at the peritoneal edge.[7] Hubbard et al. investigated the effects of different suture materials and reported that parietal peritoneal defects in dogs healed with a 40% to 60% incidence of adhesions when left unsutured, compared with an incidence of 95% to 100% when sutured using chromic catgut or silk ($p < 0.001$).[17] A recent rigorous study of sutured parietal peritoneal defects has confirmed that suture materials induce adhesions in the order catgut > polyglactin > polypropylene, all differences being statistically significant.[27] Increasing the diameter of polyglactin sutures increased adhesion rates significantly.

Peritoneal Grafts

For completeness, one should consider the outcome of grafting peritoneal defects. Singleton et al. removed 1 cm × 1 cm squares of visceral peritoneum from dog ileum.[15] Patching the defects with peritoneum led to an increased incidence of adhesions compared with nonclosure. Two subsequent studies reported increased incidences of adhesions after autografting parietal peritoneal defects.[7,18] Raftery reported adhesions to 20 of 20 autografted parietal peritoneal defects in rats compared to only 1 of 20 defects left open ($p < 0.001$).[18] Experimental use of expanded polytetrafluoroethylene (ePTFE) membrane to close pelvic peritoneal defects after radical gynecologic resection has been found to increase adhesion scores (mean, 2.8) compared with nonclosure (mean 1.5; $p = 0.01$).[28]

Clinical Studies

Trimpi and Bacon observed a low (but unspecified) incidence of small intestinal obstruction in more than 500 patients in whom the pelvic peritoneum was left unsutured following rectal resection[29]; that is, exactly the reverse of that which was predicted by Smith in 1895.[9] Later, in a prospective randomized controlled trial Irvin and Goligher found no difference in the incidence of prolonged ileus, obstruction, or reoperation after proctectomy whether the pelvic peritoneum was sutured or left open.[30] Subsequent prospective randomized controlled trials have confirmed that suturing the (visceral) peritoneal edges of the gallbladder bed after cholecystectomy,[31] or the pelvic peritoneal defect after hysterectomy,[32,33] or after radical resection for ovarian carcinoma including pelvic and paraaortic lymphadenectomy[34] offers no advantages over nonsuture. Leaving the pelvic peritoneum open after hysterectomy does not increase rates of intestinal obstruction, lymphocyst formation,[33] or dyspareunia.[32] Moreover, Kadalani et al. performed "second-look" laparoscopy after radical resection for ovarian cancer and found significantly reduced adhesion scores in patients in whom the pelvic peritoneum had been left unsutured.[34]

Conclusions

Surgically created defects in visceral and parietal peritoneum are generally best left unsutured. This approach is based on sound experimental evidence and the results of numerous prospective randomized clinical trials.

Suturing the Parietal Peritoneum During Closure of Abdominal Wounds

Although the parietal peritoneum is thin and weak, suturing it has long been considered an important part of abdominal wound closure. Indeed, as one author put it "like eating peas off your knife, . . . failure to close the peritoneum of an abdominal incision seems at first sight to be a gross deviation from what is right and proper."[35] A recent questionnaire suggested that 86% of surgeons in the United Kingdom suture the peritoneal layer during closure of laparotomy wounds.[36]

Peritoneal Suturing and Healing

Experimental studies have shown that suturing the parietal peritoneum adds nothing to the strength of midline or paramedian wound closures (determined by the force necessary to disrupt the wound).[8,37,38] In humans, the effects of peritoneal suturing on the healing of abdominal wound have been evaluated in several prospective randomized controlled clinical trials (Table 15.2).[37,39–42] Ellis and Heddle observed no significant difference in wound dehiscence or incisional hernia rates between groups in which the peritoneum was sutured with chromic catgut or left unsutured during closure of paramedian and midline wounds.[37] These observations were confirmed for midline wounds,[39] lateral paramedian wounds,[40] Pfannenstiel wounds performed for infertility surgery,[41] and Kocher's wounds for cholecystectomy.[42] Hugh et al.[39] demonstrated that peritoneal suture or nonsuture produced no significant difference in postoperative pain scores or analgesic requirements. Three prospective randomized controlled trials have examined the need to suture the parietal peritoneum after cesarean section.[43–45] In-hospital morbidity including wound-related morbidity was similar whether the peritoneum was sutured or left open. Two of these trials reported increased requirements for parenteral[45] and oral narcotics[43] with peritoneal suture. Long-term incisional hernia rates are not reported in any of these studies but are unlikely to be influenced by peritoneal suture.[35]

A special case for peritoneal suturing may be made in patients with ascites and those undergoing peritoneal dialysis. Following laparotomy such patients require a closure that is leakproof as well as strong. Suturing the peritoneum may reduce leakage through the wound[41] and is advised in these circumstances.

Peritoneal Suturing and Adhesions

Among 210 patients undergoing repeat laparotomy, Menzies and Ellis reported adhesions between the old scar and omentum in 81% and between the old scar and small intestine in 20%.[2] It is likely that the peritoneum was sutured in the majority of these patients.[36] Suturing peritoneal defects promotes adhesions, possibly because suturing under tension induces ischemia.[7] However, it cannot be assumed that such a mechanism operates when incised peritoneum is sutured with less or no tension. Hubbard was probably first to suggest, with anecdotal evidence, that suturing the peritoneum during closure of a laparotomy wound might increase the incidence of adhesions compared with nonsuture.[17] The question was investigated formally by Conolly and Stephens.[46] After midline laparotomy, they found adhesions to abdominal wounds in 18 of 32 rats (56%) in which the peritoneum had been sutured with chromic catgut compared with only 5 of 24 (21%) when the peritoneum was left unsutured ($p < 0.01$). Subsequent animal experiments (Table 15.3) have confirmed a trend to increased adhesion formation when the peritoneum was sutured, which was statistically significant ($p < 0.05$) in three of five studies.[8,37,38,46,47] Two animal studies have evaluated the effect of more or less reactive suture materials on adhesion formation. Although the numbers involved were small, the incidence of adhesions to the scar

TABLE 15.2. Is it necessary to suture the parietal peritoneum after laparotomy? Results of prospective randomized clinical trials.

Suture	n	Dehiscence (%): sutured/open	Hernia (%): sutured/open	Reference
Midline and paramedian	138	2.5/3.0	4.3/4.3	Ellis (1977)[37]
Midline	185	0.0/1.0	1.0/1.0	Hugh (1990)[39]
Lateral paramedian	152	0.0/0.0	0.0/1.3	Gilbert (1987)[40]
Pfannenstiel	333	0.0/0.0	0.0/0.0	Tulandi (1988)[41]
Kocher's	129	3.0/1.6	4.5/3.2	Dorfman (1997)[42]

No significant differences were observed between sutured or nonsutured groups in any of these studies.

TABLE 15.3. Effect of suturing the parietal peritoneum on incidence of adhesions to the scar in animal models.

Reference	Peritoneum sutured (adhesions/n)	Peritoneum open (adhesions/n)	p
Conolly (1968)[46]	18/32	5/24	<0.01
Ellis (1977)[37]	4/11	3/12	NS
Kapur (1979)[38]	8/10	2/10	<0.05
Kyzer (1986)[47]	6/12	1/11	<0.05
O'Leary (1992)[8]	11/15	6/15	0.07

Peritoneal layer sutured with catgut or left unsutured ("open"). Results expressed as number of animals per group with adhesions to the scar.

was not significantly different whether the peritoneum was sutured with catgut or nylon.[8,38]

Clinical studies of the effect of peritoneal suturing on adhesion formation are restricted to patients undergoing second laparotomies or "second-look" laparoscopy (or autopsy). Tulandi et al. performed laparoscopy on women who had previously undergone infertility surgery by laparotomy.[41] Adhesions to the scar were noted in 14 of 63 (22%) of those in whom the parietal peritoneum had been sutured with catgut versus 9 of 57 (15.8%) where it had been left unsutured; however, the difference was not statistically significant.[41]

Suturing, Sepsis, and Adhesions

Suturing parietal peritoneum promotes a fibrinous inflammatory response[48] and perhaps increased adhesion formation.[8,38,46,47] Surgical trauma and peritonitis each depress peritoneal fibrinolytic activity.[4,49] The net result of these interactions might be increased adhesion formation if the peritoneum is sutured in the presence of sepsis. This possibility was tested in rats undergoing laparotomy after intraperitoneal inoculation with pure bacterial cultures or saline.[8] In animals that had received saline inoculum, the peritoneum was sutured with nylon and the incidence of adhesions to the laparotomy scar was 3 of 10. In contrast, in the presence of intraperitoneal infection the incidence of adhesions to the laparotomy scar was 8 of 9 when the peritoneum was sutured with nylon but only 2 of 10 when it was left unsutured ($p < 0.01$). Intraperitoneal infection, independent of a particulate or chemical irritant, proved to be a potent cause of adhesions. Moreover, suturing the peritoneum and sepsis appeared to act synergistically to promote adhesions to the scar.

Conclusions

Compelling evidence from clinical trials indicates that suturing the peritoneal layer is unnecessary during abdominal wound closure. Moreover, the incidence of adhesions to the scar is likely to be lowest when the peritoneum is not sutured during abdominal wound closure, especially in the presence of peritonitis.

Incorporation of Visceral Peritoneum in Sutures

Visceral peritoneum is invariably incorporated in sutured closures or anastomoses involving peritonealized parts of the gastrointestinal tract, for example, in gastric, biliary, and intestinal operations, and it may be incorporated in gynecologic closures also.

Peritoneal Suturing and Healing

In a limited number of operations, nonsuture of visceral peritoneum may be practical (and potentially beneficial). Gynecologists have reported that the uterus may be safely sutured after cesarean section without incorporating the visceral peritoneum.[43,45] In contrast, deliberate avoidance of the peritoneum during suture placement is not considered desirable or practical during anastomoses involving the gastrointestinal or biliary tracts. Indeed, the lack of a peritoneal layer may be one factor that contributes to the less reliable healing of esophageal and low rectal anastomoses. It is also often wise to suture mesenteric defects during intestinal resection to prevent small-bowel herniation and obstruction.[12] In these instances the benefit from suturing takes priority over potential for adhesion formation.

Peritoneal Suturing and Adhesions

Adhesions are common where visceral peritoneum is incorporated in suture lines, such as around intestinal or tubal anastomoses.[50–52] Experimentally, Glucksman[20] incised the terminal 10 cm of ileum down to the mucosa in 20 dogs. The incidence of adhesions was 10 of 10 among dogs where the incision was sutured with silk versus 0 of 10 where it was left unsutured ($p < 0.01$). Meyer et al. observed, following cautery incisions in the ovary, that the degree of envelopment in adhesions, and their vascularity, was significantly greater if the incisions had been sutured with polyglactin 910 than when they had been left unsutured.[53]

In infertility surgery, tubal or ovarian adhesions are unwanted. However, in the case of gastrointestinal anastomoses it has been suggested that adhesions around the anastomosis, especially those involving omentum, might provide an additional blood supply[7,54] and help to contain minor leakage or sepsis.[55] This argument is probably overstated.[56] In a large prospective randomized controlled trial ($n = 712$), deliberate attempts to produce an adhesive seal around large-bowel anastomoses by wrapping them in omentum did not decrease leak rates significantly (4.7% wrapped vs. 5.2% control).[57]

Suture Material and Adhesions

Gastrointestinal surgeons use a variety of suture techniques and suture materials for anastomoses. The effect of these differences on adhesion formation is largely unknown. The influence of suture material has been investigated in gynecologic surgery with conflicting results. Laufer et al. observed adhesions in 11 of 12 animals undergoing uterine horn repair with polyglactin 910 versus 5 of 12 ($p < 0.01$) when polydioxanone had been used.[58] Others have found no difference in the adhesiogenic response to these materials in a broadly similar model.[59,60] Definitive assessment of the effect of suture material is hindered by difficulty in adequately controlling other variables between and within studies. These factors include suture tightness and potential for ischemia, number of suture bites, mass of suture material implanted, and incidental trauma to adjacent viscera. Evidence from suturing peritoneal defects suggests that the more reactive suture materials are more likely to induce adhesions.[27] This effect is also likely to apply to visceral suturing.[61]

Alternatives to Sutures

Fibrin glue has been used to approximate tissues and to seal suture lines and peritoneal defects with variable success. Takeuchi et al. reported improved adhesion scores using fibrin glue to close ovarian defects versus historical controls (unclosed).[62] Use of fibrin to seal the serosal layer of tubal repairs does not appear to reduce adhesions at subsequent laparoscopy or improve fertility significantly compared with polyglactin sutures.[50] Fibrin "sealing" of sutured colonic anastomoses impairs anastomotic healing and promotes adhesions to the anastomosis significantly.[52,63] Fibrin glue is based on human blood products and prompts concerns about transmission of infectious agents.[64,65]

Evidence from a randomized controlled clinical trial suggests that the biofragmentable anastomosis ring (BAR) is a practical and competitive alternative to sutured or stapled colorectal anastomoses.[66] In dogs, the incidence of peritoneal adhesions involving colonic anastomoses was similar following anastomosis with either the BAR or interrupted silk sutures, but was significantly lower using a conventional intraluminal circular stapler.[51]

Lasers offer the possibility of anastomosis without strangling tissue or leaving foreign material. In a small experimental study, CO_2 laser-assisted or laser-welded fallopian tube anastomoses offered no advantages with regard to adhesion formation, healing, or patency compared to microsurgical anastomosis.[67] However, Kuramoto et al. observed a significant reduction in adhesions to colotomies repaired using Nd:YAG laser welding (5 of 15; $p < 0.05$) compared with interrupted 5-0 monofilament polyglyconate (11 of 15).[68] Laser-welded (Nd:YAG) colonic anastomoses had a lower initial bursting strength than anastomoses sutured with 5-0 monofilament polyglyconate, but this did not lead to leakage.[69] Adhesion rates and scores were lower after laser welding but not significantly so.

Ligatures are likely to promote adhesions more as a consequence of ischemia of the ligated tissue rather than the nature of the ligature.[70] Closure of the divided cystic duct with titanium or absorbable clips[71] or closure of the divided fallopian tube with clips or chromic catgut ligatures[70] produces no significant difference in adhesion rates.

Additional Measures to Prevent Adhesions

Factors promoting adhesion formation often work synergistically.[5,8] Other adhesiogenic influences should be avoided so as to minimize the effect of suturing, for example, gentle surgical technique, fine relatively nonreactive sutures and ligatures, trimming ligatures short, avoiding excess (ischemic) tissue beyond ligatures, using wet swabs to reduce peritoneal abrasion, and removing all blood and clot at the end of abdominal operations.[26,61] The omentum may be placed beneath laparotomy wounds to prevent potentially more troublesome adhesions between intestines and the scar. Some surgical trauma is inevitable at the operative site, but injury to other peritoneal surfaces should be minimized.[22] In gastrointestinal surgery, the efficacy of pharmacologic agents in preventing adhesions around anastomoses must be weighed against potential impairment of healing; several "barriers" and chemical prophylactics have been found to promote leakage from gastrointestinal anastomoses.[72,73]

Conclusions

Incorporation of visceral peritoneum in sutures promotes adhesions. Further, research is necessary to define optimal suture materials and the role of alternative tissue-approximating techniques, with the aim of achieving satisfactory tissue healing at suture lines without excessive adhesions.

Use of Prosthetic Mesh in Hernia Repair

Polypropylene mesh is commonly employed during laparoscopic repair of groin hernias. Exposed polypropylene mesh within the peritoneal cavity may become adherent to bowel, leading to intestinal erosion or obstruction.[74] Closing the peritoneum over the mesh or use of a totally extraperitoneal approach minimizes these complications and is recommended.[75,76] Alternative prosthetic mesh materials are under investigation for repair of incisional hernias. Relative rates of adhesion formation in response to these meshes are in the order polyglycolic acid > polypropylene > polytetrafluoroethylene "Dual Mesh" (PTFEDM) (Gore-DM; W.L. Gore & Associates, Flagstaff, AZ, USA).[77–79] Intraperitoneal PTFEDM leads to relatively low adhesion scores compared with other intraperitoneal meshes,[79,80] suggesting that this material may be advantageous when an intraperitoneal repair of incisional hernias is necessary.

Economic Considerations

Several prospective clinical trials indicate that considerable savings in operating times and costs may be achieved by omitting to suture peritoneal defects and the peritoneal layer of the abdominal closure.[43–45] In addition, nonsuture of peritoneum is likely to be associated with long-term economic benefits through reduced adhesion-related illness.

Summary

Suturing peritoneum promotes adhesions whereas unsutured peritoneal defects or incisions tend to heal without adhesions. Compelling evidence from rigorous clinical trials indicates that (1) surgically created peritoneal defects do not need to be sutured and (2) the peritoneal layer does not need to be sutured during laparotomy wound closure. Omission of peritoneal suturing will reduce the incidence of adhesions and should also reduce operating times and costs.

In some circumstances (e.g., uterine surgery) it may be possible and safe to avoid incorporating visceral peritoneum in sutures. However, it is impractical and undesirable to omit the visceral peritoneal layer from gastrointestinal anastomoses or closures. Future research should be directed toward methods of preventing adhesions in relation to such suture lines, or developing less adhesiogenic tissue approximation techniques.

Acknowledgment

This chapter includes some material previously published in O'Leary DP. Role of sutures and suturing in the formation of postoperative peritoneal adhesions. In: Treutner K-H, Schumpelick V, eds. Peritoneal Adhesions. Berlin: Springer-Verlag, 1997:111–120. Reproduced with permission from the publishers.

References

1. Weibel MA, Majno G. Peritoneal adhesions and their relation to abdominal surgery. Am J Surg 1973;126:345–353.
2. Menzies D, Ellis H. Intestinal obstruction from adhesions—how big is the problem? Ann R Coll Surg Engl 1990;72:60–63.
3. Raf LE. Causes of small intestinal obstruction: a study covering the Stockholm area. Acta Chir Scand 1969;135: 67–72.
4. Buckman RF, Woods M, Sargent L, et al. A unifying pathogenetic mechanism in the aetiology of intraperitoneal adhesions. J Surg Res 1976;20:1–5.
5. Ryan GB, Grobety J, Majno G. Postoperative peritoneal adhesions: a study of the mechanisms. Am J Pathol 1971; 65:117–138.
6. Saxen L, Myllarniemi H. Foreign materials and postoperative adhesions. N Engl J Med 1968;279:200–202.
7. Ellis H. The aetiology of post-operative abdominal adhesions. An experimental study. Br J Surg 1962;50:10–16.
8. O'Leary DP, Coakley JB. The influence of suturing and sepsis on the development of postoperative peritoneal adhesions. Ann R Coll Surg Engl 1992;74:134–137.
9. Smith JG. Is the apposition of peritoneum to peritoneum a surgical error? Br Med J 1895;1:1–2.
10. Zollinger RM, Zollinger RM. Abdominoperineal resection. In Atlas of Surgical operations, 6th Ed. New York: Macmillan, 1988:144–155.
11. Williams NS. Surgical treatment of rectal carcinoma. In: Keighley MR, Williams NS, eds. Surgery of the Anus, Rectum and Colon. London: Saunders, 1993:939–1053.
12. Hawley PR, Thomson JPS. Colon. In: Kirk RM, ed. General Surgical Operations, 3rd Ed. Edinburgh: Churchill Livingstone, 1994:271–295.
13. von Dembowski T. Ueber die ursachen der peritonealen adhasionen nach chirurgischen eingriffen mit rucksicht auf die frage des ileus nach laparotomien. Arch Klin Chir 1888;37:745–748.
14. Robbins GF, Brunschwig A, Foote FW. Deperitonealization: clinical and experimental observations. Ann Surg 1949;130:466–470.
15. Singleton AO, Rowe EB, Moore RM. Failure of reperitonealization to prevent abdominal adhesions in the dog. Am J Surg 1952;18:789–792.
16. Williams DC. The peritoneum. A plea for change in attitude towards this membrane. Br J Surg 1955;42:401–405.
17. Hubbard TB, Khan MZ, Carag VR, et al. The pathology of peritoneal repair: its relation to the formation of adhesions. Ann Surg 1967;165:908–916.
18. Raftery AT. Effect of peritoneal trauma on peritoneal fibrinolytic activity and intraperitoneal adhesion formation: an experimental study in the rat. Eur Surg Res 1981;13: 397–401.
19. Thomas JW, Rhoads JE. Adhesions resulting from removal of serosa from an area of bowel; failure of oversewing to lower incidence in the rat and guinea pig. Arch Surg 1950; 61:565–576.
20. Glucksman DL. Serosal integrity and intestinal adhesions. Surgery (St. Louis) 1966;60:1009–1011.
21. Raftery AT. Regeneration of parietal and visceral peritoneum. Br J Surg 1973;60:293–299.
22. Haney AF, Doty E. The formation of coalescing peritoneal adhesions requires injury to both contacting peritoneal surfaces. Fertil Steril 1994;61:767–775.
23. Hertzler AE. The Peritoneum. St. Louis: Mosby, 1919.
24. Ellis H, Harrison W, Hugh TB. The healing of peritoneum under normal and pathological conditions. Br J Surg 1965;52:471–476.
25. Raftery AT. Regeneration of parietal and visceral peritoneum: an electron microscopic study. J Anat 1973;115: 375–392.

26. di Zerega GS. Contemporary adhesion prevention. Fertil Steril 1994;61:219–235.
27. Bakkum EA, Dalmeijer RA, Verdel MJ, et al. Quantitative analysis of the inflammatory reaction surrounding sutures commonly used in operative procedures and the relation to postsurgical adhesion formation. Biomaterials 1995; 16:1283–1289.
28. Fowler JM, Lacy SM, Montz FJ. The inability of Gore-Tex Surgical Membrane to inhibit post-radical pelvic surgery adhesions in the dog model. Gynecol Oncol 1991;43: 141–144.
29. Trimpi HD, Bacon HE. Clinical and experimental study of denuded surfaces in extensive surgery of the colon and rectum. Am J Surg 1952;34:596–602.
30. Irvin TT, Goligher JC. A controlled clinical trial of three different methods of perineal wound management following excision of the rectum. Br J Surg 1975;62:287–291.
31. Mok SD, Li AKC. Is reperitonealization of the gallbladder bed a ritual or necessity? Am J Surg 1989;157:312–314.
32. Lipscomb GH, Ling FW, Stovall TG, et al. Peritoneal closure at vaginal hysterectomy: a reassessment. Obstet Gynecol 1996;87:40–43.
33. Franchi M, Ghezzi F, Zanaboni F, et al. Nonclosure of peritoneum at radical abdominal hysterectomy and pelvic node dissection: a randomized trial. Obstet Gynecol 1997;90:622–627.
34. Kadalani S, Erten O, Kucukozkan T. Pelvic and periaortic peritoneal closure or non-closure at lymphadenectomy in ovarian cancer: effects on morbidity and adhesion formation. Eur J Surg Oncol 1996;22:282–285.
35. Anonymous. Why suture the peritoneum? Lancet 1987; 1:727.
36. Scott-Coombes DM, Vipond MN, Thompson JN. General surgeons attitudes to the treatment and prevention of abdominal adhesions. Ann R Coll Surg Engl 1993;75: 123–128.
37. Ellis H, Heddle R. Does the peritoneum need to be closed at laparotomy? Br J Surg 1977;64:733–736.
38. Kapur BM, Daneswar A, Chopra P. Evaluation of peritoneal closure at laparotomy. Am J Surg 1979;137:650–652.
39. Hugh TB, Nankivell C, Meagher AP, et al. Is closure of the peritoneal layer necessary in the repair of midline surgical abdominal wounds? World J Surg 1990;14:231–234.
40. Gilbert JM, Ellis H, Foweraker S. Peritoneal closure after lateral paramedian incision. Br J Surg 1987;74: 113–115.
41. Tulandi T, Hum HS, Gelfand MM. Closure of laparotomy incisions with or without peritoneal suturing and second-look laparoscopy. Am J Obstet Gynecol 1988;158:636–537.
42. Dorfman S, Rincon A, Shortt H. Cholecystectomy via Kocher incision without peritoneal closure. Invest Clin 1997;38:3–7.
43. Hull DB, Varner MW. A randomized study of closure of the peritoneum at Cesarean delivery. Obstet Gynecol 1991;77:818–821.
44. Pietrantoni M, Parsons MT, O'Brien WF, et al. Peritoneal closure or nonclosure at Cesarean. Obstet Gynecol 1991; 77:293–296.
45. Ohel G, Younis JS, Lang N, et al. Double-layer closure of uterine incision with visceral and parietal peritoneal closure: are they obligatory steps of routine Cesarean sections? J Mat Fet Med 1996;5:366–369.
46. Conolly WB, Stephens FO. Factors influencing the incidence of intraperitoneal adhesions: an experimental study, Surgery (St. Louis) 1968;63:976–979.
47. Kyzer S, Bayer I, Turani H, et al. The influence of peritoneal closure on formation of intraperitoneal adhesions: an experimental study. Int J Tissue React 1986;8:355–359.
48. O'Leary DP. Studies on the development of peritoneal adhesions. B.Sc. dissertation. Dublin: National University of Ireland, 1984: 12–17.
49. van Goor H, de Graaf JS, Grond J, et al. Fibrinolytic activity in the abdominal cavity of rats with faecal peritonitis. Br J Surg 1994;81:1046–1049.
50. Tulandi T. Effects of fibrin sealant on tubal anastomosis and adhesion formation. Fertil Steril 1991;56:136–138.
51. Bundy CA, Zera RT, Onstad GA, et al. Comparative surgical and colonoscopic appearance of colon anastomoses constructed with sutures, staples and the biofragmentable anastomotic ring. Surg Endosc 1992;6:18–22.
52. Byrne DJ, Hardy J, Wood RA, et al. Adverse influence of fibrin sealant on the healing of high-risk sutured colonic anastomoses. J R Coll Surg Edinb 1992;37:394–398.
53. Meyer WR, Grainger DA, DeCherney AH, et al. Ovarian surgery on the rabbit. Effect of cortex closure on adhesion formation and ovarian function. J Reprod Med 1991; 36:639–643.
54. McLachlin AD, Olsson LS, Pitt DF. Anterior anastomosis of the rectosigmoid colon: an experimental study. Surgery (St. Louis) 1976;80:306–311.
55. Morison R. Remarks on some functions of the omentum. Br Med J 1906;1:76–78.
56. O'Leary DP. Use of the greater omentum in colorectal surgery. Dis Colon Rectum 1999;42:533–539.
57. Merad F, Hay J-M, Fingerhut A, et al. Omentoplasty in the prevention of leakage after colonic or rectal resection. Ann Surg 1998;227:179–186.
58. Laufer N, Merino M, Trietsch HG, et al. Macroscopic and histological reaction to polydioxanone, a new synthetic monofilament microsuture. J Reprod Med 1984;29: 307–310.
59. Neff MR, Holtz GL, Betsill WL. Adhesion formation and histologic reaction with polydioxanone and polyglactin suture. Am J Obstet Gynecol 1985;151:20–23.
60. Scoccia B, Fortress K, Marcovici I, et al. Histology and fertility effects of polydioxanone on rat reproductive tissue. Eur J Obstet Gynecol Reprod Biol 1992;44:151–156.
61. Diamond MP, Schwartz LB. Prevention of adhesion development. In: Sutton C, Diamond M, eds. Endoscopic Surgery for Gynecologists, 2nd Ed. London: Saunders, 1998:398–403.
62. Takeuchi H, Awaji M, Hashimoto M, et al. Reduction of adhesions with fibrin glue after laparoscopic excision of large ovarian enometriomas. J Am Assoc Gynecol Laparosc 1996;3:575–579.
63. van der Ham AC, Kort WJ, Weijma IM, et al. Effect of fibrin sealant on the healing colonic anastomosis in the rat. Br J Surg 1991;78:49–53.
64. Jack D. Sticky situations: surgical adhesions and adhesives. Lancet 1998;351:118.

65. Tulandi T. How can we avoid adhesions after laparoscopic surgery? Curr Opin Obstet Gynecol 1997;9:239–243.
66. Bubrick MP, Corman ML, Cahill CJ, et al. Prospective randomized trial of the biofragmentable anastomosis ring. Am J Surg 1991;161:136–142.
67. Kao WL, Giles HR. Comparison of laser-assisted anastomosis, laser welding and microsurgical anastomosis of rabbit uterine tubes. Obstet Gynecol 1993;81:122–126.
68. Kuramoto S, Ryan P. First sutureless closure of a colotomy: short-term results of experimental laser anastomosis of the colon. Dis Colon Rectum 1991;34:1079–1084.
69. Kawahara M, Kuramoto S, Ryan P, et al. First experimental sutureless laser anastomosis of the large bowel. Dis Colon Rectum 1996;39:556–561.
70. Grainger DA, Meyer WR, DeCherney AH, et al. Laparoscopic clips. Evaluation of absorbable and titanium with regard to hemostasis and tissue reactivity. J Reprod Med 1991;36:493–495.
71. Klein RD, Jessup G, Ahari F, et al. Comparison of titanium and absorbable polymeric surgical clips for use in laparoscopic cholecystectomy. Surg Endosc 1994;8:753–758.
72. Laufman H, Method H. Effect of absorbable foreign substances on bowel anastomoses. Surg Gynecol Obstet 1948; 86:669–673.
73. Snoj M, Ar'Rajab A, Ahren B, et al. Effect of phosphatidylcholine on postoperative adhesions after small bowel anastomosis in the rat. Br J Surg 1992;79:427–429.
74. Liem MS, van Vroonhoven JM. Laparoscopic inguinal hernia repair. Br J Surg 1996;83:1197–1204.
75. McKernan JB, Laws HL. Laparoscopic repair of inguinal hernias using a totally extraperitoneal prosthetic approach. Surg Endosc 1993;7:26–28.
76. Vader VL, Vogt DM, Zucker KA, et al. Adhesion formation in laparoscopic inguinal hernia repair. Surg Endosc 1997; 11:825–829.
77. Baykal A, Onat D, Rasa K, et al. Effects of polyglycolic acid and polypropylene meshes on postoperative adhesion formation in mice. World J Surg 1997;21:579–582.
78. Bellon JM, Contreras LA, Bujan J, et al. The use of biomaterials in the repair of abdominal wall defects: a comparative study between polypropylene mesh (Marlex) and a new polytetrafluoroethylene prosthesis (Dual Mesh). J Biomater Appl 1997;12:121–135.
79. LeBlanc KA. Two-phase in vivo comparison studies of the tissue response to polypropylene, polyester, and expanded polytetrafluoroethylene grafts used in the repair of abdominal wall defects. In: Treutner K-H, Schumpelick V, eds. Peritoneal Adhesions. Berlin: Springer, 1997: 352–362.
80. Christoforoni PM, Kim YB, Preys Z, et al. Adhesion formation after incisional hernia repair: a randomized porcine trial. Am Surg 1996;62:935–938.

16

Pollutants Resulting from Intraabdominal Tissue Combustion

Douglas E. Ott

CONTENTS

Chemical changes occurring in the abdominal cavity can have direct effects by contact or through peritoneal absorption. Local and global homeostasis is influenced by the unique chemical circumstances of each event. Through its large surface area and proficient absorptive capacity, the peritoneum sustains normal physiologic activities and transfers large quantities of substances that can range from normal constituents to noxious toxins. Laparoscopy exposes the peritoneum to rapid stretching, sustained pressure, a gaseous distending medium, and the changes that occur within the abdominal cavity as a result of access, gas delivery, surgery, irrigation, instrumentation, and energy sources. Electrosurgery, laser, or harmonic scalpel devices used for their desired intentional tissue effects (vaporization, ablation, and coagulation) also can have unintended consequences: aerosol production, dissipation of straying energy, and unintended tissue injury.

Bioaerosol

The bioaerosol produced by these energy devices is composed of chemicals, blood, blood by-products, and particulates produced from tissue disruption and pyrolysis. The aerosol concentration, length of exposure, and abdominal pressure influence the peritoneum cells directly and communicate via transport with the vascular system changes that occur in the intraabdominal environment. The consequences of chemical and particulate production from tissue pyrolysis have direct and indirect effects on the peritoneum and peritoneal fluid composition; pyrolysis is an exposure consistent with smoke poisoning. Data show that patients undergoing laparoscopic procedures are exposed acutely to high levels of chemicals that have toxicologic significance. The effects of peritoneal exposure to chemicals and particles from tissue combustion during laparoscopy, its effects on the peritoneum, and the hematologic significance are neither well understood nor appreciated.

The smoke produced from human tissue combustion is a heterogeneous aerosol as a result of complete and incomplete combustion. The aerosol composition is a gas phase in which particulate matter is dispersed. This aerosol contains particles, gases, mutagens, carcinogens, and, if microbes are present, foreign DNA constituents. Smoke produced in an "open" environment (laparotomy) exerts its effects primarily through inhalation and the respiratory tract.[1,2] Smoke generated in the "closed" peritoneal cavity (laparoscopy) has specific tissue consequences and toxic hematologic significance. During combustion, tissue temperatures can reach 400°C, causing thermal decomposition (pyrolysis) and producing cellular fragments, stable chemicals, unstable chemical radicals, and elemental forms. During this process volatile substances are distilled directly into the smoke.

Recombination of these chemicals in the presence of intense heat is the process of pyrosynthesis, which allows

TABLE 16.1. Toxic chemical products resulting from pyrolysis of tissue protein and lipids.

Acrolein	Creosols	Phenol
Acetonitrile	Ethane	PAHs
Acrylonitrile	Ethene	Propene
Acetylene	Ethylene	Propylene
Alkyl benzenes	Formaldehyde	Pyridene
Benzene	Free radicals	Pyrrole
Butadiene	Hydrogen cyanide	Styrene
Butene	Isobutene	Toluene
Carbon monoxide	Methane	Xylene

molecules to combine to form and reform compounds that were originally present in the tissue or to form new compounds. This toxic chemical aerosol exposure is absorbed through the peritoneum and has local and hematologic effects. Macrophages are affected, and elevation of methemoglobin (metHb) and carboxyhemoglobin (COHb) levels represent a laparoscopic-induced hemoglobinopathy.[3, 4]

Ninety percent of the total weight of the smoke formed from tissue cauterization is in the gas phase. Most of the gases are nitrogen, oxygen, and carbon dioxide. The remaining gases and particulate matter can have toxicologic significance. Most of these substances are physiologically reactive and have local and systemic effects. Table 16.1 lists the toxic chemical products that result from the pyrolysis to tissue proteins and lipids.[3, 5] The volume of tissue mass that represents the residual of combustion and vaporization of 1 g of tissue is 284 mg; the remainder represents the change to aerosol and gaseous elements. The aerosol contains 0.3 to 3.3×10^9 particles per cubic centimeter of tissue vaporized, with a mean particulate size of 0.2 to 0.5 μm. This disrupted cellular debris becomes foreign material that must be cleared from the peritoneal cavity by macrophages, peritoneal fluid dynamics, and scavenging mechanisms.

Carbon Monoxide

Carbon monoxide (CO) is colorless, odorless, nonirritating, and tasteless gas that is produced by incomplete combustion of organic material and characterized as a toxic chemical asphyxiant.[6] High levels of CO are produced during tissue combustion during laparoscopy.[7] Two minutes after initiation of tissue combustion, the median CO concentration of the pneumoperitoneum increases to more than 425 parts per million (ppm) and ranges from 115 to 2100 ppm. The combined effects of concentration and length of exposure determine the cellular and systemic consequences of CO. The National Institute for Occupational Safety and Health (NIOSH) classifies CO as one of six pollutant categories established by the U.S. Environmental Protection Agency (EPA).[8,9] The Occupational Safety and Health Administration (OSHA) has established a danger level for CO of 50 ppm for 8 hours or an allowed accumulation of COHb level of 8%.[7–9] The EPA has established a goal of keeping danger levels of COHb for nonsmoking persons below 2%. This guideline allows a 1-hour mean maximum exposure of 35 ppm with a ceiling concentration of 200 ppm. The normal background level of COHb in a nonsmoking person is less than 1%. Normal metabolism generates a COHb level of 0.4%.[10] In contrast, a one-pack-a-day cigarette smoker has a COHb level of 5%[10] (Table 16.2).

Absorption of CO causes an acute pathophysiologic change that results in altered oxygen affinity. A predominant characteristic of CO is its affinity for hemoglobin (Hb) over oxygen by a factor of 200- to 240 fold and is defined by the Haldane equation. Thus, CO will combine with the same amount of Hb as oxygen when the CO partial pressure is 200 to 240 times lower. Because of the higher affinity of CO for Hb, exposures to low concentrations of CO cause significant COHb formation and accumulation. The CO competes with oxygen for the central iron-porphyrin-binding site of Hb. CO impairs oxygen transport and interferes with the release of oxygen from the Hb molecule, resulting in cellular hypoxia or anoxia. The Hb molecule has no intrinsic mechanism to distinguish between oxygen and CO. Therefore, adverse effects occur by limiting the amount of available oxyhemoglobin (oxyHb) because CO occupies Hb-binding sites.

Methemoglobin

Smoke absorbed via the peritoneum has also shown statistically significant elevation of metHb levels. Nearly 90 compounds are implicated in the production of MetHb,[11–13] some of which are the result of incomplete combustion of carbon-based materials. It has been shown that small but significant quantities of toxic and carcinogenic chemicals are produced by laser irradiation of tissue or electrocautery.[14] Levels of metHb compared to control patients at laparoscopy show that 76% of pa-

TABLE 16.2. Carbon monoxide threshold limit concentrations recommended by regulatory organizations and carbon monoxide concentrations found during typical surgery using laser or cautery.

	ppm
NAAQS limiting average/hour × 8	9
EPA 1 h mean maximum exposure	35
OSHA danger level	50
EPA 1 h ceiling concentration	200
Study 2 min mean	425
Study maximum concentration	2,100

tients have significant elevation at 5 minutes and 100% of patients have a statistically significant elevation at 30 minutes. Postoperatively, 64% of patients show a return to preoperative levels within 60 minutes.

Methemoglobin is the oxidative product of hemoglobin in which the reduced ferrous (Fe^{2+}) form has been converted to the ferric (Fe^{3+}) form. The difference between metHb and oxyHb in the ferric state is that metHb is formed from unoxygenated hemoglobin and is not capable of carrying either oxygen or carbon dioxide. Therefore, metHb cannot carry oxygen to tissues. Methemoglobin also decreases the oxygen affinity of the remaining normal hemoglobin by shifting the oxyHb dissociation curve to the left and further inhibiting oxygen delivery to tissues.[15] The body normally maintains a metHb level of less than 1%.[16,17] The specific chemical or component of the smoke that influences the acute metHb elevation is not known.

Methemoglobin is controlled by four mechanisms or systems to maintain levels below 1%: two are enzymatic and two act directly. The two enzymatic systems are (1) nicotine adenine dinucleotide-dependent metHb reductase (NADH-methemoglobin reductase), accounting for 67% of the in vivo reduction of metHb,[18] and (2) nicotinamide adenine dinucleotide phosphate (NADPH) - dependent metHb reductase, which is responsible for 5% of the in vivo reduction of meHb.[19] Of the two nonenzymatic mechanisms of metHb reduction, NADPH can directly regenerate reduced glutathione, which reduces metHb; this pathway accounts for 15% of the in vivo conversion. Second, an ascorbate pathway reaction clears about 12% of the endogenous metHb.[20]

Toxicity

Findings suggest that CO and metHb are independent variables and that metHb is related to specific products of combustion.[21] This smoke is toxic and dangerous. It is suspected that the variability in time to demonstrate an effect of metHb elevation caused by smoke absorption followed by a return to baseline is because the total amount of tissue combustion and resultant smoke production is user dependent.

Smoke from human tissue combustion contains components found in cigarette smoke: potent ciliotoxins, irritants, carcinogens, and impaired oxygen transport. The shared toxic materials of cigarette smoke and human tissue smoke are polynuclear aromatic hydrocarbons, creosol and phenol in the particulate phase, and hydrogen cyanide, acrolein, formaldehyde, and carbon monoxide in the gas phase[15] (Table 16.3).

A concentration of 10 ppm of CO produces a COHb of 2%; a 25-ppm exposure results in 4% saturation.[17,22] Carboxyhemoglobin levels between 5% and 10% cause acceleration of coronary artery blood flow and myocardial changes when greater than 6%.[23] Hemoglobin concentration and PO_2 may be normal, but the oxygen content under these conditions is grossly reduced. Elevation and detection of elevated COHb with tissue combustion at laparoscopy is acute and significant. The peak concentrations of CO observed during one study was equivalent to 6 times that of a cigarette smoker and 60 times the EPA 1-hour standard exposure limit recommendation of 35 ppm.

Table 16.3. Shared toxic components from human tissue combustion and cigarette smoke.

Particulate phase	Gas phase
Polynuclear aromatic hydrocarbon	Hydrogen cyanide
Creosol	Acrolein
Phenol	Formaldehyde
	Carbon monoxide

Manifestations of CO poisoning are protean, including headache, tinnitus, shortness of breath, lower extremity weakness, dyspnea, impaired judgment, clumsiness, palpitations, chest pain, abdominal pain, diarrhea, nausea, and vomiting. These effects are commonly seen postoperative symptoms in patients who have had tissue combustion during laparoscopy (Table 16.4).

Intraabdominal laparoscopic gas should be evacuated to maintain a clear field of vision and to remove products of combustion, using a dedicated gas evacuation system or suction irrigation device. Gas should never be released through a trocar directly into the operating room. Abdominal decompression for any purpose should be done using a smoke evacuator or wall suction to prevent pressurized spraying of body fluids and the toxic products of tissue combustion. Inappropriate release spews these materials under pressure into the operating room, a potential hazard to healthcare workers.

The increase in CO concentration during laparoscopic tissue combustion can be masked by general anesthesia and therapeutic agents introduced during the pre-, intra-, and postoperative recovery phases. The effects of peritoneal cavity exposure to CO are determined by the concentration in the confined abdominal space, frequency of smoke evacuation, duration of the procedure, individual oxygen requirements, degree of exertion during the exposure, and Hb concentration. CO reduces maximal oxygen consumption by the same percentage as the percentage of Hb bound by CO.[24,25] Arterial blood gases in the presence of CO have normal PO_2, decreased

Table 16.4. Manifestations of CO poisoning.

Headache	Impaired judgment
Tinnitus	Clumsiness
Shortness of breath	Nausea
Lower-extremity weakness	Vomiting
Dyspnea	

oxygen saturation, and normal to slightly decreased PCO_2. There is a shift to the left caused by CO that allows Hb to reach saturation at a lower partial pressure of oxygen. The high-affinity Hb variant produced, COHb, is associated with a lower than normal P_{50} value.

Combustion processes that occur in low-oxygen environments are characterized by elevated CO emissions,[26] which defines the laparoscopic tissue combustion circumstance. Limiting average CO exposure during laparoscopic tissue pyrolysis is necessary to reduce patient exposure from an iatrogenic hemoglobinopathy. The half-life of COHb is 5.33 hours at rest in room air. Using a face mask with 100% oxygen, the COHb half-life is 80 to 90 minutes.[10,17] Because oxygen toxicity can occur by breathing 100% oxygen for 2 hours, an intermittent breathing sample estimate of COHb is necessary.[27,28]

Absorption

Absorption of the products and by-products of pyrolysis via the peritoneum changes peritoneal cell diffusion characteristics, affects local tissue oxygenation, and causes an induced hemoglobinopathy. The effects of metHb and COHb include (1) chemical concentration of the specific tissue combustion chemical in the confined abdominal cavity resulting from tissue combustion, (2) duration of exposure, (3) rate of respiratory ventilation, (4) blood volume, (5) Hb concentration, (6) chemical diffusibility of the offering substance through the peritoneum, (7) rate of tissue combustion, and (8) volume of tissue thermally transformed.

Simultaneously measured pulse oximetry and arterial blood gas findings show a significant lack of correlation during laparoscopic procedures when tissue combustion occurs. Pulse oximetry levels were in the normal range compared to simultaneously timed arterial sample values that were significantly lower. Pulse oximetry manufactures warn about the limitation of pulse oximetry in the presence of CO. Pulse oximeters measure oxygen saturation and relate to PaO_2 by the oxyHb dissociation curve. The sensors combine COHb with oxyHb readings, resulting in a single data point. Studies show that pulse oximeter readings consistently overestimate oxygen saturation in the presence of COHb.[29] At 940 nm, COHb has minimal light absorption and at 660 nm, its absorption coefficient is very similar to oxyHb. Therefore, the two-wavelength oximeter interprets COHb and oxyHb as oxyHb and overestimates the oxyHb content.[30]

The device calculates the ratio of the transmitted intensities of the two wavelengths, creating an absorbance signal. This signal is presumed to reflect changes in the ratio of the absorbance of the two wavelengths and estimates an arterial saturation. The relationship between absorbance and arterial saturation is empirically based using data measured on healthy awake volunteers who had normal levels of COHb and metHb breathing hypoxic gas mixtures. In the presence of COHb, arterial saturation overestimates fractional saturation virtually proportional to COHb concentration. Using a pulse oximetry nomogram reference data does not include COHb exposure. Using a pulse oximeter usually overestimates the oxygen saturation in the presence of metHb and a diminished response to changes in oxygen saturation when metHb is present.[31,32]

The limitation of pulse oximetry to screen for intraoperative absorption of CO through the peritoneum, leading to COHb formation as a result of tissue combustion during laparoscopy requires awareness and vigilance. The liability of surgical smoke absorption is unrecognized hypoxia and induced hemoglobinopathy.

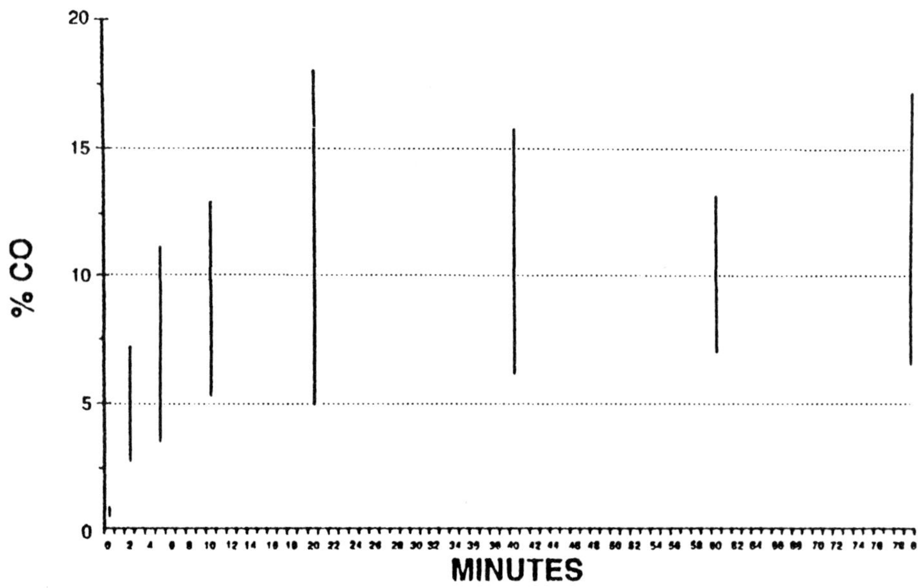

FIG. 16.1. Pre-operative and intraoperative carboxyhemoglobin levels resulting from peritoneal absorption of carbon monoxide.

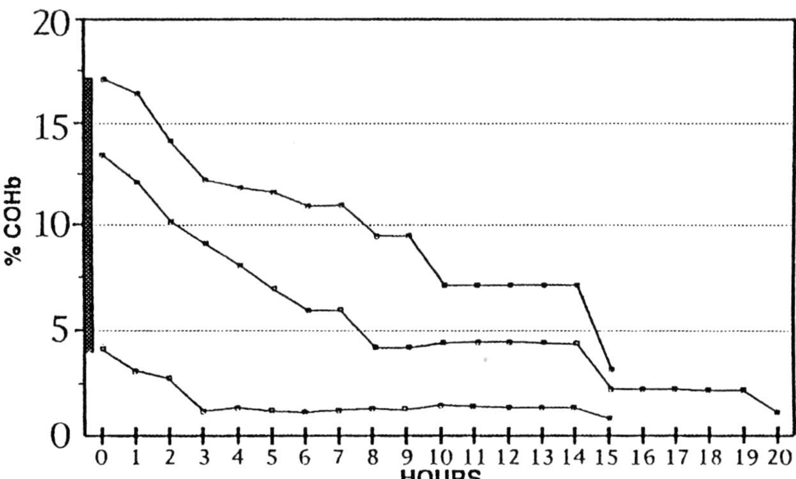

FIG. 16.2. Post-operative carboxyheoglobin levels.

Significant hypoxia is underestimated and unrecognized during laparoscopic tissue combustion exposures. Patient safety is compromised because of the coincident elevation of metHb and COHb during peritoneal smoke exposure and the inability of pulse oximetry surveillance to adequately recognize the extent of the resultant Hb changes.

Laparoscopic smoke poisoning is a chemical injury that occurs because of tissue combustion. The products of combustion when absorbed via the respiratory tract have direct systemic effects from the particulates and chemicals in the smoke. A clinical diagnosis of respiratory CO poisoning, a major component of smoke poisoning, is made by COHb determinations.[33] Systemically elevated metHb levels result in methemoglobinemia via peritoneal absorption of tissue combustion.[3] These occurrences are the result of an acute toxicologic change directly related to smoke absorption through the peritoneum. Because CO is a by-product of incomplete combustion of carbon-containing material, it is probable that elevated COHb levels should be found in blood as the result of intraabdominal tissue pyrolysis.

Carboxyhemoglobin levels ranged from 2.8 to 18.5 mg% and were elevated for as long as 16 hours after the conclusion of the procedure (Figs. 16.1 and 16.2). Patients with the highest levels postoperatively had prolonged CO poisoning symptoms of dizziness, nausea, headache, and weakness.

Summary

The importance of these findings is that smoke generated in the peritoneal cavity is absorbed and has toxicologic effects. Appropriate use of energy source instruments, their tissue effects, length of time used, and smoke removal must be appropriately controlled. Prompt, continuous, or intermittent removal of the products of tissue combustion is necessary to reduce the hazards from peritoneal smoke exposure during laparoscopy. Removal of the smoke should be coupled with correct parameter use of these devices to ensure the desired thermal effect and minimize the amount of smoke production. The change of the normal Hb:metHb ratio and formation of COHb by absorption of smoke through the peritoneal cavity leads to an induced hemoglobinopathy, a lack of correlation of pulse oximetry, and blood oxygen saturation evaluations, and establishes the toxicity and hazard of smoke at laparoscopy.

References

1. Frietag L, Chapman GA, Sielczak M, Ahmed A, Russin D. Laser smoke effect on bronchial system. Lasers Surg Med 1988;7:283–288.
2. Baggish MS, Elbakry M. The effects of laser smoke on the lungs of rats. Am J Obstet Gynecol 1987;156:1260–1265.
3. Ott DE. Smoke production and smoke reduction in endoscopic surgery: preliminary report. Endosc Surg 1993;1: 230–232.
4. Ott De. Carboxyhemoglobinemia due to peritoneal smoke absorption from laser tissue combustion at laparoscopy. J Clin Laser Med Surg 1998;16(6):309–315.
5. Kokasa JM, Eugene J. Chemical composition of laser-tissue interaction smoke plume. J Laser Appl 1989;1:59–63.
6. Kurt TL. Chemical Asphyxiants in Environmental and Occupational Medicine, 2nd Ed. New York: William N. Rom, 1996.
7. Beebe DS, Swica H, Carlson N, Palahniuk RJ, Goodale RL. High levels of carbon monoxide are produced by electrocautery of tissue during laparoscopic cholecystectomy. Anesth Analg 1993;77:338–341.
8. Environmental Protection Agency Environmental Assessment and Criteria Office. Air Quality Criteria for Carbon Monoxide. Washington, DC: EPA, 1979.
9. National Institute for Occupational Safety and Health. Occupational Exposure to Carbon Monoxide. DHEW Publ. NIOSH 73–110. Washington, DC: U.S. Government Printing Office, 1973.

10. Fraser RA, Pare JAP. Inhalation diseases caused by noxious gases and soluble aerosols. In: Diagnosis of Diseases of the Chest, Vol. 3. Philadelphia: Saunders, 1977:1529–1550.
11. Cartwright GE. Methomoglobin and sulfhemoglobin. In: Harrison TR, ed. Principles of Internal Medicine, 8th Ed. New York: McGraw-Hill, 1977:1710–1713.
12. Darling RC, Roughton FJW. The effect of methomoglobin on the equilibrium between oxygen and hemoglobin. Am J Physiol 1942;137:56–68.
13. Smith RP, Olson MV. Drug-induced methemoglobinemia. Semin Hematol 1973;10:253–268.
14. Mihashi W, Ueda S, Hirano M, Tomita Y, Hirohata T. Some problems about condensates induced by CO_2 laser irradiation. In: Proceedings of the 4th Congress of the International Society for Laser Surgery, Tokyo, Japan, 1981: 2-25–2-27.
15. West J, ed. Pulmonary Gas Exchange: Physiologic Basis of Medical Practice, 12th Ed. 546–559.
16. Stewart RD, Peterson JE, Baretta ED, Bachard RT, Hosko MJ, Herrman A. Experimental human exposure to carbon monoxide. Arch Environ Health 1970;21:154–164.
17. Masters RL. Air pollution—human health effects. In: McCormac, ed. Introduction to the Scientific Study of Atmospheric Pollution. Dordrecht: 1971:97–130.
18. Curry S. Methemoglobinemia. Ann Emerg Med 1982; 11:214–221.
19. Goldfrank LR, Price D, Kirstein RH. In: Goldfrank LR, ed. Goldfrank's Toxicologic Emergencies. Norwalk: Appleton Century Crofts, 1986:319–325.
20. Mansouri A. Review: Methemoglobinemia. Am J Med Sci 1989;289:200–209.
21. Katsumata Y, Aoki M, Oya M, Suzuki O, Yada S. Forensic application of rapid analysis of carboxyhemoglobin in blood using an oxygen electrode. Forensic Sci Int 1979; 13:151–158.
22. National Academy of Sciences and National Academy of Engineering. Effects of Chronic Exposure to Low Levels of Carbon Monoxide on Human Health, Behavior and Performance. Washington, DC: NAS-NAE, 1969.
23. Goldsmith JR, Terzaghi J, Hackney JD. Arch Environ Health 1963;7:647.
24. Ekblom B, Huot R. Response of submaximal and maximal exercise at different levels of carboxyhemoglobin. Acta Physiol Scand 1972;86:474–482.
25. Weiser PC, Morrill CG, Dickey DW. Effect of low-level carbon monoxide exposure on the adaptation of healthy young men to aerobic work at an altitude of 1610 m. In: Folinsbee LJ, ed. Environmental Stress. New York: Academic Press, 1978:198.
26. Spengler JD, Cohen MA. In: Gammage RB, Kaye SV, eds. Indoor Air and Human Health. Boca Raton: Lewis, 1985: 261–278.
27. Clark JN, Lamberson CJ. Pulmonary oxygen toxicity. Pharmacol Rev 1971:23:37–133.
28. Grim PS, Gottlieb LJ, Boddie A, Batson E. Hyperbaric oxygen toxicity. JAMA 1990;263:2216–2220.
29. Barker S, Tremer K. The effect of carbon monoxide inhalation on pulse oximetry and transcutaneous PO_2. Anesthesiology 1987;66:677–679.
30. Schnapp LM, Cohen NH. Pulse oximetry uses and abuses. Chest 1990;98:1244–1250.
31. Barker SJ, Tremper KK, Hyatt J. Effects of methemoglobinemia on pulse oximetry and mixed venous oximetry. Anesthesiology 1989;70:112–117.
32. Tremper KK, Baker SJ. Using pulse oximetry when dyshemoglobin levels are high. J Crit Ill 1988;3:103–107.
33. Zikria BA, Budd DC, Floch F, Ferrer JM. What is clinical smoke poisoning? Ann Surg 1975;181:151–156.

Section 4
Complications of Postoperative Adhesions

17

Incidence of Postsurgical Adhesions

Michael P. Diamond

In marked contrast to the clinical impression of practitioners, postoperative adhesion development occurs following most surgical procedures.[1–3] This misimpression of clinicians is most likely the result of their inability to view the intraperitoneal operative sites following a surgical procedure without a repeat operation, for which there is frequently no clinical indication. Because many of the complications these adhesions may cause can occur years or decades after the inciting event, the cause-and-effect relationship is often lost. Furthermore, the rare opportunities to perform a second operative procedure, with exceptions, result from a complication in the immediate postoperative period such as an infection or bleeding. In such situations, the finding of adhesions would not be a surprise to the surgeon.

The frequency with which intraabdominal surgical procedures are followed by the development of postoperative adhesions has been increasingly recognized over the past two decades. Most of the work to date has occurred in infertility patients because many clinicians believe that an early second-look laparoscopy would be of clinical benefit to the patient. Thus, a follow-up surgical procedure can be readily rationalized in these patients.[4] It must be recognized however that the true value of an early second-look laparoscopy in improving pregnancy outcome has never been evaluated, although several reports have suggested that early performance of a second-look laparoscopy will reduce the likelihood of finding adhesions 1 to 2 years later.

The development of postoperative adhesions has been stratified into development of adhesions at sites that underwent adhesiolysis at the initial operative procedure, and development of adhesions at sites which did not undergo adhesiolysis at the initial operative procedure.[2] These types have been referred to as adhesion reformation and de novo adhesion formation, respectively. Postoperative adhesion development has been reported to occur in 55% to 100% of patients after surgery, with an average of approximately 85% (Table 17.1). In 1984, we identified that adhesion reformation occurred in 86% of patients following the initial surgery performed at laparotomy.[5] It was hoped that laparoscopic surgery might reduce the incidence of postoperative adhesion reformation, but a decade later we reported another multicenter study in which adhesions reformed in 97% of patients undergoing initial procedure by laparoscopy.[3]

Upon further contemplation, it should probably not be surprising that lysis of adhesions, whether occurring at laparotomy or laparoscopy, might each be followed by similar rates of adhesion reformation. Regardless of the modality of entry into the abdominal cavity, the adhesions must still be lysed utilizing the same types of modalities: sutures, scalpel, electrosurgery, etc. Perhaps even more surprising was the frequency at which de novo adhesion development was observed to occur. Depending on the report, this rate ranges from 23% to 97% of patients (Table 17.2). While some may be surprised at the high frequency of de novo adhesion formation because of the expectation that laparoscopic procedures would reduce tissue trauma, recent reports have suggested that carbon dioxide insufflation in and of itself will promote de novo adhesion formation.

These categorizations of adhesions as either being de novo or reformed have further been subclassified based on whether they occurred at a site that also underwent additional surgical procedures. As a result, we have utilized four subcategories: type 1 refers to de novo adhesion formation and type 2 refers to adhesion reformation. Within each of these categories, sites with no additional surgical procedures would be given an A while sites that underwent surgical procedures (e.g., myomectomy, ovarian cystectomy) in addition to adhesiolysis would be given a B (Fig. 17.1).[14] We have previously implied that the likelihood of postoperative adhesion development would increase from 1A to 1B to 2A to 2B. A recent meta-analysis provided evidence consistent with this suggestion. If this hypothesis is correct, then it

TABLE 17.1. Pelvic adhesions noted at second-look procedures

Reference	Time from initial procedure	Total no. of patients	Total no. with adhesions	With adhesions (%)
Raj and Hulka[6]	1 wk to 2 yr	60	51	85
Diamond et al.[5]	1–12 wk	106	91	86
DeCherney and Mezer[7]	4–16 wk	20	15	75
	1–3 yr	41	31	76
Surrey and Friedman[8]	6–8 wk	31	22	71
	>6 mo	6	5	83
Pittaway et al.[9]	4–6 wk	23	23	100
Trimbos-Kemper et al.[10]	8 d	188	104	55
Daniell and Pittaway[11]	4–6 wk	25	24	96
Diamond et al.[3]	<12 wk	68	66	97

From Diamond MP.[4]

TABLE 17.2. Frequency of patients with adhesion reformation and de novo adhesion formation as assessed at early second-look surgical procedures

	Initial surgery	Patients (%)
Adhesion reformation	Laparotomy	86[2]
	Laparoscopy	97[3]
De novo adhesion formation	Laparotomy	51[12]
	Laparotomy	85[13]
	Laparoscopy	23[3]

Type 1. De novo adhesion formation; development of adhesions at sites that did not have adhesion intitally
- **A.** No operative procedure at site of adhesion formation
- **B.** Operative procedure performed at site of adhesion formation

Type 2. Adhesion reformation; redevelopment of adhesions at sites at which adhesiolysis was performed.
- **A.** No operative procedure at site of adhesion reformation (other than adhesiolysis)
- **B.** Operative procedure performed at site of adhesion reformation (in addition to adhesiolysis)

FIG. 17.1. Classification of postoperative adhesion development. (From Diamond MP, Nezhat F. Letter to the Editor: Adhesions after resection of ovarian endometriomas. Fertility & Sterility 59:934–935, 1993; with permission.)

TABLE 17.3. Frequency of postoperative adhesion development by anatomic site as assessed at early second-look surgical procedures

Anatomic site	Site (%)
Pelvic sidewall	76[16]
Pelvic sidewall	76[17]
Abdominal incision	94[18]
Ovary	75[19]
Ovary, uterus, tubes	71[20]

would be expected that reduction of postoperative adhesion development would be easiest for type 1A adhesions and hardest for type 2B adhesions, and furthermore that antiadhesion adjuvants may be efficacious only for less significant classifications of adhesions. Consistent with this suggestion is the finding that an adjuvant for reduction of postoperative adhesions, composed of a 0.4% solution of hyaluronic acid, was successful in reducing type 1A adhesions but not type 1B adhesions.[15]

In addition to consideration of de novo adhesion formation and adhesion reformation in the patient as a whole, it is important to note that observations at individual sites throughout the abdomen and pelvis provide consistent findings. The incidence of adhesions in the female reproductive tract and of different components of the abdominal wall range from 71% to 94% (Table 17.3).

Because most of the studies evaluating postoperative adhesion development have been conducted with infertile women, there remained the possibility that the observations described may in some way be limited to women with infertility and not represent the population at large. However, the recent report by Becker et al. eliminated this possibility.[18] This survey was conducted among general surgical patients undergoing colectomy for ulcerative colitis or familial polyposis. Among women in the control group for this study, adhesions to the midline abdominal incision as assessed at the time of the second-look procedure (at the time of ileostomy takedown with reestablishment of bowel continuity), 94% of patients had adhesions to the anterior abdominal wall. This patient population included noninfertile women as well as men, and in fact analysis within this population showed increased likelihood of adhesions in men as opposed to women. Thus, the observations that have been identified in infertile women appear to be generalizable to all patients, both men and women.

In a metanalysis recently completed and published by Wiseman et al., we evaluated adhesion development fol-

TABLE 17.4. Metanalysis of adhesion-free sites for de novo adhesion formation at sites with (1B) and without (1A) additional surgical procedures after surgical procedures performed by laparotomy or laparoscopy

	De novo 1A		De novo 1B	
Procedure	%	*n*	%	*n*
Laparotomy (+)	72	1245/1734	20	5/25
Laparoscopy (−)	82	14/17	37	19/51

From Wiseman DM, Trout JR, Diamond MP. The rates of adhesion development and the effects of crystalloid solutions on adhesion development in pelvic surgery. Fertility & Sterility, 70:702–711, 1998, with permission.

TABLE 17.5. Metanalysis of absence of type 1B de novo adhesions formation versus adhesion reformation after surgical procedures performed at laparotomy and laparoscopy

	De novo 1B adhesion-free		Reformed adhesion-free		
Procedure	%	*n*	%	*n*	*p*
Laparotomy (−)	45	98/217	27	105/395	<0.001
Laparoscopy (−)	37	19/51	14	3/21	0.09

From Wiseman DM, Trout JR, Diamond MP. The rates of adhesion development and the effects of crystalloid solutions on adhesion development in pelvic surgery. Fertility & Sterility, 70:702–711, 1998, with permission.

lowing pelvic surgery.[21] This report was based on a Medline search (from January 1996 to December 1996) that considered adhesion-free outcomes in patients and surgical sites. While limited by the number of studies that could be included and other factors, the report nonetheless provides the most complete analysis of this question to date. As shown in Table 17.4, adhesion-free outcome is higher for de novo 1A than for de novo 1B adhesions for procedures performed both at laparotomy or at laparoscopy. Thus, adhesions are more likely to occur at the surgical site of a myomectomy or ovarian cystectomy, for example, than incidentally at nonoperated sites. Table 17.5 compares adhesion-free outcome for de novo 1B sites as opposed to adhesion reformation; an adhesion-free outcome was more likely at both laparotomy and laparoscopy for de novo 1B adhesion than for reformed adhesion.

Table 17.6 compares the likelihood of developing de novo 1B adhesions or adhesion reformation at procedures performed by laparoscopy or laparotomy. No significant difference was noted for either of these types of adhesions; the trend for both de novo 1B adhesions and adhesion reformation was greater adhesion-free outcome if the procedures were performed at laparotomy. While this may represent variations in patients undergoing surgeries or surgeons conducting the operations, it would be consistent with an ability to handle tissues less traumatically at laparotomy. Of interest, in prior comparisons we have made in our own multicenter reports, de novo 1A adhesions do appear to be less frequent at laparoscopy than at laparotomy; however, as already stated this does not appear to extend to de novo 1B adhesions.

Several investigators have suggested that the use of crystalloids may reduce postoperative adhesion development. The length of time such fluid would remain in the peritoneal cavity, which is expected to be approximately 1 day, is however shorter than the time normally required for reperitonealization to occur, 2 to 5 days after

TABLE 17.6. Metananlysis of type 1B de novo adhesion formation and adhesion reformation after surgical procedures performed at laparotomy versus laparoscopy

	Laparoscopy		Laparotomy		
Adhesion	%	*n*	%	*n*	*p*
De novo 1B (−)	37	19/51	45	98/217	NS
Reform (−)	14	3/21	27	105/395	NS

From Wiseman DM, Trout JR, Diamond MP. The rates of adhesion development and the effects of crystalloid solutions on adhesion development in pelvic surgery. Fertility & Sterility 70:702–711, 1998, with permission.

TABLE 17.7. Metanalysis of effect of crystalloid instillation at the completion of surgical procedures on postoperative adhesion-free outcome

	No crystalloid		Crystalloid		
Adhesion	%	*n*	%	*n*	*p*
De novo 1A (O/P)	93	25/27	5	5/108	NS
De novo 1B (O/S)	45	98/217	20	5/25	0.018
Reform (O/P)	44	30/69	20	55/276	<0.001
Reform (C/P)	72	38/53	25	9/36	0.003

From Wiseman DM, Trout JR, Diamond MP. The rates of adhesion development and the effects of crystalloid solutions on adhesion development in pelvic surgery. Fertility & Sterility, 70:702–711, 1998, with permission.

the operation. When meta-analysis was conducted for the effect of crystalloid solutions as opposed to no fluids instilled in the abdominal cavity at the conclusion of the procedure, there was no suggestion that crystalloids would help reduce adhesions. In fact, type 1B adhesions and reformed adhesion occurred more frequently in individuals receiving crystalloids at the completion of the procedure (Table 17.7).

References

1. Diamond MP, DeCherney AH. Pathogenesis of adhesion formation/reformation: application to reproductive pelvic surgery. Microsurgery 1987;8:103–107.
2. Diamond MP, Daniell JF, Feste J, et al. Adhesion reformation and de novo adhesion formation following reproductive pelvic surgery. Fertil Steril 1987;47:864–866.
3. Diamond MP, Daniell JF, Johns DA, et al. Postoperative adhesion development following operative laparoscopy: evaluation at early second-look procedures. Fertil Steril 1991; 55:700–704.
4. Diamond MP. Surgical aspects of infertility. In Sciarra JJ, ed. Gynecology and Obstetrics, Vol. 5. Philadelphia: Harper & Row, 1995:1–26.
5. Diamond MP, Feste J, McLaughlin DS, et al. Pelvic adhesions at early second-look laparoscopy following carbon dioxide laser surgery. Infertility 1984;7:39–44.
6. Raj SG, Hulka JF. Second-look laparoscopy in infertility surgery: therapeutic and prognostic valve. Fertil Steril 1982;49:26.
7. DeCherney AH, Mezer HC. The nature of posttuboplasty pelvic adhesions as determined by early and late laparoscopy. Fertil Steril 1984;41:643.
8. Surrey MW, Friedman S. Second-look laparoscopy after reconstructive pelvic surgery for infertility. J Reprod Med 1982;27:658.
9. Pittaway DE, Daniell JF, Maxson WS. Ovarian surgery in an infertility patient as an indication for a short-interval second-look laparoscopy: a preliminary study. Fertil Steril 1985;44:611.
10. Trimbos-Kemper TCM, Trimbos JB, vanHall EV. Adhesion formation after tubal surgery: results of the eighth-day laparoscopy in 188 patients. Fertil Steril 1985;43:395.
11. Daniell JF, Pittaway DE. Short-interval second-look laparoscopy after infertility surgery: a preliminary report. J Reprod Med 1983;28:281.
12. Diamond MP, Daniell JF, Johns DA, et al. Postoperative adhesion development following operative laparoscopy: evaluation at early second-look procedures. Fertil Steril 1991;55:700–704.
13. Diamond MP, Seprafilm™ Adhesion Study Group. Reduction of adhesions after uterine myomectomy by Seprafilm™ (HAL-F™),* a blinded prospective, randomized, multicenter clinical study. Fertil Steril 1996;66:904–910.
14. Diamond MP, Nezhat F. Letter to the Editor: Adhesions after resection of ovarian endometriomas. Fertil Steril 1993; 59:934–935.
15. Diamond MP, Sepracoat Adhesion Study Group. Reduction of de novo postsurgical adhesions by intraoperative precoating with sepracoat (HAL-C) solution: a prospective, randomized, blinded, placebo-controlled multicenter study. Fertil Steril 1998;69:1067–1073.
16. Azziz R, Cohen S, Curole DN, et al. Pelvic sidewall adhesion reformation: microsurgery alone or with Interceed absorbable adhesion barrier. Surg Gynecol Obstet 1993; 177:135–139.
17. Sekiba K. Use of Interceed (TC7) absorbable adhesion barrier to reduce postoperative adhesion reformation in infertility and endometriosis surgery. Obstet Gynecol 1992;79:518–522.
18. Becker JM, Dayton MT, Fazio VW, et al. Prevention of postoperative abdominal adhesions by a sodium hyaluronate-based bioresorbable membrane: a prospective, randomized, double-blind multicenter study. J Am Coll Surg 1996;183:297–306.
19. Franklin RR, Diamond MP, Malinak LR, et al. Reduction of ovarian adhesions by the use of Interceed. Obstet Gynecol 1995;86(3):335–340.
20. Nordic Adhesion Prevention Study Group. The efficacy of Interceed (TC7)* for prevention of reformation of postoperative adhesions on ovaries, fallopian tubes, and fimbriae in microsurgical operations for fertility: a multicenter study. Fertil Steril 1995;63:709–714.
21. Wiseman DM, Trout JR, Diamond MP. The rates of adhesion development and the effects of crystalloid solutions on adhesion development in pelvic surgery. Fertil Steril 1998;70:702–711.

18

Classification of Adhesions

Gérard Mage, Arnaud Wattiez, Michel Canis, Jean-Luc Pouly, Florence Alexandre, and Maurice Bruhat

CONTENTS

Adhesions resulting from abdominal surgery or pelvic inflammatory disease are a very common clinical situation. Adhesions may cause infertility, pain, and bowel obstructions. Implicated in the etiology of as much as 15% to 20% of cases of infertility, adhesions are frequently associated with tubal damage[1] and are the most common pathology in patients laparoscopically controlled for pelvic pain.[2] Major abdominal surgeries are required in case of bowel obstruction caused by adhesions. Thus, the impact on healthcare costs of pelvic adhesiolysis is significant.[3]

Considering the correlation between adhesions and infertility, an inverse relationship between the degree or extent of adhesions and subsequent pregnancy rates is traditionally reported,[4,5] so that selection of patients for infertility surgery is probably a more important variable for determining success or failure than the surgical technique.[6] This finding supports the fact that in vitro fertilization (IVF) is considered as an alternative to surgery for patients with a large extent of adhesions traditionally correlated with a poor surgical prognosis. These surgical failures are explained by the high recurrence rate of adhesions that can be found at the operated site (adhesion reformation) or at another site (de novo adhesions) even after a correct surgical technique by laparotomy or laparoscopy.[7–9] Many agents have been proposed to decrease the natural tendency of adhesions to recur and are presented as a solution for adhesion prevention.[10] Despite the great variety of agents employed, there is no standard adjuvant treatment for adhesion prevention, and controlled studies have failed to identify a universally accepted agent.[11] On the contrary, it is widely accepted that the chances of surgery decrease with the increasing severity of pelvic adhesions.

To evaluate subsequent fertility, classifications of pelvic adhesions have been proposed since the beginning of microsurgery and used in clinical study and in experimental studies. A considerable amount of literature has been published on this subject. Although there is general agreement to employ a classification of adhesions, unfortunately there is no agreement on one that is universally accepted, and it is sometimes difficult to compare data from various centers and to determine the efficiency of new therapies. In a review of literature in

1995, we found about 20 systems to classify adhesions,[12] and since that date, some other scoring systems have been proposed.[13,14] It is clear that classification of adhesions is a very critical problem, characterized by the fact that everybody thinks an adhesion classification is essential but nobody uses the same scheme.

Because classification of adhesions appears sufficiently significant to be cited in most articles about adhesions, the criteria used to characterize an adhesion must be determined. In the classifications reported, the three following criteria characterize an adhesion: its type, its location, and its extent or surface. Two other criteria are sometimes mentioned: tenacity and inflammation.[13–15]

Parameters for Adhesion Classification

Types of Adhesions

It is quite clear in infertility surgery that adhesions are of different types. Sometimes, the adhesion is only a thin, avascular film between two organs that is easy to lyse. On the other hand, it is sometimes a thick vascular cohesive adhesion that requires a sharp dissection. Madelenat and Palmer[4] were probably the first, in 1979, to propose to separate adhesions into three types (a, b, and c, respectively) as type a, filmy, avascular adhesions; type b, vascular adhesions; and type c, dense, cohesive adhesions, and to evaluate success according to the different types. Hulka[16] and Mage et al.[6] proposed very similar types of adhesions. In 1988, the American Fertility Society (AFS)[17] proposed a two-type classification that considered only filmy and dense adhesions to make the method accurate. A summary of different types of adhesions reported in the literature is shown in Table 18.1.

TABLE 18.1. Types of adhesions.

2 types*	3 types†	4 types‡	5 types§
Filmy	Filmy	Filmy	Filmy
Dense	Thick	Opaque, nonvascular	Vascular
	Dense	Opaque, vascular	Cohesive a
		Dense	Cohesive b
			Cohesive c

*Young,[19] Marcovici,[20] Corson et al.,[21] Wright and Sharpe Timms,[22] West et al.,[23] American Fertility Society.[17]

†Mage et al.,[6] Yarali et al.,[24] Best et al.,[25] Luciano et al.,[26] Li and Cooke,[27] Nezhat et al.,[8] Diamond et al.,[7] Ordonez et al.,[28] Madelenat and Palmer,[4] Marana et al.,[29] Magro et al.[30]

‡Montz et al.,[31] Hershlag et al.,[1] Myomectomy Adhesion Multicenter Study Group,[14] Fiedler et al.[13]

§Adhesion Scoring Group.[18]

Sites of Adhesions

Location of adhesions is a difficult problem. Adhesions can be found in any part of the pelvic or abdominal cavity, so that the description can be not easy. The role or impact of adhesions according to location can be different in terms of pain or infertility. There is a general agreement to consider only adnexal adhesions, especially ovarian and distal tubal ones, in cases of infertility. In terms of pain, most authors prefer to evaluate all the locations. For example, the AFS classification[17] proposed only 2 sites, ovary and tube, for infertility, whereas the Adhesion Scoring Group proposed 23 locations with the aim to improve reproducibility.[18] A summary of sites of adhesions as reported in the literature is presented in Table 18.2.

Extent of Adhesions

The extent of adhesions can be quite variable, involving only a very small part of an organ or the total surface of the same organ. The surgery of lysis will be easy or difficult depending on the extent. A classification of adhesions cannot evade this characteristic. The extent can be scored by the fraction of organ involved (for example, 1/3, 2/3, 3/3) or by surface in square millimeters or square centimeters. According to classifications reported in the literature, there is no agreement about one system or another. However, in classifications proposed for clinical management of infertility, the choice of fraction of organ involved is most often reported. A summary of the extent of adhesions is presented in Table 18.3.

Tenacity of Adhesions

The tenacity of adhesions has been presented as the fourth character of an adhesion.[13–15] In fact, the type of adhesion already considers its tenacity. Filmy adhesions are easy to separate, but dense and cohesive adhesions require sharp dissection. In our opinion, these criteria are not indispensable to classify adhesions if the type is well described.

Adhesion Scores

According to the three or four criteria used to characterize an adhesion, scoring systems have been proposed. Points were allocated according to the different criteria. The overall total permits separating infertility cases by minimal, mild, moderate, and severe adhesions, with an increasing failure rate.[4,6,16,17] Pelvic surgeons hope that the use of a scoring system will facilitate the choice of surgery or IVF in case of infertility caused by adhesions.

TABLE 18.2. Sites of adhesions: Clinical studies.

2 sites*	3 sites†	5 sites‡	7 sites§	15 sites‖	23 sites¶
Ovary	Ovary	Ovary	Ovary	Anterior peritoneum	Anterior abdominal wall:
Tube	Proximal tube	Tube	Tube	Small bowel#	Left side to
	Distal tube	Omentum, bowel	Omentum	Anterior uterus	Right side to
		Anterior cul de sac	Cul de sac	Posterior uterus	Incision line to
		Posterior cul de sac	Pelvic sidewall	Omentum#	Above incision line to
			Large bowel	Large bowel#	Anterior cul de sac
			Small bowel	Cul de sac	Over uterus to
				Left pelvic sidewall	Over bladder to
				Right pelvic sidewall	Left side to
				Right ovary	Right side to
				Left ovary	Posterior uterus to**
				Right ampulla	Posterior cul de sac to**
				Left ampulla	Pelvic sidewall left-left to**
				Right ovarian fossa	Pelvis sidewall right to
				Left ovarian fossa	Posterior broad ligament left to**
					Posterior broad ligament right to**
					Round ligament to tube-left to**
					Round ligament to tube-right to**
					Ovary-left to**
					Ovary-right to**
					Tube-left to**
					Tube-right to**
					Small bowel to
					Large bowel to**
					Omentum to**

*American Fertility Society,[17]
†Mage et al.,[6] Lundorff et al.[32]
‡Nezhat et al.[8]
§Diamond et al.[7]
‖Corson et al.[21]
¶Adhesion Scoring Group [18]
No scoring for the extent of involvement.
** 13 of 23 sites that correspond to the area of the pelvis likely to be involved with tubal and ovarian adhesions.

TABLE 18.3. Extent of adhesions.

Method	Reference
By mm²	Yarali et al.[24]
	Urman et al.[33]
	Li and Cooke[27]
	Sekiba and Obstetrics and Gynecology Adhesion Prevention Committee[34]
By proportion	
1/4, 2/4, 3/4, 4/4	Mage et al. [6]
1/3, 2/3, 3/3	American Fertility Society[17]
By percentage	
<50%, >50%	Corson et al.[21]
	Adhesion Scoring Group[18]
	Mongomery Rice et al.[35]
<25%, 25%–50%, >50%	Boyers et al.[15]
	Myomectomy Multicenter Study Group[14]
<25%, <50%, <75%, >75%	Ordonez et al.[28]
	Fiedler et al.[13]

TABLE 18.4. Adhesion scoring system.

	Surface involved			
Adhesions	1/4	2/4	3/4	4/4
Ovary				
Filmy	1	1	1	1
Vascular	2	4	6	8
Dense	5	10	15	20
	1/3	2/3		3/3
Proximal Tube				
Filmy	1	1		1
Vascular	2	4		6
Dense	2	5		10
Distal Tube				
Filmy	1	1		1
Vascular	2	4		6
Dense	5	10		10

From Mage et al. (1986).[6]
Absent, 0; mild, 1–9; moderate, 10–20; severe, 20.

TABLE 18.5. Adhesion scoring system.

	Adhesions	<1/3 enclosure	1/3–2/3 enclosure	>2/3 enclosure
Ovary	R Filmy	1	2	4
	Dense	4	8	16
	L Filmy	1	2	4
	Dense	4	8	16
Tube	R Filmy	1	2	4
	Dense	4*	8*	16
	L Filmy	1	2	4
	Dense	4*	8*	16

*If the fimbriated end of the fallopian tube is completely enclosed, change the point assignment to 16.

Prognostic Classification for Adnexal Adhesions

	Left		Right
A, Minimal	________	0–5	________
B, Mild	________	6–10	________
C, Moderate	________	11–20	________
D, Severe	________	21–32	________

Prognosis for conception and subsequent viable infant (physician's judgment based upon adnexa with least amount of pathology):

________Excellent (>75%) ________Good (50%–75%)

________Fair (25%–50%) ________Poor (<5%)

From American Fertility Society.[17]

Most often, the adhesion scoring system is associated with a scoring system for the tube to make the diagnosis accurate. The principal scoring systems reported in the literature and used in clinical studies follow (Tables 18.4–18.9).

These different scoring systems, as presented by their authors, have been found to be effective in their hands. For example, we reported in 1986,[6] in mild, moderate, and severe adhesions, a subsequent pregnancy rate of 32%, 26%, and 5.5%, respectively. It is quite difficult to know exactly the efficiency of the same score in other hands and particularly in clinical studies, because in most cases adhesions and tubal damage are present in the same patient, so it has become difficult to determine the exact incidence of adhesiolysis and tubal surgery in the success rate.

Moreover, differents factors can also influence the prognosis: age, ovulatory status, and male factors. There is of course no reason for the use of a scoring system to improve the results of surgery; however, the use of one of these scoring systems is recommended to assess the development of infertility surgery.

TABLE 18.6. Adhesion scoring system.

	Description	Score
Extent	No sidewall involvement	0
	25% sidewall involvement	1
	50% sidewall involvement	2
	75% sidewall involvement	3
	>75% sidewall involvement	4
Type	None	0
	Filmy, transparent, avascular	1
	Opaque, translucent, avascular	2
	Opaque, capillaries present	3
	Opaque, larger vessels present	4
Tenacity	None	0
	Adhesions essentially fell apart	1
	Adhesions lysed with traction	2
	Adhesions require sharp dissection	3
Maximum total score		11

From Boyers et al. (1988).[15]

TABLE 18.7. More comprehensive adhesion scoring method (MCASM).

Severity	Location	Severity	Extent
0 = no adhesions present	Anterior abdominal wall (1–4)		
1 = filmy, avascular	(1) Left side to		
2 = some vascularity and/or dense	(2) Right side to		
3a = cohesive, falls apart upon touch	(3) Incision line to		
3b = cohesive, visible, dissectable planes, can be separated with minimal dissection	(4) Above incision to		
3c = cohesive, no visible dissectable planes, requires extensive dissection for separation	Anterior cul-de-sac (5–8)		
	(5) Over uterus to		
	(6) Over bladder to		
Extent	(7) Left side to		
0 = no adhesions present	(8) Right side to		
1 = mild (covering 25% total area/length)	*(9) Posterior uterus to		
2 = moderate (covering 26%–50% total area/length)	*(10) Posterior cul-de-sac to		
3 = severe (covering >51% of total area/length)	*(11) Pelvic sidewall-left to		
*Modified MCASM locations	*(12) Pelvic sidewall-right to		
	*(13) Posterior broad ligament-left to		
	*(14) Posterior broad ligament-right to		
	*(15) Round ligament to tube-left to		
	*(16) Round ligament to tube-right to		
	*(17) Ovary-left to		
	*(18) Ovary-right to		
	*(19) Tube-left to		
	*(20) Tube-right to		
	(21) Small bowel to		
	(22) Large bowel to		
	*(23) Omentum to		

*The asteriks indicate 13 of 23 sites that correspond to the area of the pelvis which are likely to be involved with tubal and ovarian adhesions. From Adhesion Scoring Group.[18]

TABLE 18.8. Adhesion scoring system: assessment of adhesions before lysis.

			If YES, specify below:					
	Adhesion present		Severity**		Extent***		If present, was adhesion lysed?	
			1 = Mild	2 = Severe	1 = Localized	2 = Extensive		
Anatomic site	Yes	No					Yes	No
Anterior peritoneum	□1	□2	□1	□2			□1	□2
Small bowel	□1	□2	□1	□2			□1	□2
Anterior uterus	□1	□2	□1	□2	□1	□2	□1	□2
Posterior uterus	□1	□2	□1	□2	□1	□2	□1	□2
Omentum	□1	□2	□1	□2			□1	□2
Large bowel	□1	□2	□1	□2			□1	□2
Cul-de-sac	□1	□2	□1	□2	□1	□2	□1	□2
Right pelvic sidewall	□1	□2	□1	□2	□1	□2	□1	□2
Left pelvic sidewall	□1	□2	□1	□2	□1	□2	□1	□2
Right ovary	□1	□2	□1	□2	□1	□2	□1	□2
Left ovary	□1	□2	□1	□2	□1	□2	□1	□2
Right ampulla	□1	□2	□1	□2	□1	□2	□1	□2
Left ampulla	□1	□2	□1	□2	□1	□2	□1	□2
Right ovarian fossa (posterior broad ligament)	□1	□2	□1	□2	□1	□2	□1	□2
Left ovarian fossa (posterior broad ligament)	□1	□2	□1	□2	□1	□2	□1	□2

**Mild = filmy, avascular; severe = organized, cohesive, vascular, dense.
***Localized = <50% of site covered; extensive = ≥50% of site covered.
From Corson et al. (1995).[21]

TABLE 18.9. Adhesion scoring system.

	Description	Score
Extent	No intraabdominal adhesions	0
	25% of abdomen involved	1
	50% of abdomen involved	2
	75% of abdomen involved	3
	>75% of abdomen involved	4
Type	No adhesions	0
	Filmy, transparent, avascular	1
	Opaque, translucent, avascular	2
	Opaque, capillaries present	3
	Opaque, larger vessels present	4
Tenacity	No adhesions	0
	Adhesions essentially fall apart	1
	Adhesions lysed with traction	2
	Adhesions require sharp dissection	3
Inflammation	None	0
	Mild erythema, localized surface involvement	1
	Moderate erythema and edema, localized surface involvement	2
	Severe erythema and edema, localized surface involvement	3
	Severe erythema and edema, widespread surface involvement	4

From Fiedler et al. (1996)[13]; modified from Boyers et al.[15]

Reproducibility of Adhesion Scoring System

The Adhesion Study Group[18] have characterized the ideal scoring system as having four parts:

1. Be predictive of the desired outcome
2. Be able to accurately portray the extent of the disease
3. Be easy to use
4. Be reproducible when used by different individuals.

For reasons already presented, it is difficult to evaluate factor 1, concerning fertility outcome. On the contrary, the reproducibility of an adhesion scoring system (ASS) can be evaluated by reviewing videotaped surgical procedures. Bowman et al.,[36] Corson et al.,[21] and the Adhesion Study Group[18] have presented data on this subject. The AFS Scoring Method (AFSSM) has been tested in these three studies because it is the most used. The Adhesion Study Group have compared the AFSSM with the MCASM (More Comprehensive Adhesion Scoring Method). Although Corson et al.[21] concluded that the intra- and interobserver variabilities were acceptable, the value of AFSSM was quite poor regarding the conclusions of Bowman et al.[36] and of the Adhesion Study Group.[18] A marked increased in reproducibility was reported with MCASM compared to AFSSM.[18] Bowman concluded "the AFSSM did not predict outcome or management decisions and the surgeon's fundamental impression of the state of the pelvis and recommendations for either surgery or IVF were more consistent and reproductible." However, these two studies did not contest that AFSSM presented some reproducibility between experienced surgeons and did not propose abandoning scoring systems.

Experimental Study

Most data about adhesions are experimental studies to test new agents assumed to reduce adhesion reformation. Because of the high variability in protocols, it is quite difficult to have a "standard" scoring system. The following recommendation can be given, however; the study's parameters should include the incidence, extent, and severity of adhesions to any anatomic site. The control must separate adhesion reformation in three parts: reformed, de novo surgical site, and de novo nonsurgical site.

Conclusion

It is a real challenge to finalize an adhesion scoring system. The best evidence is the number of systems found in the literature. On the basis of remarks developed by a selection of experienced surgeons in infertility, interviewed after the Vichy Meeting in 1995,[12] we can propose the following suggestions.

Four Types of Adhesions

A: Fine, avascular, transparent, stretched between two organs
B: Thick, vascular, opaque, stretched between two organs
C: Dense, fixing two organs one against the other with a cleavage plane at dissection; upon dissection the peritoneum or ovarian surface is intact
D: Dense, cohesive, fixing two organs one against the other with no cleavage plane at dissection; inevitably resulting in a deperitonized area after adhesiolysis

Extent of Adhesions

The choice is to separate in $0 < 1/3$; $1/3$ to $2/3$; $> 2/3$.

Sites of Adhesions

For clinical infertility prognosis, consider only the ovary and distal tube. For a clinical research study, consider anterior peritoneum, small bowel, anterior uterus, posterior uterus, omentum, large bowel, rectosigmoid portion of the large bowel, cul de sac (anterior, posterior), right pelvis sidewall, left pelvic sidewall, ovary (right, left), oviduct (right, left).

Scores must be established before and after surgery, with special attention being given to the preexisting adhesion that is not removed. The total surface deperitonized must be checked at the end of the procedure and evaluated in term of percent of organ (1/2, 2/3, 3/3).

Adhesion Reformation

In research studies or in clinical studies with a second look, adhesion reformation must be divided into reformed, de novo surgical site, and de novo nonsurgical site. No scoring points have been proposed to be allocated to these different purposes.

Acknowledgments

Special thanks to our colleagues who have given their opinion about an international adhesion scoring system:

Canis, Michel	Clermont-FD	France
Chan, Clement	Singapore	Singapore
Cooke, Ian D.	Sheffield	United Kingdom
Corson, Stephen L.	Philadelphia	USA
Diamond, Michael.	Detroit	USA
diZerega, Gere S.	Los Angeles	USA
Donnez, Jacques	Bruxelles	Belgium
Gomel, Victor	Vancouver	Canada
Jansen, Robert	Sidney	Australia
Kawakami, Seiji	Aichi	Japan
Keckstein, Jorg	Villach	Austria
Larsson, Bertil	Danderyd	Sweden
Luciano, Anthony	New Britain	USA
Lundorff, Per	Viborg	Denmark
Madelenat, Patrick	Paris	France
Mage, Gérard	Clermont-FD	France
Rock, John	Atlanta	USA
Saji, Fumitaka	Osaka	Japan
Tulandi, Togas	Montreal	Canada

References

1. Hershlag A, Diamond MP, De Cherney AH. Adhesiolysis. Clin Obstet Gynecol 1991;34(2):395–402.
2. Howard FM. The role of laparoscopy in chronic pelvic pain: promise and pitfalls. Obstet Gynecol Surv 1993;48: 357–358.
3. Fox Ray N, Larsen W Jr, Stilman R, et al. Economic impact of hospitalisation for lower abdominal adhesiolysis in the United States in 1988. Surg Gynecol Obstet 1988;176: 271–275.
4. Madelenat P, Palmer R. Etude critique des libérations percoelioscopiques des adhérences péri-annexielles. J Gynecol Obstet Biol Reprod 1979;8:347–352.
5. Hulka JF, Omran K, Berger GS. Classification of adnexal adhesions: a proposal and evaluation of its prognostic significance. Fertil Steril 1979;30:661–665.
6. Mage G, Pouly JL, Bouquet de Jolinière J, Chabrand S, Riouallon A, Bruhat MA. A preoperative classification to predict the intrauterine and ectopic pregnancy rates after distal tubal microsurgery. Fertil Steril 1986;46(5): 807–810.
7. Diamond MP, Daniell JF, Feste J, et al. Adhesion reformation and de novo adhesion formation after reproductive pelvic surgery. Fertil Steril 1987;47:864–866.
8. Nezhat CR, Nehzat FR, Metzger DA, Luciano AA. Adhesion reformation after reformation after reproductive surgery by videolaparoscopy. Fertil Steril 1990;53: 1008–1011.
9. Operative Laparoscopy Study Group. Postoperative adhesion development after operative laparoscopy: evaluation at early second look procedures. Fertil Steril 1991;55: 700–704.
10. diZerega GS. Contemporary adhesion prevention. Fertil Steril 1994;61:219–235.
11. Muzii L, Marana R. Prevention of postoperative adhesion formation in reproductive surgery. Ital J Gynaecol Obstet 1996;8/1:36–47.
12. Mage G, Canis M, Pouly JL, et al. Adhesions scores. Gynecol Obstet 1995;special issue:114–115.
13. Fiedler EP, Guzick DS, Guido R, et al. Adhesion formation from release of dermoid contents in the peritoneal cavity and effect of copious lavage: a prospective, randomized, blinded, controlled study in a rabbit model. Fertil Steril 1996;65:852–859.
14. Myomectomy Adhesion Multicenter Study Group. An expanded polytetrafluoroethylene barrier (Gore-Tex* Surgical Membrane) reduces post myomectomy adhesion formation. Fertil Steril 1995;63(3):491–493.
15. Boyers SP, Diamond MP, De Cherney AH. Reduction of post-operative pelvic adhesions in the rabbit with Gore-Tex* surgical membrane. Fertil Steril 1998;49:1066–1070.
16. Hulka JF. A prognostic staging and classification system based on a five year survey of fertility surgery results at Chapel Hill, North Carolina. Am J Obstet Gynecol 1982; 144:141–145.
17. American Fertility Society. The American Fertility Society classification of adnexal adhesions, distal tubal occlusion, tubal occlusion secondary to tubal ligation, tubal pregnancies, mullerian anomalies and intra-uterine adhesions. Fertil Steril 1988;49:444–445.
18. Adhesion Scoring Group. Improvement of interobserver reproducibility of adhesion scoring system. Fertil Steril 1994;62:984–988.
19. Young RL. The use of amniotic membrane graft to present postoperative adhesions. Fertil Steril 1991;55(3):624–628.
20. Marcovici I. Colchicine and post-inflammatory adhesions in a rabbit model: a dose response study. Obstet Gynecol 1993;82:216–218.
21. Corson SL, Batzer FR, Gocial B, et al. Intraobserver and interobserver variability in scoring laparoscopic diagnosis of pelvic adhesions. Human Reprod (Oxf) 1995;10(1): 161–164.
22. Wright JA, Sharpe Timms KL. Gonadotropin-releasing hormone agonist therapy reduces postoperative adhesion formation and reformation after adhesiolysis in rat model for adhesion formation and endometriosis. Fertil Steril 1995;63(5):1094–1100.
23. West JL, Chowdhury SM, Sawhney AS, et al. Efficacy of adhesion barriers. J Reprod Med 1996;41(3):149–154.

24. Yarali N, Zahradka BF, Gomel V. Hyaluronic acid membrane for reducing adhesion formation and reformation in the rat uterine horn. J Reprod Med 1994;39(9): 667–670.
25. Best CL, Rittenhouse D, Vasquez C, et al. Evaluation of Interceed (TCU) for reduction of postoperative adhesions in rabbits. Fertil Steril 1992;58(4):817–820.
26. Luciano AA, Maier DB, Koch EI, et al. A comparative study of postoperative adhesions following laser surgery by laparoscopy versus laparotomy in the rabbit model. Obstet Gynecol 1989;74(2):220–224.
27. Li TC, Cooke ID. The value of an absorbable adhesion barrier, Interceed, in the prevention of adhesion reformation following microsurgical adhesiolysis. Br J Obstet Gynaecol 1994;101:335–339.
28. Ordonez JL, Dominguez J, Evrard V, et al. The effect of training and duration of surgery on adhesion formation in the rabbit model. Hum Reprod (Oxf) 1997;12(12): 2654–2657.
29. Marana R, Catalano GF, Caruana P, et al. Postoperative adhesion formation and reproductive outcome using Interceed after ovarian surgery: a randomized trial in the rabbit model. Hum Reprod (Oxf) 1997;12(9):1935–1938.
30. Magro B, Mita P, Bracco GL, et al. Expanded polytetrafluoroethylene surgical membrane in ovarian surgery on the rabbit. J Reprod Med 1996;41(2):73–78.
31. Montz FJ, Holschneider CH, Bozuk M, et al. Interleukin 10: ability to minimize postoperative intraperitoneal adhesion formation in a murine model. Fertil Steril 1994; 61(6):1136–1140.
32. Lundorff P, Hahlin M, Källfelt B, et al. Adhesion formation after laparoscopic surgery in tubal pregnancy. A randomized trial versus laparotomy. Fertil Steril 1991;55(5): 911–975.
33. Urman B, Gomel V, Jetha N. Effect of hyaluronic acid in postoperative intraperitoneal adhesion formation in the rat model. Fertil Steril 1991;56(3):563–567.
34. Sekiba K, Obstetrics and Gynecology Adhesion Prevention Committee. Use of Interceed (TC7) absorbable adhesion barrier to reduce postoperative adhesion reformation in infertility and endometriosis surgery. Obstet Gynecol 1992;79(4):518–522.
35. Mongomery Rice V, Shanti A, Moghissi KS, Leach RE. A comparative evaluation of poloxamer 407 and oxidized regenerated cellulose [Interceed (TC7)] to reduce postoperative adhesion formation in the rat uterine horn model. Fertil Steril 1993;59(4):901–906.
36. Bowman MC, Li TC, Cooke ID. Interobserver variability at laparoscopic assessment of pelvic adhesions. Hum Reprod (Oxf) 1995;10(1):155–160.

19

Conventional Radiography and Cross-Sectional Imaging Modalities in the Diagnosis of Adhesions

Hans-Martin Klein

CONTENTS

The bowel is a thin-walled organ with a length of about 8 m that moves with peristalsis and respiration. The difference in x-ray absorption between the bowel and surrounding tissue makes the gastrointestinal tract, particularly the small intestines, a "worst case" for radiologic diagnostic imaging.

Peritoneal adhesions can cause a variety of abdominal complaints. In most cases, only slight functional deficits are present. For these patients, a noninvasive method is needed to exclude other pathology such as neoplasms or inflammatory disease. If adhesions cause obstruction and strangulation of the bowel, the severely ill patient must be submitted to a reliable and quick imaging method.

Abdominal Radiography

An abdominal radiograph is easy to obtain and has low risk and discomfort for the patient. In emergency cases, it can provide the most helpful information on the diagnosis and sometimes on the location of bowel obstruction.[1–5]

Methods

Abdominal radiography should always be performed in the supine and standing position or in a lateral view. The supine image is important to detect slight differences in density, subtle air collections, or fat lines. It should therefore be acquired with a tube voltage of about 65 kV. The radiograph in standing or lateral position is important to demonstrate free peritoneal air or air–fluid levels. Therefore, a tube voltage of 95 to 100 kV is adequate.

Complete obstruction of the bowel is characterized by air–fluid levels and localized dilatation (Fig. 19.1). The thickness of the abdominal wall can sometimes be determined by measuring the distance between neighboring bowel loops (Table 19.1).

Results

The sensitivity for the detection of complete bowel obstruction is reported to be about 50%.[3] For detection of incomplete obstructions caused by fibrous adhesions, the sensitivity is low. Meteorism and localized dilation of

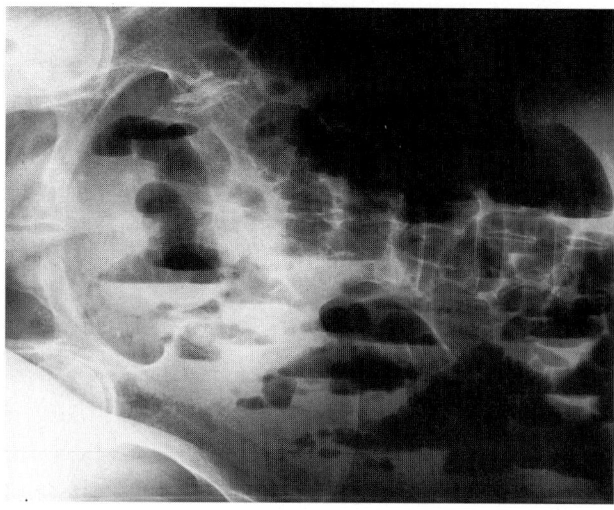

FIG. 19.1. Multiple air–fluid levels in a female patient with complete acute large-bowel obstruction.

gas-filled loops may be vague signs for a chronic incomplete obstruction. However, Kreitner and coworkers[6] reported experiences in 253 patients less than 31 years of age with unspecific abdominal complaints that might be caused partly by adhesive changes. They found radiographic images to be helpful in only 3.7% of patients, leading to a more strict indication of abdominal radiography.

Ultrasound

Ultrasound is a real-time cross-sectional imaging modality. Using a dedicated technique, ultrasound is able to demonstrate adherence of bowel loops to the peritoneal wall. Furthermore, it is well suited to detect the most important consequences of bowel obstruction in a dynamic and noninvasive way. Prestenotic dilation, wall thickening, and free peritoneal fluid are typical ultrasound signs. The empty bowel distally to the stenosis shows a "target sign." The mucosa is hyperechoic, compared to the hypoechoic muscular layer. A transition zone between pre- and poststenotic bowel can be detected (Fig. 19.1).

Methods

Abdominal ultrasound should be performed using curved or linear 3.5- to 5-MHz transducers. For regions difficult to access, a sector transducer with 3.5 to 5 Mhz is helpful. Adhesions of bowel loops to the abdominal wall can be detected best with a linear probe. The so-called visceral slide technique uses respiratory movement to detect bowel loops adherent to the abdominal wall.[7–9] Additionally, manual graded compression can be used to test the motility of the intestines.

Results

The extensive study of Truong and coworkers[5] reported 2581 patients, comprising 459 cases with surgically proven bowel obstruction. They found a sensitivity of 93.8% for the sonographic detection of obstruction. Uberoi and D'Costa[10] reported a sensitivity of 20%–42% for the detection of superficial peritoneal adhesions using the viscera slide technique (Fig. 19.2). Heistermann and coworkers[7] compared the accuracy of clinical signs and radiography with ultrasound in the detection of adhesions and found 77.1% for clinical examinations versus 89.6% for ultrasound. Borzellino et al.[11] reported a sensitivity of 100% for the detection of adhesions after laparotomy with ultrasound and a diagnostic accuracy of 88.5%. However, the specificity was only 31.5% in this study.

Fluoroscopy

To reliably detect a passage stop, a small-bowel follow-through (SBFT) examination is still frequently used (Fig. 19.3). This procedure has not only a diagnostic but sometimes also a therapeutic effect. The hyperosmolarity of iodine gastrointestinal contrast media leads to an increased filling of the bowel and activates peristalsis, which may loosen incomplete gastrointestinal occlusions. The SBFT gives an answer to the question on a passage deficit and the location of the complete or incomplete blockage. It can furthermore demonstrate di-

TABLE 19.1. Imaging signs of bowel obstruction.[1,2,4,5,15]

Imaging criterion	Radiography	Ultrasound	Fluoroscopy	CT
Dilatation	+	++	+	+
Air–fluid levels	+			+
Transition zone		+		+
Wall thickening	(+)	+	(+)	+
Abnormal peristalsis		+	+	
Target sign (empty bowel distally to obstruction)		+		+
Passage blockage			+	

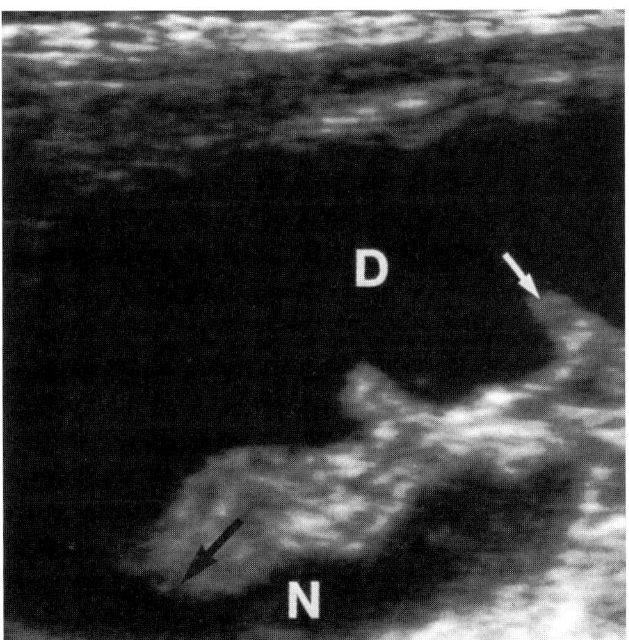

FIG. 19.2. Ultrasound image of a case with ileus shows the transition zone between dilated (*D*) and normal (N) caliber of the bowel (*arrow*). (From Jeffrey and Ralls, with permission.[23])

lation of bowel loops. A small-bowel enema is more uncomfortable for the patient, but can yield a better contrast in the intestines and is completed more quickly. The sensitivity for detection of bowel obstruction has been reported to be between 68% and 85%.[6,12]

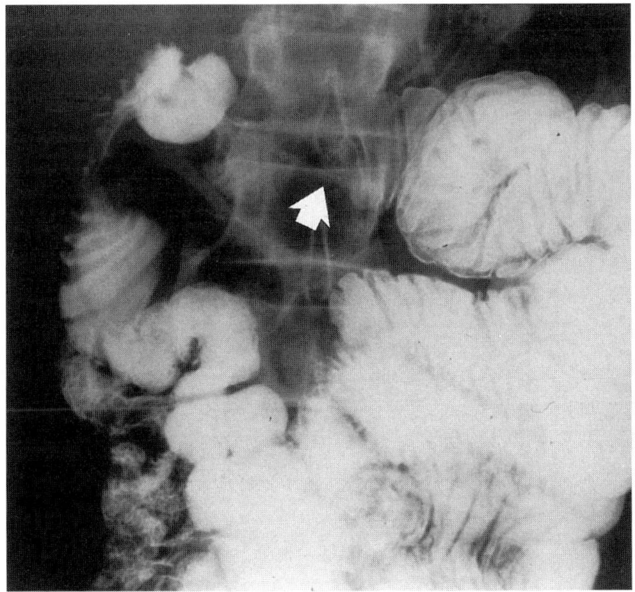

FIG. 19.3. Small-bowel follow-through with dilated bowel loops caused by peritoneal adhesions (*arrow*).

Computed Tomography

In recent years, attention has been focused on the potential of computed tomography (CT) for diagnosis of gastrointestinal disease.[1, 13–15] CT is now available nearly everywhere. It is noninvasive and can provide a complete status of the abdomen. The technical capacities of the systems have been rapidly improved. It is now possible to acquire a cross section in 0.5 seconds. The spatial resolution is reaching more than 20 line pairs/cm (minimum object size, 0.25 mm). Helical CT is facilitating three-dimensional (3D) reformatting of the cross-sectional slices. New methods such as CT-angiography and virtual endoscopy have been developed, making CT a method adequate to answer nearly every question in gastrointestinal (GI) imaging.

Incomplete obstruction is characterized by localized dilatation of bowel loops or a disharmonic displacement. These signs are vague and can be mistaken for a just-functional deficit. Signs of complete obstruction are air–fluid levels and a transition zone between dilated prestenotic and empty poststenotic bowel. A blocked passage can be appreciated if an oral contrast agent is administered. Wall thickening is a sign of bowel strangulation (see Table 19.1).[1,2,15]

Methods

CT should be performed pre- and post-intravenous injection of iodine contrast agent. For emergency indications, no oral contrast agent is necessary. A slice thickness of 3 to 5 mm should be selected. Tube current should be more than 250 mA for gas detectors and more than 200 mA for solid-state detectors. If a suitable workup of patients with chronic complaints and suspected adhesions is necessary, a CT enteroclysis can be performed.[16]

Results

Frager and coworkers[2] compared radiography and CT in a study of 85 patients. They found a sensitivity/specificity of 46/88 for radiography compared to 100/83 for CT. Megibow et al.[4] who found a sensitivity of radiography of 25% versus 94% using CT. The sensitivity of CT for detection of intestinal ischemia in strangulated bowel was reported to be 100% (no false-negative results) at a specificity of 61%.[17] Makanjuola and coworkers[18] compared the small-bowel enema to CT in 49 patients having both examinations for detection of intestinal obstruction. The sensitivity and specificity of CT were 83% and 63%, respectively. The small-bowel enema had no false-negative or false-positive findings (Table 19.1; see Fig. 19.3). Taourel et al.[16] reported a study of 57 patients in

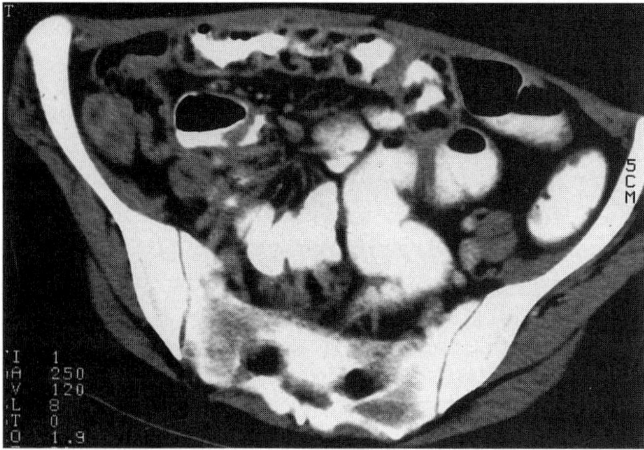

Fig. 19.4. CT of a young woman with multiple peritoneal adhesions after repeated laparotomy shows wall thickening and bowel loops adherent to the abdominal wall. Segmental dilatation is caused by fibrous peritoneal bands.

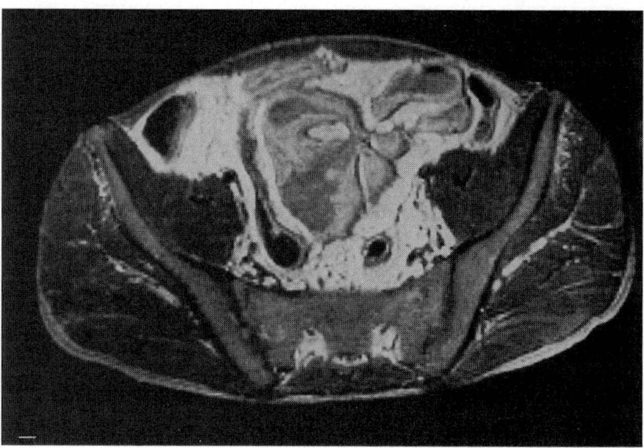

Fig. 19.5. MRI in a patient with Crohn's disease shows wall thickening and a fibrolipomatous mesenteric proliferation. Additionally, a dislocation and starlike adherence of the bowel can be appreciated.

which CT changed the patient rationale in 12 of 57 cases (21%) (Fig. 19.4).

MRI

Like CT, magnetic resonance imaging (MRI) is hampered by breathing and motion artifacts. The compromise between high imaging speed and high image quality is crucial for MRI also. However, several groups have worked intensively with gastrointestinal MRI, particularly in finding the optimal imaging strategy and the best way of distending or contrasting the bowel lumen. MRI of the gastrointestinal tract has been mainly investigated for diagnosis of inflammatory bowel disease, neoplasms, and detection of ischemia[19, 20] (Fig. 19.5). For peritoneal adhesions, no clinical experiences have been reported until now.

Gastrointestinal MRI is performed using T_1 and T_2-weighted sequences. To avoid motion artifacts caused by respiration, motion compensation is needed. In the usual spin-echo technique, this is realized using a gated acquisition. Alternatively, fast breathhold sequences can be applied, usually fast gradient-echo sequences for T_1 images, and turbo spin-echo or so-called single-shot sequences for T_2-weighted images. Gastrointestinal MRI requires a system with at least 1.0-T field strength, phase array surface coils for the abdomen, and a powerful gradient system (>20 mT/m; rise time <400 ms).

The bowel is orally contrasted with gadolinium-containing solutions (hyperintense; bright signal)[21] or ferrite-containing substances (hypointense; dark signal).[22] Intravenous gadolinium administration enables visualizing inflammatory or neoplastic changes. The imaging signs for obstruction are similar to CT criteria. MRI is superior in demonstrating wall edema and peritoneal fluid. Perfusion deficits caused by strangulation are better visualized after contrast injection.[20] However, MRI is subject to respiratory and peristaltic movement artifacts. Furthermore, the detail resolution is still inferior to that of CT. The potential use of MRI for gastrointestinal imaging requires further investigations.

Table 19.2. Diagnostic value of imaging methods in bowel obstruction.

		Radiography		Ultrasound		Fluoroscopy		CT	
Reference	*n*	Sensitivity	Specificity	Sensitivity	Specificity	Sensitivity	Specificity	Sensitivity	Specificity
Frager et al.[2]	85	46	88	—	—	—	—	100	83
Gazelle et al.[15]	75	—	—	—	—	—	—	79	—
Megibow et al.[4]	167	25	—	58	—	85	—	94<	96
Truong et al.[5]	459	90	—	93,8	—	—	—	—	—
Heistermann et al.[7]	594	77,1	—	89,6	—	—	—	—	—
Makanjuola et al.[18]	49	—	—	—	—	100	100	83	67
Borzellino et al.[11]	130	—	—	100	31,5	—	—	—	—

Perspective

With the implementation of digital storage imaging, abdominal radiographs will be more easily acquired (reduced dosage), stored, and distributed. Radiography and ultrasound will play an important role in emergency diagnostic imaging in the future also (Table 19.2).

Ultrasound is noninvasive, low in cost, widely distributed and fast and has a high relevance for functional deficits of the bowel because it is a real-time method. However, it is highly operator dependent and therefore has limited reproducibility. Improvements in ultrasound systems concerning spatial resolution, image processing, and image documentation will further increase the importance of ultrasound in clinical GI imaging.

CT development is still rapidly occurring. New multislice detectors allow the acquisition of four 5-mm slices at once in a 0.5-second scan time. The acquisition of the entire abdomen can be completed in a few seconds. Image processing tools are available that enable us to perform virtual endoscopy. Particularly for bowel examinations and emergency cases, CT will be a method of first (or at least second) choice in the diagnostic workup. Because cross-sectional methods provide the best tissue contrast resolution and have the advantage of visualization without superposition, they will play a major role in future imaging of peritoneal adhesions.

Conclusions

For subacute and chronic abdominal complaints caused by peritoneal adhesions, ultrasound is the method of first choice, and is sufficient for patient management in most cases.

For the acute abdomen, ultrasound and abdominal radiography are emergency methods.

Fluoroscopy can be useful to detect a blocked passage. If hyperosmotic contrast agents are used, this may sometimes loosen the obstruction.

If an experienced radiologist is present, CT can replace ultrasound and radiography for emergency and follow-up diagnostics.

The value of MRI for gastrointestinal imaging is not yet determined.

References

1. Frager D, Baer JW, Medwid SW, Rothpearl A, Bossart P. Detection of ischemia in patients with acute small-bowel obstruction due to adhesions or hernia: efficacy of CT. Am J Roentgenol 1996;166:67–71.
2. Frager D. Medwid SW, Baer JW, Mollinelli B, Freidman M. CT of small bowel obstruction. Am J. Roentgenol 1994; 162:37–41.
3. Gulliver DJ, Baker KA. CT of the small bowel. Appl Radiol 1994;11:39–44.
4. Megibow AJ, Balthazar EJ, Cho KC, Medwid SW, Birnbaum BA, Noz ME. Bowel obstruction: evaluation with CT. Radiology 1991;180:313–318.
5. Truong S. Arlt G, Pfingsten F, Schumpelick V, Die Bedeutung der Sonographie in der Ileusdiagnostik. Chirurg 1992;63:634–640.
6. Kreitner KF, Mildenberger P, Maurer M, Heintz A. The value of imaging techniques in the diagnosis of non-specific abdominal pain in young patients. Aktuel Radiol 1992;2(4):234–238.
7. Heistermann HP, Joosten U, Rupp KD, Holzgreve A, Horstmann R. Reliability of ultrasound ileus diagnosis. Bildgebung 1992;62:194–198.
8. Kolecki RV, Golub RM, Sigel R, et al. Accuracy of viscera slide detection of abdominal wall adhesions by ultrasound. Surg Endosc 1994;8:871–874.
9. Sigel A, Golub RM, Ioiacono IA, et al. Technique of ultrasound detection and mapping of abdominal wall adhesions. Surg Endosc 1991;5:161–165.
10. Uberoi R, D'Costa H, Brown C, Dubbins P. Visceral slide for intraperitoneal adhesions? A prospective study in 48 patients with surgical correlation. J Clin Ultrasound 1995; 23:363–366.
11. Borzellino G, De Manzoni G, Ricci F. Detection of adhesions in laparoscopic surgery: a controlled study of 130 cases. Surg Laparosc Endosc 1998;8:273–276.
12. Maglinte DDT, Gage SN, Harmon BH. Obstruction of the small intestine: accuracy and role of CT in diagnosis. Radiology 1993;188:61–64.
13. Balthazar EJ, Birnbaum BA, Megibow AJ, Gordon RB, Whelan CA, Hulnick DH. Closed-loop and strangulating intestinal obstruction: CT signs. Radiology 1992;185: 769–775.
14. Faß J, Klose KC, Raguse T. An evaluation of preoperative computed tomography for chronic inflammatory bowel disease. Coloproctology 1987;4:241–246.
15. Gazelle GS, Goldberg MA, Wittenberg J, Halpern EF, Pinkney L, Mueller PR. Efficacy of CT in distinguishing small-bowel obstruction from other causes of small-bowel dilatation. Am J Roentgenol 1994;162:43–47.
16. Taourel PG, Fabre JM, Pradel JA, Seneterre EJ, Megibow AJ, Bruel JM. Value of CT in the diagnosis and management of patients with suspected acute small bowel obstruction. Am J Roentgenol 1995;65:1187–1192.
17. Donckier V, Closset J, Van Gansbecke D, et al. Contribution of CT to decision making in the management of adhesive small bowel obstruction. Br J Surg 1988;85: 1071–1074.
18. Makanjuola D. Computed tomography compared with small bowel enema in clinically equivocal intestinal obstruction. Clin Radiol 1998;53(1):203–208.
19. Goldberg HI, Thoeni RF. MRI of the gastrointestinal tract. Radiol Clin North Am 1989;27:805–812.
20. Klein HM, Klosterhalfen B, Kinzel S, et al. CT and MRI of experimentally induced mesenteric ischemia in a porcine model. J Comput Assist Tomogr 1996;20:254–261.
21. Li KCP, Tart RP, Storm B, Rolfes R, Ang P, Ros PR. MRI contrast agents: comparative study of five potential agents

in humans. Proceedings of the Annual Meeting of the Society of Magnetic Resonance in Medicine, Book of Abstract, 1989:791.
22. Rubin DL, Muller HH, Sidhu MK, et al. Liquid oral magnetic particles as a gastrointestinal contrast agent for MRI. Efficacy in vivo. J Magn Reson Imaging 1993;3:113–118.
23. Jeffrey RS, Ralls PW, eds. Sonography of the Abdomen. New York: Raven Press, 1995.

20

Ectopic Pregnancy and Adhesion Formation

Per Lundorff

CONTENTS

During the past two decades, conservative treatment of ectopic pregnancy, including laparoscopic treatment,[1] has been focused on the fact that subsequent infertility to a certain extent may be the result of operative trauma to the fallopian tubes and the formation of new tubal and pelvic adhesions.

Periadnexal adhesion formation is an important factor in infertility after pelvic surgery, and evaluation of the etiology and prevention of adhesion formation has been the major goal for many investigations.[2,3] Normal peritoneum has an inherent fibrinolytic activity.[2,4] Peritoneal defects, if left open and vascularized, heal rapidly by fibroblast differentiation into a smooth new serosa.[5] Experimental studies in the rat show that local ischemia hampers the ability of the peritoneum to perform spontaneous fibrinolysis.[6] The inherent response to the presence of ischemic peritoneal tissue is adhesion formation, which act as vascular grafts.[5]

To avoid tissue ischemia and adhesion formation in the operative field, Levinson and Swolin[3] advocated nontraumatic techniques with bloodless entry into the abdominal cavity by use of electrosurgery, peritoneal lavage, and complete excision of diseased tissue. Peritoneal lavage with different concentrations of corticosteroids, nonsteroidal antiinflammatory agents, and high molecular weight solutions for adhesion prophylaxis has been shown to be valuable.[7,8] Efforts also are directed toward early recognition of ectopic pregnancy (EP) and thereby earlier surgical intervention with reduced damage to the pelvic organs. The value of postoperative laparoscopy at intervals from 8 days to 8 weeks or longer after conventional microsurgery for infertility has been assessed by several authors.[9–12] An early second-look laparoscopy makes adhesiolysis easier, and formation of thick and vascular adhesions is reduced.

The presence of adhesions is also suggested to be of great importance for subsequent fertility,[13] and adhesiolysis for infertility patients is recommended.[14,15] Efforts have consequently been concentrated on minimizing the formation of adhesions, for example, by using laparoscopic treatment.[16]

Clinical Studies: Ectopic Pregnancy Removal and Adhesion Formation

In a retrospective study,[17] 102 women with a strong desire for pregnancy underwent second-look laparoscopy about 6 to 10 weeks after surgery for ectopic pregnancy. The aim was to analyze whether a classification system could be applied to assess pelvic status in connection with EP surgery and whether various surgical procedures differ with respect to pelvic status at the time of second-look laparoscopy. A modification of a preoperative classification scheme was used that is based on a scoring system according to tubal damage and adhesions and intended for prediction of intrauterine pregnancy (IUP) and EP rates after distal microsurgery.[18]

The study was based on records and peroperative illustrations from these 102 women, and the scoring system of Mage was used, with minor modifications, to classify pelvic findings during and after EP surgery with respect to both tubal damage and adhesions. The analysis thus comprises: (1) a score for the contralateral tube and (2) a score for the adhesions of both sides. Furthermore, preoperative intervention such as lysis of adhesions was noted.

At the time of second-look laparoscopy, the same classification system was used and new scores were calculated, thus making it possible to determine a "score change." Tubal patency for both tubes was registered, interventions such as lysis of adhesions were noted, and the prognosis for future fertility was evaluated for all patients. The patients were separated into different groups according to the method of surgery to determine whether any method was superior with respect to patency of the oviducts or prevention of adhesions and tubal damage.

Results

Of all patients, 42% had a salpingotomy performed by laparotomy, 21% underwent expressio ovi, 21% had a salpingotomy performed by laparoscopy, 12% had a tubal resection, and 3% had a salpingectomy. Two patients underwent evacuation for a Douglas pouch hematoma. Furthermore, 2 women, who previously had a salpingectomy performed on the contralateral tube, were sterilized in connection with this EP surgery intended for future in vitro fertilization (IVF) treatment. Laparoscopic treatment, when used, was performed by electrocautery, linear salpingotomy, and suction irrigation. No women underwent a laparoscopic salpingectomy.

At the time of EP surgery, lysis of adhesions was performed in 23 patients (22.5%). Of these 23 women, 7 presented with fewer adhesions at second-look laparoscopy on the affected side. Nine patients showed improvement on the contralateral side and 5 patients were improved on both sides. At second-look laparoscopy, lysis was performed in 42 patients (41.2%). In 4 patients, advanced adhesions hampered lysis via the laparoscope. In 2 patients, sterilization was performed with the intention of future IVF treatment. Tubal patency was present on both sides in about 70% of all cases. An equal tubal score was present in 80 patients (87%); 9 patients (10%) were impaired and 3 patients (3%) were improved. Lysis of adhesions had been performed at the first surgical intervention in all 3 cases in which improvement was noted.

Adhesions

On the affected side, impairment of the adhesions between the two surgical procedures was noted in 40 patients (39%). Forty-eight patients (47%) had an unchanged status whereas 14 patients (14%) had an improved status. Seven of the latter women underwent lysis of adhesions during the first surgical intervention. On the contralateral side, 23 patients (22%) had impairment of the adhesions, 68 patients (67%) were unchanged, and 11 patients (11%) presented an improvement, that is, a lower score. Nine of the latter patients underwent lysis of adhesions during the first operation.

In 67 cases, at least one tube was classified as normal and the anatomic condition of the pelvis was considered satisfactory. These patients were not subjected to further surgical intervention during the first year of observation. In 13 cases the probability of future pregnancy was considered extremely low because of adhesions or tubal damage. These patients were therefore offered microsurgery. More advanced damage to the tubes or severe adhesions were found in 12 women, and microsurgery was considered meaningless, as it was in 2 patients sterilized at EP surgery. These 14 women were offered IVF treatment or recommended adoption. Gamete intrafallopian transfer (GIFT) was offered in one case. The remaining 7 patients were recommended to undergo hysterosalpingography for further evaluation of anatomic conditions.

Conclusion

Surprisingly, there was no correlation between surgical methods and tubal patency, and as to tubal and adhesion score, no surgical procedure was found to be correlated to improvement or impairment. Thus, a laparoscopic treatment did not imply fewer adhesions at second-look laparoscopy compared with conventional laparotomy. Subjective evaluation of the degree of adhesions by different surgeons may have contributed to a certain bias. In spite of this, it was found most valuable to study possible benefits of a second-look laparoscopy in routine clinical practice and to investigate whether there were any special conditions leading to an impairment of the pelvic status after EP surgery.

Based on results from this study, it was thus not possible to determine which patients would develop impairment of adhesions after EP surgery. As almost every second woman in this material presented an impairment of adhesions, it was suggested that all patients with a desire for pregnancy should be offered a second-look laparoscopy. These results further indicate that patency is not seen more frequently after laparoscopic treatment than after conservative treatment by laparotomy. Neither could less frequent adhesions be demonstrated after laparoscopic treatment than after conservative treatment by laparotomy. However, as this study was not a randomized prospective trial, no conclusions could be drawn in that respect.

Surprisingly, it was found that a large proportion of the patients had undergone lysis of adhesions at the EP operation. This is generally not recommended.[19] Nevertheless, it was observed that half the patients subjected to lysis of adhesions at the time of EP surgery presented an improved status at the time of the second-look laparoscopy. Nearly 40% of all the patients presented an impairment of the pelvic status at the second-look laparoscopy and as many were treated by lysis of adhesions. To what extent such adhesiolysis will contribute to a better fertility prognosis could not be stated on the basis of this study.

Clinical Studies: Ectopic Pregnancy Removal and Subsequent Fertility

Encouraged by these results, the same group initiated a randomized trial to study adhesion formation[20] and the subsequent fertility prospects[21] in women with EP treated either by laparotomy or laparoscopy. Women with tubal pregnancies fulfilling the entry criteria (see following) were stratified, on the basis of age and risk determinants[22] (previous EP, previous abdominal surgery, history of infertility, or intrauterine device [IUD] in situ) to establish comparable groups for future fertility evaluation and randomized in a prospective trial to either surgery by laparoscopy ($n = 48$) or laparotomy ($n = 57$) by sealed envelopes.[23] In case of laparotomy, vasopressin injection, 5 IU in 10 mL saline, and a salpingotomy with a similar diathermy knife as in laparoscopy were performed and the pregnancy products squeezed through the opening. Irrespective of the operative approach, the affected tube was left open for secondary healing.

Entry criteria were (1) diameter of the tubal gestation greater than 4 cm, (2) ampullary gestation accessible for laparoscopic approach, (3) a trained laparoscopist on duty, and (4) hemodynamic stability. If the preoperative human chorionic gonadotropin level was known, cases with titers greater than 10,000 IU/L were excluded. A gross anatomy evaluation of the periadnexal and tubal status was undertaken during surgery.

Second-look laparoscopy[20] was performed at a mean of 12 weeks (range, 1–29 weeks) after primary surgery in 73 cases with a desire for pregnancy (laparoscopy, n = 31; laparotomy, n = 42). Thirty-two patients had no second-look laparoscopy: 18 of these had no desire for pregnancy, 9 conceived before planned second-look laparoscopy, and 5 were recommended for in vitro fertilization (IVF) after EP surgery because of severe adhesions. Both at EP surgery and at second-look laparoscopy, the anatomic condition of the pelvis was registered on a preprinted form and lysis of adhesions was noted. At second-look laparoscopy, tubal patency was tested by dye solution.

Presentation of Adhesions

For each of the 73 woman, a score change of the presence of adhesions between the primary operation and second-look laparoscopy could be calculated (Fig. 20.1).

Laparoscopy Group

On the affected side, an impairment was noted in 5 patients (16%); 25 patients (81%) had an unchanged status and 1 patient (3%) had an improved status. On the contralateral side, 5 patients (16%) had an impaired status, 23 had an unchanged status (74%), and 3 had an improved status (10%).

Laparotomy Group

On the affected side, 22 patients (52%) had an impaired status, 18 patients (43%) had status quo, and 2 patients (5%) were improved. On the contralateral side, 13 patients had impairment of the status (31%), 29 patients status quo (69%), and no patient showed an improved status.

Patients operated on by laparoscopy developed fewer adhesions than those patients treated by laparotomy. On the operated side, the difference was statistically significant ($p < 0.001$). No statistical significant difference was

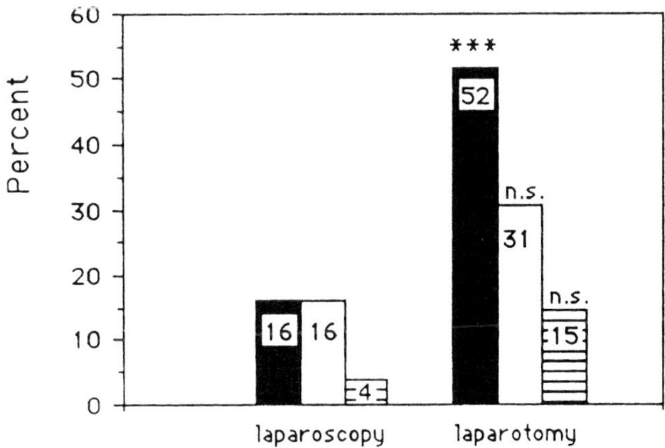

FIG. 20.1. Presentation of adhesions after laparoscopic surgery in tubal pregnancy: a randomized trial versus laparoscopy. ■, impairment of adhesions on the ipsilateral side; □, impairment of adhesions on the contralateral side; ☰, impairment of the tubal status on the contralateral side. ***, $p < 0.001$.

seen on the contralateral side. There was no statistically significant difference between the surgical methods with regard to impairment of the score and improvement or status quo. In comparison between the surgical methods, improvement of the score was classified as unchanged status, as improvement as a result of lysis of adhesions at primary surgery and not as a consequence of the surgical method per se.

Tubal Patency

In the laparoscopy group, the tube was patent in 76% and in the laparotomy group patency was found in 86%. There was no statistically significant difference between the two groups with regard to patency, neither on the operated side nor on the contralateral side.

In this controlled trial it could be demonstrated that laparoscopic surgery in tubal pregnancy causes less adhesion formation on the operated side compared to conventional surgery. On the other hand, there was no statistical significant differences in adhesion formation on the contralateral side, in tubal condition, or in tubal patency. A possible explanation is that in case of laparotomy, the Levinson and Swolin atraumatic technique was used, which could account for the favorable outcome in these patients. Nevertheless, it was found that patients in the laparoscopy group developed substantially fewer adhesions compared to the laparotomy group, although no intraperitoneal lavage/rinsing with any solution of known antiadhesion formation ability was used. From this trial, it could be concluded that adhesion formation occurs less frequently after laparoscopic treatment for tubal pregnancy compared to laparotomy using atraumatic technique. Whether this reduction of adhesion formation would increase subsequent fertility was evaluated in a life table analysis, using questionnaires to all 105 patients participating in the trial.

Fertility

Questionnaires including items such as wish for pregnancy and outcome, use of contraceptives during the study period, and time "at risk" for pregnancy were sent to all 105 patients 1 year after surgery and at the end of the study period.[21] Of these, 87 patients, 42 from the laparoscopy group and 45 from the laparotomy group, desired a pregnancy, and 50 conceived during the study period. Thirteen women were "at risk" for pregnancy for less than 18 months and 5 for more than 30 months. Seventy percent of the first subsequent pregnancies occurred within 1 year of the "at risk" period, and 95% within 18 months. After 21 months "at risk," no further successful pregnancies were seen. Only EPs were observed after 28 months "at risk." The EP/IUP ratio increased parallel to the time "at risk." The total conception rate in both surgical groups was slightly less than 60%, and the rate of first subsequent IUP as well as the ratio of EP/IUP did not differ significantly between the two surgical methods.

The possible importance of adhesions and adhesiolysis was further analyzed, regardless of the treatment group to which the patients belonged. Forty-five of the 64 patients who underwent second-look laparoscopy after EP surgery had adhesions of varying degrees. The subsequent conception rate did not differ significantly between patients with or without adhesions. In patients without adhesions and with bilateral patency, intrauterine pregnancies were observed exclusively. Furthermore, both patients with contralateral patency and patients with bilateral patency had a higher frequency of intrauterine pregnancies. Among patients with only ipsilateral patency, the intrauterine pregnancy rate was significantly lower than in all other cases. Adhesiolysis was performed at second-look laparoscopy in 10 of 29 patients in the laparoscopy group and in 23 of 35 patients in the laparotomy group (NS).

Conclusion

In this investigation, the overall conception rate of less than 60% was rather low. Initially, the follow-up period rate was rather low, but cannot explain the low fertility rate, as the conception rate did not change significantly after repeat follow-up 5 years later (unpublished data).

Adhesiolysis at second-look laparoscopy was performed in 24% of patients in the laparoscopy group and in 51% in the laparotomy group. The higher rate of adhesiolysis in the laparotomy group probably reflects increased adhesion formation after laparotomy.[20] Among all subsequent intrauterine pregnancies in the laparoscopy group, 18% had been subjected to adhesiolysis, versus 45% in the laparotomy group. To what extent the adhesiolysis contributed to subsequent fertility is difficult to say as the adhesiolysis was not randomly performed.

According to the design of the study, the surgeon's aim was to reestablish "normal anatomy" by adhesiolysis at a second-look laparoscopy. Complete adhesiolysis was achieved in 75% of cases. In the remaining cases, adhesiolysis could not be successfully performed owing to anatomic and/or technical factors. This study thus shows that the prospects for fertility are similar in the laparoscopy and laparotomy group when a second-look laparoscopy with adhesiolysis is performed. It is possible that this adhesiolysis, performed in half the laparotomy cases, compensates for the better adhesion scores after second-look laparoscopy and thus for more intrauterine pregnancies in this group.

References

1. Bruhat MA, Manhes H, Mage G, et al. Treatment of ectopic pregnancy by means of laparoscopy. Fertil Steril 1980;33:411–414.
2. Myhre-Jensen O, Larsen SB, Astrup T. Fibrinolytic activity in serosal and synovial membranes. Arch Pathol 1969;88: 623–630.
3. Levinson CJ, Swolin K. Postoperative adhesions; etiology; prevention and therapy. Clin Obstet Gynecol 1980;23: 1213–1220.
4. Porter JM, McGregor FH, Mullen DC, et al. Fibrinolytic activity of mesothelial surfaces. Surg Forum 1969;20:80–82.
5. Ellis H. Internal overhealing: the problem of intraperitoneal adhesions. World J Surg 1980;4:303–306.
6. Raftery AT. Effect of peritoneal trauma on peritoneal fibrinolytic activity and intraperitoneal adhesion formation. Eur Surg Res 1981;13:397–401.
7. Swolin K. Die Einwirkung von grossen, intraperitonealen dosen Glucokortikoid auf die Bildung von postoperativen Adhäsionen. Acta Obstet Gynecol Scand 1967;46:204.
8. Rosenberg SM, Board JA. Effectiveness of 32% high molecular weight dextran in reducing adhesions in human infertility surgery. Presented at the Thirtieth Annual Meeting of the Society for Gynecologic Investigation, March 17–20, 1983, Washington, DC.
9. Raj SG, Hulka JF. Second-look laparoscopy in infertility surgery: therapeutic and prognostic value. Fertil Steril 1982;38:325–329.
10. DeCherney AH, Mezer HC. The nature of posttuboplasty pelvic adhesions as determined by early and late laparoscopy. Fertil Steril 1984;41:643–646.
11. Trimbos-Kemper TCM, Trimbos JB, van Hall EV. Adhesion formation after tubal surgery: results of the eighth-day laparoscopy in 188 patients. Fertil Steril 1985;43:395–400.
12. Jansen RPS. Early laparoscopy after pelvic operations to prevent adhesions: safety and efficacy. Fertil Steril 1988; 49:26–31.
13. Caspi E, Halperin Y, Bukowsky I. The importance of periadnexal adhesions in tubal reconstructive surgery for infertility. Fertil Steril 1979;31:296–300.
14. Bronson RA, Wallach EE. Lysis of periadnexal adhesions for correction of infertility. Fertil Steril 1977;28:613–619.
15. Tulandi T, Collins JA, Burrows E, et al. Treatment-dependent and treatment-independent pregnancy among women with periadnexal adhesions. Am J Obstet Gynecol 1990;162:354–357.
16. Pouly JL, Mahnes H, Mage G, et al. Conservative laparoscopic treatment of 321 ectopic pregnancies. Fertil Steril 1986;46:1093–1097.
17. Lundorff P, Thorburn J, Lindblom B. Second-look laparoscopy after ectopic pregnancy. Fertil Steril 1990;53: 604–609.
18. Mage G, Pouly J-L, Bouquet de Jolinière J, et al. A preoperative classification to predict the ntrauterine and ectopic pregnancy rates after tubal microsurgery. Fertil Steril 1986;46:807–810.
19. Winston RML, Margara RA. Conservative management of ectopic pregnancy. Obstet Gynecol 1984;5:51–54.
20. Lundorff P, Thorburn J, Hahlin M, et al. Adhesion formation after laparoscopic surgery in tubal pregnancy: a randomized trial versus laparotomy. Fertil Steril 1991;55: 911–915.
21. Lundorff P. Modern management of ectopic pregnancy. Early recognition, laparoscopic treatment and fertility prospects. Thesis, University of Gothenburg, Göteburg, Sweden, 1991.
22. Thorburn J, Berntsson C, Philipson M, et al. Background factors of ectopic pregnancy. I. Frequency distribution in a case-control study. Eur J Gynecol Reprod Biol 1986;23: 321–331.
23. Lundorff P, Thorburn J, Hahlin M, et al. Short term benefits of laparoscopic surgery in ectopic pregnancy—a randomized trial versus laparotomy. Acta Obst Gynecol Scand 1991;70:341–348.

21

Ovarian Surgery and Laparoscopy

Michel Canis, Revaz Botchorishvili, Gérard Mage, Marie Claude Anton Bousquet, Patrice Mille, Jean-Luc Pouly, Arnaud Wattiez, Hubert Manhes, and Maurice Antoine Bruhat

CONTENTS

Laparoscopic Ovarian Surgery and Postoperative Adhesion

Laparoscopic ovarian cystectomy is becoming the gold standard in the treatment of benign ovarian cyst.[1] Although difficulties may be encountered, and the ovaries are generally left open, the effectiveness of this procedure and postoperative adhesion formation have been rarely studied. The ovarian nonclosure, which is used by most authors,[2,3] is highly controversial because surgical procedures that involve the ovarian cortex frequently result in periovarian adhesions and associated infertility.[4,5]

By avoiding drying of the peritoneum and decreasing the risk for infection, laparoscopy likely reduces postoperative adhesion de novo formation.[6] However, these theoretical advantages must be confirmed in clinical studies. We are reporting here three clinical studies that addressed these questions.

Study 1

Study Design

Patients who underwent a second laparoscopic procedure several months or years after the conservative laparoscopic treatment of a benign ovarian neoplasm were evaluated. Infertile patients, patients operated for a functional cyst, and patients who had adhesions or endometriosis or who were reoperated for a pelvic inflammatory disease were excluded. Twenty patients who were operated for 22 adnexal cysts were included. One studied had a previous adnexectomy, so that adhesion formation was evaluated on 22 treated adnexae and 17 contralateral adnexae. No sutures were used to close the ovary. Fifteen second-look laparoscopies were performed incidentally for another gynecologic disease, mainly an adnexal cyst discovered several years after the initial treatment. Five young patients underwent a routine second-look lapa-

TABLE 21.1. Adhesion formation after laparoscopic surgery for nonendometriotic benign ovarian cysts.

Group	*n*	Diameter (mm)	Adhesion score at second-look laparoscopy
All cases	22	70.4 ± 37 (30–180)	2.7 ± 5.9 (0–24)
Intraperitoneal cystectomy	15	68.7 ± 42 (30–180)	2.4 ± 6.1 (0–24)
Extraabdominal cystectomy	7	74.3 ± 27 (50–120)	3.3 ± 5.9 (0–16)
Teratomas[a]	13	68.4 ± 33 (30–140)	4.6 ± 7.2 (0–24)
Others pathologic diagnosis[a]	9	73.3 ± 45 (30–180)	0.0 ± 0.0
Contralateral adnexae	17	—	0.0 ± 0.0

Range is given in parentheses.
[a]All adnexae were free of adhesions before the treatment.

roscopy 6 to 9 months after the treatment of a large teratoma. Thirteen of the treated adnexae had been operated for a benign teratoma, and 9 for another benign ovarian neoplasm. The treatments were performed according to techniques previously reported.[7]

All the operative reports were reviewed retrospectively by one of the authors (M.C.). Using the American Fertility Society (AFS) adhesion classification numbering system, the adnexal adhesion score was calculated by adding the points applied to adhesions of the ovary and of the tube. Statistical analysis was performed using Wilcoxon's signed rank test and Spearman's rank correlation. The data are presented as means ± SEM.

Results

Results are summarized in Table 21.1. The mean adhesion score was 2.7 ± 5.9 on the treated adnexa. We found no adhesions on the contralateral adnexa. All the postoperative adhesions occurred in patients treated for a teratoma. Severe adhesions were the consequences of the treatment of large teratomas with severe spillage of the cyst contents. In contrast, there were no ovarian adhesions after ovarian incisions performed to remove other benign ovarian neoplasms. Postoperative adhesion formation was not related to the laparoscopic procedure used.

Study 2

Study Design

We studied spontaneous fertility after the laparoscopic treatment of adnexal cysts.[8] Laparoscopic management and treatment were performed as previously described.[7] Patients who had been using contraception since the procedure, or who were previously infertile, and patients with endometriomas were excluded. Patients were followed in our department, or the patient and her referring physician were contacted by mail with a standard questionnaire.

Results

The pathologic diagnosis and laparoscopic procedures are listed in Table 21.2. Forty-six cysts were treated in 43 patients. Twelve patients had a functional cyst (31.6%), 7 a paraovarian cyst (15.8%), and 24 a benign ovarian neoplasm (52.6%). Sixteen patients had a cyst more than 6 cm in diameter. All these patients had uneventful postoperative recovery.

The overall intrauterine pregnancy (IUP) rate was 93% (40 patients). One patient had an extrauterine pregnancy (2.4%), 37 months after an intraperitoneal cystectomy (IPC) for the treatment of a paraovarian cyst 12 cm in diameter. Two patients remained infertile (4.6%). According to the laparoscopic procedure, the IUP rates were 100% after puncture, biopsy, and resection (PBR) (10 cases), 93.3% after extraabdominal cystectomy (EAC) (14 IUPs of 15 cases), and 88.9% after IPC (16 IUPs of 19 cases) (not significant). Of the 26 patients who had an ovarian cystectomy, 25 conceived (96%). Fertility was not correlated to the pathologic diagnosis or the diameter of the cyst. Of the 16 patients who had an adnexal cyst of more than 6 cm, 13 conceived (81.3%). Of the 12 patients who had an ovarian

TABLE 21.2. Pathologic diagnosis and operative procedures.

Pathology	*n*	IUP	%	PBR	IPC	EAC
Functional	12	12	100.0	10	1	1
Serous + mucinous	10	10	100.0	—	5	5
Dermoid	14	13	92.9	—	8[a]	7
Paraovarian	7	4	57.1	—	5	2
Total	43	40	93.0	10	18	15

IUP, intrauterine pregnancy; PBR, Puncture, biopsy, and resection for functional cyst; IPC, intraperitoneal cystectomy; EAC, extraabdominal cystectomy (cystectomy by minilaparotomy without sutures).
[a]One patient with bilateral dermoid cysts.

cyst of more than 6 cm, 11 conceived (91.7%). The cumulative pregnancy rate was 70.1% and 84.2% at 12 and 24 months, respectively.

Study 3

Study Design

Forty-two patients who underwent a second-look laparoscopy within 3 to 6 months of a laparoscopic cystectomy for an ovarian endometrioma of more than 3 cm in diameter were included.[9] At both laparoscopies, the patients were staged according to the Revised American Fertility Society Classification scheme (R-AFS).[10] Fifteen patients (35.7%) had stage III endometriosis and a unilateral endometrioma greater than 3 cm. Twenty-seven patients (64.3%) had stage IV endometriosis, including 11 patients with bilateral endometriomas of more than 3 cm. Thus, 53 ovarian endometriomas greater than 3 cm were included. The mean diameter was 5.6 ± 1.9 cm (range, 3.5–11 cm). As 10 patients with stage IV endometriosis had a contralateral endometriomas smaller than 3 cm, 21 adnexae without deep ovarian endometriosis were available to study adhesion formation on a nontreated contralateral adnexa. Forty-one patients had an uneventful postoperative recovery. One patient had a retrouterine hematocoele, treated laparoscopically within the third postoperative week. Four months later, this patient underwent a third laparoscopy, which was considered as her second-look laparoscopy in this study. All laparoscopic procedures were performed as previously described. Postoperatively, all patients underwent ovarian suppression with danazol or gonadotropin-releasing hormones analogues for 3 months.

Using the R-AFS numbering system, we calculated the adnexal adhesion score, adding the points applied to adnexal adhesions. The endometriosis ovarian scores and the adnexal adhesion scores at initial and second laparoscopy were compared. Statistical analysis was performed using Wilcoxon's signed rank test and Spearman's rank correlation. The data are presented as means ± SEM (Table 21.3).

Results

The mean score of deep ovarian endometriosis was significantly reduced at second-look laparoscopy (1.7 ± 4.8; $p < 0.001$). Similar results were found in all the groups studied (data not shown). However, at second-look laparoscopy, four "persistent" deep ovarian endometriomas (7.6%) were diagnosed [two <3 cm (3.8%); two >3 cm (3.8%)].

The adnexal adhesion score at second-look laparoscopy was slightly but not significantly decreased (see Table 21.3). Among 19 adnexae with an initial ovarian adhesion score = 4, 4 adnexae (21%) had an adnexal adhesion score = 16, at second-look laparoscopy after treatment of endometriomas of 3.5, 7, 8, and 9 cm in diameter. Excluding these 4 cases, the adnexal adhesion scores at initial and second laparoscopy were 3 ± 2.6 and 3.4 ± 4.4, respectively ($p > 0.9$).

Among 34 adnexae with an ovarian adhesion score = 8 (Table 21.1), a partial or a complete recurrence occurred in 28 cases (82.4%), and a positive correlation was identified between the initial and the final adnexal adhesion score ($r = 0.41$; $p < 0.05$). Among 21 contralateral adnexae without deep ovarian endometriosis, 17 had an initial adnexal adhesion score of 4 or less. In both groups, the mean adnexal adhesion score was slightly, but not significantly, higher at second-look laparoscopy (Table 21.1). Three of 17 adnexae (17.6%) with an initial adnexal adhesion score of 4 had an adnexal adhesion score of 8 at second-look laparoscopy. One of these failures was explained by a postoperative hematocoele.

TABLE 21.3. Comparison of adnexal adhesion scores at initial and second-look laparoscopy

		Adnexal Adhesion Score		
Group	*n*	Laparoscopy treatment	Second-look laparoscopy	*p*
All cases	53	12.7 ± 10.8	10.4 ± 10	>0.1
Stage III	15	6.1 ± 5.9	5.8 ± 5.6	>0.7
Stage IV	38	15.2 ± 11.3	12.1 ± 10.8	>0.1
Diameter <6 cm	32	14.9 ± 11.3	11.3 ± 10.9	>0.07
Diameter = 6 cm	21	9.2 ± 9.3	8.9 ± 8.6	>0.8
Unilateral	31	12.6 ± 11.4	9.4 ± 9.7	>0.1
Bilateral	22	12.7 ± 10.2	11.8 ± 10.5	>0.4
Treated adnexae				
Ovarian adhesion score = 4	19	3 ± 2.4	6.5 ± 7.4	>0.1
Ovarian adhesion score = 8	34	18.1 ± 9.9	12.5 ± 10.7	<0.01
Contralateral adnexae				
All cases	21	3.9 ± 8.6	2.6 ± 4.2	>0.6
Adnexal adhesion score = 4	17	0.5 ± 1.3	1.4 ± 2.7	>0.08

Comments

From our results, fertility following laparoscopic treatment of benign adnexal cysts appeared to be normal. However, at the beginning of our experience,[1] the best cases were selected for laparoscopic treatment and included in this study. Therefore, these results need to be confirmed.

These fertility results are confirmed by the results of second-look laparoscopies reported here. We demonstrated that when treating a unilateral disease the main advantage of the laparoscopic approach is the absence of trauma of the contralateral adnexa. As the fertility of a patient who has one normal adnexa is normal, our fertility results will probably be confirmed in future studies. These results on the contralateral adnexa may explain why 13 of the 14 patients treated for a dermoid cyst conceived, including 1 patient with bilateral dermoid cysts, whereas adhesion formation was not uncommon in our experience. It should be emphasized that in study 1 the incidence of ovarian adhesions after the treatment of ovarian teratomas is probably overestimated because 5 patients were selected for a second look at the end of a difficult and unsatisfactory procedure. These adhesions are probably induced by the spillage of the cyst contents rather than by the ovarian incision.[11] This is a very strong argument to treat these patients without puncture or using large endobags.[12]

Two experimental studies showed in a rabbit model that nonclosure of an ovarian surgical incision is less adhesiogenic than microsurgical closure.[13,14] However, in both studies the ovaries were bivalved so that the shape of the ovary was spontaneously approximated at the end of the procedure, and the nonsutured ovary was free of adhesions in only 53.3% and 26.3% of the cases in the studies from Wiskind et al.[13] and Brumsted et al.,[14] respectively.

Recommendations

From these results and our experience, some rules should be proposed to improve laparoscopic cystectomy. The ovarian puncture and the ovarian incision should be performed on the antimesenteric surface of the ovary, as far as possible from the fimbria, so that the edges of the incision will be approximated when the ovary falls back in the posterior cul de sac. The cystectomy should be performed using only one incision, which should be large enough to avoid any additional tearing of the ovarian cortex. A careful hemostasis should be achieved. Finally, the shape of the ovary may be approximated using a minimal resection of the remaining ovarian tissue or a superficial coagulation of the ovarian stroma to induce an inversion of the ovary, as coagulation of the serosa is used to obtain the eversion of the distal part of the tube.[15] These rules are probably more important when treating large ovarian cysts.

Despite the advantages of laparoscopic surgery one should not consider that any procedure is valuable so far as it is performed laparoscopically. In contrast, strict guidelines should be followed when treating adnexal cysts. An adequate surgical technique should prevent adhesion formation in most cases, except in patients whose peritoneum is abnormal because of an associated condition such as endometriosis or pelvic inflammatory disease.

Fibrin Deposition

The importance of the surgical technique was further emphasized by our results obtained in the treatment of ovarian endometriomas more than 3 cm in diameter. Adhesion de novo formation occurred in 21% of the treated adnexae (4 19 cases) and in 17% of the contralateral adnexae (3 of 17 cases). In 4 of these 7 adnexae (3 patients), postoperative adhesions were likely to be related to the surgical procedure (large endometriomas, 3 cases; postoperative complication, 1 case). In the remaining 3 adnexae (2 patients), endometriomas of only 4 cm in diameter were associated with large areas of histologically "active" peritoneal endometriosis. Thus, postoperative adhesion formation might be interpreted as a consequence of the natural history of the disease. Similarly adhesion formation had been reported in patients treated with danazol.[16] These results suggest that adhesion formation is more common in patients treated for ovarian endometriomas.

Another issue of study 3 was to assess the two patients with endometriomas of only 4 cm in diameter that were associated with large areas of histologically "active" peritoneal endometriosis. Thus postoperative adhesion formation might be interpreted as a consequence of the natural history of the disease. The Operative Laparoscopy Study Group concluded that adhesion recurrence is frequent after laparoscopic adhesiolysis.[17] It has been demonstrated by both experimental and clinical studies[6,17,18] that laparoscopic surgery results in significantly reduced postoperative adhesion formation as compared to laparotomy. However, adhesion de novo formation may be observed following laparoscopic adhesiolysis,[9] and Redwine recently reported ovarian surgery as one of the predictors of adnexal adhesions found at reoperation.[19] Moreover, from these studies about ovarian surgery and from the poor fertility results obtained in patients treated for a distal tubal occlusion with severe adhesion,[20] we found that adhesion reformation is still a significant clinical problem after laparoscopic surgery.

Laparoscopic Ovarian Surgery, Adhesion Formation, Peritoneal Trauma, and Cancer Dissemination

The Questions

Because of the risks of dissemination, laparoscopic surgery remains controversial in the management of benign ovarian tumors. These risks are attributed to two problems: the puncture and the drainage required to remove the cyst,[1,21] and the complications of trocar site metastasis and peritoneal carcinomatosis that are observed in patients treated laparoscopically for an intraperitoneal cancer.[22-36]

Nowadays, the problems related to the puncture can be summarized as follows. From several multivariate analyses we know that when the tumor is immediately and entirely removed, the puncture of a cancer has no incidence on the prognosis.[37-42] These data, established after punctures or ruptures performed by laparotomy, must be confirmed after punctures performed by laparoscopy. National surveys clearly demonstrated that a laparoscopic puncture or biopsy may worsen the prognosis when the tumor is removed only several days or weeks later,[43-47] confirming that, as noted previously by laparotomy,[48-52] inadequate surgical procedures may be detrimental for the patients.

Spillage may occur during any puncture whatever the technique. These risks cannot be avoided when a conservative treatment (cystectomy) is performed. Conservative surgery without puncture or rupture is impossible; indeed, if a malignant tumor invades the cleavage plane it cannot be separated from the surrounding ovarian tissue without rupture. Because a routine adnexectomy for all adnexal masses suspicious at ultrasound is unacceptable in young patients, malignant cells may be spilled when treating adnexal masses. However, the importance of this problem should not be overestimated. When using an adequate technique for the puncture, the spillage can be minimized; the consequences of spillage on the survival rates are questionable, and this situation is uncommon because a puncture was necessary for the diagnosis of a stage Ia ovarian cancer in only 4 of 25 cancers encountered among 1200 adnexal masses diagnosed by laparoscopy in our department.[1,35]

The complications encountered after the laparoscopic treatment of cancer may be more worrying. Despite some clinical series with satisfactory results,[53-55] numerous cases of trocar site metastasis[22-33] and some cases of peritoneal dissemination[34-36] recently suggested that the laparoscopic treatment of cancer should be carefully evaluated, although some of these complications may be attributed to inadequate procedures.

Animal Studies

Many experimental studies have been designed by general surgeons and gynecologists.[56-77] Their results can be summarized in three parts.

Most studies demonstrated, using different models, that tumor growth is greater after laparotomy than after laparoscopy.[56-59,65,66] In contrast, using a nude mice model, Volz et al. found a greater tumor growth after CO_2 laparoscopy.[67] Several studies suggested that trocar site metastases are more common after laparoscopy.[56,62,63] However, three studies showed an higher incidence of wound metastases after laparotomy using an intraperitoneal injection of malignant cells (cell seeding models).[57,58,73]

Several studies suggested an increased tumor dissemination after a CO_2 pneumoperitoneum.[57,67-71] In a study by our group,[57] this difference was found by studying the score of each intraabdominal organ. Thus, we found a higher score for the peritoneum in the 10 mmHg CO_2 pneumoperitoneum group than in the laparotomy group. Moreover, in the laparotomy group, the peritoneal score was explained by the metastases found along the midline incision (60% of the score), whereas in the laparoscopy group this peritoneal score was explained by numerous small nodules of 2 mm spread on the peritoneum. Similar dissemination patterns after CO_2 laparoscopy were reported by others.[67,71] Furthermore Mathew et al.[68,69] recently published two papers suggesting that, when using a large number of cells, it seems possible to induce an aerosol of malignant cells.

These experimental data, which suggested that a laparoscopic approach may be detrimental for cancer patients, are surprising when accounting for the decreased surgical stress and trauma and for the better postoperative immunity after laparoscopy.[78-80] These experimental results should be interpreted cautiously. First, there are many important differences between the clinical and the experimental situation. In animals, a large number of highly aggressive tumor cells are used, whereas this situation is uncommon in clinical practice.[81] Moreover in humans the pressure is much lower and its consequences are treated by controlled ventilation.

Second, each detail of the experimental model, including all the parameters of the laparoscopic environment (pressure, gas, number of cells, etc.), is important and may influence the results. For instance, the experimental design may explain the results of Volz et al. concerning tumor growth. They compared a 2-cm laparotomy with an 8-mmHg pneumoperitoneum in nude mice whereas Allendorf et al. compared a 4- to 6-mmHg pneumoperitoneum to a xyphopubic laparotomy in rats.

Similarly, the increased incidence of wound metastasis after laparotomy in cell seeding models may be explained by the volume used to inject the cells. If a volume of 1 or 2 mL is used to inject the cells in the peritoneum during the procedure, the delay between the injection and a possible contamination of the scar is different in the laparotomy and in the pneumoperitoneum groups. Indeed, such volumes are large enough to induce an immediate contamination of the midline incision, but not to fill the pneumoperitoneum, so that the contamination of the trocar sites is possible only at the end of the procedure. As several studies suggested that direct contamination of the wound sites is the main mechanism of these metastases,[73–76] and Zoetmuller et al. showed that malignant cells are included inside the healing tissue within the first postoperative hour,[77] this different delay may explain the results observed with different models.

Mechanisms

Malignant cells may be found in the peritoneum during and after colon cancer surgery,[82–84] as well as during ovarian surgery. On the other hand, it is well established that surgical trauma and wound healing promote the implantation and the growth of cancer cells.[85–91]

The importance of fibrin deposition in tumor metastasis was demonstrated of Murthy et al.[87] and See,[92] who showed that the injection of plasminogen activators decreased the incidence of tumor formation at the site of trauma. Fibronectin appears to be essential in mediating cell adhesion via a cell attachment domain, L-arginyl-glycyl-L-aspartic acid (RGD), which binds to 5-β_1 integrin on malignant cells.[93] Peptides that contain the sequence Arg-Gly-Asp inhibit tumor implantation at the sites of trauma.[94–97] However, other mechanisms and extracellular matrix proteins (vitronectin, laminin) are involved in cell attachment to injured surfaces.

Mechanical Trauma

Recently, Tol et al.[91] showed that the degree of peritoneal trauma was correlated to the growth of ectopic tumors under the renal capsule and that, a few hours after the trauma, the tumor growth-promoting effects could be passively transferred to naïve nontraumatized peritoneal cavities, confirming that tumor cells benefit from the growth factors released during wound healing. Several growth factors are involved, with various effects on the growth of cancer cells.[98,99] Malignant cells included in fibrin deposits are protected from destruction by cytotoxic cells (NK, LAK), intraperitoneal chemotherapy, and postoperative low-dose irradiation.[85,87,100]

All these data explain why a peritoneal trauma such as a trocar incision may facilitate a wound metastasis; however, the dissemination observed on the parietal peritoneum in our animal study is more difficult to understand, because no direct or visible surgical trauma was induced and de novo adhesion formation has been shown to be decreased after laparoscopic procedures. Two hypotheses can be discussed.

First, the peritoneal environment facilitates the implantation and the growth of metastases. It has been suggested that the number of malignant cells required to induce a peritoneal carcinomatosis by direct contamination is much lower than that necessary to induce a metastasis by an intravenous injection.[101] The adhesion of malignant cells to the mesothelium itself without extracellular matrix could induce a peritoneal metastasis. Thereafter, the cytokines and the growth factors of the peritoneal fluid may increase tumor growth and decrease the local cellular-mediated immunity.[102,103]

Second, the concept of peritoneal trauma may have to be revised. When surgeons are discussing a peritoneal trauma, they discuss direct traumas induced by scissors and forceps. However, we have known for a long time that other events, such as drying of the serosa, are important traumas.[104] Watters and Buck described a technique to remove the mesothelial cells without damaging the underlying connective tissue.[105] Tol et al. recently reported different peritoneal damages using different surgical gauzes.[106] These occult or minimal traumas may be important for the adhesion of malignant cells. Groothuis et al. recently showed that minimal damage to the epithelium facilitates the adhesion of benign endometrial cells.[107] In an experimental model, using amnion, they confirmed that the endometrial cells are able to adhere to the extracellular matrix, but they also found that adhesion of cells to the epithelial side of the amnion was possible at locations where the epithelium was absent or only slightly damaged.[107]

Therefore, although adhesion formation is decreased after laparoscopy, the trauma induced by the environment of endoscopic surgery should not be underestimated. Several studies confirmed that, in rat models, a high intraperitoneal pressure induces a severe trauma that includes ischemia of the jejunal mucosa,[108,109] bradycardia, and respiratory acidosis.[110] This trauma has been confirmed in pigs,[111] but it has not been studied in humans. The importance of the intraabdominal pressure was probably already confirmed by the decreased dissemination observed with a gasless approach in rat models.[68,69]

Peritoneal Environment

Other parameters are important. Sahakian et al. showed that the low pH induced by CO_2 may influence postoperative adhesion formation.[112] Jacobi et al. reported that, in vitro and in vivo, a helium pneumoperitoneum decreased the growth of colon cancer cells when compared with CO_2.[113] West et al. showed that peritoneal macrophages incubated in CO_2 have lower tumor necrosis factor (TNF) and IL-1 responses to bacterial endotoxins when compared with macrophages incubated in either air or helium.[114] This again was attributed to the lower pH, which impaired macrophage functions.[115] The inhibition of IL-1 occurred within 15 minutes of CO_2 exposure whereas TNF was inhibited only after a longer incubation.[114]

Watson et al. confirmed a significant decrease in peritoneal macrophage TNF release after CO_2 laparoscopy when compared to laparotomy and air laparoscopy. In contrast, the macrophage phagocytosis was significantly decreased by laparotomy and air laparoscopy but not by CO_2 laparoscopy.[116] They suggested that an airborne endotoxin could be responsible for the altered macrophage functions. The temperature both of the gas used and of the patient may be important.[117,118] Other parameters such as the smoke induced by electrosurgery[119,120] and the fluid used for the peritoneal lavage must be studied.[121,122] Within the next few years, it may again appear essential to use frequent and copious peritoneal irrigation, when performing long surgical procedures by laparoscopy, to avoid drying of the peritoneum. This problem, which was avoided when performing short surgical procedures in infertile patients using low-flow insufflators, may again become a significant clinical problem when performing long procedures with high-flow insufflators in cancer patients.

Conclusions and Clinical Consequences

By developing laparoscopic surgery, we have decreased the trauma to the patient; however, we have created a new environment for peritoneal surgery. This environment has well-known advantages and potential disadvantages that may be clinically important when performing longer procedure or when treating malignant tumors. Obviously, further research is necessary to define the best environment for each clinical situation. These progresses will appear as a major step forward in the development of surgery for the twenty-first century.

From all the data discussed here, we conclude that, when used cautiously with an adequate surgical technique,[1] laparoscopic diagnosis is safe and reliable, whereas the laparoscopic treatment of cancer may be detrimental and should be evaluated carefully in well-designed prospective clinical trials. Consequently, we propose a very simple surgical management of adnexal masses:

TABLE 21.4. Calculated incidence of laparotomy, based on the data from the patients treated in our department between 1992 and 1994

Data used to calculate the theoretical incidence of laparotomy	
Total number of patients	516
Cancer and borderline tumors (*n*)	28
Benign masses suspicious at surgery (*n*)	59
including *n* masses >6 cm	22
including *n* masses >6 cm or with external vegetations	36
Benign masses nonsuspicious at surgery (*n*)	429
Laparotomies for technical difficulties (*n*)	9
Results: *n* and rate of laparotomy,[a] if indicated for:	
All benign masses suspicious at surgery	97 (18.8%)
Benign masses suspicious at surgery >6 cm	60 (11.6%)
Benign masses suspicious at surgery >6 cm or with external vegetations	55 (14.3%)

[a]This result includes all malignant tumors (cancer, borderline) and all laparotomies for technical reasons; among 488 benign masses the calculated incidence of laparotomy would be 14% (59 benign masses suspicious at surgery and 9 cases of technical difficulties).

- A laparoscopic diagnosis can be proposed to all patients, whatever the ultrasonographic appearance of the mass
- All masses diagnosed as suspicious or malignant at laparoscopy should removed and treated by an immediate midline laparotomy

Using the clinical and surgical data of the patients managed in our department between 1992 and 1994, we have evaluated the clinical consequences of this management, by calculating a theoretical incidence of laparotomy that included all the cases of cancer and of low malignant potential tumors, all the masses suspicious at surgery and found to be benign at pathologic examination, and all the laparotomies related to technical difficulties encountered in nonsuspicious adnexal masses (Table 21.4).

This management is simple: It can be used in all surgical departments that manage ovarian cancer, it ensures an optimal management of cancer patients, and it allows the treatment of more than 85% of benign tumors by laparoscopy, whatever the tumor diameter, the age of the patient, and the ultrasonographic appearance.

References

1. Canis M, Mage G, Pouly JL, Wattiez A, Manhes H, Bruhat MA. Laparoscopic diagnosis of adnexal cystic masses: a 12 year experience with long term follow up. Obstet Gynecol 1994;83:707–712.
2. Nezhat C, Winer WK, Nezhat F. Laparoscopic removal of dermoid cysts. Obstet Gynecol 1989;73:278–281.
3. Daniell JF, Kurtz BR, Gurley LD. Laser laparoscopic management of large endometriomas. Fertil Steril 1991;55: 692–695.

4. Pittaway DE, Maxson WL, Daniell JF. A comparison of the CO_2 laser and electrocautery on postoperative intraperitoneal adhesion formation in rabbits. Fertil Steril 1983; 40:366–368.
5. Buttram VC, Vaquero C. Post-ovarian wedge resection adhesive disease. Fertil Steril 1975;26:874–876.
6. Luciano AA, Maier B, Koch EI, Nulsen JC, Whitman GF. A comparative study of postoperative adhesions following laser surgery by laparoscopy versus laparotomy in the rabbit model. Obstet Gynecol 1990;74:220–224.
7. Bruhat MA, Mage G, Pouly JL, Manhes H, Canis M, Wattiez A. Operative Laparoscopy. New York: McGraw-Hill, 1992.
8. Canis M, Bassil S, Wattiez A, et al. Fertility following laparoscopic management of benign adnexal cysts. Hum Reprod (Oxf) 1992;4:529–531.
9. Canis M, Mage G, Wattiez A, Chapron C, Pouly JL, Bassil S. Second-look laparoscopy after laparoscopic cystectomy of large ovarian endometriomas. Fertil Steril 1992;53: 617–619.
10. American Fertility Society. Revised American Fertility Society Classification of Endometriosis: 1985. Fertil Steril 1985;43:351–352.
11. Fiedler EP, Guzick DS, Guido R, Kanbour-Shakir A, Krasnow JS. Adhesion formation from release of dermoid contents in the peritoneal cavity and effect of copious lavage: a prospective randomized, blinded, controlled study in a rabbit model. Fertil Steril 1996;65:852–859.
12. Volz J, Köster S, Melchert F. Laparoscopic treatment of ovarian cysts, experiences with different techniques to avoid spillage. Gynaecol Endosc 1995;4:177–181.
13. Wiskind AK, Toledo AA, Dudley AG, Zusmanis K. Adhesion formation after ovarian wound repair in New Zealand white rabbits: a comparison of microsurgical closure with ovarian non closure. Am J Obstet Gynecol 1990;163: 1674–1678.
14. Brumsted JR, Deaton J, Lavigne E, Riddick DH. Postoperative adhesion formation after wedge resection with and without ovarian reconstruction in the rabbit. Fertil Steril 1990;53:723–726.
15. Bruhat MA, Mage G, Manhes H. Use of CO_2 laser in neosalpingostomy. In: Kaplan I, ed. Proceedings of the 3rd Internatinal Congress for Laser Surgery. Tel Aviv: Jerusalem Academic Press, 1979:271.
16. Dmowsky WP, Cohen MR. Treatment of endometriosis with an antigonadotropin, danazol: a laparoscopic and histologic evaluation. Obstet Gynecol 1975;46:147–154.
17. Operative Laparoscopy Study Group. Postoperative adhesion development after operative laparoscopy: evaluation at early second-look procedures. Fertil Steril 1991;55: 700–704.
18. Nezhat CR, Nezhat FR, Metzger DA, Luciano AA. Adhesion reformation after reproductive surgery by videolaseroscopy. Fertil Steril 1990;53:1008–1011.
19. Redwine DB. Conservative laparoscopic excision of endometriosis by sharp dissection: life table analysis of reoperation and persistent or recurrent disease. Fertil Steril 1991;56:628–634.
20. Canis M, Mage G, Pouly JL, Manhes H, Wattiez A, Bruhat MA. Laparoscopic distal tuboplasty; report about 87 cases and a 4 years experience. Fertil Steril 1991;56(4): 616–621.
21. Nezhat F, Nezhat C, Welander CE, Benigno B. Four ovarian cancers diagnosed during laparoscopic management of 1011 women with adnexal masses. Am J Obstet Gynecol 1992;167:790–796.
22. Dobronte Z, Wittmann T, Karacsony G. Rapid development of malignant metastases in the abdominal wall after laparoscopy. Endoscopy 1978;10:127–130.
23. Stockdale AD, Pocock TJ. Abdominal wall metastasis following laparoscopy, a case report. Eur J Surg Oncol 1985; 11:373–375.
24. Hsiu JG, Given FT, Kemp GM. Tumor implantation after diagnostic laparoscopic biopsy of serous ovarian tumors of low malignant potential. Obstet Gynecol 1986;68S: 90S–93S.
25. Gleeson NG, Nicsia SV, Mark JE, Hofman MS, Cavanagh D. Abdominal wall metastases from ovarian cancer after laparoscopy. Am J Obstet Gynecol 1993;169:522–523.
26. Shepherd JH, Carter PG. Wound recurrence by implantation of a borderline ovarian tumor following laparosopic removal. Br J Obstet Gynecol 1994;101:265–266.
27. Childers JM, Aqua KA, Surwit EA, Halum AV, Hatch KD. Abdominal-wall tumor implantation after laparoscopy for malignant conditions. Obstet Gynecol 1994;84: 765–769.
28. Wexner SD, Cohen SM. Port site metastases after laparoscopic colorectal surgery for cure of malignancy. Br J Surg 1995;82:295–298.
29. Nduka CC, Monson JRT, Menzies-Gow N, Darzi A. Abdominal wall metastases following laparoscopy. Br J Surg 1994; 81:648–652.
30. Leroy J, Champault G, Risk N, Boutelier P. Metastatic recurrence at the cannula site: should digestive carcinomas still be managed by laparoscopy (abstract). Br J Surg 1994; 81(suppl):31.
31. Wang PH, Yen MS, Yuan CC, et al. Port site metastasis after laparoscopic assisted vaginal hysterectomy for endometrial cancer: possible mechanisms and prevention. Gynecol Oncol 1997;66:151–155.
32. Kruitwagen RFPM, Swinkels BM, Keyser KGG, Doesburg WH, Schijf CHPTH. Incidence and effect on survival of abdominal wall metastases at trocar or puncture sites following laparoscopy or paracentesis in women with ovarian cancer. Gynecol Oncol 1996;60:233–237.
33. Lane G, Pfau SC. Ovarian cancer presenting in a laparoscopy scar and metastatic to the spleen. Br J Obstet Gynecol 1996;103:386–387.
34. Wang PH, Yuan CC, Chao KC, Yen MS, Ng HT, Chao HT. Squamous cell carcinoma of the cervix after laparoscopic surgery. A case report. J Reprod Med 1997;42:801–804.
35. Canis M, Pouly JL, Wattiez A, Mage G, Manhes H, Bruhat MA. Laparoscopic management of adnexal masses suspicious at ultrasound. Obstet Gynecol 1997;89:679–683.
36. Cohn DE, Tamimi HK, Goff BA. Intraperitoneal spread of cervical cancer after laparoscopic lymphadenectomy. Obstet Gynecol 1997;89:864.
37. Dembo AJ, Davy M, Stenwig AE, Berle EJ, Bush RS, Kjorstad K. Prognostic factors in patients with stage I epithelial ovarian cancer. Obstet Gynecol 1990;75:263–273.

38. Sevelda P, Vavra N, Schemper M, Salzer H. Prognostic factors for survival in stage I epithelial ovarian carcinoma. Cancer (Phila) 1990;65:2349–2352.
39. Finn CB, Luesley DM, Buxton EJ, et al. Is stage I epithelial ovarian cancer overtreated both surgically and systemically? Results of a five-year cancer registry review. Br J Obstet Gynecol 1992;99:54–58.
40. Vergote IB, Kaern J, Abeler VM, Pettersen EO, De Vos LN, Trpé CG. Analysis of pronostic factors in stage I epithelial ovarian carcinoma: Importance of degree of differentiation and desoxyribonucleic acid ploidy in predicting relapse. Am J Obstet Gynecol 1993;160:40–52.
41. Sjovall K, Nilsson B, Einhorn N. Prognostic incidence of intraoperative rupture of malignant ovarian tumor with immediate surgical treatment. In: Bruhat MA, ed. Proceedings of the 1st European Congress on Gynecologic Endoscopy. London: Blackwell, 1994:107–108.
42. Kodama S, Tanaka K, Tokunaga A, Sudo N, Takahashi T, Matsui K. Multivariate analysis of prognostic factors in patients with ovarian cancer stage I and II. Int J Obstet Gynecol Obstet 1997;56:147–153.
43. Maiman M, Seltzer V, Boyce J. Laparoscopic excision of ovarian neoplasms subsequently found to be malignant. Obstet Gynecol 1991;77:563–565.
44. Blanc B, Boubli L, D'Ercole C, Nicoloso E. Laparoscopic management of malignant ovarian cysts: a 78-case national survey. Part 1: preoperative and laparoscopic evaluation. Eur J Obstet Gynecol Reprod Biol 1994;56:177–180.
45. Blanc B, D'Ercole C, Nicoloso E, Boubli L. Laparoscopic management of malignant ovarian cysts: a 78-case national survey. Part 2: Follow up and final treatment. Eur J Obstet Gynecol Reprod Biol 1994;61:147–150.
46. Kinderman G, Maassen V, Kuhn W. Laparoscopic management of ovarian malignomas. Geburtsh Frauenkeilkd 1995;55:687–694.
47. Wenzl R, Lehner R, Husslein P, Sevelda P. Laparoscopic survey in cases of ovarian malignancies: an Austria-wide survey. Gynecol Oncol 1996;63:57–61.
48. Young RC, Decker DG, Wharton JT, et al. Staging laparotomy in early ovarian cancer. JAMA 1983;250:3072–3076.
49. Soper JT, Johnson P, Johnson V, Berchuk A, Clarke-Pearson DL. Comprehensive restaging laparotomy in women with apparent early ovarian carcinoma. Obstet Gynecol 1992;80:949–953.
50. Stier EA, Barakat RB, Curtin JP, Brown CL, Jones WB, Hoskins WJ. Laparotomy to complete staging of presumed early ovarian cancer. Obstet Gynecol 1996;87:737–740.
51. Helawa ME, Krepart GV, Lotocki R. Staging laparotomy in early epithelial ovarian carcinoma. Am J Obstet Gynecol 1986;154:282–286.
52. McGowan L, Lesher LP, Norris HJ, Barnett M. Mistaging of ovarian cancer. Obstet Gynecol 1985;65:568–572.
53. Clinical Outcomes of Surgical Therapy (COST) Study Group. Early results of laparoscopic surgery for colorectal cancer. Dis Colon Rectum 1996;39:S53–S58.
54. Querleu D, Leblanc E, Castelain B. Laparoscopic lymphadenectomy in the staging of early carcinoma of the cervix. Am J Obstet Gynecol 1991;164:579–581.
55. Pomel C, Canis M, Mage G, et al. Hystérectomie élargie par laparoscopie pour cancer du col utérin: technique, indications et résultats, à propos d'une série de 41 cas. Chir 1997;122:133–136.
56. Mathew G, Watson DI, Rofe AM, Baigrie CF, Ellis T, Jamieson GG. Wound metastases following laparoscopic and open surgery for abdominal cancer in a rat model. Br J Surg 1996;83:1087–1090.
57. Canis M, Botchorishvili R, Wattiez A, Mage G, Pouly JL, Bruhat MA. Tumor growth and dissemination after laparotomy and CO_2 pneumoperitoneum: a rat ovarian cancer model. Obstet Gynecol 1998;92:104–108.
58. Bouvy ND, Marquet RL, Jeekel H, Bonjer J. Impact of gas(less) laparoscopy and laparotomy on peritoneal tumor growth and abdominal wall metastases. Ann Surg 1996; 224:694–701.
59. Jacobi CA, Ordermann J, Böhm B, et al. The influence of laparotomy and laparoscopy on tumor growth in a rat model. Surg Endosc 1997;11:618–621.
60. Hubens G, Pauwels M, Hubens A, Vermeulen P, Van Marck E, Eyskens E. The influence of a pneumoperitoneum on peritoneal implantation of free intraperitoneal colon cancer cells. Surg Endosc 1996;10:809–812.
61. Targarona EM, Martinez J, Nadal A, et al. Cancer dissemination during laparoscopic surgery: tubes, gas and cells. World J Surg 1998;22:55–60.
62. Jones DB, Guo LW, Reinhard MK, et al. Impact of pneumoperitoneum on trocar site implantation of colon cancer in hamster model. Dis Colon Rectum 1995;38: 1182–1188.
63. Wu JS, Brasfield EB, Guo LW, et al. Implantation of colon cancer at trocar sites is increased by low pressure pneumoperitoneum. Surgery (St. Louis) 1997;122:1–7.
64. Watson DI, Mathew G, Ellis T, Baigrie CF, Rofe AM, Jamieson GG. Gasless laparoscopy may reduce the risk of port-site metastases following laparoscopic tumor surgery. Arch Surg 1997;132:166–168.
65. Allendorf JDF, Bessler M, Kayton ML, et al. Increased tumor establishment and growth after laparotomy vs laparoscopy in a murine model. Arch Surg 1995;130:649–653.
66. Bouvy ND, Marquet RL, Jeekel J, Bonjer HJ. Laparoscopic surgery is associated with less tumor growth stimulation than conventional surgery: an experimental study. Br J Surg 1997;84:358–361.
67. Volz J, Köster S, Schaeff B. Laparoscopic management of gynaecological malignancies, time to hesitate. Gynaecol Endosc 1997;6:145–146.
68. Mathew G, Watson DI, Rofe AM, Ellis T, Jamieson GG. Adverse impact of pneumoperitoneum on intraperitoneal implantation and growth of tumor cell suspension in an experimental model. Aust N Z J Surg 1997;67:289–292.
69. Mathew G, Watson DI, Ellis T, De Young N, Rofe AM, Jamieson GG. The effect of laparoscopy on the movement of tumor cells and metastasis to surgical wounds. Surg Endosc 1997;11:1163–1166.
70. Chen WS, Lin WC, Kou YR, Kuo HS, Hsu H, Yang WK. Possible effect of pneumoperitoneum on the spreading of colon cancer tumor cells. Dis Colon Rectum 1997;40: 791–797.
71. Le Moine MC, Navarro F, Burgel JS, et al. Experimental assessment of the risk of tumor recurrence after laparoscopic surgery. Surgery (St. Louis) 1998;123:427–431.

72. Bouvy ND, Giuffrida MC, Tseng LN, et al. Effects of carbon dioxide pneumoperitoneum, air pneumoperitoneum, and gasless laparoscopy on body weight and tumor growth. Arch Surg 1998;133:652–656.
73. Paik PS, Misawa T, Chiang M, et al. Abdominal incision tumor implantation following pneumoperitoneum laparoscopic procedure vs standard open incision in a syngenic rat model. Dis Colon Rectum 1998;41:419–422.
74. Allardyce R, Morreau P, Bagshaw P. Tumor cell distribution following laparoscopic colectomy in a porcine model. Dis Colon Rectum 1996;39:S47–S52.
75. Hewett PJ, Thomas WM, King G, Eaton M. Intraperitoneal cell movement during abdominal carbon dioxide insufflation and laparoscopy. Dis Colon Rectum 1996;39:S62–S66.
76. Whelan RL, Sellers GJ, Allendorf JD, et al. Trocar site recurrence is unlikely to result from aerosolization of tumor cells. Dis Colon Rectum 1996;39:S7–S13.
77. Zoetmuller FAN. Cancer cell seeding during abdominal surgery: experimental studies. In: Sugarbaker PH, ed. Peritoneal Carcinosis: Principles of Management. Boston: Kluwer, 1996:155–161.
78. Redmond HP, Watson WG, Houghton T, Condron C, Watson RGK, Bouchier-Hayes D. Immune function in patients undergoing open vs laparoscopic cholecystectomy. Arch Surg 1994;129:1240–1246.
79. Griffith JP, Everitt NJ, Lancaster F, et al. Influence of laparoscopic and conventional cholecystectomy upon cell-mediated immunity. Br J Surg 1995;82:677–680.
80. Allendorf JDF, Bessler M, Whelan RL, et al. Better preservation of immune function after laparoscopic-assisted vs open bowel resection in a murine model. Dis Colon Rectum 1996;39:S67–S72.
81. Reymond MA, Wittekind CH, Jung A, Hohenberger W, Kirchner TH, Kôckerling F. The incidence of port site metastases might be reduced. Surg Endosc 1997;11: 902–906.
82. Leather AJM, Kocjan G, Savage F, et al. Detection of free malignant cells in the peritoneal cavity before and after resection of colorectal cancer. Dis Colon Rectum 1994;37: 814–819.
83. Hansen E, Wolff N, Knuechel R, Ruschoff J, Hofstaedter F. Tumor cells in blood shed from the surgical field. Arch Surg 1995;130:387–393.
84. Wong LS, Morris AG, Fraser IA. The exfoliation of free malignant cells in the peritoneal cavity during resection of colon cancer. Surg Oncol 1996;5:115–121.
85. Jones FS, Rous P. On the cause of the localization of secondary tumors at points of injury. J Exp Med 1914;20: 404–412.
86. Fisher B, Fisher ER, Feduska N. Trauma and the localization of tumor cells. Cancer (Phila) 1967;20:23–30.
87. Murthy S, Goldschmidt RA, Rao LN, Ammirati M, Buchmann T, Scanlon EF. The influence of surgical trauma on experimental metastasis. Cancer (Phila) 1989;64: 2035–2044.
88. Baker DG, Masterson TM, Pace R, Constable WC, Wanebo H. The influence of the surgical wound on local tumor recurrence. Surgery (St. Louis) 1989;106:525–532.
89. Murthy MS, Summaria LJ, Miller RJ, Wyse TB, Goldschmidt RA, Scanlon EF. Inhibition of tumor implantation at sites of trauma by plasminogen activators. Cancer (Phila) 1991;68:1724–1730.
90. Jacquet P, Elias D, Sugarbaker PH. Tumor implantation in gastrointestinal wound sites. J Chir 1996;133:175–182.
91. Tol PM, Rossen EEM, Eijck CHJ, Bonthuis F, Marquet RL, Jeekel H. Reduction of peritoneal trauma by using non surgical gauze leads to less surgical implantation metastasis of spilled tumor cells. Ann Surg 1998;227:242–248.
92. See WA. Plasminogen activators: regulators of tumor cell adherence to sites of lower urinary tract surgical trauma. J Urol 1993;150:1024–1029.
93. Ruoslathi R, Giancotti FG. Integrins and tumor cell disemination. Cancer Cells (Cold Spring Harbor) 1989;1: 119–126.
94. Humphries MJ, Olden K, Yamada KM. A synthetic peptide from fibronectin inhibits experimental metastasis of murine melanoma cells. Science 1986;233:467–470.
95. Whalen GF, Ingber DE. Inhibition of tumor-cell attachment to extracellular matrix as a method for preventing tumor recurrence in a surgical wound. Ann Surg 1989; 210:758–764.
96. Murthy MS, Weiss BD, Miller RJ, Trueheart R, Scanlon EF. Inhibition of tumor implantation at sites of trauma by Arg-Gly-Asp containing proteins and peptides. Clin Exp Metastasis 1992;10:39–47.
97. Goldstein DS, Lu ML, Hattori T, Ratliff TL, Loughlin KR, Kavoussu LR. Inhibition of peritoneal tumor-cell implantation: model for laparoscopic cancer surgery. J Endourol 1993;7:237–241.
98. Mauviel A, Uitto J. The extracellular matrix in wound healing: role of the cytokine network. Wounds 1993;1: 137–152.
99. Slooter GD, Marquet RL, Jeekel J, Ijzermans JNM. Tumor growth stimulation after partial hepatectomy can be reduced by treatment with TNF-α. Br J Surg 1995;82: 129–132.
100. Gunji Y, Gorelik E. Role of fibrin coagulation in protection of murine tumor cells from the destruction by cytotoxic cells. Cancer Res 1988;48:5216–5221.
101. Sugarbaker PH. Patient selection and treatment of peritoneal carcinomatosis from colorectal and appendiceal cancer World J Surg 1995;19:235–240.
102. Moradi MM, Carson LF, Weinberg JB, et al. Serum and ascitic fluid levels of interleukin-1, interleukin-6, and tumor necrosis factor alpha in patients with epithlial ovarian cancer. Cancer (Phila) 1993;72:2433–2440.
103. Gotlieb WH, Abrams JS, Watson JM, et al. Presence of interleukin 10 (IL-10) in the ascites of patients with epithelial and other intraabdominal cancer. Cytokine 1992;4: 385–390.
104. Ryan GB, Grobety J, Majno G. Postoperative peritoneal adhesions. Am J Pathol 1971;65:117–148.
105. Watters WB, Buck RC. Scanning electron microscopy of mesothelial regeneration in the rat. Lab Invest 1972;26: 604–609.
106. Tol MP, Stijn I, Bonthuis F, Marquet RL, Jeekel J. Reduction of intraperitoneal adhesion formation by use of non abrasive gauze. Br J Surg 1997;84:1410–1415.
107. Groothuis PG, Koks CAM, de Goeij AF, Dunselman GAJ, Arends JW, Evers JLH. Adhesion of human endometrium

to the epithelial lining and extracellular matrix of amnion in vitro: an electron microscopic study. Hum Reprod (Oxf) 1998;13:2275–2281.
108. Kotzampassi K, Kapinidis N, Kazamias P, Eleftheriadis E. Hemodynamic events in the peritoneal environment during pneumoperitoneum in dogs. Surg Endosc 1993;7: 494–499.
109. Eleftheriadis E, Kotzampassi K, Papanotas K, Heliadis N, Sarris K. Gut ischemia, oxidative stress and bacterial transplantation in elevated abdominal pressure in rats. World J Surg 1996;20:11–16.
110. Berguer R, Cornelius T, Dalton M. The optimum pneumoperitoneum pressure for laparoscopic surgery in the rat model. Surg Endosc 1997;11:915–918.
111. Volz J, Köster S, Weiβ M, et al. Pathophysiology of a pneumoperitoneum in laparoscopy. A swine model. Am J Obstet Gynecol 1996;174:132–140.
112. Sahakian V, Rogers RG, Halme J, Hulka J. Effects of carbon dioxide-saturated normal saline and Ringer's lactate on postsurgical adhesion formation in the rabbit. Obstet Gynecol 1993;82:851–853.
113. Jacobi CA, Sabat R, Bohm B, Zieren HU, Volk HD, Muller JM. Pneumoperitoneum with carbon dioxide stimulates growth of malignant colonic cells. Surgery (St. Louis) 1997;121:72–78.
114. West MA, Baker J, Bellingham J. Kinetics of decreased LPS-stimulated cytokine release by macrophages exposed to CO_2. J Surg Res 1996;63:269–274.
115. Mahiout A, Brunkhorst R. Pyruvate anions neutralize peritoneal cytotoxicity. Nephrol Dial Transplant 1995; 10:391–394.
116. Watson RWG, Redmond HP, McCarthy J, Burke PE, Bouchier-Hayes D. Exposure of the peritoneal cavity to air regulates early inflammatory responses to surgery in a murine model. Br J Surg 1995;82:1060–1065.
117. Volz J, Paolucci V, Schaeff B, Koster S. Laparoscopic surgery: the effects of insufflation gas on tumor-induced lethality in nude mice. Am J Obstet Gynecol 1998; 178:793–795.
118. Kurz A, Sessler DI, Lenhardt R. For the study of wound infection and temperature group. N Engl J Med 1996; 334:1209–1215.
119. Beebe DS, Swica H, Carlson N, Palahniuk RJ, Goodale RL. High level of carbon monoxide are produced by electro-cautery of tissue during laparoscopic cholecystectomy. Anesth Anal 1993;77:338–341.
120. Salzberg Moore S, Green CR, Wang FL, Pandit SK, Hurd WW. The role of irrigation in the development of hypothermia during laparoscopic surgery. Am J Obstet Gynecol 1997;176:598–602.
121. Morris PC, Scholten V. Osmolytic lysis of tumor spill in ovarian cancer: a murine model. Am J Obstet Gynecol 1996;175:1489–1492.

22

Peritoneal Endometriosis

Mark A. Damario and John A. Rock

CONTENTS

Peritoneal endometriosis is a relatively common disease, but its prevalence in the general population is not entirely certain. From mostly uncontrolled clinical studies, an extraordinarily wide range of prevalence (0.7%–82%) is noted.[1] This wide range of prevalence is the result of inherent differences in the particular groups of women studied ("selection biases"). Therefore, women with the least risk of having endometriosis (asymptomatic parous women undergoing tubal sterilization) have been reported to have a low incidence (2%), whereas women with a high risk of having endometriosis (teenagers with pelvic pain severe enough to warrant laparoscopic investigation) have been reported to have a much higher prevalence (>50%).[2,3] Endometriosis appears to be present in approximately 25% (range, 4.5%–82.0%) and 20% (range, 2.1%–70%) of women undergoing laparoscopy for pelvic pain and infertility, respectively.[1]

Because of our lack of complete understanding with regards to the essential factors responsible for growth and maintenance of endometrial lesions, our present forms of therapy are limited. Although medical therapy has been associated with symptom relief and lesion regression in the majority of treated patients, the chief limitation of medical therapy is that lesions are capable of regrowth after discontinuation of the drug.[4] Medical therapy also seems to play a very limited role in the enhancement of fertility. Surgical therapy, on the other hand, has been reported to be more effective in the long-term management of this disease. Fertility appears to be clearly enhanced in women following conservative surgery for severe disease.[5] It has also been shown that women undergoing laparoscopic ablative surgery for early-stage disease also have enhancement of fertility.[6,7] In addition, numerous uncontrolled studies have reported immediate relief of pelvic pain to be significant (between 70% and 100%) after conservative surgery.[8] Long-term follow-up, however, has demonstrated that maintenance of pain relief is present in a lesser percentage of patients, even after aggressive excisional resection at laparoscopy.[9] The limitation of surgical therapy appears to be that lesions frequently reappear. It has been estimated that 28% of patients within 18 months and 40% after 9 years will experience reappearance of peritoneal endometriotic lesions.[10]

Effective long-term management of peritoneal adhesions associated with endometriosis has also been historically disappointing. Peritoneal adhesions have been reported to reform in 40% to 50% of patients undergoing lysis of adhesions at time of conservative surgery for endometriosis.[11] Women with endometriosis have long been suspected to have an increased propensity for postoperative adhesion formation. It has been hypothesized that the impact of a heightened degree of peritoneal fluid inflammation on the peritoneal healing process is most responsible.

Recent studies have produced new insights into our understanding of this common, yet enigmatic, disorder. These studies have promoted development of promising therapeutic modalities. Improved surgical techniques, adjuvant barriers, and medications designed to alter the peritoneal inflammatory response all show promise in the management of peritoneal endometriosis and associated adhesions.

Pathogenesis

Multifactorial Etiology

The development of endometriosis is most likely a multifactorial event. There are numerous theories as to the etiology of endometriosis, with none fully adequate to explain all manifestations of the disease. The most widely accepted implantation theory suggests that viable endometrial cells reflux through the fallopian tubes during menstruation and subsequently implant on peritoneal surfaces or abdominal organs. To support this theory are experiments that have proven the viability of cast-off cells from shed endometrium in menstrual effluvium.[12] Viable endometrial cells have also been found in the fallopian tube[13] and peritoneal fluid.[14,15] Experiments in animals and human subjects revealed that the placement of endometrial tissue in ectopic locations results in lesions histologically similar to endometriosis.[16–18] It is known that retrograde menstruation occurs commonly. Halme et al.[19] showed that bloody peritoneal fluid was noted in 90% of women when laparoscopies were performed during the time of menstruation. Those women who are at increased risk for a higher volume of retrograde menstruation also appear to be at higher risk for peritoneal endometriosis. In a comprehensive study, women with short cycles and longer flow had more than twice the risk of endometriosis than women with longer cycles and shorter duration of flow.[20] It has also been suggested that women with endometriosis may demonstrate a greater degree of uterotubal atonia, which may be predisposing them to greater volumes of retrograde menstruation.[14] Certainly, there have also been associations between cervical stenosis[21] as well as congenital outflow tract obstruction[22] and endometriosis.

As retrograde menstruation appears to be quite common, it is not entirely known why endometriosis is actually not more prevalent. Studies on the factors involved in initial contact between endometrial cells and the peritoneal lining are just beginning. Van der Linden et al.[23,24] studied the expression of members of the integrin and cadherin family in endometriotic lesions. Cadherins are calcium-dependent transmembrane glycoproteins that predominantly mediate cell–cell interactions.[25] Integrins are a family of cell-membrane glycoproteins consisting of an α- and β-subunit that primarily mediate cell–extracellular matrix (ECM) interactions.[26] Integrins $\alpha_2\beta_1$, $\alpha_3\beta_1$, $\alpha_4\beta_1$, $\alpha_5\beta_1$, and $\alpha_6\beta_1$ and E-cadherin have been shown to be expressed in endometriotic lesions as well as in cells and tissues that are potentially involved in the development of endometriosis.[23] However, regurgitated endometrial cells obtained from peritoneal fluid showed expression of cell adhesion molecules, particularly E-cadherin and some β_1 integrins, although to a lesser extent than seen in in situ endometrium. This finding suggests that there may be some loss of cell adhesion molecules in the process of endometrial shedding during menses. Perhaps this process may be differentially regulated in endometriosis and normal patients.

A second process that may regulate the implantation of viable endometrial cells in the peritoneal cavity focuses on local immune factors normally responsible for clearance of debris and foreign cells. Peritoneal macrophages are the primary cell type in the peritoneal cavity and are the cell type most likely responsible for the removal of potentially viable refluxed endometrial cells. In studies comparing women with endometriosis to fertile and infertile women without endometriosis, differences in the cellular and biochemical composition of peritoneal fluid have been noted. Hill et al.[27] found increased concentrations of leukocytes in peritoneal fluid of patients with stages I and II endometriosis compared to fertile controls. Halme et al.[28,29] demonstrated an increased number of activated peritoneal macrophages as well as an increased rate of macrophage-derived growth factor secretion in women with endometriosis. Similarly, increased peritoneal fluid concentrations and in vitro macrophage production of interleukin-1 (IL-1),[30,31] tumor necrosis factor-α (TNF-α),[32,33] and interleukin-8 (IL-8)[34] have been described in endometriosis patients. The production of interleukin-6 (IL-6)[35] and interleukin-10 (IL-10)[36] by cultured peritoneal macrophages from patients with endometriosis has also been shown to be greater than in cultured peritoneal macrophages from fertile controls. In addition, transforming growth factor-β (TGF-β) has also been found to be in greater concentration in the peritoneal fluid from women with endometriosis.[37]

Recently, two cytokines that are predominantly monocyte chemoattractants, MCP-1[38] and RANTES,[39] have also been noted to have higher peritoneal levels in women with endometriosis compared to controls. In sum, these growth factors and cytokines are known to have specific effects on growth and differentiation of endometrial cells. It is unclear, however, whether the increased concentration of peritoneal mononuclear cells and cytokine products contribute to the histogenesis of endometriotic lesions or whether these findings are simply a result of the immunologic reaction to peritoneal endometriotic lesions. On the other hand, the increased peritoneal cytokine levels may also contribute to the formation of fibrinous adhesions, which are often found in association with peritoneal endometriotic implants.

Immune Response

There is further evidence of alterations in the immune response in endometriosis patients. Various data suggest alterations in both cell-mediated and hormonal immunity in peritoneal endometriosis. An early study by Weed and Arguembourg[40] identified the presence of the C_3 component of complement and IgG deposits in the eutopic endometrium of women with endometriosis, suggesting that the pathogenesis of endometriosis involved an alteration of the immune response. Mathur et al.[41] identified IgG and IgA autoantibodies against endometrial tissue in serum and in vaginal as well as cervical secretions of women with endometriosis. Unfortunately, these latter findings could not be confirmed by other groups.[42] Oosterlynck et al.[43] noted the intriguing finding of altered peritoneal immunity manifested by decreased cytotoxicity to endometrial cells attributable to a defect in peritoneal natural killer cells in women with advanced endometriosis. This latter study lends further support to the theory that women with endometriosis have endometrial cells that are somehow less susceptible to the normal body defense mechanisms and, as a result, implant and grow more easily in ectopic sites.

Angiogenesis

Angiogenic factors released from peritoneal macrophages may also play a role in the development of endometriosis. Utilizing glass filters impregnated with peritoneal fluid on the exposed chorioallantoic membrane of chick embryos, it was noted that the peritoneal fluid from endometriosis patients appeared to initiate more angiogenic activity than peritoneal fluid from controls.[44] In addition, the potent angiogenic factor, vascular endothelial growth factor (VEGF), is present in significantly increased levels in the peritoneal fluid of women with endometriosis.[45,46] It is somewhat unclear whether these angiogenic factors are produced by refluxed menstrual endometrial cells or endometriotic lesions themselves. It may be hypothesized, however, that because growth of endometriotic lesions requires an accessible blood supply, the increased release of these angiogenic factors may facilitate lesion development by permitting increased microvascularization of the parietal peritoneum.

Lymphatic Dissemination

Dissemination of endometrial cells through lymphatic or vascular channels has long been appreciated.[47,48] This mechanism may account for the rare findings of endometriosis at sites distant from the pelvis, such as lung and pelvic lymph nodes. Numerous accounts of endometriosis in episiotomy scars and laparotomy scars following gynecologic procedures and cesarean sections suggest that endometriosis can result from mechanical transplantation of viable endometrial tissue.[49,50] The theory of coelomic metaplasia, in which it is hypothesized that peritoneal mesothelium may dedifferentiate into endometrial-like glands and stroma, is supported by rare instances of endometriosis in women with Mullerian agenesis,[51] or the occasional presence of endometriosis in men.[52] The ability of peritoneal mesothelium to undergo such metaplastic change, however, has never been proven. Finally, the embryonic cell rest theory is based on the existence of small clusters or rests of Mullerian cells that have the potential to develop into functioning endometrial-like tissue. Because no cells of this type have been documented, this latter theory also remains speculative.

Pathophysiology

Pelvic Pain

Although endometriosis is acknowledged as a cause of pelvic pain, little is known about the exact mechanisms of pain production. Conventional thinking states that pain is related to the sequential swelling of endometriotic implants and the extravasation of blood and menstrual debris into surrounding tissues. However, ectopic endometrium does not usually appear to respond cyclically in concert with eutopic endometrium.[53] Reasons stated for this behavior include a lower hormonal receptor population in endometriotic lesions[54,55] as well as other alterations in peritoneal fluid regulatory factors.

It has been postulated that inflammatory substances may contribute to the pain associated with endometriosis. Endometriotic lesions may secrete prostaglandins,[56] and responding macrophages may secrete various inflammatory mediators such as IL-1[30,31] and TNF-α,[32,33] which may cause local inflammation, tissue damage, fibrosis, and pain. Advanced endometriosis may cause pain by leakage of endometriotic cysts and consequent peritoneal irritation, retraction of the peritoneal surface by scarring, stretching of the peritoneal surface by an enlarging mass,or invasion of other viscera.

Pelvic pain has been associated with various morphologic appearances of endometriosis, including atypical forms.[57] A substantial body of evidence is now accumulating with regards to evolution of peritoneal endometriosis and lesion type. Red peritoneal lesions represent the first stage following implantation of endometrial glands and stroma. Red peritoneal endometriotic lesions share many morphologic and morphometric features with eutopic endometrium.[58] Red peritoneal lesions have also been noted to be more active metabolically, with increased production of prostaglandins.[59] Red peritoneal lesions are present more frequently in younger patients.[60] After partial shedding, red lesions produce an inflammatory reaction that provokes scarification. Resultant scarification turns the lesions black. Subsequent fibrosis may also lead to areas of white opacification, which are believed to represent completely inactive lesions.

A significant amount of data is now accumulating associating deeply invasive endometriotic lesions with pelvic pain. Cornillie et al.[61] found that lesions penetrating deeper than 5 mm were more likely to be associated with pelvic pain. Koninckx and coworkers[62] found that the degree of pelvic pain was not related to the total surface area of endometriosis or the type of implant. These investigators noted that pain correlated most strongly with the depth of penetration of the deepest lesions. The posterior cul-de-sac and rectovaginal septum are common sites for deeply invasive lesions. Nisolle and Donnez[58] offered an opinion with regards to the histogenesis of rectovaginal nodular endometriotic lesions. Because of the many morphologic and histochemical differences from superficial peritoneal lesions, these authors have recommended considering peritoneal endometriosis and rectovaginal nodules as two different disease entities. They believe that rectovaginal nodules should be considered as adenomyomas because of the frequent presence of surrounding smooth muscle, active glandular epithelium, and scant stroma.

Infertility

In advanced stages, endometriosis can result in the formation of ovarian endometriomas and adhesions that distort normal pelvic anatomy. Peritubular adhesions and periovarian adhesions can alter the crucial tubo-ovarian relationships necessary for ovum pickup. Fimbrial distortion or destruction, the formation of fimbrial bridges, and even distal occlusion with formation of a hydrosalpinx can result. Endometriosis is also a common cause of proximal tubal occlusion, with endometriosis found as the etiologic factor in 14% of patients undergoing proximal tubal resection and reanastomosis in one series.[63] Ovarian endometriosis and endometriomas have also been associated with ovarian dysfunction and anovulation. In certain cases, fixation in the pelvis or encasement in adhesions mechanically prohibits ovum release into the abdominal cavity. In advanced cases, large volumes of ovarian stroma may also be destroyed by endometriomas.

The factors contributing to reduced fecundity associated with mild to moderate disease, in the absence of anatomic distortion, are less clear. Many mechanisms have been proposed, including toxic effects of prostaglandins, macrophage activation, altered immune responses, and abnormalities of ovulation, fertilization, and implantation.

The fallopian tubes and ovaries are naturally bathed in peritoneal fluid. The volume of peritoneal fluid varies, with a peak noted at about the time of ovulation. Some reports have noted an increased volume of peritoneal fluid in patients with endometriosis.[15] It has been suggested that peritoneal fluid volume may be a prognostic indicator as patients with a volume less than 14 mL generally have higher pregnancy rates than those with larger volumes.[64] There is some evidence that peritoneal fluid in patients with endometriosis exhibits reproductive toxicity. For instance, mouse oocyte pickup was impaired after exposure to peritoneal fluid from patients with endometriosis.[65] There is also evidence that peritoneal fluid from endometriosis patients has adverse effects on sperm motility and velocity.[66]

Prostaglandins appear to play a diverse role in reproductive functions, such as the regulation of follicular rupture, regression of the corpus luteum, tubal motility, and uterine contractility. Prostaglandins may also play a role in macrophage activation and the local immune response. Some studies have reported increased levels of prostaglandins in the peritoneal fluid of endometriosis patients,[67,68] but other studies have not.[69] One explanation for this conflicting evidence is that both peritoneal fluid volume and prostanoid concentrations vary greatly over the course of the menstrual cycle. Another hypothesis is that levels of prostaglandin synthesis may differ according to the type of endometriotic lesion. Vernon et al.[59] reported, in terms of prostaglandin F production, that reddish petechial lesions were more biochemically active than intermediate brownish lesions, which in turn were more active than powder-burn or black implants.

There have been several reports of increased numbers and activation of peritoneal macrophages in the setting of endometriosis.[28,70,71] One of the primary actions of activated macrophages is the recognition and phagocytosis of foreign antigens. It has been shown that peritoneal macrophages can phagocytose sperm in vitro. Peritoneal macrophages from patients with endometriosis exhibit greater phagocytosis of sperm than peritoneal macrophages from fertile controls or infertile women without endometriosis.[72] Macrophages are also known to modify local immune responses by the secretion of various cytokines. In addition to their known effects as primary mediators of the local immune response, certain cytokines known to be elevated in the peritoneal fluid of endometriosis patients have been suspected to have potential adverse reproductive effects. For instance, researchers have noted mouse embryo development toxicity with concentrations of IL-1 that are typically found in the peritoneal fluid of endometriosis patients.[30]

Reduced folliculogenesis has been noted in endometriosis patients. Reduced follicular growth, as assessed by follicular diameter change, has been correlated with endometriosis.[73] Other studies have also shown smaller follicles as well as lower preovulatory estradiol levels.[74] In addition, the luteinized unruptured follicle syndrome has been reported to be more common in patients with endometriosis.[75] Inadequate luteolysis and prolongation of corpus luteal function has also been suggested on the basis of estradiol and progesterone concentrations from peripheral and ovarian veins during the early follicular phase.[76] Discounting some earlier reports,[77,78] recent well-controlled studies have failed to find a relationship between endometriosis and increased pregnancy wastage.[79,80]

Peritoneal Environment in Endometriosis and Adhesion Formation

Growth factors and inflammatory mediators produced by activated peritoneal leukocytes are postulated to play a role in the pathogenesis of peritoneal endometriotic implants. The peritoneal fluid environment in endometriosis is characterized by elevated levels of inflammatory cellular products, such as prostaglandins, proteolytic enzymes, complement components, IL-1, TNF-α, IL-6, TGF-β, and VEGF, and decreased levels of IFN-γ compared to the peritoneal fluid from women without the disease (Table 22.1).[30,32–34,37,46,81–91] IL-1, TNF-α, and IL-6, which are potent proinflammatory cytokines exert a plethora of immunologic changes that accompany acute and chronic inflammation. Functions of IFN-γ include induction of major histocompatibility antigens and general inhibition of cell growth and differentiation. Interestingly, in response to GnRH-a (gonadotropin-releasing hormone agonist) therapy, IL-6 concentrations and IFN-γ concentrations have been noted to decrease and increase, respectively, in the peritoneal fluid of endometriosis patients.[83] In addition, the peritoneal fluid from endometriosis patients has also been characterized by elevated concentrations of three additional proinflammatory chemoattractant cytokines: MCP-1, IL-8, and growth-regulated α. Perhaps these proinflammatory chemical messengers may also play a role in the development of peritoneal adhesions that often accompany endometriotic lesions.

TABLE 22.1. Growth factors and cytokines known to have elevated concentrations in peritoneal fluid of patients with endometriosis.

Mediator	Concentration	Reference
TGF-β	↑	Oosterlynck et al.[37]
IGFs	↑	Giudice et al.[85]
PDGF	↑	Halme et al.[29]
IL-1	↑	Fakih et al.[30]; Taketani et al.[31]
IL-4	↑	Hsu et al.[86]
IL-6	↑	Rier et al.[81]; Koyama et al.[87]
IL-8	↑	Ryan et al.[88]; Arici et al.[89]
TNF-α	↑	Taketani et al.[31]; Eiserman et al.[32]; Halme[33]
MCP-1	↑	Akoum et al.[38]; Arici et al.[90]
GR-α	↑	Oral et al.[91]
RANTES	↑	Khorram et al.[39]

TGF, transforming growth factor; IGFs, insulin-like growth factors; PDGF, platelet-derived growth factor; IL, interleukin; TNF, tumor necrosis factor; IFN, interferon; MCP, monocyte chemotactic protein; GR, growth-regulated.

Dou et al.[92] recently proposed an important role for TGF-β_1 in regulating the growth, anchor-dependent cell aggregation, and integrin mRNA expression in human promonocytes. Using TGF-β antisense oligonucleotides, these investigators were able to downregulate TGF-β mRNA in a dose-dependent manner. Utilizing a promonocyte human cell line, the TGF-β antisense oligonucleotides inhibited the rate of DNA synthesis and proliferation of these cells. Colony formation was also suppressed under anchor-dependent culture conditions (soft agar assay), and α_2, α_3, α_4, α_6, β_1, and β_2 integrin mRNA expression was markedly reduced. Therefore, these results provided evidence for an autocrine loop of monocyte/macrophage-derived TGF-β_1 action that is essential for regulation of growth, aggregation, and expression of adhesion molecules. Perhaps the higher numbers of activated tissue macrophages (with their capacity to express excess TGF-β_1) produces an environment whereby cell–cell and cell–matrix interactions are enhanced, with subsequent development of endometriotic implants and peritoneal fibrinous adhesions.

Surgical Techniques to Limit Adhesion Formation

Emphasizing the Laparoscopic Approach

The development of improved endoscopic instrumentation, optics, and video systems has allowed more complex gynecologic operations to be performed via the laparoscope. There are many advantages emphasizing a laparoscopic approach to reproductive surgery, particularly in the treatment of peritoneal endometriosis. Besides the advantages of patient convenience, prompt recovery, and cost savings, there is a growing body of evidence that operative laparoscopy limits postoperative adhesion formation. Operative laparoscopy avoids tissue drying, exposure to cool temperatures, foreign bodies (such as lint and talc), and abrasions occurring during packing and tissue handling. Because of these advantages, many authors believe that operative laparoscopy is effective in minimizing both adhesion reformation as well as de novo adhesion formation following surgery.

Several studies in laboratory animals have concluded that significantly fewer postoperative adhesions followed surgical procedures performed laparoscopically.[93,94] One retrospective review failed to ascertain the superiority of laparotomy versus laparoscopy in improving pregnancy rates in women with endometriosis, although there was evidence suggesting that laser laparoscopy may have been superior in the setting of moderate to severe disease.[95] Fayez et al.[96] reported significantly higher pregnancy rates in endometriosis patients treated with laparoscopy (58%) than for similar patients who were treated by laparotomy (36%). Recently, a large ($n = 579$) retrospective study compared pregnancy rates of patients across all stages of endometriosis and compared outcomes following no treatment, medical therapy, operative laparoscopy, and laparotomy.[97] Utilizing a life table analysis, the authors actually reported that the laparoscopic group had approximately equal fecundity to those not receiving any treatment. Both of these latter two groups, however, had higher fecundity rates than either the medical therapy or laparotomy groups.

The approach used in the surgical management of the infertile woman with endometriosis should be based primarily on the expertise of the surgeon. If the surgeon is relatively equally proficient in both approaches, then the laparoscopic approach will provide economic and social benefits for the patient. The laparoscopic approach appears to provide a result at least equal, if not superior, to that from the utilization of microsurgical techniques at laparotomy.

Recognizing the Protean Manifestations of Peritoneal Endometriosis

To maximize results, the surgeon treating the infertile patient with endometriosis should be familiar with the various manifestations of peritoneal endometriosis. If peritoneal lesions are not properly identified, then the disease will persist and eventually progress.

Jansen and Russell[98] were the first to draw attention to some of the subtle appearances of nonpigmented endometriosis. These authors described several types of lesions including (1) white opacification of the peritoneum with or without thickening; (2) red, flamelike lesions of the peritoneum, often raised above the peritoneal surface; (3) vesicular glandular excresences on the peritoneal surface; (4) unexplained lesions between the undersurface of the ovary and the peritoneum of the ovarian fossa; (5) yellow-brown patches; and (6) circular peritoneal defects. Histologic specimens confirmed endometriosis in 81% of white, opacified lesions; 81% of red, flamelike lesions; 67% of glandular lesions; 50% of subovarian adhesions; 47% of yellow-brown patches; and in 45% of circular peritoneal defects.

Stripling and coauthors[99] noted that increased documentation of subtle nonpigmented lesions was related to the surgeon's experience and awareness of such lesions. In their series, subtle lesions were identified in 32% of patients undergoing laparoscopy during the first 5 months of the study and in 72% of patients undergoing laparoscopy during the last 5 months of the study. Martin et al.[100] also reported an increase in the diagnosis of endometriosis (from 42% to 72% of patients) occurring following increased surgeon awareness of subtle lesions.

Besides the subtle lesions of nonpigmented endometriosis, the phenomenon of microscopic endometriosis has also been described. Vasquez and colleagues described characteristics of minimal peritoneal endometriotic lesions utilizing scanning electron microscopy techniques.[101] Murphy and coworkers reported being able to identify microscopic endometriosis by scanning electron microscopy in 25% of random biopsies of visually normal peritoneum in patients with endometriosis.[102] Therefore, it appears somewhat unrealistic to believe that all disease is being treated during most surgical procedures for peritoneal endometriosis. Becoming very familiar with the various protean manifestations of peritoneal endometriosis, however, will allow one to limit the volume of residual disease and to optimize results.

Treatment Methods That Eradicate Lesions Effectively and Preserve Normal Tissue

The destruction of peritoneal implants can be achieved using one of a number of techniques. Choice of a particular technique depends on the size, extent, and location of implants as well as the surgeon's experience. All surgeons operating on infertile women with endometriosis should fully understand the basic physics and usual tissue effects of the particular modality employed (Fig. 22.1).

Lesions can be removed by sharp excision at either laparotomy or laparoscopy. The advantage of sharp excision is that it allows histologic confirmation and avoids

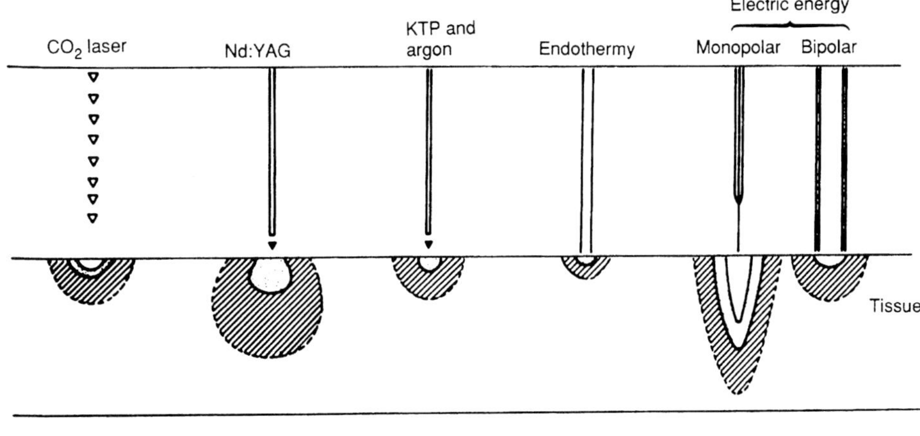

FIG. 22.1. Relative tissue damage created by various energy sources. (Reprinted with permission from ref. 109.)

any destruction of adjacent normal tissue. The main disadvantage of sharp excision is the risk of bleeding and hemorrhage. Monopolar electrocauterization permits complete and deep coagulation of nodular lesions. The advantage of monopolar cautery is its ease of use and usual absence of bleeding. Disadvantages of monopolar cautery are the risk of electrical burn injuries to viscera, destruction of tissue without biopsies, and considerable collateral tissue damage. Bipolar electrocauterization allows for a more precise coagulation of tissue. Its advantages again are primarily ease of use and usual absence of bleeding. Its main disadvantage is that it achieves only a very superficial coagulation and, therefore, presents a higher risk of disease persistence in deeper lesions.

CO_2 laser vaporization is a popular technique as it permits a complete, precise, and controlled destruction of tissue. CO_2 laser vaporization also assures the operator that lesions are treated to a proper depth because it permits visualization at the base of lesions. CO_2 laser vaporization is also associated with minimal postoperative adhesion formation.[93] The main disadvantages of the CO_2 laser are the generation of smoke and its expense. The CO_2 laser can also be utilized as an excisional tool, a preferred technique for large lesions, such as rectovaginal nodules.[103,104] Other lasers, such as the Nd-YAG, argon, and potassium-titanylphosphate (KTP) lasers, have all been used for the surgical treatment of peritoneal endometriosis. These lasers, in general, have more coagulation tendency and are usually less precise than the CO_2 laser. Their use through flexible fibers and either contact or near-contact mode, however, makes them easier to operate, and backstopping is not generally needed. The Nd-YAG laser, whose tissue effect is ordinarily characterized by a large zone of lateral thermal spread, can also be focused through the application of sapphire tips. When utilizing any laser, power settings should be set at appropriate levels so that contiguous thermal damage is minimized.

General "microsurgical" techniques should be maintained whether operating by laparotomy or laparoscopy. These principles include use of magnification, meticulous hemostasis, continuous irrigation, careful tissue handling, and use of nonreactive staples or suture materials. During adhesiolysis procedures, in general, it is best to attempt to completely excise fibrinous adhesions. Fibrinous adhesion remnants not only contain devascularized tissue but actually are often found to contain active endometriotic glands and stroma.[105]

Use of Adjunctive Medical Therapy

The use of preoperative medical therapy, either danazol or GnRH agonists, may offer some potential advantages that include suppression of functional cysts, reducing the volume of disease, and facilitating surgical treatment, as well as limiting surgical risks. The reduced pelvic vascularity may result in reduced inflammation and postoperative adhesions, although this has not been proven. Potential disadvantages of preoperative medical therapy include delay in ultimate diagnosis, the costs and potential side effects of the drug, and the potential for changed appearances of peritoneal lesions (and a subsequent more difficult diagnosis).

Postoperative medical therapy may be indicated to attain complete obliteration of disease, to treat possible microscopic or residual disease, or to treat patients who either continue to have pain or have recurrence of pain. Most studies do not report an advantage to either preoperative or postoperative medical therapy in terms of enhanced pregnancy rates with combined treatment.

Adjunctive Therapies to Prevent Adhesions

Many adjunctive therapies to prevent postoperative adhesions have been tried following surgery for peritoneal endometriosis. These modalities include high molecular weight dextran, steroids, antihistamines, antiinflammatory agents, anticoagulant agents (heparin), fibrinolytic agents, and barrier methods. Only barrier methods have had clearly proven efficacy. The goal of barriers is to prevent apposition of tissue surfaces during the early phases of healing. The main commercially available surgical barriers that have been extensively studied to date are oxidized regenerated cellulose (Interceed [TC7] Absorbable Adhesion Barrier; Johnson & Johnson Medical, Somerville, NJ, USA) and expanded polytetrafluoroethylene (PTFE; Gore-Tex Surgical Membrane, W.L. Gore and Associates, Flagstaff, AZ, USA).

Both products can be utilized at either laparotomy or laparoscopy. The TC7 barrier is absorbable, whereas the Gore-Tex Surgical Membrane is not. The Gore-Tex Surgical Membrane barrier has a history of long-term use in other surgical disciplines, such as cardiac surgery where it has served as a pericardial patch. It is inert and may not pose any long-term risks; however, most reproductive surgeons have opted to remove the Gore-Tex Surgical Membrane at second-look laparoscopy. The TC7 barrier is easy to use and adheres easily to tissue once dampened. Its main limitation appears to be limited efficacy in the presence of blood. Therefore, it is important to have a perfectly hemostatic surgical site for proper use of this barrier.

Two studies have specifically reviewed the efficacy of the TC7 barrier following conservative surgery for peritoneal endometriosis. The first was a randomized, multicenter study performed in Japan in which 63 patients from 12 treatment centers were enrolled.[106] Patients were eligible if they demonstrated bilateral pelvic sidewall adhesions. Those patients who had evidence of active infection were excluded. Twenty-nine of the 63 patients had endometriosis (20 of these patients were judged to be stage IV). Following complete lysis of adhesions at laparotomy, each patient had one pelvic sidewall treated through random assignment and the other sidewall left untreated. At second-look laparoscopy, significantly more adhesions were present on the control pelvic sidewalls (48/63; 76%) than on the treated sidewalls (26/63, 41%; $p < 0.0001$). In addition, the TC7-treated sidewalls also showed significantly less area involved with adhesions. Specifically, for the 28 endometriosis patients, the results were similar: significantly more adhesions on the control side (23/28, 82%) than the treated side (14/28, 50%; $p < 0.05$). In the second trial, 32 women with severe endometriosis and complete, cul-de-sac obliteration underwent random assignment to either laparoscopic surgery alone or laparoscopic surgery plus TC7 barrier.[107] At time of second-look laparoscopy, 12 of 16 (75%) women treated with the TC7 barrier were free of adhesions as compared to only 2 of 16 controls (12.5%; $p < 0.05$).

A number of other barriers have had some limited use in either animal trials or small clinical series. Use of fibrin glue was reported to reduce postoperative adhesions following laparoscopic resection of large ovarian endometriomas.[108] The ideal barrier as an adjunct to surgery for peritoneal endometriosis would be one that can easily be applied through laparoscopic techniques and is versatile enough to maintain efficacy in a variety of clinical circumstances.

Summary

Patients with peritoneal endometriosis are prone to adhesion formation following conservative surgical treatment. The reasons include the effects of the altered peritoneal environment and proinflammatory growth factors and cytokines on the normal tissue healing process. Our lack of complete understanding with regards to the pathogenesis of peritoneal endometriosis leaves us without a form of treatment with 100% efficacy. At the present time, methods to limit postoperative adhesions following surgical therapy for peritoneal endometriosis include emphasis on laparoscopic techniques, effective methods of lesion destruction with preservation of normal tissue, heightened surgeon awareness of atypical lesions, and adjuvant tissue barriers.

References

1. Eskenazi B, Warner ML. Epidemiology of endometriosis. Obstet Gynecol Clin North Am 1997;24:235–258.
2. Strathy JH, Molgoard CA, Coulam CB, et al. Endometriosis and infertility: a laparoscopic study of endometriosis among fertile and infertile women. Fertil Steril 1982;38:667–672.
3. Chatman DL, Ward AB. Endometriosis in adolescents. J Reprod Med 1982;27:156–160.
4. Waller KG, Shaw RW. Gonadotropin-releasing hormone analogs in the treatment of endometriosis: long-term follow-up. Fertil Steril 1993;59:511–515.
5. Buttram VC. Conservative surgery for endometriosis in the infertile female: a study of 206 patients with implications for both medical and surgical therapy. Fertil Steril 1979;31:117–123.
6. Nowroozi K, Chase JS, Check JH, et al. The importance of laparoscopic coagulation of mild endometriosis in infertile women. Int J Fertil 1987;32:442–444.
7. Marcoux S, Maheux R, Berube S, et al. Laparoscopic surgery in infertile women with minimal or mild endometriosis. N Engl J Med 1997;337:217–222.
8. Damario MA, Rock JA. Pain recurrence: a quality of life issue in endometriosis. Int J Gynecol Obstet 1995;50(suppl 1)S27–S42.

9. Redwine DB. Laparosocopic excision of endometriosis by sharp dissection: lifetable analysis of reoperation and persistent or recurrent disease. Fertil Steril 1991;56:628–634.
10. Olive DL, Schwartz LB. Endometriosis. N Engl J Med 1993;328:1759–1769.
11. Vancaillie T, Schenken RS. Endoscopic surgery. In: Schenken RS, ed. Endometriosis: Contemporary Concepts in Clinical Management. Philadelphia: Lippincott, 1989: 249–266.
12. Keetel WC, Stein RJ. The viability of the cast-off menstrual endometrium. Am J Obstet Gynecol 1951;61:440–442.
13. Novak E. The significance of uterine mucosa in the fallopian tube, with a discussion of the origin of aberrant endometrium. Am J Obstet Gynecol 1926;12:484–526.
14. Bartosik D, Jacobs SL, Kelly LJ. Endometrial tissue in peritoneal fluid. Fertil Steril 1986;46:796–800.
15. Syrop CH, Halme J. Peritoneal fluid environment and infertility. Fertil Steril 1987;48:1–9.
16. Te Linde RW, Scott RB. Experimental endometriosis. Am J. Obstet Gynecol 1950;60:1147–1173.
17. Merrill JA. Endometrial induction of endometrisosis. across Millipore filters. Am J Obstet Gynecol 1966;34: 366–398.
18. Vernon MW, Wilson EA. Studies on the surgical induction of endometriosis in the rat. Fertil Steril 1985;44:684–694.
19. Halme J. Hammond MG, Hulka JF, et al. Retrograde menstruation in healthy women and in patients with endometriosis. Obstet Gynecol 1984;64:151–154.
20. Candiani GB, Danesino V, Gastaldi A, et al. Reproductive and menstrual factors and risk of peritoneal and ovarian endometriosis. Fertil Steril 1991;56:230–234.
21. Barbieri RL, Callery M, Perez SE. Directionality of menstrual flow: cervical os diameter as a determinant of retrograde menstruation. Fertil Steril 1992;57:727–730.
22. Olive DL, Henderson DY. Endometriosis and mullerian anomalies. Obstet Gynecol 1987;69:412–415.
23. Van der Linden PJQ, de GoeiJ AFPM, Dunselman GAJ, et al. Expression of integrins and E-cadherin in cells from menstrual effluent, endometrium, peritoneal fluid, peritoneum and endometriosis. Fertil Steril 1994;61:85–90.
24. Van der Linden PLQ, de Goeij AFPM, Dunselman GAJ, et al. P-cadherin expression in human endometrium and endometriosis. Gynecol Obstet Invest 1994;38:183–185.
25. Takeichi M. Cadherins: a molecular family important in selective cell-cell adhesion. Annu Rev Biochem 1990;59: 237–252.
26. Abdelda SM. Biology of disease. Role of integrins and other cell adhesion molecules in tumor progression and metastasis. Lab Invest 1993;68:4–17.
27. Hill JA, Faris HMP, Schiff I, et al. Characterization of leukocyte subpopulations in the peritoneal fluid of women with endometriosis. Fertil Steril 1988;50:216–222.
28. Halme J, Becker S, Wing R. Accentuated cyclic activation of peritoneal macrophages in patients with endometriosis. Am J Obstet Gynecol 1984;148:85–90.
29. Halme J, White C, Kauma S, et al. Peritoneal macrophages from patients with endometriosis release growth factor activity in vitro. J Clin Endocrinol Metab 1988;66: 1044–1049.
30. Fakih J, Baggett B, Holtz G, et al. Interleukin-1: a possible role in the infertility associated with endometriosis. Fertil Steril 1987;47:213–217.
31. Taketani Y, Kuo T, Mizuno M. Comparison of cytokine levels and embryo toxicity in peritoneal fluid in infertile women with untreated or treated endometriosis. Am J Obstet Gynecol 1992;167:265–270.
32. Eiserman J, Gast MJ, Pineda J, et al. Tumor necrosis factor in peritoneal fluid of women undergoing laparoscopic surgery. Fertil Steril 1988;50:573–579.
33. Halme J. Release of tumor necrosis factor-α by human peritoneal macrophages in vivo and in vitro. Am J Obstet Gynecol 1989;161:1718–1725.
34. Rana N, Braun DP, House R, et al. Basal and stimulated secretion of cytokines by peritoneal macrophages in women with endometriosis. Fertil Steril 1996;65:925–930.
35. Rier SE, Parsons AK, Becker JL. Altered interleukin-6 production by peritoneal leukocytes from patients with endometriosis. Fertil Steril 1994;61:294–299.
36. Braun DP, Gebel H, House R, et al. Spontaneous and induced synthesis of cytokines by peripheral blood monocytes in patients with endometriosis. Fertil Steril 1996;65: 1125–1129.
37. Oosterlynck DJ, Meuleman C, Waer M, et al. Transforming growth factor-β activity is increased in peritoneal fluid from women with endometriosis. Obstet Gynecol 1994;83: 287–292.
38. Akoum A, Lemay A, McColl S, et al. Elevated concentration and biologic activity or monocyte chemotactic protein-1 in the peritoneal fluid of patients with endometriosis. Fertil Steril 1996;66:17–23.
39. Khorram O, Taylor RN, Ryan IP, et al. Peritoneal fluid concentrations of the cytokine RANTES correlate with the severity of endometriosis. Am J Obstet Gynecol 1993;169: 1545–1549.
40. Weed JC, Arguembourg PC. Endometriosis: can it produce an autoimmune response resulting in infertility? Clin Obstet Gynecol 1980;23:885–893.
41. Mathur S, Peress MR, Williamson HO, et al. Autoimmunity to endometrium and ovary in endometriosis. Clin Exp Immunol 1982;50:235–241.
42. Switchenko AC, Kauffman RS, Becker M. Are there endometrial antibodies in sera of women with endometriosis? Fertil Steril 1991;56:235–241.
43. Oosterlynck DJ, Vandeputte M, Cornillie FJ, et al. Women with endometriosis show a defect in natural killer activity resulting in a decreased cytotoxicity to autologous endometrium. Fertil Steril 1991;56:45–51.
44. Oosterlynck DJ, Meuleman C, Sobis H, et al. Angiogenic activity of peritoneal fluid from women with endometrisosis. Fertil Steril 1993;59:778–782.
45. Shifren JL, Tseng JF, Zaloudek CJ, et al. Ovarian steroid regulation of vascular endothelial growth factor in the human endometrium: implications for angiogenesis during the menstrual cycle and in the pathogenesis of endometriosis. J Clin Endocrinol Metab 1996;81:3112–3118.
46. McLaren J, Prentice A, Charnock-Jones DS, et al. Vascular endothelial growth factor (VEGF) concentrations are elevated in peritoneal fluid of women with endometriosis. Hum Reprod (Oxf) 1996;11:220–223.
47. Halban J. Metastatic hyteroadenosis. Wien Klin Wochenschr 1924;37:1205–1206.
48. Sampson JA. Metastatic or embolic endometriosis, due to menstrual dissemination of endometrial tissue into venous circulation. Am J Pathol 1927;3:93–110.

49. Rovito P, Gittleman M. Two cases of endometrioma in cesarean section scars. Surgery (St. Louis) 1986;100: 118–120.
50. Wittich AC, Endometriosis in an episiotomy scar: review of the literature and report of case. J Am Osteopath Assoc 1982;82:22–23.
51. Rosenfeld DL, Lecher BD. Endometriosis in a patient with Rokitansky-Kuster-Hauser syndrome. Am J Obstet Gynecol 1981;139:105–107.
52. Schrodt GR, Alcorn MO, Ibanez J. Endometriosis of the male urinary system: a case report. J Urol 1980;124: 722–723.
53. Metzger DA, Olive DL, Haney AF. Limited hormonal responsiveness of ectopic endometrium: histologic correlation with intrauterine endometrium. Hum Pathol 1988;19: 1417–1424.
54. Bergqvist A, Ljungberg O, Myhre E. Human endometrium and endometriotic tissue obtained simultaneously: a comparative histologic study. Int J Gynecol Pathol 1984;3: 135–145.
55. Janne O, Kauppila A, Kokko E, et al. Estrogen and progestin receptors in endometriosis lesions: comparison with endometrial tissue. Am J Obstet Gynecol 1981;141: 562–566.
56. Moon YS, Leung PCS, Yuen BH, et al. Prostaglandin F in human endometriotic tissue. Am J Obstet Gynecol 1981; 141 :344–345.
57. Vercellini P, Bocciolone L, Vendola N, et al. Peritoneal endometriosis: morphologic appearance in women with chronic pelvic pain. J Reprod Med 1991;36:533–536.
58. Nisolle M, Donnez J. Peritoneal endometriosis, ovarian endometriosis, and adenomyotic nodules of the rectovaginal septum are three different entities. Fertil Steril 1997; 68:585–596.
59. Vernon MW, Beard JS, Graves K, et al. Classification of endometriotic implants by morphologic appearance and capacity to synthesize prostaglandin F. Fertil Steril 1986; 46:801–806.
60. Redwine DB. Age-related evolution in color appearance of endometriosis. Fertil Steril 1987;48:1062–1063.
61. Cornillie RJ, Oosterlynck D, Lauweryns JM, et al. Deeply infiltrating pelvic endometriosis: histology and clinical significance. Fertil Steril 1990;53:978–983.
62. Koninckx PR, Meuleman C, Demeyere S, et al. Suggestive evidence that pelvic endometriosis is a progressive disease whereas deeply infiltrating endometriosis is associated with pelvic pain. Fertil Steril 1991;55:759–765.
63. Fortier KJ, Haney AF. The pathologic spectrum of uterotubal junction obstruction. Obstet Gynecol 1985;65: 93–98.
64. Syrop CH, Halme J. A comparison of peritoneal fluid parameters of infertile patients and the subsequent occurrence of pregnancy. Fertil Steril 1986;46:631–635.
65. Suginami H, Yano K, Watanabe K, et al. A factor inhibiting ovum capture by the oviductal fimbriae present in endometriosis peritoneal fluid. Fertil Steril 1986;46: 1140–1146.
66. Oak MK, Chantler EN, Williams CAV, et al. Sperm survival rates in peritoneal fluid from infertile women with endometriosis and unexplained infertility. Clin Reprod Fertil 1985;3:297–303.
67. Drake TS, O'Brien WF, Ramwell PW, et al. Peritoneal fluid thromboxane B_2 and 6-keto-prostaglandin $F1_\alpha$ in endometriosis. Am J Obstet Gynecol 1981;140:401–404.
68. Ylikorkala O, Viinikka L. Prostaglandins and endometriosis. Acta Obstet Gynecol Scand 1983;113(suppl):105–107.
69. Rock JA, Dubin NH, Ghodgaonkar RB, et al. Cul-de-sac fluid in women with endometriosis: fluid volume and prostanoid concentration during the proliferative phase of the cycle—days 8 to 12. Fertil Steril 1982;37:747–750.
70. Haney AF, Muscato JJ, Weinberg JB. Peritoneal fluid cell populations in infertility patients. Fertil Steril 1981;35: 696–698.
71. Halme J, Becker S, Hammond MG, et al. Increased activation of pelvic macrophages in infertile women with mild endometriosis. Am J Obstet Gynecol 1983;145:333–337.
72. Muscato JJ, Haney AF, Weinberg JB. Sperm phagocytosis by human peritoneal macrophages: a possible cause of infertility in endometriosis. Am J Obstet Gynecol 1982;144: 503–510.
73. Doody MC, Gibbons WE, Buttram VC. Linear regression analysis of ultrasound follicular growth series: evidence of an abnormality of follicular growth in endometriosis patients. Fertil Steril 1988;49:47–51.
74. Tummon IS, Maclin UM, Radwanska E, et al. Occult ovulation dysfunction in women with minimal endometriosis and unexplained infertility. Fertil Steril 1988;50:716–720.
75. Brosens IA, Koninckx PR, Corvelyn PA. A study of plasma progesterone, estradiol-17β, prolactin, and LH levels, and of the luteal-phase appearance of the ovaries in patients with endometriosis and infertility. Br J Obstet Gynecol 1978;85:246–250.
76. Ayers JWT, Birenbaum DL, Menon KNL. Luteal phase dysfunction in endometriosis: elevated progesterone levels in peripheral and ovarian veins during follicular phase. Fertil Steril 1987;47:925–929.
77. Naples JD, Batt RE, Sadigh H. Spontaneous abortion rate in patients with endometriosis. Obstet Gynecol 1981;57: 509–512.
78. Wheeler JM, Johnson BM, Malinak LR. The relationship of endometriosis to spontaneous abortion. Fertil Steril 1983;39:656–660.
79. Metzger DA, Olive DL, Stohs GF, et al. Association of endometriosis and spontaneous abortion: effect of control assay selection. Fertil Steril 1986;45:18–23.
80. Pittaway DE, Vernon C, Fayez JA. Spontaneous abortion in women with endometriosis. Fertil Steril 1988;50:711–715.
81. Rier SE, Zarmakoupis PN, Hu X, et al. Dysregulation of interleukin-6 responses in ectopic endometrial stromal cells: correlation with decreased soluble receptor levels in peritoneal fluid of women with endometriosis. J Clin Endocrinol Metab 1995;80:1431–1437.
82. Badawy SZ, Cuenca V, Marshall L, et al. Cellular components in peritoneal fluid in infertile patients with and without endometriosis. Fertil Steril 1984;42:704–708.
83. Ho H, Wu M, Chao K, et al. Decrease in interferon gamma production and impairment of T-lymphocyte proliferation in peritoneal fluid of women with endometriosis. Am J Obstet Gynecol 1996;175:1236–1241.

84. Rock JA, Hurst BS. Clinical significance of prostanoid concentration in women with endometriosis. Prog Clin Biol Res 1990;323:61–80.
85. Giudice LC, Dsupin BA, Gargosky SE, et al. The insulin-like growth factor system in human peritoneal fluid: its effect on endometrial stromal cells and its potential relevance to endometriosis. J Clin Endocrinol Metab 1994;79: 1284–1293.
86. Hsu C-C, Yang B-C, Wu M-H, et al. Enhanced interleukin-4 expression in patients with endometriosis. Fertil Steril 1997;67:1059–1064.
87. Koyama N, Matsuura K, Okamura H. Cytokines in the peritoneal fluid of patients with endometriosis. Int J Gynecol Obstet 1993;43:45–50.
88. Ryan IP, Tseng JF, Schriock ED, et al. Interleukin-8 concentrations are elevated in peritoneal fluid of women with endometriosis. Fertil Steril 1995;63:929–932.
89. Arici A, Tazuke SI, Attar E, et al. Interleukin-8 concentration in peritoneal fluid of patients with endometriosis and modulation of interleukin-8 expression in human mesothelial cells. Mol Hum Reprod 1996;2:40–45.
90. Arici A, Oral E, Attar E, et al. Monocyte chemotactic protein-1 concentration in peritoneal fluid of women with endometriosis and its modulation of expression in mesothelial cells. Fertil Steril 1997;67:1065–1072.
91. Oral E, Seli E, Bahtiyar MO, et al. Growth-regulated α expression in the peritoneal environment with endometriosis. Obstet Gynecol 1996;88:1050–1056.
92. Dou Q, Williams RS, Chegini N. Inhibition of transforming growth factor-β_1 alters the growth, anchor-dependent cell aggregation and integrin mRNA expression in human promonocytes: implications for endometriosis and peritoneal adhesion formation. Mol Hum Reprod 1997;3: 383–391.
93. Luciano AA, Maier DB, Nulsen JC, et al. A comparative study of postoperative adhesion formation following laser surgery by laparoscopy versus laparotomy in the rabbit model. Obstet Gynecol 1989;74:220–224.
94. Maier DB, Klock A, Nulsen JC, et al. Laser laparocopy versus laparotomy in lysis of dense and incidental pelvic adhesions. J Reprod Med 1992;37:965–968.
95. Gant NF. Infertility and endometriosis: comparison of pregnancy outcomes with laparotomy versus laparoscopic techniques. Am J Obstet Gynecol 1992;166:1072–1081.
96. Fayez JA, Collazo LM, Vernon C. Comparison of different modalities of treatment for minimal and mild endometriosis. Am J Obstet Gynecol 1988;159:927–932.
97. Adamson GD, Hurd SJ, Pasta DJ, et al. Laparoscopic endometriosis treatment is it better? Fertil Steril 1993;59: 35–44.
98. Jansen RPS, Russell P. Nonpigmented endometriosis: clinical, laparoscopic, and pathologic definition. Am J Obstet Gynecol 1986;155:1154–1159.
99. Stripling MC, Martin DC, Chatman DL, et al. Subtle appearance of pelvic endometriosis. Fertil Steril 1988;49: 427–431.
100. Martin DC, Hubert GD, Van der Zwaag R, et al. Laparoscopic appearances of peritoneal endometriosis. Fertil Steril 1989;51:63–67.
101. Vasquez G, Cornillie F, Brosens IA. Peritoneal endometriosis: scanning electron microscopy and histology of minimal pelvic endometriotic lesions. Fertil Steril 1984;42: 696–702.
102. Murphy A, Green W, Bobbie D, et al. Unsuspected endometriosis documented by scanning electron microscopy in visually normal peritoneum. Fertil Steril 1986;46: 696–702.
103. Nezhat C, Crowgey S, Nezhat F. Videolaseroscopy for the treatment of endometriosis associated with infertility. Fertil Steril 1989;51:237–240.
104. Reich H, McGlynn F, Salvat J. Laparoscopic treatment of cul de sac obliteration secondary to retrocervical deep fibrotic endometriosis. J Reprod Med 1991;36:516–522.
105. Jirasek JE, Henzl MR, Uher J. Periovarian peritoneal adhesions in women with endometriosis: structural patterns. J Reprod Med 1998;43:276–280.
106. Sekiba K, Obstetrics and Gynecology Adhesion Prevention Committee. Use of Interceed (TC7) absorbable barrier to reduce postoperative adhesion reformation in infertility and endometriosis surgery. Obstet Gynecol 1992;79: 518–522.
107. Mais V, Ajossa S, Marongiu D, et al. Reduction of adhesion reformation after laparoscopic endometriosis surgery: a randomized trial with an oxidized regenerated cellulose absorbable barrier. Obstet Gynecol 1995;86: 512–515.
108. Takeuchi H, Awaji M, Hashimoto M, et al. Reduction of adhesions with fibrin glue after laparoscopic excision of large ovarian endometriomas. J Am Assoc Gynecol Laparosc 1996;3:575–579.
109. Rock JA, Murphy AA, Jones HW Jr. Female Reproduction Surgery. Baltimore: Williams & Wilkins, 1992:229.

23

Prognostic Factors of Distal Tubal Occlusion

J. Donnez and M. Nisolle

CONTENTS

This chapter defines the prognostic factors associated with successful tubal surgery. New perspectives have emerged in the management of distal tubal occlusion from the tremendous advances gained in the field of assisted reproduction technology and in operative endoscopy techniques. With regard to surgery, it has been demonstrated on numerous occasions that classical microsurgery[1-3] and laparoscopic surgery[4-9] show comparable results in terms of pregnancy rates. No doubt the crucial issue in the surgical management of distal tubal occlusion is the proper selection of the patient according to a set of strict criteria, which have a prognostic value on the chances of postoperative conception.

Physiopathology of the Hydrosalpinx

To understand the physiopathologic events associated with the development of distal tubal occlusion, an experimental model has been created in the rabbit by ligating the uterotubal junction and the ampullofimbrial junction.[10] This model closely reproduces the natural clinical hydrosalpinx observed in 10% to 15% of all infertile patients. The experimental hydrosalpinx can reach 2 cm in size 6 months after the ligature. Morphologically, only the epithelium of the ampulla is affected by a significant deciliation process, appearing by 2 months after the induction of the experimental hydrosalpinx; epithelial height is seen to be decreased, and the stroma thickens because of submucosal oedema and fibrosis. After 6 months, primary mucosal folds become scarce and atrophic, whereas secondary folds completely disappear in the ampulla (Fig. 23.1).

Ampullary muscularis is typically invaded by fibrosis and the size of the capillaries in the tubal wall is significantly decreased; this decrease in the ampullary vascularization probably explains the deciliation process. It should be pointed out that the muscularis layer also shares a role in the transportation of the fertilized egg, as intrauterine pregnancies in Karthagener's syndrome have been described.[11] In addition, there is a generalized adrenergic denervation of the tubal wall, this feature being more prominent on the isthmic portion than at the level of the ampulla where the innervation is minimal in the healthy tube.[12] All these lesions induced by the hydrosalpinx in the muscularis layer are permanent and explain the high failure rate associated with the surgical restoration of tubal patency.

The increase in fluid volume of the hydrosalpinx is probably the result of the depolymerization of the fluid

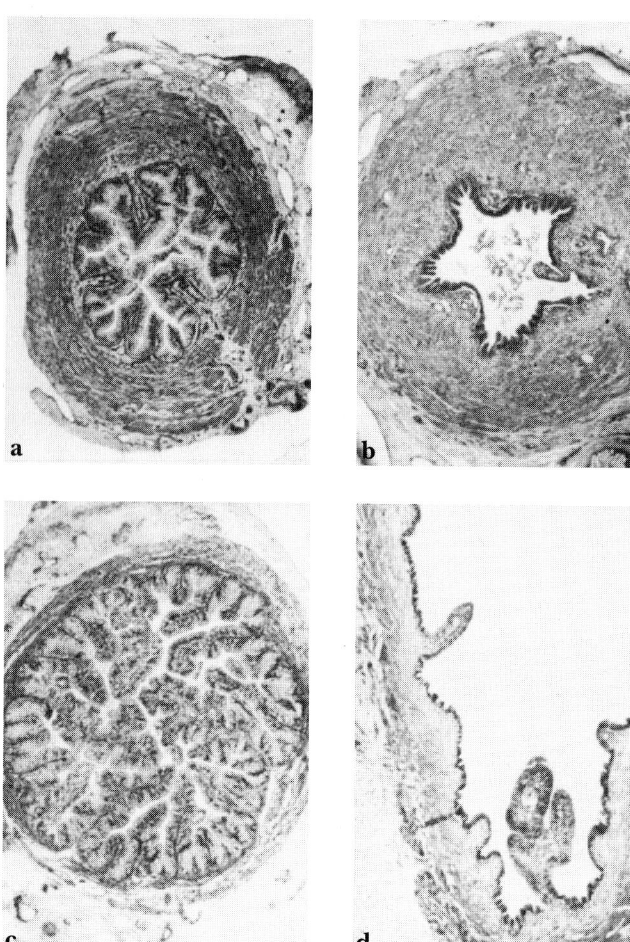

FIG. 23.1. Experimental hydrosalpinx: (a) normal isthmus; (b) dilated isthmus after induction of experimental hydrosalpinx; (c) normal ampulla; (d) dilated ampulla after induction of experimental hydrosalpinx. Reduction in number and in size of ampullary folds is shown, with flattened epithelium between the ampullary folds. *Please see insert for color reproduction of this figure.*

components and a subsequent transudation from the underlying chorion. It could also result from a slowed-down secretion of fluid by the epithelial cells combined with the complete absence of drainage.[10–12]

The experimental hydrosalpinx of the rabbit and the hydrosalpinx observed in infertile women have similar patterns: distension associated with the unfolding of the mucosal folds and degeneration of the epithelial cells. As is discussed later, the deciliation index investigated on fimbrial biopsies and the degree of dilatation are correlated, and both serve as physiopathologic prognostic factors for the success of a salpingoneostomy; indeed, from hydrosalpinx specimens obtained at hysterectomy, it seems that the occurrence of dilatation of the tube results in the adrenergic denervation and fibrosis of the muscular layer, exactly in accordance with the observations made in the experimental model.[10,11]

Diagnosis of the Hydrosalpinx

The presence of hydrosalpinx can be diagnosed by hysterosalpingogram or by laparoscopy with or without chromopertubation. A meta-analysis of all the studies comparing hysterosalpingography to the gold standard of laparoscopy with chromopertubation showed the hysterosalpingogram to have a sensitivity of 65% percent in the diagnosis of tubal obstruction and a specificity of 83%.[13,14]

Transvaginal ultrasonography (US) has also been used to evaluate pelvic structures. Normal fallopian tubes can only be recognized in the presence of pelvic fluid. Transvaginal US is very specific in the diagnosis of hydrosalpinx, but its sensitivity is poor.[15] Occasional longitudinal folds in the ampullary portion of the fallopian tube can be seen[16] by transvaginal ultrasonography. A study by Atri et al.[15] evaluated the accuracy of endovaginal sonography in the detection of fallopian tube blockage and found the specificity of transvaginal US to be 100% percent with a sensitivity of only 34%.

Methods using the passage of air or fluid to visualize the tubes sonographically have also been described. The same principle makes sonohysterosalpingography a useful tool in the diagnosis of hydrosalpinx.[17–19] Color Doppler ultrasonography has also been used in evaluating tubal patency and diagnosing hydrosalpinx.[20,21] Other diagnostic methods include salpingoscopy or falloscopy.[22–24]

Defining the Prognostic Factors for Successful Tubal Surgery

In the management of distal tubal infertility, in vitro fertilization (IVF) and tubal surgery should not be considered as competitive but rather as complementary modalities.[25] When feasible with a good chance of success, surgery should always be attempted; IVF should only be considered when the fertility prognosis associated with conservative surgery is too poor. The conditions for surgical feasibility are based on the thorough evaluation of prognostic factors, usually obtained preoperatively and at the time of laparoscopy; this will orientate the patient toward the best therapeutic alternative. Factors contributing to the establishment of a prognosis for surgery can be subdivided into two groups, tubal and extratubal factors. The information collected during the evaluation phase is usually included in various scoring systems, with the aim of better defining the chances of conception if a surgical approach is selected.

Tubal Factors

Inflammation following pelvic infection of surgery leads to a series of tubal damage that is observed, described, and eventually scored through different investigational procedures. Tubal factors to be considered are (1) ampullary dilatation, (2) preservation of the ampullary folds, (3) detection of intratubal adhesions, and (4) macroscopic and microscopic mucosal tubal status.

Ampullary Dilation

The ampullary dilatation is best assessed and measured at the time of the hysterosalpingogram. Indeed, we, like others,[26] are convinced that a well-performed hysterosalpingography (HSG) remains one of the best investigational examinations of the infertile patient. Hysterosalpingography provides clear information on the normality of the uterine cavity and the endocervical canal, the patency and status of the intramural–interstitial portion of the tube, the patency, possible dilatation, rigidity, and anatomy of the ampullar segment, and finally the suspicion of peritubal adhesions, although the predictive value of the latter remains poor compared to direct visualization by laparoscopy.

We have proposed a hysterosalpingographic classification of distal tubal occlusion[27] based on the extent of occlusion combined to the preservation of ampullary folds (Table 23.1). From a series of 215 infertile women with bilateral distal tubal disease operated on by microsurgery,[27] it was concluded that ampullary dilatation, as determined by laparoscopy and hysterosalpingography, influences the postoperative pregnancy rate. After fimbrioplasty for occlusion of degree I and salpingostomy for occlusion of degree II, the term pregnancy rate averaged 50%, whereas salpingoneostomies performed for occlusion of degree III and IV carried a term pregnancy rate of 25% and 22%, respectively. According to Singhal et al.[28] microsurgical salpingostomy results drop if the dilatation is either less or more than 2 cm. The prognostic grading system elaborated by the American Fertility Society (AFS)[29] clearly follows the same lines, stating that ampullary diameter greater than 3 cm gives a poor pregnancy outcome (Table 23.2).

A prospective study by Vasquez et al.[30] investigating tubal mucosal lesions and fertility in hydrosalpinges, recently concluded that there was a significantly better outcome following surgery of thin-walled hydrosalpinges of less than 1 cm in size, compared to moderate (1–2 cm) and large hydrosalpinges (>2 cm). Size should not be considered, however, without close examination of the thickness of the ampullary wall because thick-walled hydrosalpinges, usually a moderate dilatation, have the worst prognosis.[27]

TABLE 23.1. Classification of Donnez and Casanas.

Degree I:	phymotic ostium with preserved tubal patency
Degree II:	total distal tubal occlusion without ampullary dilatation
Degree III:	ampullary dilatation inferior to 2.5 cm; ampullary folds well preserved
Degree IV:	hydrosalpinx simplex; dilatation more than 2.5 cm; well-preserved ampullary folds
Degree V:	thick-walled hydrosalpinx; absence of ampullary folds

From Donnez and Casanas-Roux.[27]

TABLE 23.2. Distal tubal score by Mage et al.[31]

Tubal patency	Ampullary tubal mucosa (HSG)	Ampullary tubal wall (laparoscopy)
Phimosis = 2	Normal folds = 0	Normal = 0
	Decreased folds = 5	Thin = 5
Hydrosalpinx = 5	No fold, honeycomb = 10	Thick or rigid = 10

Hydrosalpinx classification by Boer-Meiseil et al.[39]

1. Normal mucosa; regular patterns of lush mucosal folds, richly vascularized
2. Hydrosalpinx with moderate attenuation of mucosal folds; patches of normal mucosa
3. Absence of ampullary folds; honeycomb aspect

Preservation of the Ampullary Folds

The presence of ampullary folds can be observed by HSG, endovaginal echography, hysterosalpingography, and falloscopy. Hysterosalpingography is still considered as a reference for the description of the inner architecture of the ampulla and is involved in several tubal scores[31] (see Table 23.2). A number of other examinations have recently been proposed as alternative investigational procedures. Endovaginal echography has the resolution power to reveal the presence of rugae in dilated tubes. Compared to HSG, endovaginal echography offers a poor sensitivity in the detection of hydrosalpinges (obviously less so in the description of the tubal wall); it is estimated to be potentially useful in detecting a combination of proximal and distal tubal blockage when HSG shows a proximal block.[15]

Hysterosalpingosonography (US-HSG)[32] was developed mainly to document tubal patency, using color Doppler imaging system,[33,34] and offers the following advantages over the classic HSG: absence of radiation, avoidance of potential allergic reactions to iodinated contrast medium, and the possibility of use in the clinician's office. If the results correlate fairly with HSG and laparoscopic findings so far as tubal patency[33,34] is concerned, it is unable to correctly delineate the inner architecture of the fallopian tube and therefore is of little prognostic interest.[26] Falloscopy is the endoscopic (transhysteroscopic) exploration of the tube,[24] an office procedure[35] that can inform on the tubal status. There is, at this stage, a definite lack of correlating studies of this procedure with HSG or laparoscopic features and with fertility outcome. A classification of luminal disease exists,[36] but it does not explicitly consider the ampullary fold preservation as a significant parameter. The obscure and narrow view provided by these endoscopes limits the quality and the reliability of the observations, thereby somewhat restricting the interest of this examination in the evaluation of ampullary fold preservation.

In addition to HSG, mucosal folds are probably best visualized at the time of the laparoscopy, combined or not with salpingoscopy[22,37] or under the magnifying microscope at microsurgery. Paucity of endotubal folds is unanimously recognized as pejorative.[10,27,29,31,38,39] Boer-Meisel et al.[39] have proposed an endosalpingeal score as part of an overall score for distal tubal occlusions (see Table 23.2); this endosalpingeal score was recently demonstrated by Dubuisson et al.[40] to correlate closely with more complex classification systems and to fairly predict the fertility outcome. In our series, complete absence of mucosal folds was often associated with thick and fibrotic tubal and was followed by no intrauterine pregnancy after microscopic repair.

Tuboscopy has the potential to provide an excellent close-up view of the tubal architecture. Abnormal findings can be revealed at tuboscopy in 20% to 30% of cases with otherwise normal HSG or laparoscopy.[41] Herschlag et al.,[42] attempting to correlate salpingoscopic findings (including the evaluation of the mucosal fold architecture) with histology, demonstrated a good correlation although only in cases of mild and severe diseases.

Our surgical approach depends on a combination of these two first prognostic factors, that is the degree of distal occlusion and the preservation of ampullary folds, as assessed by HSG.[27,43]

Intratubal Adhesions

Intratubal adhesions are detected only at falloscopy or tuboscopy. The formation of intratubal adhesions is one consequence among others of an underlying inflammatory process. It is not recognized specifically as a major prognostic factor, probably because the use of tuboscopy has not been generalized; Herschlag et al.,[42] however, include this parameter in their tuboscopic score. De Bruyne et al.[23] reported no intrauterine pregnancy in a series of 17 patients in the presence of intratubal adhesions, despite an overall intrauterine pregnancy rate of 59% percent in their study. Vasquez et al.[30] addressed this issue clearly as well; in a multicentric study grouping 50 patients, it was concluded that mucosal adhesions in thin-walled hydrosalpinges are the most important factor in determining the fertility outcome. Indeed, presence and absence of intratubal adhesions were associated with an intrauterine pregnancy rate, following surgery, of 22% and 58%, respectively, differing significantly. The rate of ectopic pregnancy was 11% if adhesions had been discovered; this condition is seriously affected by a significant risk of ectopic gestation, as was stressed also by Marana et al.[44]

Evaluation of the Tubal Mucosa

The tubal mucosa can be assessed endoscopically, and the observations are often included in various scoring classifications.[6,27,29,31,39] Apart from the several features already reviewed, the macroscopic evaluation of the tubal mucosa attempts to appreciate the tubal wall thickness[31] and, also, to distinguish areas of normal-looking mucosa on the tubal wall, the inflammatory aspect of the epithelium, and the underlying vascularization. We have pointed out[6,10] that the lesser area of normal mucosal surface observed under the operative microscope, the lesser the chance of intrauterine pregnancy; the difference was clearly significant when the cutoff level was chosen at 50% percent of normal-looking mucosal surface. Histologic data in tubal infertility are available from some authors[10,45] who have studied the histophysiopathologic factors of distal tubal occlusions and correlated it with the pregnancy outcome.

The Ciliation Index

The ciliation index was proven to be valuable in the prognosis of tubal surgery.[3,10,45] In our original study, in-

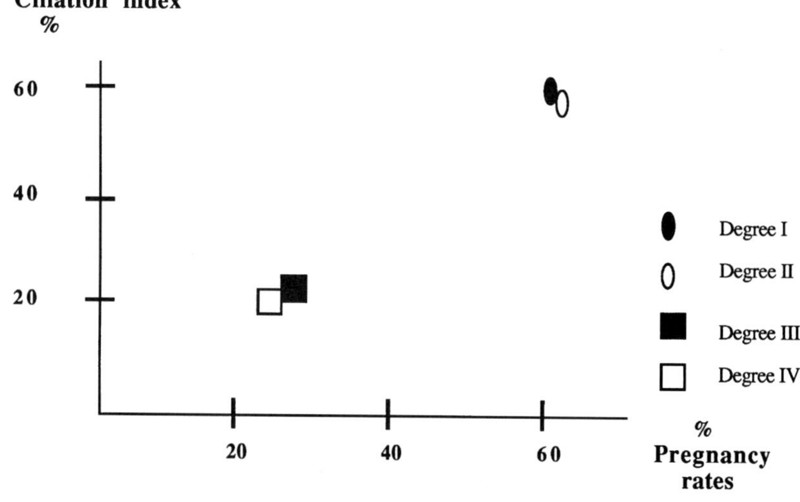

FIG. 23.2. Pregnancy rates according to classification of tubal occlusion (degree I to V).

vestigating the prognosis factors of fimbrial microsurgery on 215 patients,[27] the ciliated cell percentage, as evaluated on fimbrial microbiopsy, and the pregnancy outcome were significantly decreased in cases of degree III and IV distal occlusion when compared with degree I and II distal occlusion (Fig. 23.2). In our study, the ciliation index was related to the pregnancy rate after microsurgical correction of the distal occlusion.

Fibrosis and the Thickness of the Tubal Wall

Long-standing evolution of hydrosalpinges sometimes leads to the invasion of the muscularis by fibrosis, responsible of a significant thickening of the tubal wall and leading ultimately to the so-called thick-walled hydrosalpinx. Vasquez et al.[30] have correlated the thick-walled hydrosalpinx with histologic parameters: in thick-walled hydrosalpinges, the thickness of the tubal wall measured 2 to 10 mm at the thinnest part and 4 to 10 mm at the thickest part. The thick-walled hydrosalpinx is usually associated with other pejorative macro- and microscopic features, explaining the very poor results of fertility-promoting surgery. In our series,[27] intrauterine pregnancy rate for this type of tube is 0%, as reported by some other authors.[1–3,30,40] The recommended in this case is to perform a salpingectomy at the time of the laparoscopy in an attempt to enhance the results of IVF[46] and to limit the incidence of tubal gestation, reported to be as high as 11% percent in tubal infertility patients undergoing IVF.[47]

Extratubal Factors

Adnexal adhesions and endometriosis are sometimes included in the list of prognostic factors affecting the pregnancy rate outcome.

Periadnexal Adhesions

The significance of pelvic adhesions is controversial in the prognosis determination for the patients with tubal factors. Studies by several authors[2,28,38,39] suggest that fertility prognosis is correlated with the presence and degree of severity of tubal adhesions. Some investigators[48,49] restrict the negative influence of adhesions to severe cases only; actually, frozen pelvis is still considered as a contraindication to conservative surgery. Nevertheless, it should be noted that microsurgical or laparoscopic adhesiolysis alone has been shown to promote fertility,[28,43,50] giving credit to the implication of adhesions in mechanical infertility.

The most recent series, however, tend to challenge the role of adhesions in impairing the promotion of fertility following surgery. Dubuisson et al.,[40] in a series of 90 patients undergoing laparoscopic salpingostomy, failed to demonstrate any relation between adhesion score and pregnancy outcome. Canis et al.[9] did not note any significant difference in his group of 87 laparoscopic tuboplasties so far as crude pregnancy and monthly fecundity rates were concerned. The implication of periadnexal adhesions was also lately questioned by Vasquez et al.[30] in a prospectively designed study.

Endometriosis

Endometriosis has rarely been taken into account in the evaluation of the success of tubal surgery. The most recent study in this respect is from Dlugi et al.[49] who, treating 113 patients with tubal factors and comparing pregnancy curves, concluded that endometriosis-related tubal occlusion was less detrimental than post-PID (pelvic inflammatory disease) or postsurgical tubal distal occlusions. Treating the concomitant endometriosis at the time of tubal surgery obviously improves the fertility outcome on its own and can modulate the actual implication of endometriosis as a prognostic factor for successful tuboplasty. That statement, however, agrees with a report from Nehzat et al.,[51] who found no tuboscopic significantly abnormal findings in a population of 100 patients with endometriosis; this might suggest a better inner tubal condition in distal tubal occlusions of endometriotic origin compared to distal tubal occlusion of inflammatory etiology, where the mucosal impairment is probably more aggressive.

Therapeutic Results and Attitude

Table 23.3 describes the results we have obtained on a series of 465 laparoscopic tubal surgery cases.[43] As has been repeatedly reported in the literature, these figures are comparable to results obtained from microsurgery and from other laparoscopic series. Indeed, the pregnancy rates are significantly different after fibrioplasty for occlusion of degree I (60%), after salpingoneostomy for occlusion of degree III and IV.

Table 23.4 summarizes the results obtained in major series of laparoscopic salpingoneostomies; the intrauterine pregnancy rate ranges from 19% to 48% according to the inclusion criteria reported by the authors. These rates remain low, stressing the fact that the tubes have probably undergone irreversible damage. The degree of the lesion influences the success of fertility-promoting surgery, so it is essential to rely on prognostic factors, the evaluation of which will help in predicting the success of

TABLE 23.3. Laser laparoscopic management of distal occlusions: 18-month cumulative viable pregnancy rate.

Procedure	*n*	Pregnancies
Fimbrioplasty	380	228 (60%)
Salpingostomies	85	22 (27%)

From Donnez et al.[43]

TABLE 23.4. Intrauterine pregnancy rate (IUP, %) obtained from laparoscopic salpingoneostomies.

Reference	n	IUP (%)
Daniell and Herbert (1984)[5]	21	19
Nezhat (1984)	33	36
Bouquet (1987)	20	25
Reich (1987)	7	29
Manhes (1987)	19	48
Donnez et al. (1989)[6]	25	20
Dubuisson et al. (1990)[7]	31	26
Larue (1990)	15	20
Henry-Suchet (1991)	28	32
McComb (1991)	22	22.7
Matvienko (1991)	50	48
Canis et al. (1991)[9]	87	33.3
Audebert (1992)	142	20.4
Donnez et al. (1994)[43]	85	27
Total	585	29.03

a surgical approach. We have opted for the attitude summarized on Fig. 23.3 for the management of distal tubal occlusion. In degree II to IV, HSG is systematically performed 3 months after surgery under antibiotic prophylaxis, in the absence of pregnancy.

Reocclusion is, in our belief, an indication to laparoscopically remove the diseased tube and to direct the patient toward IVF because the presence of a hydrosalpinx is thought to impair the success rate of IVF and exposes the patient to the increased risk of ectopic gestation.[46,47] In cases of thick-walled hydrosalpinx (degree IV, according to Donnez et al.[27]), the ampullary folds are absent. The pregnancy rate after microsurgery is 0%; for this reason, there is no indication for salpingostomy. Since 1991, we have proposed a laparoscopic salpingectomy for the patient before an IVF procedure to avoid the risk of tubal pregnancy after embryo transfer and possible embryotoxicity with subsequent low pregnancy rates.

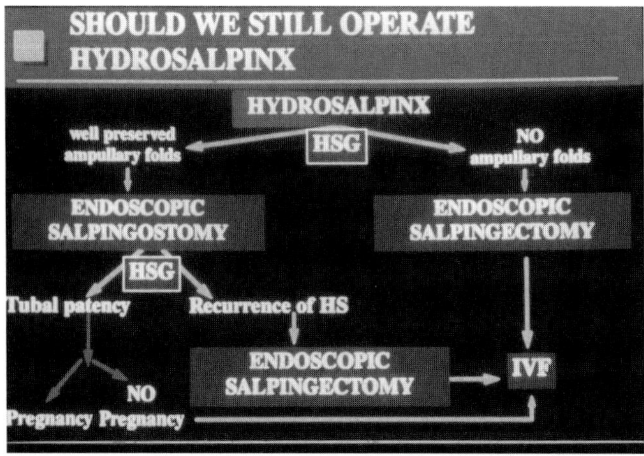

FIG. 23.3. Proposed management of hydrosalpinx in infertility.

Hydrosalpinx and IVF/ET

In a recent review, Nackley and Muasher[52] analyzed the effects of hydrosalpinx in IVF/ET (embryo transfer). Sims et al.[53] were the first to study the effect of hydrosalpinx on IVF outcome. A retrospective case-controlled study was conducted involving 118 patients with hydrosalpinx undergoing 283 stimulations and 823 patients with tubal factor infertility but without hydrosalpinx undergoing 1431 stimulations. A lower clinical pregnancy rate of 18% and a higher miscarriage rate of 42%, resulting in a lower ongoing pregnancy rate of 10%, were discovered compared to the control group. The authors suggested treatment of the hydrosalpinx, such as laparoscopic removal or peritransfer antiobiotic coverage, before IVF.

In a retrospective study, Strandell et al.[46] concluded that persistent hydrosalpinx was associated with a reduced implantation rate and increased risk for early pregnancy loss. It was hypothesized that the removal of the hydrosalpinx by salpingectomy or salpingostomy would normalize the IVF/ET rates in this group. Andersen et al.[54] reported a marked reduction in implantation rates when hydrosalpinx was visible on US. They found the rates of implantation, pregnancy, early pregnancy loss, and delivery per aspiration were significantly reduced despite a comparable number of aspirated oocytes and embryos transferred. Vandromme et al.[55] and Vejtorp et al.[56] also demonstrated a decreased pregnancy rate after IVF in women with hydrosalpinx. The significant decrease in implantation rate and pregnancy rate per transfer in the hydrosalpinx group suggests an unfavorable uterine environment.

We have suggested[57] that this unfavorable environment could possibly be attributable to hydrosalpingeal fluid drainage into the endometrial cavity. The possibility has been raised that there a connection between the hydrosalpinx and the uterine cavity allowing a direct flow of hydrosalpingeal fluid into the uterus, thus exposing the endometrium and embryo to potentially toxic fluid. It is postulated that the fluid in damaged tubes contains microorganisms, debris, lymphocytes, macrophages, and other toxic agents that flow into the uterus and exert a detrimental effect on the endometrium and developing embryo. There may also be substances such as cytokines and prostaglandins interfering with normal endometrial function.[46,54]

Freeman et al.[58] recently suggested that hydrosalpinx not only negatively affects endometrial receptivity during implantation but also exerts a negative influence over oocytes early in follicular recruitment. The presence of hydrosalpinx has also been shown to affect the implantation rates in unstimulated cycles.[59] Hydrosalpinx also predisposes to increased ectopic pregnancies after IVF/ET.[59-61] The first human pregnancy after

IVF was indeed a tubal pregnancy.[62] Zouvres et al.[63] suggested prophylactic proximal tubal occlusion to prevent tubal pregnancy after IVF. This recommendation had also been suggested by Steptoe,[64] Tucker et al.,[65] and Herman et al.[66] We did not recommend proximal tubal occlusion in cases of distal occlusion, however, because of the risk of subsequent pelvic pain and inflammation from increased intratubal pressure.[57] We prefer to recommend prophylactic salpingectomy instead of prophylactic proximal occlusion. A study by Schenk et al.[67] and Mukherjee et al.[68] examined the effect of hydrosalpingeal fluid on embryogenesis. All samples demonstrated significant embryotoxic effects.

Although the exact mechanism by which hydrosalpinx alters intrauterine receptivity remains unclear, a marker of uterine receptivity has been established. Integrins are adhesion molecules that participate in cell–cell interactions and which are present on all human cells. Lessey et al.[69] conducted an interesting study that examined endometrial integrin expression to evaluate the effects of hydrosalpinges on uterine receptivity by assessing the expression of β-integrin measured by immunohistochemical assays of endometrial biopsies. Women with hydrosalpinges expressed significantly lower levels than those without hydrosalpinges.[69]

Removal of Hydrosalpinx Before IVF/ET

The benefit of salpingectomy before IVF/ET in patients with hydrosalpinx has been debated by Puttemans and Brosens.[70] They believe that preventative salpingectomy should not be performed without demonstration of severe pathology, specifically chronic inflammation, by salpingoscopy. On the other hand, the study by Vandromme et al.[55] sought to determine whether surgical treatment would benefit those patients with hydrosalpinx attempting IVF/ET. The ongoing pregnancy rate before surgery was 10.1% whereas the postoperative group had an ongoing pregnancy rate of 31% and that in the control group the rate was 21.3%. The results revealed that surgical correction by ablation of the diseased tubes restored the normal chances of success for patients with hydrosalpinges.

Shelton et al.[71] were the first to conduct a prospective study that demonstrated a positive impact on pregnancy rates in patients with repeated IVF failures by removing the hydrosalpinges. Fifteen patients with unilateral or bilateral hydrosalpinges with a history of repeated IVF failures underwent laparoscopic excision of the affected tubes. Because the patients undergoing surgical excision served as their own control, the ongoing pregnancy rate per transfer was 0% presalpingectomy; after salpingectomy, the ongoing pregnancy per transfer rate was 25%. Improved pregnancy rates were noted for both fresh and frozen embryo transfers after surgery. Lessey et al.[69] were also successful in demonstrating an improvement of integrin status and, therefore, uterine receptivity after correction of the hydrosalpinx.

It is unclear whether salpingectomy has a detrimental effect on ovarian blood supply and neural linkage, thus affecting folliculogenesis and hormone production. Studies by Vandromme, Kassabji, and Shelton and their colleagues[55,72,73] showed no difference in ovarian response, oocyte retrieval, or fertilization rates after salpingectomy. Nevertheless, Donnez et al.[74] and McComb and Delbelke[75] addressed the importance of maintaining the integrity of the anastomotic vessels between the ovary and tube. They[75] evaluated the relationship between the ovary and oviduct using microsurgery to alter the structure of the fallopian tube. The number of ovulations was reduced by ablating the vasculature transmitted through the mesosalpinx. Preservation of the anastomotic ovarian blood supply at the time of salpingectomy must be emphasized to decrease the possible effects of radical surgery on ovarian function.[74]

The risk of interstitial pregnancy is not eliminated, and the remote chance of uterine rupture at the site of salpingectomy exists.[47,76] Pavic et al.[77] were the first to report an interstitial pregnancy after bilateral salpingectomy for hydrosalpinx and IVF Cornual resection at the time of salpingectomy does not prevent interstitial pregnancies.

Conclusion

In conclusion, the list of prognostic factors for tubal infertility is long. It stresses the major role attributable to the quality of the investigational exams performed preoperatively on the infertile patient, particularly the hysterosalpingogram, and at the time of the laparoscopy, where the exploration of the tubal mucosa must be minutious. Direct visual investigation of the tube, whether preoperatively (falloscopy) or peroperatively (tuboscopy), is able to well document the endosalpingeal features. Failure in being aware of these prognostic factors and, therefore, improperly selecting the patient for conservative surgery, would lead to an unacceptable loss of time and of illusions for our patients.

References

1. Swolin K. Electromicrosurgery and salpingostomy: long-term results. Am J Obstet Gynecol 1975;121:418–419.
2. Gomel V. Salpingostomy by microsurgery. Fertil Steril 1978;34:380–385.
3. Winston RML. Microsurgery of the fallopian tube: from fantasy to reality. Fertil Steril 1980;46:521–530.

4. Gomel V. Salpingostomy by laparoscopy. J Reprod Med 1977;18:265–267.
5. Daniell JF, Herbert CM. Laparoscopic salpingostomy utilizing the CO_2 laser. Fertil Steril 1984;41:558–563.
6. Donnez J, Nisolle M, Casanas-Roux F. CO_2 laser laparoscopy in infertile women with adnexal adhesions and women with tubal occlusion. J Gynecol Surg 1989;5:47–53.
7. Dubuisson JB, de Jolinière JB, Aubriot FX, et al. Terminal tuboplasties by laparoscopy: 65 consecutive cases. Fertil Steril 1990;54:401–403.
8. Mettler LR, Irani S, Kapamadzija A, et al. Pelviscopic tubal surgery: the acceptable vogue. Hum Reprod (Oxf) 1990;5: 971–974.
9. Canis M, Mage G, Pouly JL, et al. Laparoscopic distal tuboplasties: reports of 87 cases and a 4-year experience. Fertil Steril 1991;56:616–621.
10. Donnez J. La trompe de Fallope: hystopathologie normale et pathologique. Université Catholique de Louvain, 1984.
11. Afzelius BA, Camner P, Mossberg B. On the function of the cilia in the female reproductive tract. Fertil Steril 1978; 29:72.
12. Donnez J, Caprasse J, Casanas-Roux F, et al. Loss of adrenergic innervation in rabbit induced hydrosalpinx. Gynecol Obstet Invest 1986;21:213–216.
13. Mol BWJ, Swart P, Bossuyt PMM, et al. Reproducibility of the interpretation of hysterosalpingography in the diagnosis of tubal pathology. Hum Reprod (Oxf) 1996;11: 1204–1208.
14. Swart P, Mol BWJ, van der Veen F, et al. The accuracy of hysterosalpingography in the diagnosis of tubal pathology, a meta-analysis. Fertil Steril 1995;64:486–491.
15. Atri M, Tran CN, Bret PT, et al. Accuracy of endo-vaginal sonography for the detection of fallopian tube blockage. Ultrasound Med 1994;13(3):429–434.
16. Schiller VL, Tsuchiyama K. Development of hydrosalpinx during ovulation induction. J Ultrasound Med 1995;14: 799–803.
17. Friberg B, Joergensen C. Tubal patency studied by ultrasonography. A pilot study. Acta Obst Gynecol Scand 1994; 73:53–55.
18. Heikkinen H, Tekay A, Volpi E, et al. Transvaginal salpingosonography for the assessment of tubal patency in infertile women: methodological and clinical experiences. Fertil Steril 1995;64:293–298.
19. Volpi E, Piermatteo M, Zuccaro G, et al. The role of transvaginal sonosalpingography in the evaluation of tubal patency. Minerva Ginecol 1996;48:1–3.
20. Allahbadia GN. Fallopian tubal patency using color Doppler. Int J Gynaecol Obstet 1996;40:241–244.
21. Yarali H, Gurgan T, Erden A, et al. Colour Doppler hysterosalpingosonography: a simple and potentially useful methods to evaluate fallopian tube patency. Hum Reprod (Oxf) 1994;9:64–66.
22. Brosens I, Boeckx W, Delattin P, et al. Salpingoscopy: a new pre-operative diagnostic tool in tubal infertility. Br J Obstet Gynaecol 1987;94:768–773.
23. De Bruyne F, Puttemans P, Boeckx W, et al. The clinical value of salpingoscopy in tubal infertility. Fertil Steril 1989; 51:339–340.
24. Kerin J, Daykhovsky L, Grundfest W, et al. Falloscopy. A microendoscopic transvaginal technique for diagnosing and treating endotubal disease incorporating guide wire cannulation and direct balloon tuboplasty. J Reprod Med 1990;35:606–612.
25. Gomel V, Taylor PJ. In vitro fertilization versus reconstructive tubal surgery. J Assist Reprod Genet 1992;9:306–309.
26. Gomel V, Yarali H. Infertility surgery: microsurgery. Curr Opin Obstet Gynecol 1992;4:390–399.
27. Donnez J, Casanas-Roux F. Prognostic factors of fimbrial microsurgery. Fertil Steril 1986;46:200–204.
28. Singhal V, Li TC, Cooke ID. An analysis of factors influencing the outcome of 232 consecutive tubal microsurgery cases. Br J Obstet Gynaecol 1991;98:628–636.
29. American Fertility Society. The American Fertility Society: classifications of adnexal adhesions, distal tubal occlusion, tubal occlusion secondary to tubal ligation, tubal pregnancies, müllerian abnormalities and intrauterine adhesions. Fertil Steril 1988;49:944–955.
30. Vasquez G, Boeckx W, Brosens I. Prospective study of tubal mucosal lesions and fertility in hydrosalpinges. Hum Reprod (Oxf) 1995;10:1075–1078.
31. Mage G, Pouly JL, Bouquet de Jolinière J, et al. A preoperative classification to predict the intrauterine and ectopic pregnancy rates after distal microsurgery. Fertil Steril 1986;46:807–810.
32. Schlief R, Deichert U. Hysterosalpingo-contrast sonography of the uterus and fallopian tube: results of a clinical trial of a new contrast medium in 120 patients. Radiology 1991;178:213–215.
33. Peters AJ, Coulam CB. Hysterosalpingography with color doppler ultrasonography. Am J Obstet Gynecol 1991;164: 1530–1534.
34. Stern J, Peters AJ, Coulam CB. Color Doppler ultrasonography assessment of tubal patency: a comparison study with traditional techniques. Fertil Steril 1992;58:897–900.
35. Dunphy BC. Office falloscopic assessment in proximal tubal occlusive disease. Fertil Steril 1994;61:168–170.
36. Kerin JF, Williams DB, San Roman GA, et al. Falloscopic classification and treatment of fallopian tube lumen disease. Fertil Steril 1992;57:731–741.
37. Cornier E, Feintuch MJ, Bouccara L. Ampullafibrotuboscopy. J Gynecol Obstet Biol Reprod 1985;14:459–466.
38. Schlaff WD, Hassiakos DK, Damewood MD, et al. Neosalpingostomy for distal tubal obstruction: prognostic factors and impact of surgical technique. Fertil Steril 1990;54: 984–990.
39. Boer-Meisel ME, Te Velde ER, Habbema JDF, et al. Predicting the pregnancy outcome in patients treated for hydrosalpinx: a prospective study. Fertil Steril 1986;45:23–29.
40. Dubuisson JB, Chapron C, Morice P, et al. Laparoscopic salpingostomy: fertility results according to the tubal mucosal appearance. Hum Reprod (Oxf) 1994;9:334–339.
41. Marana R, Muscatello P, Muzii L, et al. Perlaparoscopic salpingoscopy in the evaluation of the tubal factor in infertile women. Int J Fertil 1990;35:211–214.
42. Herschlag A, Seifer DB, Carcangiu ML, et al. Salpingoscopy: light microscopic and electron microscopic correlations. Obstet Gynecol 1991;77:399–405.

43. Donnez J, Nisolle M, Casanas-Roux F, et al. CO_2 laser laparoscopic surgery: adhesiolysis, salpingostomy and fimbrioplasty. In: Donnez J, Nisolle M, eds. Atlas of Laser Operative Laparoscopy and Hysteroscopy. London: Parthenon, 1994:97–112.
44. Marana R, Muzii L, Rizzi M, et al. Salpingoscopy in patients with contralateral ectopic pregnancy. Fertil Steril 1991;55:838–840.
45. Brosens I, Vasquez G. Fimbrial microbiopsy. J Reprod Med 1976;16:171.
46. Strandell A, Waldenstrom U, Nilsson L, et al. Hydrosalpinx reduces in vitro fertilization/embryo transfer pregnancy rates. Hum Reprod (Oxf) 1994;9:861–863.
47. Dubuisson JB, Aubriot FX, Mathieu L, et al. Risk factors for ectopic pregnancy in 556 pregnancies after in vitro fertilization: implications for preventive management. Fertil Steril 1991;56:686–690.
48. Laatikainen TJ, Tenhumen AK, Venesmaa PK, et al. Factors influencing the success of microsurgery for distal tubal occlusion. Arch Gynecol Obstet 1988;243: 101–106.
49. Dlugi AM, Reddy S, Saleh WA, et al. Pregnancy rates after operative endoscopic treatment of total (neosalpingostomy) or near total (salpingostomy) distal tubal occlusion. Fertil Steril 1994;62:913–920.
50. Donnez J. CO_2 laser laparoscopy in infertile women with endometriosis and women with adnexal adhesions. Fertil Steril 1987;48:390.
51. Nehzat F, Winer WK, Nehzat C. Fimbrioscopy and salpingoscopy in patients with minimal to moderate pelvic endometriosis. Obstet Gynecol 1990;75:15–17.
52. Nackley AC, Muasher SJ. The significance of hydrosalpinx in in vitro fertilization. Fertil Steril 1998;69:373–384.
53. Sims JA, Jones D, Butler L, et al. Effect of hydrosalpinx on outcome in in vitro fertilization (IVF). Presented at the 49th annual meeting of the American Fertility Society, 1993, program supplement 1993:S95.
54. Andersen A, Yue Z, Meng F, et al. Low implantation rate after in vitro fertilization in patients with hydrosalpinges diagnosed by ultrasonography. Hum Reprod (Oxf) 1994; 9:1935–1938.
55. Vandromme J, Chasse E, Lejeune B, et al. Hydrosalpinges in in vitro fertilization: an unfavorable prognostic feature. Hum Reprod (Oxf) 1995;10:576–579.
56. Vejtorp M, Petersen K, Andersen AN, et al. Fertilization in vitro in the presence of hydrosalpinx and in advanced age. Ugeskr Laeg 1995;157:4131–4134.
57. Donnez J, Polet R, Nisolle M. Prognostic factors of distal tubal occlusion. Ref Gynecol Obstet 1993;1:94–102.
58. Freeman MR, Whitworth CM, Hill GA. Hydrosalpinx reduces in vitro fertilization-embryo transfer rates and in vitro blastocyst development. Presented at the 52nd annual meeting of the American Fertility Society, 1996, program supplement 1996:S211.
59. Akman MA, Garcia JE, Damewood MD, et al. Hydrosalpinx affects the implantation of previously cryopreserved embryos. Hum Reprod (Oxf) 1996;11:1013–1014.
60. Herman A, Ron-El R, Golan A, et al. The role of tubal pathology and other parameters in ectopic pregnancies occurring in in vitro fertilization and embryo transfer. Fertil Steril 1990;54:79–87.
61. Martinez F, Trounson A. An analysis of risk factors associated with ectopic pregnancy in a human in vitro fertilization program. Fertil Steril 1986;45:79–87.
62. Steptoe P, Edwards R. Reimplantation of a human embryo with subsequent tubal pregnancy. Lancet 1976;1:880.
63. Zouvres C, Erenus M, Gomel V. Tubal ectopic pregnancy after in vitro fertilization and embryo transfer: a role for proximal occlusion or salpingectomy after failed distal tubal surgery. Fertil Steril 1991;56:691–695.
64. Steptoe PC. Pregnancies following implantation of human embryos grown in culture. Presented at the 45th annual meeting of the American Fertility Society, 1989, program supplement 1989:S152.
65. Tucker M, Smith D, Pike I, et al. Ectopic pregnancy following in vitro fertilization and embryo transfer. Lancet 1981; 2:1278.
66. Herman A, Ron-El R, Golan A, et al. The dilemna of optimal surgical procedure in ectopic pregnancies occurring in in vitro fertilization. Hum Reprod (Oxf) 1991;6: 1167–1169.
67. Schenk LM, Ramey JW, Taylor SL, et al. Embryotoxicity of hydrosalpinx fluid. Presented at the 43rd annual meeting of the Society of Gynecologic Investigators 1996. J Soc Gynecol Invest 1996;88A.
68. Mukherjee T, Copperman AB, McCaffrey C, et al. Hydrosalpinx fluid has embryotoxic effects on murine embryogenesis: a case for prophylactic salpingectomy. Fertil Steril 1996;66:851–853.
69. Lessey BA, Castelbaum AJ, Riben M, et al. Effect of hydrosalpinges on markers of uterine receptivity and success in IVF. Presented at the 50th annual meeting of the American Fertility Society, 1994, program supplement 1994:S45.
70. Puttemans PJ, Brosens IA. Preventive salpingectomy of hydrosalpinx prior to IVF. Salpingectomy improves in vitro fertilization outcome in patients with a hydrosalpinx: blind victimization of the fallopian tube? Hum Reprod (Oxf) 1996;11:2079–2084.
71. Shelton KE, Butler L, Toner JP, et al. Salpingectomy improves the pregnancy rate in in vitro fertilization with hydrosalpinx. Hum Reprod (Oxf) 1996;11:523–525.
72. Kassabji M, Sims J, Butler L, et al. Reduced pregnancy rates with unilateral or bilateral hydrosalpinx after in vitro fertilization. Eur J Obstet Gynecol Reprod Biol 1994;56: 129–132.
73. Levy MJ, Murray D, Sagoskin A. The adverse effect of hydrosalpinges on IVF success rates are reversed equally well by salpingectomy, proximal tubal occlusion and neosalpingostomy. Presented at the meeting of the American Society for Reproductive Medicine, 1996, program supplement 1996:S64.
74. Donnez J, Wauters M, Thomas K. Luteal function after tubal sterilization. Obstet Gynecol 1982;37:38.
75. McComb P, Delbelke L. Decreasing the number of ovulations in the rabbit with surgical division of the blood vessels between the fallopian tube and ovary. J Reprod Med 1984;29:827–829.

76. Sharif K, Kaufmann S, Sharma V. Heteropic pregnancy obtained after in vitro fertilization and embryo transfer following bilateral total salpingectomy: case report. Hum Reprod (Oxf) 1994;9:1966–1967.

77. Pavic N, Neuenschwander E, Gschwind C, et al. Interstitial pregnancy following bilateral salpingectomy and in vitro fertilization-embryo transfer. Fertil Steril 1986;46: 701–702.

24

Endometriosis, Endometrioma, and the Problem of Adhesions

Ivo A. Brosens, Stephan Gordts, Rudi Campo, and Luk Rombauts

CONTENTS

Endometriosis is one of the three major causes of pelvic adhesions in women. It affects young women, causing infertility and pelvic pain, and can result in ovarian disease, compromising seriously the ovarian function. In addition, the disease develops insidiously and by time the diagnosis is established, adhesions have frequently caused severe disease. Surgery is the treatment of choice but, unfortunately, is also a cause of adhesion formation. As can be anticipated, once a vicious circle of adhesive pelvic disease and repeat surgery is established, the only road out leads to radical surgery and premature castration. Nevertheless, the disease is benign and there is a risk of undertreatment, but probably even more of overtreatment. Excessive surgery can result in loss of normal ovarian tissue and postoperative adhesions in recurrent cyst formation. Consequently, the first surgical procedure may well determine the reproductive outcome in young women affected by the disease, and therefore both the decision to operate and the performance of the procedure require the best possible consideration and care.

Although we do not know the cause and pathogenesis of endometriosis, much progress has been made in recent years in our understanding of the disease process. We first describe the appearances and pathophysiology of the disease. The phenotype of the ectopic endometrial tissue is apparently to a large extent determined by the topographic surroundings and cell-to-cell interactions. Second, laparoscopy has remained the gold standard for diagnosis, but we should be aware of the limitations of visual diagnosis and the artifacts that can be created by the inspection of the pelvic structures at laparoscopy. Finally, the surgical approach is discussed. The goal is to restore the integrity of the tuboovarian structures and preserve their function. It is fortunate that, although the disease may seem to affect severely the pelvic organs, the disease process is not invasive by destruction of the tissues. We should avoid that damage and dysfunction of the tuboovarian structures which are increased more by surgery than by endometriosis.

Appearances of Endometriosis

Active and progressive endometriosis can be defined by the presence of endometrial-like activity in the ectopic implants. These endometrial-like activities are determined by the sex steroid hormone response of the ectopic implant, which similarly as in the uterus is polarized by the topography and microenvironment. The implants or parts of the implants can cause proliferation, secretory, and decidual changes and menstrual shedding, similar to superficial endometrium, or a poor sex steroid hormone response of glands and stroma, but smooth muscle cell differentiation and proliferation, similar to basal endometrium and junctional zone endomyometrium. However, at the ectopic sites the endometrial-like tissue lacks the uterine polarization of sex steroid hormone response and, depending on the topography and microenvironment, the endometrial activities result in inflammatory reaction, fibrosis, adhesions, and endometrioma formation or in adenomyotic nodules or a combination of these lesions.

Superficial Peritoneal Endometriosis

Superficial peritoneal endometriosis has multiple appearances.[1] Scanning electron microscopy studies have shown that most superficial peritoneal implants are not growing on the surface of the mesothelium, but appear as papules, blebs, or vesicles with the endometrial-like tissue covered by mesothelium.[2–4] The mesothelial layer is frequently disrupted at biopsy, and the loose layer can be lost during histologic preparation[3] (Fig.24.1). Intramesothelial implants have been described as microscopic endometriosis, although it is not clear whether they represent the early stage of implantation or metaplasia or result from ruptured endometriotic vesicles.[2,5]

The hemorrhagic blebs result from sex steroid hormone-dependent bleeding, which can be cyclic or noncyclic (Fig. 24.2). Although these lesions represent the most typical endometrial activity, they are sometimes coined as atypical or subtle lesions.[6] Such lesions were originally described and illustrated by Sampson[7] and formed the basis of his theory of menstrual regurgitation and implantation.[8] The so-called typical, puckered, and pigmented lesions are characterized by the presence of a variable amount of fibrosis, a moderately vascularized stroma, glands with intraluminal debris, and hemosiderin-laden macrophages. White lesions have extensive fibrosis, mini-

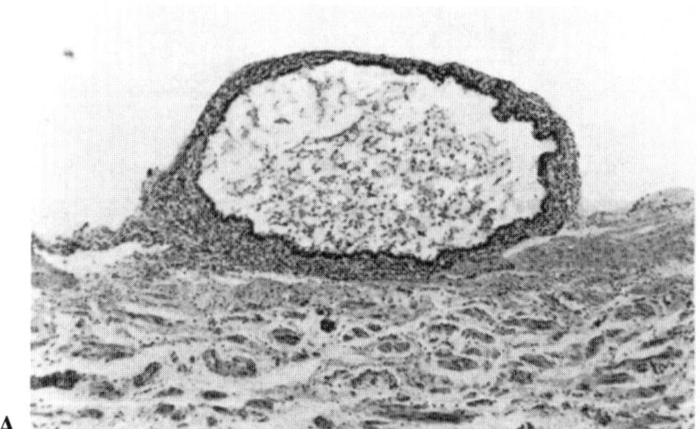
A

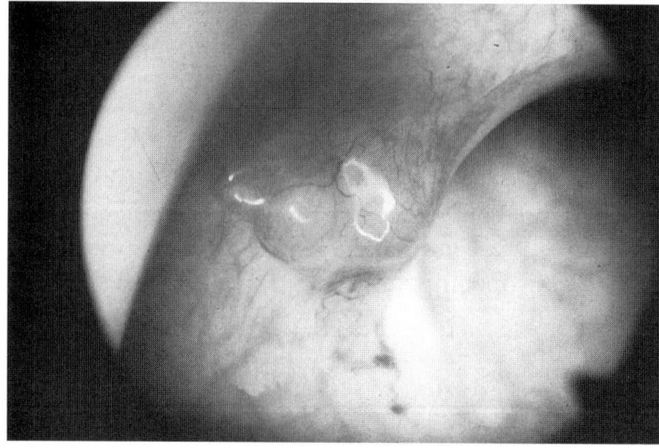
B

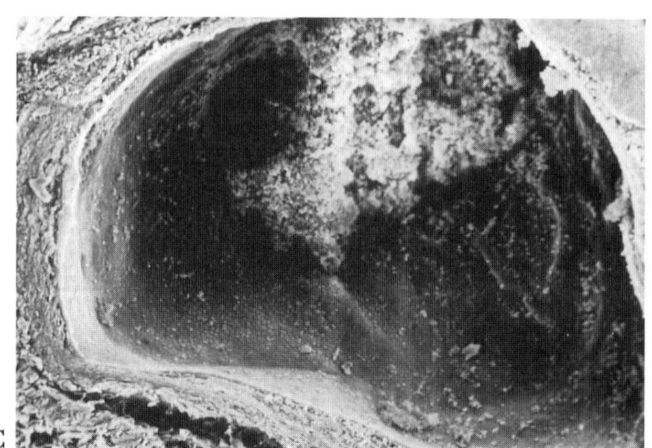
C

FIGURE 24.1. **A.** Photomicrograph of small peritoneal bleb, apparently growing on the surface. (Reproduced with permission from Sampson JA [1921]. Perforating Haemorrhagic [chocolate] cysts of ovary. Arch. Surg. 3:245–323. Copyright 1921, American Medical Association.) **B.** Glandular excrescences or blebs formed by distended glands and covered by mesothelium. **C.** Scanning electron microscopy. Section of the specimen shows a glandular excrescence covered by mesothelium. *Please see insert for color reproduction of Figures B and C.*

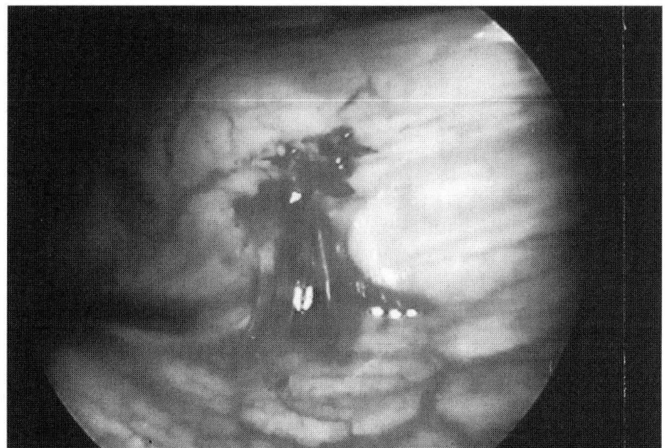

FIGURE 24.2. Hemorrhagic endometriotic vesicles during menstruation. *Please see insert for color reproduction of this figure.*

mal stroma, poor vascularization, and some glandular debris. It is now generally accepted that the chronic bleeding of the red, highly active lesions follows an evolution of resorption or inflammatory reaction that leads to increased fibrosis, decrease of stromal and glandular activity, and ultimately to healing and scarification.[9]

The petechial implant is the only type present in 20% of adolescents with endometriosis,[10] whereas the black and white lesions apparently dominate at later ages.[11] The distinction between red, black, and white peritoneal lesions has recently been included in the revised American Fertility Society (r-AFS) classification of endometriosis.[12] Many lesions, however, show a mixed appearance and visual evaluation is inadequate to exclude healthy endometrial-like tissue in the implant. It is important to note that in the primate[13] and human[14,15] the superficial peritoneal lesions of endometriosis can disappear and reappear on the peritoneal surface depending on the endocrine condition. Peritoneal endometriosis is found at laparoscopy in women with polycystic ovary syndrome when they have regular menses or oligomenorrhea, but not with amenorrhea of more than 3 months.[16] After 6 months of ovarian suppressive therapy, the peritoneal surface appears dry and clean, masking implants that reappear as soon as the menstrual cycle has resumed.[17]

Ovarian Endometriosis

The ovary is not only the most frequent site of endometriosis, but ovarian implants also show more vascularization[18] and sex steroid hormone response such as menstrual shedding[19] than at other sites. It is therefore no surprise that ovarian endometriosis is frequently associated with adhesions. Ovarian endometriomas larger than 2 cm are associated with adhesions in 86% of cases.[20] Adhesions are frequently located on the anterior side of the ovary facing the fossa ovarica or posterior side of the uterus, but can also cover part of the ovary and gyri and cause sequestration of implants with early invagination of the ovarian cortex.

The typical ovarian lesion is the chocolate cyst or endometrioma. The endometrial cyst of the ovary was discovered by Sampson[17] in 1921 when he observed in specimens obtained at the time of menstruation that the endometrial-like tissue showed evidence of menstrual shedding (Fig. 24.3). The study of the ovarian endometrioma requires the examination of in situ and not excisional specimens for an accurate and complete description. Sampson[7] studied with great care hysterec-

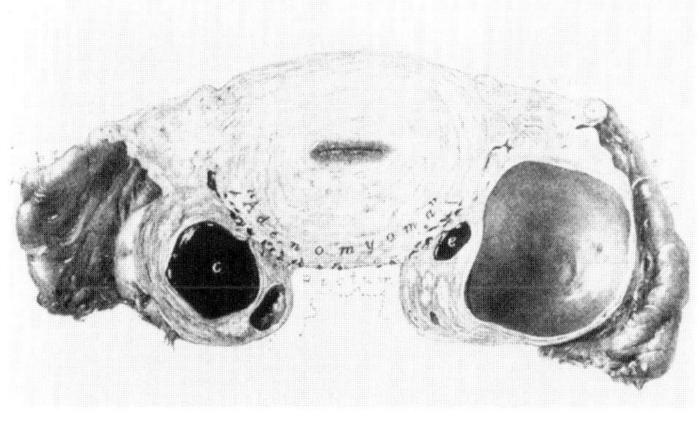

A

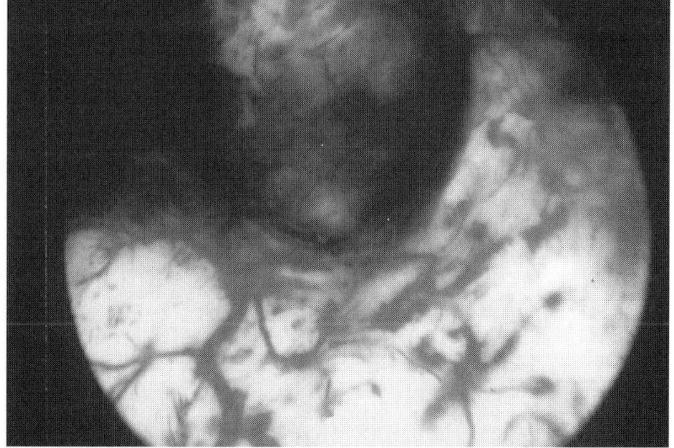

B

FIGURE 24.3. **A.** Cross section of the uterus and ovaries showing their relationship before surgery. Typical features of the ovarian endometrioma include (1) adhesions between the endometriomas (*c* and *e*) and the posterior side of the uterus; (2) the site of "perforation" sealed off by adhesions; (3) adenomyosis in the area of adhesions. Note the presence of a functional cyst on the *right side.* (Reproduced with permission from Sampson JA [1921]. perforating haemorrhagic [chocolate] cysts of ovary. Arch. Surg. 3:245–323. Copyright 1921, American Medical Association.) **B.** Endoscopic view inside the endometrioma at the time of menstruation shows the site of "invagination" and the hemorrhagic endometrial-like mucosa colonizing the inverted ovarian cortex. *Please see insert for color reproduction of Figure B.*

tomy and bilateral salpingo-ophorectomy specimens with endometriomas in the operating room and under the microscope and described four major features of the endometrioma: (1) adhesions, (2) lining of part of the wall with endometrial-like tissue with evidence of menstrual shedding, (3) a so-called site of perforation, and (4) adenomyotic lesions outside the cyst at the site of adhesions. He observed that the endometrioma was always adherent to the posterior side of the parametrium or uterus and speculated initially that the chocolate content was spilled at "the site of perforation" causing peritoneal endometriosis and adhesions. This view, however, was abandoned in 1927 when he formulated the theory of menstrual regurgitation and implantation.[8] Hughesdon[21] demonstrated on serial section of ovaries with the endometrioma in situ that in 93% of cases the wall of the endometrioma was formed by the ovarian cortex, as evidenced by the presence of primordial follicles. There was no evidence that "ectopic endometrium ate its way into the ovary like insects into an apple." He presented the theory of invagination of the ovarian cortex and that "the site of perforation" was changed into "the site of invagination."

Our observations based on endoscopic inspection in situ of the large endometriomas under fluid and selective biopsies confirmed that the wall of the typical endometrioma is formed by ovarian cortex and patchily lined by superficial endometrial-like tissue.[22] In young women, the wall has retained a pearl-white appearance; the endometrial-like tissue is partially covering the wall and consists of a thin, highly vascularized mucosa that is loosely attached to the cortex. Chronic hemorrhage is most evident at the site of invagination by the presence of old clots. In older women, the wall becomes pigmented, yellow or dark brown, and at the site of inversion the vascularization is replaced by fibrosis and dense adhesions.[23] Large endometriomas are frequently multilocular and associated with lutein cysts with which they can communicate (Table 24.1). Early colonization of the lutein cyst by endometrial-like mucosa was described by Sampson.[7] This report has caused some investigators[20,24] to suggest that endometriomas are formed by colonization of the lutein cyst, although it is as likely that lutein cysts arise in the invaginated cortical wall of the endometrioma.

TABLE 24.1. Excisional specimens of hemorrhagic cysts diagnosed as endometriomas before surgery but lutein cyst at histopathology.

Reference	Number	Percentage
Martin and Berry (1990)[103]	41	27
Nezhat et al. (1992)[20]	216	33

[a]In 8% of cases, the lutein cyst was communicating with the endometrial cyst.

An additional typical feature, but frequently not diagnosed, is the smooth muscle hyperplasia, which to a variable degree can be found focally in the deeper layers of the ovary and in the fibromuscular or uterine tissues involved in the adhesions outside the endometrioma.[21] These nodular lesions at the site of adhesions show the features of adenomyosis.[7]

Rectovaginal Endometriosis

Rectovaginal endometriosis is a deep; nodular lesion that presents at histopathologic examination the features of basal and junctional zone endomyometrium.[25–27] In contrast with superficial lesions the glands, stroma, and vessels show poor hormone response, the stroma is infiltrated with plasmolymphocytes, and at menstruation the vessels show congestion but not necrosis and menstrual shedding is absent.[28,29] Today the lesion is described as adenomyosis. Nodular lesions similar to adenomyosis have been described in other fibromuscular structures of the pelvis such as the uterosacral and uteroovarian ligaments, the vesicouterine pillars, and the wall of bladder and bowel[30] (Fig. 24.4). Nodules at the posterior fornix have, more frequently than at other sites, the histologic features of adenomyosis.[31] Rectovaginal endometriosis is focally associated with microendometriomas,[32] which

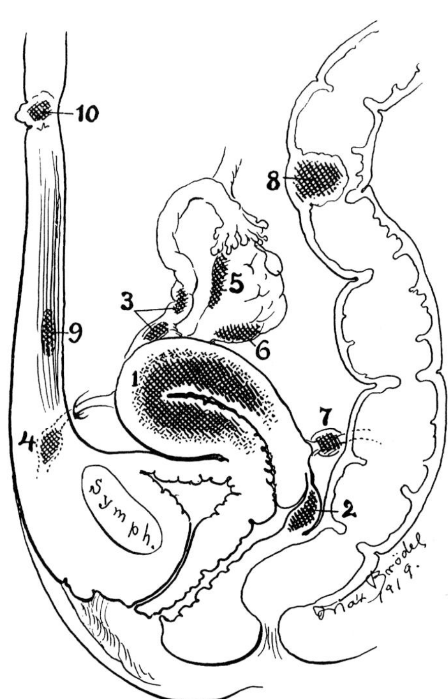

FIGURE 24.4. Diagram prepared by Cullen (1920)[30] shows the sites of nodular endometriosis or adenomyosis in the pelvic supportive structures (2,4,6,7) and muscular wall of the pelvic organs. (3,8,9,10) (Reproduced with permission from Cullen TS [1920]. The distribution of adenoma containing uterine mucosa Arch. Surg. 1:215–283. Copyright 1920, American Medical Association.)

can be much greater in the loose tissue underlying the vaginal epithelium and the rectal and vesical mucosa.

Pathophysiology

Pathogenesis

Peritoneal, ovarian, and rectovaginal endometriosis have recently been described as three distinctive pathological and clinical entities of endometriosis.[33,34] Whether they represent different pathogenetic entities or are appearances of the same endometriotic tissue in a different topographic environment remains to be elucidated. Clinical and experimental examples exist that cannot be explained unless implantation as well as metaplasia are accepted as mechanisms for the presence and development of endometrial-like tissue at ectopic sites. In a recent review[35] we presented the view that the differentiation process of the ectopic implant is closely regulated by the interaction between sex steroids and locally expressed proinflammatory cytokines.

As is the case in eutopic endometrium, the topography and the local microenvironment of the ectopic implant will determine if the endometrial-like activity resembles that of the superficial or basal layer endometrium (Table 24.2). The superficial layer shows the "classical" sex steroid hormone response and is characterized by proliferation and secretory changes of the glands, decidualization of the stroma and vessels in the late luteal phase, and menstrual shedding. This response gradually decreases toward the basalis, where both basalis and junctional zone endometrium display a different hormonal response with low secretory activity and delayed decidualization. Such polarization of the endometrium is thought to be effected by the cytokines released by T lymphocytes that are found at the endometriomyometrial junction.[36–38]

Endometriosis, a Disease Characterized by Cyclic Bleeding

In superficial peritoneal endometriosis and even more in ovarian endometriomas, the nonfibrotic implant has a surface epithelium, a highly vascularized stroma with or without glands, and like superficial endometrium a great tendency for cyclic bleeding[39,40] (Table 24.3). On histologic examination, evidence of extravasation of red blood cells and presence of hemosiderin-laden macrophages were found in 77% of biopsies of histologically verified endometriosis.[19] The mucosal vessels of these implants bleed cyclically in response to ovarian sex steroids, similar to the spiral arterioles in the superficial layer of the endometrium.[28] Cyclic bleeding is seen in the red, vesicular lesions of the peritoneum and in ovarian endometrioma. These lesions, but not the black peritoneal or rectovaginal lesions, have been shown to express MMP-1 mRNA[41,42] (Table 24.4).

In eutopic endometrium, the MMP-1 expression is restricted to the superficial stromal compartment in the premenstrual period.[43] This confined temporal expression is thought to be mediated through potent inhibition of MMP-1 gene transcription by estradiol and progesterone.[44,45] In ectopic implants, focal expression of MMP-1 mRNA can be detected irrespective of the phase of the menstrual cycle.[42] This observation indicates that, although ectopic implants express estrogen and progesterone receptors, the biologic activity of these steroid hormone receptors on gene transcription is impaired.

Superficial lesions of peritoneal and ovarian endometriosis are associated with adhesion formation. A number of peritoneal factors have been implicated in pathogenesis of adhesions, such as growth factors released from macrophages, fibronectin that promotes cellular growth, cytokines such as tumor necrosis factor, epidermal growth factors, and finally iron and free radical

TABLE 24.3. Vascularization of endometriotic implants.

Site of implant	Capillary/stroma area (mean value in %)	Cyclic changes
Peritoneal		
Red lesion	4.5	Present
Black lesion	2.3[a]	Absent
Ovarian endometrioma	3.4	Present
Rectovaginal	1.8[a]	Absent
Superficial endometrium	4.3	Present

[a]Different from eutopic superficial endometrium.
Adapted from Nisolle (1996).[39]

TABLE 24.2. Zonal differentiation of the sex steroid hormone (SSH) response in the uterus during the menstrual cycle.

Superficial endometrium:
- Proliferation, secretory changes, decidual reaction
- Zonal-specific gene expression (e.g., MMP-1), menstrual shedding

Basal endometrium
- Low SSH response
- T lymphocytes

Junctional zone:
- Smooth muscle cell differentiation
- SSH-dependent contractility

Outer myometrium

TABLE 24.4. MMP-1 expression in endometriotic foci with matrix breakdown.

Endometriotic lesion	MMP-1 mRNA	Matrix breakdown present: MMP-1 mRNA positive foci	Matrix breakdown present: MMP-1 mRNA negative foci
Superficial peritoneal			
Red lesion	4/13	2/3	2/7
Black lesion	0/12		1/10
Ovarian endometrioma	4/11	3/3	1/7
Rectovaginal	0/11		1/7

Adapted from Kokerine et al. (1997).[42]

reactions, but their exact role remains unclear.[46–50] Unfortunately, early adhesion formation tends to be masked at standard laparoscopy by the intraperitoneal pressure. It is not routine to inspect the ovary and fossa ovarica under fluid for detection of filmy adhesions (Fig. 24.5). These small, free-floating adhesions are not addressed in any adhesion classification system. No correlation has been made between early adhesion formation and the presence of inflammatory cytokines in the peritoneal fluid in endometriosis.

Adenomyosis

The nodular adenomyotic lesion is infiltrated by lymphoid aggregates that are characteristically found in the endomyometrial junctional zone. The stromal cell compartment is, similarly as in the basal layer of eutopic endometrium, characterized by poor sex steroid hormone response. Studies in vitro have shown that immune cell cytokines such as interferon-γ, interleukin-1, and tumor necrosis factor-α induce HLA-DR expression in glandular epithelial cells and inhibit their proliferation, consistent with the phenotype of the basalis.[51,52] Some genes, such as the interstitial collagenase, are expressed in the superficial but not in the basal endometrial layer.

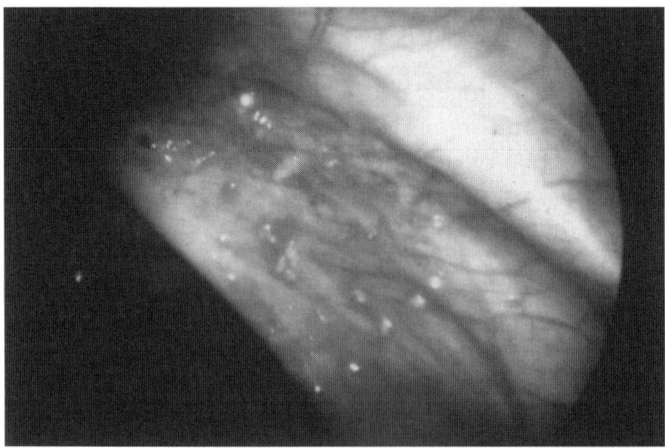

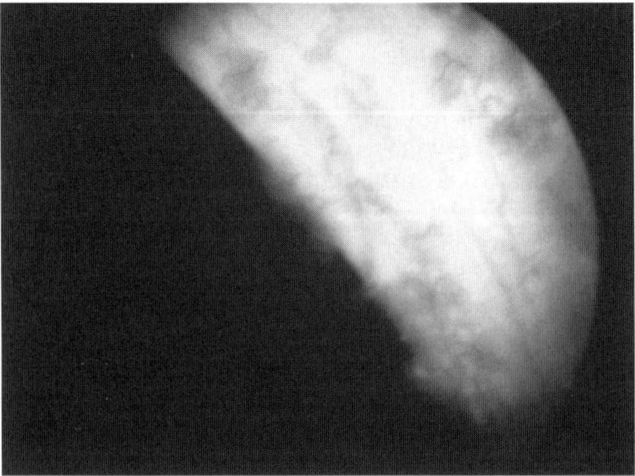

FIGURE 24.5. Superficial peritoneal endometriosis as seen at standard laparoscopy (*top*) and under fluid (*bottom*). Note the small, vascularized, free-floating adhesions seen on the peritoneum under fluid. *Please see insert for color reproduction of this figure.*

The phenotype of the ectopic endometrial tissue appears to be largely determined by the topography and local microenvironment. As the posterior fornix is derived from uterine mesenchymal cells,[53] it is not surprising that lesions resembling uterine adenomyosis are found at this site. If our view is correct then rectovaginal endometriosis is not endometriosis of the rectovaginal septum but rather vaginal or cerviacl adenomyosis.[35]

Symptomatology

Although chronic pelvic pain, dysmenorrhea, deep dyspareunia, and infertility are considered to be the main symptoms of pelvic endometriosis, many women with endometriosis are completely asymptomatic.

Chronic Pelvic Pain

A large prospective study[54] has shown that women with endometriosis experience dysmenorrhea more frequently than women with sequelae of pelvic infection or laparoscopically normal pelvis, however, the same study demonstrated that 32% of women with endometriosis did not have dysmenorrhea.

Deep dyspareunia and chronic pelvic pain affect one in three and one in two women with endometriosis, respectively.[54,55] There has been a surprising lack of correlation between the stage of the disease as determined by the revised American Fertility Society (r-AFS) classification[12] and the prevalence and severity of symptoms.[55] Sites of focal tenderness on examination are strongly associated with the presence of disease in the uterosacral ligaments and cul-de-sac and are associated significantly with deep and larger volumes of the implants.[56] However, no relationship is found between size and adenomyotic features such as the presence of T lymphocytes.[57] The majority of lesions at the posterior fornix but not at the uterosacral ligaments present features of adenomyosis, indicating that the site rather than the size is indicative of an adenomyotic lesion.[31]

Pain in endometriosis had been related to adhesions and restricted mobility of the organs, but treatment regimens have often produced relief of pain without affecting the adhesion score. Pain relief is usually achieved by ovarian suppressive therapy as soon as amenorrhea is installed.[40,58]

Infertility

The relationship between endometriosis and infertility has been suggested by the prevalence of the disease in fertile and infertile couples. The incidence of endometriosis in the female partner of infertile couples undergoing laparoscopy is currently estimated to range

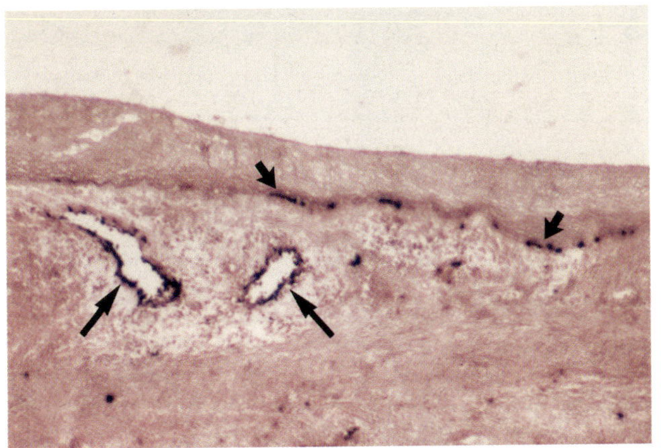

Fig. 9.6. Plasminogen activator inhibitor-1 production localized to mesothelial (*small arrows*) and submesothelial endothelial (*large arrows*) cells in inflamed human peritoneum using mRNA in situ hybridization.

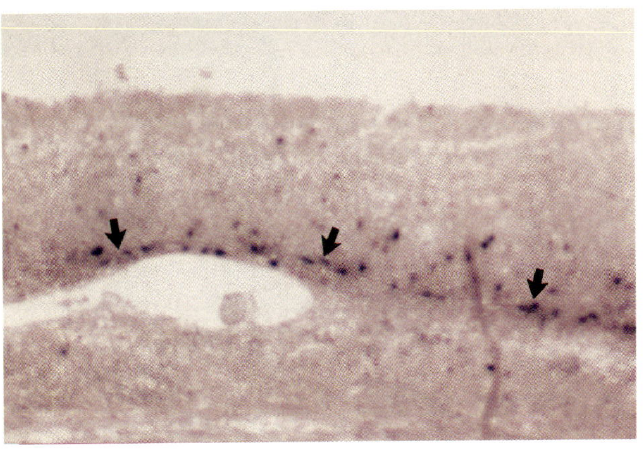

Fig. 9.7. Plasminogen activator inhibitor-2 production localized to mesothelial cells (*arrowed*) on the surface of an inflamed appendix using mRNA in situ hybridization.

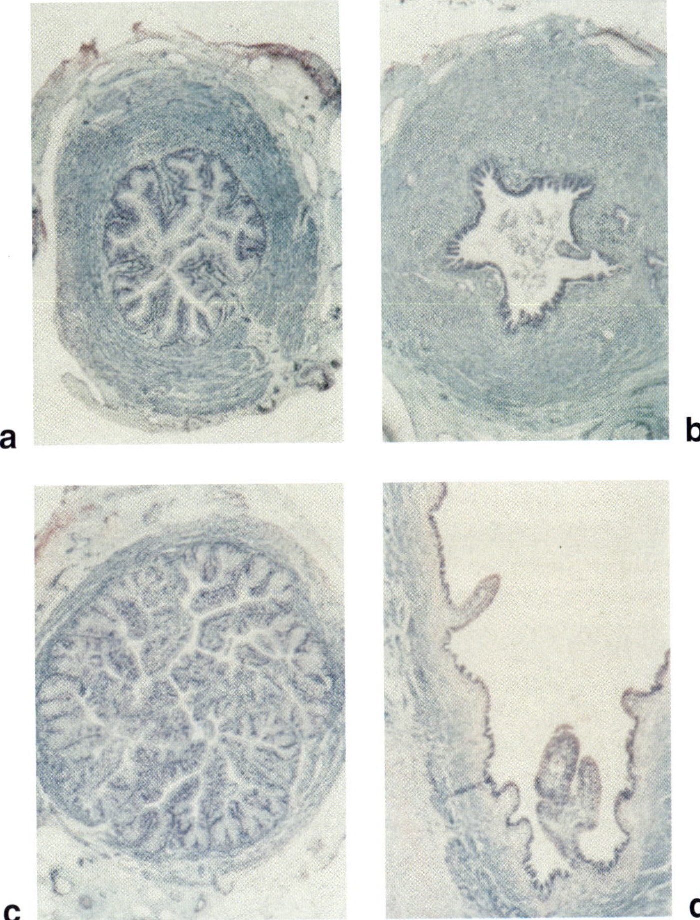

Fig. 23.1. Experimental hydrosalpinx: (**a**) normal isthmus; (**b**) dilated isthmus after induction of experimental hydrosalpinx; (**c**) normal ampulla; (**d**) dilated ampulla after induction of experimental hydrosalpinx. Reduction in number and size of ampullary folds is shown, with flattened epithelium between the ampullary folds.

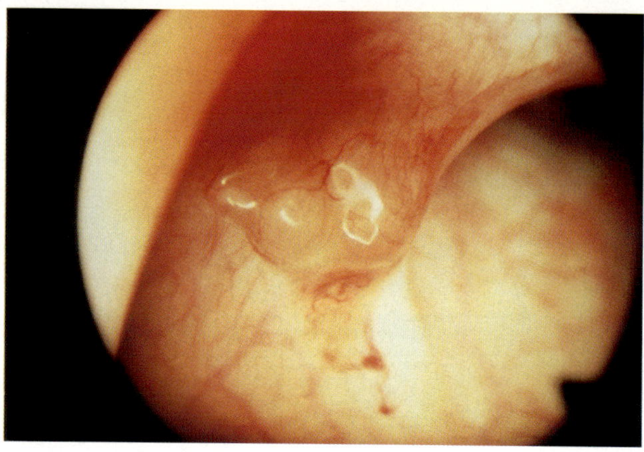

FIG. 24.1. B. Glandular excrescences or blebs formed by distended glands and covered by mesothelium.

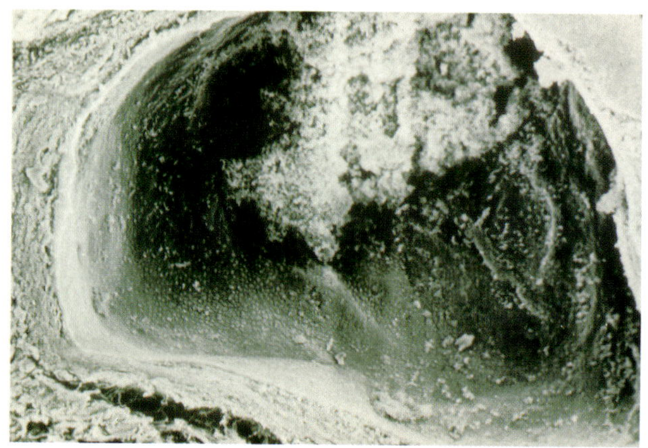

FIG. 24.1 C. Scanning electron microscopy. Section of the specimen shows a glandular excrescence covered by mesothelium.

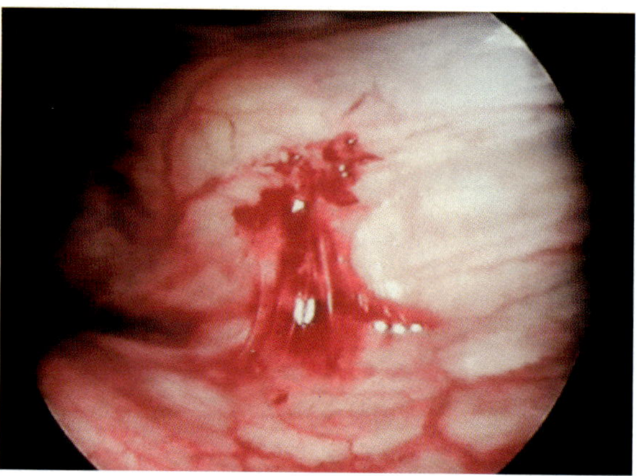

FIG. 24.2. Hemorrhagic endometriotic vesicles during menstruation.

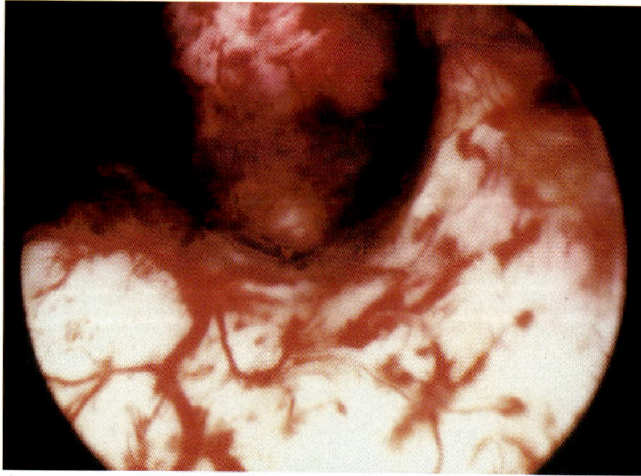

FIG. 24.3. B. Endoscopic view inside the endometrioma at the time of menstruation shows the site of "invagination" and the hemorrhagic endometrial-like mucosa colonizing the inverted ovarian cortex.

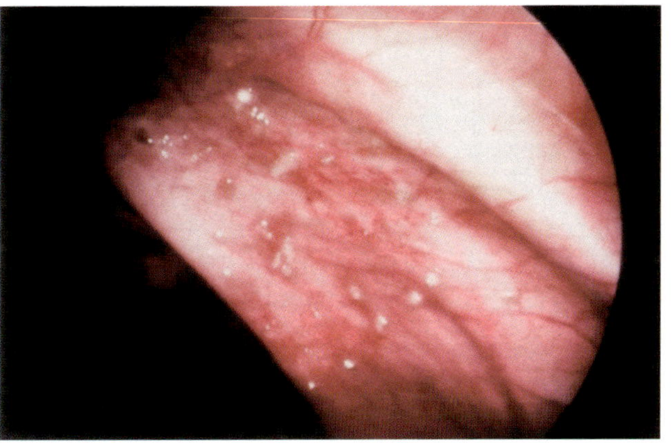

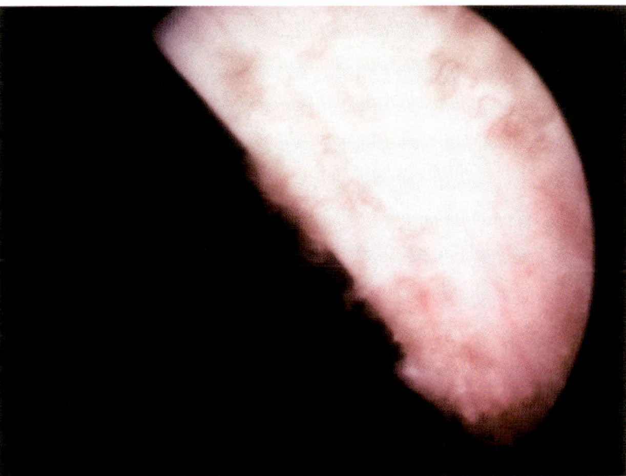

FIG. 24.5. Superficial peritoneal endometriosis as seen at standard laparoscopy (*top*) and under fluid (*bottom*). Note the small, vascularized, free-floating adhesions seen on the peritoneum under fluid.

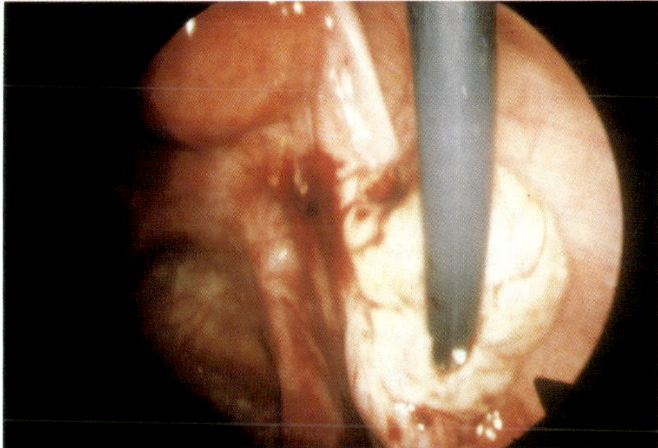

FIG. 24.6. At laparoscopy, the ovary is lifted to expose the fossa ovarica. Adhesions between the ovary (showing slight invagination of the cortex) and the fossa ovarica are disrupted by the maneuver, causing diffuse bleeding.

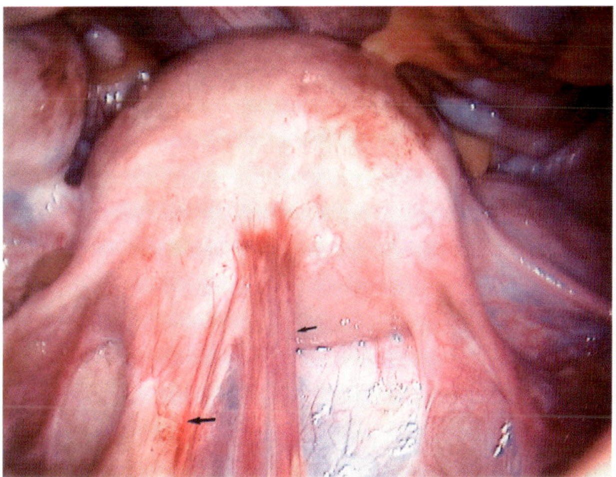

FIG. 25.1. Adhesions from the anterior uterine wall 1 year after a laparoscopic myomectomy (filmy adhesions, *small arrow;* dense adhesions, *large arrow*).

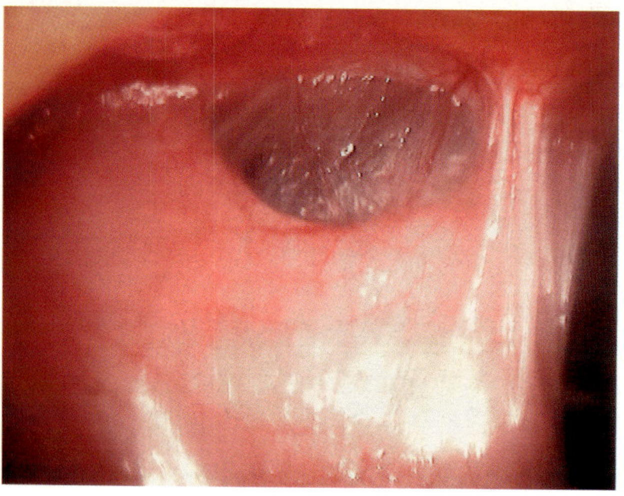

Fig. 25.2. Intestinal adhesions to the previous abdominal incision after myomectomy by laparotomy.

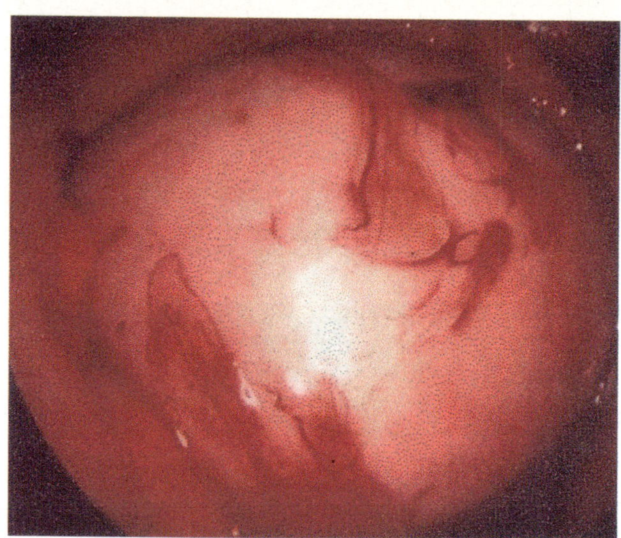

Fig. 39.2. Large endometrioma at right side.

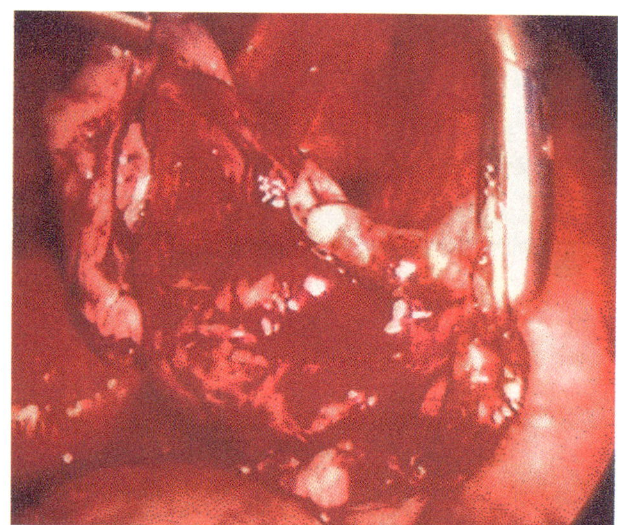

Fig. 39.3. Wide-open capsule after excision of ovarian cyst.

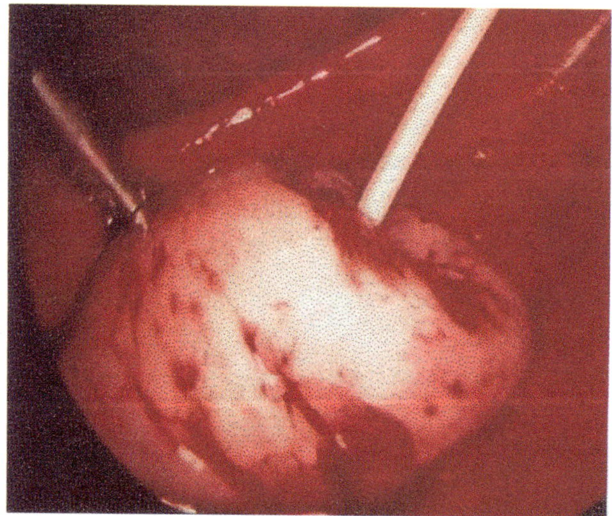

Fig. 39.4. Endoscopic application of fibrin glue to close the ovary.

from 20% to 50%, while the incidence of endometriosis in the general population of women of reproductive age is between 2% and 22%.[59] This fact had led many clinicians to consider the endometriosis implants to be responsible in some way for the concurrent infertility, despite the absence of a defined mechanism. However, these data can only serve to support the notion of an association, but not a causal relationship.[60] As it has never been proven that the implants themselves are the cause of infertility, it is therefore no surprise that the treatment of endometriosis in infertility remains one of the most controversial issues in gynecology. Until a causal relationship can be established, it remains just as plausible that infertility causes endometriosis as it does that endometriosis causes infertility or that both are caused by an unknown factor.

For the moment endometriosis-associated infertility is usually divided into infertility in women with peritoneal implants alone and infertility in women with adhesive disease. This distinction is largely conceptual as there are no data correlating the site, extent, and type of adhesions and infertility in endometriosis. The role of adhesive disease in endometriosis tends to be evaluated in analogy with pelvic inflammatory disease as a mechanical factor, although the pathophysiology of these two conditions is fundamentally different.

Peritoneal Inflammation

Endometriosis is apparently associated with peritoneal fluid inflammation, and this has led to the suggestion that the intraperitoneal inflammation rather than the endometrial implants may be responsible for reduced fecundity. The intraperitoneal inflammation is manifested by an increase in peritoneal fluid volume, macrophage number, degree of activation of macrophages, and the concentrations of macrophages secretory products, that is, prostaglandins, proteolytic enzymes, cytokines, and growth factors.[61] The level of these factors shows usually a wide variation. Controversy exists whether these factors are secreted by regurgitated endometrial fluid, ectopic endometrial tissue, or peritoneal macrophages. The changes are rather consistent with a proinflammatory condition and suggest that in women with endometriosis the physiologic role of peritoneal fluid exudate removing regurgitated menstrual debris is quantitively increased. The concept that the peritoneal fluid in endometriosis is responsible for reduced fertility is based on data showing, in experimental conditions, a detrimental effect of some factors on the reproductive process, such as phagocytosis of sperms, reduced sperm motility, and embryo toxicity.

Ovarian Dysfunction

Mild and minimal endometriosis are associated with abnormal follicular development as manifested by reduced granulosa cell steroidogenesis[62] and reduced follicular fluid luteinizing hormona (LH) concentration.[63] Implantation rates have been shown to be lower after oocyte donation when endometriosis was the donor's cause of infertility, suggesting an abnormal development of the oocyte in patients with endometriosis.[64,65] The luteal function as evaluated by the dating of the endometrial biopsies in relationship with the LH peak is apparently normal in patients with endometriosis.[66] However, endometriosis as well as patients with unexplained infertility are characterized by a delay in the rise of the plasmaprogesterone following the LH peak and the absence of an ovulatory stigma at laparoscopy.[67] The occurrence of the luteinized unruptured follicle has remained controversial because it is difficult in clinical practice to establish the diagnosis reliably by the present endoscopic and imaging techniques. Two investigators reported on cycles in which conception had occurred and identified the presence of an ovulatory stigma up to day 24 but not thereafter.[68,69] Recently, Mio and collaborators[70] found that endometriosis was associated as well in terms of patients as cycles with a significant increase of luteinized unruptured follicles, from which in 43% the oocyte cumulus could be aspirated.

Failure of the follicle to rupture has also been described to occur in repeat cycles in patients with laparoscopically proven sequelae of pelvic inflammatory disease, and microsurgery did not seem to change the ovulatory disturbance.[71] When periovarian adhesions cover more than half the ovarian surface, the prognosis after microsurgery is extremely poor.[72] Subclinical oophoritis has been described in patients with unexplained infertility.[73] The inspection of the ovaries under fluid in transvaginal hydrolaparoscopy showed 50% more filmy ovarian adhesions in minimal and mild endometriosis than at standard laparoscopy, indicating that subclinical adhesive disease of the ovaries may be underestimated at standard laparoscopy.[74]

At present we can only speculate on the role of adhesions in endometriosis. However, more and more data cast doubt on the concept that ovarian adhesions are only a mechanical factor of infertility in endometriosis. Our present endoscopic and imaging techniques are inadequate for the investigation of the process of ovum release in subclinical ovarian adhesive disease. Standard laparoscopy changes the tuboovarian architecture and provokes collapse of the fine tuboovarian structures such as the folds of fimbriae, the ovulatory ostium, the cumulus mass, and the filmy adhesions. In addition, the technique is too invasive for repeat procedures. Further progress by ultrahigh-resolution imaging techniques and less traumatic microendoscopic techniques is awaited to allow the visualization of the process of release of the cumulus mass and the reliable diagnosis of subclinical ovarian adhesive disease.

Tubal Dysfunction and Disease

It has been speculated that peritoneal prostaglandins, presumably produced by active surface implants,[75] may alter tubal transport of the gametes or embryo. It is however unclear to which extent the implants contribute to the changes of the peritoneal fluid in endometriosis. In the human, the oocyte pickup and transport in the ampullary segment is effected by ciliary activity, which is apparently not altered by potent prostaglandin analogs.[76] The process of ovum retrieval by the fimbriae in the human still remains elusive but has recently been visualized by transvaginal endoscopy under fluid.[77] The technique shows the normal fimbrial architecture and the close approximation of the distended fimbriae with the caudal pole of the ovary. During the process of retrieval, the cumulus mass is firmly adherent to the fimbriae and is released from the site of rupture by the sweeping movements of the congested and tumescent fimbrial folds. One can speculate that adhesions in the fossa ovarica immobilizing the ovary may prevent the ovary from rotating with the corpus luteum into a caudal position. On the other hand, there is clinical evidence that an indirect retrieval from the cul-de-sac or intervisceral spaces exists in the human, but judging from the finding of the oocyte in the tube contralateral to the corpus luteum the frequency of this phenomenon is less than 5% in normal fertile women.[78]

Endometriosis can be associated with an extensive degree of pelvic adhesions, and the tube is frequently involved in severe endometriosis. In severe endometriosis, hydrosalpinx can be caused by compression or serosal stricture of the distal tubal segment. Tubal distension, flattening of the folds, and deciliation are found in the ampullary segment. These changes are seen in a mechanical hydrosalpinx in experimental conditions and are reversible at salpingostomy.[79] In contrast with pelvic inflammatory disease, the tubal mucosa is not affected by adhesions or fibrosis in endometriosis.[80,81] Clinically, endometriosis with or without adhesions is not associated with an increased risk of tubal pregnancy. Unfortunately, in clinical practice tubal disease is evaluated by laparoscopic inspection and not tubal endoscopy, although it has been demonstrated that mucosal adhesions are a more reliable marker than peritubal serosal adhesions for the outcome of tubal disease in terms of pregnancy and risk of ectopic pregnancy.[82–85]

Diagnosis and Classification

Laparoscopy is the gold standard for the diagnosis of endometriosis. Visual inspection by laparoscopy has increased the awareness of the multiple, subtle, and typical appearances of endometriosis. However, the risk exists that the clinical significance of endometriosis is overestimated if whatever looks like endometriosis at laparoscopy or even represents some endometrial-like tissue at histopathology is considered as presence of the disease. The visual concept of endometriosis has several pitfalls, making endometriosis sometimes an illusive disease.

Peritoneal Endometriosis

Peritoneal surface endometriosis has been shown to have a variable and changing appearance that is likely to be related to the irregular hormonal response. Failure to recognize the relationship between the hormonal status and the appearance of the implants has led to the visual illusion of efficacy that has been shown to occur when in normally cycling women the effect of medical therapy is evaluated by a second-look laparoscopy at the end of a period of amenorrhea and compared with the pretreatment findings. The peritoneum will appear dry and clean when for a period of 6 months recurrent bleeding in the implant has been suppressed. Evers[17] has shown that as soon as menstruations resume the "beneficial" effect disappears. Because the peritoneum is more clean after 6 months than after 3 months of amenorrhea, it has also been assumed that the minimal duration of medical therapy is 6 months. At microscopy, however, there is no evidence that the prolonged use of medication results in a greater loss of endometriotic cells.[86] In clinical practice there is no difference in the outcome of pain relief between 3 and 6 months GnRH-analog therapy.[87]

Ovarian Endometriosis

Ultrasonography is frequently the initial modality by which the ovarian endometrioma is detected in young women. Its diagnostic accuracy can be improved by combination with color Doppler ultrasonography. The vascular pattern of an endometrioma is typically focal and located in the caudal pole of the cyst. Low impedance and high diastolic flow are present when there is hemorrhage during the menstrual phase of the cycle.[88]

The visual diagnosis of the typical endometrioma remains the most accurate method for detecting and diagnosing the endometrioma, with a sensitivity, specificity, and accuracy of 97, 95, and 96, respectively.[89] The typical gross features include (1) diameter not more than 12 cm; (2) adhesions to the pelvic side wall or the posterior leaf of the broad ligament; (3) "powder burns" and minute red or blue spots with adjacent puckering on the surface; and (4) tarry, thick, chocolate-colored fluid content. In the absence of the typical features, the diagnosis should not be based on the aspiration of chocolate content, which can be present in an old lutein cyst or even a cystadenoma. There is always a need for biopsy and histopathologic confirmation. Unfortunately, the endometriotic cyst is not lined uniformly by endometrial-like tissue, and in approximately one-third of cases the histopathology is not diagnostic but is compatible with that of endometriosis.

Adhesions

Severity of endometriosis as diagnosed at laparoscopy largely depends on the presence, extent, and type of tuboovarian adhesions and the presence and size of ovarian endometriomas. Laparoscopy is at present the gold standard but unfortunately not a perfect technique for the accurate exploration of the tuboovarian structures and the presence of adhesions. First, the normal position and the architecture of the fimbriae and the tuboovarian relationship are modified by the Trendelenburg position and the CO_2 pneumoperitoneum. Second, the access from the umbilicus requires rotation of the adnexa to expose the fossa ovarica and the anterior surface and hilus of the ovary. Filmy adhesions between the ovary and fossa ovarica can rupture and cause diffuse bleeding before they are inspected and recorded (Fig. 24.6). Finally, the intraabdominal pressure by the CO_2 pneumoperitoneum tends to mask filmy adhesions by flattening them against the surface and by compressing the capillary vascularization (see Fig. 24.5). After previous pelvic surgery, particularly of the ovaries, the adhesion score can increase because of postoperative adhesion formation. The resultant increase in the r-AFS score is frequently seen as evidence of progression of disease, but can reflect postsurgical adhesive disease as much as true progression of the disease. More ovarian surgery results in more adhesive disease with cyst formation and recurrent pelvic pain. The ultimate hysterectomy and salpingo-oophorectomy in such patients is not so much evidence of progressive endometriosis as the result of surgical failure.

It is no surprise that a high interobserver variation is noted at the diagnosis of extensive endometriosis, which reflects the difficulties in evaluating depth and extent of lesions.[90] In addition, some endoscopists systematically examine the tuboovarian structures under fluid. This technique allows them to detect filmy adhesions, which otherwise are flattened and made invisible by the pneumoperitoneum. Recently, Gordts and coworkers[74] have described a new technique of transvaginal hydrolaparoscopy that is performed under local anesthesia and uses saline as the distension medium. The access via the posterior fornix under fluid allows inspection of the tuboovarian structures in their natural position. The architecture of the fimbriae and the relationship with the ovary are maintained. Filmy adhesions are easy to detect while they are floating in the fluid. Preliminary results show 50% more ovarian adhesions in patients with minimal and mild endometriosis when inspected under fluid in comparison with CO_2 pneumoperitoneum.

Laparoscopic Surgical Techniques

Superficial Peritoneal Endometriosis

Superficial peritoneal endometriosis can be excised surgically to provide pathologic proof of the presence of the disease, but this is time consuming and laborious; therefore, most surgeons prefer bipolar electrocoagulation or laservaporization.

Ovarian Endometrioma

The typical endometrioma can be described as a hematometria that is formed by the invaginated ovarian cortex and sealed off by adhesions. As such the endometrioma is not a cyst in the ovary, but an extraovarian

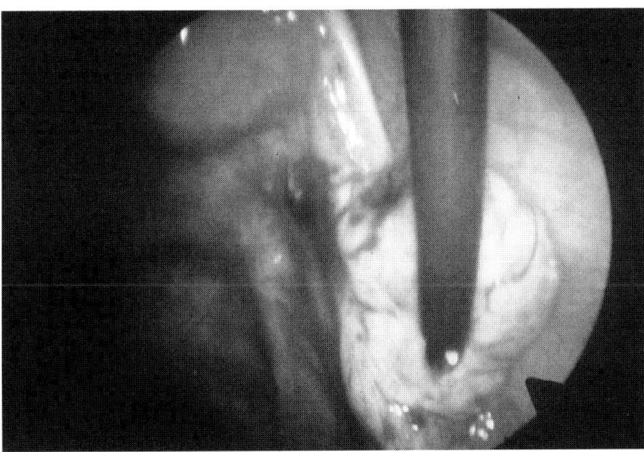

FIGURE 24.6. At laparoscopy, the ovary is lifted to expose the fossa ovarica. Adhesions between the ovary (showing slight invagination of the cortex) and the fossa ovarica are disrupted by the maneuver, causing diffuse bleeding. *Please see insert for color reproduction of this figure.*

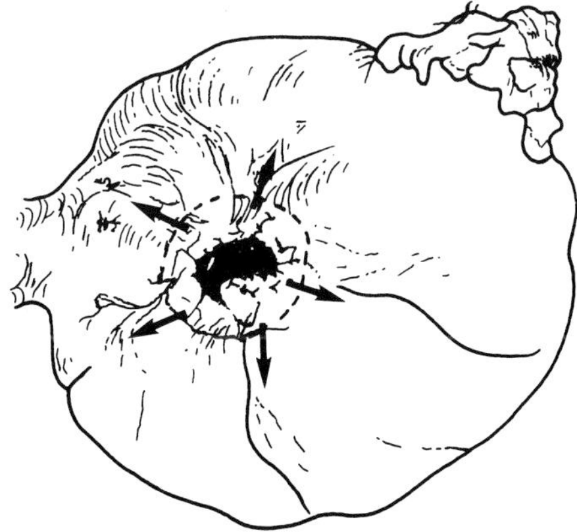

FIGURE 24.7. The eversion is performed after complete adhesiolysis and mobilization of the ovary. The site of inversion is identified and the fibrotic ring is resected. In contrast with cystectomy, the walls stay usually open, and superficial coagulation of the edges results in a wide opening.

pseudocyst, and therefore we first describe the technique which is based on reconstruction of this particular surgical pathology.

Eversion Technique

The technique for extraovarian reconstruction by eversion has recently been described by our group and is proposed as the first choice in young women to maximally preserve ovarian tissue and minimize ovarian damage.[91] The technique should not be confused with fenestration, which tends to close and cause recurrence, in much the same way as an hydrosalpinx treated by salpingotomy tends to close while a salpingostomy stays open (Fig. 24.7)

The first, most important step is the complete adhesiolysis of the ovary, allowing full mobilization and identification of the site of inversion. The adhesiolysis is performed following the plane of cleavage along the ovarian surface to avoid entering the peritoneum. It is most important to perform the adhesiolysis with perfect hemostasis. The endometrioma can be densily adherent to the pelvic sidewall at the site of inversion, sometimes requiring sharp dissection at this stage. The dissection should be carried out with great care during this step because the ureter is very close. During the adhesiolysis the endometrioma almost invariably "ruptures" at the site of inversion and the thick hemosiderin-loaden content escapes. It is vital to have an efficient suction-irrigator system to remove all the chocolate fluid and to irrigate with warm Hartmann solution until the effluent runs clear.

In the second step, the stigma of inversion is identified and the pseudocyst is widely opened by resecting the fibrotic ring. It is typical for the endometrioma that, in contrast with true ovarian cysts, the opening does not cause collapse of the walls as they remain rigid. The opening of the cystic structure is indeed not done by fenestration but by eversion. The third step is the coagulation of the thin layer of superficial endometrial-like mucosa lining the cortex, which as on the outer cortex can be identified by its vascularization. Representative biopsies are always taken from vascularized and suspected areas. Using the technique of eversion, there is obviously no need of suturing, as this would result in invagination of the ovarian cortex.

It is also important to identify endometriotic lesions on the opposing pelvic sidewall to which the endometrioma was adherent. At this site the implants may be nodular and adenomyotic, and excision may be required for full removal. Very large (more than 12 cm) or multilocular endometriomas are preferably treated by a two-step laparoscopy technique for two reasons. First, they occur frequently in combination with hemorrhagic, dysfunctional cysts and, second, full inspection and superficial coagulation can be difficult if not impossible. The initial laparoscopy consists in diagnosing the endometrioma, performing the first step of the eversion technique, and taking the biopsies. The second laparoscopy is then performed 2 to 3 months after the first procedure. During this period the cystic structures regress and the ovary resumes an almost normal configuration; this avoids excessive surgical trauma to the ovary.

The use of ovarian suppressive therapy during this period has been recommended.[92,93] This therapy may have the advantage of avoiding at surgery the presence of a developing follicle or corpus luteum and theoretically of reducing the inflammatory condition of the peritoneum and therefore the risk of postoperative adhesion formation. However, the primary prevention of postoperative adhesion formation is achieved by atraumatic manipulation of the tissues, avoiding any unnecessary surgical procedure such as incision of normal ovarian cortex or excision of functional structures, and using the greatest care for complete hemostasis. The eversion technique is proposed as the primary approach for reconstructive surgery in young women. The technique is not applicable in the fibrotic, encapsulated, or recurrent endometrioma.

Excision Technique

Endometriosis that are adherent to the pelvic wall first need to be teased away from the adhesions binding to the fossa ovarica in the same way as in the eversion technique. The endometrioma is entered at the site of spontaneous rupture or where the wall appears more thin. Aspiration and flushing of the tarry, chocolate content is performed as previously described. The wall of the cyst is carefully inspected, preferably under water, and selective biopsies are taken from the red or suspected lesions.

The fibrotic capsule is resected and any bleeding is coagulated. It seems illogical to us to induce ischemia with surgical knots, and we leave the ovarian defect open or use a fibrin glue to close the walls. We always leave 1 L of warm Hartmann's solution in the peritoneal cavity in the hope of preventing the initial phase of fibrinous adhesion formation, which occurs in the first 24 hours following surgery.[94] The beneficial effect of oxidized regenerated cellulose absorbable barrier in the prevention of postoperative adhesions has been reported.[95]

Risks, Complications, and Recurrence

Incomplete surgery and recurrence occur when the adhesiolysis is not complete. For this reason, fenestration that is performed at the most accessive part of the cyst without full adhesiolysis of the ovary is to be avoided: first, small endometriomas present at the hilus of the ovary can be missed, and second, nodular implants at the site of adhesions are not identified and destroyed.

Excessive surgery can result for two main reasons. First, not all chocolate cysts are of endometrial origin. Although peroperative inspection is supposedly reliable, excisional specimens reveal luteal lining in approximately one-third of cases (see Table 24.1). Recurrent cysts and large multilocular endometriomas are likely to be associated with dysfunctional cysts. Second, excision specimens frequently reveal ovarian cortex with primordial follicles at microscopic examination. Therefore, eversion rather than excisional technique should be used in young women. Ovarian resistance during stimulation for in vitro fertilization is reportedly more frequent after excision of ovarian endometriomas than after conservative techniques.[96] Premature menopause has also been reported after repeat excision of endometriomas.

Specific complications include profuse bleeding from the ovarian hilus vessels; ovarian atrophyl caused by excessive coagulation; and ureter damage during dissection. The most frequent complication is the formation of postoperative adhesions,[97] resulting in tubal infertility, chronic pelvic pain, and recurrent cyst formation.

Comparison of laparoscopy with laparotomy has shown that most endometriomas can be treated safely and efficiently by laparoscopic surgery.[98] The recurrence rate and the pregnancy rates are, as expected, similar. We reported a recurrence rate of 3% after microsurgery[99,100] and 6% after laparoscopic eversion.[91]

Rectovaginal Endometriosis

Rectovaginal endometriosis and other adenomyotic lesions of the pelvic structures are deep lesions and show no plane of cleavage with the surrounding tissue. Coagulation and vaporization techniques are inadequate, and excisional techniques are required to assess the depth of penetration and achieve full resection.[101]

Conclusions

Pelvic endometriosis is best treated by surgery, preferably laparoscopically. In a randomized double-blind controlled study comparing the efficacy of laparoscopic surgery for peritoneal endometriosis stages 1 through 3 with a control arm receiving no surgery, Sutton and coworkers[102] were the first to show convincingly superior results as far as pelvic pain was concerned. Recently, a randomized trial by Marcoux et al.[103] showed that laparoscopic resection or ablation of minimal and mild endometriosis enhanced fecundity in infertile women. Although this study provides the best evidence we have today on surgical treatment of minimal and mild endometriosis in infertile patients, the question remains whether the results of this study are valid and can be generalized. The collaborative study was performed by surgeons who may have a vested interest in the outcome. The study included a significant number of cases with pelvic adhesions, the monthly fecundity after surgery remained much lower than the rate expected in fertile women, and in contrast with medical trials no second-look laparoscopy was performed to provide data on postoperative adhesion formation.

Because ovarian endometriomas can respond to medical therapy, but almost always recur,[104] reconstruction of the ovary and prevention of adhesions are the most important steps to restore and preserve the ovarian function. As rectovaginal endometriosis and other deep lesions of the adenomyotic type are in the long term poorly responsive to medical therapy, the argument for surgical excision is also convincing in this condition.

References

1. Martin DC, Hubert GD, Van der Zwaag R, El-Zeky FA. Laparoscopic appearances of peritoneal endometriosis. Fertil Steril 1989;51:63–67.
2. Vasquez G, Comillie F, Brosens IA. Peritoneal endometriosis: scanning electron microscopy and histology of minimal pelvic endometriotic lesions. Fertil Steril 1984;42:696–703.
3. Cornillie FJ, Brosens IA, Vasquez G, Riphagen I. Histologic and ultrastructural changes in human endometriotic implants treated with the antiprogesterone steroid ethylnorgestrienone (gestrinone) during 2 months. Int J Gynecol Pathol 1986;5:95.
4. Nakamura M, Katzabuchi H, Tohya T, Fukumatsu Y, Matsuura K, Okamura H. Scanning electron microscopic and immunohistochemical studies of pelvic endometriosis. Hum Reprod (Oxf) 1993;8:2218–2226.
5. Murphy AA, Green WR, Bobbie D, de la Cruz ZC, Rock JA. Unsuspected endometriosis documented by scanning electron microscopy in visually normal peritoneum. Fertil Steril 1987;46:522–524.
6. Stripling MC, Martin DC, Chatman DL, Van der Zwaag R, Poston WM. Subtle appearances of pelvic endometriosis. Fertil Steril 1988;49:427–431.
7. Sampson JA. Perforating haemorrhagic (chocolate) cysts of the ovary. Arch Surg 1921;3:245–323.
8. Sampson JA. Peritoneal endometriosis due to the menstrual dissemination of endometrial tissue into the peritoneal cavity. Am J Obstet Gynecol 1927;14:422–469.
9. Brosens I, Puttemans P, Deprest J, Rombauts L. The endometriosis cycle and its derailments. Hum Reprod (Oxf) 1994;9:770–771.
10. Goldstein DP, deCholnoky C, Emans SJ, et al. Laparoscopy in the diagnosis and management of pelvic pain in adolescents. J Reprod Med 24:251–256.
11. Redwine DB. Age-related evolution in color appearance of endometriosis. Fertil Steril 1987;48:1062–1063.
12. American Fertility Society. Revised classification of endometriosis. Fertil Steril 1985;43:351–352.
13. D'Hooghe TM, Bambra CS, Comillie FJ, Isahakia M, Koninckx PR. Prevalence and laparoscopic appearance of spontaneous endometriosis in the baboon (*Papio anubis, Papio cynocephalus*). Biol Reprod 1991;45:411–416.
14. Hoshiai H, Ishikawa M, Sawatari Y, Noda K, Fukaya T. Laparoscopic evaluation of the onset and progression of endometriosis. Am J Obstet Gynecol 1993;169:714–719.

15. Wiegerinck MAHM, Van Dop PA, Brosens IA. The staging of peritoneal endometriosis by the type of active lesion in addition to the revised American Fertility Society classification. Fertil Steril 1993;60:461–464.
16. Singh KB, Patel YC, Wortsman J. Coexistence of polycystic ovary syndrome and pelvic endometriosis. Obstet Gynecol 1989;74:650–652.
17. Evers J. The second look laparoscopy for the evaluation of the results of controlled trials in endometriosis-associated infertility. Fertil Steril 1987;47:502–504.
18. Nisolle M, Casanas-Roux F, Anaf V, et al. Morphometric study of the stromal vascularization in peritoneal endometriosis. Fertil Steril 1993;59:681–684.
19. Metzger DA, Olive DL, Haney AF. Limited hormonal responsiveness of ectopic endometrium: histologic correlation with intrauterine endometrium. Hum Pathol 1988; 19:1417–1424.
20. Nezhat F, Nezhat C, Allan CJ, Metzger DA, Sears DL. A clinical and histologic classification of endometriomas: implications for a mechanism of pathogenesis. J Reprod Med 1992;37:771–776.
21. Hughesdon PE. The structure of endometrial cysts of the ovary. J Obstet Gynaecol Br Emp 1957;44:481–487.
22. Brosens IA, Puttemans PJ, Deprest J. The endoscopic localisation of endometrial implants in the ovarian chocolate cyst. Fertil Steril 1994;61:1034–1038.
23. Brosens IA. Classification of endometriosis. Endoscopic exploration and classification of the chocolate cysts. Hum Reprod (Oxf) 1994;9:2213–2214.
24. Nezhat C, Nezhat F, Nezhat C, Seidman DA. Classification of endometriosis. Improving the classification of endometriotic ovarian cysts. Hum Reprod (Oxf) 1994;9: 2212–2213.
25. Koninckx PR, Martin D. Deep endometriosis: a consequence of infiltration or retraction or possible adenomyosis externa? Fertil Steril 1992;58:924–928.
26. Brosens I. Classification of endometriosis revisited. Lancet 1993;341:603.
27. Donnez J, Nisolle M, Casanas-Roux F, Bassil S, Anaf V. Rectovaginal septum, endometriosis or adenomyosis: laparoscopic management in a series of 231 patients. Hum Reprod (Oxf) 1995;2:630–635.
28. Nieminen J. Studies on the vascular pattern of ectopic endometrium with special reference to cyclic changes. Acta Obstet Gynecol Scand 1962;41(suppl 3):1–81.
29. Nisolle M, Donnez J. Peritoneal endometriosis, ovarian endometriosis, and adenomyotic nodules of the rectovaginal septum are three different entities. Fertil Steril 1997;68: 585–596.
30. Cullen TS. The distribution of adenomyoma containing uterine mucosa. Arch Surg 1920;1:215–283.
31. Brosens IA. New principles in the management of endometriosis Acta Obstet Gynecol Scand Suppl 1994;159: 18–21.
32. Cornillie FJ, Oosterlynck D, Lauwereyns JM, et al. Deeply infiltrating pelvic endometriosis: histology and clinical significance. Fertil Steril 1990;53:978–983.
33. Donnez J, Nisolle M, Casanas-Roux F, Smoes P, Gillet N, Beguin S. Peritoneal endometriosis and "endometriotic" nodules of the rectovaginal septum are two different entities. Fertil Steril 1996;66:362–368.
34. Donnez J, Nisolle M. Peritoneal endometriosis, ovarian endometriosis, and adenomyotic nodules of the rectovaginal septum are three different entities. Fertil Steril 1997;68: 585–596.
35. Brosens JJ, Brosens IA. Ovarian, peritoneal and rectovaginal endometriosis: a unifying hypothesis. In: Vercellini P, Evers H. Endometriosis: Basic Research and Clinical Practice. Camforth: Parthenon Press (in press).
36. Fox HS, Bond BL, Parslow TG. Estrogen regulates the INF-γ promoter. J Immunol 1991;146:4362–4367.
37. Brosens J, deSouza N, Barker F. Uterine junction zone function and disease. Lancet 1995;346:558–560.
38. Brosens J, Brosens I. Adenomyosis. In: Cameron I, Fraser I, Smith S, eds. Clinical Disorders of the Menstrual Cycle and Endometrium. Oxford: Oxford University Press, 1998: 297–312.
39. Nisolle M. Peritoneal, ovarian and rectovaginal endometriosis are three distinct entities. (Thèse d'Agrégation de l'Enseignement Supérieur.) Louvain, Belgium: Université Catholique de Louvain, 1996.
40. Brosens I. Endometriosis—a disease because it is characterized by bleeding. Am J Obstet Gynecol 1997;176: 264–267.
41. Kokorine I, Marbaix E, Henriet P, et al. Focal cellular origin and regulation of interstitial collagenase (matrix matalloproteinase-1) are related to menstrual breakdown in the human endometrium. J Cell Sci 1996;109: 2151–2160.
42. Kokorine I, Nisolle M, Donnez J, et al. Expression of interstitial collagenase (matrix metalloproteinase-1) is related to the activity of human endometriotic lesions. Fertil Steril 1997;68:246–251.
43. Hampton AL, Salamonsen LA. Expression of messenger ribonucleic acid encoding matrix metalloproteinases and their tissue inhibitors is related to menstruation. J Endocrinol 1994;141:R1–R3.
44. Marbaix E, Kokorine I, Henriet P, et al. The expression of interstitial collagenase in human endometrium is controlled by progesterone and by oestradiol and is related to menstruation. Biochem J 1995;305:1027–1030.
45. Singer CF, Marbaix E, Kokorine I, et al. Paracrine stimulation of interstitial collagenase (MMP-1) in the human endometrium by interleukin 1 alpha and its dual block by ovarian steroids. Proc Natl Acad Sci USA 1997;94: 10341–10345.
46. Halme J, White C, Kauma S, Estes J, Haskill S. Peritoneal macrophages from patients with endometriosis release growth factor activity in vitro. J Clin Endocrinol Metab 66:1044–1049.
47. Kauma S, Clark MR, White C, Halme J. Production of fibronectin by peritoneal macrophages, concentrations of fibronectin in peritoneal fluid from patients with and without endometriosis. Obstet Gynecol 1988;72:13–18.
48. Halme J. Release of tumor necrosis factor by human peritoneal macrophages in vivo and in vitro. Am J Obstet Gynecol 161:1718–1725.
49. Simms JS, Chegini N, Williams RS, Rossi AM, Dunn WA Jr. Identification of epidermal growth factor, transforming growth factor, and epidermal growth-factor receptor in

surgically induced endometriosis in rats. Obstet Gynecol 1991;78:850–857.
50. Arumugam K, Yip YC. De novo formation of adhesions in endometriosis: the role of iron and free radical reactions. Fertil Steril 1995;64:62–64.
51. Tabibzadeh SS, Geber MA, Satyaswaroop PG. Induction of HLA-DR antigen expression in human endometrial epithelial cells in vitro by recombinant gamma-interferon. Am J Pathol 1986;125:656–663.
52. Tabibzadeh S, Sun XZ, Kong OF, et al. Induction of a polarized micro-environment by human T cells and interferon-gamma in three-dimensional spheroids cultures of human endometrial epithelial cells. Hum Reprod (Oxf) 1993;8:182–193.
53. O'Rahilly R. Prenatal human development. In: Wynn RM, ed. Biology of the Uterus. New York: Plenum Press, 1977.
54. Mahmood TA, Templeton A. Prevalence and genesis of endometriosis. Hum Reprod (Oxf) 1991;6:544–549.
55. Fedele L, Bianchi S, Bocciolone L, et al. Pain symptoms associated with endometriosis. Obstet Gynecol 1992;79: 767–769.
56. Koninckx PR, Meuleman C, Demeyere S, Lesaffre E, Cornillie FJ. Suggestive evidence that pelvic endometriosis is a progressive disease whereas deeply infiltrating endometriosis is associated with pelvic pain. Fertil Steril 1991;55:759–765.
57. Oosterlynck DJ, Cornillie FJ, Waer M, et al. Immunohistological characteristics of leucocyte subpopulations in endometriotic lesions. Arch Gynecol Obstet 1993;253:197–206.
58. Telimaa S, Puolakka J, Rönnberg L, Kauppila A. Placebo-controlled comparison of danazol and high-dose medroxyprogesterone acetate in the treatment of endometriosis. Gynecol Endocrinol 1987;1:13–23.
59. Moen MH. Endometriosis in women at interval sterilization. Acta Obstet Gynecol Scand 1987;66:451–454.
60. Haney AF. Endometriosis-asociated infertility. Bailliere's Clin Obstet Gynecol 1993;7:791–810.
61. Haney AF. Endometriosis-associated infertility. Reprod Med Rev 1997;6:145–161.
62. Harlow CR, Cahill DJ, Maile LA, et al. Reduced preovulatory granulosa cell steroidogenesis in women with endometriosis. J Clin Endocrinol Metab 1996;81:426–429.
63. Cahill DJ, Wardle PG, Maile LA, Harlow CR, Hull MGR. Ovarian dysfunction in endometriosis-associated and unexplained infertility. J Assoc Reprod Gen 1997;14: 554–557.
64. Simon C, Gutierrez A, Vidal A, et al. Outcome of patients with endometriosis in assisted reproduction: results from in-vitro fertilization and oocyte donation. Hum Reprod (Oxf) 1994;9:725–729.
65. Pellicer A, Oliveira N, Ruiz A, et al. Exploring the mechanism(s) of endometriosis-related infertility: an analysis of embryo development and implantation in assisted reproduction. Hum Reprod (Oxf) 1995;10:91.
66. Koninckx PR, Goddeeris PG, Lauwereyns JM, De Hertogh RC, Brosens IA. Accuracy of endometrial biopsy dating in relation to the midcycle luteinizing hormone peak. Fertil Steril 1977;28:443–445.
67. Brosens IA, Koninckx PR, Corveleyn PA. A study of plasma progesterone, oestradiol-17β, prlacti and LH levels, and of the luteal phase appearance of the ovaries in patients with endometriosis and infertility. Br. J Obstet Gynaecol 1978;85:246–250.
68. Portuondo JA, Peña J, Otaloa C, et al. Absence of ovulation stigma in the conception cycle. Int J Fertil 1983;28:51.
69. Brosens IA. Diagnostic et traitement de la stérilité des femmes avec syndrome du follicule lutéinisé non rompu. In: Buvat J, Bringer J, eds. Progrès en Gynécologie. Induction et Stimulation de l'Ovulation. Paris: Doin, 1986: 209–217.
70. Mio Y, Toda T, Harada T, Terakawa N. Luteinized unruptured follicle in the early stages of endometriosis as a cause of unexplained infertility. Am J Obstet Gynecol 1992;167: 271–273.
71. Hamilton CJCM, Evers JLH, Hoogland HJ. Ovulatory disorders and inflammatory adnexal damage: a neglected cause of the failure of fertility microsurgery. Br J Obstet Gynaecol 1986;93:282.
72. Hulka JF. Adnexal adhesions: a prognostic staging and classification system based on a five-year survey of fertility surgery results at Chapel Hill, North Carolina. Am J Obstet Gynecol 1982;144:141.
73. Toth A. Asymptomatic oophoritis discovered during infertility workup. In: Scientific program and abstracts. Thirty-first Annual Meeting of the Society for Gynecologic Investigation, March 21–24, San Francisco, CA, USA, 1984:186.
74. Gordts S, Campo R, Rombauts L, Brosens I. Transvaginal hydrolaparoscopy as an outpatient procedure for infertility investigation. Hum Reprod (Oxf) 1998;13:99–103.
75. Vemon MW, Beard SJ, Graves K, et al. Classification of endometriotic implants by morphologic appearance and capacity to synthesize prostaglandin F. Fertil Steril 1986;46: 801–806.
76. Croxatto HB, Ortiz ME, Guiloff E, et al. Effect of 15(S)-15-methylprostaglandin F_{2a} on human oviductal motility and ovum transport. Fertil Steril 1978;30:408.
77. Gordts S, Campo R, Rombauts L, Brosens I. Endoscopic visualization of the process of fimbrial ovum retrieval in the human. Hum Reprod (Oxf) 1998;13:1425–1428.
78. Croxatto HB, Ortiz ME. Oocyte pickup and oviductal transport. In: Capitano GL, Asch RH, De Cecco L, Croce S, eds. GIFT from Basics to Clinics. New York: Raven Press, 1989:137–147.
79. Karbowski B, Vasquez G, Boeckx W, Brosens I, Schneider H. An experimental study of tubo-ovarian function following restoration of patency in hydrosalpinges. Eur J Obstet Reprod Biol 1988;28:305–315.
80. Nezhat F, Winer WK, Nezhat C. Fimbrioscopy and salpingoscopy in patients with minimal to moderate pelvic endometriosis. Obstet Gynecol 1990;75:15–17.
81. Heylen SM, Brosens IA, Puttemans P. Clinical value and cumulative pregnancy rates following salpingoscopy during laparoscopy in infertility. Hum Reprod (Oxf) 1995; 10:2913–2916.
82. Vasquez G, Boeckx W, Brosens I. No correlation between peritubal and mucosal adhesions in hydrosalpinges. Fertil Steril 1995;64:1032–1033.
83. Vasquez G, Boeckx W, Brosens I. Prospective study of tubal lesions and fertility in hydrosalpinges. Hum Reprod (Oxf) 1995;10:1075–1078.

84. Surrey ES, Surrey MW. Correlation between salpingoscopic and laparoscopic staging in the assessment of the distal fallopian tube. Fertil Steril 1996;65:267–271.
85. Marana R, Rizzi M, Muzii L, Catalano GF, Caruana P, Mancuso S. Correlation between the American Fertility Society classifications of adnexal adhesions and distal tubal occlusion, salpingoscopy and reproductive outcome in tubal surgery. Fertil Steril 1995;64:924–949.
86. Brosens IA, Verleyen A, Cornillie F. The morphologic effect of short-term medical therapy of endometriosis. Am J Obstet Gynecol 1987;157:1215–1221.
87. Hornstein MD, Yuzpe AA, Burry KA, Heinrichs LR, Buttram VL, Orwoll ES. Prospective randomized double-blind trial of 3 versus 6 months of nafarelin therapy for endometriosis associated pelvic pain. Fertil Steril 1995;63: 955–962.
88. Kurjak A, Kupesic S. Scoring system for prediction of ovarian endometriosis based on transvaginal color and pulsed Doppler sonography. Fertil Steril 1994;62:81–88.
89. Vercellini P, Vendola N, Bocciolone L, Rognoni M, Carinelli S, Candiani G. Reliability of the visual diagnosis of ovarian endometriosis. Fertil Steril 1990;53:1198–1200.
90. Hornstein MD, Gleason RE, Orav J, et al. The reproducibility of the revised American Fertility Society classification of endometriosis. Fertil Steril 1993;59:1015–1021.
91. Brosens IA, Van Ballaer P, Puttemans P, Deprest J. Reconstruction of the ovary containing large endometriomas by an extraovarian endosurgical technique. Fertil Steril 1996;66:517–521
92. Donnez J, Nisolle M, Clerckx F, et al. The ovarian endometrial cyst: the combined (hormonal and surgical) therapy. In: Brosens I, Jacobs HS, Runnebaum B, eds. LNRH-Analogues in Gynaecology. Carnforth: Parthenon, 1990: 165–175.
93. Donnez J, Nisolle M, Gillet N, Smets M, Bassil S, Casanas-Roux F. Large ovarian endometriomas. Hum Reprod (Oxf) 1996;11:641–646.
94. Sutton CJG, MacDonald R. Laser laparoscopic adhesiolysis. J Gynaecol Surg 1990;6:155–160.
95. Mais V, Aiossa S, Marongiu D, Peiretti RF, Guerriero S, Melis GB. Reduction of adhesion formation after laparoscopic endometriosis surgery a randomized trial with an oxidized regenerated cellulose absorbable barrier. Obstet Gynecol 1995;86:512–515.
96. Maruyama M, Yano T, Morita Y, et al. Effect of ovarian cystectomy on outcome of IVF-ET treatment in endometriosis patients. In: Proceedings of Vth World Congress on Endometriosis, 21–24 October, Yokohama, Japan, Abstracts 1996:118.
97. Fayez JA, Vogel MF. Comparison of different treatment methods of endometriomas by laparoscopy. Obstet Gynecol 1991;78:660–665.
98. Adamson GD, Subak LL, Pasta DU, Hurd SJ, von Fraque O, Rodriguez BD. Comparison of CO_2 laser laparoscopy with laparotomy for treatment of endometriomata. Fertil Steril 1992;57:965–973.
99. Gordts S, Boeckx W, Brosens I. Microsurgery of endometriosis in infertile patients. Fertil Steril 42:520–525.
100. Brosens I, Boeckx W, Page G. Microsurgery of ovarian endometriosis. Hum Reprod (Oxf) 1986;3:365–366.
101. Donnez J, Nisolle M, Gillerot S, Smets M, Bassil S, Casanas-Roux F. Rectovaginal septum adenomyotic nodules: a series of 500 cases. Br J Obstet Gynaecol 1997;104: 1014–1018.
102. Sutton CJG, Ewen SP, Whitelaw N, Haines P. Prospective, randomized double-blind, controlled trial of laser laparoscopy in the treatment of pelvic pain associated with minimal, mild and moderate endometriosis. Fertil Steril 1994;62(4):696–700.
103. Marcoux S, Maheux R, Bérubé S. Canadian Collaborative Group on Endometriosis. Laparoscopic surgery in infertile women with minimal or mild endometriosis. N Engl J Med 1997;337:217–222.
104. Martin DC, Berry JD. Histology of chocolate cysts. J Gynecol Surg 1990;6:43–46.

25

Myomectomy and Adhesion Formation

Susie Lau and Togas Tulandi

CONTENTS

Leiomyoma is the most common benign tumor occurring in the uterus and female pelvis. It is estimated that 25% of women over the age of 35 years have leiomyoma.[1] Symptomatic leiomyoma embellishes the spectrum of pelvic pain, pressure, and bleeding, as well as unexplained infertility or recurrent pregnancy losses. As women continue to delay their childbearing until the third and fourth decades of life, symptomatic leiomyoma will be encountered more frequently. Myomectomy is advocated for the treatment of symptomatic leiomyoma in women wishing to preserve their reproductive potential.

Incidence of Postmyomectomy Adhesions

Myomectomy can be accomplished via laparoscopy or laparotomy or via a combination of the two techniques known as laparoscopically assisted myomectomy.[2,3] Unfortunately, all these techniques cause adhesion formation. The best method to evaluate adhesion formation and reformation is by a second-look laparoscopy. It is inappropriate and biased to evaluate adhesion formation during a cesarian section. It is obvious that those who did conceive and subsequently required a cesarian section have a lesser degree of adnexal adhesions than those who did not.

Using a second-look laparoscopy as a tool, Tulandi et al.[4] found adnexal adhesions in 93.7% of women after an abdominal myomectomy with a posterior uterine incision and in 55.5% of women after myomectomy with anterior or fundal uterine incisions (Fig. 25.1). Ugur et al.[5] found that, following an abdominal myomectomy, 83.3% of patients had adhesions between the uterus and omentum or intestines. In their study, adnexal adhesions occurred with a frequency of 64.6% after myomectomy. Adhesion formation after laparoscopic myomectomy appears to be less than after myomectomy by laparotomy.[7,11–16] The incidence of adhesions is approximately 48% after laparoscopic myomectomy (Table 25.1) and 70% after myomectomy by laparotomy (Table 25.2). Adhesion after laparotomy is often found between the intestines and the site of previous abdominal incision (Fig. 25.2).

Factors Involved in Postmyomectomy Adhesion Formation

Nothing replaces good surgical technique. However, besides operative technique, other factors influence the occurrence of adhesion after myomectomy. Suturing of the

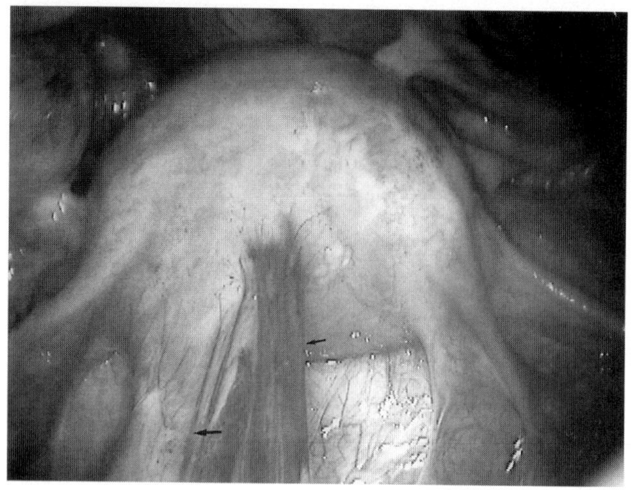

FIG. 25.1. Adhesions from the anterior uterine wall 1 year after a laparoscopic myomectomy (filmy adhesions, *small arrow;* dense adhesions, *large arrow*). *Please see insert for color reproduction of this figure.*

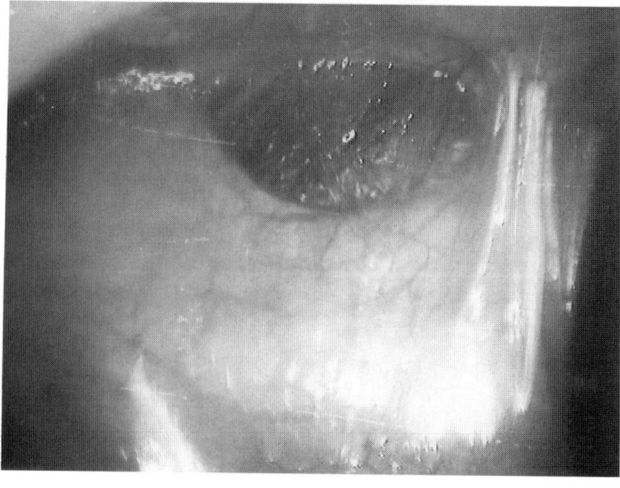

FIG. 25.2. Intestinal adhesions to the previous abdominal incision after myomectomy by laparotomy. *Please see insert for color reproduction of this figure.*

uterine incision produces good approximation of the uterine defect and promotes better healing, but the presence of suture material may produce more adhesion formation.[6] It seems that the presence of adhesions at the initial myomectomy is correlated with an increased adhesion formation at second-look laparoscopy.[7] Posterior uterine incision is also associated with more and a higher degree of adnexal adhesions than that with fundal or anterior uterine incisions.[4] In addition, a transverse uterine incision and treatment with LHRH-a (luteinizing hormone releasing hormone agonist) may promote more adhesions.[12]

Mechanism of Adhesion Formation After Myomectomy

Perhaps no other gynecologic surgery causes more adhesion formation than a myomectomy. This occurs for several reasons: the uterine defect is relatively large and the incision could be multiple, and hemostasis at the myomectomy incision is rarely absolute and this predisposes to adhesion formation. Blood itself does not cause adhesion, but a combination between blood and raw peritoneal surfaces predisposes adhesion formation. Be-

TABLE 25.1. Adhesion formation following laparoscopic myomectomy.

Reference	Total number of patients	Myoma size (cm)	Incidence of adhesions at second-look laparoscopy
Nezhat et al. (1991)[6]	154	3–15	30/56 sites (54%)
Hasson et al. (1992)[7]	56	3–16	16/24 patients (67%)
Dubuisson et al. (1991)[8]	43	1–11	1/6 patients (17%)
Daniell and Gurley (1991)[9]	17	3–7	1/1 patient (100%)
Dubuisson et al. (1994)[10]	102	NA	2/17 patients (11.8%)
Bulletti et al. (1996)[11]	16	4.2–10.9	4/14 patients (29%)
Stringer et al. (1997)[12]	50	4–11	7/12 patients (58%)

TABLE 25.2. Adhesion formation following abdominal myomectomy.

Reference	Total number of patients	Myoma or uterine size	Incidence of adhesions at a second-look procedure or at subsequent operation
Berkeley et al. (1983)[13]	50	283 g (average)	4/4 patients at laparoscopy (100%)
Starks (1988)[14]	32	4–18 cm	10/10 patients at cesarean and 10/10 patients at laparoscopy (100%)
Fayez and Dempsey (1993)[15]	148	10–16 weeks or more sized uterus	3/32 patients at laparoscopy (9%)
Gehlbach et al. (1993)[16]	37	8.2 ± 0.9 cm (pregnant) and 7.8 ± 0.6 cm (nonpregnant)	13/19 patients at laparoscopy (68%)
Tulandi et al. (1993)[4]	25	18.2 ± 0.6 weeks sized uterus 388.1 ± 71.1 g, myoma weight	20/25 patients at laparoscopy (80%)
Bulletti et al. (1996)[11]	16	5.1–10.6 cm	9/14 patients at laparoscopy (64%)

cisions. Overall, the adhesion scores were significantly lower in the covered incisions. Other investigators have similarly found favorable outcomes with the use of Gore-Tex surgical membrane.[37,39,40]

A case of fistula to the bladder after implanting a PTFE membrane was recently reported.[41] Whether it was solely caused by the membrane itself is unknown. PTFE is highly effective, but it is not popular among gynecologists because of the fear of leaving a foreign body in the abdominal cavity. The widely publicized malpractice suits by some women with breast implants have heightened this concern.

Seprafilm Bioresorbable Membrane

Seprafilm is a relatively new adhesion prevention barrier composed of chemically derivatized sodium hyaluronate and carboxymethylcellulose. Resorption from the peritoneal cavity occurs within 7 days and excretion from the body occurs within 28 days. In a multicenter trial, Diamond et al.[42] randomized 127 women undergoing myomectomy by laparotomy to receive Seprafilm or nothing to cover the sutured uterine incisions. Two sheets of Seprafilm were used to cover the incisions by wrapping the uterus anteriorly and posteriorly leaving an excess margin of 2.5 cm or more. The Seprafilm was then molded to the contours of the uterus. A second-look laparoscopy was performed 1 to 10 weeks after the initial surgery. In patients with at least one anterior incision, 39% of the women treated with Seprafilm were free of adhesions, compared to 6% in the control group. However when the incision was on the posterior uterine wall, only 13% of patients were free from adhesions in the Seprafilm group versus 8% in the control group. At least one adnexa was totally free of adhesions to the posterior uterus in 48% of the Seprafilm group, compared to 31% of the control group. Currently, this material cannot be utilized by laparoscopy.

Conclusions

With the trend of women delaying childbearing to a later age, the frequency of women requiring myomectomy for symptomatic leiomyoma will increase. In general, myomectomy is associated with severe adhesion formation. Adhesions to the intestines may cause abdominal pain and bowel obstruction, while adnexal adhesions may hamper future fertility. For these reasons, attempts to decrease postmyomectomy adhesion formation are very important. It appears that myomectomy by laparoscopy is associated with less adhesion formation than by laparotomy. However, because uterine rupture can occur after laparoscopic myomectomy,[43-45] the uterine defect should be sutured in layers as is usually done by laparotomy. Accordingly, only surgeons who have expertise in laparoscopic suturing should perform myomectomy by laparoscopy.

Fundamental practices for preventing postmyomectomy adhesions involve strict adherence to the principles of gentle tissue handling, meticulous hemostasis, and copious irrigation. It is important not to use reactive materials such as catgut sutures. The location of the uterine incision is also important. Minimizing the number of incisions and avoiding posterior uterine incisions when possible will reduce the incidence of adnexal adhesions.

The choice of adhesion preventive agents rests with the adhesion barrier. These materials have been shown to decrease adhesion formation, specifically in the myomectomy population. However, it is not that simple. Oxidized regenerated cellulose may reduce adhesion formation, but its efficacy is decreased in the presence of blood, and hemostasis at myomectomy incision is rarely absolute. Expanded polytetrafluoroethylene is highly effective, but it is a permanent implant that is concerning to most gynecologists, and Seprafilm cannot be used by laparoscopy. Today there is no adhesion-preventing substance that is unequivocally effective to decrease postmyomectomy adhesion. Developing a vehicle to deliver a high concentration of active material (perhaps NSAID or others) to the myomectomy incision may be beneficial.

References

1. Tulandi T. The role of laparoscopy in the management of leiomyoma uteri. Journal of the Society of Obstetricians and Gynecologists of Canada 1994;16:1903–1908.
2. Nezhat C, Nezhat F, Bess O, et al. Laparoscopically assisted myomectomy: a report of a new technique in 57 cases. Int J Fertil 1994;39:39–44.
3. Tulandi T, Youseff H. Laparoscopy-assisted myomectomy of large uterine myomas. Gynecol Endosc 1997;6: 105–108.
4. Tulandi T, Murray C, Guralnick M. Adhesion formation and reproductive outcome after myomectomy and second-look laparoscopy. Obstet Gynecol 1993;82:213–215.
5. Ugur M, Turan C, Mungan T, et al. Laparoscopy for adhesion prevention following myomectomy. Int J Gynaecol Obstet 1996;53:145–149.
6. Nezhat C, Nezhat F, Silfen SL, et al. Laparoscopic myomectomy. Int J Fertil 1991;36:275–280.
7. Hasson HM, Rotman C, Rana N, et al. Laparoscopic myomectomy. Obstet Gynecol 1992;80:884–888.
8. Dubuisson JB, Lecuru F, Foulot H, et al. Myomectomy by laparoscopy: a preliminary report of 43 cases. Fertil Steril 1991;56:827–830.
9. Daniell JF, Gurley LD. Laparoscopic treatment of clinically significant symptomatic fibroids. J Gynecol Surg 1991;7: 37–40.
10. Dubuisson JB, Chapron C. Laparoscopic myomectomy. Operative procedure and results. Ann N Y Acad Sci 1994; 734:450–454.

11. Bulletti C, Polli V, Negrini V, et al. Adhesion formation after laparoscopic myomectomy. J Am Assoc Gynecol Laparosc 1996;3:533–536.
12. Stringer NH, McMillen MA, Jones RL, et al. Uterine closure with the endo stitch 10 mm laparoscopic suturing device—a review of 50 laparoscopic myomectomies. Int J Fertil Womens Med 1997;42:288–296.
13. Berkeley AS, De Cherney AH, Polan ML. Abdominal myomectomy and subsequent fertility. Surg Gynecol Obstet 1983;156:319–322.
14. Starks GC. CO_2 laser myomectomy in an infertile population. J Reprod Med 1988;33:184–186.
15. Fayez JA, Dempsey RA. Short hospital stay for gynecologic reconstructive surgery via laparotomy. Obstet Gynecol 1993;81:598–600.
16. Gehlbach DL, Sousa RC, Carpenter SE, et al. Abdominal myomectomy in the treatment of infertility. Int J Gynaecol Obstet 1993;40:45–50.
17. DiZerega GS. Contemporary adhesion prevention. Fertil Steril 1994;62:219–235.
18. Murray C, Tulandi T. Prevention of postmyomectomy adhesions. Infertil Reprod Med Clin North Am 1996;7: 169–177.
19. Tulandi T. How can we avoid adhesions after laparoscopic surgery? Curr Opin Obstet Gynecol 1997;9:239–243.
20. Luijendijk RW, de Lange DC, Wauters CC, et al. Foreign material in postoperative adhesions. Ann Surg 1996;223: 242–248.
21. Grow DR, Coddington CC, Hsiu JG, et al. Role of hypoestrogens or sex steroid antagonism in adhesion formation after myometrial surgery in primates. Fertil Steril 1996; 66:140–147.
22. Montanino-Oliva M, Metzger DA, Luciano AA. Use of medroxyprogesterone acetate in the prevention of postoperative adhesions. Fertil Steril 1996;65:650–654.
23. Holtz G. Failure of a non-steroidal anti-inflammatory agent (ibuprofen) to inhibit peritoneal adhesion reformation after lysis. Fertil Steril 1982;37:582–583.
24. Jansen RPS. Early laparoscopy after pelvic operations to prevent adhesions safety and efficacy. Fertil Steril 1988; 49:26–40.
25. Magyar DM, Hayes MF, Spirtos JN, et al. Is intraperitoneal dextran 70 safe for routine gynecologic use? Am J Obstet Gynecol 1985;152:198–204.
26. Adoni A, Addatto-Levy R, Mogle P, et al. Postoperative pleural effusion caused by dextran. Int J Gynecol Obstet 1980;18:243–247.
27. Borton M, Seibert CP, Taymor ML. Recurrent anaphylactic reaction of intraperitoneal dextran 70 used for prevention of postsurgical adhesions. Obstet Gynecol 1983;61: 755–757.
28. Ahmed N, Falcone T, Tulandi T, et al. Anaphylactic reaction because of intrauterine 32% dextran-70 instillation. Fertil Steril 1991;55:1014–1016.
29. Diamond MP, DeCherney AH, Linsky CB, et al. Assessment of carboxymethylcellulose and 32% dextran 70 for prevention of adhesions in a rabbit uterine horn model. Int J Fertil 1988;33:278–282.
30. Oelsner G, Graebe RA, Pan SB, et al. Chondroitin sulphate. A new intraperitoneal treatment for postoperative adhesion prevention in the rabbit. J Reprod Med 1987; 32:812–814.
31. Burns JW, Skinner K, Colt MJ, et al. A hyaluronate-based gel for the prevention of postsurgical adhesions: evaluation of two animal species. Fertil Steril 1996;66:814–821.
32. Pagidas K, Tulandi T. Effects of Ringer's lactate, Interceed (TC7) and GoreTex surgical membrane on postsurgical adhesion formation. Fertil Steril 1992;57:199–201.
33. Dunn DL, Barke RA, Ahrenholz DH, et al. The adjuvant effect of peritoneal fluid in experimental peritonitis. Ann Surg 1984;199:37–42.
34. Shear L, Swartz C, Shinaberger JA, et al. Kinetics of peritoneal fluid absorption in adult man. N Engl J Med 1965; 272:123–127.
35. diZerega GS. Use of adhesion prevention barriers in ovarian surgery, tuboplasty, ectopic pregnancy, endometriosis, adhesiolysis, and myomectomy. Curr Opin Obstet Gynecol 1996;8:230–237.
36. Mais V, Ajossa S, Piras B, et al. Prevention of de novo adhesions formation after laparoscopic myomectomy: a randomized trial to evaluate the effectiveness of an oxidized regenerated cellulose absorbable barrier. Hum Reprod (Oxf) 1995;19:3133–3135.
37. Surgical Membrane Study Group. Prophylaxis of pelvic sidewall adhesions with Gore-Tex surgical membrane: a multicenter clinical investigation. Fertil Steril 1992;57: 921–923.
38. Myomectomy Adhesion Study Group. An expanded polytetrafluoroethylene barrier (Gore-Tex Surgical Membrane) reduces post-myomectomy adhesion formation. Fertil Steril 1995;63:491–493.
39. March CM, Boyers S, Franklin R, et al. Prevention of adhesion formation/reformation with the Gore-Tex Surgical Membrane. Prog Clin Biol Res 1993;381:253–259.
40. Haney AF. Removal of surgical barriers of expanded polytetrafluoroethylene at second-look laparoscopy was not associated with adhesion formation. Fertil Steril 1997;68: 721–723.
41. Monteforte CA, Queirazza R, Franceschetti P, et al. Fistula formation after implanting an ePTFE membrane. A case report. J Reprod Med 1997;42:184–187.
42. Diamond MP. Reduction of adhesions after uterine myomectomy by Seprafilm membrane (HAL-F): a blinded, prospective, randomized, multicenter clinical study. Seprafilm Adhesion Study Group. Fertil Steril 1996;66: 904–910.
43. Harris WJ. Uterine dehiscence following laparoscopic myomectomy. Obstet Gynecol 1992;80:545–546.
44. Dubuisson JB, Chavet X, Chapron C, et al. Uterine rupture during pregnancy after laparoscopic myomectomy. Hum Reprod (Oxf) 1995;10:1475–1477.
45. Pelosi MA III, Pelosi MA. Spontaneous uterine rupture at thirty-three weeks subsequent to previous superficial laparoscopic myomectomy. Am J Obstet Gynecol 1997;177: 1547–1549.

Section 5
Outcome Measures and Adhesion Formation

26

The Magnitude of Adhesion-Related Problems

Harold Ellis

CONTENTS

Since the earliest days of abdominal surgery, surgeons have encountered examples of postoperative intestinal obstruction caused by adhesions. Nowadays, adhesions are the commonest cause of intestinal obstruction in the western world. McEntee and colleagues[1] reviewed 228 patients in four neighboring district general hospitals in the United Kingdom who required a total of 236 admissions over a 12-month prospective period. Adhesions accounted for 75 admissions (32%), malignant disease for 61 (26%), strangulated hernias for 59 (25%), and volvulus for 10 (4%). Other causes were all in single figures. Adhesive obstruction is essentially confined to the small intestine, and numerous large series have been reported showing that this cause accounts for some 60% or more of all small-bowel obstructions.[2,3]

Intraabdominal adhesions may occasionally be congenital or inflammatory in origin, but most result from previous surgery. Systematic studies at either postmortem examination or laparotomy are surprisingly few. Weibel and Majno[4] reviewed 298 subjects at autopsy who had had previous laparotomies, and 67% of these showed adhesions; after multiple operations, the incidence rose to 93%. In our prospective analysis[5] of 210 patients undergoing laparotomy who had previously had one or more abdominal operations, 195 (93%) were found to have adhesions attributed to previous surgery. In addition, 2 had adhesions from their current disease alone, and 1 had adhesions that were considered to be congenital. Seven of the 12 patients with no adhesions had undergone previous appendicectomy and 3 had undergone gynecologic procedures through a Pfannenstiel incision. In contrast, of 115 patients undergoing first-time laparotomy, only 12 (10.4%) were found to have adhesions. Of these, 11 were considered to be inflammatory and 1 to be congenital.

Until recently, because it seemed that nothing could really be done to prevent the formation of adhesions following surgery, a sense of fatalism seems to have affected the surgical community. It must be something like the attitude of surgeons to wound infection in the days before Lister. Because of this pessimistic attitude, surprisingly little research, pro rata, has been carried out on this subject at either the clinical or experimental level. If you do not believe this statement, a glance through any recent volume of the major surgical journals shows how few papers appear on this topic. It is only now, when we realize that there are precautions we can take at the time of surgery to prevent the development of unwanted adhesions, and also with the development of pharmacologic methods to prevent the formation of adhesions and of their recurrence following division, that at last surgeons are becoming interested in identifying the magnitude of adhesion-related problems.

There are four problems produced by intraabdominal adhesions:

First, and by far the most important, as a cause and indeed the commonest cause of small-bowel obstruction
Second, as a difficulty encountered on reoperating on a patient's abdomen after previous surgery
Third, pelvic adhesions as a problem in female fertility
Fourth, as a cause, again in women, of pelvic pain

Taking the first and second problems alone, which are the problems to be addressed in this chapter, many questions are present that are now the subject of active research. These include the following:

1. What is the burden of cases of intestinal obstruction caused by adhesions?
2. Can we define which abdominal operations are at special risk of obstruction?
3. Can we distinguish between simple and strangulated obstruction? This, of course, is of immense importance in deciding on whether to treat a patient conservatively or operatively or when to abandon conservative treatment.
4. What is the time scale between the initial operation and the risk of adhesion obstruction?
5. What is the risk of recurrent obstruction when the patient has been treated either conservatively or by operation for adhesive obstruction?
6. Finally, in these days of commercialism, can we work out the workload and costs to a health service of these problems? This last question may be of considerable importance when we have to justify economically the value of what might be quite an expensive prophylactic measure or measures.

Burden of Cases in the Community

We know from our own studies that 93% of patients who had undergone previous laparotomy were found to have adhesions at second operation.[5] Abdominal surgery is now extremely common, so there are vast numbers of people in our communities, usually and fortunately quite symptom free, who we know must have intraabdominal adhesions. Only recently has there been an attempt to quantify this problem. There is a fascinating study, as yet unpublished, by Dr. Robert Beart and his colleagues in Los Angeles, who reviewed the autopsy records of 2645 patients of which only 4% were under the age of 21. Evidence of surgery included the presence of an abdominal surgical scar on external examination, a record of past surgery within the clinical history, or documentation of a surgically removed organ in the autopsy report. No less than 32% of the individuals had evidence of previous abdominal surgery, and the rate in the over-60 age group, comprising 32% of the subjects, was 43.8%. The incidence of abdominal surgery was higher in women than in men. One can imagine that similar high figures would be obtained in studies in other Western countries so that a staggeringly large percentage of our symptomless adult population, perhaps 30% to 40%, are walking around with abdominal adhesions. We know that a proportion of these, at some time, will develop intestinal obstruction.

Which Operations Are at Especial Risk of Obstruction?

It would be useful and indeed important to document the percentage risk of obstruction of the various major operations. Our own studies[5,6] have confirmed the general impression that operations in the lower abdominal compartment are at especial risk of producing small-bowel obstruction. The type of surgery originally performed in 80 consecutive cases is shown in Table 26.1. A high proportion of these involved the left side of the colon or rectum (25%). Other common procedures were appendicectomies (15%), gynecologic operations (14%), or total colectomies (9%). Sixty-one patients had operations involving the peritoneal cavity below the transverse mesocolon (76%). Eleven had surgery above the transverse mesocolon (14%), of whom 4 had generalized peritonitis at operation.

Similar findings were reported in a recent study of 144 admissions of patients with adhesive obstruction by Cox and his colleagues.[7] Previous appendicectomy accounted for 23% of the cases, colorectal resection for 20%, gynecological surgery, 12%, upper gastrointestinal surgery, 9.2%, and small-bowel resection, 8.3%. Patients who had undergone more than one previous laparotomy amounted to 23.6% of the series. Interestingly, adhesions ac-

TABLE 26.1. Type of previous surgery producing adhesive intestinal obstruction (80 consecutive cases).

Original surgery	Number
Appendicectomy	12
Rectal surgery	12
Left colon	8
Total colectomy	7
Gynecologic	11
Right colon	4
Cholecystectomy	4
Perforated duodenal ulcer	4
Unknown	8
Others	10
Total	80

From Menzies and Ellis.[5]

counted for no less than 79% of all small-bowel obstructions in this group of patients.

Total colectomy has a bad reputation for subsequent adhesive obstruction. In 1967 Lockhart-Mummery,[8] reviewing his cases of total colectomy for polyposis coli, pointed out the high incidence of this complication, and even wondered if these patients had a special diathesis for adhesion formulation.

Fazio and his colleagues at the Cleveland Clinic[9] have reported their figures from a review of 1500 patients undergoing proctocolectomy with ileal pouch anal anastomosis from 1983 to 1993. The majority of patients (812) had ulcerative colitis. Other diagnoses were familial adenomatous polyposis (62), indeterminate colitis (54), Crohn's disease (67), and a miscellaneous group (10). The mean follow-up time was 35 months (range, 1–125 months). Of this large series, 25% (254 patients) developed small-bowel obstruction (7.5% within 30 days of the initial surgery), and of these 27.6% (70 patients) underwent reoperation. Early intestinal obstruction occurred in 15% of 1193 patients who underwent this operation at the Mayo Clinic,[10] which confirms the high risk of adhesive obstruction after this procedure, and one-third of these required reoperation. Fazio pointed out that a higher incidence of small-bowel obstruction caused by adhesions must be expected with longer follow-up.

Neonates are not immune from this problem. Wilkins and Spitz[11] from Great Ormond Street Hospital, London, followed up 649 neonatal (first 28 days of life) abdominal operations for a period between 6 months and 10 years. Of these, 54 (8.3%) required surgery for adhesive obstruction, 16 in the early postoperative period and 38 later; 90% of the operations took place within 1 year of surgery. Operations at particularly high risk were surgery for malrotation (15%) and for gastroschisis (15.4%).

Can We Distinguish Between Strangulated and Nonstrangulated Obstruction?

Most patients with a diagnosis of obstruction caused by adhesions are treated initially with conservative measures of intravenous drip and nasogastric suction, first popularized in the 1930s by Owen Wangensteen.[12] Indeed, a proportion (and the exact proportion remains to be documented accurately), responds entirely to conservative treatment. Of course, the danger is that a loop of obstructed bowel is strangulated and, under this conservative treatment, is going to progress to gangrene over the next few hours, with eventual perforation. If only we could be certain of the diagnosis between simple and strangulated obstruction! However, although certain clinical features are somewhat suggestive of strangulation, any experienced surgeon knows that the distinction between the two is extremely difficult or even impossible. When series of cases of simple and strangulated obstruction were compared, a similar incidence of pain, vomiting, distension, tachycardia, pyrexia, and abdominal tenderness was found, although the finding of a mass on abdominal examination is more suggestive of strangulation.[13,14] The claim that an elevated white cell count denotes strangulation is not found to be true in practice. In one study, a white cell count greater than 15,000 was present in 27% of simple cases and in 38% of strangulated cases.[14] A detailed breakdown of the cases in two large series is shown in Table 26.2.

There are no diagnostic laboratory tests that will accurately confirm or refute the diagnosis of small-bowel ischemia. The white blood cell count, as we have already noted, may be normal or slightly elevated in uncomplicated small-bowel obstruction, but high counts ($>15.0 \times 10^9$/L) or very low counts (4.0×10^9/L) are suspicious and should alert the clinician to the possibility of bowel ischemia. The hematocrit and serum urea will be elevated in individuals suffering from dehydration. Serum electrolytes often remain normal in distal small-bowel obstruction. A proximal obstruction will create a pattern of metabolic alkalosis with hypokalemia and hypochloremia, similar to that seen in gastric outlet obstruction. A raised serum amylase is unusual in small-bowel obstruction and is more suggestive of pancreatitis. Serum phosphate, creatine kinase, and glutamate oxalotransferase (SGOT) have been suggested as possible markers of complicated small-bowel obstruction but have not been of proven help.

Can the computer help us in differentiation between strangulated and nonstrangulated bowel in small intesti-

TABLE 26.2. Clinical features of simple and strangulated obstructions.

New Orleans[a]	324 simple cases (%)	88 strangulated cases (%)
T 37.7°C+	16	23
P 100+	15	23
Abdominal or pelvic tenderness	73	82
Mass	5	10
Leucocytosis	44	50
All these signs absent	12	7
Columbus, Ohio[b]	**387 simple cases (%)**	**45 strangulated cases (%)**
T 37.2°C+	38	45
P 100+	38	52
Mass	22	32
Constant pain	18	20
WBC 15,000+	27	38

[a]From Becker (1952).[13]
[b]From Zollinger and Kinsey (1964).[14]

nal obstruction? Pain and colleagues[15] have carried out an interesting retrospective study of 120 patients with simple small-bowel obstruction that resolved on conservative treatment, 38 patients with viable strangulated bowel subjected to adhesiolysis and 39 with nonviable strangulation which required resection. For multivariate computer analysis of the presenting data of these patients, they used the following:

1. Presence of continuous pain
2. Clinical features of peritonism
3. Presence of an abdominal mass
4. Reduced or absent bowel sounds
5. Tachycardia
6. Pyrexia or hypothermia
7. Leucocytosis

The computer diagnosed accurately 85% of patients with simple, 61% with viable, and 74% with nonviable strangulation. More importantly, it allocated correctly 82% of those with viable and 97% of those with nonviable strangulation to categories in which strangulation was present or would occur. That is to say, the computer predicted that surgical intervention was mandatory in these patients. This result contrasts with the diagnostic accuracy of the surgeons, because only 66% of the viable and 46% of the nonviable strangulations were diagnosed prospectively as requiring immediate surgery, with resultant delay in their surgical treatment. These authors noted that they are employing their computer program in a prospective trial, and the result of this will be interesting.

Meagher and colleagues[16] in Adelaide have recently reviewed five large series of cases of adhesive obstruction. In these, conservative treatment was given a trial for 27% to 83% of the patients, surgery was required for 22% to 54%, the bowel resection rate ranged from 5% to 14%, and mortality following resection varied from 15% to 20%. Can we identify any particular clinical features that would suggest conservative or surgical management? An interesting observation was made by these authors. They noted that patients presenting with small-bowel obstruction whose only previous surgery was for appendicectomy or operation on the ovary or tube only rarely settled down with nonoperative management. When laparotomy is undertaken in such patients, a closed loop of intestine is typically found to be caught by a band adhesion, and it is this type of obstruction that is highly unlikely to resolve without operative intervention. To confirm this, they examined 330 admissions for small-bowel obstruction. In 40 cases, the only previous laparotomy was appendicectomy or operation on the tube or ovary. In 38 (95%) of these, division of adhesions was undertaken as compared with 154 operations (53%) in the remaining 290 cases. In the former group, band adhesions were commoner (86% compared with 45%) and bowel resection was required more frequently (22% against 10%). They concluded that a trial of conservative management may be unsafe or not worthwhile in patients with obstruction following these particular operations. In contrast, patients presenting with recurrent intestinal obstruction after several previous laparotomies for this condition are more likely to have intestinal loops so matted together that they are unlikely to become strangulated. Partial obstruction, and previous success with conservative treatment, might also indicate probable resolution with a conservative regime.

Patients who develop signs and symptoms of intestinal obstruction within days of their laparotomy behave in a somewhat different manner from those who present at a later date. Bowel ischemia is uncommon, the adhesions are likely to be filmy and fibrinous, and the obstruction will resolve in 80% to 90% of cases provided, of course, that the patient receives appropriate nasogastric suction and is parenterally nourished and hydrated.[17] An important exception to this is early obstruction following abdominoperineal excision of the rectum. Here the obstruction may well be caused by a loop of bowel herniating through the pelvic floor with strangulation.[18] In other cases, the small bowel may snare around the colostomy if the lateral space adjacent to the sigmoid colon has not been closed.

The lesson is, of course, to undertake conservative treatment in adhesive obstruction with the greatest care. The patient requires repeated examinations, as often as every half hour, and the slightest clinical evidence of deterioration, whether this be increasing distension, tenderness, or a rise in pulse rate or temperature, is an indication for immediate surgical intervention.

What Is the Time Scale Between the Initial Operation and the Risk of Adhesion Obstruction?

Very few studies have addressed the question of the lag period between initial surgery and subsequent adhesive obstruction, and as yet figures are not available for individual types of abdominal surgery. Stewart and colleagues,[19] in a collected series of 8098 patients who had undergone abdominal surgery, found that 0.63% developed postoperative adhesive obstruction within 4 weeks of their surgery.

We had the opportunity[5] of studying this problem as a result of our long-term review of wound healing in a prospective study of 2708 patients undergoing major laparotomy (appendicectomy through a muscle-split incision being excluded). An accurate record was kept of information including the initial diagnosis, the operative procedure, postoperative complications, and their timing. From January 1976 to December 1988, 2708 major

TABLE 26.3. Time to obstruction from postoperative adhesions.

Time from surgery	Number
<1 month	17 (21.25%)
1 month–1 year	14 (17.5%)
1–5 years	17 (21.25%)
5–10 years	5 (6.25%)
>10 years	17 (21.25%)
Unknown	10 (12.5%)
Total	80

From Menzies and Ellis (1990).[5]

TABLE 26.4. The incidence of recurrent intestinal obstruction following initial division of adhesions.

Reference	Total cases	Recurrences (%)	Follow-up (years)
Krook (1947)[20]	135	14	4–24
Brightwell et al. (1977)[21]	30	13	4–7
Close and Christensen (1979)[22]	107	11	0.5–12
Bizer et al. (1986)[23]	103	21	3–13

laparotomies were performed. Follow-up was for a mean period of 14.5 months (range, 0–91 months), with 94% follow-up at 1 month and 76% at 1 year. Of these patients, 26 (0.96% of all laparotomies) developed adhesive obstruction requiring surgical intervention within 1 year of our initial major abdominal surgery. Of these 26 patients, 14 developed their obstruction within 1 month of the initial operation (0.52% of all laparotomies), a figure similar to the collected series of Stewart et al.[19]

What of the time scale of later obstruction? We tabulated[5] the time between initial surgery and later operation for adhesive obstruction in 80 consecutive patients (Table 26.3). Unfortunately, 10 patients could not recall the date of their initial laparotomy. Thirty-one of these 80 patients presented within a year of surgery (39%); the distribution of the others is shown in Table 26.3. Note the high number of 17 cases (21.25%) whose initial operation took place more than 10 years before their obstruction. My own longest interval was a man who presented at the age of 38 with adhesive obstruction whose initial operation (for intussusception) took place when he was a baby of 1 year of age. It may be that the time scale in neonates differs from adults. In a study of 649 neonates undergoing laparotomy, 54 (8.3%) required subsequent surgery for adhesive obstruction, 75% of these within 6 months and 90% within 1 year of the initial operation.[11]

Risk of Recurrent Obstruction

The one statistic that we all wish to have would allow us to tell our patient, after treatment for an episode of adhesive obstruction, the risk of further episodes of obstruction. We know that the likelihood is high, but, once again, as it is a lifetime risk, an entirely accurate figure cannot be given.

In 1947, Krook[20] reported a recurrence rate of 14% in a group of 135 patients who had undergone adhesiolysis for the first time; 16% of these patients required subsequent surgery for repeated obstruction and 25% required a third laparotomy. Overall recurrence rates following simple division of adhesions in published series, followed up from 4 to 24 years, range from 11% to 21% (Table 26.4). Even when various plication methods have been used at intial adhesiolysis, or long tube intubation of the lysed intestine was employed, recurrences are still common, and range from 3% to 32% (Table 26.5). Obviously, more statistical studes are required on this, as with so many other aspects of adhesion-related problems. In the last section of this chapter, work is described that will produce accurate figures on a national scale on postoperative adhesion problems.

The Workload

There is no doubt that the formation of adhesions is a serious, common, and costly complication of surgery. However, the exact cost to the health service of a country, in terms of both workload and actual cost, has until now received little documentation.

In 1990, we reviewed[5] the workload of a single surgical academic unit in London. Over the years 1964 to 1988, 28,297 adult patients were admitted. The number of major laparotomies (excluding appendicectomy) was 4,502. A diagnosis of large- or small-bowel obstruction from any cause accounted for 514 admissions (1.8% of all admissions). Of these, 261 were caused by adhesions (0.9% of all admissions, 51% of all cases of intestinal obstruction).

TABLE 26.5. Incidence of recurrent intestinal obstruction following plication and intubation procedures.

Reference	n	Plication (%)	Long tube (%)	Follow-up (years)
Brightwell et al. (1977)[21]	28		32	4–7
Close and Cristensen (1979)[22]	65	14	8	0.5–12
Weigelt et al. (1980)[24]	140		8.6	0–5
Hollender et al. (1983)[25]	51	4		1–17
Jones and Munro (1985)[26]	123		3.3	0.25–11

A total of 148 admissions for adhesive obstruction required laparotomy and division of adhesions (3.3% of all laparotomies, 29% of all cases of obstruction), while 113 further patients were treated conservatively. Of the remaining small- and large-bowel obstructions from other causes, 211 (83%) required surgery. In 1997, Schoffel and colleagues[27] reported from Freiburg, Germany, a series of 5,000 laparotomies in their department; 64 of 171 cases operated on for intestinal obstruction were caused by adhesions (1.3% of all laparotomies and 37.4% of all cases of obstruction).

The first attempt at a national review of adhesion-related problems was carried out in 1993 by Scott-Coombes and colleagues.[28] They sent a questionnaire to one-third (randomly selected) of the approximately 1200 general surgeons of the United Kingdom (England, Scotland, and Wales). A total of 416 questionnaires were sent, with 350 responses (84%). In most cases the surgeons' replies were estimates rather than material obtained from formal audited records. It appeared from this survey that general surgeons operated upon, on average, 3 to 4 patients each year for small-bowel adhesive obstruction. Assuming a total of 1200 general surgeons, this amounts to between 3,600 and 4,800 laparotomies. The average number of patients admitted under each surgeon for suspected adhesive obstruction and treated conservatively amounted to a further 7 to 8 per year, accounting for 8,400 to 9,600 admissions annually. An additional estimated average of 3 patients per surgeon each year (3,600) were found to have adhesions that caused a significant problem during laparotomy for non-adhesion-related disease. Thus, intraabdominal adhesions were estimated to cause clinical problems in between 12,000 and 14,000 patients treated by general surgeons in the U.K. (population roughly 50 million) each year. The mean duration of hospital stay for patients operated on for adhesion obstruction was found by McEntee and colleagues[1] to be in excess of 15 days, partly related to a high postoperative morbidity.

An important nationwide study in the United States, covering the year 1988, was carried out by Ray and colleagues.[29] Using data from the National Hospital Discharge Survey, which represents a national stratified sample of all discharges from short-stay acute-care hospitals exclusive of military and Veterans Administration facilities. Approximately 9% of U.S. hospitals are included in the sample. Estimates of charges incurred per hospital day were obtained from the 1988 Medicare Provider Analysis and Review data file; this allowed an estimate of the number of hospital admissions, inpatient days of care, and health care expenditures associated with lower abdominal adhesiolysis in 1988. In that year, 281,982 hospital admissions took place in which division of abdominal adhesions was performed. These procedures accounted for 948,727 days of inpatient care; the economic burden, including hospital costs and surgeons' fees, was $1,179.9 million. This estimate did not include outpatient direct medical costs and indirect morbidity and mortality costs. An important follow-up study by the same group[30] reviewed the year 1994. Adhesiolysis was responsible for 303,836 hospital admissions during that year, primarily for procedures on the digestive and female reproductive systems. These procedures accounted for 846,415 days of inpatient care and $1.3 billion in hospital and surgeons' fees. Although the admission rate for adhesion surgery had remained almost the same as in 1988, inpatient expenditure had decreased by nearly 10% because of a 15% decrease in average length of inpatient hospital stay. It is interesting that the increased use of laparoscopy during this 6-year period did not appear to be associated with a concomitant reduction in hospital admission rate for adhesiolysis.

An estimate of workload and costs in Sweden has been carried out by Ivarsson and colleagues.[31] During a 5-month period in 1992–1993, 34 patients over the age of 15 were admitted to the Ostra Hospital in Goteburg with small-bowel obstruction caused by adhesions, accounting for 85% of all cases of small-bowel obstruction. Of these, 10 (45%) had to be operated upon, 2 of them on two occasions. Major complications occurred in 6, and 1 patient died. The population served by the hospital is approximately 250,000 people, and the total population of Sweden 16 years or older is 7.1 million. To extrapolate these figures nationally, these authors estimate that adhesive obstruction may cause 2,330 hospital admissions annually, associated with an estimated direct cost of about U.S. $13 million.

Jeekel[32] carried out an important study on the cost of patients admitted to a single university surgical unit with clinical symptoms of adhesions. Direct costs were calculated for a single year, 1992, at the Department of Surgery in the University Hospital Diijkzigt, Rotterdam and included those for hospitalization, surgery, special investigations, specialist staff, etc. A total of 20 patients required surgery for abdominal adhesions, which resulted in a mean hospital stay of 24.5 days, far higher than the average mean hospital stay of 11 to 12 days in the department. The complication rate was high, with 4 patients having surgical complications and 3 other complications. The operative mortality was 10%, unusually high when compared with general operative mortality. The total costs associated with these patients was 348,930 Dutch guilders (U.S.$210,000). The need for intensive therapy was a major contributor to these costs.

This study led to a prospective investigation to secure more accurate data. All patients admitted to the University Hospital during an 18-month period (1994–1995) in which adhesions were responsible for clinical symptoms were entered into the study. A total of 59 patients were identified, of which 35 required surgery for division of adhesions and the others were managed conservatively. Complication rate during surgery was high (70%) with a 13% operative mortality. The total costs associated with these cases were 1,209,433 Dutch guilders (approximately U.S.$720,000). These costs are high given that this is a single 18-month period in a single hospital. Once again most of the costs were for general surgery (47.2%) and intensive care (26.5%). Other costs identified were for operative time (10.5%), laboratory and diagnostic tests (7.6%), outpatient care (4.8%), and medication (3.4%).

Information from the Scottish National Health Service Database

A research tool has recently become available that should provide the answers to many of the questions raised in this chapter concerning the short-term and long-term morbidities produced by postoperative intra-abdominal adhesions, which is based on a large population survey. This study, by a small committee of surgeons, gynecologists, and health economists, with myself as chairman uses data from the Information and Statistics Division (ISD) of the Common Services Agency, which is part of the National Health Service (NHS) in Scotland. Situated in Edinburgh, this government body captures all hospital records from population of more than Scotland's 5 million. With low migration and distinct physical borders, Scotland provides a sufficiently large, stable, yet not unwieldy study group. The Scottish Medical Record Linkage Database held by the ISD, which holds data from 1981, contains information on all NHS hospital admissions in Scotland, together with details of the Registrar General's Death Certificates in Scotland. At the time of discharge from hospital, the patient's clinical notes are abstracted on a special form, the Scottish Morbidity Record, by centrally trained coders. ISD has a Quality Assessment and Accreditation Team that carries out a routine 1% stratified audit, which compares the hospital records returns against the patient's original notes. This check is carried out by a professional team of assessors. Record linkage enables readmission of patients to be identified and indexed, thus allowing follow-up over time of individual patients. This care has enabled ISD to achieve a remarkable accuracy of 90% to 95% for diagnostic and procedure coding and 99% for linkage of an individual patient's records. Our committee has used information supplied by ISD to provide actual event details on the incidents and time scale of complications caused by adhesions following abdominal surgery over a 10-year period.[33]

The total number of patients in NHS hospitals in Scotland undergoing abdominal surgery (open, laparoscopic, and endoscopic) in 1986 was 64,731. Patients with disease (ICD 9) and procedure (OPCS 3/4) codes for adhesion-related problems or operations that might be complicated by adhesions were identified and followed over the succeeding 10 years. Of these 64,731 abdominal procedures performed in 1986, a total of 27,952 individuals required one or more admissions either related to adhesions or requiring an abdominal reoperation that could potentially be complicated by the presence of adhesions (43.2%). To limit the potential impact of adhesions from previous surgery, all patients who had undergone surgery in the 5 years before 1986 were identified. This patient group, which would influence the eventual results because of a preexisting adhesion burden, amounted to 12,538 patients. This left 52,192 patients having selected abdominal procedures in 1986, of which 20,418 patients were to have subsequent readmissions (39.2%) over the next 10 years. These 20,418 patients were to have a total of 42,557 admissions either related to adhesions or complicated by the presence of adhesions. Of these readmissions, 2,002 (4.5%) were identified as directly attributable to adhesions, of which 465 admissions had intestinal obstruction, treated either surgically or conservatively, which amounted to 1.1% of total readmissions during the 10-year period. Of the 12,539 patients who had undergone previous surgery in 1981–1986, a total of 7,494 (59.8%) were readmitted for surgical or medical procedures related to or potentially complicated by adhesions, compared with the 39.2% in the main study cohort.

We have broken down the total of abdominal operations into upper abdominal procedures, involving the foregut and its adnexae, lower abdominal procedures, involving mid- and hindgut, and abdominal gynecological surgery. The breakdown of patient readmissions of the 52,192 patients in 1986 who had not had any abdominal surgery in the preceding 5 years, followed up over the next 10-year period, is shown in Table 26.6. The breakdown of readmissions directly related to adhesions divided into these subgroups is shown in Table 26.7. The incidence is highest in the mid- and hindgut, where readmissions directly related to adhesions during 10 years amounted to 7.1% of 13,704 operations, 2.1% being small-bowel obstruction. The first year showed a peak for the majority of outcome groups, but readmissions continued throughout the 10-year period. Outcomes over time are shown in Table 26.8. From our knowledge of the daily costs of inpatient care and of operations, we can make a cost assessment of this 10-year burden of admissions for adhesive obstruction at more than £4.5 million.

Further studies in progress are aimed at documenting the specific risks of adhesive obstruction from each of the major groups of abdominal operations (for example, appendicectomy, hysterectomy) over a 10-year period.

TABLE 26.6. Number of patient readmissions during 10 years.

Site of initial surgery	Patients with 1 or more readmissions (% total patients)	Total number of hospital readmissions	Average number of readmissions per patient
Mid- and hindgut—open (n = 12,584)	4,101 (32.6%)	8,861	2.2
Colorectal endoscopy (n = 263)	139 (52.4%)	325	2.3
Abdominal wall endoscopy (n = 3,917)	2,106 (53.8%)	4,518	2.1
Female reproductive tract—open (n = 8,489)	2,931 (34.5%)	5,433	1.9
Female reproductive tract—endoscopic (n = 7,869)	2,498 (31.7%)	4,479	1.8
Foregut/other abdominal—open (n = 8,714)	3,293 (37.8%)	7,048	2.1
Foregut/other abdominal—endoscopic (n = 10,354)	5,390 (52.1%)	11,893	2.2
Total	20,458 (39.2%)	42,557	2.1

TABLE 26.7. Readmissions directly related to adhesions during 10 years.

Site of initial surgery	Total readmissions that were directly adhesion related	Small-bowel obstruction: surgery/medical	Other adhesions: surgery/medical	Gynecologic adhesiolysis
Midgut/hindgut (n = 13,704)	968 (7.1%)	289 (2.1%)	611 (4.5%)	68 (0.5%)
Foregut (n = 18,941)	644 (3.4%)	134 (0.7%)	509 (2.7%)	1 (0%)
Female reproductive tract (n = 9,912)	390 (3.9%)	42 (0.4%)	316 (3.2%)	32 (0.3%)
Total (n = 42,557)	2,002 (4.7%)	465 (1.1%)	1,436 (3.4%)	101 (0.24%)

These studies well establish the risks of recurrent bowel obstruction treated both operationally and medically, as well as the mortality and morbidity of such treatment including more details of its financial burden on the National Health Service.

Adhesions As Problems at Reoperation

To date there has been little documentation of the consequences of adhesions at reoperation on the abdomen, that is, the increased time required to perform the abdominal exposure and the risks of perforation or damage to adherent viscera. At the June 1998 Malmo meeting of the International Society of University Colon and Rectal Surgeons, two contributors addressed these problems.

B. Moran (personal communication) reported a comparison of the time taken on his surgical unit at Basingstoke UK to open the abdomen and to divide relevant adhesions in first-time (55 patients) and repeat laparotomies (65 patients). The average incision time was prolonged by 5 minutes and the division of relevant adhesions required a mean of 19 minutes (0–120 minutes).

H. Van Goor (personal communication) reported a study at Nijmegen, Holland, of patients who underwent a repeat laparotomy, calculated the incidence of iatro-

TABLE 26.8. Outcomes over time.

Year	Adhesiolysis with or without small-bowel obstruction (%)	Adhesions with or without small-bowel obstruction treated medically (%)	Surgery possibly related to adhesions (%)	Medical intervention possibly related to adhesions (%)	Gynecologic adhesions treated surgically (%)	Gynecologic surgery possibly related to adhesions (%)	Repeat surgery complicated by adhesions (%)	Total (%)
1	348 (26.8)	99 (16.5)	466 (13.1)	1,762 (19.2)	20 (19.8)	157 (4.6)	7,024 (28.8)	9,876 (23.2)
2	173 (13.3)	65 (10.8)	170 (4.8)	1,053 (11.5)	14 (13.9)	151 (4.4)	4,089 (16.8)	5,715 (13.4)
3	125 (9.6)	55 (9.2)	367 (10.3)	911 (9.9)	18 (17.8)	370 (10.8)	2,532 (10.4)	4,378 (10.3)
4	102 (7.9)	55 (9.2)	465 (13.1)	927 (10.1)	7 (6.9)	461 (13.5)	1,636 (6.7)	3,653 (8.6)
5	84 (6.5)	55 (9.2)	417 (11.8)	964 (10.5)	9 (8.9)	480 (14.0)	1,508 (6.2)	3,517 (8.3)
6	106 (8.2)	50 (8.3)	377 (10.6)	919 (10.0)	6 (5.9)	471 (13.7)	1,507 (6.2)	3,436 (8.1)
7	98 (7.5)	60 (10.0)	385 (10.9)	766 (8.4)	13 (12.9)	422 (12.3)	1,731 (7.1)	3,475 (8.2)
8	126 (9.7)	66 (11.0)	393 (11.1)	895 (9.8)	7 (6.9)	412 (12.0)	1,909 (7.8)	3,808 (9.0)
9	110 (8.5)	78 (13.0)	394 (11.0)	761 (8.3)	7 (6.9)	398 (11.6)	2,010 (8.2)	3,758 (8.8)
10[a]	28 (2.2)	18 (3.0)	114 (3.2)	204 (2.2)	0 (0.0)	105 (3.1)	472 (1.9)	941 (2.2)
Total	1,300	601	3,548	9,162	101	3,427	24,418	42,557

[a]Full year data for year 10 are not yet available from the Information and Statistics Division (National Health Service Scotland).

genic bowel perforation, and analyzed the risk factors and the consequences of these bowel perforations. In this study, 274 patients underwent 291 repeat laparotomies between June 1995 and September 1997. A repeat laparotomy was defined as a laparotomy via a prior incision line. Patients with emergency relaparotomies for complications of a prior laparotomy in the same admission period were excluded. Medical records were reviewed to collect data including age, number of previous laparotomies, indication for operation, level of surgical experience, occurrence of bowel perforation, ICU admittance, parental feeding, postoperative complications such as intraabdominal sepsis, wound infection, and postoperative mortality. These data were compared between the groups of patients with and without adhesion-related iatrogenic bowel perforation, using univariate and multivariate analyses.

In the elective surgery group who had no previous surgery, the incision time was a mean of 5 minutes with a range of 3 to 9 minutes for the 47 cases; 44 of 46 had no intraabdominal adhesions, and 2 patients required 4 minutes and 15 minutes, respectively, for division of relevant intraperitoneal adhesions. In the elective group who had undergone previous surgery, the mean incision time was 10 minutes, and the mean time for division of adhesions was 19 minutes, with a range of 0 to 120 minutes. However, 19 of 48 (40%) had insignificant adhesions in that 11 had zero adhesion division time and in 8 patients the division time was less than 5 minutes. In a separate analysis of the 28 with significant adhesions, the mean adhesion division time was 30 minutes. Similarly, the incision time for the 18 patients who had emergency surgery and had previous abdominal surgery was 10 minutes with a division of relevant adhesions time of 31 minutes.

In summary, in a colorectal surgical practice half the patients having elective surgery will have had previous intraabdominal surgery and 60% of these will have significant intraabdominal adhesions, resulting in prolonged incision time and substantial division of adhesions time. For all patients with previous surgery, on average the incision time is prolonged by 5 minutes and the division of relevant adhesions requires a mean of 19 minutes, with a range of 0 to 120 minutes. In this series of patients, small-bowel obstruction accounted for a substantial proportion of emergency surgery. Adhesions pose major problems for the colorectal surgeon, and cost-effective strategies to reduce adhesions would significantly benefit patients, surgeons, and healthcare providers.

At 61 of 291 repeat laparotomies (21%), one or more bowel perforations occurred. The number of previous laparotomies and age were significantly higher ($p < 0.05$) in patients with bowel perforation compared to those without bowel perforations. With multivariate analysis, the number of previous laparotomies and patient age appeared to be independent risk factors for bowel perforation. The skill level of the surgeon, the urgency of the operation, and the time period from the previous laparotomy were not risk factors, nor was the indication for operation, although there was a tendency that bowel perforations occurred more frequently at surgery for small-bowel obstruction (33%). Of 291 patients, 23 (8%) died during hospital stay, 11% of patients with bowel perforations and 7% of those without a perforation (p = NS). The rate of postoperative complications (anastomotic leak, wound infection, hemorrhage, organ failure) was a significantly higher ($p < 0.05$) in patients with bowel perforation (54%) compared to patients without bowel perforation (36%). Moreover, there was significant difference ($p < 0.05$) in ICU admittance, the number of urgent relaparotomies, need for parental feeding, and duration of hospital stay (mean, 13 days with perforation versus 10 days without perforation).

Van Goor concluded that in reoperated patients the risk of adhesion-related bowel perforation is about 20%. A patient of greater age and with more previous laparotomies has an increased risk of bowel perforation. In terms of morbidity and duration of hospital stay, the consequences of adhesion-related iatrogenic bowel perforation are serious.

Conclusions

Only recently have serious attempts been made to document the clinical and financial burdens consequent upon postoperative intraabdominal adhesions. These studies, some of which are ongoing and others not yet published, have demonstrated the high incidence of adhesions in the western world population, the high frequency of this as a cause of small-bowel obstruction, the lifetime risk of this complication following abdominal surgery, its high incidence following certain types of abdominal procedures, the difficulty of distinguishing between simple and strangulated obstruction, the increased difficulties and time loss in reoperations on patients with adhesions, and, finally, the very heavy financial burden these problems place on healthcare systems.

References

1. McEntee G, Pender D, Mulvin D, et al. Current spectrum of intestinal obstruction. Br J Surg 1987;74:976–980.
2. Raf LE. Causes of abdominal adhesions in cases of intestinal obstruction. Acta Chir Scand 1969;135:73–76.
3. Stewardson RH, Bombeck T, Nyhus LM. Critical operative management of small bowel obstruction. Ann Surg 1978; 187:189–193.
4. Weibel MA, Majno G. Peritoneal adhesions and their relation to abdominal surgery. Am J Surg 1973;126:345–353.
5. Menzies D, Ellis H. Intestinal obstruction from adhesions—how big is the problem? Ann R Coll Surg Engl 1990;72:60–63.

6. Ellis H. The clinical significance of adhesions: focus on intestinal obstruction. Eur J Surg 1997;577(suppl):5–9.
7. Cox MR, Gunn IF, Eastman MC, et al. The operative aetiology and types of adhesions causing small bowel obstruction. Aust N Z J Surg 1993;63:848–852.
8. Lockhart-Mummery HE. Intestinal polyposis: the present position. Proc R Soc Med 1967;60:381–384.
9. Fazio VW, Ziv Y, , et al. Ileal pouch—anal anastomoses, complications and function in 1,005 patients. Ann Surg 1995;222:120–127.
10. Kelly KA. Anal sphincter—saving operations for chronic ulcerative colitis. Am J Surg 1992;163:5–11.
11. Wilkins BM, Spitz L. Incidence of post-operative adhesion obstruction following neonatal laparotomy. Br J Surg 1986;73:762–764.
12. Wangensteen OH, Paine JR. Treatment of acute intestinal obstruction by suction with the duodenal tube. JAMA 1933;101:1532–1539.
13. Becker WF. Acute adhesive ileus. Surg Gynecol Obstet 1952;95:472–476.
14. Zollinger RM, Kinsey DL. Diagnosis and management of intestinal obstruction. Am Surg 1964;30:1–5.
15. Pain JA, Collier D, Hanka R. Small bowel obstruction: computer-assisted prediction of strangulation at presentation. Br J Surg 1987;74:981–983.
16. Meagher AP, Moller C, Hoffmann DC. Non-operative treatment of small bowel obstruction following appendicectomy or operation on the ovary or tube Br J Surg 1993;80:1310–1311.
17. Pickleman J, Lee RM. Management of patients with suspected early postoperative small bowel obstruction. Ann Surg 1989;210:216.
18. Sannella NA. Early and late obstruction of the small bowel after abdominoperineal resection. Am J Surg 1975;130: 270–272.
19. Stewart RM, Page CP, Brender J, Schwesinger W, Eisenhut D. The incidence and risk of early post-operative small-bowel obstruction: a cohort study. Am J Surg 1987;154: 643–647.
20. Krook SS. Obstruction of the small intestine due to adhesions and bands. Acta Chir Scand 1947;95(suppl)125: 1–200.
21. Brightwell NL, McFee AS, Aust JB. Bowel obstruction and the long tube stent. Arch Surg 1977;112:505–511.
22. Close MB, Christensen NM. Transmesenteric small bowel plication or intraluminal stenting. Am J Surg 1979;138: 89–96.
23. Bizer LS, Delaney HM, Gerut Z. Observations on recurrent intestinal obstruction and modern non-operative management. Dig Surg 1986;3:229–231.
24. Weigelt JA, Snyder WH, Norman JL. Complications and results of 160 Baker tube plications. Am J Surg 1980; 140:810–815.
25. Hollender LF, Meyer C, Keller D, Bahnini J. Plication operations for recurrent obstruction. In: Ellis H, Lennox M, eds. Adhesions: The Problems. London: Westminster Medical School, 1983:31–35.
26. Jones PF, Munro A. Recurrent adhesive small bowel obstruction. World Med 1985;9:868–875.
27. Schoffel U, Sendt W, Haring R, Farthmann EH. Indications and therapeutic strategy for intestinal obstruction due to intra-abdominal adhesions. In: Treutner K-H, Schumpelick V, eds. Peritoneal Adhesions. Berlin: Springer, 1997:271–277.
28. Scott-Coombes DM, Vipond MN, Thompson JN. General surgeon's attitudes to the treatment and prevention of abdominal adhesions. Ann R Coll Surg Engl 1993;75: 123–128.
29. Ray NF, Larsen JW, Stillman RJ, et al. Economic impact of hospitalizations for lower abdominal adhesiolysis in the United States in 1988. Surg Gynecol Obstet 1993;176: 271–276.
30. Ray NF, Denton WG, Thamer M, et al. Abdominal adhesiolysis: inpatient care and expenditure in the United States in 1994. J Am Coll Surg 1998;186:1–9.
31. Ivarsson ML, Holmdahl L, Franzen G, et al. Cost of bowel obstruction resulting from adhesions. Eur J Surg 1997; 163:679–684.
32. Jeekel H. Cost implications of adhesions as highlighted in a European study. Eur J Surg 1997;579(suppl):43–45.
33. Wilson MS, Ellis H, Parker MC, et al. The surgical implication of adhesions. Br J Surg 1998;85(suppl 1):34.

27

Prevalence of Adhesions and the Associated Costs in General Surgery

D.C.D. de Lange and J. Jeekel

CONTENTS

The formation of adhesions in the peritoneal cavity is a frequently occurring problem. Intraabdominal adhesions may lead to symptoms varying from abdominal discomfort to obstructive ileus. In women, 15% to 20% of all infertility is secondary to adhesions involving the internal female reproductive organs.[1–5] In addition, the presence of adhesions complicates further abdominal surgery.

By far the most common cause of intraabdominal adhesions is previous surgical treatment. Intestinal obstructions that are caused by adhesions (about 30%)[6–8] are postsurgical in approximately 70% to 90% of cases and are caused by previous inflammatory disease in the remaining 10% to 30%. Congenital bands account for a much lower percentage (~3%).[7–9] Weibel and Majno[10] autopsied 752 cadavers and found an incidence of adhesions of 67% in those that had undergone previous surgery, compared to 28% in those with no previous surgery. More recently, Menzies and Ellis[11] studied 210 patients undergoing a relaparotomy and 115 patients undergoing a first-time laparotomy, and found that of these 93% and 10.4%, respectively, had adhesions.

Adhesions may be regarded as the most frequent complication of the surgeon, with a high impact on healthcare problems. The long-term implication of adhesions should be investigated taking into account the complications and costs. In a retrospective survey in our hospital in 1992, all patients with complaints of obstructive bowel disease and adhesions at operation that were held responsible for clinical symptoms were investigated. A considerable percentage (0.85%) of the total expenditure for our surgical department was caused by treatment of the investigated group. We found a high overall morbidity (30%) and a postsurgical mortality of 10%. Because complications are the most important reason for a prolonged hospitalization, efforts should be directed toward prevention of complications of surgery.

In recent literature, comprehensive studies are reported on the etiology of adhesion. A number of studies relate to the incidence and prevention of adhesions, and a few studies have been performed to show the costs in the hospital resulting from the treatment of adhesions.[12,13] This is an additional way to show the effects of adhesions, not only on morbidity and mortality but also on budgets and costs.

Etiology and Incidence

Etiology of Adhesion Formation

Adhesions that develop after abdominal operations represent a response to the stimulus of ischemic tissue or foreign-body material within the peritoneal cavity and are not, as was previously thought, the healing mechanism of extensive serosal defects.[14] Large defects, left open and bleeding, heal within a few days without adhesion formation. Adhesions carry vessels from adjacent viable organs into the damaged tissue and provide what can be an essential additional blood supply to jeopardized tissues. The vast majority of postoperative adhesions represent an important component of the inflammatory (walling-off) and healing process and are harmless.[6,14–19] The incidence of unnecessary adhesion formation, however, must be reduced to avoid the risk of subsequent intestinal obstruction and infertility.

There is a growing appreciation of the dynamic nature of adhesions. Early after surgery or an inflammatory process, adhesions tend to be filmy, diffuse, extensive, and well vascularized. After about 3 months, the vascularity of adhesions is decreased, and the adhesions become less extensive and more defined.[19]

TABLE 27.1. Macroscopic classification according to Zühlke et al.[20]

I	Filmy and easy to separate by blunt dissection
II	Blunt dissection possible, partly sharp dissection necessary, beginning vascularization
III	Lysis possible by sharp dissection only, clear vascularization
IV	Lysis possible by sharp dissection only, organs strongly attached with severe adhesions, damage of organs hardly preventable

TABLE 27.2. Histological classification according to Zühlke et al.[20]

I	Loose connective tissue, cell-rich, old and new fibrin, fine reticulin fibers
II	Connective tissue with cells and capillaries, few collagen fibers
III	Connective tissue more firm, fewer cells, more vessels, few elastic and smooth muscle fibers
IV	Old firm granulation tissue, cell-poor, serosal layers hardly distinguishable

Classifications According to Zühlke

In addition, adhesions can be scored using the macroscopic classification according to Zühlke et al.[20] (Table 27.1). Furthermore, adhesions can be scored microscopically, using the histologic classification according to Zühlke et al.[20] (Table 27.2).

Incidence of Adhesions and Recurrence

The volume of general surgical effort for treatment of adhesions is large. Menzies and Ellis[11] demonstrated that, during a 25-year period, the proportion of general surgery adult admissions as the result of adhesive obstruction was 0.9% and that 3.3% of all laparotomies were for adhesions causing obstruction. Bevan[21] has reported an approximate figure of 1.5% of all admissions for intestinal obstruction (from any cause). Bizer et al.[22] showed that, of 405 patients with mechanical small intestinal obstruction, 74% was caused by adhesions.

Adhesions are the most common cause of small-bowel obstruction in the western world. In addition, there is a high recurrence rate of intestinal obstruction following lysis of the adhesions. Brightwell et al.[23] found a recurrence rate of 13% following enterolysis alone and a 32% recurrence rate following the use of an intraluminal long tube stent. After reproductive pelvic surgery, Diamond et al.[24,25] found a de novo adhesion formation of approximately 50%. Laparoscopic adhesiolysis followed by a second operative procedure within 90 days revealed adhesion reformation in 66 of 68 women (97%). Other complications following lysis are the development of postoperative fistulas and intraabdominal abscesses. In 448 patients with adhesions at laparotomy. Luijendijk et al.[26] found significantly fewer adhesions in patients with a history of only one minor operation or one major operation, compared with those with multiple laparotomies. Also, the number of adhesions was significantly higher in patients with adhesions at previous laparotomy, compared with those without. Several operations have a higher risk of postoperative adhesions. Appendectomy, for instance, presents with adhesions in 68% of cases.[27] Although postoperative adhesions may involve any of the viscera within the abdominal cavity, the small intestine is usually implicated, especially the ileum.[6,8]

Incidence of Bowel Obstruction

Stewart et al.[28] studied 8098 patients undergoing various types of abdominal surgery and found an incidence of early postoperative small-bowel obstruction (evident within 4 weeks) of 0.69%. Adhesions accounted for 92% of all obstructions. Stewart demonstrated that operations performed below the transverse mesocolon impose an increased risk, whereas those limited to the upper abdomen (where contact with the small bowel is limited to exploration only) are virtually free of risk. The operations most frequently associated were operations on the left side of the colon or rectum (2.9%; $n = 378$), small-bowel operations (2.3%; $n = 256$), penetrating trauma with associated small-bowel injury (2.3%; $n = 215$), and perforated appendicitis (1.7%, $n = 354$). Menzies,[11] in a study of 4502 laparotomies, found an incidence of 0.52% at 1 month and 0.96% at 1 year of adhesive obstruction requiring surgery and demonstrated that especially large bowel (24%), rectal (15%), appendiceal (15%), and gynecologic surgery (14%) accounted for the majority of the obstructions confirming the observations of Nemir,[7] Perry et al.,[8] Becker,[9] Colett and Bossart,[29] Räf,[30] Sykes and Schofield,[31] and Quatromoni et al.[32]

In addition, Brightwell et al.[23] found penetrating abdominal trauma to account for 24% of early and late bowel obstruction. Stewart confirmed the high risk of colorectal procedures, but appendectomies, although accounting for a high percentage of the total postoperative obstructions, were not particularly prone to producing obstruction (0.35%; $n = 844$). The high total amount occurs because appendectomy is the most frequent indication to laparotomy. In conclusion, the majority of operations producing intestinal adhesive obstruction are lower abdominal, principally involving the intestine.

Menzies[11] studied the onset of postoperative adhesive obstruction following laparotomy and found that 21% occurred within 1 month, 39% occurred within 1 year, and 60% occurred within 5 years. In addition, 21% occurred more than 10 years after the preceding surgery.

Adhesions and Foreign-Body Reactions

The effect of the extent of previous abdominal operations, or in other words the effect of the extent of peritoneal damage, on the occurrence of foreign-body reactions was analyzed by Myllärniemi.[33] The frequency of granulomas was highest in the group subjected to multiple operations (70%), the number rising with the number of previous operations, followed by those subjected to extensive operations (66%) and those subjected to minor operations (49%). The lowest rate of granulomas pertained to the group subjected to gynecologic and obstetric procedures (30%). Operations on the digestive tract significantly increased the rate of granulomatous cases (74%), probably on one hand because of the risk of peritoneal contamination by intestinal contents and on the other hand the long duration of such operations.

Granulomas were also investigated by Luijendijk[26] in 424 patients with adhesions at laparotomy, finding granulomas in 26% of all patients. Suture granulomas were found in 25% and starch granulomas in 5% of the patients operated upon with starch-containing gloves. When suture granulomas were present, the median interval between the current and the most recent previous laparotomy was 13 months. When suture granulomas were absent, this interval was significantly longer, 30 months. The percentage of patients with suture granulomas decreased gradually, from 37% if the previous laparotomy had occurred up to 6 months before the present operation to 18% if the previous laparotomy had occurred more than 2 years ago. Because suture granulomas occur in a large percentage in recent adhesions, this suggests that the intraabdominal presence of foreign material is an important cause of adhesion formation.

Inflammatory Diseases

Following inflammatory disease, the strands that are present are localized to those areas where intense tissue anoxia can be assumed to have occurred.[14] Intestinal obstruction following inflammatory disease is mainly caused by appendicitis and diverticulitis. Perry[8] found these to account for 42% and 14.5%, respectively. Raf,[30] in his series, found 9% and 10%, respectively, and 14% caused by pelvic inflammatory disease. In 39% of his cases there was no cause demonstrable. Less common causes were regional enteritis, cholecystitis, ulcerative colitis, and tuberculous peritonitis.

Luijendijk[26] found significantly more adhesions in patients with a history of adhesions at previous laparotomy, with presence of abdominal abscess, hematoma, and intestinal leakage as complications after former surgery, and a history of an unoperated inflammatory process. No influence was found from prosthetic material used intraabdominally or in those who had received abdominal radiotherapy.

Distribution of Adhesions

Menzies[11] also studied the distribution of adhesions. In 210 laparotomies the commonest sites for adhesions were from omentum to the laparotomy scar (170). Other locations were site of surgery alone (57), from omentum to site of surgery (47), from small bowel to laparotomy scar (42), from small bowel to site of surgery (33), and from small bowel to small bowel (17).

Myllärniemi,[33] in his series, found adhesions to be most frequent in the areas of laparotomy scars (88%; $n = 271$), followed by the areas of visceral scars (59%;

$n = 181$). In other sites, the frequency was 39% ($n = 121$). In 448 patients studied, Luijendijk[26] found the adhesions most frequently attached to omentum (68%) and small bowel (67%). Furthermore, he found the laparotomy scar attached to one or more of the following organs in 71% of patients: omentum, small bowel, colon, or abdominal wall. The site of previous surgery was attached to one or more of these organs in 53%.

TABLE 27.4. Causes of peritoneal injury.

Operative trauma
Bacterial infection
Foreign bodies
Desiccation/drying
Irradiation
Allergic reactions
Chemical injury
Ischemic injury

Preventive Measures

Many substances and procedures have been used to prevent the formation of adhesions.[34,35] The aim of all studies has been to interfere with one or several of the pathogenetic steps of adhesion formation. Ellis[16] has classified those (Table 27.3).

Initial promising results have usually been followed by further investigations that questioned or even abandoned that particular material or procedure. The most promising substance so far is recombinant tissue plasminogen activator (rtPA).[36] Enthusiasm for this approach must be tempered, however, because of the importance of the adhesive process in healing and localizing intraabdominal inflammatory processes.[19] To prevent the high incidence of adhesion formation between organs and the laparotomy scar, a bioabsorbable membrane that forms a mechanical barrier has been developed to prevent adhesion formation without causing damage to the intestine or abdominal wall.[37] At the present time, no agent seems to be overwhelmingly suitable for general use in the abdominal cavity. Therefore, most important will be the role of the surgeon to operate in a nontraumatizing fashion to prevent peritoneal injury[38] (Table 27.4)

In conclusion, unnecessary intraabdominal adhesions remain a significant cause of postoperative morbidity despite a century[39] of investigation of etiology and many preventative and curative attempts. Further study is needed to reduce the incidence of adhesions in future surgery.

TABLE 27.3. Measures of adhesion prevention.

1. Prevention of fibrin deposition
   - Anticoagulants (sodium citrate, heparin, dicoumarol, dextran)
   - Antiplasmin agent (Trasylol)
2. Removal of fibrin exudate
   - Intraperitoneal lavage
   - Enzymes (pepsin, trypsin, papain)
   - Fibrinolytic agents (streptokinase, actase, urokinase, tissue plasminogen activator
3. Separation of surfaces
   - Distension (oxygen)
   - Peristalsis stimulation (prostygmine)
   - Separating substances (olive oil, liquid paraffin, amniotic fluid, membranes of fish bladder, ox peritoneum, amniotic membrane, oiled silk, silver or gold foil, free grafts of omentum, silicone)
4. Inhibition of fibroblastic proliferation
   - Antihistamines, steroids, cytotoxic drugs

Etiology in Detail

Adhesion Formation

Following abdominal surgery, a fibrin-rich exudate is released into the abdominal cavity. The resulting delicate fibrinous adhesions are either lysed by the plasminogen-plasmin cascade or organized into permanent fibrous adhesions with ingrowth of capillaries and fibroblasts and subsequent incorporation of collagen.[40,41] Those fibrinous attachments that persist for 3 days or more invite fibroblastic proliferation. What determines whether or not the fibrinous exudate becomes absorbed or organized? The pathway of adhesion formation is extensively studied and has recently been altered[42–45]; the major steps in the formation of adhesions are displayed in Fig. 27.1.

Adhesions and Reduced Fibrinolytic Activity

The normal peritoneum has an inherent fibrinolytic activity[46] that is capable of absorbing large volumes of clot-

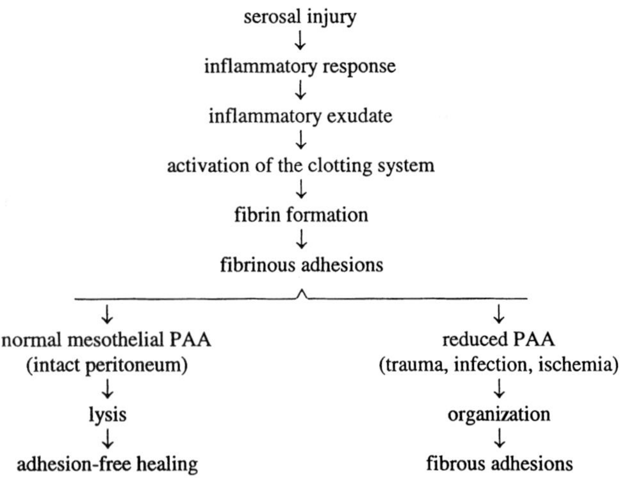

FIG. 27.1. The pathogenesis of permanent fibrous adhesions.

ted blood within 48 hours.[47] Plasmin is the principal agent of the fibrinolytic system. The fibrinolytic capacity of the peritoneum resides in plasminogen activators present in the mesothelium, the submesothelial blood vessels, and in peritoneal macrophages.[48–53] Recently, tissue plasminogen activator (tPA) has been determined as the principal physiologic plasminogen activator.[52] tPA is several hundredfold more effective as an activator of the fibrinolytic system in the presence of fibrin than urokinase-type plasminogen activator (UPA). Inactivators of plasmin such as α_2 antiplasmin and α_2 macroglobulin are ubiquitous and can rapidly inhibit plasmin's activity. However, due to the ability of tPA to bind to the fibrin surface and then induce proteolytic cleavage of plasminogen to plasmin, the plasmin thus formed is protected from inactivation.[54,55] This sequestration of plasmin after activation by tPA on the fibrin surface protects it from plasma or peritoneal inactivators, allowing for only slow degradation of its fibrinolytic effect (Fig. 27.2). In contrast, free-formed plasmin is rapidly cleared by inactivators.[56]

The critical event in the formation of permanent fibrous adhesions is the failure of the injured peritoneum to remove deposited fibrin before it is invaded by fibroblasts.[14] This failure is caused by a local depression of fibrinolytic activity of the peritoneum, resulting from a reduction in peritoneal plasminogen activator activity (PAA) at the site of trauma. Vipond et al.[46] demonstrated that levels of tPA were similar in both normal and inflamed human peritoneum but that the PAA was much lower in inflamed peritoneum. Thompson et al.[57] found similar results in inflamed and ischemic peritoneum.

Merlo et al.[58] showed significant variations in the fibrinolytic activity of normal human peritoneum taken from different sites using the Gelfilm disk technique. The activity of the omentum majus was significantly higher

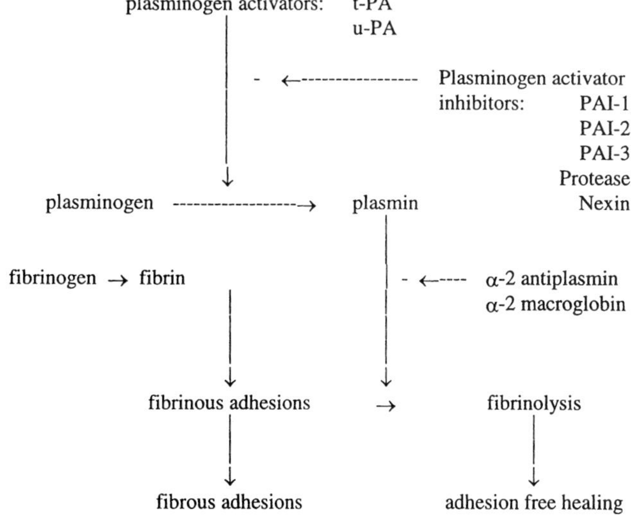

FIG. 27.2. The fibrinolytic system.

compared to almost all the other areas of the peritoneum, such as the gallbladder, duodenum, ascending and transverse colon ($p < 0.05$), sigmoid appendices epiploicae, stomach, small bowel, and parietal peritoneum of the anterior wall ($p < 0.01$). The omentum majus, therefore, has the highest fibrinolytic activity among the different peritoneal areas studied.

All kinds of serosal damage, such as thermal and mechanical trauma, chemical injury, foreign bodies (starch), ischemia, inflammation, and infection, can result in a PAA reduction. As a consequence, fibrin deposits are not lysed, allowing for the conversion of fibrinous bands to fibrous adhesions. Deperitonealized surfaces that have not otherwise been traumatized, however, heal within 5 days without permanent adhesions because they retain their ability to lyse fibrinous adhesions before organization can occur[42–44]; this may be the result of the reduced but significant PAA level in the submesothelial tissue.[59] This activity is lost in peritoneum that has been rendered ischemic. Moreover, such ischemic tissue may actively inhibit fibrinolysis by normal tissues. This phenomenon also explains the failure of intact peritoneum to lyse fibrinous adhesions to adjacent ischemic tissue.

Animal studies in rats revealed that fibrinolytic activity is not maximally depressed at the time of operation and that further depression occurs for at least 24 hours postoperatively.[44] PAA stays low for several days, and the time course of return of PAA varies with different forms of injury.[42] Ryan et al.[60] showed that a partial return of activity occurred at 3 days after injury, and by the fifth day the level of activity was greater than normal. The increased fibrinolytic activity remained relatively unchanged for another 2 to 3 weeks and then gradually fell to lower levels, although even at 2 months the activity was still greater than normal. Buckman et al.[42] studied this aspect in detail and observed an effect similar to that by Ryan; they observed that ischemic damage resulted in the most delayed restoration of fibrinolysis when, even at 4 days after injury, it had only risen to one-third of the normal activity. Raftery[44,61] also found this delay, and confirmed Ryan's observation of increased fibrinolytic effect with the passage of sufficient time (8 days). This prolonged local failure of peritoneal fibrinolysis accounts for the fibrous organization that begins around the third postoperative day.[40,41]

Locally active preparations of tPA can prevent adhesion formation. Topical recombinant tPA, by replacing the lower PAA of peritoneum under conditions producing adhesions, appears to be an effective deterrent of adhesion formation and reformation in a rabbit model.[36,62–64] Theoretically, the presence of rtPA may alter parietal and visceral wound healing and may affect hemostasis,[55] but in a rabbit model no statistically significant difference could be found.[59]

Vipond[46] found that the reduction of PAA seen in inflammation is mediated by plasminogen activator inhibitor-1 (PAI-1), PAI-1 was not detectable in normal peritoneum, but was present in inflamed tissue and might be the reason for the reduction in functional fibrinolytic activity. He suggested that topical tPA might prevent adhesion formation, possibly by competitive inhibition of PAI-1.

It is generally stated that adhesion reformation occurs by the same mechanisms as those which initiate their formation following a peritoneal injury. However, there are no experimental data confirming this, and a large number of experimental and clinical studies have established that there is a greater propensity for adhesion reformation. Dense vascular adhesions tend to reform despite the employment of meticulous technique during lysis. There may be reduced fibrinolytic activity present in adhesions, or perhaps there is simply a greater tendency for apposition of traumatized tissues to occur in these patients.[35] PAA can be determined by fibrin plate technique; tPA and PAI-1 can be measured by enzyme-linked immunosorbent assay.

In conclusion, a reduction of PAA of visceral and parietal peritoneum is believed to be the underlying pathogenetic mechanism in adhesion formation. The discovery of the role of tPA/PAA/PAI-1 is only a very recent one, and further research in this field is necessary.

Disturbing the Fibrinolytic System

Surgical Injuries

Surgical injuries to the peritoneum (abrasion, suture placement, ligations, cautery, and desiccation) are the main causes of serosal damage and formation of postoperative adhesions. These injuries implicate the development of local tissue ischemia, which in turn diminishes PAA. Thus, the local fibrinolytic potential is reduced and fibrin deposits are not lysed, allowing for the conversion of fibrinous bands to fibrous adhesions. The adhesions that form to the line of a bowel anastomosis or a laparotomy scar, for example, can be explained by the strangulating effect of sutures in these situations.[14]

Foreign-Body Materials

More than 30 years ago, Myllärniemi reported that 61% of 309 patients with postoperative adhesions showed reactions to foreign material.[33] Substances identified included talc (31%), gauze lint (16%), a combination of talc and gauze lint (11%), starch (1%), and sutures (less than 1%). Foreign materials such as glove powder,[65] fluff from surgical packs (gauze lint),[66] sutures,[67,68] and material extruded from the digestive tract cause a peritoneal inflammatory reaction.[69] This reaction potentiates adhesion formation, especially with concomitant peritoneal damage, as has been demonstrated in various animal models.[10,16,65,67,69–71] Such adhesions often contain multiple foreign-body granulomas,[33,70–76] strongly suggesting a relation between foreign material, foreign-body granulomas, and adhesion formation. Foreign bodies contaminating the peritoneal tissues might also be a cause of adhesion formation in humans.

Other Factors

Blood and bile alone will not induce adhesions. In combination with tissue ischemia or bacteria, however, they invariably induce adhesions.[71,77–79] Ryan[60,77] also evaluated the prophylactic efficacy of several physiologic fluids, including normal saline and Ringer's solution, in preventing drying injury of the serosa. With no other treatment, adhesions did not subsequently develop, but when fresh blood was dripped intraperitoneal immediately after the wetting procedure, adhesions formed identical to those found after serosal drying plus blood.

Abdominal infections also represent a considerable multifactorial reason for adhesion formation. Bacteria will contribute more or less directly to damage of the serosa and activation of various cascade systems, including the coagulation cascade, for example, by the release of endotoxin.[53] Additionally, they secrete substances that may limit tissue blood flow and attract inflammatory cells.[35] Again, the coexistence of tissue ischemia or foreign bodies will intensify the response.[80]

The effect of radiation on intraabdominal adhesions has not been well investigated. It is known, however, that radiation induces two changes in the intestinal wall that will aggravate intestinal adhesions. Radiation produces a change in terminal small arteries (endarteritis), resulting in poorly vascularized tissues with decreased intrinsic healing ability. This change is coupled with the fibrotic response seen in the wall of the intestine after radiation. In patients who have had previous intraabdominal procedures followed by high-dose radiotherapy, adhesions tend to be more vascular (even after considerable time), extensive, and fibrotic.[19]

Foreign-Body Granulomas

In recent series, 25% of 424 patients with abdominal adhesions at laparotomy had suture granulomas, and 5% of 309 patients being operated upon with starch-containing gloves had starch granulomas, while in other studies almost no suture granulomas were found.[26] Foreign-body granulomas (suture) were more often found in patients who had recently undergone surgery, but this was not true of starch granulomas. An explanation for this difference might be the ability of the body to resorb starch and suture materials. The largest extent of this resorption of suture materials seems to take place during the first year. This resorption of foreign material, however, occurs too late to prevent adhesion formation; the organization of fibrinous adhesions starts at 3 days.[40]

The resorption rate strongly influences the chance of finding foreign material. The resorption rate of starch powder is not known, but will depend on the glove powder used (kind, composition, amount, clumping) and the host (intraabdominal conditions, individual inflammatory reaction or sensitivity).[33] Experiments on animals suggest that powder can be resorbed within 24 hours, leaving granulomas and firm adhesions long thereafter.[70] At the latest, starch granulomas were still present at 15 months in experimental studies[65] and at 23 months, up to 32 years, after the last operation in clinical studies.[26,81]

Surgical Glove Powder

Contamination of the peritoneal cavity at the time of operation with various materials such as glove powder, gauze fluff, suture material, and cellulose derived from disposable gowns and drapes can induce an inflammatory foreign-body reaction, with consequent formation of granulomas and adhesions or both. Glove powder, especially, has been under suspicion. The numerous reports on the hazards of surgical glove dusting powders have been recently reviewed by Ellis.[65]

Starch powder has been used as a glove lubricant since 1948, following numerous reports of granulomatous reactions produced by surgical talc. The current powder is prepared from cornstarch by etherification with epichlorohydrin and is mixed with 2% of magnesium oxide as a desiccating agent to help prevent clumping.[80,82] In addition, it contains small amounts of sodium sulfate and sodium chloride. Initially it was said to be completely absorbed and to be biologically inert (Lee and Lehman 1947),[83] but soon reports on the pathologic changes that may follow the introduction of starch glove powder into the peritoneal cavity were published (Lee et al. 1952).[80] Provided all other factors conducive to inflammatory reaction and adhesion or granuloma formation are excluded, starch powder appears to be completely absorbed and leaves the serosal surfaces and soft tissues undamaged. Until absorption takes place, however, the starch granules constitute as much of a foreign body as would any other powder of comparable particulate size[80]; this is also true for absorbable suture material.[84]

Three pathologic situations of clinical significance were noted[81]: first, the formation of foreign-body granulomas, which are macroscopically indistinguishable from metastatic malignant or tuberculous nodules[82]; second, the association of these granulomas caused by starch with the formation of peritoneal adhesions; and finally, the development of starch peritonitis, a rather rare disease occurring 10 days to 4 weeks after operation with low-grade fever, vomiting, distension, abdominal pain, and starch-containing fluid in the abdomen. There are strong indications that hypersensitivity to starch may be responsible for the clinical features of this starch peritonitis.[73] In addition, Jaffray and Nade[85] found that the presence of surgical glove powder reduced the inoculum of bacteria required to produce an abscess by a factor of 10.

In summary, adhesion-free surgery demands the prevention of serosal injury, tissue ischemia, foreign bodies, postoperative bleeding, high-dose radiotherapy, and infectious complications.[86]

Prevention of Foreign Material Contamination

As a consequence of these findings, the use of suture material should be minimized so as to avoid its intraabdominal presence as well as the ischemia it causes. Closure of the peritoneum, for instance, is unnecessary,[16,40] and in the context of the foregoing, unwanted. A meticulous technique can limit foreign-body contamination and subsequent granuloma formation, as well as peritoneal damage; this might reduce adhesion formation.[87]

Prevention of Starch Contamination

To prevent the occurrence of starch powder contamination, washing of gloves has been recommended by several authors.[71,87–89] Jagelman and Ellis[71] demonstrated however that careful washing of the gloves in two successive bowls of saline solution fails to remove all the starch and results in clumping of residual starch granules. This, unfavorably, is more likely to result in significant foreign-body reaction, with the formation of more granulomas and adhesions, because the increased size of the clumps makes them less rapidly absorbed.[71,80] Lavage with a 1% solution of cetrimide greatly reduces the amount of residual starch.[88] A 1-minute cleansing with 10 mL of povidone-iodine followed by a 30-second rinse under sterile water leaves no residual powder.[89] Although these techniques are effective, they are costly and tiresome and few surgeons make any attempt to remove the glove surface powder (Table 27.5). As a consequence, starch contamination of the peritoneal cavity is inevitable when using starch-containing gloves.

TABLE 27.5. Operative techniques to prevent adhesions as used by surgical specialists in the Netherlands.

Procedure	Routine[a]	Sometimes[a]	Never[a]
Small intestine protection	207 (64)	84 (27)	30 (9)
Peritoneal lavage	60 (18)	237 (70)	39 (12)

	Yes[a]	No[a]
Selective instead of total adhesiolysis	313 (93)	35 (7)
Omentum placement at closure	302 (87)	46 (13)
No peritoneal closures	278 (20)	60 (80)
Powder-free gloves	174 (50)	174 (50)
Washing out powder-contaminated gloves	104 (30)	244 (70)

[a]Percentages in parentheses.

The length and type of the foreign-body reaction depends on the amount of powder introduced, the time lapsed before absorption, hypersensitivity to starch (individual variation), whether the starch occurs in grains or clumps, and the degree of cross-linkage of the particular starch. In addition, the powder composition is of influence. Apart from pure starch itself, the 2% concentration of magnesium oxide used in most surgical gloves can produce an additional foreign-body reaction.[72]

Powder-Free Gloves

In 1982, a starch-free, powderless glove was developed. It is produced by a process that binds a film of Biogel to the inner surface of the glove. Biogel has been determined in numerous studies to be entirely nonreactive.[65] The question is to what extent adhesions should be prevented by avoiding the use of starch-containing powder. Weibel and Majno[10] studied 55 adhesions histologically and found foreign-body granulomas in 69% (talc, 68%, lint or thread from gauze, 18%, other foreign bodies 13%). Myllärniemi[33] reported that 61% of 309 cases of postoperative adhesions showed foreign-body reactions (51% talc, 26% lint, 2% starch, 3% other, 18% mixture of materials). The high incidence of such adhesions reported in the early literature is partly explained by the then-prevalent use of talc as a glove lubricant. In addition, because of its absorbability, it is understandable that starch is seldom found in connection with reoperations with a long relaparotomy interval.[33] Cooke[81] showed starch granulomas in 10 of 12 patients undergoing a relaparotomy within 2 years of the previous operation. Numerous animal experiments support these findings. McEntee[70] injected 144 rats intraperitoneally with a suspension of washing from starched gloves, starch-free, gloves and starch-poor washed gloves following laparotomy. The incidence of adhesions was 78%, 37%, and 33%, respectively, confirming an advantage for thoroughly washing gloves or switching to starch-free gloves.

The easiest and possibly the safest option, however, is to avoid completely the use of starch gloves. Inadvertent glove puncture can still release starch powder from the gloves, and the risks of introducing infection through the use of rinsing processes are not insignificant.[89] Starch can be identified by recognition of a rounded particle showing specific "Maltese cross" birefringence (=doubly refractile) under polarized light. In addition, starch granules can be detected by periodic acid-Schiff (PAS) staining.[90]

Cost of Treatment of Adhesions

Economic Background

Healthcare practitioners are under continuous pressure to control surgical expenditure. One major recurrent problem in surgery is the presence of abdominal adhesions, which leads to large expenditure. The treatment of patients with complaints of abdominal adhesions still is a large problem. Options are an operative intervention or a conservative regimen.

We sent a questionnaire to 500 surgical specialists in the Netherlands; 348 of the queried specialists replied (73%), noting that they operate annually on three to five patients for small-bowel obstruction based on adhesions. Furthermore, each specialist hospitalizes annually three to five patients with the diagnosis of small-bowel obstruction caused by adhesions, who are treated nonoperatively. These figures reflect the findings of Scott-Coombes et al.,[91] who performed a similar survey in the United Kingdom.

To determine the actual cost impact on the department budget, concurrent studies have been undertaken for patients operated with signs of adhesive bowel obstruction in the hospital. Ray et al.[12] analyzed all hospitalizations for adhesions using the 1988 National Hospital Discharge Survey, in which 9% of a representative cross section of the hospitals in the United States were analyzed, using a random sampling of 240,243 discharge-stratified hospitalizations. Costs were determined by Medicare provider analysis review diagnosis using the International Classification of Diseases, 9th Revision Clinical Modification, and procedures using the current procedural technology. Overall, 281,982 hospitalizations were assessed; 51,100 of these hospitalizations were precipitated by adhesions that required a mean stay of 11.24 days and a total stay of 608,084 days. During an additional 227,882 hospitalizations that were not precipitated by adhesions, adhesions were one of the problems treated during the index hospitalization, accounting for an additional total stay of 340,643 days. In total, therefore, more than 948,000 hospital-days of care were required during 1988 in the United States, for the treatment of adhesions, at a cost of approximately $1.18 billion.

Holmdahl performed a postal study in Sweden, sending a survey to all surgeons and using the Swedish population of 8.5 million[13]; 4700 patients were admitted on an annual basis to relieve small bowel obstruction: 2200 of whom required laparotomy, and an additional 1500 laparotomies were complicated by previous adhesions. Overall, 6200 patients required hospitalizations for adhesion-related problems, accounting for 3.5% of all laparotomies in Sweden. The annual impact included 150 deaths at a laparotomy cost of U.S.$4.1 million per year in Sweden translating to 1 million dollars per million Swedish inhabitants to treat the problem of adhesions.

The questionnairy survey we sent to 500 surgical specialists in the Netherlands using the population of 15 million showed us similar results. On an average each specialist operates on 3 to 5 patients each year with adhesional small-bowel obstruction, and 3 to 5 patients are admitted each year to the hospital for nonoperative treatment of small-bowel obstruction caused by adhesions. These figures suggest hospitalization and/or operation because of abdominal adhesions in 8,000 to 14,000 patients each year for all specialists in the Netherlands.

Surgical Treatment of Adhesions: Actual Cost in a Surgical Department

A retrospective investigation was performed in 1992 to determine the actual cost impact on the department budget associated with patients operated with signs of adhesive bowel obstruction in the University Hospital Rotterdam, Dijkzigt, the Netherlands. All patients with complaints of obstructive bowel disease and adhesions at operation that were held responsible for clinical symptoms were selected. Based on costs used by the Department of Finance Administration of the hospital, calculations of costs were made.[92] These real cost figures are calculated based on cost-center methods.[93] The stay in the hospital was regarded the main group, and consisted of direct costs and indirect costs.

Direct costs are all costs made in the Department of Surgery (outside investments) to perform tasks: personnel (staff included) and materials costs. Indirect costs were costs caused in other departments, for example, food supplies and laundry. Subgroups were indirect costs of other departments that could be accounted separately and were not included in the main group. These subgroups were costs of operations, laboratory investigations, diagnostic survey, consulted specialists, and visits to the outpatient clinic; 20 patients with adhesions found at laparotomy held responsible for clinical symptoms were included. Hospitalizations accounted for 486 hospital days of which 48 days were on intensive care and/or high-care units (10%). The mean length of hospital stay was 24.5 days.

Adhesions found perioperatively were held responsible for the clinical symptoms in all cases. Additionally, a strangulated small intestine was found in 13 patients. Postoperative complications were recorded in 6 of the 20 patients (30%). Two patients experienced a persisting ileus, 1 of whom had further complications and eventually died. One patient experienced a platzbauch and after a further complicated treatment died after surgery. Other patients had complications such as needing a relaparotomy (1), a sepsis (1), and a wound infection (1). Two of these patients also had other minor complications such as urinary tract infections. Therefore, postoperative mortality was recorded as high as 10%.

Costs of Treatment

Total cost of treatment of patients during the period of study (1 year) was Fl 348,595 (U.S.$175,000). The stay in the hospital accounted for 78% of costs, of which 25% were incurred because of treatment on intensive- or high-care units. Costs of operations accounted for 16%, costs of diagnostic investigations accounted for 5%, and costs of laboratory investigations for 1% of the costs. Visits to the Outpatient department and consulted specialists together accounted for less than 1% of the costs. The mean costs per patients were Fl 17,430 (U.S.$8,700). The mean hospital stay for average patients in 1992 was 14.4 days with a mean cost of Fl 12,597 (U.S.$6,300).

The expenditure of the Department of Surgery in 1992 was Fl 41,178,600 (U.S.$20,589,300), based on 125 beds in the Department of General Surgery and 22 intensive- and/or high-care beds. Therefore, the investigated group accounted for 0.85% of the annual expenditure of the entire Department of Surgery.

Conservative and Surgical Treatment: Cost Impact

To investigate prospectively the protocolized treatment of patients with complaints of abdominal (strangulating) adhesions and the related real costs and complications, all patients admitted with signs of intestinal bowel obstruction were investigated during a period of 19 months in the University Hospital Rotterdam, Dijkzigt, The Netherlands. When adhesions were responsible for clinical symptoms, patients were included in the study group. Follow-up was performed during hospitalization and visits to the outpatient clinic. Patients were put in two treatment groups, conservative or operative; morbidity and mortality were documented.

During the study period, 57 patients were hospitalized a total of 70 times: 2 patients were seen only in the outpatient department, and 5 patients were hospitalized more than one time (2–6). The hospitalizations accounted for 1395 hospital days, of which 204 days were on intensive- and/or high-care units (15%). The mean length of hospital stay was 20 days. Of the 59 patients, 30 underwent primary surgery for adhesiolysis, being operated 1 to 6 times. All other patients (29) were managed on a conservative basis, which led to a morbidity of 10% and no mortality. The overall postoperative morbidity rate was 70%, and the overall postoperative mortality rate was 13%.

Costs accounted for were divided in separate groups. The largest costs factor was the number of days admitted to the hospital, irrespectively of performed diagnostics. The overall stay in hospital accounted for 73.7% of costs, which includes a subgroup of 26.5% that were attributed to intensive- and/or high-care unit costs. Operative costs accounted for 10.5%, costs of medications 3.4%, costs of various diagnostic and laboratory investigations accounted for 7.6%, and visits to the outpatient clinic 4.8%. The mean cost for each hospitalization was Fl 21,163. Total treatment costs for patients during the period of study (19 months) were Fl 1,209,433 (U.S.$604,716), which is an annual Fl 763,852 (U.S.$381,926). Total costs of the study group accounted for 1.5% of annual expenditure allocated for the entire Department of Surgery. This total can be drawn from the total expenditure for the Department of Surgery in 1 year (1993), which was Fl 49,330,200 (US$24,665,100). These expenditures included 116 beds in the Department of General Surgery, 17 Intensive- and/or high-care beds, and the outpatient surgical department. The mean hospital stay for patients in 1993 was 13.3 days with a mean cost of Fl 12,110 per patient. In 1993, there were 3656 surgical hospitalizations in our hospital. Compared to this, the study group with 44 hospitalizations in 1 year is responsible for 1.2% of all surgical hospitalizations.

Conclusions on Costs Prevention

Prophylactic risk reduction measures that minimize intraoperative contamination by foreign materials will help reduce the number of adhesions.[16,87,94] For prevention, the intraabdominal use of foreign-body materials should be minimized. Intraperitoneal placement of stitches should be minimized although it cannot altogether be avoided. Glove powder can and should be avoided in surgery. In a recent study by Lnyendijk, starch granulomas, with typical Maltese cross, were present in 5% of adhesions.[26] Reducing the incidence of adhesions may reduce the incidence of abdominal complications caused by adhesions. Intraoperatively performed adhesiolysis is still counteracted by the reformation of adhesions in 55% to 100% of the cases.[95]

Mortality and Morbidity

The mortality and complication rate in this category of patients equals only those found after major surgery such as pancreatic or esophageal surgery. The high mortality rate (13%–30%) in the above-mentioned Dutch studies calls for a restrictive behavior and experienced surgical care. Furthermore, a morbidity rate of 30% to 70% was found in the operated group. The postsurgical complications identified in these studies are the primary reason of prolonged hospital stay. We found that the hospital stay is the single most important cost figure in the patient group (74%–78%), and therefore efforts should be made to shorten this period. The duration of the hospital stay also influences the quality of life of hospitalized patients.[96]

Prevention of Adverse Events

A strict treatment protocol should be used to improve results. Obstructional bowel disease is defined as a period of continuous or intermittent complaints of the patient consisting of pain, nausea, and a distended abdomen. In these cases treatment must be focused on the resolution of these complaints, irrespective of the origin, whether adhesional or nonadhesional. Relief without surgical intervention must be obtained in the first 24 hours of observation under a strict diet of no oral intake and intravenous infusion of 0.9% saline. If there is no relief or if the condition of the patient deteriorates, surgical intervention should take place. If the patient is presented to the surgeon with signs of an acute abdomen, with peritoneal irritation or the signs of bowel perforation (free air visible on plain X-abdomen), an acute intervention with no delay must take place. In our studies there was no record of time between arrival in the hospital and the time of operation. Therefore, we could not correlate the observation period with the high mortality rate we found. A high percentage of patients with critical ischemia of the intestine was found (7 of 30 patients, 23%). Many patients also had to be reoperated (27%, 8/30), 7 of which because of a persisting ileus.

Impact of Adhesions on Admissions

The literature reveals that small-bowel obstruction is caused by adhesions in the majority of patients.[22] Menzies and Ellis investigated the patients admitted to general surgery because of intestinal obstruction. Of all admissions during a 25-year period, 0.9% were caused by intestinal obstruction by adhesions, while 3.3% of all laparotomies were for adhesive obstruction.[11]

In the Department of Surgery of the University Hospital Rotterdam, Dijkzigt, 1.2% of the surgical admissions was caused by adhesions. The percentage of total departmental expenditures generated by these patients was 1.5%. An explanation for this difference lies in the mean hospitalization period, which was longer for patients from the study group compared to all patients (20 days against 13.3 days). This also explains the differences in related costs for the mean hospitalization periods (Fl 21,163 compared to 12,110).

Cost Reduction

As already stated, the majority of costs are created by the number of days the patient stays in the hospital. One method of earlier intervention and possible cost reduction is laparoscopic inspection and adhesiolysis, which can be performed in patients with an uncomplicated history of abdominal operations. Laparoscopic adhesiolysis has been successfully used in gynecologic surgery and has been shown to reduce surgical trauma while limiting length-of-stay. Such measures to prevent adverse outcomes will benefit the patient, and at the same time will minimize costs associated with hospitalization. Our surgical department involves 133 beds, which is 2% of the total number of surgical beds in the Netherlands during the period of study (6559 beds).[97] Therefore, we must face an annual expenditure of 50 times the costs on an national scale (more than Fl 38,000,000, or U.S.$19,000,000). In an era of cost containment and reduction, efforts should be undertaken to lower this extremely high figure and significantly decrease the costs of healthcare.

Using Preventive Measures

To prevent adverse events resulting from adhesions, measures should be taken. As adhesions form merely as a result of operative procedures, preoperative measures are most important.[6] Prevention of serosal damage should be done on a routine basis.[16] The use of peritoneal lavage is not mandatory, for it has not been proven to prevent adhesion formation. It may damage the peritoneum, but it also may lower the concentration of bacteria, wash away foreign material, and minimize the inflammatory reaction. Addition of drugs such as calcium antagonists, steroids, or nonsteroids can inhibit fibrin depositions and by addition of streptokinase the fibrin depositions can be removed.[6,16,87,98] The use of peritoneal lavage is not a routine in the surveyed specialist group. It may be considered important in selected cases in which there has been contamination or infection. In a recent study, we showed a higher number of adhesions in patients with a history of an abdominal operation complicated by an abdominal abscess, hematoma, or intestinal leakage.[26]

Studies in patients undergoing relaparotomy has shown adhesions to be present between the small intestine and the laparotomy scar in a high percentage (71%–78%).[26,99] Therefore, the omentum majus placed beneath the laparotomy wound at closure of the abdomen can prevent adhesions between wound and the bowel. Suturing of the peritoneum at closure of the abdomen does not add to a successful healing. Several studies showed that the peritoneum should not be sutured to prevent local ischemia and to minimize the intraabdominal usage of suturing material, which causes a higher incidence of adhesions.[6,26,99,100] Intraabdominal foreign-body materials (suture, starch, gauze) cause a foreign-body reaction with the formation of granulomas. In the presence of granulomas the incidence of adhesions is higher.[26,99] Since the invention of starch-free gloves in 1982, these have been used by half the surveyed specialists in the Netherlands (see Table 27.5). If powder-containing gloves are used, they should be rinsed in an iodine-containing solution followed by rinsing with sterile water to remove all starch particles.[89]

Recurrent adhesions causing obstruction form a complex problem. Besides relieving the moment of obstruction by selective adhesiolysis, several methods have been developed to approach the recurrent nature of adhesions. It must be stated that it is probably needles to perform total adhesiolysis with possible serosal damage and the risk of leakage and formation of fistula or abscesses.[98] Possible techniques for prevention of recurrence of obstructive adhesions are the small intestine intubation and plication techniques, which focus on keeping the intestine in place while adhesions develop postoperatively, without causing an obstructive moment. There seems no advantage in these techniques compared to selective adhesiolysis in patients with adhesional obstructive bowel disease,[6,98] although in case of recurrent severe adhesions there might be an advantage.[100,101]

A new method is the use of a membrane to separate adjacent organs and preventing the formation of adhesions. The membrane (Seprafilm) consists of hyaluronic acid. In a recent prospective randomized study, Seprafilm was found to reduce the incidence of postsurgical adhesions.[37]

To be able to prevent adverse events resulting from abdominal adhesions and to cut back expenditures, the use of preventive measures is of utmost importance. The value of most of the measures mentioned is, however, not proven. Some preventive measures are used with high frequency; in spite of lack of proof for most of these measures, a few rules could be advocated. In elective surgery one should not close or damage the peritoneum and should avoid leaving foreign materials in the abdominal cavity. The high incidence of abdominal complaints from adhesions will be reduced only if such a routine is followed and further methods are developed to prevent the formation of adhesions. These measures will benefit the patients and at the same time significantly reduce expenditure in overall healthcare.

References

1. Palmer R. Laparoscopy in diagnosis and treatment of endometriosis and pelvic adhesions: symposium laparoscopie in de gynecologie. Ned Tijdschr Verloskd Gynaecol 1970; 70:295.
2. Fayez JA. An assessment of the role of operative laparoscopy in tuboplasty. Fertil Steril 1983;39:476–479.
3. Trimbos-Kemper T, Trimbos B, van Hall E. Etiologic factors in tubal infertility. Fertil Steril 1982;37:384–388.
4. Gomel V. An odyssey through the oviduct. Fertil Steril 1983;39:144–156.
5. Gomel V. Laparoscopic tubal surgery in infertility. Obstet Gynecol 1975;46:47.
6. Ellis H. The causes and prevention of intestinal adhesions. Br J Surg 1982;69:241–243.
7. Nemir P. Intestinal obstruction; ten-year statistical survey at the Hospital of the University of Pennsylvania. Ann Surg 1952;135:367.

8. Perry JF, Smith GA, Yonehiro EG. Intestinal obstruction caused by adhesions; a review of 388 cases. Ann Surg 1955; 142:810.
9. Becker WF. Acute adhesive ileus; a study of 412 cases with particular reference to the abuse of tube decompression in treatment. Surg Gynecol Obstet 1952;95:472.
10. Weibel MA, Majno G. Peritoneal adhesions and their relation to abdominal surgery. Am J Surg 1973;126:345–353.
11. Menzies D, Ellis H. Intestinal obstruction from adhesions—how big is the problem? Ann R Coll Surg Engl 1990;72:60–63.
12. Ray NF, Larsen JW, Stillman RJ. Economical impact of hospitalisations for lower abdominal adhesiolysis in the United States in 1988. Surg Gynecol Obstet 1993;176: 271–276.
13. Holmdahl L, Risberg B. Adhesions: prevention and complications in general surgery. Eur J Surg 1997;163: 169–174.
14. Ellis H. The aetiology of postoperative abdominal adhesions. Br J Surg 1962;50:10.
15. Ellis H, Harrison W, Hugh TB. The healing of peritoneum under normal and abnormal conditions. Br J Surg 1965; 52:471.
16. Ellis H. The cause and prevention of postoperative intraperitoneal adhesions. Surg Gynecol Obstet 1971;133: 497–511.
17. Ellis H. Wound repair—reaction of the peritoneum to injury. Ann R Coll Surg 1978;60:219–221.
18. Ellis H. Internal overhealing: the problem of intraperitoneal adhesions. World J Surg 1980;4:303–306.
19. Fabri PJ, Rosemurgy A. Reoperation for small intestinal obstruction. Surg Clin North Am 1991;71(1):131–146.
20. Zühlke HV, Lorenz EMP, Straub EM, Savvas V. Pathophysiologie und Klassifikation von Adhäsionen. Langenbecks Arch Chir Suppl II (Kongressbericht 1990):1009–1016.
21. Bevan PG. Adhesive obstruction. Ann R Coll Surg Engl 1984;66:164–169.
22. Bizer LS, Liebling RW, Delaney HM, Gliedman ML. Small bowel obstruction: the role of nonoperative treatment in simple intestinal obstruction and predictive criteria for strangulation obstruction. Surgery (St. Louis) 1981;89: 409–413.
23. Brightwell NL, McFee AS, Aust JB. Bowel obstruction and the long tube stent. Arch Surg 1977;112:505–511.
24. Diamond MP, Daniell JF, Feste J, et al. Adhesion reformation after reproductive pelvic surgery. Fertil Steril 1987; 47:864.
25. Diamond MP, Daniell JF, Alan Johns D, et al. Postoperative adhesion development after operative laparoscopy: evaluation at early second-look procedures. Fertil Steril 1991; 55(4):700–704.
26. Luijendijk RW, Lange DC, Wauters CC, et al. Foreign material in postoperative adhesions. Ann Surg 1996;3: 242–248.
27. Lehmann-Willenbroek E, Mecke H, Riedel HH. Sequelae of appendectomy, with special reference to intra-abdominal adhesions, chronic abdominal pain, and infertility. Gynecol Obstet Invest 1990;29:241–245.
28. Stewart RM, Page CP, Brender J, Schwesinger W, Eisenhut D. The incidence and risk of early postoperative small bowel obstruction: a cohort study. Am J Surg 1987;154: 643–647.
29. Coletti L, Bossart PA. Intestinal obstruction during the early postoperative period. Arch Surg 1964;88:774–778.
30. Raf LE. Causes of abdominal adhesions in cases of intestinal obstruction. Acta Chir Scand 1969;135:73–76.
31. Sykes PA, Schofield PF. Early postoperative small bowel obstruction. Br J Surg 1974;61:594–600.
32. Quatromoni JC, Rosoff L, Halls JM, Yellin AE. Early postoperative small bowel obstruction. Ann Surg 1980;191: 72–74.
33. Myllärniemi H. Foreign material in adhesion formation after abdominal surgery. A clinical and experimental study. Acta Chir Scand Suppl 1967;377:1–48.
34. Holtz G. Prevention of postoperative adhesions. J Reprod Med 1980;24:141.
35. Holtz G. Prevention and management of peritoneal adhesions. Fertil Steril 1984;41:497–507.
36. Menzies D, Ellis H. Intra-abdominal adhesions and their prevention by topical tissue plasminogen activator. J R Soc Med 1989;82:534–535.
37. Becker JM, Dayton MT, Fazio VW, et al. Prevention of postoperative abdominal adhesions by a sodium hyaluronate-based bioabsorbable membrane in the prevention of post-operative abdominal adhesions: a prospective, randomized, double-blind multicenter study. J Am Coll Surg 1996;183:297–306.
38. Thompson J. Pathogenesis and prevention of adhesion formation. Dig Surg 1998;15:153–157.
39. Dembowski T von. Ueber die Ursachen der peritonealen Adhäsionen nach chirurgischen Eingriffen mit Rücksicht auf die Frage des Ileus nach Laparotomieen. Arch Klin Chir 1888;745–766.
40. Raftery AT. Regeneration of parietal and visceral peritoneum. A light microscopical study. Br J Surg 1973;60: 293–299.
41. Milligan DW, Raftery AT. Observations on the pathogenesis of peritoneal adhesions: a light and electron microscopic study. Br J Surg 1974;61:274.
42. Buckman RF, Woods M, Sargent L, Gervin AS. A unifying pathogenic mechanism in the actiology of intraperitoneal adhesions. J Surg Res 1976;20:1–5.
43. Buckman RF, Maj MC, Buckman D, Hufnagel HV, Gervin AS. A physiologic basis for the adhesion-free healing of deperitonealized surfaces. J Surg Res 1976;21:67–76.
44. Raftery AT. Effect of peritoneal trauma on peritoneal fibrinolytic activity and intraperitoneal adhesion formation. An experimental study in the rat. Eur Surg Res 1981;13: 397–401.
45. Hau T, Payne D, Simmons RL. Fibrinolytic activity of the peritoneum during experimental peritonitis. Surg Gynecol Obstet 1979;148:415–418.
46. Vipond MN, Whawell SA, Thompson JN, Dudley HA. Peritoneal fibrinolytic activity and intra-abdominal adhesions. Lancet 1990;335:1120–1122.
47. Benzer von H, Blumel G, Piza F. Uber Zusammehange zwischen Fibrinolyse und intraperitonealen Adhesionen. Wien Klin Wochenschr 1963;75:881.
48. Hertzler AE. The Peritoneum. St. Louis: Mosby, 1919: 20–22.

49. Myhre-Jensen O, Larsen SB, Astrup T. Fibrinolytic activity in serosal and synovial membranes. Arch Pathol 1969;88: 623.
50. Porter JM, McGregor FH, Mullen DC, Silver D. Fibrinolytic activity of mesothelial surfaces. Surg Forum 1969; 20:80.
51. Gervin AS, Puckett CL, Silver D. Serosal hypofibrinolysis, a cause of postoperative adhesions. Am J Surg 1973;125: 80.
52. Unkeless JC, Gordon S, Reich E. Secretion of plasminogen activator by stimulated macrophages. J Exp Med 1974; 139:834.
53. Chapman HA Jr, Vavrin Z, Hibbs JB Jr. Coordinate expression of macrophage procoagulant and fibrinolytic activity in vitro and in vivo. J Immunol 1983;130:261–266.
54. Matsuo O, Rijken DC, Collen D. Comparison of the relative fibrinogenolytic, fibrinolytic and thrombolytic properties of tissue plasminogen activator and urokinase in vitro. Thromb Haemostasis 1981;45(3):225–229.
55. Ferres H. Preclinical pharmacological evaluation of anisoylated plaminogen streptokinase activator complex. Drugs 1987;33(3):33–50.
56. Wiman B, Collen D. Molecular mechanism of physiological fibrinolysis. Nature (Lond) 1978;272:549–550.
57. Thompson JN, Paterson-Brown S, Harbourne T, Whawell SA, Kalodiki E, Dudley HA. Reduced human peritoneal plasminogen activating activity: possible mechanism of adhesion formation. Br J Surg 1989;76:382–384.
58. Merlo G, Fausone G, Barbero C, Castagna B. Fibrinolytic activity of human peritoneum. Eur Surg Res 1980; 12: 433–438.
59. Menzies D, Ellis H. The role of plasminogen activator in adhesion prevention. Surg Gynecol Obstet 1991;172: 362–366.
60. Ryan GB, Groberty J, Majno G. Mesothelial injury and recovery. Am J Pathol 1973;71:93.
61. Raftery AT. Regeneration of peritoneum: a fibrinolytic study. J Anat 1979;129:659.
62. Doody KJ, Dunn RL, Buttram VC. Recombinant tissue plasminogen activator reduces adhesion formation in a rabbit uterine horn model. Fertil Steril 1989;51:509–512.
63. Dunn RC, Buttram VC. Tissue-type plasminogen activator as an adjuvant for post surgical adhesions. Prog Clin Biol Res 1990;358:113–118.
64. Dorr PJ, Vemer HM, Brommer EJP, Willemsen WNP, Veldhuizen RW, Rolland R. Prevention of postoperative adhesions by tissue-type plasminogen activator (t-PA) in the rabbit. Eur J Obstet Gynecol Reprot Biol 1990;37:287–291.
65. Ellis H. The hazards of surgical glove dusting powders. Surg Gynecol Obstet 1990;171:521–527.
66. Down RHL, Whitehead R, Watts JMcK. Do surgical packs cause peritoneal adhesions? Aust N Z J Surg 1979;49: 379–382.
67. Holtz G. Adhesion induction by suture of varying tissue reactivity and caliber. Int J Fertil 1982;27:134–135.
68. Elkins TE, Stovall TG, Warren J, et al. A histologic evaluation of peritoneal injury and repair: implications for adhesion formation. Obstet Gynecol 1987;70:225–228.
69. Saxén L, Myllärniemi H. Foreign material and postoperative adhesions. N Engl J Med 1968;279:200–202.
70. McEntee GP, Stuart RC, Byrne PJ, Leen E, Hennessy TP. Experimental study of starch-induced intraperitoneal adhesions. Br J Surg 1990;77:1113–1114.
71. Jagelman DG, Ellis H. Starch and intraperitoneal adhesion formation. Br J Surg 1973;60:111–114.
72. Myllärniemi H, Frilander M, Turunen M, Saxén L. The effect of glove powders and their constituents on adhesion and granuloma formation in the abdominal cavity of the rabbit. Acta Chir Scan. 1966;131:312–398.
73. Nordstrand K, Melhus O, Eide TJ, Larsen T, Giercksky KE. Intra-abdominal granuloma reaction in rats after introduction of maize-starch powder. Acta Pathol Microbiol Immunol Scand 1937;95:93–98.
74. Davies JD, Neely J. The histopathology of peritoneal starch granulomas. J Pathol 1972;107:265–278.
75. Postlethwait RW, Howard HL, Schanher PW. Comparison of tissue reaction to talc and modified starch glove powder. Surgery (St. Louis) 1949;25:22–29.
76. Postlethwait RW, McRae J, Williams RW, Deaton WR, Cornatzer WE. Absorbable starch glove powder. Am J Surg 1949;78:510–513.
77. Ryan GB, Grobety J, Majno G. Postoperative peritoneal adhesions. A study of the mechanisms. Am J Pathol 1971; 65:117–148.
78. Walker EM. Effects of blood, bile and starch in the peritoneal cavity of the rat. J Anat 1978;126:495–507.
79. Nisell H, Larsson B. Role of blood and fibrinogen in development of intraperitoneal adhesions in rats. Fertil Steril 1978;30:470–473.
80. Lee CM, Collins WT, Largen TL. A reappraisal of absorbable glove powder. Surg Gynecol Obstet 1952;95: 725–728.
81. Cooke SAR, Hamilton DG. The significance of starch powder contamination in the aetiology of peritoneal adhesions. Br J Surg 1977;64:410–412.
82. Cox KR. Starch granuloma (pseudo-malignant seedlings). Br J Surg 1979;57:650–653.
83. Lee CM, Lehman EP. Experiments with non-irritating glove powder. Surg Gynecol Obstet 1947;84:689–695.
84. Storey BG, Lawrence KB, Chant S, et al. Factors influencing the incidence of postoperative abdominal adhesions: an experimental study. Aust N Z J Surg 1971;40:388.
85. Jaffray DC, Nade S. Does surgical glove powder decrease the inoculum of bacteria required to produce an abscess? J R Coll Surg Edinb 1983;28(4):219–222.
86. Almdahl SM, Burhol PG. Peritoneal adhesions: causes and prevention. Dig Dis 1990;8:37–44.
87. Keeman JN. Recurrent obstructive ileus due to adhesions. Neth J Med 1987;131:1509–1512.
88. Kent SJS, Burnand KG, Owen DA. A method of removing starch powder from surgeon's gloves. Ann R Coll Surg Engl 1975;57:212–214.
89. Fraser I. Simple and effective method of removing starch powder from surgical gloves. Br Med J 1982;284:1835.
90. Davies JD, Neely J. The histopathology of peritoneal starch granulomas. J Pathol 1972;107:265–278.
91. Scott-Coombes, Thompson JN, Vipond MN. General surgeons' attitudes to the treatment and prevention of abdominal adhesions. Ann R Coll Surg Engl 1993;75: 123–128.

92. Boerrighter OJ. Organische Bedrijfsrekening. University Hospital Rotterdam: Dijkzigt and Sophia Childrens Hospital, 1993.
93. Horngren CT, Foster G. Cost Accounting and Managerial Emphasis, 7th Ed. London: Prentice Hall, 1991.
94. Christen D, Buchmann P. Peritoneal adhesions after laparotomy: prophylactic measures. Hepato-Gastroenterology 1991;38:283–286.
95. Hershlag A, Diamond MP, DeCherney AH. Adhesiolysis. Clin Obstet Gynecol 1991;34:395–402.
96. Buschbach JJ. The Validity of QUALY's. Arnhem, The Netherlands: Gouda Quint, 1994.
97. National Hospital Institute. Intramural Healthcare The Netherlands: Utrecnt, 1994.
98. Menzies D. Peritoneal adhesions, incidence, cause and prevention. Surg Annu 1992;24:27–45.
99. Luijendijk RW, Wauters CCAP, Jeekel J. Intra-abdominal adhesions and foreigh-body granulomas after previous laparotomy. Neth J Med 1994;138:717–720.
100. Wittens C, Munting J, Lens J. Intraluminal Miller-Abbott tube stenting as treatment and profylaxis of recurrent intestinal obstruction. Neth J Surg 1990;42(5):123–127.
101. Ramsey-Stewart G, Shun A. Nasogastrointestinal intraluminal tube stenting in the prevention of recurrent small bowel obstruction. Aust N Z J Surg 1983;53:7–11.

28

Outcome Measures and Adhesion Formation: Pain and Postsurgical Adhesion

David M.B. Rosen and Christopher J.G. Sutton

CONTENTS

Adhesions within the peritoneal cavity may occur secondary to endometriosis, pelvic inflammatory disease, the presence of foreign material (such as sutures) or any other cause of pelvic inflammation such as perforated appendix, or, most commonly, following intraabdominal surgery. Adhesions are known to be associated with infertility,[1] and acute bowel obstruction, and they can deleteriously alter the efficacy of intraperitoneal chemotherapy. In addition, a major impact is their supposed association with chronic pain of the abdominal and pelvic cavities. Most surgeons and gynecologists no doubt have performed laparotomy or laparoscopy and adhesiolysis for patients with known or suspected adhesions and chronic pain, and indeed many of these patients may have had symptomatic improvement following their surgery. We are uncertain if this results from the surgery itself or is a placebo effect. The aim of this chapter is to consider the available evidence and to try to determine if adhesions do indeed cause pain.

Mechanism of Formation of Postsurgical Adhesions

To answer the question as to whether adhesions are associated with abdominal and pelvic pain, we must first decide if there exists a pathophysiologic mechanism by which they *can* cause pain. To do this, let us examine the mechanism for postsurgical adhesion formation. It is thought that adhesions represent a breakdown in the normal process of intraperitoneal healing and repair. Although this has been covered elsewhere in this volume, let us briefly summarize the known process.

Following surgical disruption of the delicate peritoneal surfaces, a coagulum of exudated peritoneal fluid forms at the site,[2] with release of chemotactic factors responsible for the recruitment of a variety of white blood cells, mesothelial cells, and fibrin. As in the normal process of healing macrophages soon replace these leukocytes, and they in turn are responsible for recruiting mesothelial cells from deeper layers toward the surface. In contrast to healing of skin wounds, the peritoneum is repaired by proliferation from these islands of mesothelial cells, with reepithelialization completed by 5 to 7 days.[1] The fibrin mesh thus formed is normally dissolved by these infiltrating cells once reepithelialization is complete. Fibrinolysis occurs by the conversion of fibrin to fibrin degradation products after stimulation by plasmin. Anything adversely affecting fibrinolysis at any stage of the process is likely to result in adhesion formation. Factors implicated include those events that cause tissue ischemia—suturing, diathermy injury, or peritoneal tissue grafts—all associated with the postsurgical environment.[1]

In the absence of adequate fibrinolysis it is thought that the adhesions persist. One theory holds that adhesion formation represents a continuous process commencing with weak filmy adhesions. These become organized with proliferation of fibroblasts, which lay down collagen, eventually leading to the formation of more permanent adhesions.[3] Kligman et al.[4] took this process a step further. They examined adhesions taken from 17 patients, 10 with chronic pelvic pain (CPP) and 7 without, and found evidence of nerve fibers within the adhesions of 10 of the 17 cases studied. While not proving the association between pain and adhesions, because these nerve fibers were distributed evenly between the two groups of patients, this finding does provide an explanation for one possible mechanism by which pain could be caused by adhesions. The authors hypothesized that the final stage of adhesion maturation is represented by organization of the adhesion with vascularization and establishment of their own innervation. Unfortunately, no mention was made in this paper of the length of time the adhesions were thought to have been present, nor how long this process of organization and maturation need be. Presumably, however, the process requires months to years, and as such we need to bear this in mind when analyzing studies that concern the link between adhesions and pain or pain relief following adhesiolysis, because it may be that only older adhesions (and therefore the ones more likely to be innervated) are the only ones associated with pain.

A second theory linking pain and adhesions is that of Kresch et al., published in 1984.[5] They compared laparoscopic findings in a study of 100 women with a history of CPP in the same location for at least 6 months with 50 asymptomatic women undergoing laparoscopy for tubal ligation. They found demonstrable pelvic pathology in 83% of the former group, of whom 38% had adhesions and 32% endometriosis, compared with only 29% in the asymptomatic group (12% adhesions, 15% endometriosis). Their finding of greatest significance was that the nature of adhesions differed between the symptomatic and asymptomatic groups. Adhesions in the group of patients complaining of chronic pain were more likely to restrict the motion of pelvic organs, specifically bowel expansibility, than the looser adhesions found in asymptomatic patients. This then represents a second mechanism for pain caused by adhesions, one that may complement the earlier theory of adhesion innervation. Again, it is a factor we must keep in mind when analyzing those studies claiming an association (or lack thereof) between adhesions and pain.

Adhesion Formation: Laparotomy or Laparoscopy?

Before examining the question of whether adhesions cause postsurgical pain, we should briefly look at their etiology. It is known that laparotomy is associated with postsurgical adhesion formation, occurring in 60% to 100% of women after major gynecologic surgery.[6,7] Does the more recent introduction of laparoscopic surgery mean we shall see a reduction in the extent of postoperative adhesion formation? Theoretically, a reduction in the air-drying effect on the peritoneal surfaces, reduced handling of the bowel and peritoneum, and meticulous hemostatsis should lead to a reduced incidence of postsurgical adhesion formation. Diamond et al.[2] found that the incidence of adhesions at a second-look procedure within 90 days after operative laparoscopy was 97.1%. These 68 women underwent adhesiolysis at the primary laparoscopy, although no mention was made of the origin of the adhesions in these women. Despite the high rate of recurrence of adhesions, the mean adhesion scores were reduced by 52% (from 11.4% to 5.5%) and, most significantly, de novo adhesion formation at sites not known to have adhesions at the time of laparoscopic adhesiolysis was only 12%. That is, while adhesion formation and reformation after operative laparoscopy are high, the extent and severity of those adhesions are decreased. Unfortunately, the short time scale for second-look procedures may bias the results, as we have already discussed; namely, the reformed thin filmy adhesions may be on the path to becoming organized, dense adhesions. Nevertheless, we may make the following conclusions: laparoscopy is less likely to cause adhesions within a previously untouched peritoneal cavity than is laparotomy, and once adhesions are present there seems very little we can do about eradicating them permanently. This realization highlights the need for a reliable method of adhesion prevention.

Adhesions and Pain

There are few gynecologists or surgeons who have not performed an adhesiolysis on a patient under their care to alleviate chronic pain of unknown cause. Many have found surgery to be of help with a resultant reduction in chronic pain, and it would be advantageous if we were able to confidently predict freedom from pain in all such cases. Unfortunately, the association between chronic pain and adhesions remains incompletely proven at best, and many have challenged the accepted notion that adhesions cause pain. The oft-quoted editorial by J. Alexander-Williams, an eminent surgeon from Birmingham, England, in the British Medical Journal of March 1987 summarizes this argument. He believed "it to be a poorly substantiated myth that adhesions cause abdominal or pelvic pain".[8] In the face of such skepticism we must address the issue from a more scientific rather than an anecdotal viewpoint. As most of the studies in the literature on this subject are concerned with the association between chronic *pelvic* pain and adhesive disease, we shall use this as the model for our study of the association between adhesions and pain.

To conclusively demonstrate that adhesions, postsurgical or otherwise, are a cause of chronic pelvic pain (CPP), one would need to show:

1. That some patients with CPP have adhesions and that some patients with adhesions have CPP
2. That patients without CPP have no adhesions
3. That in those patients with adhesions and CPP, lysis of adhesions results in reduced levels of pain
4. That adhesiolysis reduces pain in these patients better than placebo

Studies on Patients with Chronic Pelvic Pain

Although there is no strict definition of CPP, making analysis of the literature difficult, in broad terms CPP refers to the presence of symptomatic, intractable noncyclic pelvic pain of at least 6 (some studies say 3) months in duration, causing functional disability.[9] Some authors add the proviso that it is not treatable by simple analgesia. A number of pathologic entities have been implicated as a cause for CPP, including endometriosis, chronic pelvic inflammatory disease, pelvic congestion, and ovarian pathology among other causes. Although some conditions, such as the pelvic congestion syndrome, have been suspected of bearing a tenuous relationship at best to CPP,[9] pain associated with adhesions has advocates both for and against.

Cunanan et al.[10] retrospectively reviewed the records of 1194 women who had undergone diagnostic laparoscopy for CPP. Of these, 229 (19.2%) had adhesions as the primary pathology, and 96.5% gave a history of previous surgery (with only 34% of patients having an abnormal preoperative pelvic examination). They also found 355 patients (29.7%) with no pelvic pathology at laparoscopy despite a history of pelvic pain. These findings support those of Rapkin,[11] who retrospectively reviewed 100 laparoscopies for CPP and compared them to 89 undertaken for infertility. She found pelvic adhesions in 26% of the group of patients with CPP and 39% of those with infertility but no pain. Perhaps this discrepancy may be explained by referring to the previous section on possible pain mechanisms, it being the *nature* of the adhesions that defines the difference in pain reported, rather than merely the presence or absence of adhesions themselves. This theory however is not supported by Rapkin. Unlike the study by Cunanan et al. (which described only the presence or absence of adhesions), Rapkin classified these adhesions with respect to their characteristics, finding dense adhesions in 50% of those with CPP and in 53% of the infertility patients with no pain. Furthermore, no significant differences between the two groups were found in either the site of these adhesions or the density of the adhesions.

Does this put to rest any connection between CPP and adhesions? Surely if the incidence of adhesions in those with CPP is the same as those without reported pain, then some pathology other than adhesions is causing the pain? MacDonald and Sutton[3] believed these findings to be inherently biased in that infertility patients are likely to have adhesions and were selected by the design of the study to a group not reporting pain. They suggested a more accurate study would be to compare a group of CPP sufferers with women undergoing, for example, tubal ligation.

Fortunately, this study has been done. In a 1997 paper from the United Kingdom, 297 women were prospectively studied at laparoscopy for sterilization (105), infertility (61), or CPP (132) defined as pain of at least 3 months duration.[12] Photographs of five pelvic regions were taken before any surgical procedure and were then independently reviewed by two gynecologists unaware of the indication for laparoscopy. A single "pelvic pathology score" was then agreed upon, which was compared to the surgeons' intraoperative diagnosis. The study failed to show any correlation between a preoperative diagnosis of CPP and the presence of adhesions, finding 6.7% of those undergoing laparoscopic sterilization having adhesive disease compared with 4.5% of those with CPP (and 6.6% in the infertility group). Unfortunately, even this information, although a group of symptomatic and one of asymptomatic patients were compared, is not definitive. The lack of real-time analysis (by videotape, for example) makes accurate description of pelvic pathology more difficult on two-dimensional photographs alone, and the adhesions in this study were not classified according to site or characteristics. Nonetheless the evidence presented suggests that adhesions are found as often in patients without pain as in those with it.

The argument however does not end there. Kontoravdis et al.[13] prospectively analyzed the laparoscopic findings of 2365 women under their care who had undergone laparoscopy for acute or chronic pelvic pain. They found adhesions in 35.4% of those with CPP as the primary diagnosis, compared with no pathologic findings in 24% of these women. Similarly, Kresch et al.[5] found pain associated with adhesions of the bowel or reproductive organs in 48% of those with CPP, compared with 14% in those with adhesions but no pain. Most significantly, Kresch et al. believed the quality of these adhesions differed, with those patients reporting pain having adhesions that restricted the motion or distension of pelvic organs compared with looser, filmy adhesions in those not reporting pain. Unfortunately, no breakdown of the results was provided to support this latter contention.

Perhaps the best way of determining if adhesions are causing the pain experienced by the patient is for the patient herself to tell us. Almeida and Val-Gallas[14] found that 80.6% (25 of 31) of women with adhesions undergoing conscious pain mapping reported tenderness on manipulation of these adhesions. The adhesions were described as "significant" although no details of site or nature were provided. Furthermore, the degree of conscious sedation may have compromised self-reporting under the influence of the anesthetic agents used, especially Fentanyl (dosage, 250–500 μg), and many patients had combined pathology. We cannot therefore be certain that the pain reported on mobilization of the adhesions was the result of the adhesion alone or identical to that experienced while the patient was fully conscious. Nonetheless, the results do lend weight to the argument that some adhesions at least are associated with pain. On the basis of the evidence available, therefore, the best we can say is that adhesions *may* cause CPP.

Studies on Chronic Pelvic Pain After Adhesiolysis

It is important to keep in mind, when looking at these studies, that despite laparoscopic or microsurgical techniques reformation of adhesions occurs in as many as 95% of cases.[7] Thus, any study of pain relief after adhesiolysis must be analyzed with regard to the time that has elapsed between the adhesiolysis and reassessment of pain. As previously, it would also be useful to know the nature of the adhesions lysed to determine whether lysis of all adhesions brought symptomatic relief (or otherwise), or whether it is only the denser adhesions whose removal brings benefit.

Peters et al.[15] divided women with CPP and anything more severe than thin filmy adhesions into two groups. Twenty-four women underwent laparotomy via a low midline incision and adhesiolysis, while an equal number were controls who had no surgery other than the initial diagnostic laparoscopy before randomization. The groups were comparable in terms of preoperative pain score and stage of adhesions. They were then assessed by a blinded observer 9 to 12 months after surgery. No significant difference between the two groups at the postoperative assessment of pain or daily lifestyle disturbance was found by objective and subjective analyses; however, those with stage 4 adhesions (dense vascularized adhesions involving one or more peritoneal organs or serosa of the small or large intestine) showed a beneficial effect after adhesiolysis, a benefit not seen in those with a lesser degree of adhesive disease.

Chan and Wood also followed up their infertility patients, 43 of whom had reported chronic abdominal pain, after microsurgical adhesiolysis.[16] The minimum duration of follow-up was 6 months. They found 65.1% of their patients reported (subjective) improvement or cure of their pain, although 11.6% reported more severe pain. They believed the improvement may be the result of a correction of subacute bowel obstruction, correction of fixed uterine retroversion, mobilization of pelvic organs including the ovaries or bowel in the pouch of Douglas, or removal or abnormal organs such as cysts or hydrosalpinges. Although the severity of adhesions in the infertility patients was hinted at (described as enveloping the ovaries, thus preventing ovum pickup), no mention was made of the degree of adhesions in those women with CPP.

The review of laparoscopic adhesiolysis shows more promising results. Sutton and MacDonald[17] reported 84% pain relief at least 1 year (range, 1–5 years) after adhesiolysis via the CO_2 laser using probes with back stops to stop onward transmission of laser energy (Figs. 28.1 and 28.2), with only seven patients showing no improvement, two of whom had residual adhesions at a second-look procedure. Unfortunately the study was retrospective, the cases were not controlled, and the assessment of pain relief or relapse was symptomatic; also, no mention was made of the severity of pelvic adhesions. They did, however, make the observation that symptomatic improvement was more likely if the adhesions were tight bands immobilizing a segment of bowel and if the site correlated with the described site of maximal pain (Fig. 28.3). Similar findings, reported by Nezhat et al.[18] in an abstract to the American Association of Gynecology and Laparoscopy (AAGL), indicated complete pain relief in approximately half of those women ($n = 48$) followed up for 6 to 24 months following laparoscopic adhesiolysis for "severe" adhesions. Steege and Stout,[19] in a prospective uncontrolled trial of a laparoscopic adhesiolysis for 34 women with CPP for at least 6 months, found not only that pain location overlapped with the location of adhesions in 90% of cases, but also that 19 of 30

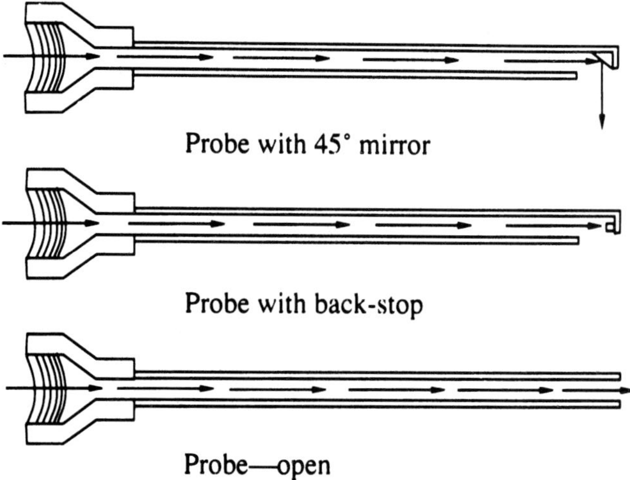

FIGURE 28.1. Probes used with CO_2 laser at the Royal Surrey County Hospital.

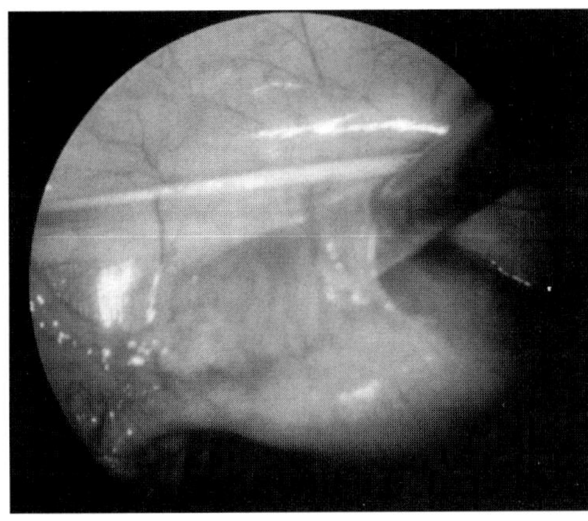

FIGURE 28.2. Use of laser probe with backstop for adhesiolysis.

(63%) patients reported improvement of daily pain or dyspareunia at their 6- to 12-month follow-up. It should be noted however that pain returned to at least 50% of preoperative levels within 2 to 5 months post adhesiolysis in 7 patients despite initial improvement. These patients were more likely to have bowel adhesions, although numbers were insufficient to confirm this statistically. Nezhat et al. concluded that adhesions involving the intestine may be more likely to be implicated in causing CPP than adhesions at other sites, in concordance with the theories of Kresch et al. Furthermore, they subdivided patients with CPP into two groups, one with CPP alone (20) and one with "chronic pelvic syndrome." The latter is defined as consisting or more of the following:

1. Pain at least 6 months in duration
2. Incomplete relief from previous treatment (either surgery or analgesia)

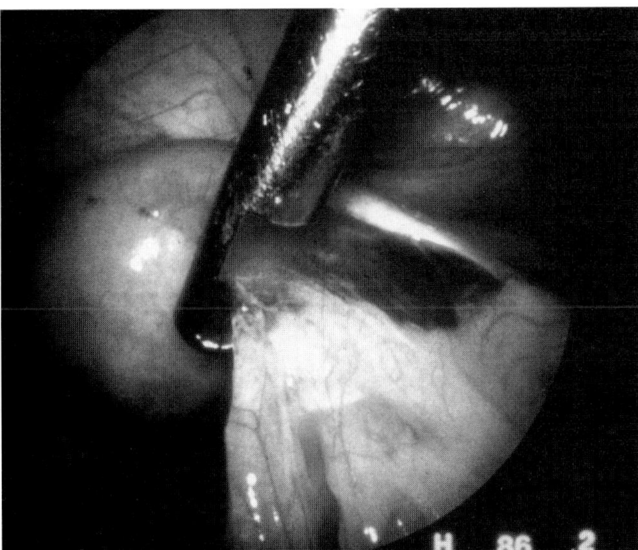

FIGURE 28.3. Adhesion restricting bowel mobility.

3. Impaired physical functioning
4. At least one vegetative sign of depression (loss of appetite, sleep disturbance, psychomotor retardation)
5. Altered family role

When patients falling within this category were excluded, adhesiolysis resulted in pain relief in up to 75% of women. This finding may point to the future direction we should take in our management of patients suffering from chronic pain.

Who Will Benefit from Adhesiolysis?

The Foregoing evidence suggests that some but not all patients with adhesions may benefit from adhesiolysis. Can we predict which patients these will be? Stovall et al.[20] Stated that we cannot. They attempted to detect links between preoperative historical and physical findings and pelvic adhesions. Of 273 patients having laparoscopy, 176 had no historical predictors (previous abdominopelvic surgery, pelvic inflammatory disease, endometriosis, etc.). Of these, 47 (26.7%) had adhesions, that is, a false-negative rate greater than 25% on history alone. On the other hand, a single historical predictor was associated with adhesions in 50% of patients, although the nature of these adhesions was not detailed. Two or more historical predictors did not significantly increase the chance of adhesive disease being present. The only significant associations on physical examination were with right adnexal tenderness, a right adnexal mass, and uterine immobility. Seventy-six of 247 patients with a normal preoperative examination had adhesions at laparoscopy, a false-negative rate of 32%. The presence of two or more positive physical findings was associated with adhesions in 74% of patients at laparoscopy. Further, of 168 patients with both negative physical examination and history, 43 had adhesions, a 25.6% false-negative rate for this combination.

Looking at the positive aspects of this study, the implication is that in 50.8% of cases a positive historical factor or two or more positive physical findings will be associated with adhesions at laparoscopy. Unfortunately, however, it provides little clinical assistance because one-quarter of those without either historical features or physical signs still will have adhesive disease. More importantly, it gets us no closer to deciding whether adhesions are associated with CPP because only 20 patients (7.4%) underwent laparoscopy for CPP, and although 12 of these (60%) had adhesions compared with 83 of 243 undergoing laparoscopy for sterilization (34%), 80% (4 of 5) of those with infertility as a primary diagnosis had adhesions.

Conclusions

This review of the available research and scientific literature enables us to draw the following conclusions:

1. Adhesions can contain nerve fibers and appear to undergo a process of maturation from filmy to dense, vascularized, and possibly innervated adhesions.[4]
2. Adhesions are present in women with CPP and no other pathology, but not consistently and not always.[5,10,11]
3. Women with adhesions complain of CPP in approximately 25% of cases; however, about 17% of those with no pain also have adhesions.[9]
4. Adhesiolysis reduces pain in 50% to 80% of women with CPP and adhesions.[17–19]
5. Those patients with severe adhesions achieve better long-term relief from pain than those with a lesser degree of adhesions, suggesting the former may be more likely to be associated with CPP.[15]
6. Those adhesions restricting distension and movement of pelvic organs, especially bowel, are more likely to be associated with CPP.[5,17]

To formulate a coherent plan of management for such patients remains difficult. Perhaps we are closer now to an understanding of the significance of severe versus coincidental and insignificant adhesions. We know that once formed adhesions tend to reform, although perhaps at an earlier stage than those that were removed before progression and maturation. We also know that the incidence of new adhesion formation after laparoscopic surgery is low (12%) compared with laparotomy. Thus our strategies for the future should include the following measures:

1. Replacing laparotomy with laparoscopy when possible to reduce the formation of adhesions in the first place
2. Finding a suitable adhesion barrier to reduce the de novo formation of adhesions, a subject covered at length elsewhere in this volume
3. Approaching the issue of CPP and adhesions from a more holistic viewpoint

It is interesting to quote Kresch[5] from 1984, deriding ". . . the temptation to ascribe chronic pelvic pain to a psychogenic origin, (resulting in) some patients (being) referred for psychotherapy . . ."

Within 9 years this attitude had completely reversed. In a 1993 review article, Punch and Roth concluded that a multidisciplinary approach may be required in the face of equivocal data on the association of adhesions with CPP and thus the potential benefits of adhesiolysis.[21] They suggested the goal should be pain "management" rather than the "painfree state." As we have seen, in the absence of a definitive association between CPP and adhesive disease, it may be wise to resist the temptation to tell our patients who have CPP and adhesions that surgery alone is the answer. Finally, it may be worthwhile to keep the paper by Steege and Stout in mind[19] and to be on the lookout for those patients with a preoperative diagnosis of chronic pain syndrome, in whom preoperative counseling and adjuvant therapy may be warranted to achieve the best possible outcome at surgery.

We have concentrated on pelvic pain because that is where the bulk of evidence in the medical literature lies, but there is no reason to assume that this information cannot be extrapolated to include postsurgical adhesions in the upper abdomen and also to men as well as women. Our initial work on laparoscopic laser adhesiolysis was rejected in a peer review process conducted by the British Medical Journal on the grounds that the subjects were entirely women. This statement ignored the fact that it would be impossible for gynecologists to recruit male patients but not that general surgeons regularly perform laparoscopic adhesiolysis. The time has surely come to conduct well-designed randomized prospective trials in men and women who present with pain believed to be caused by intraabdominal adhesions.

References

1. diZerega GS. Biochemical events in peritoneal tissue repair. Eur J Surg 1997;S577:10–16.
2. Diamond MP, De Cherney AH. Pathogenesis of adhesion formation/reformation: application to reproductive surgery. Microsurgery 1987;8:103–107.
3. MacDonald R, Sutton CJG. Adhesions and laser laparoscopic adhesiolysis. In: Sutton CJG, ed. Lasers in Gynaecology. London: Chapman & Hall, 1992:95–113.
4. Kligman I, Drachenberg C, Papadimitriou J, Katz E. Immunohistochemical demonstration of nerve fibers in pelvic adhesions. Obstet Gynecol 1993;82:566–568.
5. Kresch AJ, Seifer DB, Sachs LB, Barrese I. Laparoscopy in 100 women with chronic pelvic pain. Obstet Gynecol 1984; 64:672–674.
6. Monk BJ, Berman ML, Montz FJ. Adhesions after extensive gynecologic surgery: clinical significance, etiology and prevention. Am J Obstet Gynecol 1994;170: 1396–1403.
7. Operative Laparoscopy Study Group. Postoperative adhesion development after operative laparoscopy: evaluation at early second-look procedures. Fertil Steril 1991;55: 700–704.
8. Alexander-Williams J. Do adhesions cause pain? Br Med J 1987;294:659–660.
9. Howard FM. The role of laparoscopy in chronic pelvic pain: promise and pitfalls. Obstet Gynecol Surv 1993;48: 357–387.
10. Cunanan RG, Courey NG, Lippes J. Laparoscopic findings in patients with pelvic pain. Am J Obstet Gynecol 1983; 146:587–591.
11. Rapkin AJ. Adhesions and pelvic pain: a Retrospective Study. Obstet Gynecol 1986;68:13–15.

12. Thornton JG, Morley S, Lilleyman J, Onwude JL, Currie I, Crompton AC. The relationship between laparoscopic disease, pelvic pain and infertility; an unbiased assessment. Eur J Obstet Gynaecol Reprod Biol 1997;74:57–62.
13. Kontoravdis A, Chryssikopoulos A, Hassiakos D, Liapis A, Zourlas PA. The diagnostic value of laparoscopy in 2635 patients with acute and chronic pelvic pain. Int J Gynecol Obstet 1996;52:243–248.
14. Almeida OD, Val-Gallas JM. Conscious pain mapping. J Am Assoc Gynecol Laparosc 1997;4:587–590.
15. Peters AAW, Trimbos-Kemper GCM, Admiraal C, Trimbos JB, Hermans J. A randomized clinical trial on the benefit of adhesiolysis in patients with intraperitoneal adhesions and chronic pelvic pain. Br J Obstet Gynaecol 1992;99: 59–62.
16. Chan CLK, Wood C. Pelvic adhesiolysis—the assessment of symptom relief by 100 patients. Aust N Z J Obstet Gynaecol 1985;25:295–298.
17. Sutton C, MacDonald R. Laser laparoscopic adhesiolysis. J Gynecol Surg 1990;6:155–159.
18. Nezhat CR, Nezhat FR, Swan AE. Long-term outcome of laparoscopic adhesiolysis in women with chronic pelvic pain after hysterectomy. J Am Assoc Gynecol Laparosc 1996;3:S33–S34.
19. Steege JF, Stout AL. Resolution of chronic pelvic pain after laparoscopic lysis of adhesions. Am J Obstet Gynecol 1991; 165:278–283.
20. Stovall TG, Elder RF, Ling FW. Predictors of pelvic adhesions. J Reprod Med 1989;34:345–348.
21. Punch MR, Roth RS. Adhesions and chronic pain: an overview of pain and a discussion of adhesions and pelvic pain. Prog Clin Biol Res 1993;381:101–120.

29

Infertility and Adhesions

Riccardo Marana and Ludovico Muzii

CONTENTS

Pelvic adhesions may be the cause of bowel obstruction, pelvic pain, and infertility. Tubal factor infertility accounts for approximately 40% of the cases of female infertility.[1] Identifiable causes of tubal infertility are postinfectious tubal damage, endometriosis-related adhesions, and postsurgical adhesion formation.

Adhesion formation in the abdominal cavity can result from direct tissue trauma, drying of the serosa, ischemia, hemorrhage, presence of foreign bodies, raw surfaces, and infection. All these factors may contribute to the formation of adhesions after pelvic surgery. Even when surgery is properly performed, in strict adherence to microsurgical principles, postoperative adhesions develop de novo in more than 50% of cases.[2] Adhesion reformation may occur at 40% to 71% of the operated sites.[2] Postoperative adhesion formation may therefore plague the results of infertility surgery and is thus a major concern for the reproductive surgeon.

The aim of reproductive surgery is to restore normal anatomic relationships between the fimbriae and the ovary to allow ovum pickup. However, although reproductive surgery may be successful in restoring normal anatomy, it may not be able to provide a normal function to the tubal mucosa. An inverse correlation between the degree of adhesions and subsequent pregnancy rates has traditionally been reported.[3,4] Recently, however, as is discussed later, the status of the tubal mucosa, regardless of the presence of peritubal adhesions, has been reported to be of major prognostic significance.[5-9]

Classifications of Adhesions

In 1979, Caspi et al.[3] proposed a classification of periadnexal adhesions, and reported a 71% pregnancy rate in patients with grade I adhesions (localized, fine adhesions, mostly avascular, limited to small areas of the tubes or ovaries), 50% in grade II adhesions (extensive, fine adhesions, mostly avascular, involving large portions of the tubes and ovaries), 29% in grade III adhesions (localized, fibrous, mostly vascular adhesions, limited to small areas of the tubes or ovaries), and 20% in grade IV adhesions (extensive, fibrous, mostly vascular adhesions, involving large portions of the tubes and ovaries). The authors concluded that the pregnancy rate was inversely related to the grade of periadnexal adhesions, although differences in pregnancy rates were not statistically significant.

In 1982, Hulka et al.[4] proposed a staging system for adnexal adhesions based both on the extent (stage I and stage II) and nature (type A and type B) of the adhesions. The authors reported a significant correlation between adhesion extent and subsequent pregnancy rates, with a 46% term pregnancy rate in patients with stage I adhesions (more than 50% of the ovarian surface visible) versus 4% in patients with stage II adhesions (less than 50% of the ovarian surface visible). As to the nature of the adhesions, however, they found no difference in term pregnancy rate between patients with type A (filmy, avascular adhesions with good potential organ separation) and patients with type B adhesions (dense, vascular adhesions with minimal potential organ separation).

Also in cases of distal tubal occlusion (DTO), pregnancy outcome after reconstructive tubal surgery is thought to be related to the extent of tubal disease and of pelvic adhesions.[5] Based on various parameters, several classification systems have been proposed to assess the extent of tubal disease so as to predict pregnancy outcome.[10–12] However, none of the devised classifications has included a direct evaluation of the status of the ampullary mucosa among the parameters, although the status of the endosalpinx could be the most important prognostic factor in terms of reproductive outcome.

The American Fertility Society (AFS; now the American Society for Reproductive Medicine) proposed a scoring system in 1988[13] that is today the classification system most used. The scoring system is based on the following parameters: extent and type of adhesions in case of pelvic adhesions, and, in addition for the classification of DTO, thickness and rigidity of the tubal wall, distal ampullary diameter, and percentage of muscosal folds preserved at the neostomy site. The importance of intraoperative salpingoscopy to visualize the entire length of the ampullary mucosa as an important prognostic parameter was recognized. However, salpingoscopic findings were not included in the score system because salpingoscopy was being practiced in very few centers at that time.

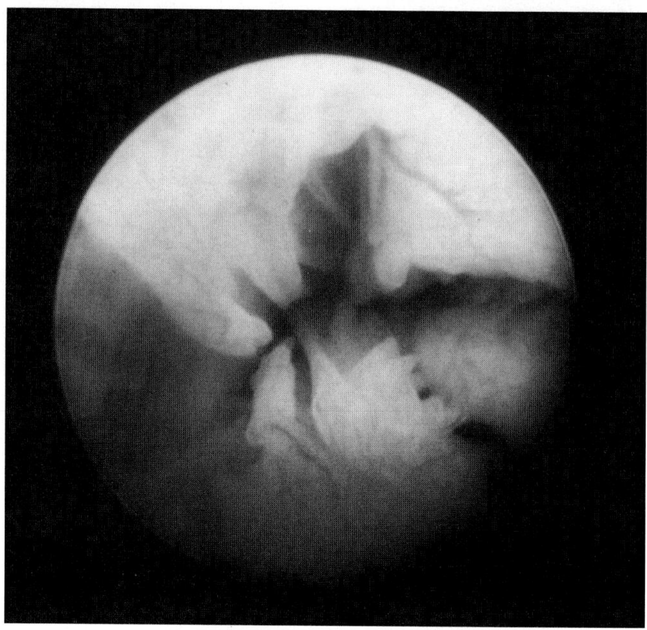

FIG. 29.1. Normal tubal mucosa as seen at salpingoscopy.

Salpingoscopy in the Evaluation of Infertility

At our institution, intraoperative salpingoscopy has been performed since 1989, in the early years of our experience at microsurgery by laparotomy,[8] and then also at operative laparoscopy for adnexal disease (Marana et al., in manuscript), for the evaluation of ampullary tubal mucosa as a prognostic factor in terms of subsequent pregnancy outcome.

To perform salpingoscopy we use a rigid salpingoscope that, when utilized during operative laparoscopy, is introduced into the abdominal cavity through the operating channel of a laser laproscope. The instruments used consist of the 2.8-mm rigid salpingoscope with an outer sheath and a 2.8-mm obturator with a rounded tip. The outer sheath is connected through an intravenous infusion set to a Ringer's lactate solution flask placed approximately 1 m above the patient's level. Under laparoscopic vision, the tube to be examined is aligned with the axis of the laparoscope. The abdominal ostium of the tube is then identified and cannulated with the outer sheath of the salpingoscope containing the rounded-tip obturator. The distal end of the tube is clamped around the outer sheath by means of an atraumatic tube holding forceps introduced through the suprapubic trocar sleeve. The obturator is withdrawn and replaced by the salpingoscope. The connection with the Ringer's lactate is opened so that the flow of the solution moderately distends the tubal wall; the salpingoscope is advanced under direct vision allowing a clear view of the mucosa.

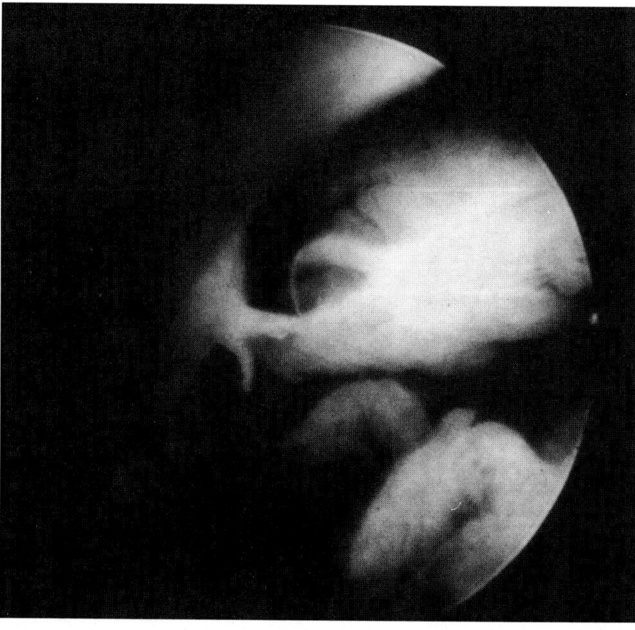

FIG. 29.2. A grade III tube with focal adhesions between the mucosal folds.

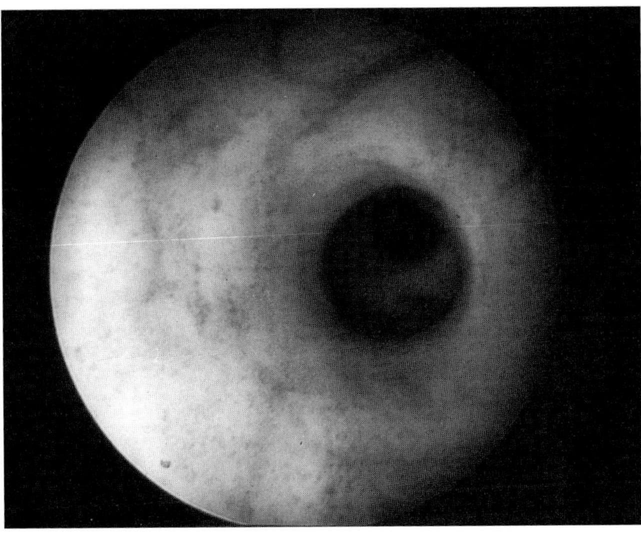

Fig. 29.3. A grade V tube with complete loss of the mucosal folds.

The status of the tubal mucosa is classified according to the classification proposed by Puttemans et al.[14] as follows: grade I, normal mucosal folds are seen (Fig. 29.1); grade II, the major folds are separated, flattened, but otherwise normal (in fact, this might be considered a grade I tube distended by an increased intraluminal hydrostatic pressure); grade III, focal adhesions between the mucosal folds are seen (Fig. 29.2); grade IV, extensive adhesions between the mucosal folds and/or disseminated flat areas are present; and grade V, complete loss of the mucosal fold pattern has occurred (Fig. 29.3).

Studies on Salpingoscopy: Prognostic Value and Correlation with Peritubal Adhesions

In 1995, we reported a prospective study[8] comparing the prognostic value of salpingoscopy with the AFS scoring systems for adnexal adhesions and DTO in patients with tubal infertility undergoing reconstructive tubal surgery, mostly by laparotomy. Fifty-five patients operated upon for salpingo-ovariolysis (29 patients) and salpingoneostomy (26 patients) underwent concomitant salpingoscopy. In all cases, tubal infertility was caused by prior pelvic inflammatory disease (PID). The mean age of the patients was 30 years (range, 22–38 years), and the mean length of infertility was 53 months (range, 12–168 months). Infertility was primary in 33 patients and secondary in 22 patients.

At the time of surgery, we evaluated the adnexal adhesions or the DTO according to the AFS classifications,[13] and at the same time assessed the status of the tubal mucosa by salpingoscopy according to the Puttemans classification.[14] Patients with asymmetric tubal lesions were classified according to the least affected adnexa. In the salpingo-ovariolysis group, 16 patients had bilateral adnexal adhesions, 6 patients had adnexal adhesions involving the only remaining tube, and 7 patients had unilateral adnexal adhesions and contralateral hydrosalpinx. In the salpingoneostomy group, hydrosalpinx was bilateral in 21 patients, and unilateral (of the only remaining tube) in 5 patients. No patient was lost to follow-up. The mean length of follow-up was 54 months (range, 29–71 months).

Statistical analysis demonstrated a positive correlation between salpingoscopic grades and the AFS classification for both the salpingo-ovariolysis ($p < 0.01$) and the salpingoneostomy ($p < 0.01$) groups. However, mucosal damage was noted at salpingoscopy in 23 of 50 tubes (46%) included in the minimal–mild class according to the AFS classification, and conversely a normal ampullary mucosa was present in 10 of 22 tubes (45%) classified as severe according to the AFS score.

Thirty-three pregnancies occurred in these 55 patients. Twenty-seven patients conceived an intrauterine pregnancy and carried it to term. In 2 patients, the term pregnancy was preceded or followed by a spontaneous abortion, and 2 patients had a second term pregnancy. Two extrauterine pregnancies occurred, 1 in a patient with an apparently normal mucosa in the salpingo-ovariolysis group, and 1 in a patient with an abnormal mucosa (class IV) in the salpingoneostomy group.

In the salpingo-ovariolysis group of patients, the term pregnancy rate was 66% (19/29), whereas this rate was 86% (19/22) for those patients with a normal ampullary mucosa (salpingoscopic grades I and II). In the salpingoneostomy group of patients, the term pregnancy rate was 31% (8/26), whereas it was 73% (8/11) for those patients with a normal ampullary mucosa. At statistical analysis, using the Fisher's exact test, there was a significant correlation between salpingoscopic grade (grades I and II versus grades III to V) and the achievement of a term pregnancy for both the salpingo-ovariolysis ($p < 0.001$) and the salpingoneostomy ($p < 0.001$) groups of patients. There was no significant correlation between the AFS scores and the achievement of a term pregnancy for both groups of patients: minimal–mild (12/19, 63%) versus moderate–severe (7/10, 70%) scores for the salpingo-ovariolysis group, and mild (6/18, 33%) versus moderate–severe (2/8, 25%) scores for the salpingoneostomy group.

In a recent prospective study (Marana et al., in manuscript) we reported on salpingoscopy used at the time of operative laparoscopy in 51 patients submitted to laparoscopic salpingo-ovariolysis (24 patients) and salpingoneostomy (27 patients). Similar evidence on the status of the tubal mucosa as the most powerful prognostic factor in reproductive outcome was obtained.

At variance with the previous study,[8] in the laparoscopic series statistical analysis demonstrated a lack of correlation between salpingoscopic grades and the AFS classification for both the salpingo-ovariolysis ($r = -0.029$; $p = 0.864$) and salpingoneostomy ($r = 0.056$; $p = 0.684$) groups.

As to pregnancy outcome, 25 pregnancies occurred in these 51 patients. Nineteen patients conceived an intrauterine pregnancy (IUP) and carried it to term. In 1 patient, the term pregnancy was preceded by a spontaneous abortion, and 2 patients had a second term pregnancy. Three extrauterine pregnancies occurred, 1 in a patient with a class III mucosa in the salpingo-ovariolysis group and 2 in 2 patients with a class IV mucosa in the salpingoneostomy group.

In the salpingo-ovariolysis group of patients, the term pregnancy rate was 50% (12/24), whereas this rate was 71% (12/17) for those patients with a normal tubal mucosa (classes I and II). In the salpingoneostomy group of patients, the term pregnancy rate was 26% (7/27), whereas it was 64% (7/11) for those patients with a normal tubal mucosa. In this study, no IUP was observed in patients with class III, IV, or V ampullary mucosa.

When the reproductive outcome was analyzed according to the AFS score, one could notice that the IUPs were distributed throughout the different classes. For salpingo-ovariolysis, the term pregnancy rate was 45% (5/11) in patients with minimal–mild disease and 54% (7/13) in patients with moderate–severe disease. For salpingoneostomy, the term pregnancy rate was 30% (3/10) in patients with mildly affected tubes and 24% (4/17) in patients with moderately and severely affected tubes.

Results reported by other groups are consistent with these findings. Since the first report by Henry-Suchet et al.[5] on the value of salpingoscopy at the time of tubal microsurgery, there has been increasing interest in the salpingoscopic technique to detect intraluminal lesions that may be inversely correlated with pregnancy outcome.

De Bruyne et al.,[6] in a series of 22 patients with bilateral hydrosalpinx, obtained a 59% (10/17) IUP rate following microsurgery when mucosal adhesions were absent at preoperative salpingoscopy. One ectopic pregnancy occurred in 1 of the 5 patients with intraluminal adhesions. The authors stated that "there was no correlation between the presence or extent of pelvic adhesions and the presence or extent of intraluminal adhesions."

Dubuisson et al.,[7] in a retrospective study, reported the fertility outcome of a series of 81 patients who underwent laparoscopic salpingoneostomy or, in some cases, fimbrioplasty. These authors reported a correlation between mucosal appearance at the neostomy site as evaluated using the criteria proposed by Boer-Meisel et al.[11] and pregnancy outcome (44% IUP rate for groups I and II, that is, normal mucosa or moderate attenuation of the mucosal folds versus 0% for group III, with no folds or honeycomb appearance). In this study there was no correlation with the adhesion stage. In fact, IUP rates in patients without adhesions (29%) were not significantly different from those in patients with adhesions (32%). According to Dubuisson, laparoscopic assessment of the tubal mucosa at neostomy site performs just as well as the distal tube score of Mage et al.[12] in providing a prognosis.

Vasquez et al.[15] examined the correlation between the presence and extent of peritubal adhesions, scored according to the AFS classification,[13] and the presence and extent of mucosal adhesions, evaluated at salpingoscopy, in 46 patients with bilateral hydrosalpinges and 14 with a hydrosalpinx of the single tube. Peritubal adhesions were absent in 7, mild in 46, moderate in 28, and severe in 9 hydrosalpinges. Of 7 hydrosalpinges without peritubal adhesions, 1 showed intratubal adhesion; in 83 hydrosalpinges with peritubal adhesions, including 37 cases with moderate or severe degrees of peritubal adhesions, mucosal adhesions were absent in 31 (37%). The correlation between the extent of peritubal and mucosal adhesion was not statistically significant.

Heylen et al.,[16] in a recent study, reported on the relation between salpingoscopic findings and pelvic adhesion at the ipsilateral side using the AFS classification for pelvic adhesions and DTO in patients with nonendometriotic pelvic disease. Of 71 tubes available for comparison, in 30 tubes no intraluminal adhesions were found (42%), and in 41 intraluminal adhesions were found (58%). These results are consistent with our findings[8] in 91 tubes with post-PID periadnexal adhesions or DTO: 46 tubes were free of intraluminal adhesions (51%) and 45 tubes had intraluminal adhesions (49%). The incidence of intraluminal adhesions in patients with post-PID pelvic disease is in sharp contrast with the presence of intraluminal adhesions found at salpingoscopy in patients with endometriosis-related pelvic adhesions. Of 370 tubes available for comparison from the three larger series available in the literature,[16–18] only 2 cases of intraluminal adhesions (class III) were found.

In a recent, prospective study, De Bruyne[9] evaluated the prognostic value of salpingoscopy in patients undergoing salpingo-ovariolysis (130 patients) or salpingoneostomy (96 patients) by microsurgical laparotomy for post-PID tubal disease. There were no other causes of infertility in these patients. The authors found a significant difference when the cumulative intrauterine pregnancy rates for salpingoscopic class I or II versus III to V were compared both in the salpingo-ovariolysis ($p = 0.015$) and salpingoneostomy groups ($p = 0.004$).

Dunphy and Greene[19] in 1995 evaluated which type of abnormalities detected at falloposcopy are the best prognostic indicators in terms of reproductive outcome. Sixty-two infertile women were examined falloposcopically in the office using the linear everting catheter. All women were subsequently examined by hysteroscopy and laparoscopy. No patient required surgery to correct DTO. Epithelial abnormalities, adhesions, vascular abnormalities, and abnormalities of luminal diameter were recorded as present or absent, and as minor or major, according to the classification by Kerin et al.[20]. When evaluating the reproductive outcome at follow-up, the authors concluded that although four or five descriptive variables, including dilatation and vascularity, have been included in the falloposcopic scoring system, a much simpler visual assessment can be whether the epithelium is normal or adhesions are present.

Summary

There is now growing evidence that the extent of intraluminal tubal damage does not necessarily correlate with the extent and nature of visible pelvic adhesions. The results from prospective studies on the prognostic value of salpingoscopy from different centers show that the status of the tubal mucosa is the most important factor determining the pregnancy outcome. Cumulative pregnancy rates in patients with normal ampullary mucosa at salpingoscopy are equal or higher than 60% for both salpingo-ovariolysis and salpingoneostomy. On the basis of these data and considering that operative laparoscopy allows us today to avoid laparotomy, the role of tubal reconstructive surgery should be reconsidered.[21] Mucosal assessment should become an integral part of the preoperative and perioperative investigation.

References

1. Westrom L. Incidence, prevalence, and trends of acute pelvic inflammatory disease and its consequences in industrialized countries. Am J Obstet Gynecol 1980;138: 880–892.
2. Diamond MP, Daniell JF, Feste J, et al. Adhesion reformation and de novo adhesion formation after reproductive pelvic surgery. Fertil Steril 1987;47:864–866.
3. Caspi E, Halperin Y, Bukovsky I. The importance of periadnexal adhesions in tubal reconstructive surgery for infertility. Fertil Steril 1979;31:296–300.
4. Hulka JF. Adnexal adhesions: a prognostic staging and classification system based on a five-year survey of fertility surgery results at Chapel Hill, North Carolina. Am J Obstet Gynecol 1982;144:141–148.
5. Henry-Suchet J, Loffredo V, Tesquier L, et al. Endoscopy of the tube (=tuboscopy): its prognostic value for tuboplasties. Acta Eur Fertil 1985;16:139–145.
6. De Bruyne F, Puttemans P, Boeckx W, et al. The clinical value of salpingoscopy in tubal infertility. Fertil Steril 1989; 51:339–340.
7. Dubuisson JB, Chapron C, Morice P, et al. Laparoscopic salpingostomy: fertility results according to the tubal mucosa appearance. Hum Reprod (Oxf) 1994;9:334–339.
8. Marana R, Rizzi M, Muzii L, et al. Correlation between the American Fertility Society classification of adnexal adhesions and distal tubal occlusion, salpingoscopy, and reproductive outcome in tubal surgery. Fertil Steril 1995;64: 924–929.
9. De Bruyne F, Hucke J, Willers R. The prognostic value of salpingoscopy. Hum Reprod (Oxf) 1997;12:266–271.
10. Rock JA, Katayama KP, Martin, EJ, et al. Factors influencing the success of salpingostomy techniques for distal fimbrial occlusion. Obstet Gynecol 1978;52:591–596.
11. Boer-Meisel ME, te Velde ER, Habbema JDF, et al. Predicting the pregnancy outcome in patients treated for hydrosalpinx: a prospective study. Fertil Steril 1986;45:23–28.
12. Mage G, Pouly JL, de Joliniere JB, et al. A preoperative classification to predict the intrauterine and ectopic pregnancy rate after distal tubal microsurgery. Fertil Steril 1986;46:807–810.
13. American Fertility Society. The American Fertility Society classifications of adnexal adhesions, distal tubal occlusion, tubal occlusion secondary to tubal ligation, tubal pregnancies, Mullerian anomalies and intrauterine adhesions. Fertil Steril 1988;49:944–955.
14. Puttemans P, Brosens IA, Delattin PH, et al. Salpingoscopy versus hysterosalpingography in hydrosalpinges. Human Reprod (Oxf) 1987;2:535–540.
15. Vasquez G, Boeckx W, Brosens I. No correlation between peritubal and mucosal adhesions in hydrosalpinges. Fertil Steril 1995;64:1032–1033.
16. Heylen SM, Brosens IA, Puttemans PJ, Clinical value and cumulative pregnancy rates following rigid salpingoscopy during laparoscopy for infertility. Hum Reprod (Oxf) 1995;10:2913–2916.
17. Marana R, Muzii L, Rizzi M, et al. Salpingoscopy in patients with endometriosis-associated infertility. Acta Eur Fertil 1990;21:247–249.
18. Nezhat F, Winer WK, Nezhat C. Fimbrioscopy and salpingoscopy in patients with minimal to moderate pelvic endometriosis. Obstet Gynecol 1990;75:15–17.
19. Dunphy BC, Greene CA. Falloposcopic cannulation of oviducts: mucosal appearances and prediction of treatment independent intrauterine pregnancy. Hum Reprod (Oxf) 1995;10:3313–3316.
20. Kerin JF, Williams DB, San Roman GA, et al. Falloposcopic classification and treatment of fallopian tube lumen disease. Fertil Steril 1992;57:731–741.
21. Gomel V. From microsurgery to laparoscopic surgery: a progress. Fertil Steril 1995;63:464–468.

30

Contributions of Adhesions to the Cost of Healthcare

Isay Moscowitz and Steven D. Wexner

CONTENTS

Postoperative abdominal adhesions are associated with numerous complications, including small-bowel obstruction,[1] difficult and dangerous reoperations, infertility, and chronic pain.[2–5] The healthcare industry has changed dramatically in the past decade. Historically, quality of care was the primary determinant of change in healthcare; however, cost has become a major motivating force in clinical decision making. Despite continued efforts to optimize outcomes, adverse sequelae ensue in all aspects of medicine and surgery. As technology advances, new drugs, devices, and procedures spawn new concerns relating to adverse outcomes. The costs of these unwanted effects contribute significantly to the global costs of healthcare.

Until anesthesia and antiseptic surgical technique made laparotomy a fairly routine and safe procedure, intraabdominal adhesions were relatively rare and invoked little interest among clinicians, even though adhesions were recognized findings at postmortem examinations for patients with tuberculous peritonitis and intraabdominal inflammatory disease. Beginning in the 1880s, more and more patients began undergoing abdominal operations; these early laparotomies were soon followed by reports of postoperative adhesions. Bryant[6] in 1872 described fatal intestinal obstruction resulting from adhesion to a ligature after an ovarian cystectomy. As far back as 100 years ago, the first ancillary therapeutic measures were considered, when Battle[7] in 1883 reported a woman who succumbed to intestinal obstruction caused by dense adhesions following the removal of bilateral ovarian cysts 4 years previously. Vast sums of money have been spent to treat adhesions and their sequelae. Until recently, however, most of the effort, technique, and money was directed toward treatment of symptomatic adhesions rather than their prevention.

Historical Perspective

Before the 1960s, most adhesion studies were epidemiologic in nature, trying to estimate incidence and prevalence rates and associations by diagnosis and procedure.[8–11] Colorectal surgery was found to be associated with intraabdominal adhesions in as many as 95% of cases and was responsible for up to 25% of cases of bowel obstruction. During the 1960s, surgeons such as Ellis and Jagelman[12–14] and others[15–17] evaluated the etiology of adhesions; ischemia was found to be the common component of most adhesiogenic cascades.[18–20] During the 1970s and 1980s, most authors concentrated on the timing and results of enterolysis and described adjunct techniques such as internal stenting.[21–24] Moreover, the cost-conscious ideology of the medical community during the 1990s led to several studies outlining the cost of treatment of adhesions.[25–27] Most recently, data have been produced documenting potential methods of reducing the incidence and severity of adhesions.[28–30]

Incidence of Intraabdominal Adhesions

As many as 93% of patients develop abdominal adhesions after laparotomy.[1,25] Specifically, Menzies and Ellis[25] reviewed the causes of intestinal obstruction and found that adhesions were responsible for between 54% and 74% of these obstructions. They further classified the types of surgery that produced adhesions, and found that 25% of patients after either rectal or left-sided colonic surgery developed adhesions as compared with 15% after appendectomy and 9% after total colectomy. These data were similar to those data reported by Raf,[15] who assessed 1477 adults with adhesions treated between 1954 and 1965. Of these individuals, 86% had undergone a prior laparotomy, most commonly either an appendectomy or a gynecologic procedure; 44% of the obstructions developed within 5 years after surgery, although obstructions secondary to postoperative adhesions occurred as long as 56 years after operative intervention.

In a similar postmortem study by Weibel and Majno,[31] 752 autopsies performed during a 1-year period revealed that almost 70% of patients had surgery. Ninety-one percent of patients who had undergone colorectal surgery and 93% of patients who had multiple prior operations had intraabdominal adhesions as compared with 60% after exploratory laparotomy alone and only 47% after appendectomy. Similarly, Menzies and Ellis[25] estimated that 93% of patients with intraabdominal adhesions had undergone at least one prior laparotomy. The latter authors performed a 25-year longitudinal study in which it was discovered that 261 of 28,297 adult general surgery admissions (0.9%) and 148 of 4,502 (3.3%) laparotomies were performed primarily for adhesions. The majority of operations that produced adhesions were lower abdominal procedures, mostly interventions upon the colon.

Ellis et al.[32] sought to determine the long-term morbidity associated with postoperative adhesions following abdominal surgery in Scotland. Patients with disease (ICD9) and procedure (OPC3/4) codes for adhesion-related problems or reoperations that may be complicated by the presence of adhesions were identified and followed during a 10-year period from 1986; 29,788 patients had abdominal surgery by laparotomy. During the next 10 years, 10,325 individuals (34.7%) required one or more readmission for conditions either related to adhesions or involving a reoperation that could be complicated by adhesions; 21,342 readmissions were identified for these patients, and 1,169 (5.5%) of these admissions were identified as a direct result of abdominal adhesions (3.9% of all initial operations). The medical and surgical impact is considerable, with 5.5% of readmissions over a 10-year period after initial surgery directly attributable to adhesions.

Scott-Coombes et al.[33] surveyed 416 general surgeons practicing in the United Kingdom. Of the queried surgeons, 362 (87%) responded, noting that 76% operate on at least two patients per year for small-bowel obstruction and 31% operate upon more than 5 such patients each year. More than 5 patients were admitted each year with suspected adhesive bowel obstruction by 64% of surgeons, and 35% of surgeons found adhesions to be a problem during a nonadhesion-related laparotomy in more than 5 patients each year. Thus, the estimated annual incidence was between 12,000 and 14,000 adhesion-related clinical problems in the United Kingdom. A number of preventative measures such as the use of starch-free gloves (78% of surgeons), peritoneal lavage (68%), and placement of the omentum beneath the wound closure (90%) were generally accepted, whereas routine moistening of swabs (39%) and nonessential adhesiolysis (49%) were mere controversial. Routine small-bowel plication (1%) and intubation (2%) were rarely used. This survey gives an indication of the large burden on patients and the health services caused by abdominal adhesions, and demonstrates the wide variety of approaches to both the treatment and prevention of adhesions.

Economic Impact of Intraabdominal Adhesions

To document the incidence of adhesion-related problems and the current concepts on the prevention of adhesions among Swedish surgeons, a postal questionnaire was sent during 1992.[34] At least 4700 patients were admitted annually with symptoms of adhesive small bowel obstruction, 2200 of whom were operated on to relieve obstruction. No consistent methods were in use to minimize formation of adhesions. Surgical gloves were not washed before the operation by surgeons in 49 of the 84 surgical units that replied, and only 12 of those centers always used powder-free gloves. Interestingly, only 13 (16%) of the units consistently avoided separately suturing the peritoneum. Annually, at least 1500 laparotomies were complicated by previously formed adhesions. The annual medical expenditure for adhesive small-bowel obstruction was more than U.S.$6 million per year or $1,000,000 per million Swedish inhabitants.

Ivarsson et al.,[35] in a prospective study, evaluated 57 patients with bowel obstruction. In 34 of the 57 patients (60%), bowel obstruction was caused by adhesions; 22 of the 42 patients who required a hospital stay of more than

24 hours had adhesive obstruction, and 10 of these 22 patients had to be operated on (2 of them twice). Major complications occurred in 60%, including 1 death. In Sweden, adhesive bowel obstruction causes 2330 hospital admissions annually, which is associated with an estimated direct cost of approximately U.S.$13 million.

Beck,[29] to establish the incidence of small-bowel obstruction and adhesiolysis following colorectal surgery, conduced a retrospective cohort study using patient-specific Health Care Financing Administration (HCFA) data to evaluate a random 5% sample of all Medicare patients undergoing surgery in 1993. Follow-up data were available for all patients through 2 years after the index procedure, which was categorized as excision and anastomosis of the intestine (ICD-9 code 45), other operations upon the intestine (code 46), operations upon the rectum, rectosigmoid, or perirectal tissues (code 48), and other operations within the abdominal region (code 54). Outcomes included hospitalizations with (1) obstruction, (2) adhesions with obstruction, (3) adhesiolysis, and (4) adhesiolysis with obstruction. Small-bowel obstruction was very frequent, ranging from 18.6% to 25% over 2 years postoperatively, and adhesiolysis ranged from 6.9% to 9.5%.

Ray et al.,[26] in their first report, described the number of hospitalizations and days of care attributable to adhesiolysis in the United States and estimated the costs associated with these stays. The cost per hospital day and associated surgeon's fees was based on prevailing nationwide charges. During 1988 there were 281,982 hospitalizations during which adhesiolysis was performed, accounting for 948,727 days of inpatient care. These hospitalizations were responsible for an estimated $1,179.9 million in expenditures, of which $925.0 million was associated with hospital costs and indirect costs. The results of this study demonstrated substantial costs are associated with hospitalizations for adhesiolysis.

Ray et al.[27] updated their data by assessing 303,836 hospitalizations during 1994. They noted that 19% of these hospitalizations were for primary adhesiolysis while the additional 81% included secondary adhesiolysis. Overall, adhesiolysis was performed during 1% of hospitalizations in the United States that year. The incidence was 117.3 per 100,000 U.S. population with a ratio of 188.8 females to 41.8 males. Interestingly, although 83% of adhesiolysis patients were female, only 60% of the inpatients that year were female. The overall financial package was very similar to that noted in the earlier study by Ray, with an annual price tag of $1.3 billion. The paper also assessed adhesiolysis of the gastrointestinal system versus adhesiolysis of digestive organs, at a cost of $1.1 billion for that year.

The National Hospital Discharge Survey (NHDS), conducted by the National Center for Health Statistics (NCHS), is a multistage random sample of discharge records from a stratified random sample of noninstitutional short-stay hospitals, excluding federal, military, and Veteran's Administration facilities, in the United States. The sample of hospitals included 478 respondents to the survey with a total sample of 276,533 discharge records.[36] Hospitalization costs, which are not available in the NHDS, can be estimated from the Medical Provider Analysis and Review (MEDPAR) data file, which includes approximately 11.8 million discharge records from all Medicare participating institutions in the United States.[36]

Economic Impact of Intraabdominal Adhesions in the United States

Using the Medicare database (Table 30.1) to assess hospital discharge between 1990 and 1996, two separate categories were analyzed;[22] first, Diagnosis-Related Group (DRG) 150 and 151, representing peritoneal adhesiolysis, and second, DRG 180 and 181, correlating to medical treatment of bowel obstruction. The total number of hospitalizations per year during which time peritoneal adhesiolysis was required in the Medicare population increased 8% in that 7-year time period from 26,466 to 28,899. Furthermore, if secondary adhesiolysis was factored into the equation between 1990 and 1994, the number of operations during which adhesiolysis was required as either the primary or secondary procedure increased 15.6%, from 91,107 to 107,929. The total length of hospitalization in this population (surgical and medical treatment) during that 7-year period decreased 8% from 962,642 in 1990 to 885,396 in 1996 (Fig. 30.1); however, the total charges increased from $924,124,796 in 1990 to $1,463,830,771 in 1996, representing 0.92% of the total Medicare reimbursement for this year and a total expenditure in 7 years (1990–1996) of $8,691,281,221 (Fig. 30.2).

Separately analyzing the medical treatment of bowel obstruction, the number of hospitalizations increased by 25% from 88,601 during 1990 to 110,817 in 1996. Reimbursement for the nonsurgical treatment of bowel obstruction increased 48%, from $261,989,036 to $386,874,429, over the same 7-year period (Fig. 30.3). The total annual Medicare expenditure for both medical and surgical treatment of bowel obstruction increased 40%, from $506,370,991 to $709,392,959 in 1996. These increasing costs were not at all surprising, considering that the incidence of peritoneal adhesiolysis in patients in the Medicare population increased 8% between 1990 and 1996, rising from 26,466 procedures per year to 28,899 annually performed procedures.

Twenty-seven percent of all peritoneal adhesiolysis procedures were performed on Medicare patients. Nearly 40% (28,500) of the 74,000 hospitalizations dur-

TABLE 30.1. Resource Utilization Due to Adhesiolysis Based on DRG Categorization from the Health Care Financing Administration Bureau of Data Management and from the 100% MEDPAR Inpatient Hospital Fiscal Year 1990–1996.

DRG	Total charges	Covered charges	Medicare	Total days	Number of cases	Total avg. days
1990						
150	$ 380,428,665	$ 357,617,386	$ 218,933,054	299,536	21,019	14.3
151	$ 43,735,319	$ 43,232,936	$ 25,448,901	43,669	5,447	8.0
180	$ 421,705,235	$415,943,643	$ 222,542,242	510,977	65,386	7.8
181	$ 78,255,577	$ 77,368,561	$ 39,446,794	108,460	23,215	4.7
Total	$ 924,124,796	$ 894,162,526	$ 506,370,991	962,642	115,067	
1991						
150	$ 427,979,933	$ 423,323,048	$ 222,171,315	306,611	22,038	13.9
151	$ 41,805,195	$ 41,357,584	$ 22,186,154	39,643	4,763	8.3
180	$ 505,822,783	$ 498,654,112	$ 250,348,521	543,488	71,031	7.7
181	$ 82,358,034	$ 81,274,661	$ 38,907,201	101,076	22,076	4.6
Total	$1,057,965,945	$1,044,609,405	$ 533,613,191	990,818	119,908	
1992						
150	$ 478,695,474	$ 472,974,367	$ 237,963,161	315,806	22,901	13.8
151	$ 44,012,135	$ 43,562,007	$ 21,762,948	33,277	4,669	7.1
180	$ 593,340,420	$ 585,249,176	$ 288,522,383	570,863	77,962	7.3
181	$ 87,112,025	$ 85,772,155	$ 40,162,295	95,290	21,591	4.4
Total	$1,203,160,054	$1,187,557,705	$ 588,410,787	1,015,236	127,123	
1993						
150	$ 514,721,551	$ 509,581,202	$ 257,923,801	296,662	23,034	12.9
151	$ 42,401,701	$ 42,070,854	$ 20,435,234	29,086	4,270	6.8
180	$ 635,446,183	$ 627,793,979	$ 306,036,548	564,942	79,570	7.1
181	$ 85,919,079	$ 85,029,579	$ 38,069,496	85,717	20,223	4.2
Total	$1,278,488,514	$1,264,475,614	$ 622,465,079	976,407	127,097	
1994						
150	$ 556,902,299	$ 553,160,303	$ 268,242,269	294,409	23,888	12.3
151	$ 44,173,653	$ 43,883,877	$ 19,259,397	27,122	4,190	6.4
180	$ 677,073,787	$ 670,073,154	$ 316,172,124	543,647	83,944	6.4
181	$ 86,064,256	$ 85,313,944	$ 35,314,300	79,018	20,031	3.9
Total	$1,364,213,995	$1,352,431,278	$ 638,988,090	944,196	132,053	
1995						
150	$ 575,956,908	$ 571,306,674	$ 279,752,510	285,143	24,445	11.6
151	$ 42,485,050	$ 42,052,434	$ 18,635,451	24,322	4,024	6
180	$ 694,862,485	$ 688,284,533	$ 324,717,453	523,587	86,877	6
181	$ 86,192,703	$ 85,385,523	$ 34,136,159	73,129	19,547	3.7
Total	$1,399,497,146	$1,387,029,164	$ 657,241,573	906,181	134,893	
1996						
150	$ 592,800,926	$ 588,879,462	$ 300,137,320	273,524	24,615	11.1
151	$ 48,526,139	$ 48,245,226	$ 22,381,210	26,225	4,284	6.1
180	$ 723,177,923	$ 717,536,292	$ 346,120,208	506,089	89,427	5.7
181	$ 99,325,783	$ 98,275,789	$ 40,754,221	79,558	21,390	3.7
Total	$1,463,830,771	$1,452,936,769	$ 709,392,959	885,396	139,716	
Total:	$8,691,281,221	$8,583,202,461	$4,256,482,670	6,680,876	895,857	

DRG, diagnosis-related group
150, peritoneal adhesiolysis with complications and/or comorbidity; 151, peritoneal adhesiolysis without complications and/or comorbidity; 180, GI obstruction with complications and/or comorbidity; 181, GI obstruction without complications and/or comorbidity.

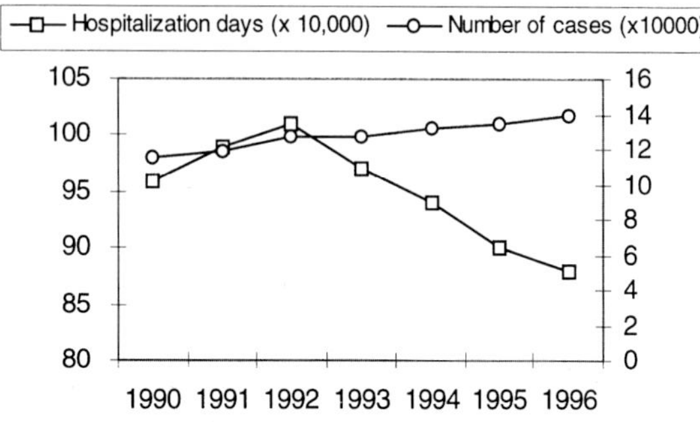

FIGURE 30.1 Number of cases and hospitalization days. Health Care Financing Administration, MEDPAR Database, 1990–1996.

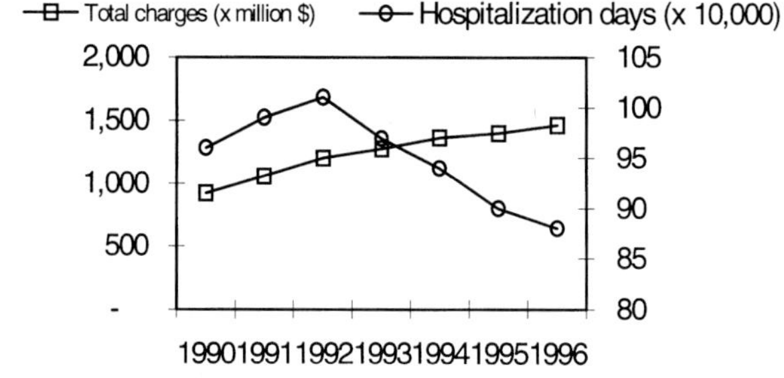

FIGURE 30.2 Total charges for procedures involving adhesiolysis for patients aged more than 65 years. Health Care Financing Administration, MEDPAR Database, 1990–1996.

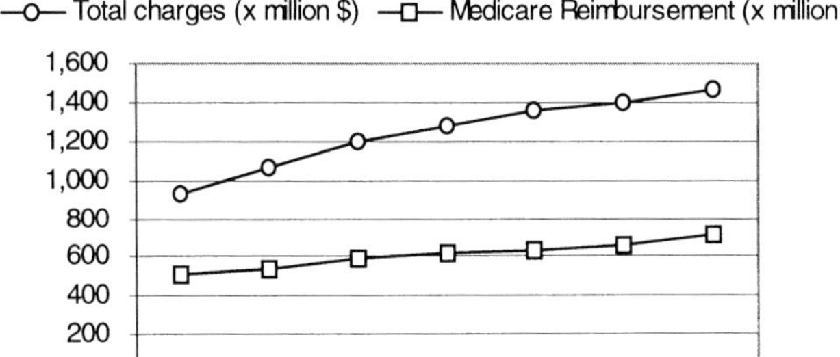

FIGURE 30.3 Total Medicare reimbursement, diagnosis-related groups (DRG) 150, 151, 180, and 181. Health Care Financing Administration, MEDPAR Database, 1990–1996.

ing which peritoneal adhesiolysis was the primary surgical procedure were performed in Medicare patients, and Medicare patients accounted for 52% (175,200) of approximately 340,000 hospitalizations for major colorectal surgical procedures. Finally, Medicare patients accounted for 60% (106,600) of the 177,400 hospitalizations for medical treatment of bowel obstruction, representing a growth of 26% over the 7-year period discussed.

Clearly, in addition to the obvious perioperative morbidity and mortality, the problem is financially significant. However, one must remember that expenditure is undoubtedly greater, as these figures did not include disability, lost revenue, the treatment of morbidity after initial discharge from hospital, and recurrent bowel obstruction. Additional costs associated with adhesiolysis are not represented, such as laboratory tests, endoscopy procedures including gastroenterologist consultation fees, computed tomography images, x-rays, drugs ordered by the primary care physician or surgeon before hospitalization, ambulance services, inpatient medical care provided by other physicians (i.e., anesthesiologist and patient's primary care physician), and home health care or community support services after discharge. Indirect costs, such as patient's loss of workdays or productivity because of short- or long-term morbidity and premature mortality, and costs associated with problems secondary to adhesions, such as infertility and the psychological impact of long-term illness, were also not included in the estimated total cost. Inclusion of work-loss days resulting from hospitalization and outpatient care, time spent by family members caring for adhesiolysis patients, pain and suffering of the patient, and impact on family members would substantially increase the economic impact of adhesiolysis. Furthermore, many surgeons do not code for adhesiolysis (CPT code 44005) because such coding is considering "unbundling" and is not eligible for separate reimbursement unless it is the main focus of the operation. Therefore, the only assumption that can be made is indeed much higher.

Risk and Morbidity of Intraabdominal Adhesions

Malcolm,[37] in the Surgical and Clinical Adhesions Research study (SCAR), determined the long-term morbidity associated with postoperative adhesions following abdominal and pelvic surgery; 52,192 patients were assessed with follow-up over 10 years. This study indicated that 1 in 3 patients undergoing a laparotomy will be readmitted during the next 10 years, with an average of 2.1 readmissions per patient; 2,002 patients readmitted were directly related to adhesions (4.7%), and adhesion-related admissions continued to occur throughout the 10-year period studied with little evidence of any decline in rate. This ongoing burden is reflected in the annual prevalence of 4,199 admissions that were directly adhesion related.

McGuire[38] assessed the same group of patients and classified them into three categories: category 1 identified all subsequent surgery directly attributable to prior adhesions; and category 2 identified those who had subsequent surgery possibly attributable to adhesions. The cumulative discount cost of surgical adhesions in the category 1 patients during the 10-year follow-up period was calculated to be more than £4.5 million. The average cost per readmission over the follow-up period was approximately £2,500. For the category 2 patients, the total accumulative discounted cost was less than £30 million over the follow-up period, with readmission cost of £2,225.

Moran,[39] in a prospective study, assessed 120 patients undergoing laparotomy, 93 elective cases and 27 emergencies. Information was collected concerning previous surgery, indications for the operations, and the incision time (from skin incision to complete opening of the peritoneal cavity). The adhesion division time was recorded as the time taken to divide the relevant intraabdominal adhesions. In the elective surgery group who had no previous surgery, the incision time was a mean of 5 minutes with a range of 3 to 9 minutes in 47 cases. In the elective group who had previous surgery, the mean incision time was 10 minutes, while the mean division of adhesions time was 19 minutes with a range of 0 to 120 minutes. However, in a separate analysis of the 28 patients with significant adhesions, the mean adhesion division time was 30 minutes. Similarly the incision time for the 18 patients who had emergency surgery and had previous abdominal surgery was 10 minutes, with a division of relevant adhesions time of 31 minutes. Moran concluded that in a colorectal surgical practice half the patients had previous surgery, and 60% of them will have significant intraabdominal adhesions resulting in prolonged incision and division time.

van Goor[40] assessed 274 patients who underwent 291 repeat laparotomies. Patients who required an emergency repeat laparotomy for complications of a prior laparotomy were excluded. In 61 (21%) of the repeat laparotomy cases, one or more bowel perforations occurred. The rate of postoperative complications (anastomotic leak, wound infection, hemorrhage, and organ failure) was significantly higher ($p < 0.05$) in patients with bowel perforation (54%) compared to patients without bowel perforation (36%). The authors concluded that the risk of adhesion-related bowel perforation is about 20% and carried significant postoperative morbidity and an obvious financial impact.

Efforts to Decrease the Morbidity and Symptoms of Adhesions

In a effort to decrease the morbidity and symptoms of adhesions, a multicentered, surgeon-blinded, prospective, randomized clinical study was designed to prospectively assess the incidence of adhesions following a standardized major abdominal operation using direct laparoscopic peritoneal imaging to determine the safety and effectiveness of Seprafilm®, a carboxymethylcellulose/sodium hyaluronate membrane (Genzyme Corporation, Cambridge, MA, USA), in preventing postoperative adhesions to the site of application.[30] Eleven centers enrolled 183 patients with mucosal ulcerative colitis or familial adenomatous polyposis scheduled for colectomy and ileal pouch–anal anastomosis with diverting loop ileostomy. Before abdominal closure, patients were randomized to receive or not receive Seprafilm® under the midline incision. At ileostomy closure 8 to 12 weeks later, laparoscopy was used to evaluate the incidence, extent, and severity of adhesion formation to the midline incision.

Data were analyzed on 175 evaluable patients. Although only 6% of control patients had no adhesions, no adhesions were observed in 51% of patients who received Seprafilm® ($p < 0.00000000001$). Moreover, a mean of 63% of the incision involved adhesions in the control group, significantly greater than the 23% observed in the Seprafilm® patients ($p < 0.001$). Moreover, dense adhesions were observed in 58% of the control patients but in only 15% of those individuals who received Seprafilm® ($p < 0.0001$). Comparison of the incidence of specific adverse events between the groups did not identify any differences ($p < 0.05$). In this study, Seprafilm® was safe and significantly reduced the incidence, extent, and severity of postoperative abdominal adhesions.

Subsequent to that prospective randomized trial, a compassionate use study was undertaken between August 1995 and August 1996.[41] Surgeons various of sites enrolled a total of 15 patients who had undergone a minimum of two prior hospitalizations during the preceding year for either medical or surgical treatment of bowel obstruction. These 13 female and 2 male patients were of mean age of 46.9 years (range, 20–36) and had undergone a mean of 7.2 laparotomies (range, 1–13) per patient. After extensive lysis of adhesions undertaken during a mean of 3.4 hours (range, 1–9) all patients underwent placement of as many as 10 sheets of Seprafilm®. At the initial follow-up of a mean of 13 months (range, 10–19), 1 patient died remote to the time of surgery of multisystemic organ failure. She had undergone hemodialysis pending renal failure for a long period of time before surgery. However, 10 of the 14 remaining patients (71%) were symptom free. One patient had undergone repeat laparotomy for enterolysis of the previously unlysed bowel area. One patient developed recurrent obstruction and fistulas. However, 2 additional patients were reexplored for nonobstructive indications and both were found to be free of adhesions.

Salum et al.[42] compared 100 patients who received Seprafilm® between August 1996 and August 1997 to 100 patients who did not receive Seprafilm® before the time of its availability in August 1996. Patients were matched for age, gender, diagnosis, type of procedure, midline incision, and incidence of prior operations; the 1996 Medicare reimbursement rates were utilized as medical treatment of bowel obstruction for $3,500 per patient and surgical treatment for $12,000 per patient. Although 5 patients in the Seprafilm® group did develop small-bowel obstruction during the follow-up period, all 5 were successfully medically treated (for a reimbursement rate of $17,500). Interestingly, although this rate was not significantly different from the 3 bowel obstructions that occurred in the control group, 2 of the 3 patients in the latter group required surgery (for a Medicare reimbursement rate of $27,500). There were no differences in postoperative septic sequelae between the two groups. Thus, in conclusion, as had been shown in the prospective randomized multicenter trial, although Seprafilm® did not eliminate formation of adhesions or obstruction it did significantly reduce their severity, allowing the patients to undergo less costly, less invasive, and less morbidity-associated treatment.

Moreira et al.[44] designed a study to evaluate the safety of Seprafilm® after bowel injury in a prospective randomized trial on a rabbit model. Sixty rabbits underwent laparotomy with equal distribution to 1 of 3 groups: creation of either 3 repaired or 3 unrepaired myotomies, or 3 repaired enterotomies. Thus, a total of 180 defects were created in the same anatomic positions in these 60 animals. In one-half of the rabbits in each group, the surface of the myotomies or enterotomies was covered by Seprafilm® and not in the other half. The presence of intraabdominal abscess, adhesions, and the integrity of the suture line were evaluated 14 days later by examination by a surgeon blinded to the use of Seprafilm® and also by standard radiographic isobaric contrast study. The incidence of adhesions for both repaired and unrepaired myotomy sites was significantly reduced by the application of Seprafilm® ($p < 0.05$). Specifically, in the 60 repaired myotomy sites, the incidence of adhesions fell from 30% in the non-Seprafilm® group to 6.6% at the sites that had been covered with Seprafilm®.

Similarly, in the unrepaired myotomy group, the incidence of adhesions fell from 33% without the use of Seprafilm® to 6.6% when Seprafilm® was utilized. However, in sites of enterotomy, adhesions were noted in 97% of the untreated sites and 94% of the treated sites. In terms of safety, the single phlegmon in the myotomy group occurred at a Seprafilm® site (1.6% vs. 0%; p = NS), and the incidence of phlegmon and leaks in the enterotomy with and without Seprafilm® was 30% and 7% versus 26.6% and 10%, respectively (p = NS). The use of Seprafilm® on injured bowel allowed the normal septic process to occur through the formation of a contained abscess. Importantly, Seprafilm® did not increase septic mortality in any groups while it still reduced adhesions in the myotomy groups.

It appears that after decades of the inability to successfully treat adhesions, we are finally able to actually try to prevent them. The future includes new and more facile forms of Seprafilm®. This substance seems safe and effective in a substantial number of patients.

Summary

Postoperative adhesions clearly are very vexing from numerous aspects. They are costly in financial terms, cause considerable morbidity and disability to the patients, and recur despite traditional treatment. The economic impact, discounting the disability feature, is staggering. Recent advances in our understanding of the economic impact of adhesions have shown a tremendous financial burden in terms of time to reenter an abdomen, the cost of treatment of complications associated with adhesiolysis, and charges for hospitalization for medical and surgical treatment of bowel obstruction. Fortunately, one recent major technologic advance has finally enabled the potential vision of adhesion prevention rather than treatment. Seprafilm® has been shown to significantly reduce adhesions to the site of application. Subsequent to that initial very powerful prospective, randomized, surgeon-blinded trial, more recent scientific studies have indeed confirmed the initial findings. Specifically, it appears that we may now be able to offer hope to patients by significantly reducing the incidence, severity, and therefore financial burden secondary to postoperative intraabominal adhesions.

Acknowledgment

This work was supported in part by a generous educational grant from Genzyme Surgical Products Inc., Cambridge, MA.

References

1. Menzies D. Peritoneal adhesions: incidence, cause and prevention. Ann Surg 1992;24(part 1):29–45.
2. Caspi E, Halpern Y, Bukosky I. The importance of peritoneal adhesions in tubal reconstructive surgery for infertility. Fertil Steril 1979;31:296–300.
3. Diamond E. Lysis of postoperative pelvic adhesions in infertility. Fertil Steril 1979;31:287–295.
4. Frantzen C, Schlosser HW. Microsurgery and postinfectious tubal infertility. Fertil Steril 1982;38:397–420.
5. Tulandi T. Salpingo-ovariolysis: a comparison between laser surgery and electrosurgery. Fertil Steril 1986;45: 489–491.
6. Bryant T. Clinical lectures on intestinal obstruction. Med Times Gazette 1872;1:363.
7. Battle WH. Intestinal obstructions coming 4 years after the operation of ovariotomy. Lancet 1883;1:818.
8. Vick RM. Statistics of acute intestinal obstruction. Br Med J 1932;2:546–548.
9. Waldron GW, Hampton JM. Intestinal obstruction: a half century comparative analysis. Ann Surg 1961;153: 839–850.
10. P. Nemir Jr. Intestinal obstruction: ten year survey at the hospital of the University of Pennsylvania. Ann Surg 1952; 135:367–375.
11. Perry JF, Smith GA, Yonehiro EG. Intestinal obstruction caused by adhesions: a review of 388 cases. Ann Surg 1955; 142:810–816.
12. Ellis H. The etiology of post-operative abdominal adhesions. An experimental study. Br J Surg 1962;50:10–16.
13. Ellis H. The cause and prevention of post-operative intraperitoneal adhesions. Surg Gynecol Obstet 1971;133 (3):497–511.
14. Jagelman DG, Ellis H. Starch and intraperitoneal adhesion formation. Br J Surg 1973;60(2):111–114.
15. Raf EL. Causes of abdominal adhesions in cases of intestinal obstruction. Act Chir Scand 1969;135:73.
16. Myllarniemi H. Foreign material in adhesion formation after abdominal surgery. Acta Chir Scand 1967;(suppl)377: 13–48.
17. Goldman IL, Rosemond PG. Fluorouracil inhibition of experimental peritoneal adhesions. Am J Surg 1967;113(4): 491–493.
18. Buckman R, Buckman PD, Hufnagel HV, Gervin AS. A physiological basis for the adhesion-free healing of deperitonealized surfaces. J Surg Res 1976;21(2):67–76.
19. Buckman R, Woods M, Sargeant I, Gerwin SA. A unifying mechanism in the etiology of intraperitoneal adhesions. J Surg Res 1976;20(1):1–5.
20. Raftery TA. Effect of peritoneal trauma on peritoneal fibrinolytic activity and intraperitoneal adhesion formation. An experimental study in the rat. Eur Surg Res 1981; 13(6):397–401.

21. Playforth RH, Holloway JB, Griffin WO. Mechanical small bowel obstruction: a plea for early surgical intervention. Ann Surg 1970;171:783–788.
22. Laws HL. Management of small bowel obstruction. Am Surg 1978;44:313–317.
23. Stewardson RH, Bombeck CT, Nyhus LM. Critical operative management of small bowel obstruction. Ann Surg 1978;189–193.
24. Munro A, Jones PF. Operative intubation in the treatment of complicated small bowel obstruction. Br J Surg 1978; 65(2):123–127.
25. Menzies D, Ellis H. Intestinal obstruction from adhesions—how big is the problem? Ann R Coll Surg Engl 1990;72:60–63.
26. Ray NF, Larsen JW Jr, Stillman RJ, Jacobs RJ. Economic impact of hospitalizations for lower abdominal adhesiolysis in the United States in 1988. Surg Gynecol Obstet 1993; 176(3):271–276.
27. Ray NF, Denton WG, Thamer M, Henderson SC, Perry S. Abdominal adhesiolysis: inpatient care and expenditures in the United States in 1994. J Am Coll Surg 1998;186(1): 1–9.
28. Wiseman D. Polymers for the prevention of surgical adhesions. In: Domb AJ, ed. Polymeric Site-Specific Pharmacotherapy. New York: Wiley, 1994:370–421.
29. Beck DE. The role of Seprafilm™ bioresorbable membrane in adhesion prevention. Eur J Surg 1997;7:49–55.
30. Becker MJ, Dayton LM, Fazio WV, et al. Prevention of postoperative abdominal adhesions by sodium hyaluronate-based bioresorbable membrane: a prospective, randomized, double-blind multicenter study. J Am Coll Surg 1996;183:297–306.
31. Weibel MA, Majno G. Peritoneal adhesions and their relation to abdominal surgery. Am Chir Scand 1969;135: 73–76.
32. Ellis H, Parker MC, Menzies D, et al. The surgical impact of adhesions. American Society of Colon and Rectal Surgeons (ASCRS) 97th Annual Convention, 1998, San Antonio, TX, Abstract C75.
33. Scott-Coombes DM, Thompson JN, Vipond MN. General surgeon's attitudes to the treatment and prevention of abdominal surgery. Am J Surg 1973;126:345–353.
34. Holmdahl L, Risberg B. Adhesions: prevention and complications in general surgery. Eur J Surg 1997;163: 169–174.
35. Ivarsson ML, Holmdahl L, Franzjen G, Reisberg B. Cost of bowel obstruction resulting from adhesions. Eur J Surg 1997;163(9):679–684.
36. Health Care Financing Administration. MEDPAR Database www.hcfa.gov/stats/medpar/medpar.htm 1990–1996.
37. Malcolm W. The surgical impact of adhesions. The surgical and clinical adhesions research study (SCAR). Abstract presented at the annual scientific meeting of Association of Surgeons of Great Britain and Ireland (ASGBI), 13th–15th May, Scotland, 1998.
38. McGuire A. The economic impact of post-operative adhesions. In: Clinical and epidemiological perspectives on post-operative adhesions. Abstract presented at the annual scientific meeting of Association of Surgeons of Great Britain and Ireland (ASGBI), 13th–15th May, Scotland, 1998.
39. Moran BJ. The workload from adhesions in re-operative surgery. In: Clinical and epidemiological perspectives on post-operative adhesions. Abstract presented at the annual scientific meeting of Association of Surgeons of Great Britain and Ireland, 13th–15th May, Scotland, 1998.
40. van Goor H. Complications in re-operated patients. Prevention and treatment of adhesive complications in colorectal surgery. Abstract presented at the International Society of University Colon and Rectal Surgeons (ISURS). XVIIth Biennial Congress, 7th–11th June, Malmo, Sweden, 1998.
41. Wexner S, Beck D, Seprafilm® Compassionate Use Study Group. Clinical resolution of life-threatening recurrent adhesive disease by Seprafilm®: a compassionate use treatment series (Abstract). Dis Colon Rectum 1998;41:A58.
42. Salum M, Weiss EG, Nogueras JJ, Wexner SD. Early obstructive and septic complications with hyaluronate-based membrane in colorectal surgery (Abstract). Dis Colon Rectum 1998;41:A45.
43. Salum MR, Batista O, Baig MK, et al. Does the sodium hyaluronate and carboxymethylcellulose membrane (HCM) reduce the incidence and/or severity of small bowel obstruction (SBO)? (Abstract) Colorectal Disease 1999;1(suppl 1):59.
44. Moreira H Jr, Yamaguchi T, Choi J, Sardinha C, Billoti V, Wexner S. Safety of sodium hyaluronate-based membrane (Seprafilm™) after bowel injury: a prospective randomized trial (Abstract). Dis Colon Rectum 1998;41:A6.

31

Clinical Significance of Adhesions in Patients with Chronic Pelvic Pain

John F. Steege

CONTENTS

Chronic pelvic pain (CPP) is one of the most common and most difficult disorders encountered by the practicing gynecologist and primary care physician. Pain is generally defined as "chronic" when it has persisted for 6 months or more. The causes are multiple, including structural and functional disorders of the reproductive, urinary, gastrointestinal, neurologic, and musculoskeletal systems.[1] This chapter reviews the available information regarding the role of pelvic adhesions in the generation of CPP.

The prevalence of CPP has been examined in both referral and primary care settings. In two nongynecologic clinics in a university medical center, 12% of women reported current CPP and 33% had experienced it at some point of their lives.[2] Among 581 women of reproductive age attending primary care practices, 39.1% had pelvic pain other than dysmenorrhea, dyspareunia, or bowel-related pain at least some of the time, and 11.7% had pain more than 5 days per month or lasting a full day or more each month.[3] Further, a nationwide Gallup poll of 5325 women discovered that 16% of women reported problems with pelvic pain.[4] In this group, 15.8% took medication and 4% missed at least 1 day of work per month because of the pain problem.

Medical resource utilization for the care of pelvic pain is incompletely assessed, but it is no doubt substantial. Of the 600,000 hysterectomies performed annually in the United States, approximately 12% were performed for the primary indication of pelvic pain.[5] Approximately 40% of laparoscopies performed in the United States are done to evaluate a pain problem.[6] The direct dollar cost per annum for the care of CPP in the United States has been roughly estimated as $2.8 billion.[4]

There is no gynecologic pathologic condition that causes pain in every patient afflicted with that disorder. This generalization applies especially to endometriosis and to pelvic adhesions, perhaps the two most commonly discovered forms of pathology in women undergoing laparoscopy for pelvic pain. In many instances, organic reproductive system pathology may interact with functional disorders of the bowel, bladder, and musculoskeletal systems. The total pain syndrome may thus have several contributing factors, only one of which might be the pathology of the reproductive organs. The clinical assessment of the role of adhesions in the production of pelvic pain and reports of pain treatment with adhesiolysis should be assessed with these complexities in mind.

Before the development of laparoscopy, the entire concept of the role of adhesions in pain production was almost a moot point. Traditional teaching has held that laparotomy for lysis of adhesions is indicated only in the presence of true intestinal obstruction and is not a useful therapy for chronic pain. The absence of effective treatment for adhesions, together with the observation of some painfree patients with extensive adhesions, often led physicians to discount the importance of adhesions altogether. Now that a surgical approach to the treatment of adhesions is more feasible, reports of successful relief of pain following adhesiolysis are accumulating. Further work is necessary to define the appropriate niche for these approaches in the overall management of pain seen in the presence of adhesive disease. This process requires a consideration of the basic mechanisms of pain perception.

Pain Perception

Chronic pain appears to be qualitatively different from acute pain in terms of the physiologic and psychologic mechanisms involved. The theoretic constructs needed to explain acute pain are relatively simple: centrally perceived pain results from painful stimuli from damaged or irritated tissues; pain intensity is roughly proportional to tissue damage. Laboratory tests and other diagnostic tools commonly reveal the tissue damage, and appropriate therapy follows.

In the case of chronic pain, it is most often difficult to find "enough" pathology to explain the pain. In fact, pain is not directly proportional to the amount of documented tissue damage. Clinical confusion results when relentless attempts are made to search for "enough" tissue damage.

This qualitative difference in chronic pain is currently best described by the Gate Control theory.[7] In contrast to the specificity (Cartesian) theory, the Gate Control theory allows for communication of information in two directions: both from the periphery to the central nervous system and from higher centers in the central nervous system to spinal cord interneurons. The interneurons in this "gate" system may be up- or downregulated by a host of neurotransmitters and humoral factors. A large body of experimental evidence in animals suggests that sensitization of spinal cord interneurons can serve to amplify the intensity of peripheral nociceptive signals as well as to maintain signal transmission to higher centers even in the virtual absence of peripheral nociception. These data have prompted extrapolation to the clinical situation of chronic pain to explain the frequent observation of persistent pain syndromes even when peripheral tissue damage has been optimally treated. In a word, the nervous system is described as having "neuroplasticity"[8] rather than being an entirely static and hardwired system. The plasticity of this system allows for the experience of pain to modify the perception of pain on a physiologic basis, as well as for heretofore designated "psychological" states to physiologically influence pain perception. These interactions make any arbitrary dichotomy between "physical" and "psychological" pain indistinct and clinically unproductive.

For the practicing clinician, this formulation is both good news and bad news. The bad news is that endless treatment of peripheral tissue abnormalities can sometimes be fruitless; the good news is that this formulation may both provide a mechanism to explain the therapeutic benefits of drugs active on a central nervous system and promote the development and testing of medications aimed at modifying the sensitization of spinal cord intraneuronal mechanisms. Indeed, composite treatment of the pain perception mechanisms at the peripheral, spinal cord, and central levels may ultimately provide the best hope for effective pain management.

Superimposed on these more standard neurologic considerations are, of course, the additional layers of complexity provided by the genetic background, both recent and distant past experiences, social support, and the nuances of personality. These factors are of obvious importance in clinical management, but current theorization as outlined may stress their role as modulators of pain and factors that may impact on a functional level, as opposed to playing a role in the generation of the pain in the first place. As different centers of care may recruit patient populations who vary in these dimensions, they are also of importance when comparing reports from different authors when considering surgical therapies for pain attributed to gynecologic pathology, including the treatment of adhesions.

Studies of Adhesiolysis for Pelvic Pain

Approximately 60% to 90% of women who have had a previous laparotomy have some form of intraabdominal adhesions, most often involving the adherence of the omentum to the anterior abdominal wall.[9] Indeed, autopsy studies reveal a 30% prevalence of adhesions in women who have never had pelvic surgery.[10] Kresch and colleagues[11] found a 12% incidence of adhesions in women undergoing laparoscopy for tubal sterilization and a threefold higher prevalence of adhesions in women with pelvic pain. When pain is unilateral, adhesions are most commonly found on the side of the pelvis that is symptomatic.[12]

A number of clinical series have suggested that lysis of adhesions through the laparoscope may be helpful. Sutton and MacDonald[13] reported 85% of patients relieved after laparoscopic lysis of adhesions. Another study[14] reported 67% of women experiencing pain relief after laparoscopic adhesiolysis. However, this same group found that only 40% of women who had a behaviorly defined chronic pain syndrome were improved. Several other series suggest similarly optimistic results.[15,16]

There are currently no published randomized clinical trials of laparoscopic lysis of adhesions. Peters and colleagues[17] diagnosed adhesions laparoscopically, but then randomized patients to lysis of adhesions by laparotomy versus no surgical therapy. At 9 to 12 months postoperatively, no difference in pain level was found between the two groups, except for those who were noted to have severe bowel adhesions at the time of the initial procedure. In view of the documented superiority of laparoscopy compared to laparotomy in avoiding adhesion reformation, these results are not surprising.

In a similar vein, it would appear that laparoscopy by itself may often be insufficient treatment for chronic pain seen in the presence of adhesions. Peters and colleagues[18] demonstrated that laparoscopy in a traditional gynecologic setting was no more effective than a multifactorial nonsurgical approach to CPP. This study may only partially apply to the adhesion problem, as the patient population involved had a variety of gynecologic conditions. It would make good clinical sense to combine a multifactorial pain management approach with operative laparoscopy in selected cases.

In summary, reported clinical series suggest that laparoscopic adhesiolysis is a useful procedure. However, the evidence published so far is virtually all in the form of clinical case series as opposed to well-structured clinical trials.

How Would We Know If Adhesions Really Cause Pain?

The obstacles to convincing investigation of the role of adhesions as pain generators are myriad. The intrinsic complexities of the pain perception mechanism, as outlined here, readily give rise to a long list of factors to be considered. Listed briefly (and incompletely) these might include the following:

1. How do we know when pain has become centralized?
2. How do we know when peripheral nociception is still going on?
3. Is the presence or absence of neutral tissue or inflammatory tissue changes in adhesions or other forms of pelvic pathology relevant to the generation of nociceptive signals from this tissue, or is nociception rather the result of the constraints these adhesions may place on surrounding organs?
4. Given that the sum total of this pain experience, the relative contributions of peripheral nociception, spinal cord upregulation, and the central nervous system factors may vary, how does one develop a homogeneous population of patients who might be entered into a treatment trial for any particular therapeutic technique, for example, adhesiolysis?
5. Most treatment trials originate from referral centers. How can we be certain that these patient populations are comparable to those seen in primary care settings? Do patients not tend to allow themselves to be referred to physicians whose approach to diagnosis and treatment they can believe in?
6. Patients appear to have the ability to find sources of care that are in philosophic agreement with their own self-perception. Those who place more faith in surgical approaches tend to find physicians who share those beliefs. How do we manage to convince such patients to be entered into a randomized clinical trial of adhesiolysis, and indeed is it difficult to do so?

The uncertainties involved in assessing the relationship between gynecologic pathology and symptoms have been underlined by Thornton et al.[19] They diagnosed and photographed the pathologic findings seen at laparoscopy in women both with and without pain as their primary indication for the surgical exploration. Physician reviewers blinded to the clinical symptoms rated the likelihood that the pathology observed would produce clinical pain. The only form of pathology consistently predictably related to pelvic pain was deep infiltrative endometriosis. Specifically, the raters were unable to predict the association of pain with adhesive disease. However, the number of patients who had adhesive disease was small, and the clinical biases of the raters were not described. Specifically, it was not noted whether the raters looked for the degree of restriction of motion of the abdominal viscera by the adhesions.

Placebo Effect of Surgery

The intensity of the placebo effect seems to be related to the magnitude of the treatment offered. Specifically, surgery may have a stronger and possibly more long-lasting placebo effect when compared with medical or other less traumatic treatment options. The most vivid example of this is a controlled study of cardiac revascularization using the internal mammary artery, in which patients undergoing a sham thoracotomy experienced relief of chest pain in 73% of cases.[20] In studies of adhesiolysis, it is difficult to know whether the return of pain after the procedure is the attenuation of the placebo effects for the reformation or perhaps reinnervation of adhesions.

To confound the matter further, many gynecologists sufficiently motivated to publish their series of laparoscopic adhesiolysis cases are also those who would readily prescribe other forms of treatment both pre- and postoperatively in recognition of the multifactorial nature of pain. Stratification of patient populations or statistical covarying of these potential confounds is extremely difficult.

Second-Look Clinical Trial Design

With these considerations in mind, a true randomized clinical trial of laparoscopic adhesiolysis will be extraordinarily difficult. Most physicians likely to conduct such a study have spent years developing referral practices based on their laparoscopic expertise. These investigators and their patients are likely to be most disinclined to randomize surgical treatment versus medical therapy. Alternatively, it may be feasible to evaluate the impact of laparoscopic adhesiolysis by performing second-look diagnostic procedures, perhaps using microlaparoscopic techniques. Ideally, such trials should include careful standardization of patient assessment, including evaluation of gastrointestinal, musculoskeletal, and urinary tract contributions to pelvic pain. Subjects should most likely also be stratified according to the level of psychopathology documented.

Meanwhile, what is a reasonable clinical role for adhesiolysis and the overall management of pelvic pain in the presence of adhesions? While encouraging and attempting further clinical research in this important area, I take here the chapter author's prerogative of describing my own clinical practice.

A Practical Approach to the Treatment of Pain in the Presence of Adhesions

As a physician practicing in a referral setting, I have noticed a clear shift in the type of patients referred during the past 10 years. In the early days of operative laparoscopy, a substantial proportion of referred patients had pain that was of relatively briefer duration, a more precisely focused location, and less confounded by the simultaneous presence of other contributing factors. In these cases, when laparoscopy revealed adhesions whose location corresponded nicely to the location of the pain, straightforward adhesiolysis was in general a rewarding experience for patient and surgeon alike. With the acquisition of laparoscopic skills by more and more practicing gynecologists, this type of patient is now less frequently referred for tertiary care. Presently, the more typical referral patient has had pain for a longer period of time, has gradually accrued contributions from other organ systems, has declined emotionally and psychologically, and had one or more previously unsuccessful laparoscopic adhesiolysis procedures. Clearly, proceeding immediately to yet another laparoscopy is a less productive enterprise in this latter type of patient.

Rehabilitation

The more a patient presents with this more complex disorder, the more patient education and preoperative pain management must be employed. The patient and her family must come to understand that treating the adhesions surgically is only one component of an overall treatment plan. Further, they must learn that as pain may become more centralized, and spinal cord disregulation may be involved, that the recovery from pain is a more long-term process of rehabilitation. For example, some patients experiencing pelvic pain for a long period of time may develop muscular components including spasm of the pelvic floor levator muscles, piriformis muscles, and lumbar paraspinous muscles. In many cases, treatment by a physical therapist may be helpful in reducing a person's discomfort substantially. In other instances such involvement with other organ systems may diminish spontaneously after successful laparoscopic treatment of adhesions. It is a difficult matter of clinical judgment to determine the appropriate sequence of therapies, but a reasonable general principle is to employ the less expensive and less intrusive treatments first.

Consistent with a general plan for rehabilitation, postoperative visits should be planned before the surgery. Regular visits at relatively closely spaced intervals may be required to carefully monitor ongoing therapies such as bowel management and psychotropic and analgesic management, as well as continuing education regarding return to full activities.

Surgical Considerations

The surgical technique employed for adhesiolysis may be important to success in terms of pain relief. Consistent with comments made in other chapters in the volume, gentle tissue handling, pursuit of avascular planes, and copious irrigation reflect the methods traditionally employed in microsurgery. Whenever possible, direct grasping of the fallopian tubes is to be avoided. In many situations it is difficult to successfully lyse all the involved adhesions, especially those that are more dense and cohesive. The information from the literature is consistent with the notion that the more involved the dissection becomes, and the more bleeding that occurs, the more likely that adhesions will simply reform. It then becomes a matter of judgment as to whether it remains useful to pursue every last adhesion. Sometimes, it may be that "better is the enemy of good."

At times, the extent and density of adhesions makes a laparoscopic approach impractical altogether. In these instances, I have on occasion carried out a laparotomy with complete lysis of adhesions, followed by a second-look laparoscopy. Although there is fragmentary support in the literature for a second-look approach,[21–23] both of these studies involved infertility patients, not patients seeking relief of pain. It would appear that adhesions are already substantially formed by 2 weeks after surgery.[24] When second-look laparoscopy is planned, I schedule it for no more than 7 to 10 days after the first one.

A particular note of caution must be sounded on this account. Especially when the original dissection involved substantial enterolysis, the involved loops of bowel remain more vulnerable to injury 7 to 10 days after that procedure. In several instances, enterotomies have occurred in the course of gentle repeat adhesiolysis while doing second-look laparoscopy.

These considerations (together with the obvious discomfort, inconvenience, and difficulties with reimbursement involved with second-look procedures) invite the development of more effective methods of adhesion prevention (see Chapters 32, 34, 37, and 41), as well as less intrusive methods of evaluating the success of adhesiolysis.

Future Directions

In view of the multiple potential confounds involved in studying the outcome of the studies involving the treatment of pain in the presence of pelvic adhesions, future studies need to be carried out by like-minded and comparably skilled physicians who enroll subjects in carefully designed protocols involving detailed screening and proactive stratification. Such studies will be labor intensive and require prolonged follow-up (at least 1–2 years) before therapeutic success can be declared.

Previous studies of adhesiolysis, including those involving the agents aimed at preventing adhesion reformation, have most often tested the efficacy of a single intervention. It would seem, given the complexity of adhesion formation, that the ultimately successful regimen might involve a combination of efforts, such as meticulous laparoscopic surgical technique, the installation of an adhesion preventive agent, perhaps a postoperative reinstallation of adhesion-preventing agents at intervals via a transabdominal catheter, or one or more second-look laparoscopies for repeated mechanical disruptions of new adhesions as they are forming. A pilot study has been performed demonstrating the feasibility of this latter approach.[25]

Conclusions

Taken as a whole, the available clinical evidence suggests that adhesions play a role in generating nociceptive signals. These signals are subject to substantial modification at both the spinal cord and higher levels. Surgical treatment of the adhesions may therefore be more successful in instances in which such amplification is less prominent; therapeutic success in more involved cases may involve the substitution of medical approaches for surgical management or using the two methods together. The more complicated the patient problems involved, the more preoperative education must take place concerning the multifactorial nature of chronic pain and the need for an overall treatment plan. The potentials for therapeutic success of any measure employed must be employed fairly and conservatively, as patients with chronic pelvic pain who are in substantial distress are often propelled by their desperation into placing unrealistic degrees of hope upon a new surgical approach. As a rule of thumb, referral for a consultation at a pain management center, preferably involving a gynecologist skilled at such an assessment, should take place when either the patient situation is obviously complex at first glance or when a first attempt at laparoscopic adhesiolysis fails to produce the desired result. The growing interest in pain research, and the development of professional groups (International Pelvic Pain Society, IPPS) focusing on pelvic pain represent hopeful signs that may lead to more extensive future research and ultimately better treatment methods.

References

1. Steege JF, Metzger DA, Levy BS. Chronic Pelvic Pain: An Integrated Approach. Philadelphia: Saunders, 1998.
2. Walker EA, Katon WJ, Jemelka R, et al. The prevalence of chronic pelvic pain and irritable bowel syndrome in two university clinics. J Psychosom Obstet Gynecol 1991; 12(suppl):65–75.
3. Jamieson DJ, Steege JF. The prevalence of dysmenorrhea, dyspareunia, pelvic pain, and irritable bowel syndrome in primary care practices. Obstet Gynecol 1996;87:55–58.
4. Mathias SD, Kupperman M, Liberman RF, et al. Chronic pelvic pain: prevalence, health-related quality of life, and economic correlates. Obstet Gynecol 1996;87:321–327.
5. National Center for Health Statistics, Graves EJ. National Hospital Discharge Survey: Annual Summary, 1990. Vital and Health Statistics. DHHS (PHS) 92-1773. Series 13, No. 112. Washington, DC: U.S. Government Printing Office, 1992.
6. Hulka JF, Peterson HB, Phillips JM, Surrey MW. Operative laparoscopy: American Association of Gynecologic Laparoscopists 1991 membership survey. J Reprod Med 1993; 38:569–571.
7. Melzack R. Neurophysiologic foundations of pain. In Sternbach RA, ed. The Psychology of Pain. New York: Raven Press, 1986:1.

8. Coderre RJ, Katz J, Vaccarino AL, Melzack R. Contribution of central neuroplasticity to pathological pain: review of clinical and experimental evidence. Pain 1993;52: 259–285.
9. Monk BJ, Berman ML, Montz FI. Adhesions after extensive gynecologic surgery: clinical significance, etiology, and prevention. Am J Obstet Gynecol 1994;170: 1396–1403.
10. Weibel MA, Majno G. Peritoneal adhesions and their relation to abdominal surgery. Am J Surg 1973;126:345–353.
11. Kresch AJ, Seifer DB, Sachs LB, et al. Laparoscopy in 100 women with chronic pelvic pain. Obstet Gynecol 1984;64: 672–674.
12. Stout AL, Steege JF, Dodson WC, et al. Relationship of laparoscopic findings to self-report of pelvic pain. Am J Obstet Gynecol 1991;164:73–79.
13. Sutton C, MacDonald R. Laser laparoscopic adhesiolysis. J Gynecol Surg 1990;6:155–159.
14. Steege JF, Stout AL. Resolution of chronic pelvic pain after laparoscopic lysis of adhesions. Am J Obstet Gynecol 1991;165:278–283.
15. Mueller MD, Tschudi J, Herrmann U, Klaiber C. An evaluation of laparoscopic adhesiolysis in patients with chronic abdominal pain. Surg Endosc 1995;9(7):802–804.
16. Saravelos HG, Li TC, Cooke ID. An analysis of the outcome of microsurgical and laparoscopic adhesiolysis for chronic pelvic pain. Hum Reprod (306) 1995;10(11): 2895–2901.
17. Peters AAW, Trimbos-Kemper GCM, Admiraal C, Trimbos JB. A randomized clinical trial on the benefit of adhesiolysis in patients with introperitoneal adhesions and chronic pelvic pain. Br J Obstet Gynaecol 1992;99:59–62.
18. Peters AAW, van Dorst E, Jellis B, et al. A randomized clinical trial to compare two different approaches in women with chronic pelvic pain. Obstet Gynecol 1991;77: 740–744.
19. Thornton JG, Morley S, Lilleyman J, Onwude JL, Curri I, Crompton AC. The relationship between laparoscopic disease, pelvic pain and infertility; an unbiased assessment. Eur J Obstet Gynecol Reprod Biol 1997;74(1):57–62.
20. Turner JA, Dayo RA, Loeser DJ, Von Korff M, Fordyce WE. The importance of placebo effects in pain treatment and research. JAMA 1994;271:1609–1614.
21. Raj SG, Hulka JF. Second-look laparoscopy in infertility surgery: therapeutic and prognostic value. Fertil Steril 1982;38:325–329.
22. Trimbos-Kemper TCM, Trimbos JB, van Hall EV. Adhesion formation after tubal surgery: results of the eighth-day laparoscopy in 188 patients. Fertil Steril 1985;43:395–400.
23. Jansen RPS. Failure of peritoneal irrigation with heparin during pelvic operations upon young women to reduce adhesions. Surg Gynecol Obstet 1988;166:154–160.
24. Malinak RL. Interceed (TC7) as an adjuvant for adhesion reduction: clinical studies. In: diZerega GS, Malinak LR, Diamond MP, Linsky CP, eds. Treatment of Postoperative Surgical Adhesions. New York: Wiley, 1990:193–206.
25. Steege JF. Repeated clinic laparoscopy for the treatment of pelvic adhesions: a pilot study. Obstet Gynecol 1994;83: 276–279.

Section 6
Adhesion Prevention Adjuvants for Clinical Use

32

Development and Clinical Evaluation of Intergel Adhesion Prevention Solution for the Reduction of Adhesions Following Peritoneal Cavity Surgery

Douglas B. Johns and Gere S. diZerega

CONTENTS

Adhesion formation after peritoneal surgery is a major cause of postoperative bowel obstruction, infertility, and chronic pelvic pain.[1–7] Therefore, a method by which postsurgical adhesion formation could be reduced or prevented would be of great benefit in reducing postoperative morbidity and failed surgical therapy. Studies have indicated that placement of an absorbable barrier of oxidized regenerated cellulose (Interceed® [TC7] Absorbable Adhesion Barrier; Ethicon), expanded polytetrafluoroethylene (Preclude® Surgical Membrane; W.L. Gore), or hyaluronic acid/carboxymethylcellulose (Seprafilm® Surgical Membrane; Genzyme) between injury sites or addition of a viscous solution (dextran, Hyskon® Solution, Pharmacia; hyaluronic acid, Sepracoat®, Genzyme) into the peritoneal cavity during or after surgery can reduce postoperative adhesion formation.[8–20] In the case of Interceed barrier, Preclude membrane, or Seprafilm membrane, the surgeon must predict potential sites of adhesion formation to determine placement and optimize barrier benefit. Sepracoat, a dilute solution of hyaluronic acid (HA), has only been shown to be effective at reducing the number of de novo adhesions at sites remote from the surgical trauma, while the use of Hyskon in clinical practice has shown some undesirable side effects resulting from the accumulation of intraperitoneal ascites from oncotic properties.[21] In addition, several reports indicate that Hyskon is ineffective in pelvic surgery because of gravitational pooling in the cul-de-sac.[22–26]

Hyaluronic Acid

HA is a linear polysaccharide with repeating disaccharide units composed of sodium D-glucuronate and *N*-acetyl-D-glucosamine. It is a major component of many body tissues and fluids, providing mechanically protective and physically supportive roles.[27,28] It undergoes degradation and replacement (turnover) and has been extensively studied in animal and human disease. Aqueous solutions of this polymer have a water-like or viscous consistency depending upon the concentration of HA.

Viscous HA solutions were shown to reduce adhesion formation in several situations including subcutaneous tissue, arthritic joints, tendons, and peritoneal tissues.[29–35]

The viscosity and intraperitoneal residence time of an HA solution can be dramatically increased by chelation or cross-linking with ferric ion (FeHA). Cross-linking between the carboxylate groups on the hyaluronate and the trivalent iron (Fe^{3+}) is ionic in nature, and produces a significant increase in solution viscosity compared to the starting sodium hyaluronate solution.[36] Simple exchange of the ferric ion regenerates the native hyaluronate molecule.

This chapter summarizes the development of Intergel Adhesion Prevention Solution, the first clinical product derived from FeHA. The next section discusses various FeHA gels and their preclinical evaluation.[36] Then, the effect of a single administration of Intergel solution in randomized controlled clinical studies is examined in peritoneal cavity surgery.[37,38] Together, these studies show that Intergel solution is safe and effective in reducing the incidence, extent, and severity of adhesions after pelvic surgery in women. Reduction is found in both reformed and de novo adhesions, as well as those at the site of direct surgical trauma.

Preclinical Evaluation of Ferric Hyaluronate Gels (FeHA)

Two animal models for evaluating adhesion prevention were extensively utilized during the preclinical development of Intergel Adhesion Prevention Solution.

Sidewall Model

Rabbits were prepared for surgery with intramuscular anesthesia followed by hair removal from the abdominal area. The animals were placed in a dorsal recumbent position and the abdomen was exposed through a ventral midline incision. The cecum was then exteriorized and abraded by applying digital pressure with gauze (approximately 40 times) until punctate bleeding occurred. A 10-cm area of the large bowel was scraped (approximately 40 times) using a #10 scalpel blade until punctate bleeding occurred. The right sidewall was then exposed and a 3×5 cm lesion was created by scoring the sidewall with a scalpel blade and removing the peritoneum and transverse abdominis muscle. If a test material was used, a small amount of the material was applied to each of the injured sites (approximately 8 mL). The remaining test material (approximately 7 mL) was applied to the abdominal cavity just before closing the abdominal muscle layer. The skin was closed with 3-0 Vicryl running sutures. Seven days after surgery, the animals were sacrificed and the following parameters were assessed: (a) area (percent) of the sidewall study site with adhesions, (b) length (cm) of the cecum with adhesions, (c) length (cm) of large bowel with adhesions, and (d) number of adhesion-free sidewalls. The area of the sidewall study site was the primary efficacy parameter.

Uterine Horn Model

Rabbits were prepared for surgery with intramuscular anesthesia followed by hair removal from the abdominal area. The animals were placed in the dorsal recumbent position and the abdomen was entered through a ventral midline incision. The uterine horns were exposed and the diameter measured on a French catheter scale. Only those animals whose uterine horn size was French catheter scale 9–16 were utilized. The uterine horns were scraped with a #10 scalpel blade until punctate bleeding occurred (approximately 20–30 times). A small amount (approximately 5 mL) of the test sample was applied to both injured uterine horns before closure. The remaining sample (approximately 10 mL) was injected via a syringe (directed toward the pelvis) through the peritoneal muscle layer just before closure. The abdomen, subcutaneous, and subcuticular layers were closed using Prolene or Vicryl suture (4-0). The skin was closed with skin staples. After 14 ± 1 days following surgery, the animals were sacrificed and the extent of uterine horn adhesions was assessed by estimating the length of uterine horn with adhesions (maximum, 5 cm). Group means and variances were calculated from the average extent of adhesions for each animal. The extent (cm) of horns involved with adhesions was used as the primary measurement parameter.

Preparation of FeHA Gels

Intergel Adhesion Prevention Solution, 0.5% ferric hyaluronate gel, an FeHA gel, is an aqueous solution of sodium hyaluronate that has been ionically cross-linked by the addition of a ferric chloride solution via a proprietary process which avoids precipitation of insoluble ferric hyaluronate and results in a gel formation. Cross-linking between the carboxylate groups on the hyaluronate and the trivalent iron (Fe^{3+}) is ionic in nature, but results in a significant increase in solution viscosity compared to the starting sodium hyaluronate solution.[36] Simple exchange of the ferric ion regenerates the native hyaluronate molecule. FeHA gels with a wide range of viscosity profiles can be prepared. Increasing either the sodium hyaluronate or the ferric iron concentration leads to higher viscosity formulations. The clinical formulation, Intergel Adhesion Prevention Solution, is prepared from a 0.5% sodium hyaluronate solution that has been cross-linked by ferric ion to 90% of the theoretical maximum. The theoretical maximum is based on one ferric ion per three disaccharide units.

Efficacy of FeHA Versus HA

In the rabbit sidewall model, 15 mL (5–7.5 mL/kg) of a 90% cross-linked FeHA gel or HA solution was applied to each of the injured sites. Surgical control animals received no treatment. The HA formulation was not effective in reducing adhesions to the sidewall area (55%) compared with controls (67%), whereas FeHA effected a significant reduction in adhesions to the sidewall area (<1%) (Table 32.1). A similar pattern was noted in the secondary efficacy parameters, that is, the extent of adhesions to the cecum and large bowel. The two formulations contained similar concentrations of HA (approximately 1%), but were different in viscosity.

In the rabbit uterine horn model, higher concentrations of HA that have similar viscosity to FeHA were still not as effective (Table 32.2). A 32,600 cps FeHA gel (1% HA, 90% cross-linked) significantly reduced adhesions compared with surgical controls (mean extent of uterine horn involvement in adhesions, 1.84 cm vs. 4.28 cm, respectively), while HA at a similar concentration (1%) with a viscosity of 1,000 cps, or HA at a higher concentration (2.75%) and similar viscosity, 30,000 cps, was not effective compared with surgical controls (3.82 cm vs. 3.67 cm and 3.83 cm vs. 3.94 cm, respectively).

Further increasing the concentration of HA to prepare more viscous materials did not improve its efficacy (Table 32.3). HA with a viscosity of 99,600 cps (3.65%) was not effective in preventing adhesion formation (3.71 cm), while FeHA gel with viscosities of 146,000 and 57,200 cps (HA concentrations of 1.43% and 1%, respectively) significantly reduced the extent of adhesions (2.27 cm and 2.42 cm) compared with surgical controls (4.64 cm). Thus, while efficacy may be independent of HA concentration or formulation viscosity, it directly correlates with the presence of ionic cross-linking.

Optimal Cross-Linking Determination

The optimum degree of cross-linking was evaluated in several studies, and efficacy was found to improve with increasing cross-link density. In the rabbit uterine horn model, the efficacy of 5% cross-linked FeHA, 25% cross-linked FeHA, or 50% cross-linked FeHA was evaluated. The concentration of HA was decreased as cross-linking was increased to keep formulation viscosity relatively constant. Of each formulation, 15 mL was applied to the injured area. Surgical control animals did not receive any treatment. As shown in Table 32.4, the 50% cross-

TABLE 32.2 Average extent of adhesions in the rabbit uterine horn "Adhesion Formation" and "Bleeding" models.

	Adhesion formation (cm)		
Treatment group	*n*	Mean	SEM
Part I[a]			
Surgical control	6	3.67	0.85
HA (1,000 cps)	7	3.82	0.63
Part II[b]			
Surgical control	8	4.28	0.41
FeHA (90% cross-linked, 32,600 cps)	8	1.84*	0.38
Part III[c]			
Surgical control	4	3.94	0.66
HA (30,000 cps)	3	3.83	0.73

[a]HA = 1% HA, 1,000 cps, 15 mL

[b]FeHA = 1% HA, 90% cross-linked, 55,000 cps, 10 mL.

[c]HA = 2.75% HA, 30,000 cps, 15 mL.

*Significantly different from control value, < 0.05; Student's *t*-test.

TABLE 32.3. Average extent of adhesions in the rabbit uterine horn adhesion model.

	Extent (cm)		
Treatment group	*n*	Mean	SEM
Surgical control	7	4.64	0.17
FeHA (146,000 cps)[a]	6	2.27*	0.83
FeHA (57,200 cps)[b]	7	2.42*	0.53
HA 3.65% (99,600 cps)[c]	6	3.71	0.62

[a]FeHA, 1.43% HA, 90% cross-linked, 146,000 cps.

[b]FeHA, 1% HA, 90% cross-linked, 57,200 cps.

[c]HA, 3.65% H, 99,600 cps.

*Significantly different from control value, $p = 0.05$; Student's *t*-test.

TABLE 32.1. Efficacy of hyaluronic acid (HA) and ferric ion-linked HA (FeHA) in the rabbit sidewall adhesion model.

Treatment group	*n*	Cecum length adherent (cm)	Bowel length adherent (cm)	Total sidewall adherent (%)
Surgical control	8			
Mean		10.13	4.94	67.25
SEM		2.20	0.83	11.88
HA[a]	8			
Mean		6.63	4.63	55.25
SEM		1.18	0.65	11.28
FeHA[b]	7			
Mean		0.93*	0.93*	0.29*
SEM		0.58	0.40	0.14

[a]HA = 1.13% HA, 1,285 cps.

[b]FeHA = 1% HA, 90% cross-linked, 55,000 cps.

*Significantly different from control value, $p < 0.05$; Student's *t*-test.

TABLE 32.4. The effects of cross-linking in the rabbit uterine horn adhesion model.

Treatment group	n	Mean extent (cm)
Surgical control	6	4.17 ± 0.36
5% Cross-linked FeHA[a]	7	4.25 ± 0.31
25% Cross-linked FeHA[b]	6	2.04* ± 0.75
50% Cross-linked FeHA[c]	7	1.11* ± 0.43

[a]HA = 1.2% HA, 1970 cps.
[b]HA = 0.9% HA, 7660 cps.
[c]HA = 0.675% HA, 8840 cps.
*Significantly different from control value, $p < 0.05$; Student's t-test.

linked FeHA significantly reduced adhesion formation compared with controls (1.11 cm vs. 4.17 cm); 25% cross-linked FeHA also significantly reduced the extent of adhesions (2.04 cm) compared with controls (4.17 cm), although the magnitude of the reduction was not as marked as that achieved with 50% cross-linked FeHA. The 5% cross-linked FeHA was not effective in this model (4.25 cm). Thus, of the three FeHA samples tested, 50% cross-linked FeHA was most effective in reducing adhesions.

In a separate study, a similar trend toward improved efficacy with increasing cross-linked density was evident when the degree of cross-linking and the viscosity were evaluated in the rabbit sidewall model. Four groups of animals received 15 mL of the assigned test sample (Table 32.5). A fifth group of animals served as the surgical control and did not receive any treatment. High-viscosity HA (56,800 cps) significantly reduced adhesions to the sidewall compared with controls (19% vs. 73%, respectively), whereas both 90% cross-linked FeHA at high (47,800 cps) and low viscosity (6,300 cps) and high-viscosity 50% cross-linked FeHA (88,000 cps) completely prevented adhesions to the sidewall (0%). The FeHA groups demonstrated a similar pattern in the extent of adhesions to the cecum and large bowel. However, the magnitude of adhesion reduction, especially in the large bowel, was greater in the 90% cross-linked FeHA groups than in the 50% cross-linked FeHA group. These data demonstrate that 90% cross-linked FeHA, at high and low viscosity, was slightly more efficacious in reducing adhesions in the sidewall model than high-viscosity 50% cross-linked FeHA.

Evaluation of 90% Cross-Linked FeHA

The effect of the different viscosities of 90% cross-linked FeHA formulations on adhesion formation was evaluated. Previous studies had shown that 90% cross-linked FeHA was effective at both high and low viscosities in reducing adhesions in either the rabbit uterine horn model or the rabbit sidewall model. Additional studies were conducted to further evaluate the effect of viscosity on FeHA performance with regard to the volume administered, the method of application, the presence of lavage fluid, and handling properties.

In the rabbit sidewall model, the efficacy of both high- and low-viscosity 90% cross-linked FeHA was evaluated at

TABLE 32.5. The effects of cross-linking in the rabbit sidewall adhesion model.

Treatment group	n	Cecum length adherent (cm)	Bowel length adherent (cm)	Total sidewall adherent (%)
Surgical control	6			
Mean		8.75	4.83	73.33
SEM		1.78	0.69	4.59
HA[a] high viscosity	6			
Mean		4.50	4.92	19.17*
SEM		1.45	1.28	9.70
50% Cross-linked FeHA,[b] high viscosity	3			
Mean		1.00*	1.33	0.00*
SEM		1.00	1.09	0.00
90% Cross-linked FeHA,[c] high viscosity	5			
Mean		0.40*	0.60*	0.00*
SEM		0.40	0.37	0.00
90% Cross-linked FeHA,[d] low viscosity	4			
Mean		0.75*	0.00*	0.00*
SEM		0.75	0.00	0.00

[a]HA = 3% HA, 56,800 cps.
[b]HA = 1.5% HA, 88,000 cps.
[c]HA = 1% HA, 47,800 cps.
[d]HA = 0.45%, HA, 6,300 cps.
*Significantly different compared with control value, $p < 0.05$; Student's t-test.

volumes less than the 15-mL regimen. In this study, only the injured sites were coated with test materials. In some animals, 5 mL of test material was applied and 10 mL in other animals. Control animals did not receive treatment. Both high- and low-viscosity FeHA significantly reduced adhesions to the sidewall and to the cecum when administered at 5-mL and 10-mL, but only the 10-mL volume of either viscosity significantly reduced adhesions to the large bowel as well (data not shown). The number of sidewalls with zero adhesions was also evaluated; the 10-mL volume of either viscosity completely prevented adhesions to the sidewalls, while the 5-mL volumes prevented adhesions to the sidewalls in three of four and four of five animals for the high- and low-viscosity FeHA, respectively. Only one of five surgical control animals had no sidewall adhesions.

In a separate study, the effect of a 5-mL volume of a high- or low-viscosity 90% cross-linked FeHA gel on adhesion formation was evaluated in the rabbit sidewall model. Test material was applied either directly to the injured site with 15 mL saline (applied in a remote location) to mimic a residue of lavage fluid, or at a site remote from the injury without saline to test the ability of the material to flow throughout the abdomen. Surgical control animals did not receive any treatment. As shown in Table 32.6, both the low-viscosity (10,000 cps) and the high-viscosity (48,000 cps) FeHA gels prevented sidewall adhesions when applied directly to injured sites at the same time 15 mL saline was applied to a remote site. Thus, the presence of saline did not interfere with the effectiveness of FeHA in this model. When 5 mL of the same FeHA formulation was applied to a remote location without saline, adhesions to the sidewall were reduced but not prevented in all animals as previously. The latter result demonstrates the ability of FeHA gel to flow throughout the abdomen, but also indicates the importance of applying a volume sufficient to treat the entire abdomen if maximal results are to be achieved.

In addition to safety studies to support the clinical use of Intergel solution, wound healing and infection potentiation studies were performed to directly address the intended clinical use as surgical adjuvant. Wound healing studies, including breaking strength of the skin closure site and bursting strength of bowel anastomotic sites, were tested in four groups (Intergel solution at 5 and 15 mL/kg, saline at 15 mL/kg, and sham control). The results of these studies demonstrated that i.p. administration of Intergel solution at dose volumes up to 15 mL/kg following surgery does not affect healing of colonic anastomoses or incisional wounds in rats.

Based on these studies, a formulation was identified for further development. Intergel Adhesion Prevention Solution (0.5% HA, 90% cross-linked) solution was tested against a low-viscosity HA formulation (1.28% HA, 1350 cps) in the rabbit sidewall model. Animals received 15 mL of Intergel solution; again, those in the surgical control group did not receive treatment. Adhesions to the sidewall were prevented in all animals treated with Intergel solution, whereas in animals treated with HA, 40% of the sidewall was involved in adhesions compared with 66% in control animals. The number of sidewalls with no adhesions was also evaluated. Intergel Adhesion Prevention Solution completely prevented adhesions to all sidewalls (six of six animals), whereas HA completely

TABLE 32.6 The effects of saline and remote application in the rabbit sidewall adhesion model.

Treatment group	Method of application	n	Cecum length adherent (cm)	Bowel length adherent (cm)	Total sidewall adherent (%)	Number of sidewalls with no adhesions/ total animals
Surgical control		5				
Mean			7.00	6.60	54.0	1/5
SEM			2.22	0.62	16.8	
5 mL low-viscosity FeHA[a]	Direct +15 mL saline applied remote	5				
Mean			2.30	4.00	0.00*	5/5
SEM			1.09	1.22	0.00	
5 mL high-viscosity FeHA[b]	Direct +15 mL saline applied remote	5				
Mean			0.95	3.60*	0.00*	5/5
SEM			0.83	0.51	0.00	
5 mL low-viscosity FeHA[a]	Applied remote	5				
Mean			5.90	6.60	13.0	3/5
SEM			2.09	0.60	11.8	
5 mL high-viscosity FeHA[b]	Applied remote	3				
Mean			4.17	4.33	16.7	2/3
SEM			3.44	0.73	16.7	

[a]FeHA = 90% cross-linked, 0.5% HA, 10,000 cps.
[b]FeHA = 90% cross-linked, 1.0% HA, 48,000 cps.
*Significantly different compared with control value, $p < 0.05$; Student's t-test.

prevented adhesions to the sidewall in only two of seven animals compared to zero of seven untreated, surgical control animals.

Effects of Infection Potentiation

The ability of Intergel Adhesion Prevention Solution to potentiate infection caused by implantation of fecal material into the abdomen was evaluated in a model described by Weinstein et al.[39] Peritonitis was induced in 140 female Sprague-Dawley rats weighing 150 to 200 g by implanting a double-walled gelatin capsule containing a mixture of cecal/fecal contents from hamburger-fed rats, peptone yeast broth, glucose, and barium sulfate in the peritoneum on the right side through a midline incision. Before closure of the wound, the assigned test material (Table 32.7) was applied to the area surrounding the capsule. Animals in the surgical control group received the capsule only. Twenty animals were evaluated in each treatment regimen. The animals were observed daily for 11 days for signs of morbidity and mortality. Those that died during the observation period were necropsied to confirm the presence of acute bacterial infection. Those that survived the acute infection were killed 11 days following surgery and examined for transcutaneous palpability of the abscesses. Upon opening, the odor of the peritoneal cavity was recorded, the presence of splenomegaly was recorded, and abscess formation at the liver, spleen, abdominal wall, retrohepatic gutter, colonic gutter, bowel, and omentum was graded by two separate observers in a blinded randomized manner based on a 5-point scale as follows: 0 = no abscesses present at site, 0.5 = one very small abscess present at site, 1 = several small abscesses present at site, 2 = medium to large abscesses present at site, and 3 = one very large abscess present at site.

The mortality and abscess formation data (Table 32.7) showed no significant differences in mortality between the surgical control group, Ringer's lactate control groups, Intergel solution-treated groups, or the low-dose-volume Hyskon group. In contrast, administration of 15 mL/kg Hyskon significantly increased the mortality associated with the induced bacterial peritonitis (1 survivor vs. 11–17 in the other groups). No significant differences in abscess scores for the liver, bowel, omentum, or "Other" sites (combined scores for spleen, retrohepatic gutter, and colonic gutter) were observed between any of the treatment groups. In contrast, treatment with Intergel solution (both volumes) produced significant decreases in the number of abscesses in the abdominal wall and in total abscess formation relative to the surgical control group. (The low-volume Intergel Adhesion Prevention Solution group also had a significantly lower total abscess score than the low-volume Ringer's lactate control group.)

The results of this study demonstrate that intraperitoneal administration of Intergel Adhesion Prevention Solution at dose volumes up to 15 mL/kg does not potentiate mortality or abscess formation following bacterially induced peritonitis.

TABLE 32.7. Median (range) abscess score following implantation of fecal matter into the abdominal cavity.

		Abscess score					
Treatment group	No. animals dead (n = 20 per group)	Liver	Abdominal wall	Bowel	Omentum	Other	Total
Surgical control	5						
Mean		1.53	3.07	0.80	2.20	0.33	7.93
SD		0.62	0.57	1.17	0.54	0.87	2.24
Ringer's lactate,[a] 5 mL/kg	3						
Mean		1.33	1.87*	0.33	2.53	0.27	6.33
SD		1.19	1.31	0.70	0.50	0.68	2.39
Ringer's lactate,[a] 15 mL/kg	5						
Mean		0.93	1.60*	0.20	2.27	0.00	5.00*
SD		1.12	1.25	0.75	0.68	0.00	2.45
Hyskon,[b] 5 mL/kg	6						
Mean		0.93	0.86*	0.14	2.00	0.00	3.93*
SD		1.03	1.25	0.52	0.65	0.00	1.75
Hyskon,[c] 15 mL/kg	19	2	0	0	2	0	4
Intergel, 5 mL/kg	5						
Mean		0.93	1.00*	0.00	1.80	0.00	3.73*
SD		0.93	0.97	0.00	0.54	0.00	1.65
Intergel, 15 mL/kg	9						
Mean		1.22	1.07*	0.15	2.03	0.00	4.41*
SD		0.80	0.83	0.53	0.79	0.00	1.95

[a]Manufactured by Baxter.
[b]Manufactured by Abbott Laboratories, Inc.
[c]Abscess score data are based on 1 surviving animal.
*Significantly different from the surgical control value, $p \leq 0.05$; rank analysis.

Preclinical Perspective

Previous studies have shown HA to be effective in reducing adhesions in a rabbit uterine horn devascularization and abrasion model.[35] In that model, the lower adhesion scores typically resulted from a reduction in the extent of adhesions involved with tissues adjacent to the site of surgical trauma. These data show that ionic cross-linking of HA increased the efficacy compared to noncross-linked HA in two standardized animal models. In addition, the more highly cross-linked the FeHA was, the more efficacious the material became in the reduction of adhesion formation. When the concentration of the HA preparations was increased to provide formulations with similar viscosity, FeHA was still more efficacious than noncross-linked HA, especially in the sidewall model. The lower adhesion scores in these models resulted from a reduction of adhesions at the site of surgical trauma in addition to adjacent tissues.

The only difference between the FeHA and HA formulations appears to be a longer residence time at the site following intraperitoneal administration of FeHA. This delay in absorption of FeHA relative to HA from the peritoneal cavity may result from a greater tendency of FeHA to adhere to tissue surfaces or a delayed dilution with peritoneal fluids compared to HA. The lymphatic absorption rates of HA and FeHA in rats were determined to be 0.38 and 0.19 mg equivalents per gram of tissue per hour, respectively.[36] Considering that the intraperitoneal clearance of HA is the rate of total lymph turnover per unit body weight, and that the average flow rates of lymph through the thoracic duct in humans is 125 mL/hour,[40,41] the elimination half-life ($T_{1/2}$) of HA from the peritoneum would be expected to be approximately 25.5 hours. It follows that the expected half-life of FeHA from the peritoneal cavity would be approximately twice that of HA, or 51 hours.

Summary

In summary, ionically cross-linked HA (FeHA) was highly effective in reducing adhesion formation in two standardized animal models. Intergel Adhesion Prevention Solution, a formulation with the critical variables optimized, was identified for further evaluation in clinical studies.

Clinical Evaluation of Intergel Adhesion Prevention Solution

The clinical safety and effectiveness of Intergel Adhesion Prevention Solution was initially demonstrated in a single center study.[37] In the pilot, 23 patients were studied (Intergel solution, 13; lactated Ringer's solution, 10). After laparotomy, 300 mL of study device was instilled. At second-look laparoscopy, 4 to 12 weeks after the laparotomy, patients treated with Intergel solution had significantly fewer adhesions than control patients. When adhesions did form they were significantly less extensive and severe. Accordingly, a multicenter study was performed to confirm and extend the results of the pilot.

Clinical study

The study was a randomized, third-part-blinded, placebo-controlled, parallel-group design conducted at 15 centers throughout the United States and Europe (Table 32.8). The study plan was approved for human evaluation by all investigational review boards. Patients were 18 to 46 years old, requiring peritoneal cavity surgery via laparotomy, and expected to undergo a second-look laparoscopy as part of their treatment plan from 6 to 12 weeks after the initial surgery.

Patients

Patients with diabetes, hemochromatosis, hepatic, renal, autoimmune, lymphatic, hematologic, or coagulation disorders, or those presenting with pelvic or abdominal infection were excluded from the study. Also excluded from the study were patients receiving cancer therapy, postoperative hydrotubation, anticoagulants, fibrin glue, or other thrombogenic agents at the initial surgical procedure. Patients receiving any adhesion prevention adjuvant such as Interceed (TC7) Absorbable Adhesion Barrier, Seprafilm Membrane, or Preclude Surgical Membrane, or those receiving any peritoneal instillate containing corticosteroid, nonsteroidal antiinflammatory agents or Hyskon, or those in whom any absorbable hemostat was left in the abdominal or peritoneal cavity, were excluded from the study. Patients undergoing peritoneal grafting or any surgical procedure involving opening of the gastrointestinal or urinary tract, or those

TABLE 32.8. Investigators of multicenter clinical trial to evaluate efficacy of Intergel® Adhesion Prevention Solution in peritoneal cavity surgery.

C.L. Cook, University of Louisville, KY
D.A. Johns, Texas Health Care, Fort Worth, TX
L.M. Kettel, San Diego Fertility Center, La Jolla, CA
O. Lalos, University Hospital, Umea Sweden
B. Larsson, Karolinska Institutet, Danderyd Hospital, Sweden
P. Lundorff, Viborg Sygehus, Denmark
R.L. Malinak, Baylor College of Medicine, Houston, TX
M.G. Martens, Hennepin County Medical Center, Minneapolis, MN
B. Stewart, Pacific Gynecology Specialists, Seattle, WA
M.H. Thornton, USC School of Medicine, Los Angeles, CA
S.E. Tronstad, Skovde Hospital, Skovde, Sweden
R. Valle, Prentice Women's Hospital, Chicago, IL
H.J. van Geldorp, University Hospital, Rotterdam, The Netherlands
C. Witz, University of Texas Health Science Center at San Antonio, TX
P. Young, IGO Medical Group, San Diego, CA

undergoing tubal implantation, reversal of previous surgical sterilization only, or tubal sterilization only did not participate.

Within 2 weeks before the initial surgical procedure, the following baseline data were collected: demographic, medical and surgical history, current medications, physical examination, vital signs, and laboratory evaluations (hematology, blood chemistries, urinalysis, and urine pregnancy test). Hematologic evaluations consisted of hemoglobin, hematocrit, RBC, WBC, and differential. Blood chemistries consisted of BUN, creatinine, phosphorus, calcium, uric acid, total protein, albumin, total bilirubin, SGOT (AST), SGPT (ALT), alkaline phosphatase, sodium, potassium, and chloride.

Study Design

At the time of the initial surgical procedure, patients were assigned the next available study number corresponding to study device or control solution as determined by the randomization schedule. Before any adhesiolysis, the investigator assessed the overall presence, extent, and severity of adhesions at each of the following 23 anatomic sites: the anterior peritoneum (three quadrants), small bowel, anterior uterus, posterior uterus, omentum, large bowel, rectosigmoid portion of the large bowel left and right, cul-de-sac (posterior), right pelvic sidewall, left pelvic sidewall, right ovary medial aspect, right ovary lateral aspect, left ovary medial aspect, left ovary lateral aspect, right tube, right ampulla, left tube, right ovarian fossa (posterior broad ligament), and left ovarian fossa (posterior broad ligament). The extent of adhesions was classified as localized (i.e., <1/3 of the site covered with adhesions), moderate (1/3 to 2/3 of the site covered), or extensive (i.e., >2/3 of the site covered with adhesions) for these 23 sites except for the following 4 sites: large bowel left and right (difficult to visualize entire structure), and omentum and small bowel (the size precludes adequate evaluation of the extent), which are termed "not evaluable" and given an intermediate score (moderate) in the calculation of an adhesion score as discussed next. The severity of adhesions was classified as Mild (i.e., filmy, avascular) or Severe (i.e., organized, cohesive, vascular, dense).

Each patient who met all inclusion and exclusion criteria received 300 mL of either Intergel solution (Treatment) or lactated Ringer's solution (Control). The assigned study solution was administered into the peritoneal cavity by the surgeon after the primary surgical procedure, completion of hemostasis, aspiration of all irrigants, and the removal of all packs and sponges. Six to 12 weeks after the initial surgical procedure, a second-look laparoscopic procedure was performed to reevaluate the 23 anatomic sites as previously described during the initial surgery. A 24th site, the anterior peritoneum incision (from the first operation), was also evaluated.

Study Endpoints

The number and proportion of sites with adhesions were determined. The mean proportion was based on the number of sites with adhesions divided by the number of possible adhesion sites, which equals 24 except when sites are not present (e.g., a missing tube or ovary). The severity and extent of adhesions were evaluated: severity was scored on a three-point scale (0 = None, 1 = Mild, and 2 = Severe), and extent was scored on a four-point scale (0 = None, 1 = Localized, 2 = Moderate, and 3 = Extensive). A total adhesion score using the Adhesion Scoring Method of the American Fertility Society (AFS) applied to 24 anatomic sites was determined.[42] Adhesions occurring at each of the 24 potential adhesion sites were scored as follows:

No adhesion; 0
Severity: Mild; Extent: Localized; 1
Severity: Mild; Extent: Moderate; 2
Severity: Mild; Extent: Extensive; 4
Severity: Severe; Extent: Localized; 4
Severity: Severe; Extent: Moderate; 8
Severity: Severe; Extent: Extensive; 16

Scores from all potential adhesion sites were averaged to yield a total adhesion score.

Safety evaluation was based on concomitant medications and conditions as well as on the type and severity of adverse events recorded throughout the study. Safety was also based on gross evaluation at second-look laparoscopy and on clinical laboratory tests performed within 2 weeks before the initial surgery, immediately before discharge from the hospital, and 7 to 28 days after the initial surgery. Length of hospital stay was also evaluated. The Treatment and Control groups were compared using Student's *t*-test for continuous variables and Fisher's exact test for categoric variables. Additional analyses using the Wilcoxon rank-sum test did not suggest any difference in the conclusions to be drawn.

Study Results

A total of 213 patients were treated, 109 in the 0.5% Intergel Adhesion Prevention Solution (Treatment) group and 104 in the lactated Ringer's solution (Control) group. As shown in Table 32.9, patients in the two groups were comparable in terms of age, height, race, and vital signs, and the type and frequency of surgical procedures were similar for the two groups (Table 32.10). There were no statistically significant differences between the two groups in the number of nights spent at the hospital (3.1 ± 1.6 vs. 3.2 ± 1.7, respectively), the number of days to second-look laparoscopy (58.9 ± 20 vs. 58.5 ± 21, respectively), or the operative time (1.87 ± 0.86 vs. 1.85 ± 0.85 hours, respectively) for the Treatment and Control groups. In both groups, bowel

TABLE 32.9. Patient demographic characteristics.

Factor	Intergel Adhesion Prevention Solution (n = 109)	Control (n = 104)
Age (yr)		
Mean ± SD	33.4 ± 5.9	33.7 ± 5.6
Range	18.8–44.9	18.6–45.9
Height (in.)		
Mean ± SD	64.5 ± 2.5	64.6 ± 2.8
Range	57–71	57–71.7
Weight (lb)		
Mean ± SD	149.4 ± 31.6	149.3 ± 31.2
Range	104–252	100–264
Race (% of patients)		
Caucasian	57.8	57.7
Hispanic	17.4	20.2
Black	19.3	17.3
Oriental	3.7	2.9
Other	1.8	1.9
Endometriosis	19	22
Stage I	7	5
Stage II	4	8
Stage III	4	4
Stage IV	4	4

TABLE 32.10. Type and frequency of surgical procedures.

Procedure	Intergel solution	Control
Myomectomy	71	65
Adhesiolysis	58	54
Tuboplasty	18	20
Ablation of endometriosis	9	10
Ovarian cystectomy	24	30
Simple	11	12
Dermoid	3	8
Endometrioma	10	10

function returned to normal within 3 days, there was no evidence of ascites, and there were no cases of postoperative sepsis.

Adverse Events

There were no serious or potentially serious adverse events reported in this study. No deaths occurred during this study, and there were no study discontinuations because of an adverse event. At least one adverse event was reported by all patients in both study groups. However, no comparisons reached conventional levels ($p = 0.05$) of significance. The three body systems with the highest patient incidence of adverse events were body as a whole with 98% of patients in both groups, digestive with 70% of patients in the Treatment group versus 73% in the Control group, and nervous system with 25% versus 27% respectively. Of events affecting the body as a whole, the largest proportions were attributable to pain. Digestive system disorders were frequently attributable to nausea and constipation while the nervous system disorders were mostly attributable to dizziness and insomnia. These expected events (given that patients were undergoing anesthesia and surgery) were generally mild to moderate and resolved spontaneously or with standard postoperative care.

Efficacy

As shown in Table 32.11, the mean number of sites at baseline with adhesions, number of adhesions that were lysed, and the number of surgical sites (which includes adhesiolysis, surgical treatment of endometriosis, and

TABLE 32.11. Number and proportion of adhesions.

	Intergel solution		Lactated Ringer's solution			
	n	Mean ± SD	n	Mean ± SD	p	Reduction (%)
Baseline						
Number of sites with adhesions	109	3.8 ± 4.35	104	4.03 ± 4.65	0.799	
Number of sites with adhesions lysed	109	3.26 ± 2.94	104	3.39 ± 4.29	0.808	
Number of primary surgical sites	109	5.67 ± 3.55	104	5.86 ± 3.73	0.710	
Extent	109	0.31 ± 0.4	104	0.35 ± 0.43	0.504	
Severity	109	0.41 ± 0.49	104	0.40 ± 0.4	0.939	
Modified AFS score	109	1.13 ± 1.70	104	1.24 ± 1.7	0.589	
Second-look						
Adhesions	109	6.22 ± 4.86	104	8.23 ± 5.57	.005	24
Proportion	109	0.271 ± 0.214	104	0.364 ± 0.246	.004	26
Modified AFS score	109	1.22 ± 1.50	104	2.48 ± 2.76	.000	51
Severity score	109	0.49 ± 0.44	104	0.81 ± 0.66	.000	40
Extent score	109	0.45 ± 0.45	104	0.69 ± 0.6	.001	35
De novo adhesions	109	4.52 ± 4.29	104	5.88 ± 4.77	.029	23
Proportion	109	0.229 ± 0.203	104	0.308 ± 0.239	.010	26
Surgical site adhesions	109	2.50 ± 2.68	104	3.55 ± 3.27	.011	30
Proportion	109	0.352 ± 0.295	104	0.479 ± 0.298	.002	27
Surgical site de novo	109	0.630 ± 0.678	104	1.01 ± 1.01	.003	38
Proportion	109	0.263 ± 0.310	104	0.389 ± 0.359	.007	32
Reformed adhesions	58	3.19 ± 2.81	54	4.52 ± 3.24	.022	29
Proportion	58	0.491 ± 0.344	54	0.730 ± 0.305	.000	33

AFS, American Fertility Society.

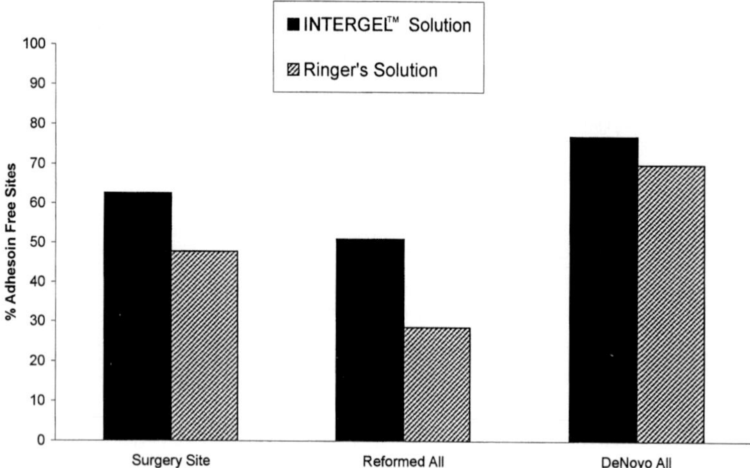

FIG. 32.1 Percent of anatomic sites that were adhesion free at second-look laparoscopy in patients who received 300 mL of an intraperitoneal instillate of Intergel Adhesion Prevention Solution (*black bars*) or lactated Ringer's solution (*shaded bars*) at the end of surgery. Data are summarized for the primary surgical site, reformed adhesions, and de novo adhesions. Patients who received Intergel solution had a statistically significant increase in adhesion-free sites at the surgical site ($p = 0.001$), as well as in reformation ($p = 0.019$) and de novo adhesion ($p = 0.003$).

other surgical procedures) were comparable for the two groups. However, at second-look laparoscopy, the mean number of sites with adhesions (excluding sites with adhesions that were not lysed at the first procedure) as well as the proportion of possible adhesion sites was significantly reduced in the Intergel Adhesion Prevention Solution group compared to Control ($p = 0.005$ and 0.005, respectively).

Patients treated with Intergel solution had a significantly lower number of sites with reformed as well as de novo adhesions than control patients at second-look laparoscopy ($p < 0.001$) (Fig. 32.1). Further, the number of adhesions at the primary surgical site was significantly reduced with Intergel solution ($p < 0.01$). The severity and extent of adhesions at baseline and at second-look

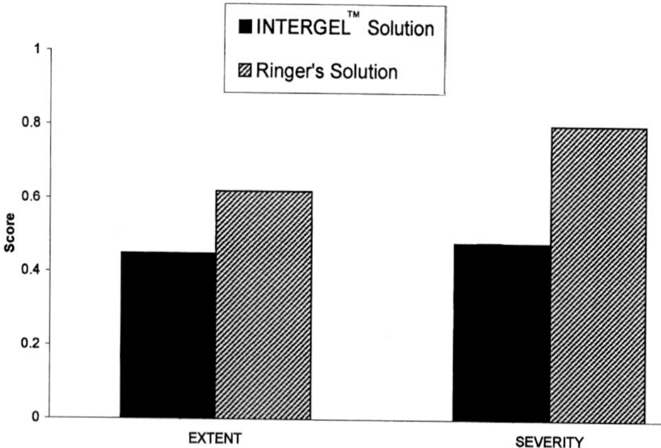

FIG. 32.2. Severity and extent of adhesions at second-look laparoscopy in patients who received a 300-mL intraperitoneal instillate of either Intergel Adhesion Prevention Solution (*shaded bars*) or lactated Ringer's solution (*black bars*). Patients treated with Intergel solution had significantly lower adhesion severity and extent scores compared to patients who received lactated Ringer's solution ($p < 0.01$ for all groups; error bars are $x \pm$ SEM).

laparoscopy were also evaluated. Although the two groups were comparable at baseline (Fig. 32.2), Intergel solution significantly reduced the severity and extent of adhesions that did form following peritoneal cavity surgery ($p < 0.01$).

The effect of Intergel solution on reducing adnexal adhesions was shown by a significant reduction in the AFS score compared to control (Fig. 32.3). The minimum score of both the right and left adnexa was significantly reduced by administration of Intergel solution. In addition, the proportion of patients with minimal scores (AFS score 0–5) increased in the patient group that received Intergel solution; in contrast, the proportion of patients who received lactated Ringer's solution who had minimal AFS scores decreased at second-look laparoscopy. Similarly, the proportion of patients with mild, moderate, or severe AFS scores (6–10, 11–10, and 21–32, respectively) decreased in the group that received Intergel and increased in the control groups (Table 32.12).

Adhesion formation was also assessed via a composite score adopted from the method proposed by the AFS and modified as applied to all 24 anatomic sites.[42] Baseline adhesion scores were comparable, and Intergel solution significantly reduced the total adhesion score at second-look laparoscopy compared to control ($p < 0.001$).

When patients were subgrouped into those who underwent myomectomy (Table 32.13) or adhesiolysis (Table 32.14), into those patients with endometriosis (Table 32.15) or who had ovarian surgery (Table 32.16), including those patients with ovarian dermoids or endometriomas (Table 32.17), Intergel solution was found to significantly reduce second-look adhesion formation, reformation, adhesion formation at the surgical site, and the modified AFS score in all groups. Intergel solution was also effective at reducing adhesion reformation when adhesiolysis was performed using sharp dissection, blunt dissection, or cautery (Table 32.18) and at sites where tissue was sutured (Table 32.19).

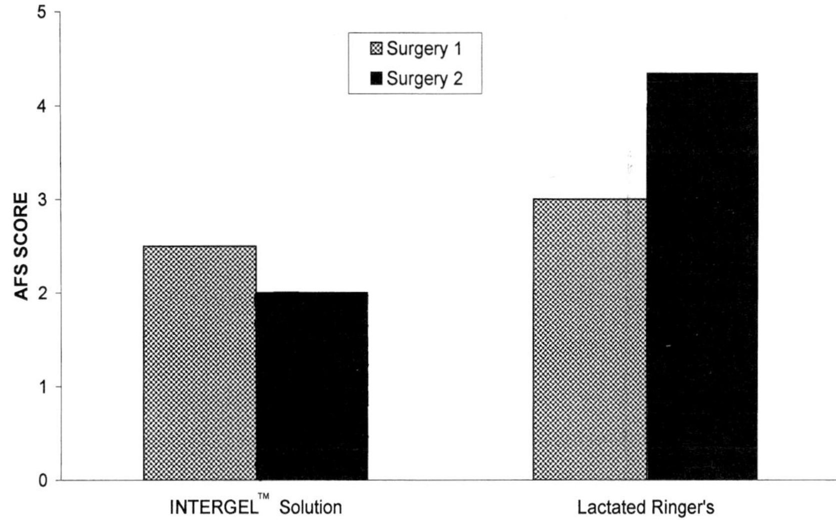

FIG. 32.3. American Fertility Society (AFS) adhesion score determined at the time of initial laparotomy (*striped bars*) and second-look laparoscopy (*black bars*) in patients who received 300 mL of an intraperitoneal instillate of Intergel solution. Patients who received Intergel solution (*left*) had a statistically significant reduction in AFS score compared to patients who received lactated Ringer's solution (*right*) ($p < 0.001$).

TABLE 32.12. American Fertility Society score.

	Intergel solution			Lactated Ringer's solution				
Variable	*N*	Mean	(SD)	*N*	Mean	(SD)	*p*	Reduction (%)
Mean Values								
Baseline	109	2.54	(5.58)	104	3.37	(6.50)	0.321	
Second -look	109	1.86	(3.54)	104	5.01	(7.90)	0.000	63%

Minimum score of right and left adnexa

		Intergel solution			Lactated Ringer's solution			
Variable		*n*	*N*	%	*n*	*N*	%	*p*
Proportion baseline	0–5 (minimal)	90	109	82.6	81	104	77.9	0.491
	6–15 (mild)	12	109	11.0	8	104	7.7	0.485
	11–20 (moderate)	5	109	4.6	11	104	10.6	0.121
	21–32 (severe)	2	109	1.8	4	104	3.8	0.437
Second-look	0–5 (minimal)	100	109	91.7	74	104	71.2	0.000
	6–15 (mild)	6	109	5.5	12	104	11.5	0.141
	11–20 (moderate)	2	109	1.8	13	104	12.5	0.003
	21–32 (severe)	1	109	0.9	5	104	4.8	0.112

TABLE 32.13. Patients with myomectomy.

	Intergel solution		Lactated Ringer's solution			
	n	Mean ± SD	*n*	Mean ± SD	*p*	Reduction (%)
Baseline						
Adhesions	71	2.48 ± 3.49	65	2.06 ± 3.40	0.482	
Second-look						
Adhesions	71	6.35 ± 4.99	65	8.05 ± 5.83	0.070	19
Proportion	71	0.272 ± 0.213	65	0.347 ± 0.254	0.064	21
Modified AFS score	71	1.25 ± 1.62	65	2.63 ± 3.05	0.001	52
Severity score	71	0.49 ± 0.46	65	0.80 ± 0.70	0.003	38
Extent score	71	0.44 ± 0.44	65	0.68 ± 0.64	0.012	35
De novo adhesions	71	5.18 ± 4.55	65	6.71 ± 5.11	0.068	22
Proportion	71	0.247 ± 0.205	65	0.319 ± 0.250	0.069	22
Surgical site adhesions	71	2.07 ± 2.40	65	2.71 ± 2.54	0.135	23
Proportion	71	0.337 ± 0.289	65	0.457 ± 0.312	0.022	26
Surgical site de novo	71	0.72 ± 0.74	65	1.12 ± 0.94	0.006	34
Proportion	71	0.290 ± 0.300	65	0.408 ± 0.331	0.032	27
Reformed adhesions	29	2.86 ± 2.81	24	3.63 ± 2.34	0.294	22
Proportion	29	0.498 ± 0.341	24	0.788 ± 2.91	0.002	36

TABLE 32.14. Patients with adhesiolysis.

	Intergel solution		Lactated Ringer's solution			
	n	Mean ± SD	n	Mean ± SD	p	Reduction (%)
Baseline						
Adhesions	58	7.12 ± 3.54	54	7.61 ± 3.80	0.481	
Second-look						
Adhesions	58	7.26 ± 4.40	54	9.83 ± 5.24	0.006	24
Proportion	58	0.324 ± 0.201	54	0.445 ± 0.233	0.004	27
Modified AFS score	58	1.55 ± 1.50	54	3.15 ± 2.90	0.000	51
Severity score	58	0.61 ± 0.43	54	1.01 ± 0.66	0.000	40
Extent score	58	0.54 ± 0.42	54	0.87 ± 0.60	0.001	37
De novo adhesions	58	4.07 ± 3.39	54	5.31 ± 4.01	0.078	23
Proportion	58	0.244 ± 0.194	54	0.337 ± 0.244	0.027	27
Surgical site adhesions	58	3.81 ± 2.95	54	5.41 ± 3.42	0.009	29
Proportion	58	0.417 ± 0.282	54	0.567 ± 0.258	0.004	26
Surgical site de novo	58	0.45 ± 0.57	54	0.72 ± 0.81	0.040	34
Proportion	58	0.220 ± 0.293	54	0.340 ± 0.380	0.064	32
Reformed adhesions	58	3.19 ± 2.81	54	4.52 ± 3.24	0.022	29
Proportion	58	0.491 ± 0.344	54	0.730 ± 0.305	0.000	32

TABLE 32.15. Sites with endometriosis.

	Intergel solution		Lactated Ringer's solution			
	n	Mean ± SD	n	Mean ± SD	p	Reduction (%)
Baseline						
Adhesions	19	1.68 ± 2.21	22	1.82 ± 2.24	0.849	
Second-look						
Adhesions	19	1.05 ± 1.47	22	2.05 ± 1.96	0.078	44
Proportion	19	0.409 ± 0.444	22	0.751 ± 0.370	0.010	45
Modified AFS score	19	1.95 ± 3.14	22	5.58 ± 5.84	0.020	65
Severity score	19	0.72 ± 0.96	22	1.49 ± 1.10	0.023	57
Extent score	19	0.82 ± 1.08	22	1.65 ± 1.14	0.023	50
De novo adhesions	11	0.64 ± 0.67	16	0.94 ± 0.68	0.267	31
Proportion	11	0.347 ± 0.437	16	0.622 ± 0.461	0.134	44
Surgical site adhesions	18	0.94 ± 1.51	22	2.00 ± 1.95	0.068	53
Proportion	18	0.417 ± 0.462	22	0.764 ± 0.351	0.010	45
Surgical site de novo	10	0.40 ± 0.52	15	0.93 ± 0.70	0.052	57
Proportion	10	0.350 ± 0.474	15	0.622 ± 0.448	0.159	43
Reformed adhesions	11	1.18 ± 1.78	12	2.50 ± 2.32	0.143	52
Proportion	11	0.445 ± 0.472	12	0.972 ± 0.96	0.001	54

TABLE 32.16. Patients with ovarian surgery.

	Intergel solution		Lactated Ringer's solution			
	n	Mean ± SD	n	Mean ± SD	p	Reduction (%)
Baseline						
Adhesions	27	6.33 ± 4.60	32	5.59 ± 4.51	0.537	
Second-look						
Adhesions	27	6.44 ± 4.51	32	9.22 ± 4.93	0.029	30
Proportion	27	0.287 ± 0.212	32	0.430 ± 0.227	0.016	33
Modified AFS score	27	1.34 ± 1.43	32	2.74 ± 2.45	0.012	51
Severity score	27	0.50 ± 0.40	32	0.93 ± 0.63	0.004	46
Extent score	27	0.53 ± 0.51	32	0.82 ± 0.55	0.043	35
De novo adhesions	27	3.67 ± 3.80	32	5.88 ± 3.79	0.030	37
Proportion	27	0.207 ± 0.197	32	0.354 ± 0.217	0.009	41
Surgical site adhesions	27	3.41 ± 3.05	32	4.69 ± 3.46	0.141	27
Proportion	27	0.373 ± 0.291	32	0.567 ± 0.251	0.008	34
Surgical site de novo	27	0.48 ± 0.94	32	1.19 ± 1.20	0.016	59
Proportion	27	0.191 ± 0.326	32	0.401 ± 0.349	0.021	52
Reformed adhesions	21	3.57 ± 3.04	22	4.86 ± 3.43	0.199	26
Proportion	21	0.460 ± 0.348	22	0.809 ± 0.217	0.000	43

TABLE 32.17. Patients with dermoids or endometriomas.

	Intergel solution		Lactated Ringer's solution			
	n	Mean ± SD	*n*	Mean ± SD	*p*	Reduction (%)
Baseline						
Adhesions	13	5.85 ± 4.06	18	4.28 ± 4.27	0.311	
Second-Look						
Adhesions	13	5.46 ± 4.82	18	8.44 ± 5.44	0.125	35
Proportion	13	0.251 ± 0.249	18	0.408 ± 0.256	0.097	38
Modified AFS score	13	0.97 ± 1.20	18	2.45 ± 2.32	0.044	60
Severity score	13	0.39 ± 0.38	18	0.77 ± 0.61	0.053	49
Extent score	13	0.44 ± 0.55	18	0.81 ± 0.61	0.096	45
De novo adhesions	13	3.46 ± 3.60	18	6.44 ± 4.53	0.059	46
Proportion	13	0.194 ± 0.222	18	0.367 ± 0.254	0.059	47
Surgical site adhesions	13	2.54 ± 3.02	18	3.78 ± 2.88	0.256	32
Proportion	13	0.324 ± 0.325	18	0.537 ± 0.260	0.052	39
Surgical site de novo	13	0.38 ± 0.77	18	1.61 ± 1.24	0.004	76
Proportion	13	0.141 ± 0.271	18	0.491 ± 0.306	0.003	71
Reformed adhesions	11	2.36 ± 3.04	10	3.60 ± 2.37	0.315	34
Proportion	11	0.383 ± 0.432	10	0.828 ± 0.176	0.007	53

TABLE 32.18. Adhesiolysis techniques and adhesion reformation.

	Intergel solution		Lactated Ringer's solution			
	n	Mean ± SD	*n*	Mean ± SD	*p*	Reduction (%)
Sites lysed using sharp dissection						
Adhesions	29	2.90 ± 2.41	30	3.90 ± 2.20	0.100	25
Proportion	29	0.607 ± 0.358	30	0.772 ± 0.287	0.055	21
Sites lysed using cautery						
Adhesions	34	2.59 ± 2.55	32	4.41 ± 3.25	0.014	41
Proportion	34	0.409 ± 0.346	32	0.691 ± 0.313	0.001	40
Sites lysed using blunt dissection						
Adhesions	26	2.31 ± 2.00	17	3.06 ± 1.64	0.204	24
Proportion	26	0.605 ± 0.399	17	0.951 ± 0.141	0.001	36

TABLE 32.19. Adhesion formation at sites with sutures.

	Intergel solution		Lactated Ringer's solution			
	n	Mean ± SD	*n*	Mean ± SD	*p*	Reduction (%)
Adhesions	109	0.94 ± 0.94	104	1.30 ± 1.26	0.021	25
Proportion	109	0.337 ± 0.309	104	0.435 ± 0.361	0.033	22

Clinical Perspective

Previous studies of adhesion prevention adjuvants where effectiveness has been demonstrated by second-look laparoscopy are primarily limited to site-specific barriers such as INTERCEED barrier and Seprafilm membrane. While these products reduce adhesions, their benefit is limited to the site of placement of the membrane or film. This study was designed to evaluate safety and efficacy of Intergel solution in humans after peritoneal cavity surgery for reduction of adhesion formation at 24 sites throughout the entire abdomen. The Intergel Adhesion Prevention Solution was shown to be easy to use and significantly reduced the number, severity, and extent of adhesions after laparotomy throughout the abdominal cavity. The safety profile of Intergel solution was comparable to that of lactated Ringer's solution (Control). There were no statistically significant differences between treatment groups as to concomitant medications or adverse events. There were no clinically meaningful changes in laboratory values in either treatment group. There were no statistically significant differences between treatment groups in hospital stay.

Coating the abdominal surfaces with solutions to inhibit adhesive contact of injured tissues has previously met with moderate success. Although this approach appears to be convenient and uncomplicated, no solution has provided universal benefit. A substantial body of clinical data is available to assess the benefit of crystalloid instillates, such as saline and lactated Ringer's solution, in adhesion prevention. During the early 1980s four clinical studies were published which compared dextran to crystalloid used as instillates. A combination of these studies showed an adhesion reformation rate of approximately 80% in patients who received crystalloid instillates.[43] This high rate of adhesion formation with the use of intraperitoneal instillates was confirmed by Fayez and Schneider.[44]

Recently, reports appeared describing the use of crystalloid solutions to reduce adhesion formation after laparoscopic ovarian surgery. Naether and Fischer instilled 300 to 500 mL of saline into the peritoneal cavity after laparoscopic coagulation of the ovarian surface in patients with polycystic ovarian disease.[45] When compared to a previous series treated in a similar fashion by these authors without the crystalloid instillation, they found no difference in the incidence of adhesions (17% vs. 19%, respectively). Gurgan et al. instilled 150 mL of lactated Ringer's solution into the pelvis after laparoscopic electrocautery or laser vaporization of the ovarian surface in polycystic ovarian disease patients; 82% were found to have adhesions to the ovarian surface at second-look laparoscopy.[46] More recently, Tulandi et al.[47] and Gurgan et al.[48] both reconfirmed the failure of crystalloid (lactated Ringer's solution, 500 mL) to reduce adhesion formation in patients undergoing laparoscopic ovarian surgery (see Chapter 34). To significantly reduce adhesion formation and reformation, the device must effectively separate damaged surfaces during the crucial phases of postsurgical repair. The rapid rate of absorption of crystalloid solution from the peritoneal cavity (35 mL/h) may preclude its residence during the crucial time of adhesion formation.[49–51] Meta-analysis of clinical studies using crystalloid solution conclusively showed no reduction in adhesion with instillation of lactated Ringer's solution or saline.[52]

Hyaluronic acid is a naturally occurring component of peritoneal fluid.[27] Peritoneal mesothelial cells were shown to synthesize HA in vitro, and HA is thought to play a role in lubrication of cells and maintenance of the structural integrity of tissues as well as regulation of fluid retention.[28] A number of investigators previously studied the efficacy of HA solutions in adhesion prevention. Urman and Gomel evaluated the effectiveness of HA solution in preventing intraperitoneal adhesions in rats after CO_2 laser injury of the serosa.[29] Although precoating of the serosa reduced de novo adhesion formation, no significant reduction of adhesions was seen when HA was added at the end of the procedure, that is, post treatment.[29] The effectiveness of reducing de novo adhesions by precoating before injuring the serosa of rats was confirmed by West et al.[32] A similar reduction of de novo adhesions in rats after serosal abrasion was noted by Shushan et al. following administration of HA as an instillate as well as application of an HA membrane after laser injury to the rat uterine horn.[34] Diamond et al. reported the clinical effectiveness of Sepracoat Hyaluronic Acid Coating Solution used as a precoating solution in 245 patients undergoing laparotomy.[15] The solution was applied upon entry into the abdominal cavity and periodically thereafter.

The results reported here are with HA ionically cross-linked by ferric chloride to produce a viscous gel. In animal studies, ferric hyaluronate gel was more efficacious than HA, even when the concentration of HA was increased to produce a viscosity similar or greater than ferric hyaluronate gel.[36] In addition, Intergel solution reduced adhesion formation not only at sites of application but throughout the abdominal cavity of laboratory animals, suggesting widespread distribution by the intra-abdominal circulation. The results reported from a multicenter clinical trial confirm and extend those data from a pilot clinical trial reported by Thornton et al.[37] In that study, Intergel solution was found to be more than twice as effective as Ringer's lactate in reducing adhesion formation. The efficacy difference between the ferric hyaluronate gel and HA formulations appears to result primarily from a longer residence time for ferric hyaluronate gel relative to HA in the peritoneal cavity. This difference may result from a greater tendency of ferric hyaluronate gel to adhere to the tissue or a delayed dilution with peritoneal fluids compared to HA.

In summary, Intergel Adhesion Prevention Solution was shown to be easy to use in this multicenter, international study and significantly reduced the number, severity, and extent of adhesions after laparotomy at 24 sites throughout the abdominal cavity. A significant reduction in the AFS score (adnexal adhesions) as well as a modified AFS score (applied to 24 anatomic sites throughout the abdominal–pelvic cavity) was also demonstrated. The safety profile of Intergel solution was comparable to that of lactated Ringer's solution (Control). There were no statistically significant differences between treatment groups as to concomitant medications and adverse events. There were also no clinically meaningful changes in laboratory values in either treatment group. In conclusion, Intergel Adhesion Prevention Solution provides a new, clinically proven intraperitoneal surgical therapy for reduction of adhesions that is both broad in coverage and easy to use.

References

1. Howard FM. The role of laparoscopy in chronic pelvic pain: promise and pitfalls. Obstet Gynecol Surv 1993;48: 357–358.
2. Steege JF, Stout AL, Somkuti SG. CPP in women with: toward an integrative model. Obstet Gynecol 1991;165: 278–283.
3. Kresch AJ, Seifer DB, Sachs LB, et al. Laparoscopy in 100 women with CPP. Obstet Gynecol 1984;64:672–674.

4. Strickler B, Blanco J, Fox HE. The gynecologic contribution to intestinal obstruction in females. J Am Coll Surg 1994;178:617–621.
5. Miller EM, Winfield JM. Acute intestinal obstruction secondary to postoperative adhesions. Arch Surg 1959;78: 148–153.
6. Bronson RA, Wallach EE. Lysis of periadnexal adhesions for correction of infertility. Fertil Steril 1977;28:613–619.
7. Tulandi T, Chen MF, Al-Took S, et al. A study of nerve fibers and histopathology of postsurgical, postinfectious, and endometriosis-related adhesions. Obstet Gynecol 1988;92:766–768.
8. Azziz R. Microsurgery alone or with INTERCEED absorbable adhesion barrier for pelvic sidewall adhesion reformation. Surg Gynecol Obstet 1993;177:135–139.
9. Keckstein J, Ulrich U, Sasse V, et al. Reduction of postoperative formation after laparoscopic ovarian cystectomy. Hum Reprod (Oxf) 1996;11:579–582.
10. Nordic Adhesion Prevention Study Group. The efficacy of Interceed (TC7) for prevention of reformation of postoperative adhesions on ovaries, fallopian tubes, and fimbriae in microsurgical operation for fertility: a multicenter study. Fertil Steril 1995;63:709–714.
11. Franklin RR, Malinak RL, Larsson B, et al. Reduction of ovarian adhesions by the use of Interceed. Obstet Gynecol 1995;86:335–338.
12. Mais V, Ajossa SA, Piras B, et al. Prevention of de novo adhesion formation after laparoscopic myomectomy: a randomized trail to evaluate the effectiveness of an oxidized regenerated cellulose absorbable barrier. Hum Reprod (Oxf) 1995;12:3133–3135.
13. Mais V, Ajossa SA, Marongiu D, et al. Reduction of adhesion formation after laparoscopic endometriosis surgery; a randomized trial with an oxidized regenerated cellulose absorbable barrier. Obstet Gynecol 1995;86:512–515.
14. Sekiba K. Use of Interceed (TC7) absorbable adhesion barrier to reduce postoperative adhesion reformation in infertility and endometriosis surgery. Obstet Gynecol 1992;79:518–522.
15. Diamond MP, Sepracoat Adhesion Group. Reduction of de novo postsurgical adhesions by intraoperative precoating with Sepracoat (HAL-C) solution: a prospective, randomized, blinded, placebo-controlled multicenter study. The Sepracoat Adhesion Study Group. Fertil Steril 1998;69:1067–1074.
16. Myomectomy Adhesion Study Group. An expanded-polytetrafluoroethylene barrier (Gore-Tex surgical membrane) reduces postmyomectomy adhesion formation. Fertil Steril 1995;63:491–493.
17. Diamond MP, Seprafilm Adhesion Study Group. Reduction of adhesions after uterine myomectomy by Seprafilm® membrane (HAL-F®): a blinded, prospective, randomized, multicenter clinical study. Fertil Steril 1996;66: 904–910.
18. Wallwiener D, Meyer A, Bastert G. Adhesion formation of the parietal and visceral peritoneum: an explanation for the controversy on the use of autologous and alloplastic barriers? Fertil Steril 1998;68:132–137.
19. Haney AF, Doty E. Expanded polytetrafluoroethylene but not oxidized regenerated cellulose prevents adhesion formation and reformation in a mouse uterine horn model of surgical injury. Fertil Steril 1993;60:550–554.
20. diZerega GS. Use of adhesion prevention barriers in pelvic reconstructive and gynecologic surgery. In diZerega GS, DeCherney AH, eds. Pelvic Surgery Adhesion Formation and Prevention. New York: Springer-Verlag, 1997:188–209.
21. Gauwerky JF, Heinrich D, Kubli F. Complications of intraperitoneal dextran application for prevention of adhesions. Biol Res Pregnancy Perinatol 1986;7:93–97.
22. diZerega GS. Contemporary adhesion prevention. Fertil Steril 1994;61:219–235.
23. Adhesion Study Group. Reduction of postoperative pelvic adhesions with intraperitoneal 32% dextran 70: a prospective, randomized clinical trial. Fertil Steril 1983;40: 612–619.
24. Larsson B. Effect of intraperitoneal instillation of 32% dextran 70 on postoperative adhesion formation after tubal surgery. Acta Obstet Gynecol Scand 1985;64: 4437–441.
25. Rosenberg SM, Board JA. High-molecular weight dextran in human infertility surgery. Am J Obstet Gynecol 1984; 148:380–385.
26. Jansen RP. Failure of intraperitoneal adjuncts to improve the outcome of pelvic operations in young women. Am J Obstet Gynecol 1985;153:363–371.
27. Yung S, Coles GA, Williams JD, et al. The source and possible significance of hyaluronan in the peritoneal cavity. Kidney Int 1994;46:527–533.
28. Asplund T, Vershel MA, Luarent TC, et al. Human mesothelioma cells produce factors that stimulate the production of hyaluronan by mesothelial cells and fibroblasts. Cancer Res 1993;53:388–392.
29. Urman B, Gomel V. Effect of hyaluronic acid on postoperative intraperitoneal adhesion formation and reformation in the rat model. Fertil Steril 1991;56:568–570.
30. Weiss C, Levy HJ, Delinger J, et al. The role of Na-Hylan in reducing postsurgical tendon adhesions. Bull Hosp Joint Dis Orthop Inst 1986;45:9–15.
31. Weiss C, Suros JM, Michalow A, et al. The role of Na-hylan in reducing postsurgical tendon adhesions: Part 2. Bull Hosp Joint Dis Orthop Inst 1987;47:31–39.
32. West JL, Chowdhury SM, Sawhney AS, et al. Efficacy of adhesion barriers: resorbable hydrogel, oxidized regenerated cellulose and hyaluronic acid. J Reprod Med 1996; 41:149–154.
33. Thomas SC, Jones LC, Hungerford DS. Hyaluronic acid and its effects on postoperative adhesions in the rabbit flexor tendon. Clin Orthop 1982;206:281–289.
34. Shushan A, Mor-Yosef S, Avgar A, et al. Hyaluronic acid for preventing experimental postoperative intraperitoneal adhesions. J Reprod Med 1994;39:398–402.
35. Rodgers KE, Johns DB, Girgis W, et al. Reduction of adhesion formation with hyaluronic acid following peritoneal surgery in rabbits. Fertil Steril 1997;67:553–538.
36. Johns DB, Rodgers KE, Donahue WD, et al. Reduction of adhesion formation by postoperative administration of ionically cross-linked hyaluronic acid. Fertil Steril 1997; 68:37–42.
37. Thornton MH, Johns DB, Campeau JC, et al. Clinical evaluation of 0.5% ferric hyaluronate adhesion prevention gel

for the reduction of adhesion following peritoneal cavity surgery: open-label pilot study. Hum Reprod (Oxf) 1998; 13:1480–1485.

38. Lundorff P, diZerega GS, Johns DB, et al. Clinical evaluation of Intergel adhesion prevention solution for the reduction of adhesion following peritoneal cavity surgery: an international multicenter study of safety and efficacy. Abstract No. 0-069. European Society of Hormones and Reproductive Endocrinology (ESHRE), Goteborg, Sweden, 1998.
39. Weinstein WM, Onderdonk AB, Barlett JG, et al. Experimental intraabdominal abscesses in rats: development of an experimental model. Infect Immun 1974;10: 1250–1255.
40. Bowen DL, Manning TA, eds. The Lymphatic System. Anatomy and Physiology. St. Louis: Mosby, 1983:483.
41. Gowens JL. The effect of the continuous re-infusion of lymph and lymphocytes on the output of lymphocytes from the thoracic duct of unanesthetized rats. Br J Exp Pathol 1967;38:67–78.
42. American Fertility Society. The American Fertility Society classifications of adnexal adhesions, distal tubal occlusion, tubal occlusion secondary to tubal ligation, tubal pregnancies, Mullerian anomalies and intrauterine adhesions. Fertil Steril 1998;49:944–955.
43. diZerega GS, Campeau JD. Use of instillates to prevent intraperitoneal adhesions: crystalloids and dextran. Infertil Reprod Med Clin North Am 1994;5:463–478.
44. Fayez JA, Schneider PJ. Prevention of pelvic adhesion formation by different modalities of treatment. Am J Obstet Gynecol 1987;157:1184–1188.
45. Naether OGJ, Fischer R. Adhesion formation after laparoscopic electrocoagulation of the ovarian surface in polycystic ovary patients. Fertil Steril 1993;60:95–98.
46. Gurgan T, Kisnisei H, Yarali H, et al. Evaluation of adhesion formation after laparoscopic treatment of polycystic ovarian disease. Fertil Steril 1991;56:1176–1178.
47. Tulandi T, Murray C, Guralnick M. Adhesion formation and reproductive outcome after myomectomy and second-look laparoscopy. Obstet Gynecol 1993;82:213–215.
48. Gurgan T, Urman B, Yarali H, et al. Adhesion formation and reformation after laparoscopic removal of ovarian endometriomas. J Am Assoc Gynecol Laparosc 1996;82: 213–215.
49. Shear L, Swartz C, Shinaberger J, et al. Kinetics of peritoneal fluid absorption in adult man. N Engl J Med 1965; 272:123–127.
50. Sites CK, Jensen BA, Jacob BS, et al. Transvaginal ultrasonographic assessment of Hyskon or lactated Ringer's solution instillation after laparoscopy: randomized, controlled study. J Ultrasound Med 1997;16:195–199.
51. Hart R, Magos A. Laparoscopically instilled fluid: the rate of absorption and the effects on patient discomfort and fluid balance. Gynaecol Endosc 1996;5:287–291.
52. Wiseman DM, Trout JR, Diamond MP. The rates of adhesion development and the effects of crystalloid solutions on adhesion development in pelvic surgery. Fertil Steril 1998;70:702–711.

33

Laparoscopic Treatment of Peritoneal Adhesions

Christine H. Holschneider and Alan H. DeCherney

CONTENTS

Peritoneal adhesions are common, although the true prevalence of adhesions in the general population can only be deduced from indirect evidence. In asymptomatic women undergoing laparoscopic tubal sterilization, pelvic adhesions are found in 12% to 14%.[1,2] Similarly, in general surgery patients with no history of prior laparotomies there is a 10% prevalence of adhesions.[3] In symptomatic patients, adhesions are seen even more frequently. A retrospective review of 100 consecutive laparoscopies performed for chronic pelvic pain found that 26% of patients had pelvic adhesions as the only pathologic finding. In the same study, the comparison group of infertility patients undergoing laparoscopy had pelvic adhesions in 39% of cases.[4] Patients who have undergone surgery following one or more prior laparotomies are found to have adhesions in up to 93% of cases.[3]

Adhesion formation is at times life saving, for example, in aiding the omentum to seal off a perforation of the gastrointestinal tract or an infectious process. In most cases, however, intraperitoneal adhesions are a major source of morbidity, such as infertility, pelvic pain, and bowel obstruction. Adhesions also increase the technical difficulty and risk of intraoperative complications at subsequent surgery. Adhesion-related morbidity poses a substantial drain on limited healthcare resources, accounting for almost 282,000 hospitalizations in 1988 in the U.S. alone. The cost of the resulting adhesiolysis was $1.18 billion, which did not take into account outpatient care and indirect costs from loss of productivity and consumer spending.[5] In a more recent study by the same investigators, which was based on the 1994 National Hospital Discharge Survey, females constituted 83% of all patients undergoing adhesiolysis. The female reproductive system was the primary site of most adhesiolysis performed, most of which was carried out as outpatient procedures. In contrast, more than 90% of days of inpatient care resulted from adhesiolysis of the digestive tract.[6] These numbers reflect the current practice pattern that gynecologic adhesiolysis is largely being performed as a laparoscopic outpatient procedure, whereas bowel obstruction typically requires inpatient care and adhesiolysis is generally performed via laparotomy. However, such statistics do not address the outcome of laparoscopic adhesiolysis.

Minimizing the risk of adhesion reformation challenges any physician performing adhesiolysis. Laparoscopy is replacing laparotomy as the method of choice for lysing most pelvic adhesions because laparoscopy is associated with less de novo adhesion formation than laparotomy. In addition, laparoscopy has the advantage of being a minimally invasive outpatient procedure with short associated recovery time and high patient acceptance. While laparoscopy may be the treatment modality of choice for many pelvic adhesions, it carries a significant potential for damage to adjacent organs, depending largely on location and character of the adhesions as well as on surgical technique.

In the following sections, we review the literature on the laparoscopic management of peritoneal adhesions and discuss the laparoscopic approach to adhesiolysis.

Preoperative Diagnosis of Adhesions

Establishing a preoperative diagnosis of adhesions is difficult. Stovall and colleagues prospectively examined 273 women in an attempt to identify predictors of pelvic adhesions encountered at laparoscopy. Previous pelvic surgery was the only significant historical predictor of adhesions in these women. Findings on physical examination such as uterine immobility, adnexal mass, and tenderness were also associated with adhesions. However, history and physical examination in combination still failed to predict 26% of patients found to have adhesions at the time of surgery.[7]

Although laparoscopy remains the gold standard in the diagnosis of adhesions, hysterosalpingography and ultrasound have been evaluated as noninvasive diagnostic techniques in an attempt to reduce the number of low-yield laparoscopies. In some reports, hysterosalpingographic findings of a convoluted fallopian tube, loculation of spillage of contrast medium in the peritoneal cavity, ampullary dilatation, peritubal halo effect, and vertical fallopian tube have demonstrated a positive predictive value of 0.75 for adhesions.[8] However, most studies find that hysterosalpingography has very poor sensitivity for detecting adhesions.[8,9] Thus, in routine screening hysterosalpingography lacks effectiveness as a method for detecting peritubal adhesions.[10]

Few papers address the usefulness of ultrasonography in the diagnosis of abdominopelvic adhesions. Based on a study by Guerriero and colleagues,[11] certain transvaginal ultrasound findings are strongly associated with the presence of pelvic adhesions. These findings include fixation of the ovary to the uterus, blurring of the margins of the ovary, and an increased distance of the ovary from the transvaginal ultrasound probe. When these findings are combined with a history of prior surgery they increase the probability of adhesions to 93%. However, investigators who included cases of filmy adhesions reported it difficult to accurately characterize adhesions with ultrasound.[12]

Ultrasound has also been used to locate abdominal wall adhesions in patients with previous surgeries to aid in the safe placement of the initial laparoscopic access. The underlying principle is to scan for spontaneous viscera slide caused by respiratory excursions of the diaphragm, as well as viscera slide induced by manual pressure. Using this technique in the assessment of an existing abdominal scar, the periumbilical region, and the remaining abdominal quadrants, Caprini and colleagues were able to ultrasonographically identify all abdominal wall adhesions present in 30 patients undergoing laparoscopy following prior laparotomy.[13] Similar encouraging results have been found in a number of other studies.[14–16]

Some of these advances in the noninvasive imaging of adhesions are promising, but the studies are small and preliminary. It remains unclear how these results translate to the general practice setting. At present, laparoscopy and laparotomy remain the only definitive diagnostic procedures of abdominopelvic adhesions.

Adhesiolysis Via Laparoscopy Versus Laparotomy

Success of adhesiolysis can be evaluated principally in two ways: (1) absence or presence of adhesions following surgical adhesiolysis as determined during a second-look procedure or (2) resolution or improvement of the patient's adhesion-related complaint, such as infertility, pain, or bowel obstruction. In this section, we discuss the outcome of adhesiolysis by laparoscopy versus laparotomy as assessed at second look. The subsequent sections evaluate adhesiolysis on a disease-specific basis.

Adhesions reform in a substantial number of patients after adhesiolysis via laparotomy/microsurgery or laparoscopy, with 68% to 76% and 38% to 61% of patients, respectively, having recurrent adhesions at second-look surgery; this holds true whether the surgery is performed mainly for other procedures (Table 33.1) or for adhesiolysis alone (Table 33.2). While overall recurrence of adhesions seems to be somewhat reduced following laparoscopic adhesiolysis, direct comparison of these retrospective studies is limited by inherent selection bias and lack of controls for the approach to adhesiolysis. Despite these limitations, a few conclusions seem valid. In carefully designed animal studies[17,18] and human trials,[19] laparoscopy does appear to be associated with fewer inci-

TABLE 33.1. Adhesion formation in women after laparotomy or laparoscopy surgery as assessed by second look.

		Laparotomy ± microsurgery		Laparoscopy	
Reference	Study design	*n*	Adhesions at second look	*n*	Adhesions at second look
Lundorff (1991)[19]	Randomized, controlled	42	33/42 (79%)	31	19/31 (58%)
Keckstein (1996)[87]	Prospective, randomized	—	—	17	11/17 (65%)
Trimbos-Kemper (1985)[49]	Prospective, controlled	188	104/188 (55%)	—	—
Jansen (1988)[89]	Prospective, controlled	256	210/256 (82%)	38	23/38 (61%)
DeCherney (1984)[88]	Prospective, uncontrolled	61	46/61 (75%)	—	—
Operative Laparoscopy Study Group (1991)[20]	Retrospective, uncontrolled	—	—	68	66/68 (97%)
Surrey (1982)[90]	Retrospective, uncontrolled	37	27/37 (73%)	—	—
Barbot (1987)[82]	Retrospective, uncontrolled	172	53/172 (31%)	—	—
Total		756	473/756 (63%)	154	118/154 (77%)

TABLE 33.2. Outcome after adhesiolysis in women treated via laparotomy or laparoscopy as assessed by second look.

		Laparotomy ± microsurgery		Laparoscopy		
Reference	Study design	*n*	Adhesions at second look	*n*	Adhesions at second look	Time of second look
Azziz (1993)[91]	Prospective, randomized	134	102/134 (76%)	—	—	10–14 days postoperatively
Trimbos-Kemper (1985)[49]	Prospective, controlled	—	—	104	39/104 (38%)	8 days postoperatively
Perez (1991)[92]	Prospective, uncontrolled	—	—	30	16/30 (53%)	7 days postoperatively
Serour (1989)[93]	Prospective, uncontrolled	—	—	22	12/22 (55%)	9–12 months postoperatively
Jansen (1988)[94]	Prospective, uncontrolled	—	—	38	23/38 (61%)	12 days postoperatively
Tulandi (1989)[50]	Retrospective, uncontrolled	19	13/19 (68%)	—	—	1 year postoperatively
Total		153	115/153 (75%)	194	90/194 (46%)	

sional and de novo adhesions than laparotomy as seen at second look. In a report of 68 women undergoing laparoscopic adhesiolysis, de novo adhesion formation, defined as adhesions at initially uninvolved sites, occurred in only 12% of cases.[20] This rate is substantially less than the 51% rate of de novo adhesions found in a similar study after laparotomy.[21] Two well-designed animal trials support the concept that, if the technique of tissue handling is kept exactly the same, the degree of adhesion formation at the operative site is equal for laparoscopy and laparotomy, whereas incisional adhesions are significantly more common after laparotomy than laparoscopy.[18,22]

This trend is further supported by a study by Levrant and colleagues who prospectively scored adhesions in a cohort of 215 infertility patients. Adhesions were present in none of the 91 patients with no prior surgery, nor in 45 patients who had undergone prior laparoscopies. Adhesions were found, however, in 28 of 68 women (41%) who were operated by laparotomy in the past.[23] Certain risk factors for adhesions are more likely encountered at laparotomy. These conditions include the use of retraction and packing rougher handling of the tissue, drying of serosal surfaces in room air, and the introduction of foreign bodies such as glove talc and lint during laparotomy. In addition, close-up magnification of the entire operative field at laparoscopy may confer a distinct advantage in minimizing tissue damage.

In summary, while there may not be objective evidence that laparoscopy is superior to conventional laparotomy or microsurgery for adhesiolysis per se, there is a decreased risk of incisional and de novo adhesion formation with laparoscopy. Thus, overall adhesions formation is decreased with the laparoscopic approach. Furthermore, the fact that laparoscopy allows for simultaneous diagnosis and treatment in an outpatient setting, with minimal recovery time and good cosmetic results at lower cost, make it the preferred surgical approach to the diagnosis and treatment of most pelvic adhesions.

Laparoscopic Adhesiolysis in the Management of Chronic Pelvic Pain

The relationship of adhesions to abdominopelvic pain continues to be controversial. Numerous investigators have implicated adhesions as a cause of acute and chronic pelvic pain.[1,24–26] The incidence of adhesions is higher in women undergoing laparoscopy for chronic pelvic pain (26%–48%)[1,4,7,24] than in asymptomatic women undergoing tubal sterilization (12%–14%).[1,2] However, a higher incidence of adhesions in chronic pelvic pain patients does not establish a causal relationship. Generally, the duration and severity of pain correlates poorly with the extent of adhesions, whereas the location of adhesions found at laparoscopy tends to coincide with consistently localized areas of pain.[25,26] Lysis of adhesions may not always improve chronic pelvic pain. Rather than being causally related, adhesions and pain are both frequently manifestations of an underlying disease process such as endometriosis or pelvic inflammatory disease. What then is the evidence that adhesions cause pain and that lysis of adhesions improves pain? Rapkin did not find any difference in character or distribution of adhesions in patients who were symptomatic with pain compared to infertility patients who did not experience any pain,[4] which supports the view of some that the notion that adhesions cause abdominal or pelvic pain is "a poorly substantiated myth."[27] Others contend that adhesions cause pain through the entrapment of distensible viscera, which may result in the activation of nociceptors through tension and traction. Kresch and colleagues found a higher prevalence of restrictive adhesions (i.e., adhesions limiting the motion or expansibility of one or more organs) in women with complaints of chronic pelvic pain compared to loose adhesions (i.e., adhesions allowing unrestricted movement of organs) in an asymptomatic control group.[1] Similarly, in a prospective laparoscopic assessment study Stout and colleagues found significantly higher adhesion scores in women with self-reported pain than in women without pain.[26]

Because the causality of adhesions and chronic pelvic pain is unclear, it has been difficult to demonstrate that adhesiolysis relieves chronic pelvic pain. In some uncontrolled studies, lysis of adhesions lead to relief of symptoms in a substantial number of patients.[25,26,28] Controlled studies are scant. In a recent randomized controlled trial, Peters and colleagues demonstrated that women with severe, dense vascularized bowel adhesions had a significant reduction in pain after adhesiolysis. Women with mild or moderate pelvic adhesions did not benefit from adhesiolysis compared to women managed expectantly.[29] In this study adhesiolysis was performed via laparotomy in all patients. Thus, for women with mild or moderate adhesions the possibility needs to be considered that any potential benefit of adhesiolysis may have been masked by the risk of incisional and de novo adhesion formation associated with laparotomy. Overall, results of adhesiolysis via laparoscopy versus laparotomy (with or without microsurgery) appear similar, with an overall improvement rate of 61% to 89% with laparoscopy and 46% to 71% with laparotomy and microsurgery (Table 33.3). It is important to remember that these procedures are not directly comparable because these nonrandomized studies have inherent differences in case selection, in addition to variable duration of follow-up and symptom assessment.

Laparoscopic Adhesiolysis in the Management of Infertility

Pelvic adhesions are recognized as a common cause of infertility. In 15% to 20% of cases infertility is thought to be secondary to peritubal and periovarian adhesions without true occlusion of the tube as the principal cause.[30–32] The degree to which adhesions interfere with fertility depends on the extent, location, density, and underlying cause of the adhesions. Several studies have found a correlation between the severity of adhesions and infertility.[33–35] In addition, more recent studies have implied that pelvic adhesions and high-grade tubal damage may impair the reproductive prognosis by interfering with the results of assisted reproductive technologies.[36–38] A greater understanding is needed of the role pelvic adhesions play for oocyte development and the success of in vitro fertilization, particularly because tubal factor infertility is one of the major indications for in vitro fertilization.

Impairment of Fertility by Adhesions

Pelvic adhesions may impair fertility by any one or more of the following mechanisms. Enclosure of the fallopian tube or distortion of the anatomic and functional tubo-

TABLE 33.3. Outcome of adhesiolysis via laparotomy or laparoscopy for chronic pelvic pain.

		Laparotomy		Laparoscopy	
Reference	Study design	n	Improved	n	Improved
Peters (1992)[29]	Prospective, randomized	—	—	24	11/24 (46%)
Saravelos (1995)[95]	Retrospective, controlled	72	51/72 (71%)	51	31/51 (61%)
Steege (1991)[25]	Prospective, uncontrolled	—	—	30	19/30 (63%)
Miller (1996)[96]	Prospective, uncontrolled	—	—	19	16/19 (84%)
Goldstein (1990)[28]	Retrospective, uncontrolled	—	—	18	16/18 (89%)
Sutton (1990)[97]	Retrospective, uncontrolled	—	—	65	53/65 (82%)
Chan (1985)[98]	Retrospective, uncontrolled	43	28/43 (65%)	—	—
Total		115	79/115 (69%)	207	146/207 (71%)

ovarian relationship may lead to disruption of ovum pickup and transport. Aboulghar and colleagues studied 42 women with laparoscopically proven tuboovarian adhesions but at least one patent fallopian tube in an ovarian superstimulation program. They found a strong correlation between decreasing pregnancy rates and increasing severity of adhesions.[39] Periovarian adhesions—or diseases that lead to formation of such—may interfere with the ovulatory mechanism, as suggested by Hamilton and colleagues. These authors, using ultrasound and midluteal progesterone measurements, found luteinized unruptured follicles in more than half of 25 women previously diagnosed with and treated for adhesions and hydrosalpinges caused by pelvic inflammatory disease.[40] Similarly, Levinson and colleagues found that coating of the ovary by adhesions led to interference with the ovulatory mechanism.[41]

Data on the effects of periovarian adhesions on ovarian folliculogenesis are controversial. Bowman et al. found adhesions to be associated with compromised ovarian function.[42] Furthermore, Mahadevan and colleagues retrieved significantly fewer oocytes from ovaries with adhesions than from adhesion-free ovaries.[43] In a case control study of patients undergoing in vitro fertilization with a "frozen pelvis," Molloy and colleagues found a significantly higher number of canceled oocyte retrievals, lower rates of rise and peak serum estradiol values, slower response to hyperstimulation, and fewer follicles with lower numbers of oocytes retrieved than in the control group of patients without adhesions.[44] Poor folliculogenesis may result from the underlying disease process that led to dense adhesions, or one may speculate that the cause is ovarian entrapment by the dense adhesions, not allowing enough space for the optimal follicular diameter to develop. The observation of compromised ovarian folliculogenesis in the presence of pelvic adhesions is, however, not universally confirmed. In a study of 49 women Diamond and colleagues did not find periovarian adhesions as scored by laparoscopy to be a major determinant of either the ovarian response to gonadotropin stimulation or the number of mature oocytes recovered in an in vitro fertilization setting.[45]

Adhesiolysis for Fertility Enhancement

While it appears universally accepted that adhesions frequently interfere with spontaneous conception, only a few investigators have addressed the question whether adhesiolysis improves conception rates in a controlled fashion. Tulandi and colleagues compared fertility outcome following either adhesiolysis or continued expectant management. In their case control study of 147 women with documented periadnexal adhesions, Tulandi and colleagues found a 45% pregnancy rate at 24 months among the 69 women who underwent salpingo-ovariolysis, compared with 16% for the 78 women who were managed expectantly.[46] In support of their findings there is evidence from several, nonrandomized, noncontrolled, retrospective studies that conception rates following adhesiolysis are about 50% to 60%. Operative laparoscopy and laparotomy with or without microsurgery appear to be comparable in terms of improved fertility outcome, although reported results from individual studies vary widely (Table 33.4). For a number of reasons only a very limited direct comparison of these data is feasible. One has to assume an inherent selection bias for patients undergoing laparoscopy versus laparotomy. The patient populations vary widely in the severity of adhesions and the underlying disease processes. Follow-up is different, as are surgical techniques, power settings, instrumentations used, and operative experience.

Attempts have been made to further distinguish those patients who are likely to benefit from adhesiolysis from those who are not. Pelvic adhesiolysis is unlikely to help the patient with significant intraluminal tubal pathology. Bowman and colleagues have recommended tubal intraluminal assessment for all patients in whom adhesiolysis for fertility is considered, which appears to be par-

TABLE 33.4. Laparotomy versus laparoscopy for infertility: pregnancy outcomes after salpingo-ovariolysis.

Laparotomy/microsurgery				Laparoscopy			
Reference	*n*	Conception rate	Viable pregnancy rate	Reference	*n*	Conception rate	Viable pregnancy rate
Reich (1987)[75]	12	10/12 (83%)	9/12 (75%)	Reich (1987)[75]	27	23/27 (87%)	21/27 (78%)
Fayez (1982)[99]	32	21/32 (66%)	19/32 (60%)	Fayez (1983)[84]	50	30/50 (60%)	23/50 (46%)
Jansen (1980)[100]	37	20/37 (54%)	n/a	Serour (1989)[93]	25	n/a	3/25 (12%)
Kelly (1983)[101]	21	5/21 (24%)	4/21 (19%)	Donnez (1987)[108]	54	31/54 (57%)	31/54 (57%)
Frantzen (1982)[102]	49	22/49 (45%)	19/49 (39%)	Gomel (1983)[109]	92	62/92 (67%)	54/92 (59%)
Hulka (1982)[103]	47	15/47 (32%)	12/47 (26%)	Tulandi (1990)[46]	69	41/65 (59%)	—
Luber (1986)[104]	13	9/13 (69%)	7/13 (54%)	—	—	—	—
Diamond (1979)[105]	140	86/140 (61%)	80/140 (57%)	—	—	—	—
Wallach (1983)[106]	94	52/94 (55%)	43/94 (46%)	—	—	—	—
Marana (1995)[48]	29	17/29 (59%)	n/a	—	—	—	—
Caspi (1981)[107]	101	46/101 (46%)	36/101 (36%)	—	—	—	—
Totals	575	303/575 (53%)	229/575 (40%)		317	187/292 (64%)	132/248 (53%)

ticularly important in cases of pelvic inflammatory disease because correlation between external and internal tubal pathology in these cases was high.[47] Although the reproductive outcome was not addressed in Bowman's report, a more recent study by Marana and colleagues found a significant correlation between intraluminal tubal integrity and conception following salpingo-ovariolysis.[48]

Adhesion Reformation

Recurrence of adhesions after adhesiolysis is high. Some authors have recommended second-look laparoscopy to lyse reformed as well as de novo adhesions. Trimbos-Kemper and colleagues evaluated the effectiveness of the initial lysis of adhesions via second-look laparoscopy, and employed third-look laparoscopy to evaluate the effectiveness of adhesiolysis during second-look laparoscopy, which had been performed in half the study patients. Second-look laparoscopy significantly reduced permanent adhesions, but fertility rates remained similar in both groups.[49] The failure of adhesiolysis at second-look laparoscopy to improve fertility rates has been further confirmed by Tulandi and colleagues. In a randomized study of 74 women who had failed to conceive 1 year following initial infertility surgery, these authors found second-look laparoscopy of no benefit to subsequent conception rates compared with expectant management in the control patients.[50]

Conclusion

In conclusion, therapeutic considerations for women with infertility caused by tuboovarian adhesions include laparoscopy for adhesiolysis and in vitro fertilization. Several authors prefer laparoscopy before employing assisted reproductive technologies to confirm the diagnosis and treat those adhesions that may impair spontaneous or assisted reproduction.[11] Depending on the degree of adhesions, adhesiolysis can be an effective treatment of infertility, as in cases of mild filmy adhesions it is associated with a cumulative 2-year pregnancy rate similar to that reported after five cycles of in vitro fertilization.[51] Although there is no objective evidence that laparoscopy is superior to conventional laparotomy or microsurgery for adhesiolysis per se, there is a decreased risk of de novo adhesion formation with the laparoscopic approach.[20,21] Laparoscopy allows for simultaneous diagnosis and treatment of adhesions in an outpatient setting with minimal recovery time and good cosmetic results at lower cost. It is therefore the preferred surgical approach to the diagnosis and treatment of most pelvic adhesions. At present, there is no evidence that second-look laparoscopy for lysis of reformed adhesions has any fertility-enhancing effect.

Laparoscopic Adhesiolysis in the Management of Bowel Obstruction

Bowel obstruction secondary to adhesions accounts for nearly 1% of all general surgical and gynecologic adult admissions with approximately 3% of all laparotomies being for isolated adhesive bowel obstruction.[3,52] Adhesions are the most common cause of bowel obstruction in the industrialized world, being responsible for 30% of bowel obstructions in general and 60% to 75% of small intestinal obstructions.[53] Following division of adhesions, recurrence of intestinal obstruction is common, in some series as high as 13%.[54]

After an appropriate trial of conservative management, the standard approach to acute small-bowel obstruction is laparotomy and adhesiolysis with or without bowel resection. Laparoscopy in such patients is considered dangerous because of the increased risk of damaging dilated loops of bowel with the insufflating needle or trochar or during intraoperative manipulation. Appropriate visualization and exposure of the operative field is frequently technically difficult because distended bowel loops fill the peritoneal cavity. In recent years, however, laparoscopy has been used successfully for the management of acute and recurrent small-bowel obstruction caused by postoperative adhesions.[55,56] In a retrospective case-control study of 139 patients requiring surgery for small-bowel obstruction (65 open laparoscopies, 74 laparotomies), Bailey and colleagues successfully treated 46 of 65 (71%) patients laparoscopically for small-bowel obstruction. Laparoscopically treated patients were discharged home significantly earlier, but had a higher number of unplanned reoperations than patients treated via laparotomy.[57] Laparoscopic management of small-bowel obstruction may be feasible in selected cases, that is, with mild abdominal distension and a relatively proximal obstruction, and if a single adhesive band is encountered during diagnostic laparoscopy. However, laparoscopic division of multiple adhesions or broad-based adhesions involving larger segments of small bowel may be not only time consuming and technically demanding but also dangerous.

Effects of Surgical Technique on Adhesion Formation

Studies on tissue repair following surgery have provided insight into the process of peritoneal healing and adhesion formation. Following peritoneal injury, an exudate of fibrin and inflammatory cells forms. In principle, wherever fibrin is degraded, normal peritoneal repair ensues, whereas adhesions form in areas where the fibrin matrix persists, being invaded by collagen-producing fibroblasts. Decreases in plasminogen activator activity, which is central to fibrin degradation, are thought to play a central role in the pathophysiology of adhesion formation. Peritoneal ischemia as well as inflammation result in a significant decrease in plasminogen activator activity,[58] which may explain the association between tissue ischemia[59] or abrasion[60] and adhesion formation. Foreign bodies, such as powder, lint, or suture materials have been found in a large proportion of postoperative adhesions after laparotomy.[61] Different suture materials have been studied comparatively by Holtz,[62] who found a lack of correlation between microscopic reactivity evoked by the suture material and the adhesions formed. Holtz further confirmed that suture placement per se infrequently induced adhesions so long as there was no coexisting peritoneal injury. The effects of drying of serosal surfaces and bleeding were studied by Ryan et al., who found that drying alone had little effect, but that the combination of drying and bleeding consistently induced adhesions to the dried area.[63] The fact that fresh blood alone also induced adhesions may explain why the pelvis and especially the posterior cul-de-sac, where blood tends to collect, are so frequently involved in adhesion formation.

Trochar Placement in a Patient with Suspected Adhesions

While pelvic adhesions are commonly an unpredictable finding at laparoscopy, some patients may be suspected to have adhesions, especially those who underwent prior abdominopelvic surgeries. Intraabdominal adhesions between the abdominal scar and underlying viscera, in particular omentum and bowel, are a common consequence of laparotomy. At operative laparoscopy of 360 women who had laparotomies in the past, Brill and colleagues found incisional adhesions in significantly more women with prior midline incisions (58/102, =57%) than with prior Pfannenstiel incisions (70/258, =27%).[64]

Thus, whenever laparoscopy is to be performed in a patient in whom adhesions are suspected, the laparoscopist must be mindful during trochar placement that the underlying intraabdominal anatomy may be altered. Bowel injury during placement of the insufflating needle or trochar is generally estimated to occur with a frequency of 1.6–1.8/1000.[65] In Brill's study focusing on laparoscopy in 360 women who had undergone at least one previous laparotomy, the incidence of injury during trochar insertion was substantially increased by anterior abdominal wall adhesions. There were 15 (4.2%) omental injuries associated with significant bleeding and 6 (1.6%) bowel injuries.[64] Hasson introduced the open laparoscopy technique in 1971 in the hope that it would avoid trochar injuries to the underlying viscera.[66] While many gynecologists and surgeons think of open laparoscopy as the entry procedure of choice in patients suspected to have adhesions, it is important to remember that trochar injuries still occur.[64,67] Direct trochar insertion without antecedent pneumoperitoneum has been reported to not increase morbidity in a number of studies that excluded[68] or included[69,70] patients with prior abdominal surgeries. As most fatalities of laparoscopic bowel injury occur not because of the injury itself but as the result of its frequently delayed diagnosis, it is imperative with either trochar insertion technique to inspect the entry site carefully to recognize any potential injury promptly.

Patients who have umbilical hernias or abdominal incisions that extend to or past the umbilicus pose a particular problem as the umbilicus usually serves as the primary laparoscopic access site. For these patients, left-upper quadrant placement of the insufflating needle and primary trochar has been recommended.[71] This technique has gained increasing acceptance because the left-upper quadrant is a relatively adhesion-free and safe entry site. Before placement of the insufflating needle or trochar the stomach should be decompressed using an oral or nasal gastric tube. The insufflating needle can be placed in the left 9th intercostal space in the anterior axillary line "wandering" over the cephalad aspect of the 10th rib. This location is well below the diaphragm. After generation of the pneumoperitoneum, a 5-mm trochar can then be inserted just beneath the left costal margin in the midclavicular line. Alternatively, the trochar for the 2-mm laparoscope can be inserted directly beneath the left costal margin in the midclavicular line. Once the peritoneal cavity has been explored and adhesions lysed as needed, the umbilical port can be established under direct visualization.

Techniques for Laparoscopic Adhesiolysis

In principle, laparoscopic techniques for adhesiolysis include blunt dissection, hydrodissection, sharp dissection with scissors, unipolar or bipolar electrosurgery, and laser dissection or evaporization. The following is a general review of these techniques and a discussion of their advantages and disadvantages.

Whenever extensive adhesions are suspected preoperatively, the patients should undergo a mechanical bowel preparation the day before the planned operation. Certain surgical principles apply to laparoscopic adhesiolysis regardless of the ultimate dissection instrument used. After identification, the adhesion should be stretched using an uterine manipulator or a sponge stick in the vagina in opposing directions to a blunt probe or atraumatic grasping forceps introduced through one of the laparoscopic ancillary ports. Adhesions should be divided individually. Some separate easily along the correct anatomic cleavage plains with gentle blunt traction;

others require to be taken down in layers with either endoscopic scissors, laser, or electrosurgery. Using traction and countertraction is very important throughout the adhesiolysis procedure, as it thins out the adhesion and allows identification of blood vessels and underlying tissues, minimizing the risk of bleeding or damage to bowel and urinary tract. Blunt dissection, hydrodissection, and sharp dissection with scissors should be used and thermal energy sources avoided whenever surrounding vital structures cannot be clearly identified and dissection carried out at a safe distance. In all cases with some degree of cul-de-sac obliteration caused by adhesions, Reich and colleagues recommend the use of a sponge or ring forceps in the posterior vaginal fornix, an 81-French rectal probe placed in the rectum, and a solid uterine manipulator to help define the posterior vaginal fornix and rectum.[72] While dissection with a blunt probe is unidirectional, hydrodissection may be advantageous at times because it cleaves planes multidirectionally following the path of least resistance.[73]

Vascular adhesions are best approached with a thermal energy source to allow for hemostatic dissection. Monopolar "cutting" current should be used for cutting, desiccation, and coagulation, and "coagulation" current avoided. This is due to the fact that with cutting current (100% duty cycle) the voltage is low enough that the risk of arching of the current to adjacent tissues can be minimized, whereas coagulation current, with typically only 6% duty cycle, is associated with very high peak voltages that allow arcing of current to adjacent tissues over several millimeters. Another determinant of arching is the surrounding medium: CO_2 gas is only 70% as effective at transmitting a charge as room air, whereas argon gas promotes conduction of electrical current, a feature that is exploited in the argon-beam coagulator.[74] Bipolar forceps using "cutting" current may be helpful for compressing dense vascular adhesions and thus facilitating complete desiccation.[75]

The CO_2 laser is the laser type most commonly used for gynecologic surgery. The neodymium:yttrium laser (Nd:YAG laser)[76] and the argon laser[77] have also both been used successfully for laparoscopic adhesiolysis. It is important to note that the scatter and depth of penetration are different for the CO_2, argon, and Nd:YAG lasers; the CO_2 laser offers the distinct advantage of less than 0.1 mm tissue penetration, provided small spot size, adequate power, and limited time of tissue exposure. The depth of thermal damage is even less with superpulse or ultrapulse modes.[74] Adhesion formation appears similar for the continuous and superpulse mode of the CO_2 laser.[78] Furthermore, the inability of the CO_2 laser beam to traverse through water may provide some additional protection against damaging adjacent bowel, bladder, ureter, or blood vessels.[73]

Numerous authors find electromicrosurgery and laser equally effective in the lysis of adhesions, both in animal models[79] and in humans as assessed by second look.[80–82] Similarly, Luciano and colleagues found no difference between laser and electrocautery with regards to depth of thermal damage, extent of collagen deposition, or postoperative adhesion formation in rabbits.[83] In a randomized controlled trial of 63 patients undergoing salpingo-ovariolysis, Tulandi and colleagues compared the CO_2 laser with the microdiathermy needle. Pregnancy rates at 2-year follow-up were not significantly different, 53.3% and 51.5%, respectively.[84] Diamond and colleagues of the Intraabdominal Laser Study Group examined tubal patency and pelvic adhesions at second-look laparoscopy after intraabdominal use of the CO_2 laser.[81] An equivalent rate of adhesion recurrence was found when their results were compared with those of the Adhesion Study Group, who utilized nonlaser reconstructive pelvic surgery.[85] Although the comparison of two large multicenter trials may have limitations, it is the best evidence we have short of randomized controlled trials.

Thus, at present neither laser nor electromicrosurgery can be recommended as superior to the other in respect to adhesion reformation and postadhesiolysis pregnancy rates. In particular, there is no evidence to indicate that laser offers any biologic advantage over electrosurgery.

Complications of Laparoscopic Adhesiolysis

The association of preexisting adhesions with complications during trochar placement has been discussed earlier. Complications related to endoscopic adhesiolysis itself are generally considered to be rare, and incidence data are difficult to obtain. Several of the publications reviewed addressing laparoscopic adhesiolysis make no mention of complications. Redwine[86] reported 20 complications during 1467 laparoscopies performed for endometriosis and other conditions and involving adhesiolysis, which would give an estimated complication rate of 1.4%. All these complications occurred among the 546 patients with stage III and IV endometriosis or severe abdominopelvic adhesions. Reported complications included the need for transfusion in 2 of 4 cases of significant bleeding, the need for reoperation in 3 cases, and 1 clinically suspected deep venous thrombosis. The 1 reported postoperative ileus and 5 cases of postoperative infection all occurred in patients who in addition to adhesiolysis underwent a laparoscopy-assisted vaginal hysterectomy, which independently carries morbidity.[86] While not encountered in Redwine's series, the risk of injury to the ureter or bladder increases in any surgery where the anatomy is distorted by prior surgery or the disease process.

Adjuvant Therapy After Laparoscopic Adhesiolysis

Superior surgical technique with minimal tissue compromise and meticulous hemostasis during adhesiolysis are crucial to minimize adhesion reformation. In addition, numerous agents have been used in an attempt to reduce adhesion formation, both at initial surgery and at the time of adhesiolysis. These methods include the instillation of crystalloids, dextran, and corticosteroids or the application of barriers such as Interceed, Gore-Tex Surgical Membrane, and Sepracoat. The effectiveness of these agents is reviewed in detail elsewhere in this volume (Chapter 34).

Summary

Adhesions are commonly associated with infertility, chronic pelvic pain, and bowel obstruction. Adhesiolysis leads to improvement or resolution of these conditions in a substantial number of patients. Laparoscopic adhesiolysis is generally safe and well tolerated. Because laparoscopy allows for simultaneous diagnosis and treatment of adhesions in an outpatient setting with minimal recovery time, it is the preferred surgical approach to the diagnosis and treatment of pelvic adhesions in most patients.

References

1. Kresch AJ, Seifer DB, Sachs LB, et al. Laparoscopy in 100 women with chronic pelvic pain. Obstet Gynecol 1984; 64:672–674.
2. Trimbos JB, Trimbos-Kemper GCM, Peters AAW, et al. Findings in 200 consecutive asymptomatic women, having a laparoscopic sterilization. Arch Gynecol Obstet 1990; 247:121–124.
3. Menzies D, Ellis H. Intestinal obstruction from adhesions—how big is the problem? Ann R Coll Surg Engl 1990;72:60–64.
4. Rapkin AJ. Adhesions and pelvic pain: a retrospective study. Obstet Gynecol 1986;68:13–15.
5. Ray NF, Larsen JW Jr, Stillman RJ, et al. Economic impact of hospitalizations for lower abdominal adhesiolysis in the United States in 1988. Surg Gynecol Obstet 1993;176: 271–276.
6. Ray NF, Denton WG, Thamer M, et al. Abdominal adhesiolysis: inpatient care and expenditures in the United States in 1994. J Am Coll Surg 1998;186:1–9.
7. Stovall TG, Elder RF, Ling FW. Predictors of pelvic adhesions. J Reprod Med 1989;34:345–348.
8. Karasick S, Goldfarb AF. Peritubal adhesions in infertile women: diagnosis with hysterosalpingography. AJR 1989; 152:777–779.
9. Swart P, Mol BWJ, van der Veen F, et al. The accuracy of hysterosalpingography in the diagnosis of tubal pathology: a meta-analysis. Fertil Steril 1995;64:486–491.
10. Bateman BG, Nunley WC, Kitchin JD, et al. Utility of the 24-hour delay hysterosalpingogram film. Fertil Steril 1987; 47:613–617.
11. Guerriero S, Ajossa S, Lai MP, et al. Transvaginal ultrasound in the diagnosis of pelvic adhesions. Hum Reprod (Oxf) 1997;12:2649–2653.
12. Ubaldi F, Wisanto A, Camus M, et al. The role of transvaginal ultrasonography in the detection of pelvic pathologies in the infertility workup. Hum Reprod (Oxf) 1998;13: 330–333.
13. Caprini JA, Arcelus JA, Swanson J, et al. The ultrasonic localization of abdominal wall adhesions. Surg Endosc 1995; 9:283–285.
14. Sigel B, Golub RM, Loiacono LA, et al. Technique of ultrasonic detection and mapping of abdominal wall adhesions. Surg Endosc 1991;5:161–165.
15. Kolecki RV, Golub RM, Sigel B, et al. Accuracy of viscera slide detection of abdominal wall adhesions by ultrasound. Surg Endosc 1994;8:871–874.
16. Kodama I, Loiacono LA, Sigel B, et al. Ultrasonic detection of viscera slide as an indicator of abdominal wall adhesions. J Clin Ultrasound 1992;20:375–380.
17. Luciano AA, Maier DB, Koch EI, et al. A comparative study of postoperative adhesions following laser surgery by laparoscopy versus laparotomy in the rabbit model. Obstet Gynecol 1989;74:220–224.
18. Jorgensen JO, Lalak NJ, Hunt DR. Is laparoscopy associated with a lower rate of postoperative adhesions than laparotomy? A comparative study in the rabbit. Aust N Z J Surg 1995;65:342–344.
19. Lundorff P, Hahlin M, Källfelt B, et al. Adhesion formation after laparoscopic surgery in tubal pregnancy: a randomized trial versus laparotomy. Fertil Steril 1991;55: 911–915.
20. Operative Laparoscopy Study Group. Postoperative adhesion development after operative laparoscopy: evaluation at early second look procedures. Fertil Steril 1991;55: 700–704.
21. Diamond MP, Daniell JF, Feste J, et al. Adhesion reformation and de novo adhesion formation after reproductive pelvic surgery. Fertil Steril 1987;47:864–866.
22. Tittel A, Schippers E, Treutner KH, et al. Laparoscopy versus laparotomy. An animal experiment study comparing adhesion formation in the dog. Langenbecks Arch Chir 1994;379:95–98.
23. Levrant SG, Bieber EJ, Barnes RB. Anterior abdominal wall adhesions after laparotomy or laparoscopy. J Am Assoc Gynecol Laparosc 1997;4:353–456.
24. Kontoravdis A, Chryssikopoulos A, Hassiakos D, et al. The diagnostic value of laparoscopy in 2365 patients with acute and chronic pelvic pain. Int J Obstet Gynecol 1996;52: 243–248.
25. Steege JF, Stout AL. Resolution of chronic pelvic pain after laparoscopic lysis of adhesions. Am J Obstet Gynecol 1991; 165:278–283.
26. Stout AL, Steege JF, Dodson WC, et al. Relationship of laparoscopic findings to self-report of pelvic pain. Am J Obstet Gynecol 1991;164:73–79.

27. Alexander-Williams J. Do adhesions cause pain? BMJ 1987; 294:659–660.
28. Goldstein DP, deCholnoky C, Emans SJ, et al. Laparoscopy in the diagnosis and management of pelvic pain in adolescents. J Reprod Med 1980;24:251–256.
29. Peters AAW, Trimbos-Kemper GCM, Admiraal C, et al. A randomized clinical trial on the benefit of adhesiolysis in patients with intraperitoneal adhesions and chronic pelvic pain. Br J Obstet Gynecol 1992;99:59–62.
30. Gomel V. Laparoscopic tubal surgery in infertility. Obstet Gynecol 1975;46:47–48.
31. Drolette CM, Badawy SZA. Pathophysiology of pelvic adhesions: modern trends in preventing infertility. J Reprod Med 1992;37:107–122.
32. Hershlag A, Diamond MP, DeCherney AH. Adhesiolysis. Clin Obstet Gynecol 1991;34:395–402.
33. Hulka JF, Omran K, Berger GS. Classification of adnexal adhesions: a proposal and evaluation of its prognostic value. Fertil Steril 1978;30:661–665.
34. Fayez JA. An assessment of the role of operative laparoscopy in tuboplasty. Fertil Steril 1983;39:476–479.
35. Caspi E, Halperin Y, Bukovsky I. The importance of periadnexal adhesions in tubal reconstructive surgery for infertility. Fertil Steril 1979;31:296–300.
36. Al-Shawaf T, Ah-Moye M, Fiamanya W, et al. Gamete intrafallopian transfer in non-endometriotic adhesions. Hum Reprod (Oxf) 1990;5:434–438.
37. Fakih H, Marshall J. Subtle tubal abnormalities adversely affect gamete intrafallopian transfer outcome in women with endometriosis. Fertil Steril 1994;62:799–801.
38. Csemiczky G, Landgren BM, Fried G, et al. High tubal damage grade is associated with low pregnancy rate in women undergoing in-vitro fertilization treatment. Hum Reprod (Oxf) 1996;11:2438–2440.
39. Aboulghar MA, Mansour RT, Serour GI. Ovarian superstimulation in the treatment of infertility due to peritubal and periovarian adhesions. Fertil Steril 1989;51: 834–837.
40. Hamilton CJCM, Evers JLH, Hoogland HJ. Ovulatory disorders and inflammatory adnexal damage: a neglected cause of failure of fertility microsurgery. Br J Obstet Gynecol 1986;93:282–284.
41. Levinson CJ, Swolin K. Postoperative adhesions: etiology, prevention, and therapy. Clin Obstet Gynecol 1980;23: 1213–1220.
42. Bowman MC, Cooke ID, Lenton EA. Investigation of impaired ovarian function as a contributing factor to infertility in women with pelvic adhesions. Hum Reprod (Oxf) 1993;8:1654–1656.
43. Mahadevan MM, Wiseman D, Leader A, et al. The effects of ovarian adhesive disease upon follicular development in cycles of controlled stimulation for in vitro fertilization. Fertil Steril 1985;44:489–492.
44. Molloy D, Martin M, Speirs A, et al. Performance of patients with a "frozen pelvis" in an in vitro fertilization program. Fertil Steril 1987;47:450–455.
45. Diamond MP, Pellicer A, Boyers SP, et al. The effect of periovarian adhesions on follicular development in patients undergoing ovarian stimulation for in vitro fertilization-embryo transfer. Fertil Steril 1988;49:100–103.
46. Tulandi T, Collins JA, Burrows E, et al. Treatment-dependent and treatment-independent pregnancy among women with periadnexal adhesions. Am J Obstet Gynecol 1990;162:354–357.
47. Bowman MC, Cooke ID. Comparison of fallopian tube intraluminal pathology as assessed by salpingoscopy with pelvic adhesions. Fertil Steril 1994;61:464–469.
48. Marana R, Rizzi M, Muzii L, et al. Correlation between the American Fertility Society classification of adnexal adhesions and distal tubal occlusion, salpingoscopy, and reproductive outcome in tubal surgery. Fertil Steril 1995;64: 924–929.
49. Trimbos-Kemper TCM, Trimbos JB, van Hall EV. Adhesion formation after tubal surgery: results of the eighth-day laparoscopy in 188 patients. Fertil Steril 1985;43:395–400.
50. Tulandi T, Falcone T, Kafka I. Second-look operative laparoscopy 1 year following reproductive surgery. Fertil Steril 1989;52:421–424.
51. Oelsner G, Sivan E, Goldenberg M, et al. Should lysis of adhesions be performed when in-vitro fertilization and embryo transfer are available? Hum Reprod (Oxf) 1994;9: 2339–2341.
52. Krebs HB, Goplerud DR. Mechanical intestinal obstruction in patients with gynecologic disease: a review of 368 patients. Am J Obstet Gynecol 1987;157:577–583.
53. Menzies D. Peritoneal adhesions: incidence, cause and prevention. Surg Ann 1992;24:27–45.
54. Brightwell NL, McFee AS, Aust JB. Bowel obstruction and the long tube stent. Arch Surg 1977;112:505–511.
55. Silva PD, Cogbill TH. Laparoscopic treatment of recurrent small bowel obstruction. Wis Med J 1991;90:169–170.
56. Adams S, Wilson T, Brown AR. Laparoscopic management of acute small bowel obstruction. Aust N Z J Surg 1993;63: 39–41.
57. Bailey IS, Rhodes M, O'Rourke N, et al. Laparoscopic management of acute small bowel obstruction. Br J Surg 1998;85:84–87.
58. Thompson JN, Paterson-Brown S, Harbourne T, et al. Reduced human peritoneal plasminogen activator activity: possible mechanism of adhesion formation. Br J Surg 1989;76:382–384.
59. Ellis H. The cause and prevention of postoperative intraperitoneal adhesions. Surg Gynecol Obstet 1971;133: 497–511.
60. Gervin AS, Puckett CL, Silver D. Serosal hypofibrinolysis: a cause of postoperative adhesions. Am J Surg 1973;125: 80–88.
61. Weibel MA, Majno G. Peritoneal adhesions and their relation to abdominal surgery: a postmortem study. Am J Surg 1973;126:345–353.
62. Holtz G. Adhesion induction by suture of varying tissue reactivity and caliber. Int J Fertil 1982;27:134–135.
63. Ryan GB, Grobéty J, Majno G. Postoperative peritoneal adhesions: a study of the mechanisms. Am J Pathol 1971; 65:117–138.
64. Brill AI, Nezhat F, Nezhat CH, et al. The incidence of adhesions after prior laparotomy: a laparoscopic appraisal. Obstet Gynecol 1995;85:269–272.
65. Metzger DA. Trochar injuries to the small intestine. In: Corfman RS, Diamond MP, DeCherney AH, eds. Compli-

cations of Laparoscopy and Hysteroscopy. Malden: Blackwell, 1997:38–42.
66. Hasson HM. A modified instrument and method for laparoscopy. Am J Obstet Gynecol 1971;110:886–887.
67. Hasson HM. Open laparoscopy: a report of 150 cases. J Reprod Med 1974;12:234–258.
68. Nezhat FR, Silfen SL, Evans D, et al. Comparison of direct insertion of disposable and standard reusable laparoscopic trochars and previous pneumoperitoneum with the veress needle. Obstet Gynecol 1991;78:148–150.
69. Dingfelder JR. Direct laparoscope trochar insertion without prior pneumoperitoneum. J Reprod Med 1978;21: 45–47.
70. Byron JW, Fujiyoshi CA, Miyazawa K. Evaluation of the direct trochar insertion technique at laparoscopy. Obstet Gynecol 1989;74:423–425.
71. Childers JM, Brzechffa PR, Surwit EA. Laparoscopy using the left upper quadrant as the primary trochar site. Gynecol Oncol 1993;50:221–225.
72. Reich H, McGlynn F, Salvat J. Laparoscopic treatment of cul-de-sac obliteration secondary to retrocervical deep fibrotic endometriosis. J Reprod Med 1991;36:516–22.
73. Reich H. Lysis of adhesions. In: Hulka JF, Reich H, eds. Textbook of Laparoscopy, 3rd Ed. Philadelphia: Saunders, 1998:257–267.
74. Munro MG. Energy sources for operative laparoscopy. In: Gomel V, Taylor PJ, eds. Diagnostic and Operative Gynecologic Laparoscopy. St. Louis: Mosby, 1995:26–56.
75. Reich H. Laparoscopic treatment of extensive pelvic adhesions, including hydrosalpinx. J Reprod Med 1987;32: 736–742.
76. Yanagibori A, Kojima E, Ohtaka K, et al. Nd:YAG laser therapy for infertility with a contact-type probe. J Reprod Med 1989;34:456–460.
77. Diamond MP, DeCherney AH, Polan ML. Laparoscopic use of the argon laser in nonendometriotic reproductive pelvic surgery. J Reprod Med 1986;31:1011–1013.
78. Badawy SZA, El Bakry MM, Baggish MS. Comparative study of continuous and pulsed CO_2 laser on tissue healing and fertility outcome in tubal anastomosis. Fertil Steril 1987;47:843–847.
79. Filmar S, Gomel V, McComb P. The effectiveness of CO_2 laser and electromicrosurgery in adhesiolysis: a comparative study. Fertil Steril 1986;45:407–411.
80. Tulandi T. Adhesion reformation after reproductive surgery with and without the carbon dioxide laser. Fertil Steril 1987;47:704–706.
81. Diamond MP, Daniell JF, Martin DC, et al. Tubal patency and pelvic adhesions at early second-look laparoscopy following intraabdominal use of the carbon dioxide laser: initial report of the Intraabdominal Laser Study Group. Fertil Steril 1984;42:717–723.
82. Barbot J, Parent B, Dubuisson JB, et al. A clinical study of the CO_2 laser and electrosurgery for adhesiolysis in 172 cases followed by early second-look laparoscopy. Fertil Steril 1987;48:140–142.
83. Luciano AA, Whitman G, Maier DB, et al. A comparison of thermal injury, healing patterns, and postoperative adhesion formation following CO_2 laser and electromicrosurgery. Fertil Steril 1987;48:1025–1029.
84. Tulandi T. Salpingo-ovariolysis: a comparison between laser surgery and electrosurgery. Fertil Steril 1986:45: 489–491.
85. Adhesion Study Group. Reduction of postoperative pelvic adhesions with intraperitoneal 32% dextran 70: a prospective, randomized clinical trial. Fertil Steril 1983:40: 612–619.
86. Redwine DB. Complications of sharp and blunt adhesiolysis. In: Corfman RS, Diamond MP, DeCherney AH, eds. Complications of Laparoscopy and Hysteroscopy. Malden: Blackwell, 1997:78–81.
87. Keckstein J, Ulrich U, Sasse V, et al. Reduction of postoperative adhesion formation after laparoscopic ovarian cystectomy. Hum Reprod (Oxf) 1996;11:579–582.
88. DeCherney AH, Mezer HC. The nature of posttuboplasty pelvic adhesions as determined by early and late laparoscopy. Fertil Steril 1984;41:643–646.
89. Jansen RPS. Early laparoscopy after pelvic operations to prevent adhesions: safety and efficacy. Fertil Steril 1988; 49:26–31.
90. Surrey MW, Friedman S. Second-look laparoscopy after reconstructive pelvic surgery for infertility. J Reprod Med 1982;27:658–660.
91. Azziz R, Interceed (TC7) Adhesion Barrier Study Group II. Microsurgery alone or with Interceed absorbable adhesion barrier for pelvic sidewall adhesion reformation. Surg Gynecol Obstet 1993;177:135–139.
92. Perez RJ. Second-look laparoscopy adhesiolysis: the procedure of choice for preventing adhesion recurrence. J Reprod Med 1991;36:700–702.
93. Serour GI, Badraoui MH, El Agizi HM, et al. Laparoscopic adhesiolysis for infertile patients with pelvic adhesive disease. Int J Obstet Gynecol 1989;30:249–252.
94. Jansen RPS. Failure of peritoneal irrigation with heparin during pelvic operations upon young women to reduce adhesions. Surg Gynecol Obstet 1988;166:154–160.
95. Saravelos HG, Li TC, Cooke ID. An analysis of the outcome of microsurgical and laparoscopic adhesiolysis for chronic pelvic pain. Hum Reprod (Oxf) 1995;10: 2895–2901.
96. Miller K, Mayer E, Moritz E. The role of laparoscopy in chronic and recurrent abdominal pain. Am J Surg 1996; 172:353–357.
97. Sutton C, MacDonald R. Laser laparoscopic adhesiolysis. J Gynecol Surg 1990;6:155–159.
98. Chan CLK, Wood C. Pelvic adhesiolysis—the assessment of symptom relief by 100 patients. Aust N Z J Obstet Gynecol 1985;25:295–298.
99. Fayez JA, Suliman SO. Infertility surgery of the oviduct: comparison between macrosurgery and microsurgery. Fertil Steril 1982;37:73–78.
100. Jansen RPS. Surgery-pregnancy time intervals after salpingolysis, unilateral salpingostomy, and bilateral salpingostomy. Fertil Steril 1980;34:222–225.
101. Kelly RW, Roberts DK. Experience with the carbon dioxide laser in gynecologic microsurgery. Am J Obstet Gynecol 1983;146:585–588.
102. Frantzen C, Schlösser HW. Microsurgery and postinfectious tubal infertility. Fertil Steril 1982;38:397–402.
103. Hulka JF. Adnexal adhesions: a prognostic staging and classification system based on a five-year survey of fertility

surgery results at Chapel Hill, North Carolina. Am J Obstet Gynecol 1982;144:141–148.
104. Luber K, Beeson CC, Kennedy JF, et al. Results of microsurgical treatment of tubal infertility and early second-look laparoscopy in the post-pelvic inflammatory disease patient: implications for in vitro fertilization. Am J Obstet Gynecol 1986;154:1264–1270.
105. Diamond E. Lysis of postoperative pelvic adhesions in infertility. Fertil Steril 1979;31:287–295.
106. Wallach EE, Manara LR, Eisenberg E. Experience with 143 cases of tubal surgery. Fertil Steril 1983;39:609–617.
107. Caspi E, Halperin Y. Surgical management of periadnexal adhesions. Int J Fertil 1981;26:49–52.
108. Donnez J. CO_2 laser laparoscopy in infertile women with endometriosis and women with adnexal adhesions. Fertil Steril 1987;48:390–394.
109. Gomel V. Salpingo-ovariolysis by laparoscopy in infertility. Fertil Steril 1983;40:607–611.

34

Use of Adhesion Prevention Barriers in Pelvic Reconstructive and Gynecologic Surgery

Gere S. diZerega

CONTENTS

Minimization of peritoneal injury forms the basis of modern surgical and microsurgical techniques and is the most important component in the prevention or reduction of postoperative adhesions.[1-3] However, despite strict adherence to these principles, serosal trauma inevitably occurs, resulting in adhesion formation. Adhesions after peritoneal surgery are a major cause of postoperative bowel obstruction, infertility, and chronic pelvic pain.[4-6] Therefore, a method by which postsurgical adhesion formation could be reduced or prevented would be of great benefit in reducing postoperative morbidity. Studies have indicated that placement of an absorbable barrier of oxidized regenerated cellulose (Interceed® [TC7]) Absorbable Adhesion Barrier; Ethicon, Somerville, NJ, USA), expanded polytetrafluoroethylene (Preclude® Surgical Membrane; W.L. Gore & Associates, Flagstaff, AZ, USA), or hyaluronic acid/carboxymethylcellulose (Seprafilm® Bioresorbable Membrane; Genzyme, Cambridge, MA, USA; Intergel® Adhesion Prevention Solution; Ethicon) between injured sites or addition of a viscous solution (Hyskon® 32% dextran 70; Pharmacia, Piscataway, NJ, USA; Sepracoat® Hyaluronic Acid Coating Solution; Genzyme) to the peritoneal cavity during or after surgery can reduce postoperative adhesion formation.[7-11] In the case of Interceed, Preclude, or Seprafilm, the surgeon must predict potential sites of adhesion formation to determine placement site and optimize barrier benefit. A dilute solution of hyaluronic acid (HA; Sepracoat) has only been shown to be effective at reducing the number of de novo adhesions at sites remote from the surgical trauma,[10] while reports indicate that Hyskon is ineffective in several types of pelvic surgery because of gravitational pooling in the cul-de-sac.[7] In addition, the use of Hyskon in clinical practice has shown some undesirable side effects resulting from the accumulation of intraperitoneal ascites from oncotic properties.[12] Intergel, the device most recently released for adhesion prevention, showed promising results in a pilot[11] and multicenter study[13] as a viscoelastic gel that reduces both de novo and reformed adhesions at both nonsurgical as well as surgical sites. This new technology is extensively discussed in Chapter 32 of this volume.

This chapter reviews the use of devices for adhesion reduction that are currently available to the practicing surgeon.

Peritoneal Irrigants

Prolonged drying of the peritoneum was shown by Ryan et al. to induce significant injury.[14] Immediately after drying, intact mesothelial cells were found to be absent in a rat cecal preparation. Four hours later, no mesothelial cells were seen; most of the surface contained only an irregular thin coating of fibrin without cells. Continuous irrigation minimizes tissue desiccation and either dilutes or washes away fibrinous exudates. However, the temperature of the irrigating solution is important. Kappas et al.[15] demonstrated an increase in adhesion formation in rats when the temperature of saline exceeded 37°C. Concern arises over the use of nonbuffered peritoneal irrigating solutions because of the elevated level of hydrogen ions (i.e., acidic) that form in peritoneal fluid after surgery. Serosal damage with swelling of the underlying tissue and cell damage can occur with hypotonic and many nonbuffered irrigating solutions. For this reason, many clinicians perform intraoperative irrigation with lactated Ringer's solution. Yaacobi et al.[16] recently reported that neither saline nor Ringer's lactate may be an ideal intraperitoneal irrigant because in some cases both may promote adhesions in animal models.

Although antibiotics are frequently added to intraperitoneal lavage solutions, their efficacy is unproven. The efficacy of antibiotic peritoneal lavage in the formation of postoperative adhesions is controversial. When the role of intraperitoneal cefazolin and tetracycline in the formation of adhesions was studied in a rodent model,[17] rats treated with antibiotics demonstrated significantly more adhesions than controls. The histologic appearance of the antibiotic-irrigated groups showed mesothelial thickening with presence of fibroblasts and collagen. Cefazolin and tetracycline irrigation of the abdominal cavity contributes to the formation of peritoneal adhesions in the rat; however, clinical data are not available.

Peritoneal Instillates

Hyaluronic Acid

Sodium hyaluronate is a naturally occurring high molecular weight mucopolysaccharide comprising sodium D-glucuronate and *N*-acetyl-D-glucosamine, which are linked as disaccharides by β_1–β_3 linkages. The subunits are joined by β_1–β_4 glycosidic bonds. Sodium hyaluronate is hydrolyzed to disaccharide or tetrasaccharide units by the action of the enzyme hyaluronidase.

Hyaluronic acid is a naturally occurring component of peritoneal fluid.[18] Peritoneal mesothelial cells were shown to synthesize HA in vitro, and HA is thought to play a role in lubrication of cells and maintenance of the structural integrity of tissues as well as regulation of fluid retention.[19] A number of investigators previously studied the efficacy of HA solutions in adhesion prevention. Urman et al.[20] evaluated the effectiveness of HA solution in preventing intraperitoneal adhesions in rats after carbon dioxide laser injury of the serosa. Although precoating of the serosa reduced de novo adhesion formation, no significant reduction of adhesions was seen when HA was added at the end of the procedure, that is, post treatment.[20] The effectiveness of reducing de novo adhesion by precoating before injuring the serosa of rats was confirmed by West et al.[21] A similar reduction of de novo adhesions after serosal abrasion was noted by Shushan et al.[22] following administration of HA as an instillate as well as application of an HA membrane after laser injury to the rat uterine horn. Diamond et al.[10] reported the clinical effectiveness of Sepracoat as a precoating solution in 245 patients undergoing laparotomy. The solution was applied upon entry into the abdominal cavity and periodically thereafter. However, the clinical effectiveness of Sepracoat, limited to nonsurgical site de novo adhesions, was not considered sufficient by the U.S. Food and Drug Administration to warrant approval for human use.

Crystalloid Solutions

The adjuvant most commonly used to reduce adhesion formation is crystalloid solution, such as lactated Ringer's solution, phosphate buffered saline, or normal saline, which is administered as an instillate at the end of the surgical procedure. Absorption of water and electrolytes from the peritoneal cavity is rapid. The 10,000-cm^2 surface area of the peritoneum absorbed crystalloid at the rate of 35 mL per hour[18] with up to 500 mL of physiologic saline absorbed in less than 24 hours.[23] Because the peritoneal surface requires 5 to 8 days to remesothelialize following surgical injury,[24–28,33] crystalloid solution should be absorbed well before the process of fibrin deposition and adhesion formation is completed. Hart and Magos[29] confirmed the short intraperitoneal residence time of crystalloid in a prospective study of patients undergoing laparoscopic surgery for conservative gynecologic indications. At the end of the procedure, 1 L of saline was instilled into the cul-de-sac and a drain was placed that remained clamped for varying periods of time following surgery. The residual fluid in the peritoneal cavity, measured from the drainage, became nondetectable by 29 hours (Fig. 34.1). Different patients were used to establish the variable time points.

Similar observations were made using ultrasound to assess the volume of crystalloid (12 mL) remaining in the cul-de-sac 24 hours after instilling 250 mL.[30] From a theoretical point of view intraperitoneal crystalloid would

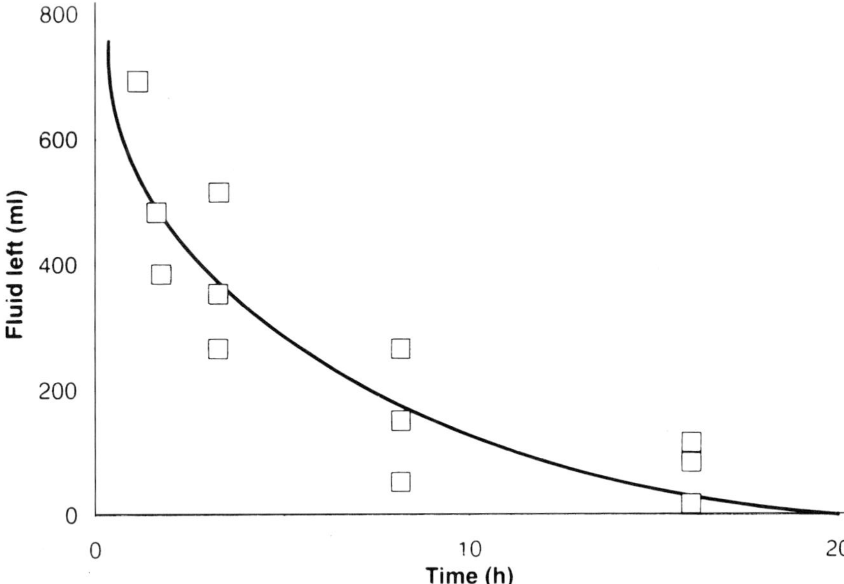

FIG. 34.1. At the end of the procedure, 1 L of saline was instilled into the peritoneal cavity, and a drain was placed into the cul-de-sac that remained clamped for varying periods of time following surgery. The residual fluid in the peritoneal cavity, measured from drainage, became nondetectable by 29 hours. Data from ref 29.

not be expected to prevent adhesion formation. Although some preclinical studies found a benefit of lactated Ringer's solution,[31,32] a number of animal studies have directly shown that lactated Ringer's solution and saline administered as an instillate at the end of surgery do not reduce adhesion formation.[6,7]

A substantial body of clinical data is available to assess the benefit of crystalloid instillate in adhesion prevention. During the early 1980s four clinical studies were published that compared dextran to crystalloid used as instillates as control solutions in Hyskon clinical trials.[12] A combination of these studies showed an adhesion reformation rate of approximately 80% in patients who received crystalloid instillates.[6,7] This high rate of adhesion formation with the use of intraperitoneal instillates was confirmed by Fayez and Schneider[34] as well as by Jansen.[35]

Reports have recently appeared describing the use of crystalloid solutions to reduce adhesion formation after laparoscopic ovarian surgery. Naether and Fischer[36] instilled 300 to 500 mL of saline into the peritoneal cavity after laparoscopic coagulation of the ovarian surface in patients with polycystic ovarian disease. When compared to a previous series they had treated in a similar fashion without the crystalloid instillation, these authors found no difference in the incidence of adhesions (17% vs. 19%, respectively). Gurgan et al.[37] instilled 150 mL of Ringer's lactate into the pelvis after laparoscopic electrocautery or laser vaporization of the ovarian surface in polycystic ovarian disease patients: 82% were found to have adhesions to the ovarian surface at second-look laparoscopy. More recently, Gurgan et al.[38] reconfirmed the failure of crystalloid (Ringer's lactate, 500 mL) to reduce adhesion formation in patients undergoing laparoscopic removal of endometriosis. When Tulandi initiated a pilot study evaluating the efficacy of crystalloid solutions for postmyomectomy adhesion prevention, the study was terminated because of the lack of benefit for his patients. A recent meta-analysis to summarize the results of clinical papers reporting on postoperative adhesion formation and the use of crystalloid instillates found that the only effect of crystalloid instillate was to increase adhesion formation.[39]

Cross-Linked Hyaluronic Acid

Sodium hyaluronate has been shown to significantly reduce adhesion formation in animal models and is believed to function through a physical effect by providing a viscous, lubricious coating on the peritoneal surfaces.[40] Although recent clinical studies have demonstrated safety when sodium hyaluronate was administered as a precoat throughout surgery and was left as an instillate, it has only been shown to be effective at reducing the number of de novo adhesions at sites remote from the surgical trauma.[10]

Ferric hyaluronate gel is an aqueous solution of sodium hyaluronate that has been cross-linked by the addition of a ferric chloride solution. Cross-linking between the carboxylate groups on the sodium hyaluronate and the trivalent iron (Fe^{3+}) is ionic in nature, resulting in a significant increase in solution viscosity and in the intraperitoneal residence time compared with that of the starting sodium hyaluronate solution. Ferric hyaluronate gel was shown to prevent or reduce adhesion formation in preclinical animal models in which sodium hyaluronate had little or no effect.[41] In addition, ferric hyaluronate gel reduced adhesion formation not only at sites of application but throughout the abdominal cavity of laboratory animals, suggesting widespread distribution by the intraabdominal circulation.

A pilot clinical study was performed to assess safety and to make a preliminary assessment of the efficacy of 0.5% ferric hyaluronate adhesion prevention gel (Intergel, 300 mL) used as an instillate in patients undergoing peritoneal cavity surgery by laparotomy as determined by a subsequent second-look laparoscopy.[11] Intergel was found to be easy to use (Table 34.1). Efficacy was based on the number of sites with adhesions divided by the number of possible adhesion sites, and the severity and extent of adhesions were evaluated. A total adhesion score using a modification of the adhesion scoring method of the American Fertility Society applied to 18 anatomic sites was determined.[42]

At second-look laparoscopy, the mean number of sites with adhesions as well as the proportion of possible adhesion sites was significantly reduced in the Intergel-treated group compared with those of the control (Fig. 34.2). In addition, patients treated with Intergel had fewer sites with adhesions than control patients at second-look laparoscopy irrespective of the adhesion status at initial laparotomy. The severity and extent of the adhesions at baseline and at second-look laparoscopy were also evaluated. While the two groups were comparable at baseline, Intergel significantly reduced the severity and extent of adhesions that did form following surgery. Adhesion formation was also assessed via a composite score adopted from the method proposed by the American Fertility Society.[42] As shown in Fig. 34.3, baseline adhesion scores were comparable, and Intergel significantly reduced the total adhesion score at second-look laparoscopy compared with that of the control. These results were recently confirmed in an international, multicenter study[13] (see Chapter 32).

The difference in effectiveness between the Intergel and HA formulations appears to result primarily from a longer residence time in the peritoneal cavity of ferric hyaluronate gel relative to HA, which may result from a greater tendency of ferric hyaluronate gel to adhere to the tissue or to its delayed dilution with peritoneal fluids compared with that of HA. The elimination half-life ($t_{1/2}$) of HA from the peritoneum in humans was estimated to be about 25.62 hours.[39] When comparing the lymphatic absorption rates of HA or ionically cross-linked HA in rats (0.38 and 0.19 μg equivalents per gram of tissue per hour, respectively), it appears that the time needed to eliminate ionically cross-linked HA from the peritoneum is approximately twice that of HA. The expected elimination half-life ($t_{1/2}$) of 0.5% ferric hyaluronate adhesion prevention gel from the peritoneal cavity of women is approximately twice that of HA, or about 51 hours.[41]

TABLE 34.1. Directions for use: Intergel® Adhesion Prevention Solution.

Intergel solution, 300 mL, is administered into the peritoneal cavity following peritoneal cavity surgery, after the surgeon has completed the surgical procedure(s), aspirated all irrigants, and removed all packs and sponges.

Intergel solution may be warmed to body temperature before use. Prolonged storage, in excess of 24 hours, at temperatures greater than 30°C is not recommended.

1. Transfer the Intergel solution bellows-type bottle to the sterile field using standard aseptic operating room techniques.
2. Remove the tab from the bottle by twisting, instill the Intergel solution directly into the peritoneal cavity by collapsing the bellows bottle (some excess, 10–20 mL, will remain in the bottle).
3. For endoscopic procedures, attach the tube that has been designed to fit directly into most 5-mm-diameter trocars. Alternatively, the Intergel solution can be dispensed into a sterile basin, and applied by means of a syringe and 5-mm cannula.
4. Direct the Intergel solution to cover all operative sites, and distribute the remainder of the 300 mL of Intergel solution throughout the abdomen.
5. Special attention should be given to ensure the gel has covered sites such as the ovarian fossa or rectosigmoid where peritoneal circulation may be limited. Distribution can be facilitated by the surgeon's hand or probe.

Dextran

Dextran is a water-soluble glucose polymer originally used as a plasma expander. It can be manufactured in a variety of molecular weights; however, most of the research in adhesion prevention has focused on a 32% solution of dextran 70 (average, 70,000 daltons) suspended in 10% dextrose (Hyskon; Pharmacia, Uppsala, Sweden).

The basis for the effects of dextran on adhesion formation relates hypothetically to a variety of activities.[41,42] Dextran may cause a mechanical separation of serosal surfaces. Tissues are held apart by the heavy fluid in the peritoneal cavity, resulting in "hydroflotation." This effect is further enhanced by the osmotic gradient created by dextran, which draws fluid into the peritoneal cavity. The osmotic gradient caused by application of 32% dextran 70 into the peritoneal cavity can draw in 2.5 to 3 times the volume instilled from the vascular space.[43–45] Dextran may have antithrombotic activity that retards adherence of blood clot and deposition of fibrin matrix. Furthermore, dextran can modify the fibrin network and thereby facilitate fibrinolysis; 32% dextran 70 was shown to reduce the ability of intraperitoneal trauma to depress plasminogen activator activity, and dextran can cause plasminogen activation in vitro.[46] In cells isolated from patients undergoing laparoscopy, lymphocyte proliferation and macrophage phagocytosis were reduced in vitro following incubation with 32% dextran 70, suggesting a role for dextran in immunosuppression.[47]

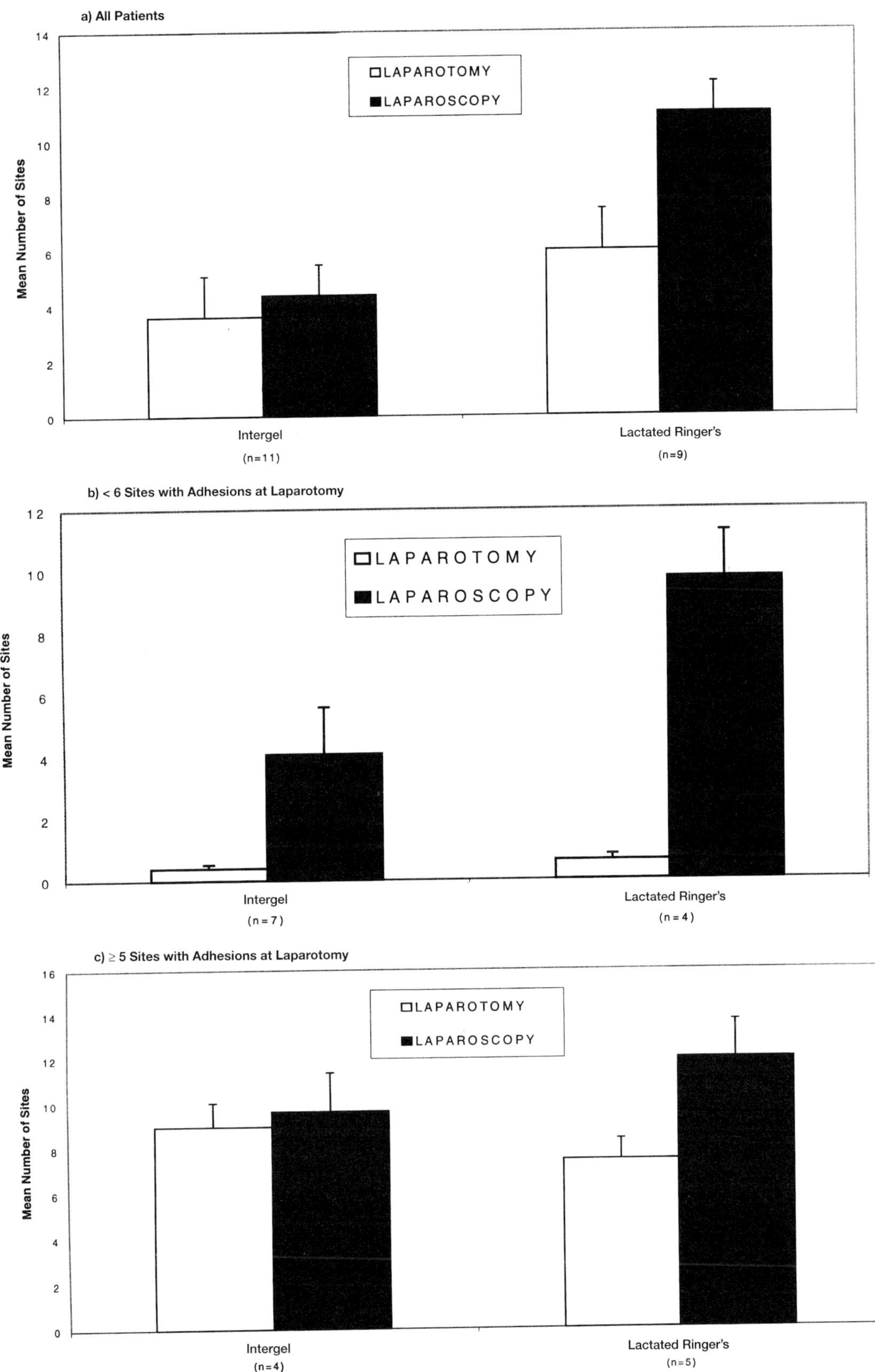

FIG. 34.2. Number of anatomic sites with adhesion seen at initial laparotomy (*open bars*) and second-look laparoscopy (*black bars*) in patients who received 300 mL of an intraperitoneal instillate of 0.5% ferric hyaluronate adhesion prevention gel (Intergel® solution, *left*) or lactated Ringer's solution (*right*) at the end of surgery. The data are summarized for all patients (**A**), and for those patients with <5 (**B**) and those patients with ≥5 (**C**) anatomic sites with adhesions at initial laparotomy (error bars, $\bar{X} \pm$ SEM). An *asterisk* indicates a statistically significant difference ($p < 0.05$; Student's *t*-test) between adhesion prevention gel and lactated Ringer's solution. Data from ref 11.

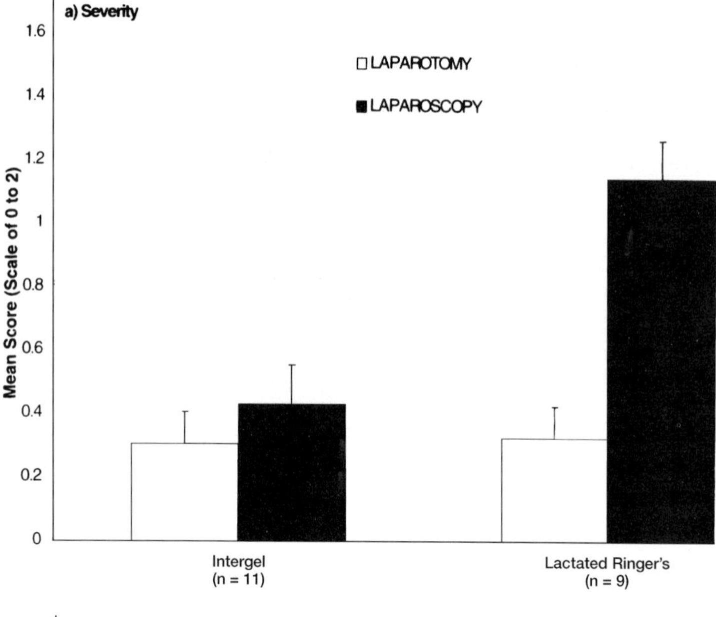

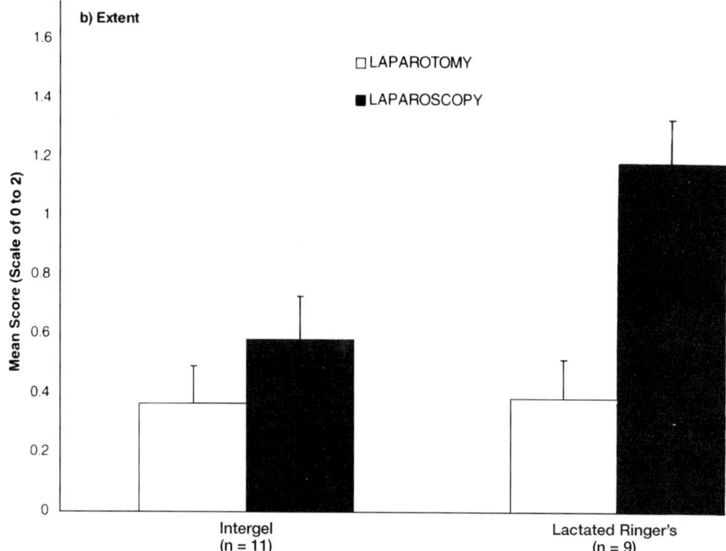

FIG. 34.3. Severity (**A**) and extent (**B**) of adhesions seen at initial laparotomy (*open bars*) and second-look laparoscopy (*black bars*) in patients who received a 300-mL intraperitoneal instillate of either 0.5% ferric hyaluronate adhesion prevention gel (Intergel® solution, *left*) or lactated Ringer's solution (*right*). Patients treated with Intergel had significantly lower adhesion severity and extent scores compared with patients who received lactated Ringer's solution ($p < 0.01$ for significant difference, $p < 0.05$, Student's t-test) between adhesion prevention gel and lactated Ringer's solution. Data from ref 11.

There is a positive relationship between dextran molecular weight and prolonged absorption rate.[45,48,49] The greater the molecular weight, the longer the intraperitoneal residence. In general, the higher molecular weight dextrans provide a greater and longer-lasting hydroflotation effect than lower molecular weight dextran, resulting in a greater reduction in adhesion formation. For example, Ruiz Navas et al.[50] reported that dextran 70 was significantly more effective than dextran 40 in reducing the incidence of adhesion formation in a rat uterine horn model. Beneficial effects of dextran 70 (either 6% or 32%) on the incidence or severity of adhesion formation are usually observed in animal models.[49] Failures to observe any beneficial effect with dextran 70 in animal studies were also reported.[51,52]

Two prospective, controlled, clinical studies in patients undergoing infertility surgery reported a significant beneficial effect of 32% dextran 70 on adhesion formation. In one study, in a total of 102 patients undergoing surgery for distal tubal disease, endometriosis, or pelvic adhesions, 250 mL of 32% dextran 70 ($n = 55$) or 250 mL saline ($n = 47$) was instilled intraperitoneally before closure of the abdomen.[7] Although prophylactic antibiotics were given to all patients, no other therapeutic adjuvants were used. The extent and severity of adhesions were evaluated at the time of the initial laparotomy and at a second-look laparoscopy performed 8 to 12 weeks later. Patients with severe adnexal adhesions at the time of the initial laparotomy had a greater reduction in adhesions if they received 32% dextran 70 than if they received saline. Furthermore, a marked reduction in adhesion formation was observed in more of the patients treated with 32% dextran 70 (50%) than in saline-treated patients (30%). Adhesions were found to occur significantly more frequently at the time of the second-look laparoscopy in control patients than in 32% dextran 70 patients at the ovary, cul-de-sac, and pelvic sidewall.

In the second prospective study, patients undergoing infertility surgery were randomized to receive 200 mL 32% dextran 70 ($n = 23$) or 200 mL Ringer's lactate ($n = 21$) intraperitoneally before closure.[53] Four to 12 weeks after the initial surgery, a second-look laparoscopy was performed. There was a significant difference between the two groups with respect to the net change in patient adhesion scores at the time of the initial surgery and at laparoscopy. Adhesion scores tended to worsen after receiving Ringer's lactate but improved after receiving 32% dextran 70. When 39 patients underwent lysis of adhesions at the time of the original surgery, the same pattern of results was evident: no improvement or worsening in the control group but improvement in the 32% dextran 70 group.

Not all clinical evaluations reported a therapeutic benefit of 32% dextran 70 on adhesion formation. In a prospective, controlled evaluation of 250 mL of 32% dextran 70 versus saline in 39 patients undergoing salpingoneostomy, fimbrioplasty, or adhesiolysis, Larsson et al.[54] reported no difference between the two treatments in reducing the adhesions at follow-up laparoscopy 4 to 10 weeks later. Jansen[35] also reported no benefit from the addition of 100 to 200 mL 32% dextran 70 on adhesion scores at follow-up laparoscopy performed 12 days later in patients after infertility surgery.

The clinical use of 32% dextran 70 is associated with side effects. Ascites is commonly observed following administration of 32% dextran 70. Cleary et al.[55] reported that serum dextran levels gradually increase during the initial days after surgery and that clinical ascites was resolved by the 4-week follow-up visit in each of the five patients. A transient weight gain is usually observed with 32% dextran 70.[56] Perhaps the most common clinical complication after intraperitoneal instillation of 32% dextran 70 is vulvar edema, which may occur in 2% of cases.[12,56] In addition to vulvar edema, Tulandi[57] reported edema of the leg and pleural effusion. Pleural effusion[58] and coagulopathy[59] are less frequent in patients receiving intraperitoneal 32% dextran 70; all these side effects resolve either spontaneously or with supportive therapy. Anaphylactic shock or allergic symptoms occur in a small percentage of patients given 32% dextran 70 intraperitoneally[60,61] or as a hysterescopic distension media.[62,63] Stangel et al.[44] reported that two patients treated with intraperitoneal 6% dextran 70 developed disseminated intravascular coagulation and anaphylactoid shock.

Gauwerky et al. performed a prospective evaluation of complications that occur after repeated use of intraperitoneal dextran.[64] In 47 patients (dextran group, 32 patients; control group, 15 patients) undergoing laparotomy for microsurgical removal of adhesions and tuboplasty, the complications of a repeated postoperative intraperitoneal instillation of 6% dextran 70 (5 days) were monitored. In the dextran-treated group, abdominal pain and dyspnea occurred significantly more frequently than in the control group. In six cases edema of the vulva developed and edema of the thigh in two cases. During intraperitoneal irrigation with dextran, a significant increase of body weight and central venous pressure were noted. Bradycardia was observed between the third and sixth postoperative days; blood pressure remained unchanged. Seventy-five percent of the patients in the dextran group had pleural effusions containing dextran when sampled on the fifth postoperative day. The use of 32% dextran 70 in combination with corticosteroids or halothane (or halogenized drugs) was reported to transiently increase hepatic transminases.[65]

There appears to be a disparity between in vitro data and clinical experience with dextran in cases of pelvic infection; Dextran 70 at 32% was reported to support bacterial and fungal growth in vitro.[66] We partially confirmed this report in that gram-positive anaerobic cocci were found to proliferate in dextran. Infectious complications of dextran use are very uncommon in clinical practice, although King[67] reported the case history of a patient who developed a *Candida albicans* pelvic infection after intraperitoneal administration of 32% dextran 70. Although infection-related complications of 32% dextran 70 are uncommon, its use in the presence of pelvic infection is unwarranted.

Heparinized Solutions

Because of its effects on inhibiting thrombosis and fibrin formation, heparinized solutions are often used in an attempt to prevent postoperative adhesions. Adhesion formation was reported to be significantly reduced following addition of heparinized saline (25 IU/2 mL) before peritoneal closure in rats after uterine reanastomosis or surgical trauma.[68] Subcutaneous administration of heparinized saline 30 minutes before either surgical procedure had no significant effect on adhesion formation relative to saline-treated controls.

Cohen et al.[69] compared the effect of heparin in a fixed volume of various intraperitoneal solutions infused before tissue closure on reducing adhesion formation in the rat uterine horn model. They found significant reduction in adhesion formation after infusion of Ringer's lactate alone, with human albumin, with ampicillin, with heparin, with dexamethasone, and with the combination of dexamethasone, hydrocortisone, and ampicillin. The reduction in adhesion formation was similar following the first three solutions, while the greatest reduction was seen with the solution containing steroids and ampicillin.

Heparin per se actively reduces adhesions in human and animal studies. However, in the early studies utilizing heparin, the dose required to reduce adhesion formation resulted in hemorrhagic diathesis. There are many mechanisms by which heparin may exert its beneficial effects. Heparin in combination with antithrombin III inhibits clotting by enhancing serine esterase activity,[70] thus reducing the deposition of fibrin strands that form the scaffold for fibroblast ingrowth. Second, heparin directly stimulates plasminogen activator activity,[71,72] which in turn enhances fibrinolysis. Third, heparin binds to fibroblast growth factor, which stimulates wound healing.[73]

In clinical studies, Fayez and Schneider[34] and Jansen[74] reported no significant reduction in adhesions by the use of heparinized Ringer's lactate (2500–5000 IU/L) compared to Ringer's lactate alone in patients undergoing infertility surgery. Jansen reported no adverse effects of the heparin solution on blood loss or wound healing. High-dose heparin given intraperitoneally was associated with hemorrhage and delayed wound healing.[75] Diamond et al.[76] evaluated the use of Interceed as a local delivery device for heparin. They found that a significant reduction in adhesion formation was observed with the combination of a oxidized cellulosic fabric (Interceed) plus heparin. In additional studies, heparin delivery by intraperitoneal (i.p.) lavage, intravenous injection, or intraabdominal instillation failed to demonstrate efficacy. A recent clinical study of Interceed used as a delivery device for heparin demonstrated clinical efficacy of Interceed but no additional benefit from heparin.[77]

Barrier Agents

Ideally, a physical barrier for adhesion prevention should not affect healing, should persist during the critical stages of reepithelialization, and then should undergo absorption. Further, a physical barrier for adhesion prevention should not potentiate infection, but should be completely absorbable and nonreactive; further, it should be deliverable via laparoscopy and stay in place within the body without the use of sutures or staples.

Oxidized Regenerated Cellulose

Oxidized regenerated cellulosic (ORC) barriers appear to satisfy these criteria (Interceed Absorbable Adhesion Barrier; Gynecare Division of Ethicon, Sommerville, NJ). Initial studies with ORC evaluated the use of Surgicel, an absorbable material that is used extensively in maintaining hemostasis. When left in the body, Surgicel is converted into a gelatinous mass and absorbed within a few days in the majority of animals (e.g., rabbits[78]). A significant reduction in adhesion formation was demonstrated in the rat multiple peritoneal trauma and ischemic peritoneal models,[79] rabbit uterine horn trauma model,[78,80] and rabbit bowel reanastomosis model.[80]

However, not all studies demonstrated efficacy of Surgicel Absorbable Hemostat in preventing adhesions. Schroder et al.[81] and Yemini et al.[82] evaluated Surgicel among other modalities and failed to demonstrate a reduction in cecal adhesions in rats. Soules et al.[83] found that Surgicel offered no advantage over no treatment after a standardized cut or scrape of the rabbit uterine horn. Hixson et al.[84] studied the ability of Surgicel to prevent postsurgical adhesions to the fimbria and ovaries; Surgicel did not reduce adnexal adhesions.

A modification of Surgicel was found to be more effective in preventing adhesion formation in the rabbit.[85,86] This newer material (Interceed) is also an oxidized regenerated cellulose. The difference is that the knitted pattern was changed so that Interceed has a longer intraperitoneal residence time than Surgicel. A significant reduction in adhesion formation was observed following use of Interceed after uterine or peritoneal sidewall trauma in the rabbit.[85–87]

A prospective, multicenter, randomized clinical evaluation of Interceed was conducted to evaluate clinical efficacy.[88,89] Infertility patients (n = 148) in 13 investigational centers underwent lysis of bilateral pelvic sidewall adhesions. Following adhesiolysis, the area of the deperitonealized surface was measured. Interceed was applied in an amount sufficient to completely cover deperitonealized surfaces on the sidewall; the contralateral sidewall was left uncovered, thereby serving as control. A second-look laparoscopy was performed between 10 days and 14 weeks after the laparotomy; the Interceed barrier was found to significantly reduce the incidence, extent, and severity of postoperative adhesions (Table 34.2). Interceed also significantly reduced adhesion formation between ovaries and peritoneal sidewall and prevented the reformation of adhesions in more than twice as many patients as did the control. These observations were confirmed by a similar multicenter study performed in Japan[90] and a more recent laparoscopic study of Interceed application to visceral peritoneal surfaces performed in Germany.[91] In October 1989, Interceed received approval by the U.S. Food and Drug Administration as the first surgical adjuvent specifically indicated for the reduction of postsurgical adhesions.

Larsson et al. suggested that oxidized regenerated cellulose prevents adhesion formation by its transformation into a gelatinous mass that covers the damaged peritoneum and thereby protects it from involvement in adhesion formation.[92] This gelatinous "cocoon" seems to provide a protective coating over healing tissue during the initial postoperative interval.[85,86] During this time, reepithelialization of damaged peritoneal surfaces is com-

TABLE 34.2. Clinical studies with barriers confirm efficacy.

Procedure	Barrier	Patients (n)	Reference
Laparotomy:			
Ovarian surgery			
Cystectomy	Interceed	66	Nordic Adhesion Prevention Study Group[94]
	Interceed	52	Franklin et al.[93]
	Interceed	20	Van Geldorp[95]
	Interceed	31	Reid et al.[77]
Pelvic sidewall adhesiolysis	Interceed	74	Interceed Adhesion Barrier Study Group[88]
	Interceed	134	Azziz et al.[113]
	Interceed	63	Sekiba et al.[90]
	Interceed	35	Reid et al.[77]
	Interceed	28	Li and Cooke[102]
	Preclude/Interceed	32	Haney et al.[103]
Tubal surgery:			
Adhesiolysis	Interceed	66	Nordic Adhesion Prevention Study Group[94]
Salpingostomy	Interceed	21	Curto et al.[99]
Myomectomy	Preclude	16	Surgical Membrane Study Group[108]
	Interceed	50	Mais et al.[105]
	Seprafilm	54	Diamond et al.[9]
Endometriosis:			
Resection stage III–IV	Interceed	28	Sekiba et al.[90]
Endometrioma	Interceed	14	Van Geldorp[95], Wiseman et al.[112]
Severe disease	Interceed	32	Mais et al.[100]
Pelvic surgery	Preclude	18	Surgical Membrane Study Group[108]
Laparoscopy	Preclude	57	Korell[114]
Ovarian cystectomy	Interceed	17	Keckstein et al.[98]
Ovarian drilling	Interceed	20	Giannacodimos et al.[97]
Endometriosis	Interceed	32	Mais et al.[100]

pleted (7–10 days).[24–28] In preclinical studies, the presence of blood significantly reduced the efficacy of ORC barriers such as Interceed.[87] To obtain maximum benefit, it is essential to achieve adequate hemostasis before applying the Interceed, which means that the barrier should not turn brown or black after application; this color change is indicative of inadequate hemostasis.

Ovarian Surgery

Efficacy of Interceed after ovarian surgery was evaluated in multiple clinical studies (see Table 34.2). Franklin et al.[93] conducted a prospective, multicenter, randomized study to assess the efficacy of Interceed as a barrier to the reformation of ovarian adhesions after surgery involving the ovaries in which 52 patients with bilateral ovarian disease were treated at initial laparotomy. At the end of the procedure, one ovary was wrapped with Interceed and the other was left uncovered. Treatment with Interceed eliminated the formation of adhesions in nearly twice as many ovaries compared to surgery alone (control ovaries) as determined by second-look laparoscopy. This difference represents an 86% improvement over control in preventing adhesion formation or reformation.

The Nordic Adhesion Prevention Study Group[94] studied 66 women with infertility caused, at least in part, by bilateral adnexal adhesions. Adhesiolysis was performed through laparotomy with microsurgical techniques. Interceed was applied to one ovary while the contralateral ovary served as the untreated control. The results indicated that microsurgical techniques alone resulted in a significant reduction of postoperative adhesions to the adnexa (Fig. 34.4). Further, the number of ovaries without adhesions at the time of second-look laparoscopy was significantly increased by approximately twofold when the ovaries were covered with Interceed. When combined with microsurgical techniques, Interceed reduced adhesion reformation scores by 70%.

Van Geldorp[95] evaluated the use of Interceed as an ovarian wrap. Twenty patients underwent bilateral ovarian surgery including cystectomy, removal of endometriosis, and endometriomas as well as adhesiolysis via laparotomy. At the end of the procedure one ovary was chosen on a random basis for wrapping with Interceed while the other served as an unwrapped control. Estimation of the ovarian surface with adhesions (damaged area left after adhesiolysis) was made at laparoscopy 4 to 8 weeks later; 11 treated (55%) and 3 control (15%) ovaries had no adhesions. Overall, 17 of the treatment (85%) and only 5 (25%) of the control ovaries had a reduction in the size of the initial area of injury at second look; 10 of the other control ovaries had an increase in area involved in adhesions compared with only 1 of the Interceed-treated ovaries. Wrapping the ovary with Interceed after ovarian surgery significantly reduced the area

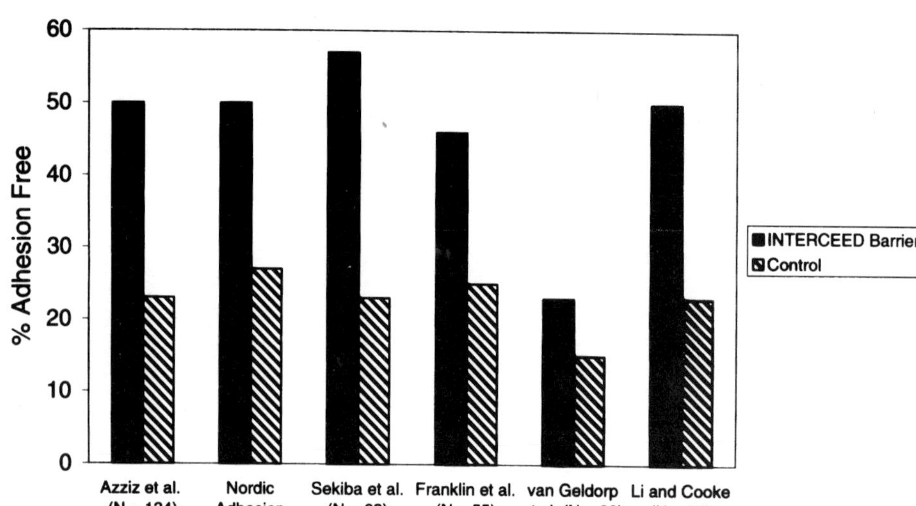

FIG. 34.4. A meta-analysis, based on six clinical studies, was conducted to evaluate the efficacy and safety of Interceed® barrier (*black bars*) for the prevention of postoperative adhesion formation following gynecologic surgery performed by laparotomy. Although no study demonstrated 100% effectiveness, Interceed was in general twice as effective as good surgical technique alone in achieving adhesion-free outcome (controls, *striped bars*). Data from ref 112.

involved with adhesions to the ovary as well as the adjacent attachment sites from which adhesions had been removed. Although no clinical data are available regarding pregnancy outcome, Marana et al.[96] showed an increase in nidation index in rabbits treated with Interceed. Swada reported a significant increase in pregnancy rates in a general infertility population using a randomized, prospective clinical design.[106]

Giannacodimos et al.[97] used a CO_2 laser to perform ovarian drilling in 40 patients with polycystic ovarian disease. Vaporization was performed on 10 to 30 follicles per ovary. After complete hemostasis, cut pieces of Interceed (average size, 3 × 3 cm) were applied in a single layer covering the entire ovarian surface. Within 2 years, 24 patients became pregnant; 20 of these were delivered by cesarean section, at which time the frequency and severity of adhesion formation were evaluated. Postoperative adhesion development was observed in 3 patients (15%), consisting of fine, filmy adhesions, and in 17 patients (85%) no adhesions were present. However, the study had no control group, and the second-look data were collected at cesarean section, which occurred as much as 2 years after the initial laparoscopic procedure. Thus, the interpretation of their results is limited.

Keckstein et al.[98] evaluated the efficacy of Interceed in 17 patients following removal of 16 cysts (5 mucinous, 11 serous) and 22 endometriomas. The ovaries were equally distributed between Interceed-treated and control ovaries. At second-look laparoscopy, 13 of 17 Interceed-treated ovaries (76%) and 6 of 17 control ovaries (35%) were free of adhesions. Five of the 8 Interceed-treated ovaries that had endometriomas were adhesion free at second look (62%) compared to 4 of 11 control ovaries (36%). All the adhesions that formed were classified as filmy. De novo adhesions were found in 4 of 16 possible ovaries in the Interceed-treated group (25%) and 7 of 12 ovaries in the control group (58%). Wrapping the ovary with Interceed after ovarian surgery significantly reduced the area involved with adhesions to the ovary, as well as the adjacent attachment site from which adhesions had been removed (Fig. 34.5).

Tubal Surgery

Curto et al.[99] reported a 100% incidence of adhesion-free fimbria when Interceed was used to cover the fimbria after salpingostomy. However, their series was uncontrolled and reported results in only 21 of their 54 patients. Larsson et al.[94] evaluated the efficacy of Interceed as an adjuvant in the prevention of postoperative adhesion reformation to the fallopian tube and fimbria. Adhesiolysis was performed in infertility patients (n = 66) with bilateral adhesions attached to both fallopian tubes. The side of Interceed application was randomly assigned. Follow-up laparoscopy after 4 to 10 weeks indicated that twice as many fallopian tubes were free of adhesions after the use of Interceed compared to microsurgery alone (see Fig. 34.2).

Endometriosis

Interceed was also effective in preventing adhesion formation after removal of severe endometriosis in 28 patients (American Fertility Society Endometriosis grade IV, 25 patients; grade III, 3 patients). After completion of all operative procedures, including lysis of pelvic sidewall adhesions, one side was randomly assigned coverage with Interceed. In 28 patients with severe endometriosis, significantly fewer Interceed-treated sidewalls contained adhesions compared to the control side as determined by second-look laparoscopy.[90]

Mais et al.[100] evaluated the effectiveness of Interceed in the reduction of adhesion reformation after laparoscopic surgery for endometriosis. Thirty-two women with endometriosis and complete posterior cul-de-sac obliter-

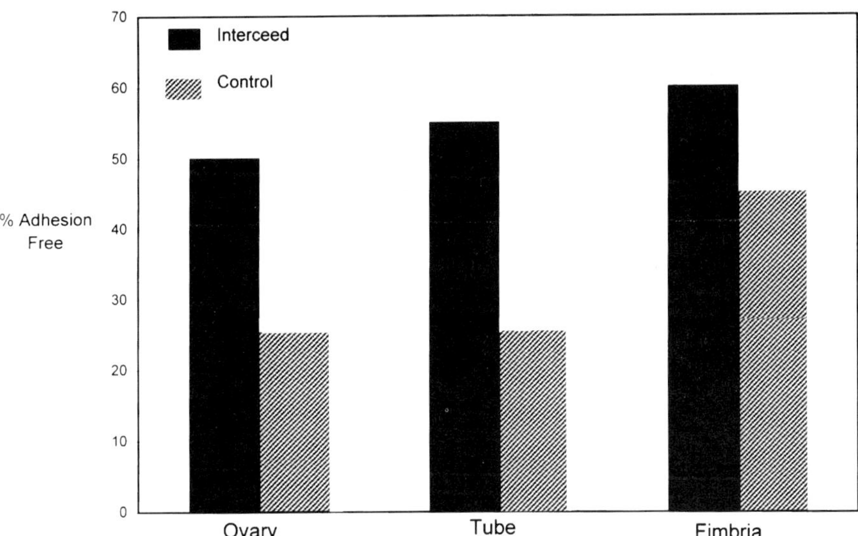

FIG. 34.5. Bilateral adnexal surgery was performed on infertility patients including removal of adhesions from ovaries, fimbria, and the Fallopian tube. Interceed® barrier use (*left bars*) on the surgical site prevented adhesion reformation compared to surgery-only control (*right bars*) (ovary: 65% vs. 31%, $p < 0.02$; fimbria: 38% vs. 21%, $p < 0.01$; fallopian tube: 18% vs. 24%). (Adapted from Larsson et al.[94])

ation were randomly assigned to either surgery alone or surgery and Interceed after laparoscopic removal of endometriosis. Second-look laparoscopy was performed after 12 to 14 weeks by an investigator blinded to the treatment, and the incidence of adhesion-free subjects was assessed. Twelve of 16 (75%) women treated with the oxidized regenerated cellulose barrier were free of adhesions, compared with 2 of 16 (12.5%) controls. Thus, Interceed significantly reduced adhesion reformation after laparoscopic surgery for endometriosis.

Adhesiolysis

The initial clinical evaluation of Interceed was conducted in fertility patients who underwent lysis of bilateral pelvic sidewall adhesions.[101] Following adhesiolysis, the area of the deperitonealized surface was measured. Interceed was applied in an amount sufficient to completely cover deperitonealized surfaces on the sidewall; the contralateral sidewall was left uncovered, thereby serving as control. At second-look laparoscopy, Interceed barrier was found to significantly reduce the incidence, extent, and severity of postoperative adhesions. A similar study was published by Sekiba et al.,[90] confirming the efficacy of Interceed in preventing sidewall adhesions in 63 infertility patients.

Li and Cooke[102] reported the results of Interceed together with intraperitoneal hydrocortisone in the prevention of adhesion reformation. Twenty-seven women underwent pelvic microsurgery for infertility or chronic pelvic pain as well as bilateral pelvic adhesions and deperitonealized areas following adhesiolysis. After microsurgical adhesiolysis, one side of the pelvis was randomized to cover the deperitonealized surface with Interceed, whereas the contralateral side served as control. Both groups of patients received hydrocortisone administered into the peritoneal cavity (30 mL) at the time of surgery. The amount of adhesion reformation at second-look laparoscopy was compared with the amount of deperitonealized area exposed following microsurgical adhesiolysis. The area of adhesion reformation found at second-look laparoscopy was twice as great on the control side compared to the Interceed-treated side.

Another confirmatory clinical study[77] on reduction of peritoneal sidewall adhesions after adhesiolysis using a similar protocol was reported from Canada ($n = 35$ patients; 80% reduction in adhesions). Similar demonstrations of Interceed efficacy at the pelvic sidewall after adhesiolysis were reported in two clinical studies in which Preclude Surgical Membrane was used as a comparison on the contralateral sidewall. Haney et al.[103] reported a significant reduction of sidewall adhesions with Interceed use in 29 patients in contrast to reports by the same authors in rodents.[104] Importantly, none of these studies nor any other clinical study reported any adverse reaction of surrounding organs or tissues attributable to Interceed use in women.

Myomectomy

In a prospective, randomized study Interceed was evaluated for prevention of de novo adhesion formation after laparoscopic myomectomy.[105] Patients were randomized to surgery alone (control group; $n = 25$) or surgery followed by Interceed coverage of the uterine incision (Interceed group; $n = 25$). The incidence of adhesion-free patients was assessed at second-look laparoscopy by an investigator not informed of the treatment. There were 3 adhesion-free patients of 25 (12%) in the control group and 15 of 25 (60%) in the treatment group. In this study, Interceed significantly reduced de novo adhesion formation after laparoscopic myomectomy. The reduction of adhesions after myomectomy with the use of Interceed was confirmed in a recent study[106] that also preliminarily

TABLE 34.3. Directions for use: Interceed® Absorbable Adhesion Barrier.

1. Apply at the end of the procedure.
2. Hemostasis must be achieved before application.
3. Place patient in reverse Trendelenburg and remove as much of the irrigation fluid as possible from the cul-de-sac.
4. Cut to size to allow at least a 5-mm margin around area at risk.
5. Apply Interceed.
   If Interceed turns black upon application, then blood is present and may reduce efficacy. Remove Interceed and achieve hemostasis. Then apply new piece of Interceed.
6. Apply Interceed dry and in a single layer.
   If more than one piece is required, allow the pieces to overlap by a margin of 3–5 mm to ensure contiguous coverage of the area at risk.
7. No sutures needed.
8. Moisten with up to 2 mL of irrigant per 7.6 cm × 10.2 cm piece.

reported significant increased pregnancy rates in women who received Interceed (78%) compared to surgical controls (46%; $p < 0.05$).

Recommendations for Use

Attention to technical detail is important in any surgical technique (Table 34.3). Interceed should be applied at the end of the surgical procedure just before closure. The most important steps to maximize efficacy of Interceed barrier are (1) removal of intraperitoneal irrigants, which usually requires aspiration of all residual fluid remaining in the cul-de-sac with the patient in reverse Trendelenburg position; (2) inspection to ensure that adequate hemostasis has been achieved (as evidenced by Interceed not turning black); and (3) use of a sufficiently large piece of Interceed to completely cover the area of interest, leaving at least a 5-mm border. If hemostasis has not been achieved, Interceed will develop a black spot discoloration which will rapidly expand in size. In these cases the material must be removed, hemostasis achieved, and a new piece of Interceed applied.

Ovarian Surgery

The ovary may be completely wrapped with Interceed by (1) lifting the ovary away from the ovarian fossa and placing a corner of Interceed (one-half piece) up into the ovarian fossa; (2) allowing the ovary to return to normal position, thereby holding the Interceed in place; and (3) lifting the opposite corner laterally over the ovary, then moistening with a few drops of irrigating solution to ensure adherence of the barrier to the ovary (Fig. 34.6).

Tubal Surgery

The Interceed barrier is suspended by two grasping instruments and brought into contact with the salpingostomy site (Fig. 34.7). The barrier is then folded over the surgical site until the four corners of the barrier are in contact with the isthmic portion of the fallopian tube. Irrigating solution (3–5 mL) is placed over the Interceed, thereby "sealing" an Interceed bag around the fimbria. In the event the surgeon prefers the fimbria not to come into contact with the barrier, the fimbria should be wrapped with a "cuff" of Interceed followed by moistening of the cuff to ensure that the Interceed covers the outer portion of the ampulla. Concerns over fimbrial contact with the barrier are reduced by the recent report of safe application of an Interceed "bag" over the fimbria with good results following salpingostomy.[94]

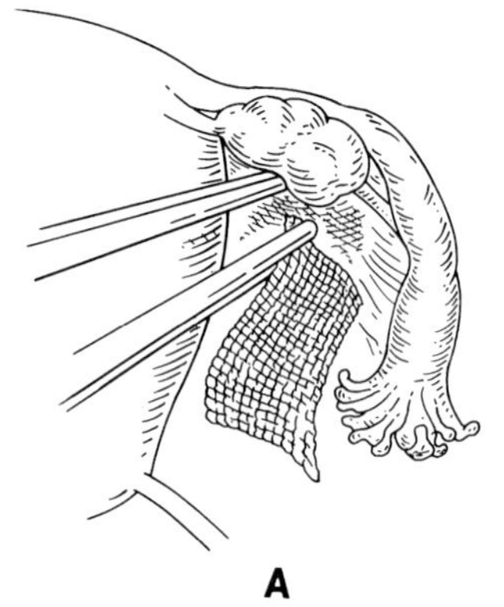

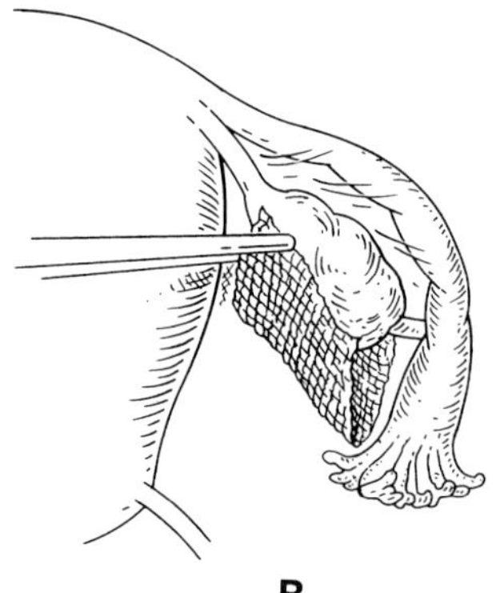

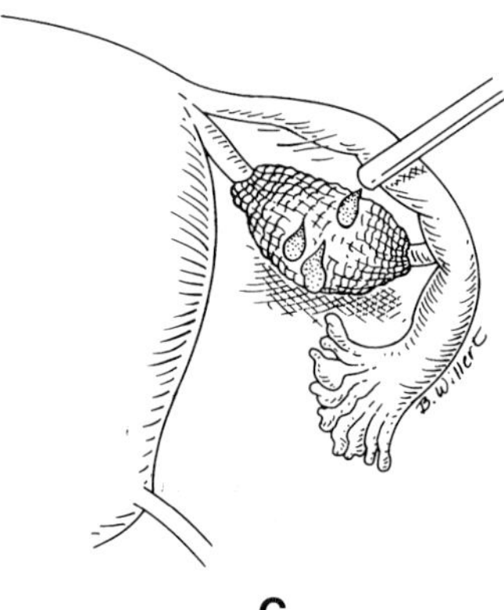

FIG. 34.6. The ovary is completely wrapped with Interceed® barrier **(A)** by lifting the ovary away from the ovarian fossa and placing a corner of Interceed (1/2 piece) up into the ovarian fossa; **(B)** allowing the ovary to return to normal position thereby holding the Interceed in place; **(C)** then moistening with a few drops of irrigating solution to ensure adherence of the barrier to the ovary. Reproduced with permission from ref. 111.

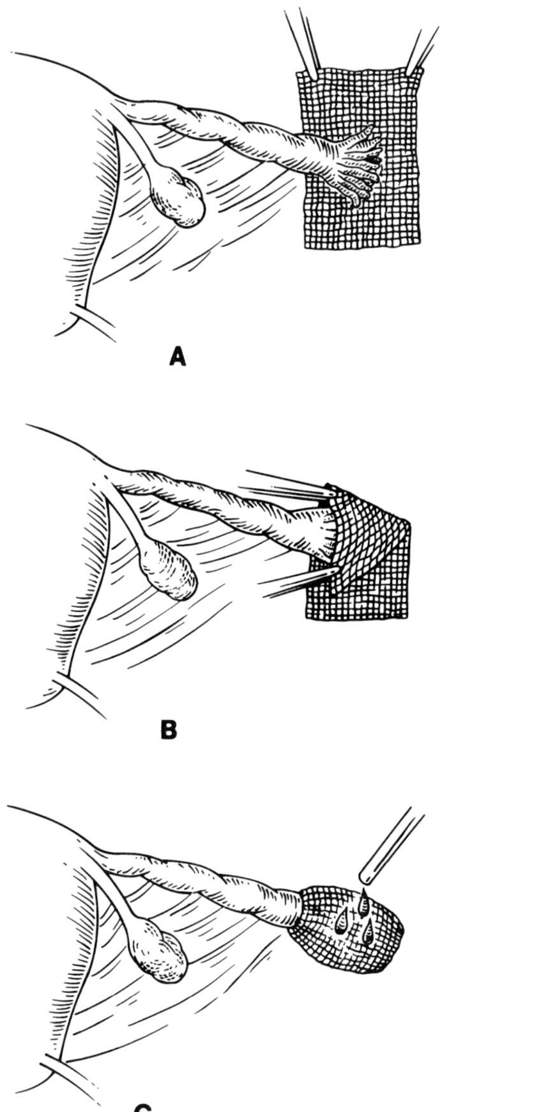

FIG. 34.7. For use after salpingostomy, the Interceed® barrier is suspended by two grasping instruments and brought into contact with the salpingostomy site **(A)**. The barrier is then folded over the surgical site until the four corners of the barrier are in contact with the isthmic portion of the fallopian tube **(B)**. Irrigating solution (3–5 mL) is dripped over the Interceed **(C)**, thereby "sealing" an Interceed bag around the fimbria. Reproduced with permission from ref. 111.

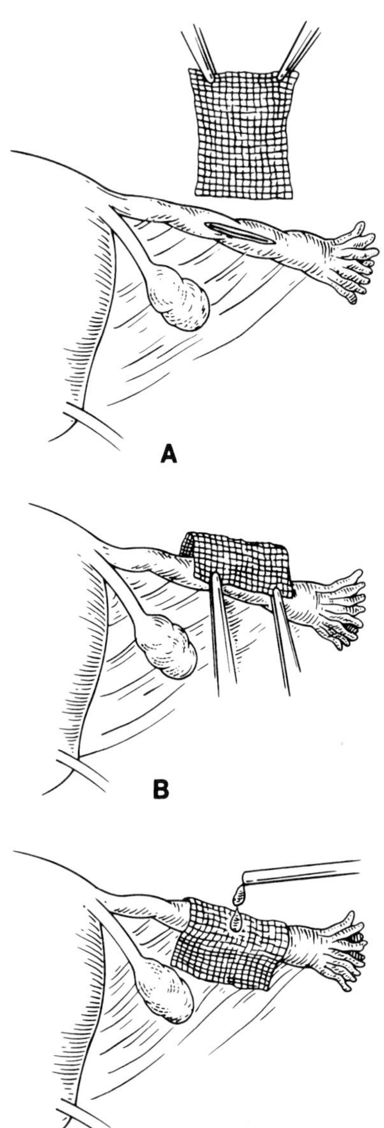

FIG. 34.8. After the ectopic pregnancy has been removed from the tube hemostasis is controlled, which often requires 3–10 mL of pitressin (5000 U in 10 mL of aqueous solution) injected into the tubal muscularis. The Interceed® barrier is cut to size (at least 5-mm border around ectopic site), grasped by forceps and brought into contact with the mesosalpinx **(A)**. The remaining Interceed is wrapped over the ectopic site and layered over the Fallopian tube **(B)**. Hydrostatic bonding is accomplished with the use of 3–5 mL of irrigation solution applied directly onto the barrier **(C)**. Reproduced with permission from ref. 111.

Ectopic Pregnancy

After the ectopic pregnancy has been removed from the tube, hemostasis is controlled, which often requires 3 to 10 mL of pitressin (5 units in 10 mL of aqueous solution) injected into the tubal muscularis. The Interceed is cut to size (at least a 5-mm border around ectopic site), grasped by forceps, and brought into contact with the mesosalpinx. The remaining Interceed is wrapped over the ectopic site and laid over the Fallopian tube (Fig. 34.8). Hydrostatic bonding is accomplished with the use of 3 to 5 ml of irrigation solution applied directly onto the barrier.

Seprafilm

Seprafilm® (Genzyme, Cambridge, MA, USA) is a flexible membrane composed of hyaluronic acid and carboxymethyl cellulose. Hyaluronic acid (HA) is a naturally occurring glycosaminoglycan consisting of repeating units, β1,3-linked *N*-acetyl-D-glucosamine and β1, 4-linked D-glucuronic acid. It is a major component of the extracellular matrix, including connective tissue, skin, cartilage, vitreous, and synovial fluid. it is purified following bacterial fermentation into a high molecular weight polymer that is biocompatible, nonimmunogenic, and bioabsorbable. Carboxymethylcellulose (CMC) is a derivative of cellulose in which the glucosidic hydroxyl groups have been carboxymethylated, making the polymer more hydrophilic. HA is combined with CMC and chemically modified to produce a compound with a longer in vivo residence time compared with unmodified HA and CMC. The resulting longer residence time of the polymer at the site of the application enhances its ability to prevent adhesion formation. Seprafilm adheres well to moist tissue surfaces, then turns into a gel approximately 24 hours after placement. It is cleared from the body and does not require a second operation for removal. Its use is not restricted in the presence of blood.

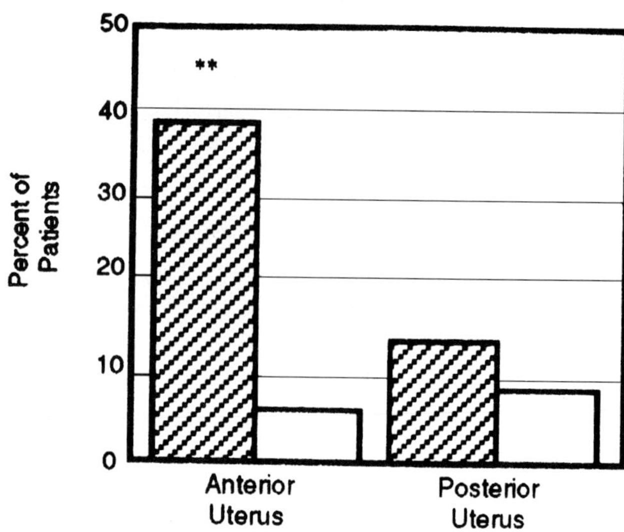

FIG. 34.9. Percentage of patients with no adhesion at second-look laparoscopy (*shaded bars*, Seprafilm; *open bars*, no treatment). **, $p < 0.0001$.[9]

Gynecologic Surgery

A prospective, randomized, double-blind, multicenter trial examined the efficacy of Seprafilm in reducing adhesion formation in patients undergoing myomectomy.[9] All patients had at least one posterior uterine incision of 1 cm or more in length. Patients were randomly assigned to receive either Seprafilm (59 treatment patients) or nothing (68 controls). Seprafilm was wrapped on both the anterior and posterior uterine surfaces, ensuring that all uterine incisions were completely covered following the myomectomy. Approximately two 5 × 6 inch membranes of Seprafilm were applied in each treatment patient. Of the 127 patients who completed the trial, 117 were evaluable for analysis; 54 received Seprafilm and 63 controls.

The development of postsurgical uterine adhesions was recorded at laparoscopy when patients returned for second-look surgery 7 days to 10 weeks after the initial myomectomy. The entire uterus and the individual anterior and posterior uterine surfaces were evaluated. The mean number of locations adherent to the entire uterine surface in the Seprafilm recipients was 4.98 compared with 7.88 in the controls (Fig. 34.9). A statistically

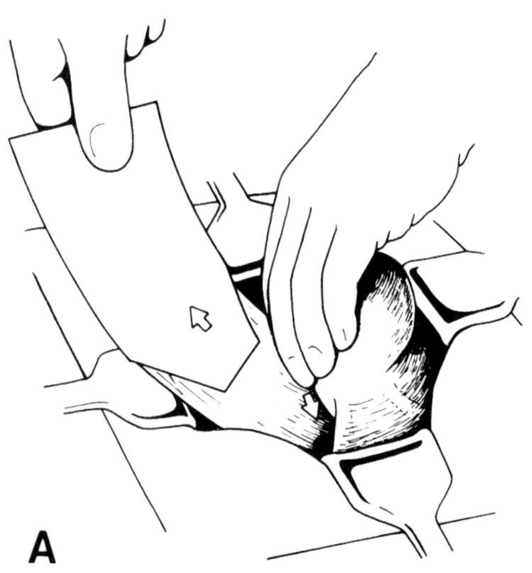

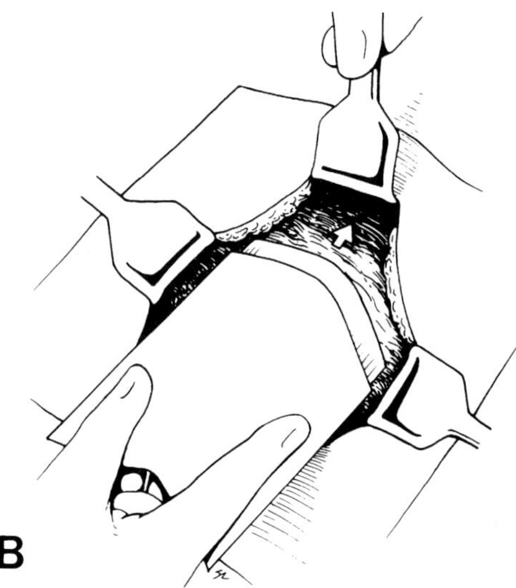

FIG. 34.10. Seprafilm membrane application is shown **(A)** to the posterior uterus and **(B)** beneath an anterior abdominal wall incision. To apply Seprafilm, a 2-cm leading edge of the membrane is advanced beyond the holder. The membrane is applied to the posterior side of the uterine surface. Entry into the abdominal cavity and placement beneath the abdominal wall can be facilitated by slightly arching the membrane and holder. Reproduced with permission from ref. 111.

significant reduction in adhesions was evident on the anterior uterine surfaces (1.45 vs. 2.88). However, adhesion reduction was only significantly reducedt on the anterior surface of the uterus in contrast to the posterior. This difference may have been the result of the self-adherence of Seprafilm, which requires careful application with a paper sleeve (Fig. 34.10; Table 34.4). In the Seprafilm group, 39% of patients had no adhesions compared with only 6% in the control group. Patients who received Seprafilm had fewer locations adherent to the uterine surface when compared with patients who received no treatment. Thus, Seprafilm significantly reduced adhesion formation following myomectomy.

General Surgery Studies

A prospective, randomized, double-blind, multicenter trial examined the efficacy of Seprafilm in reducing adhesion formation in patients (106 male, 77 female) undergoing colectomy and ileal pouch–anal anastomosis with temporary diverting loop ileostomy for ulcerative colitis or familial polyposis.[107] They were randomized to receive Seprafilm (91 treatment patients) following initial surgery or no further treatment (92 control patients). Seprafilm was applied directly over the omentum and bowel to separate tissues from the abdominal wall and the midline incision. Approximately two 5 × 6 inch membranes of Seprafilm were applied in each treatment patient.

This trial was the first prospective general surgical study of postsurgical abdominal adhesion formation using second-look laparoscopy (8–12 weeks after initial surgery). During the second surgery, a laparoscope was inserted through the abdominal wall opening of the ileostomy to make a quantitative assessment of the adhesions to the midline incision. A total of 175 patients were evaluable, 85 Seprafilm-treated patients and 90 controls. No adhesions were seen in 51% of Seprafilm patients compared with only 6% of controls. The incidence of patients with one or more adhesions to the midline incision was significantly reduced from 94% among the control patients to 49% among the Seprafilm-treated patients. In conclusion, Seprafilm significantly reduced the incidence of postsurgical adhesion formation between the abdominal wall and the underlying viscera, including the omentum, small bowel, bladder, and stomach. When adhesions were present in treatment patients, they were less extensive and less severe than those in control patients.

TABLE 34.4. Directions for general use: Seprafilm® Bioresorbable Membrane.

1. Seprafilm should be applied immediately before abdominopelvic cavity closure following laparotomy.
2. Membrane must be kept dry before application.
3. The surgical field, especially the desired site of application, should be as dry as possible. Thoroughly aspirate excess fluid with the patient in reverse Trendelenburg position.
4. Open the pouch immediately before application and drop the interior sterile sleeve containing Seprafilm onto the dry sterile field.
5. Remove the holder containing Seprafilm from the polyolefin sleeve.
6. Where applicable, cut membrane and holder with scissors to desired size and shape.
7. The membrane should be handled gently with dry instruments and/or gloves.
8. Expose 1–2 cm of the membrane through the open end of the holder.
9. When necessary, facilitate entry into abdominopelvic cavity by slightly curving or arching the membrane/holder.
10. When applying, avoid contact with tissue surfaces until directly at site of application. If contact occurs, moderate application of standard irrigation solution may be used to gently dislodge membrane from unintended tissue surfaces.
11. Allow exposed membrane to first adhere to desired position on the tissue or organ by gently pressing the membrane down with a dry glove or instrument and then withdraw the holder.
12. Extend membrane significantly beyond the margins of incision and associated surgical trauma to achieve adequate coverage.
13. When necessary, lightly moisten membrane with standard irrigation solution to facilitate its coverage around the contours of tissue or organs.
14. Allow sufficient overlap of individual membranes to ensure complete, continuous coverage of traumatized tissue surface.

After placement:
1. Discard holder(s) following application.
2. Care should be taken not to disturb the membrane once it is placed on the tissue.
3. Do not suture the membrane in place.
4. Abdominopelvic cavity should be closed according to the standard technique of the surgeon.

Polytetrafluoroethylene

Preclude™ (W.L. Gore, Flagstaff, AZ, USA) is a thin sheet (0.1 mm) of expanded polytetrafluoroethylene (PTFE) that is used as a substitute for the pericardium. Experience in cardiovascular surgery has shown that use of PTFE results in minimal adhesion formation when used as a pericardial substitute. Preclude has a small pore size (≤1 μm) that retards cellular penetration. The membrane must be fixed in place within the body and is nonabsorbable. It is antithrombogenic, noninflammatory, nonreactive, and easy to handle at laparotomy.

Clinical Studies: Gynecology

A multicenter, noncontrolled study evaluated Preclude in patients treated for one of the following conditions: (1) moderate to severe pelvic adhesive disease, (2) significant deperitonealization, or (3) leiomyomata.[108] Adhesions were lysed and/or a myomectomy was performed. The area covered by the Preclude had significantly lower adhesion scores than those before surgery. There was no morbidity (i.e., infection, inflammation) attributable to the use of the PTFE barrier. At second look, all the Preclude was removed by cutting the sutures and withdrawing the barrier through an operating trocar. Histologic analysis of the retrieved barrier showed no tissue adherence to the material and mild to no foreign-body response. Third-look laparoscopy of a single sidewall site showed no adhesion formation subsequent to Preclude removal.

Recently a multicenter clinical study confirmed the efficacy of Preclude in preventing adhesions. This study was a randomized, paired comparison of Interceed and Preclude applied to pelvic sidewalls after adhesiolysis in infertility patients.[103] The Preclude was attached to the pelvic sidewall by nonabsorbable sutures, and 1 to 6 weeks later a second-look laparoscopy demonstrated a marked reduction in adhesions by both barriers.

Clinical Studies: Myomectomy

The Myomectomy Adhesion Group[109] performed myomectomies in 28 patients via laparotomy. All patients had two uterine incisions located on the fundus and posterior uterus. All incisions were sutured closed and randomly assigned coverage with Preclude or left as uncovered controls. Suturing of the Preclude was performed with 7-0 nylon or polypropylene (Fig. 34.11). The number of adhesion-free sites covered by Preclude was significantly greater when compared to the control (Fig. 34.12) as determined by a second-look laparoscopy. Adhesions to the Preclude sites were found mainly at the edges of the barriers. In situ the PTFE was covered by a thin layer of tissue that readily separated during removal of the material. The surgical membrane was easily removed by cutting the sutures and applying gentle traction. Histologic examination of the barrier revealed no tissue attachment to the material. The interstices were filled with proteinaceous fluid, and the surface occasionally showed the presence of fibroblasts, histocyte, erythrocytes, and mesothelial cells. Because of the permanent nature of PTFE, the use of Preclude may require removal at a subsequent surgical procedure (Table 34.5).[110]

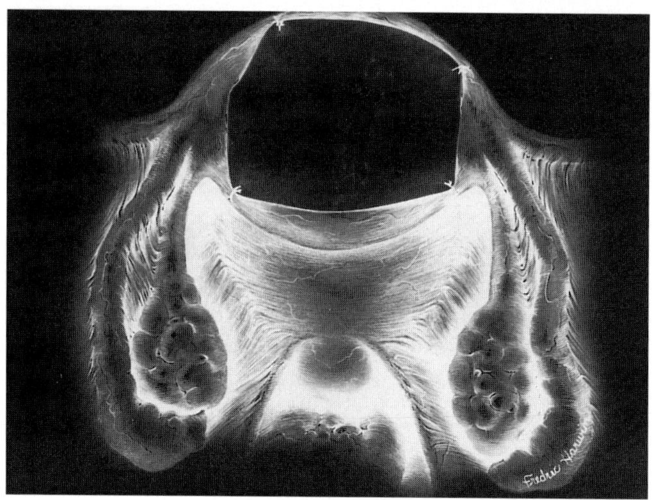

Fig. 34.11. Application of Preclude over a myomectomy incision. Permanent sutures are used to ensure positioning of the barrier, which was cut to cover the entire area at risk for adhesion formation.[109]

Perspective

Although all solid barriers were shown to be safe and effective in all human clinical trials (see Table 34.2), their use did not eliminate adhesions in all patients. Many investigators are incorporating adhesion prevention barriers into their routine clinical practice and achieving good results, even in difficult clinical settings. Because of multiple demonstrations of barrier efficacy, adhesion prevention adjuvants have received widespread acceptance in appropriate surgical settings. Efficacy of the barriers is limited to surgical situations in which the area in question can be completely covered. Physician acceptance is constrained by technical difficulties, including the need for hemostasis and removal of excess peritoneal fluid (Interceed; Table 34.3) as well as fixation techniques and concerns regarding subsequent removal of the barrier (Preclude; Table 34.5) and limitations in application and handling properties within the surgical field (Seprafilm; see Table 34.4). Perhaps the recent availability of Intergel, a viscoelastic gel, will provide generalized peritoneal coverage that can be accomplished by device administration via either laparoscopy or laparotomy (see Table 34.1).

Systemic administration of medicaments requires adequate blood supply to the site of potential adhesion for-

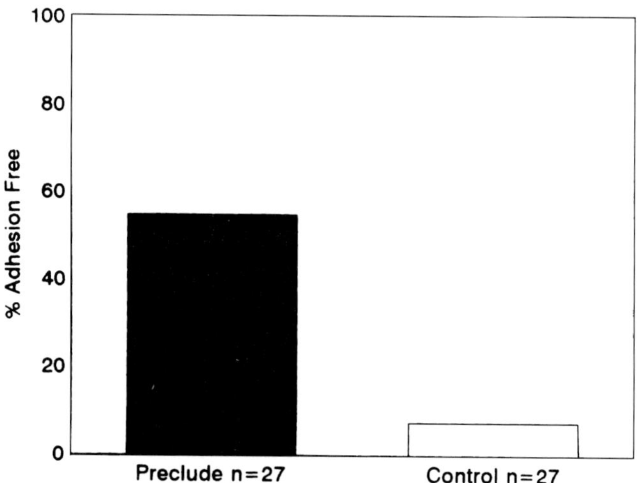

Fig. 34.12. Prevention of adhesion formation with the use of Preclude™ membrane (*left, black bar*) to cover suture sites after myomectomy (55.6% adhesion-free sites) compared to suture-only site (*right,* control; 7.4%, $p < 0.01$). (Adapted from Becker et al.[107])

TABLE 34.5. Directions for use: Preclude™ Adhesion Prevention Membrane.

1. Cut to proper size. Ensure that the repair site is completely covered by the Preclude membrane, including overlap of the edges of the repair site.
   - If the Preclude membrane is cut too small, excessive stress may be placed on the tissue by Preclude membrane and sutures may pull out.
   - If the Preclude membrane is sized too large, excessive wrinkling may occur, possibly resulting in undesired tissue attachment.
2. Suturing
   - Use nonabsorbable suture with a tapered, piercing point (or reverse cutting needle) of appropriate size to anchor the material.
   - Absorbable sutures can be used once the material is adequately anchored.
   - If ONLY absorbable sutures are used with Preclude membrane, the repair may fail, possibly resulting in detachment from the implant site.
   - For best results, use monofilament sutures.
   - Use the minimum number of sutures required to maintain adequate anchoring of the Preclude membrane.
   - Do not use a conventional cutting needle.
   - Do not allow excessive wrinkles in the Preclude membrane.
   - Do not use ONLY absorbable sutures to anchor the Preclude membrane.

mation so that sufficient tissue levels of medicament are available to achieve pharmacologic effects. Many postsurgical sites become devoid of blood supply during the course of surgery. These ischemic areas, which are likely candidates for adhesion formation, are also not available to systemically administered pharmaceuticals. Accordingly, one of the major challenges to the pharmacotherapy of adhesion prevention is the development of appropriate drug delivery systems.

The multifactoral nature of infertility and pain necessarily limits the utility of trials designed to assess the clinical efficacy of adhesion prevention agents. Accordingly, the clinical problems associated with adhesion formation were not evaluated in any of the aforementioned studies. Studies of "clinical efficacy" have only assessed the presence or absence of adhesions and not the clinical benefits of adhesion prevention per se. The first study demonstrating increased pregnancy rates with use of a barrier (Interceed) was recently presented.[106]

What constitutes sufficient benefit from an adhesion prevention adjuvant or regimen to justify its use in clinical practice? What clinical response to a new device or drug is necessary and sufficient to justify USFDA approval for an adhesion prevention indication? The outcome of the adhesion that is responsible for the patient's symptomatology, whether it is prevented from reforming or persists, may well determine the clinical benefit or failure. Adhesion formation to the rest of the peritoneum may have no clinical significance and as a result may be irrelevant to the patient's wellbeing. Unfortunately, clinical problems caused by adhesions are multifactorial in nature and consequently necessitate large patient studies to address clinical benefits.

Conclusion

Adhesions are not required for peritoneal repair. They are a major cause of postoperative morbidity and failure of surgical therapy and cannot be prevented by surgical technique alone. The development of adjuvants to prevent postsurgical adhesion formation is encumbered by differences between the process of peritoneal healing and that of tissues not covered by mesothelium, access to the peritoneal cavity, interspecies differences in peritoneal physiology, limitations of animal models, and the complexities of transperitoneal transport. Clinical utilization of adhesion prevention regimens is slowed by the ambiguities of efficacy assessment. Clinical benefits of adhesion prevention are only a part of the multifactorial problems of pain, bowel obstruction, and infertility. A direct cause-and-effect relationship between adhesion prevention and amelioration of disease is difficult to establish.

To date no treatment has proven uniformly effective in preventing postoperative adhesion formation. The use of surgical techniques that limit tissue ischemia, as well as the use of absorbable, nonreactive mechanical barriers, provides clinical benefits to patients today. Ongoing evaluations of liquid and nonabsorbable barriers, drugs that modify the local inflammatory response (e.g., nonsteroidal antiinflammatory drugs), and agents that promote plasminogen activator activity (e.g., recombinant tissue plasminogen activator) show promise for limiting adhesion formation in the future (see Chapter 37).

References

1. Stone K. Adhesions in gynecologic surgery. Curr Opin Obstet Gynecol 1993;5:322–327.
2. Gomel V, Urman B, Gürgan T. Pathophysiology of adhesion formation and strategies for prevention. J Reprod Med 196;41:35–41.
3. Damario MA, Rock JA. Methods to prevent postoperative adhesion formation in gynecologic surgery. J Gynecol Tech 1995;1:77–88.
4. Strickler, B Blanco J, Fox HE. The gynecologic contribution to intestinal obstruction in females. J Am Coll Surg 1994;178:617–621.
5. Howard FM. The role of laparoscopy in chronic pelvic pain: promise and pitfalls. Obstet Gynecol Surv 1993;48: 357–361.
6. Ratcliff JB, Kapernick P, Brooks G, et al. Small bowel obstruction and previous gynecologic surgery. S Med J 1983; 76:1349–1360.
7. Adhesion Study Group. Reduction of postoperative pelvic adhesions with intraperitoneal 32% dextran 70: a prospective, randomized clinical trial. Fertil Steril 1983;40: 612–619.
8. diZerega GS. Contemporary adhesion prevention. Fertil Steril 1994;61:210–235.
9. Diamond MP, Seprafilm Adhesion Group. Reduction of adhesions after uterine myomectomy by Seprafilm® mem-

brane (HAL-F®): a blinded, prospective, randomized, multicenter clinical study. Fertil Steril 1996;66:904–910.
10. Diamond MP, Sepracoat Adhesion Study Group. Reduction of de novo postsurgical adhesions by intraoperative precoating with Sepracoat (HAL-C) solution: a prospective, randomized, blinded, placebo-controlled multicenter study. Fertil Steril 1998;69:1067–1074.
11. Thornton M, Johns DB, Campeau JD. Clinical evaluation of 0.5% ferric hyaluronate adhesion prevention gel for the reduction of adhesion following peritoneal cavity surgery: open-label pilot study. Hum Reprod (Oxf) 1998;13:1480–1485.
12. diZerega GS, Campeau JD. Use of instillates to prevent intraperitoneal adhesions: crystalloid and dextran. Infertil Reprod Med Clin North Am 1994;5:463–478.
13. Lundorff P, diZerega GS, Johns DB, et al. Clinical evaluation of INTERGEL® adhesion prevention solution for the reduction of adhesions following peritoneal cavity surgery: an international multicentre study of safety and efficacy. Abstract No. 0-069 European Society of Human Reproduction and Endocrinology (ESHRE), Goteborg, Sweden, 1998.
14. Ryan GB, Grobety J, Majno G. Mesothelial injury and recovery. Am J Pathol 1973;71:93–112.
15. Kappas AM, Fatouros M, Papadimitriou K, et al. Effect of intraperitoneal saline irrigation at different temperatures on adhesion formation. Br J Surg 1988;75:854–856.
16. Yaacobi Y, Goldberg EP. Effect of Ringer's lactate irrigation on the formation of postoperative abdominal adhesions. J Invest Surg 1991;4:31–36.
17. Rappaport WD, Holcomb M, Valente J, Chvapil M. Antibiotic irrigation and the formation of intraabdominal adhesions. Am J Surg 1989;158:435–437.
18. Yung S, Coles GA, Williams JD, et al. The source and possible significance of hyaluronan in the peritoneal cavity. Kidney Int 1994;46:527–533.
19. Asplund T, Vershel MA, Luarent TC, et al. Human mesotheleoma cell produce factors that stimulate the production of hyaluronan by mesothelial cells and fibroblasts. Cancer Res 1993;53:388–392.
20. Urman B, Gomel V, Jetha N. Effect of hyaluronic acid on postoperative intraperitoneal adhesion formation in the rat model. Fertil Steril 1991;56:563–567.
21. West JL, Chowdhury SM, Sawhney AS, et al. Efficacy of adhesion barriers: resorbable hydrogel, oxidized regenerated cellulose and hyaluronic acid. J Reprod Med 1996;41:149–154.
22. Shushan A, Mor-Yosef S, Avgar A, et al. Hyaluronic acid for preventing experimental postoperative intraperitoneal adhesions. J Reprod Med 1994;39:398–402.
23. Shear L, Swartz C, Shinaberger J, et al. Kinetics of peritoneal fluid absorption in adult man. N Engl J Med 1965;272:123–127.
24. Ellis H, Harrison W, Hugh TB. The healing of peritoneum under normal and pathological conditions. Br J Surg 1965;52:471–476.
25. Hubbard TB, Khan MZ, Carag VR, et al. The pathology of peritoneal repair: its relation to the formation of adhesions. Ann Surg 1967;165:908–916.
26. Glucksman D. Serosal integrity and intestinal adhesions. Surgery (St. Louis) 1966;60:1009–1011.
27. Ellis H. The aetiology of post-operative abdominal adhesions. An experimental study. Br J Surg 1962;50:10–16.
28. Eskeland G, Kjærheim Å. Regeneration of parietal peritoneum in rats. I. A light microscopical study. Acta Pathol Microbiol Scand 1966;68:353–378.
29. Hart R, Magos A. Laparoscopically instilled fluid: the rate of absorption and the effects on patient discomfort and fluid balance. Gynaecol Endosc 1996;5:287–291.
30. Sites CK, Jensen BA, Jacob BS, et al. Transvaginal ultrasonographic assessment of Hyskon or lactated Ringer's solution instillation after laparoscopy: randomized, controlled study. J Ultrasound Med 1997;16:195–199.
31. Pagidas K, Tulandi T. Effects of Ringer's lactate, Interceed (TC7) and Gore-Tex Surgical Membrane on postsurgical adhesion formation. Fertil Steril 1992;57:199–201.
32. Caballero J, Tulandi T. Effects of Ringer's lactate and fibrin glue on postsurgical adhesions. J Reprod Med 1992;37:141–143.
33. Harris ES, Morgan RF, Rodeheaver GT. Analysis of the kinetics of peritoneal adhesion formation in the rat and evaluation of potential antiadhesive agents. Surgery (St. Louis) 1995;117:663–669.
34. Fayez JA, Schneider PJ. Prevention of pelvic adhesion formation by different modalities of treatment. Am J Obstet Gynecol 1987;157:1184–1188.
35. Jansen RPS. Failure of intraperitoneal adjuncts to improve the outcome of pelvic operations in young women. Am J Obstet Gynecol 1985;153:363–371.
36. Naether OGJ, Fischer R. Adhesion formation after laparoscopic electrocoagulation of the ovarian surface in polycystic ovary patients. Fertil Steril 1993;60:95–98.
37. Gurgan T, Kisnisci H, Yarali H, et al. Evaluation of adhesion formation after laparoscopic treatment of polycystic ovarian disease. Fertil Steril 1991;56:1176–1178.
38. Gurgan T, Urman B, Yarali H. Adhesion formation and reformation after laparoscopic removal of ovarian endometriomas. J Am Assoc Gynecol Laparosc 1996;3:389–392.
39. Wiseman DM, Tout JR, Diamond MP. The rates of adhesion development and the effects of crystalloid solutions on adhesion development in pelvic surgery. Fertil Steril 1998;70:702–711.
40. Rodgers KE, Johns DB, Girgis W, et al. Reduction of adhesion formation with hyaluronic acid following peritoneal surgery in rabbits. Fertil Steril 1997;67:553–558.
41. Johns DB, Rodgers KE, Donahue WD, et al. Reduction of adhesion formation by postoperative administration of tonically cross linked hyaluronic acid. Fertil Steril 1997;68:37–42.
42. American Fertility Society. The American Fertility Society classifications of adnexal adhesions, distal tubal occlusion, tubal occlusion secondary to tubal ligation, tubal pregnancies, Mullerian anomalies and intrauterine adhesions. Fertil Steril 1988;49:944–955.
43. Cleary RE, Howard T, diZerega GS. Plasma dextran levels after abdominal installation of 32% dextran 70: Evidence for prolonged retention. Am J Obstet Gynecol 1985;152:78–82.

44. Stangel JJ, Nisbet JD II, Settles H. Formation and prevention of postoperative abdominal adhesions. J Reprod Med 1984;29:143–156.
45. Krinsky AH, Haseltine FP, DeCherney A. Peritoneal fluid accumulation with dextran 70 instilled at time of laparoscopy. Fertil Steril 1984;41:647–649.
46. Wagaman R, Ingram JM, Rao PS, Saba HI. Intravenous versus intraperitoneal administration of dextran in the rabbit: effects on fibrinolysis. Am J Obstet Gynecol 1986;155: 464–470.
47. Rein MS, Hill JA. 32% Dextran 70 (hyskon) inhibits lymphocyte and macrophage function in vitro: a potential new mechanism for adhesion prevention. Fertil Steril 1989;52:953–957.
48. diZerega GS, Rodgers K. Peritoneal fluid. In: The Peritoneum. New York: Springer-Verlag, 1990:26–56.
49. Dlugi AM, DeCherney AH. Prevention of postoperative adhesion formation. Sem Reprod Endocrinol 1984;2: 125–129.
50. Ruiz Navas MT, Lopez E, Flores DP, Romeroz JA. Comparative experimental study of the effectiveness of different types of macromolecules carboxymethylcellulose dextran 40 and dextran 70 in the prevention of adhesions. Rev Exp Obstet Gynecol 1988;47:43–50.
51. Holtz G. Prevention of postoperative adhesions. J Reprod Med 1980;24:141–146.
52. ten Kate-Booij MJ, van Geldorp HJ, Drogendijk AC, et al. Dextran and adhesions in guinea-pigs. J Reprod Fertil 1985;75:183–188.
53. Rosenberg SM, Board JA. High-molecular weight dextran in human infertility surgery. Am J Obstet Gynecol 1984; 148:380–385.
54. Larsson B, Lalos O, Marsk L, et al. Effect of intraperitoneal instillation of 32% dextran 70 on postoperative adhesion formation after tubal surgery. Acta Obstet Gynecol Scand 1985;64:437–441.
55. Cleary RE, Howard T, diZerega GS. Plasma dextran levels after abdominal instillation of 32% dextran 70: evidence for prolonged intraperitoneal retention. Am J Obstet Gynecol 1985;152:78–79.
56. Magyar DM, Hayes MF, Spirtos NJ, et al. Is intraperitoneal dextran 70 safe for routine gynecologic use? Am J Obstet Gynecol 1985;152:198–204.
57. Tulandi T. Adhesion formation after reproductive surgery with and without the carbon dioxide laser. Fertil Steril 1987;47:704–706.
58. Adoni A, Adatto-Levy R, Mogle P, Palti Z. Postoperative pleural effusion caused by dextran. Int J Gynecol Obstet 1980;18:243–247.
59. Rose BI. Safety of hyskon for routine gynecologic surgery. A case report. J Reprod Med 1987;32:134–136.
60. Borten M, Seibert CP, Taymor ML. Recurrent anaphylactic reaction to intraperitoneal dextran 75 used for prevention of postsurgical adhesions. Obstet Gynecol 1983;61: 755–757.
61. Bailey G, Strub R, Klein RC, Salvaggio F. Dextran-induced anaphylaxis. JAMA 1967;200:185–189.
62. Trimbos-Kemper TC, Veering BT. Anaphylactic shock from intracavitary 32% dextran-70 during hysteroscopy. Fertil Steril 1989;51:1053–1054.
63. Ahmed N, Falcone T, Tulandi T, Houle G. Anaphylactic reaction because of intrauterine 32% dextran-70 instillation. Fertil Steril 1991;55:1014–1016.
64. Gauwerky JF, Heinrich D, Kubli F. Complications of intraperitoneal dextran application for prevention of adhesions. Biol Res Pregnancy Perinatol 1986;7:93–97.
65. Weinans MJN, Kauer FM, Klompmaker IJ, et al. Transient liver function disturbances after the intraperitoneal use of 32% dextran 70 as adhesion prophylaxis in infertility surgery. Fertil Steril 1990;53:159–161.
66. Bernstein J, Mattox J, Ulrich J. The potential for bacterial growth with dextran. J Reprod Med 1982;27:77–79.
67. King IR. *Candida albicans* pelvic abscess associated with the use of 32% dextran-70 in conservative pelvic surgery. Fertil Steril 1989;51:1050–1052.
68. Al-Chalabi HA, Otubo JAM. Value of a single intraperitoneal dose of heparin in prevention of adhesion formation: an experimental evaluation in rats. Int J Fertil 1987;32(4):332–335.
69. Cohen BM, Heyman T, Mast D. Use of intraperitoneal solutions for preventing pelvic adhesions in the rat. J Reprod Med 1983;28:649–653.
70. Lane DA, MacGregor JR, Michalski R, Kakkar VV. Anticoagulant activities of four unfractionated and fractionated heparins. Thromb Res 1973;12:257–271.
71. Rosenberg RD. Heparin antithrombin and abnormal clotting. Annu Rev Med 1978;29:367–378.
72. Andrade-Gordon P, Strickland S. Interaction of heparin with plasminogen activators and plasminogen: effects on the activations of plasminogen. Biochemistry 1986;5: 4033–4040.
73. Markwardt F, Klocking HP. Heparin induced release of plasminogen activator. Haemostasis 1977;6:370–374.
74. Jansen RPS. Failure of peritoneal irrigation with heparin during pelvic operations upon young women to reduce adhesions. Surg Gynecol Obstet 1988;166:154–160.
75. Tarvady S, Anguli VC, Pichappa CV. Effect of heparin on wound healing. J Biosci 1987;12:33–40.
76. Diamond MP, Linsky CB, Cunningham T, et al. Adhesions reformation reduction by the use of Interceed TC7 plus heparin. J Gynecol Surg 1991;7:1–6.
77. Reid RL, Lie K, Spence JE, et al. Clinical evaluation of the efficacy of heparin-saturated Interceed for prevention of adhesion reformation in the pelvic sidewall of the human. Prog Clin Biol Res 1993;381:261–264.
78. Nishimura K, Nakamura RM, diZerega GS. Evaluation of oxidized regenerated cellulose for prevention of postoperative intraperitoneal adhesions. Jpn J Surg 1983;13: 159–163.
79. Raftery AT. Absorbable haemostatic materials and intraperitoneal adhesion formation. Br J Surg 1980;67: 57–58.
80. Shimanuki T, Nishimura K, diZerega GS. Localized prevention of postsurgical adhesion formation and reformation with oxidized regenerated cellulose. J Biomed Mater Res 1987;21:173–185.
81. Schroder M, Willumsen H, Hart Hansen JP, et al. Peritoneal adhesion formation after the use of oxidized cellulose (Surgicel) and gelatin sponge (Spongostan) in rats. Acta Chir Scand 1982;148:595–596.

82. Yemini M, Meshorer A, Katz Z, et al. Prevention of reformation of pelvic adhesions by "barrier" methods. Int J Fertil 1984;29:194–196.
83. Soules MR, Dennis L, Bosarge A, et al. The prevention of postoperative pelvic adhesions: an animal study comparing barrier methods with dextran 70. Am J Obstet Gynecol 1982;143:829–834.
84. Hixson C, Swanson LA, Friedman CI. Oxidized cellulose for preventing adnexal adhesions. J Reprod Med 1986;31: 58–60.
85. Linsky CB, Diamond MP, Cunningham T, et al. Adhesion reduction in the rabbit uterine horn model using an absorbable barrier, TC-7. J Reprod Med 1987;32:17–20.
86. Diamond MP, Linsky CB, Cunningham T, et al. A model for sidewall adhesions in the rabbit: reduction by an absorbable barrier. Microsurgery 1987;8:197–200.
87. Linsky CB, Diamond MP, Cunningham, T, et al. Effect of blood on the efficacy of barrier adhesion reduction in the rabbit uterine horn model. Infertility 1989;11:273–280.
88. Interceed (TC7) Adhesion Barrier Study Group. Prevention of postsurgical adhesions by Interceed (TC7), an absorbable adhesion barrier: a prospective, randomized multicenter clinical study. Fertil Steril 1989;51:933–938.
89. Malinak LR. Interceed (TC7) as an adjuvant for adhesion reduction: clinical studies. In: diZerega GS, Malinak LR, Diamond M, Linsky C, eds. Treatment of Postoperative Surgical Adhesion. New York: Wiley-Liss, 1990:193–206.
90. Sekiba K, Obstetrics and Gynecology Adhesion Prevention Committee. Use of Interceed (TC7) absorbable adhesion barrier to reduce postoperative adhesion reformation in infertility and endometriosis surgery. Obstet Gynecol 1992;79:518–522.
91. Wallwiener D, Meyer A, Bastert G. Adhesion formation of the parietal and visceral peritoneum: an explanation for the controversy on the use of autologus and alloplastic barriers? Fertil Steril 1998;68:132–137.
92. Larsson B, Nisell H, Granberg I. Surgicel—an absorbable hemostatic material—in prevention of adhesions in rats. Acta Chir Scand 1978;144:375–378.
93. Franklin RR, Malinak RL, Larsson B, et al. Reduction of ovarian adhesions by the use of Interceed. Obstet Gynecol 1995;86:335–338.
94. Nordic Adhesion Prevention Study Group. The efficacy of Interceed (TC7) for prevention of reformation of postoperative adhesion on ovaries, fallopian tubes, and fimbria in microsurgical operation for fertility: a multicenter study. Fertil Steril 1995;63:709–714.
95. Van Geldorp H. Interceed absorbable adheson barrier reduces the formation of postsurgical adhesions after ovarian surgery (abstract). In: 50th Annual Meeting, American Fertility Society, 1994:273.
96. Marana R, Gatalano GF, Caruana P, et al. Postoperative adhesion formation and reproductive outcome using Interceed after ovarian surgery: a randomized trial in the rabbit model. Hum Reprod (Oxf) 1997;12:101–104.
97. Giannacodimos G, Dluligeris N, Lappas K. Prevention of postsurgical adhesions by Interceed (TC7) in polysystic ovary syndrome treated by CO_2 laser vaporization laparoscopy (abstract). In: Proceedings, Eighth Annual Meeting of the European Scoiety of Human Reproduction and Embryology, the Netherlands, 1992:61.
98. Keckstein J, Ulrich U, Sasse V, et al. Reduction of postoperative formation after laparoscopic ovarian cystectomy. Hum Reprod (Oxf) 1996;11:579–582.
99. Curto JM, Bentolia D, Villois G, Torresgarsa G, Etchegaray M. Adhesions (abstract). In: XIV World Congess on Fertility and Sterility, Caracas, Venezuela, 1992:46.
100. Mais V, Ajossa SA, Marongiu D, et al. Reduction of adhesion reformation after laparoscopic endometriosis surgery: a randomized trial with an oxidized regenerated cellulose absorbable barrier. Obstet Gynecol 1995;86: 512–515.
101. Azziz R, Murphy AA, Rosenberg SM, et al. Use of an oxidized regenerated cellulose absorbable adhesion barrier at laparoscopy. J Reprod Med 1991;36:479–482.
102. Li TC, Cooke ID. The value of an absorbable adhesion barrier, Interceed, in the prevention of adhesion reformation following microsurgical adhesiolysis. Br J Obstet Gynecol 1994;101:335–339.
103. Haney AF, Hesla J, Hurst BS, et al. Expanded polytetrafluoroethylene (Gore-Tex Surgical Membrane) is superior to oxidized regenerated cellulose (Interceed TC7) in preventing adhesions. Fertil Steril 1995;63:1021–1028.
104. Haney AF, Doty E. Expanded polytetrafluoroethylene but not oxidized regenerated cellulose prevents adhesion formation and reformation in a mouse uterine horn model of surgical injury. Fertil Steril 1993;60:550–558.
105. Mais V, Jossa SA, Piras B, et al. Prevention of de novo adhesion formation after laparoscopic myomectomy: a randomized trial to evaluate the effectiveness of an oxidized regenerated cellulose absorbable barrier. Hum Reprod (Oxf) 1995;12:3133–3135.
106. Swada T, Satoh M, Tsukada K, et al. Evaluation of postoperative adhesion prevention effect using oxidized regenerated cellulose adhesion barrier (Interceed TC7) in infertile patients. Abstract No. P-609, 16th World Congress on Fertility and Sterility, San Francisco, CA, 1998.
107. Becker JM, Beck DE, Dayton MT, et al. Prevention of postoperative abdominal adhesions by a sodium hyaluronate-based bioresorbable membrane: a prospective, randomized, double-bind multicenter study. J Am Coll Surg 1996; 183:297–306.
108. Surgical Membrane Study Group. Prophylaxis of pelvic side wall adhesion formation with Gore-Tex surgical membrane: a multicenter clinical investigation. Fertil Steril 1992;57:921–923.
109. Myomectomy Adhesion Study Group. An expended-polytetrafluoroethylene barrier (Gore-Tex surgical membrane) reduces post-myomectomy adhesion formation. Fertil Steril 1995;63:491–493.
110. Haney AF. Removal of surgical barriers of expanded polytetrafluoroethylene at second-look laparoscopy was not associated with adhesion formation. Fertil Steril 1997;68: 721–723.
111. diZerega GS. Use of adhesion prevention barriers in pelvic reconstructive and gynecologic surgery. In: diZerega GS, DeCherney AH, eds. Pelvic Surgery. New York: Springer-Verlag:188–209.

112. Wiseman DM, Trout JR, Franklin RR, et al. Metaanalysis of the safety and efficacy of an adhesion barrier (Interceed TC7) in laparotomy. J Reprod Med 1999;44: 325–331.
113. Azziz R and the Interceed (TC7) Adhesion Barrier Study Group 11. Microsurgery alone or with Interceed absorbable adhesion barrier for pelvic sidewall adhesion reformation. Surg Gynecol Obstet 1993;177:135–139.
114. Korell M (ed). Moglichkeiten der Adhasionsprophtylaxe. 1995, ML Services, Landsberg, Germany, P-103-121.

35

Adhesion Prevention: Past the Future

David M. Wiseman

CONTENTS

Only recently has the prophylactic treatment of adhesions begun to gain acceptance by surgeons. Data continue to accumulate regarding the efficacy of film and fabric barriers (Interceed™, Seprafilm™, Preclude™), and are beginning to emerge regarding liquids such as Sepracoat™ and Intergel™ solutions. Newer film, gel, and liquid materials are in advanced stages of development and should be available for patients in the near future. These products represent advances in adhesion prevention. They have required innovation in biomaterials as well as creative clinical studies to demonstrate efficacy and to obtain regulatory approval. Despite these innovations, most products that become available in 2004 will have been developed by using materials designed for other purposes and optimizing them for adhesion prevention.

Shortcomings remain in terms of product efficacy and scope of use. There is a limit to how much more efficacy can be squeezed out of a polymer by cross-linking, copolymerization, blending, or derivatization. To date, no product has completely prevented adhesions. Justifiably, patients and doctors are not satisfied with these incremental advances in biomaterials, important although they may be. We must therefore focus past the future on technologies that will advance the art of adhesion prevention in a quantum fashion. Accordingly, the purpose of this chapter is to look "past the future" by reviewing and proposing some avenues for future adhesions research that will result in such quantum advances.

The Six Epochs of Adhesion Prevention

To define the future and beyond, it is helpful to understand the present from the perspective of the past. Much of this perspective can be gained by consulting the valuable historical reviews of Richardson,[1] Boys,[2] Krook,[3] Connolly and Smith,[4] and Ellis.[5] Occasionally, as we shall see, we find ideas that were conceived before their time, waiting for technologic advances to facilitate their birth. Arbitrarily, the history of adhesion prevention may be divided into six "epochs," each marked by important milestones (Table 35.1).

Ancient History

The earliest description of adhesions and their relationship to functional organ impairment appears to be recorded in the Babylonian Talmud. Completed around 440 C.E., the Talmud is the compendium of Jewish law

TABLE 35.1. The six epochs of adhesion prevention.

Year	Material	Brand	Company
Ancient History			
1886	Hydroflotation (Müller[1])[6]		
1888	Viable omental grafts[7]		
1889	Colloidion (Stern in[1])		
1892	Fibrinolysin[2]		
1904	Phosphorus[6]		
1905	Peritoneal graft	Cargile membrane[9]	Johnson & Johnson
1910	Liquid petrolatum,[10] foils, fats, oils, membranes		
Dark and Middle Ages			
1936	Papain[11]		Parke Davis & Co.
1931–1957	Aminiotic fluid extract	Amfetin[12]	E. Lilly
1942	Heparin[13]		
1949	Dicumarol[14]		
Renaissance			
1960s	Streptokinase,[15] steroids[16]		
1980s	Dextran 70[17–19]	Hyskon®[20]	Pharmacia
	Ibuprofen		Upjohn
Industrial Revolution			
1989	Oxidized regenerated cellulose	Interceed®[21]	Ethicon
	Hyaluronic acid[22]	Tenalure®[23]	Ethicon/Lifecore
	ePTFE	Preclude®[24]	W.L. Gore
1996	HA/CMC	Seprafilm®[25–27]	Genzyme
	Hyaluronic acid	Sepracoat®[28]	Genzyme
1998	Iron hyaluronate[29]	Intergel®[30]	Lifecore
The Future			
	HA/CMC	Sepragel®[31]	Genzyme
	HA	Hylagel®	Biomatrix
	HA	Incert®[32]	Anika
	HA	ACP®[33]	Fidia
	nTC7	Interceed[34]	Ethicon
	PLA/PEG	Repel®[35–37]	Life Medical
	PLA/PEG	Relieve, Resolve®[38]	Life Medical
	Photopolymers (PEO/PLA)	FocalGel®[39]	Focal
	Pluronics (PEO/PPO)	FloGel®[40]	Alliance
	Collagen film	ColCys®	Flamel
	Fibrin glue		Various
	NOCM Chitosan[41]		Chitogenics
	Icodextin[42]		M.L. Laboratories
	NaCMC		Fziomed
Past the Future			
	Dextran sulfate	Adcon® L,[43] T/N[44]	Gliatech
	Dextran Sulfate	Adcon® A, P[23,45]	Gliatech
	Pericardial patch	PHB[46]	Astra
	Elastin peptides		Bioelastics[47]
			Protein Polymer[48]
	Collagen peptides		Protein Polymer[49]
Tissue engineering, spatial/temporal targeting, macrophage modulation, cell, gene, antsense, and cytokine therapy			

transmitted orally since it was given to Moses (1313 B.C.E.). Tractate Chullin (Fig. 35.1) includes pleural perforation in its list of 18 defects that invalidate a carcass for human consumption. Because the presence of pleural adhesions may indicate actual or potential perforation, procedures are described for their assessment.

The debate about whether pleural adhesions are a consequence or cause of perforation continued among the rabbis of the Middle Ages.[49] This debate has modern parallels in discussions of the causes of adhesions due to inflammation or the consequences of adhesions such as the damage incurred during adhesiolysis. Depending, inter alia, on the location of adhesions (between adjacent or nonadjacent lobes or the chest wall) and their severity (separable by gentle finger dissection vs. sharp dissection), meat may be acceptable for consumption.[49] However the complete absence of pleural adhesions indicated by the term "*glatt* [smooth] *kosher*" is the highest standard.

It is a sobering thought that, recorded more than 1500 years ago (and used for another 1800 years before then) this system of evaluation, which is still in use today, lays out three principles of interest to all those concerned with postsurgical adhesions:

חולין　　　פרק שלשי　　　אלו טריפות　　92

Rashi, a לית להו French scholar of the 11th century, holds that an adhesion results from a puncture of the lung and is a response to injury. Where היינו רביתייהו adjacent lungs are adherent, the adhesion will provide an effective covering for the perforation.

ואמר רבא הני תרתי אוני דסריכן להדדי לית להו בדיקה ולא אמרן אלא שלא כסדרן אבל כסדרן היינו רביתייהו

Rava further said. "If two lobes of the lungs adhere to each other [by fibrous tissue], no examination can avail [to render the animal permitted]. This is so, however, only if the lobes were not adjacent, but if they were adjacent [it is permitted for] this is their natural position." *

אבל Scholars of the 12th and 13th centuries hold that pleural adhesions form naturally without an existing puncture. If present between surfaces that are not normally adjacent, the adhesions will eventually work apart, causing the pleura to tear and perforate. Where adhesions form between adjacent lobes, there is no such concern. היינו

FIG. 35.1. Tractate Chullin, page 46b, Babylonian Talmud. Rendering of a Talmudic passage about pleural adhesions, and quoting Rava, a sage who lived c. 340 C.E. The margins contain the comments of medieval scholars. (Translation from Soncino Talmud, Soncino Press, London, 1938. See also 48a et seq. and Sherman and Zlotowitz.[49])

1. No adhesions are preferable to some adhesions.
2. Filmy adhesions are better than cohesive ones.
3. Some adhesions are clinically (legally) tolerable depending on their location (i.e., between adjacent lobes but not between nonadjacent lobes).

Adhesions in humans may have been known to the ancient Egyptians because, in their "Archeological Survey of Nubia," Smith and Jones (cited by Carson[50]) described a case of pelvic adhesions, although it is unknown whether the Egyptians recognized its significance.

Although clinically adhesions caused by peritonitis and infection had been known at least since Hunter (1728–1793), it was only when more invasive surgery was facilitated by antisepsis and anesthesia that an appreciation of the problem of postsurgical adhesions began in earnest. An anecdotal account exists[51] of rubbing oil being used to avert adhesions sometime in the 1880s. The first published report of the use of an agent for adhesion prevention seems to be in 1886 when Müller proposed the use of normal salt solutions (cited in[1]). Shortly thereafter, Malcolm[6] advocated preventing adhesions by distending the abdominal cavity with fluid to float the intestines "up towards the highest level of the cavity." Colloidion was used for covering pedicle stumps to prevent adhesions (Stern, 1889, cited in[1]).

With an understanding of the role of fibrin, "fibrinolysin," a preparation of "liquor thiosinamine with sodium salicylate,"[2] was introduced in 1892 with the claim of effecting the resorption of fibrin and scar tissue. By 1905 this drug was not held in great regard (Offergeld, cited in[1]). Oral phosphorus was another agent claimed to destroy fibrinogen.[8] Both naturally occurring polymers and organic polymers were soon advocated. Vogel in 1902[52] recommended that gum Arabic (a complex polysaccharide) solution be used "as a lubricant between the viscera," together with the cholinesterase inhibitor, physostigmine, to increase bowel motility. From a small study in cats, Claypool et al.[10] proposed the use of liquid petrolatum in 1910. Based on experiments done as early as 1894 by Baum (cited in[1]), Cargile (Baum) Membrane, a fixed preparation of bovine (Danish ox) cecal peritoneum, was marketed in 1905 by Johnson & Johnson[9] to prevent adhesions in abdominal surgery. This product was still available as recently as 1993, despite Richardson's prediction in 1910 that since "these membranes . . . [are] nothing more nor less than a true foreign body. . . . It seems inevitable, therefore, that these substances will gradually fall into disuse." In addition to viable omental grafts, studied by Senn[7] in 1888, a variety of other approaches were tried including foils, gold-beater's skin, shark peritoneum, lanolin, chyme, amniotic membrane, and fish bladder.

Thus, before the first decade of the twentieth century had concluded, direct ancestors of almost every major class of materials in use or development today had been proposed for the prevention of adhesions: liquids, gels, barriers, fibrinolytic drugs, water-soluble polymers, and organic polymers. In addition, most of the principles generally referred to as "good surgical technique" had been laid down.[1] The first indications of disappointment were expressed by Richardson[1]: "It is very evident from the reports that none of these substances can be relied upon to furnish more than a small percentage of successful results, and on this account, cannot be recommended for general use." With this disappointment came another sentiment: "It is futile to search for some agent that will banish adhesions from the realm of abdominal surgery, inasmuch as the processes involved in their formation are identical with those involved in peritoneal repair." Fortunately this message was not taken to heart by the clinicians and scientists who followed.

Dark and Middle Ages

By 1940, the etiology of adhesions, essentially as it is understood today, was well described: serosal and subserosal injury; fibrinous exudation; formation of fibrinous adhesions; and, unless resolved, progression to fibrous adhesions.[2] Efforts at this time centered around the prevention or removal of fibrin deposits. Hirudin had been tested as early as 1890 (cited by Boys[2]), and later efforts using sodium citrate were not followed up. A more comprehensive series conducted in animals by Lehman and Boys[4,13] showed that heparin was effective in adhesion reformation. Later clinical work with 40,000 units of heparin given over 3 days was at best inconclusive with some problems of hemorrhage and other toxicity, possibly caused by an impure preparation of heparin. This work provided important clues about the time course of heparin's action, but was soon discontinued. The removal of fibrinous deposits by the instillation of proteases (pepsin and trypsin) had been attempted from the early 1920s, but because of their instability, stimulation of peritonitis, and neutralization by antitrypsins, these were abandoned. The latter problem did not apply to papain, a protease of vegetable origin marketed by Parke Davis & Co., in 1936. An uncontrolled clinical study[11] showed that the product was safe, but with contradictory data from other laboratories,[2] the use of papain was short lived. An early study in rabbits using a preparation of streptokinase and streptodornase was encouraging.[53]

Based on an impression that peritoneal adhesions formed less frequently after cesarean section than other laparotomies, amniotic fluid and its extracts were evaluated in adhesion prevention. Initially it was thought that the product acted via fibrinolytic proteases, or through the stimulation of a mild hyperleukocytosis, which in turn would lead to proteolysis.[54] As with other modalities, initial animal experiments were promising[12] and a product, Amfetin, was marketed by Eli Lilly from approximately 1931 to 1957. Clinical series demonstrated the safety of the product, but without controls proof of Amfetin's efficacy was not forthcoming.

Renaissance

The development of specific drugs and more rigorous clinical investigation characterizes this "epoch." Noteworthy are the fibrinolytics. A concept that had waited for technologic advancement was revived by Ellis et al,[15] who reduced adhesions in rats and rabbits using highly purified streptokinase, but the idea was reshelved because of the need for more specific agents and methods of delivery.[55] Representing advances in pharmaceutical synthesis at that time are the corticosteroids. Following observations on the effects of corticoids on granulation tissue, a series of animal studies on adhesions ensued.[4] Success in reducing adhesions using steroids was demonstrated clinically by Swolin[16] in 1967, but because other data suggested deleterious[20] or equivocal[56] effects, steroids are not routinely used for adhesion prevention.

If clinical usage of adhesion prevention agents in earlier epochs was predicated on assorted animal data and clinical anecdotes, the "Renaissance" saw the requirement of hypothesis testing via controlled clinical trials. Results for Ibuprofen (Upjohn) did not warrant further study and results for Hyskon (dextran 70, Pharmacia) were conflicting.[17–20] These regrettable failures do however represent milestones in the development of clinical trial methodology. They are also important because they involved pharmaceutical companies who, realizing the market potential, were now willing to invest in costly clinical programs.

Industrial Revolution

At this time, companies not only invested in clinical programs but also to began to allocate resources toward customizing materials for adhesion prevention, even if that approach was limited to the modification of products already marketed for other indications. One such product was oxidized cellulose, used as an absorbable haemostat. The intraperitoneal response to it was published in 1948[57] and its use as an adhesion barrier was first proposed by Frantz[58]:

> "It is hoped that . . . this may be employed . . . in protecting injured surfaces where a smooth membrane is desired in final healing. For this latter use further work must be undertaken to determine the length of time the material maintains its physical properties. . . . when it is interposed between two surfaces where adhesions are to be avoided."

A softer and more uniform fabric, Surgicel® Absorbable Hemostat, composed of oxidized regenerated cellulose (ORC), was introduced by Johnson & Johnson in about 1959. Animal studies[59–62] involving Surgicel met with varying degrees of success, and the optimization of the product adhesion prevention resulted in Interceed® (TC7) Absorbable Adhesion Barrier, with demonstrated efficacy in animal[63] and human[21,64] studies.

Expanded polytetrafluoroethylene (ePTFE), because of its low reactivity, has found a variety of medical uses. As a patch, it is used in reconstructive surgery. Preclude® (W.L. Gore and Associates, Inc.) is indicated for "the reconstruction or repair of passive biological membranes, specifically the pericardium or peritoneum." It does not have a specific indication for the "reduction of adhesions" but, based on limited pelvic[24] and cardiac (reviewed by Wiseman[65]) clinical data, is nonetheless used by a small number of surgeons for this purpose. Being hydrophobic, ePTFE does not stick well to tissue, making laparoscopic handling and positioning difficult (with suturing required).

Hyaluronic acid (HA) is a naturally occurring glycosaminoglycan found in connective tissue, synovial fluid, the umbilical cord, and vitreous humor. It had been developed for as a replacement for vitreous humor and synovial fluid and as a skin moisturizer. In adhesion prevention, animal studies involving the administration of noncross-linked HA before injury, as Sepracoat® (Genzyme Corp.)[66] or after injury as Tenalure® (Lifecore Biomedical, Inc.)[22] appeared promising. However clinical studies for Tenalure[23] failed to demonstrate convincing efficacy, and Sepracoat[28] displayed only moderate efficacy against type 1a de novo adhesions. These disappointments were repeated in tendon surgery.[67,68] It was soon appreciated that plain HA did not persist long enough for it to reduce adhesions. The success in animals[27] and in human pelvic[25] and general[26] surgery of Seprafilm® (Genzyme Corporation), a film consisting of HA complexed with carboxymethylcellulose, marked the realization that merely reformulating existing materials would be unlikely to yield the desired levels of efficacy. Similarly, Intergel® Adhesion Prevention Solution (formerly Lubricoat), ionically cross-linked ferric hyaluronate,[29,30] was developed.

Along with the understanding on the part of medical companies regarding the market potential and design of adhesion prevention products came an increasing acceptance by surgeons of the need for and the utility of these products. This realization is reflected in the proliferation of reported clinical studies for various products (Table 35.2). In the case of Interceed barrier, a meta-analysis has been reported confirming its efficacy in a number of studies.[21]

The (Near) Future

Many products in development represent incremental improvements of previously tested materials. Thus, the plasticized and more flexible Seprafilm II is expected to be useful in laparoscopy. Two spongelike membranes (Hylagel®, Incert®[32]) consisting of cross-linked HA fibers are under development, as well as gels consisting of cross-linked (ACP® Gel[33]) or complexed (Sepragel®[31]) HA. A neutralized version (nTC7; neutralized Interceed) of the acidic Interceed Barrier awaits development and has superior efficacy in animals. Unlike its parent, it functions in the presence of bleeding.[34]

Several products under development are based on synthetic absorbable polymers used in other medical devices such as sutures and orthopaedic implants. These include a polylactic acid/polyethylene glycol (PLA/PEG) copolymer formulated as Repel® Film[35] (gynecology), Repel CV® Film [36] (cardiac surgery), Resolve® viscous gel[38] (gynecology/general surgery), and Relieve® (orthopaedic surgery). A more sophisticated relation of this technology (FocalGel®[39]) incorporates photopolymerizable moieties that allow the gel to be delivered to a surgical site laparoscopically and then "bonded" to it by exposure to a light source. Also containing polyethylene oxide (PEO) (as well as polyproplylene oxide) poloxamers, (Pluronics), one of which has been formulated as FloGel®.[40] Stored cold, it gels when body temperature is reached. Polyethylene glycol has itself been evaluated for adhesion prevention, at least in animals.[69]

Naturally occurring polymers have also been investigated. Collagen has undergone experimental evaluation as a gel in tendon surgery[70] and as a film in abdominal surgery.[71] It is now in development in the form of a film (ColCys®). Fibrin glue, either as commercially prepared tissue adhesive[72,73] (and Wiseman et al., unpublished data; see ref. 90) or as blood bank cryoprecipitate,[74] has been shown useful in animals and in a limited human series.[75] More recently, commercially produced fibrin sealant reduced adhesiogenesis after laparoscopic excision of endometriomas.[76] Several products (fibrin glue, FocalGel, and nTC7) are worth highlighting because they should promote hemostasis in addition to reducing adhesions. Other products (Sepragel, ACP Gel, FloGel, and Resolve) are noteworthy because of their utility in laparoscopic surgery. These products represent necessary advances in the development of the materials themselves as well as the methodology used to demonstrate ef-

TABLE 35.2. The number of clinical studies for adhesion prevention products.

Product	Company	Year	Indication	Number of studies
Interceed	J&J/Ethicon	1989	GYN	>15[21]
Preclude	W.L. Gore	1980s	Peritoneal/pericardial reconstruction	2 + >6 case series[24,65]
Seprafilm	Genzyme	1996	GYN, GEN	2[25,26]
Sepracoat	Genzyme	1997	GYN, GEN, CT	1[28]
Adcon L	Gliatech	1996	Neurosurgery	1[43]
Adcon T/N	Gliatech	1996	Tendon surgery	1[44]
Adcon P	Gliatech	1996	Pelvic surgery	2[45]
Intergel	Lifecore	1998	GYN	1[29]

TABLE 35.3. Current and future products: advantages and areas for improvement.

Product	Advantages	Areas for Improvement
Interceed	Easy to handle	Blood sensitive
	Efficacious	Site specific only
		No laparoscopy indication in USA
Preclude	Blood insensitive	Non degradable
		May need removal
		Needs suturing
		Site specific only
		Difficult to apply via laparoscope
Seprafilm	Blood insensitive	Brittle
	Efficacious in GYN and GEN	Laparotomy only
		Site specific only
		Almost impossible to apply via laparoscope
Sepracoat	Easy to use	Efficacy limited to type 1a de novo adhesions
	Generalized application	Not available in USA
Intergel	Easy to use	Blood sensitive?
	Generalized application, de novo and reformed	Viscous
	Laparotomy and laparoscopy	
Repel	Blood insensitive	Requires suture
		Site specific only
FloGel	Easy to apply	Requires refrigeration
		Site specific only
FocalGel	Easy application	Requires specific light source
	Formation in situ	Site specific only

ficacy in animals and humans. These products are also important because they are likely to act as platforms for drug delivery.

Related in part to the fact that most of these materials are adaptations of materials designed for other uses, there are still areas for improvement. For current products and products in development for which some data are available, these areas are listed in Table 35.3. This list should not be used reactively to design antiadhesion agents: to do so would only result in incremental advances in therapy. Rather, it is imperative to consider continuing needs (Table 35.4) in adhesion prevention, chief among which is efficacy. Available data suggest that despite recent advances, we will not be able to prevent adhesions entirely in the near future. By considering these continuing and unmet needs, appropriate avenues for research and development may be identified that will advance the adhesion prevention "Past the Future," the sixth epoch.

TABLE 35.4. Continuing needs in adhesion prevention: past the future.

Efficacy:	Complete adhesion prevention vs. de novo and reformed adhesions
	In the presence of blood and infection vs. site-specific and site-nonspecific adhesions
Utility:	Usable in endoscopic surgery
Indications:	Gynecology, general surgery, cardiothoracic surgery
	Tendon surgery, neurosurgery, cranial surgery
Clinical endpoints:	Reduced pain
	Reduced bowel obstruction
	Increased fertility
	Improved quality of life
	Reduced cost of adhesion-related sequelae
	Noninvasive assessment
Basic and polymer science:	Cellular mechanisms in adhesiogenesis
	Are there patient subpopulations?
	Bioactive materials
	Tissue engineering approaches

Past the Future

I highlight here just a few of the many fertile areas for further research.

A Few Basics: Technique, Glove Powder, Crystalloids, and Endoscopic Delivery

Journeying "Past the Future" implies internalization of lessons delivered expertly elsewhere in this volume. Advanced technology should supplement, not substitute for, good surgical technique (see Gomel, "The Role of Surgical technique in Peritoneal Repair"). Glove powder, whether talc or starch based, can clearly influence adhesiogenesis (see Holmdahl, "Foreign Materials and Adhesion Formation"), and soft nonlinting gauze is preferred over plain gauze.[77]

Ringer's lactate solution and other crystalloids continue to enjoy widespread use in the belief, first promulgated in 1886 (see "Ancient History"), that they will reduce adhesions by hydroflotation. That they are ineffective had been concluded as early as 1889 (Stern, cited in[1]) and 1906 (Morris[51]), and reiterated in 1940 (Boys[2]). A recent analysis[78] suggested that in some cases adhesions may be worsened by crystalloids. Supported by animal data from studies involving hyperosmolar glucose solutions[79] as well as clinical observations from patients undergoing continuous ambulatory peritoneal dialysis, an osmotically neutral polymer solution of icodextrin is under development.[42] This polymer degrades slowly to yield glucose in a manner that maintains hyperosmolarity, with associated ascites, over a period sufficiently long to reduce adhesions and overcome the problem of rapid absorption inherent in simple crystalloids. Given that the growth in endoscopic surgery is likely to continue, it is imperative that developers of antiadhesion agents consider how they are to be delivered endoscopically in a manner that is rapid, simple, and cost-effective. Instruments have been designed[80,81] that can fill this important need.

Noninvasive Assessment of Adhesions

Critical to the development and adoption of adhesion prevention products is the ability to image adhesions noninvasively, a subject reviewed extensively elsewhere (see Klein, Chapter 19, "Conventional Radiography and Cross-Sectional Imaging Modalities in the Diagnosis of Intestinal Adhesions" and Klein et al.[82]). Other than in selected instances outside the abdomen or pelvis, adhesions may only be assessed in procedures that require a second-look examination. Noninvasive assessment of adhesions is also critical as a diagnostic tool in cases of pelvic pain or bowel obstruction. Although some limited success has been achieved using CT (and MRI) in cardiac surgery,[83] the use of CT to detect abdominal adhesions has not yet yielded the same results.[84] Ultrasound is claimed to be fairly accurate in the detection of anterior abdominal wall adhesions, using a technique known as "visceral slide."[85-87] Other workers have recently claimed success in using transvaginal ultrasonography in the diagnosis of pelvic adhesions.[88] The development of techniques involving small-bore laparoscopes under local anesthesia may provide opportunities for assessment of adhesions that have hitherto been unavailable.

Tissue Engineering

The paradigm on which most currently available or developing materials are based involves the placement of an absorbable barrier material between two demesothelialized surfaces likely to adhere. Once remesothelialization is complete, the barrier is no longer needed and may absorb without consequence. A more sophisticated version of this paradigm involves the use of materials whose surfaces can modify cellular behavior, preventing adhesions and optimizing wound healing. Specifically designed polymers based on critical oligomeric amino acid sequences of elastin[47,48] or collagen[48] offer the opportunity to achieve these goals. Preliminary data using an elastin polypentapeptide in a model of adhesiogenesis[89] indicate that this concept may be a sound one.

TABLE 35.5. Past the future: paradigms in tissue engineering.

Current Paradigm: Barriers needed to protect against adhesions until mesothelial regeneration.
Future Paradigm: Barriers provide temporary protection and a scaffold for neoserosal regeneration.

However sophisticated these materials, this approach nonetheless follows the barrier paradigm. A better functional result might be obtained if the biologic membrane (e.g., peritoneum, pericardium) were to be reconstituted or newly formed where none existed (Table 35.5). In this paradigm of "functionally regenerative repair," meshes of synthetic absorbable materials provide scaffolds for the formation of this neomembrane. This concept is supported by examples in dermal, cranial, and pelvic surgery (reviewed by Wiseman[90]) and illustrated most clearly by work involving a polyhydroxybutyrate (PHB) patch in cardiac surgery. PHB has a long degradation time which in the conventional "barrier paradigm" would be rejected as a candidate material. However, during its degradation in sheep, a PHB patch was replaced by a neopericardium with physical and biochemical properties similar to native pericardium[91] in addition to reducing adhesions.[46] A reduction in pericardial adhesions was also observed in preliminary human studies.[83]

Spatial Targeting

The concept of spatial targeting—"targeting of agents to specific anatomic sites to achieve superior therapeutic performance"—is being used to develop agents for adhesion prevention past the future.

Spatial Targeting: Anatomic Synergy

Membrane or film barriers, while reasonably efficacious at specific sites, cannot be used over extensive and disparate areas at risk of adhesiogenesis. Liquids, which cover large areas, may not be as efficacious as site-specific barriers. Thus the simultaneous use of liquids and barriers may achieve "anatomic synergy": "Two agents, directed against different types of adhesions at separate sites reducing the total extent of adhesions in a way that cannot be obtained by the use of either agent alone."

To illustrate this concept we developed a rabbit model in which adhesions were induced at distinct anatomic sites.[92] For severe and localized adhesions (amenable to reduction by Interceed), the cecum was abraded and a patch of sidewall muscle excised. For more diffuse and less severe adhesions (amenable to reduction by HA), uterine horns were abraded and their mesouterine supply removed. When both treatments were used together, adhesions were reduced at the anatomically distinct sites that required different therapeutic interventions.

Spatial Targeting: Local Drug Delivery

The theoretical advantages of drug delivery to a specific anatomic site are well known, and a simple intraperitoneal injection may have advantages over systemic administration. The numerous polymers that have been developed for adhesion prevention provide a wide choice of delivery platforms. Many drugs, principally nonsteroidal antiinflammatory drugs and heparin, have been evaluated for adhesion prevention, as have steroids.[90] The limited positive, equivocal, or negative results may have been caused less by intrinsic inactivity on the part of the drugs and more by the failure to target them properly.

Steroids. Early work[16] indicated that intraperitoneal steroids reduced adhesions. In other work, they increased adhesions,[20] had no effect on reformed adhesions, and had some effect on de novo (possibly type 1b adhesions).[56] A combination of systemic and local steroids,[20] or systemic steroids given chronically[26] (to patients with bowel disease), may reduce adhesions. Studies in rats[93] hint that a local and controlled release applied of dexamethasone may be beneficial.

Nonsteroidal Antiinflammatory Drugs (NSAIDs). Despite encouraging animal data, widely known clinical studies with NSAIDs such as tolmetin and ibuprofen were unsuccessful. An analysis of animal data seems to indicate that there is no clear advantage of sustained local delivery over single-dose administration.[90] However, the animal models used in those studies may have been insufficiently sensitive to detect any differences between the two methods of delivery.

Heparin. Lehman and Boys[2,13] laid the foundation for the widespread use of heparin in irrigation and instillate solutions. Jansen[94] has suggested that this practice is ineffective, although it does not appear to be detrimental. Heparin delivered locally via Interceed barrier was highly effective in rabbit uterine horn formation[95] and reformation[96] models and reversed the inactivation of Interceed barrier by blood.[34] In a clinical trial, the percentage of ovaries free of adhesions increased from 35% to 47.5% when heparin was added to the Interceed used to wrap the ovary.[97] This difference did not reach statistical significance, possibly because of the small sample size.

Studies in dogs,[98] rabbits,[98] and rats[99] indicate that multiple intraperitoneal doses of heparin may be effective in reducing adhesions, whereas single doses are not. Because this type of dosing is largely impractical in humans, the use of a local delivery device is preferred, and would also alleviate concerns about bleeding. This concept was proven when osmotic minipumps, directing low doses of heparin to a surgical site for several days, reduced adhesions in rabbits.[100] As a further refinement, heparin may be bonded to a biomaterial to produce an athrombogenic surface. Heparin, ionically linked to cross-linked amnion via protamine, inhibited adhesions and scarring after placement over colonic serosal defects in dogs.[101] Similarly prepared porcine pericardia invoked less fibrosis than nonheparinized patches in a canine pericardial model.[102]

Fibrinolytic Drugs. Single doses of fibrinolytic drugs are effective (peritoneal or pericardial adhesions), delivered in simple solution, on a fabric,[103] or in a gel.[104] In rats, three doses of fibrinolysin (plasmin) were more effective than one.[99]

Because fibrin deposition is critical in hemostasis, these drugs carry a risk of bleeding, observed in some studies[103] but not others.[104,105] Tissue plasminogen activator (tPA) analogs may promote less bleeding while still being effective in adhesion prevention.[105] Spatially targeted fibrinolytics may also overcome this problem, a concept supported by work with osmotic minipumps in which no more than 2 days of therapy were required to eliminate adhesions in rabbits.[106] Much lower doses were required than in studies involving single i.p.[104] or pericardial[103] doses. Extending this concept, Hill-West et al.[55] showed that (in rats) t-PA, streptokinase, and urokinase produced superior results when delivered locally by via a hydrogel rather than when administered by daily i.p. injection.

Other Drugs. Aprotinin has opposing actions of inhibiting fibrinolysis and other proteases. This may account for the conflicting positive[107,108] and negative[109] data. Oxygen free radicals, superoxide, and peroxide are believed to mediate a number of inflammatory processes including fibrosis and adhesiogenesis.[110,111] Exposure to CO_2 during laparoscopy may also reduce levels of free radical scavengers in peritoneal tissue. Adhesions may be reduced by limiting the levels of reactive oxygen. Drugs that can do this include ascorbic acid,[112] vitamin E,[113] allopurinol,[114] methylene blue,[115] trimetazidine,[116] superoxide dismutase,[114,117] catalase,[114] and tirilazad.[118] Increased iron levels may be involved in the generation of reactive oxygen species.[111] Thus a chelating agent, mangan-desferrioxamin, was able to reduce adhesions in rats.[119] Nitric oxide has been shown to modulate a number of inflammatory and vascular disease processes,[120–122] with effects on macrophages[123,124] and endothelial cells.[125] Its natural precursor, L-arginine, is used to increase levels of nitric oxide in tissues and was shown to reduce adhesions in rats after i.p. administration.[126]

Certain drugs may be incorporated within polymeric devices as structural participants. *cis*-Hydroxyproline is a proline analog that is assembled into collagen, inhibiting its accumulation and maturation. To avoid systemic effects, *cis*-hydroxyproline has been conjugated with PEG or PEG lysine. When placed locally these polymers degrade to yield the active moiety.[127]

Spatial Targeting: Smart Coatings/Magic Carpets

Current liquid approaches (e.g., Intergel) require the instillation of large quantities of viscous material to coat disparate surfaces at risk of adhesiogenesis. Uninjured surfaces, by their release of fibrinolytic activity, may aid in the control of adhesions. Thus, by coating them that benefit is reduced. An agent that selectively ("smartly") targets only those tissues at risk of adhesions may be preferable and might be designed using the following premises:

- Serosal surfaces contain lipid elements, which prevent tissue adhesion.
- Serosal lipid elements are removed in surgical trauma, leading to adhesions.
- Replacement of serosal lipid elements reduces adhesions.
- Simple tissue lavage sufficient for efficacy. Only tissues in need are coated.

Support for this idea comes from work done in rabbits using phosphatidylcholine, sphingolipid, and glycolipid[128] and the extensive work in rats done by Bengmark using phosphatidylcholine.[129]

To enhance the selectivity of the agent used in this approach, a novel "brush copolymer" has been recently evaluated.[130] This material consists of a backbone of positively charged poly-L-lysine (PLL), which adheres to denuded serosal tissue. Pendant groups of PEG protrude, forming "brushes" that form a nonadhesive surface. In a rat uterine horn model, treatment with this "brush copolymer" yielded results that were superior to treatment with PEG, PLL, or a nonbrush version of the copolymer (Table 35.6).

Temporal Targeting

Few studies have examined the temporal and spatial relationships between pathology, dose, and reduction of adhesions. Such studies provide insight into the design of polymer-based drug delivery devices for adhesion prevention and add mechanistic detail to the overall picture of adhesiogenesis. Indeed, timing of drug delivery is crucial for efficacy. To illustrate this, single intraperitoneal doses of the NSAID tolmetin were given at various times relative to the abrasion and devascularization of uterine horns of rabbits.[131] The best effects were obtained in animals treated within 1 hour of surgery; mild effects seen up to 4 hours (Fig. 35.2 lower panel). Corroborating results come from other studies involving a 10-dose systemic (i.m.) regime of ibuprofen (1 hour before, 8 or 12 hours after, then every 6 hours), in which the change in timing of the second dose from 8 to 12 hours resulted in some loss of efficacy.[132] Mechanistic explanations for these observations are discussed next.

Macrophage Modulation

The suppression of peritoneal fibrinolytic activity (tPA, uPA, elastase, etc.), and the surge in plasminogen activator inhibition (α_2 macroglobulin, antiplasmin, PAI-1, PAI-2, PAI-3, etc.) following surgery is well described (see Thompson, "Peritoneal Fibrinolysis and Adhesion Formation") and is the basis for most current paradigms regarding adhesiogenesis (Table 35.7) and prevention (but see Bakkum et al.[133] for an alternate theory). This paradigm focuses on promoting mesothelial regeneration, or on reconstituting mesothelial fibrinolytic activity using exogenous tPA. Worthy as these approaches might be, they deny the role of other cell types in the repair process and our ability to affect adhesions through them.

Much is known about the biology of macrophages in peritoneal repair.[135] Empirical evidence that macrophages (more correctly, "peritoneal exudate cells," PEC) may be manipulated to reduce adhesions comes from an elegant study[136] in which elicitation of PEC 3 days before surgery was sufficient to reduce adhesions. This effect could be abrogated by lavage of PEC from "primed" animals just before surgery. These same cells were then capable of reducing adhesions after transfer to "unprimed" animals before surgery (Fig. 35.3). Changes in macrophage secretion of a variety of products might account for these observations. Changes in fibrinolytic and related activities are all the more interesting when data regarding the effect of tolmetin on macrophage fibrinolytic activity as well as adhesiogenesis are taken into account.

The temporal effect of tolmetin on adhesiogenesis in rabbits has been described.[131] In a related study[137] in the same animal model, protease secretion of peritoneal lavage cells was measured after harvesting at various

TABLE 35.6. Spatial targeting: smart coatings/magic carpets: PEG-b-PLL, brush copolymer in a rat uterine horn model

	Adhesion extent (%)	
Group	Mean	SEM(*n*)
Buffer control	77.9	6.6 (7)
MPEG	34.4	3.8 (6)
PLL	26.0	4.8 (7)
PEG + PLL	20.3	8.1 (7)
PEG-b-PLL	8.8	4.1 (7)

PEG, polyethylene glycol; PLL, positively charged poly-L-lysine.

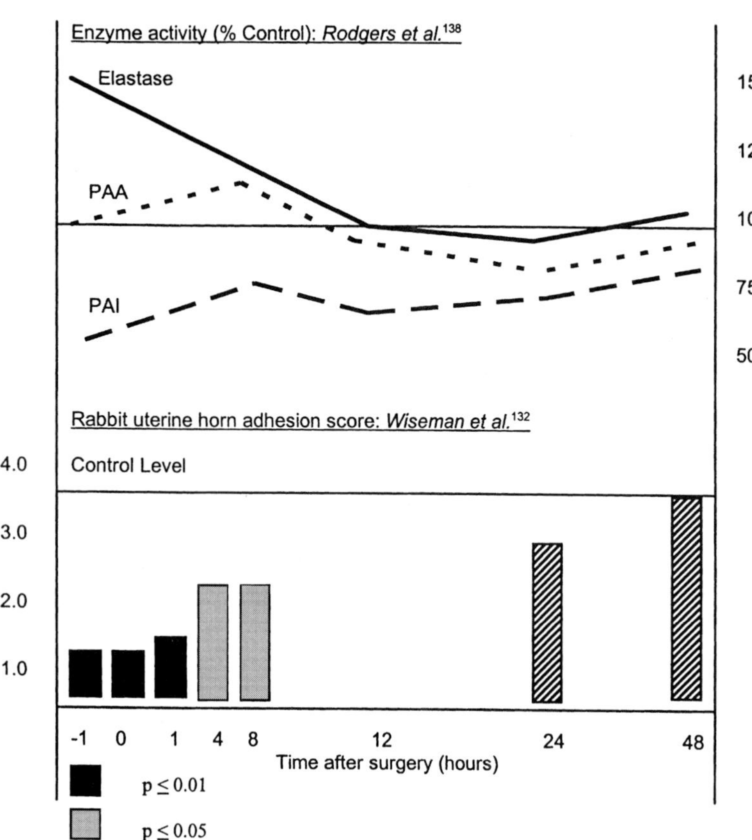

FIG. 35.2. Change in macrophage enzymic activity after treatment with tolmetin: correlation with temporal effect of tolmetin on adhesion formation in a rabbit devascularization uterine horn model.

TABLE 35.7. Current and future paradigms in adhesion prevention.

Current paradigm
1. Compromising the integrity of the mesothelium and submesothelial tissues reduces their ability to lyse fibrin
2. Failure to lyse fibrin deposited between two surfaces leads to fibrous adhesions.[134]

Future paradigm
1. Biochemical and functional differences exist between early and late postsurgical macrophages
2. Increasing fibrinolytic activity of early postsurgical macrophages reduces adhesions

times relative to surgery and exposure to tolmetin in vitro. The findings were as follows:

Resident and early postsurgical macrophages produce PAA and little PAI.
Late postsurgical macrophages produce less PAA and more PAI.
Resident and early postsurgical macrophages respond to tolmetin by producing more PAA and even less PAI.
Late postsurgical macrophages do not respond to tolmetin by changing their production of PAA and PAI.

In response to tolmetin, resident and early (0–6 hours) but not late (>12 hours) postsurgical macrophages produced a net gain in fibrinolytic activity. This pattern corresponds (see Fig. 35.2) to the time-dependent effect of tolmetin on adhesiogenesis in the same animal mode.[131]

Taken with other work,[136] it seems that there is a population of peritoneal cells (presumably macrophages) whose numbers and fibrinolytic function may be enhanced before surgery to protect a patient from adhesiogenesis. This idea of inducing a peritoneal hyperleukocytosis has existed since the turn of the century with observations that fibrin did not form in the presence of pus.[2] Induction of hyperleukocytosis was believed to be the mechanism of action of amniotic fluid,[54] and of colibactragen, advocated in the 1940s for infected cases.[2]

The inflammatory response to biomaterials is well known. Adhesion prevention materials may modulate macrophage activity, suggesting that their effectiveness may at least in part be the result of a biologic action. Degradation products of Interceed barrier interact with scavenger receptors and decrease production of interleukin-1β (IL-1β)[138] (known to reduce tPA and PAI production by mesothelial cells[139]) in macrophages. Thus, the observations that ORC (Interceed barrier)[140,141] and Seprafilm[141] increase the number of active macrophages after intraperitoneal implantation in mice or rats may be interpreted quite positively. Our own work on degradation products of ORC also confirms biologic activity.[142,143] Subtle differences in the phenotypic profiles

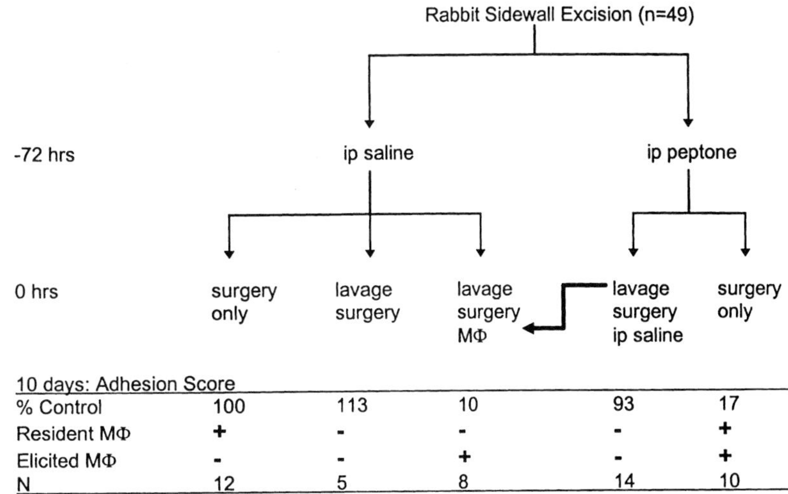

FIG. 35.3. Effect of elicted macrophages on adhesiogenesis in rabbits. (From Ar'Rajab et al.,[136] with permission.)

of the populations elicited[144] may account for some differences in barrier activity.

Cell, Gene, Antisense, and Cytokine Therapy

The arsenal of adhesion prevention approaches is not exhausted. Research into the cellular mechanisms of adhesiogenesis is providing clues about the role of mesothelial cells and macrophages in adhesiogenesis. Other interventions may be derived from work on tissue factor pathways,[145] cell adhesion molecules such as the integrins,[146,147] and manipulation of estrogen and progesterone receptors in adhesion tissue.[148] Although supported by data in rats[149] and monkeys,[150] other indirect data in humans[25] run counter to this idea.

The study of particular patient subpopulations who appear to have a propensity for forming problematic adhesions may yield information about targets for gene or antisense therapy. The nutritional state of patients undergoing surgery may well play a role in their propensity to adhesion formation.[112,113]

A few of many other promising areas worthy of further pursuit are summarized next.

Cellular Modulation by Biomaterials: "Bioactive Devices"

It is clear that biomaterials[141,144] may reduce adhesions by affecting macrophage function.[138] Other pathways too may be affected. For example, *N,O*-carboxymethyl chitosan (NOCC) suppressed the levels of a serum inhibitor of cell proliferation when administered to rats before surgery as well as the increase in growth inhibitory activity in the immediate period (1–4 hours) after injury. This action does not appear to involve transforming growth factor-β (TGF-β).[151] Interceed barrier, or its degradation products, may also bind growth factors and may have direct heparin-like activity, as suggested by work on restenosis.[142] Dextran sulfate (Adcon L) is a device indicated for use in spinal surgery.[43] It has inhibitory actions on fibroblasts and is under development for abdominal adhesions.[23,45]

Transforming Growth Factor-β (TGF-β)

TGF-β is an important mediator in wound healing and fibrosis, affecting macrophage migration,[152] expression of angiogenic activity,[153] mesothelial secretion of tPA and PAI,[139] and modulation[154] of MMP-1 and TIMP-1 levels.[155] Through the work of Chegini[156] (see Growth Factors in Peritoneal Wound Repair) and others, the role of this cytokine in adhesiogenesis is now clearer. In one study,[157] anti-TGF-β_1, but not anti-TGF-β_2 or panspecific antibodies, reduced adhesiogenesis in rats.

Antivascular Permeability Factor (VPF)/VEGF

VPF is a potent stimulator of vascular leakage. In mice, antibodies to VPF reduced adhesiogenesis,[158] presumably by inhibition of posttraumatic vascular leakage and exudation of fibrinogen, required for initial adhesion formation.

Interleukin-10 (IL-10)

IL-10 is a cytokine that inhibits macrophages and lymphocyte synthesis of a number of cytokines, several of which (IL-1, TNF-α, TGF-β) are known to be involved in adhesiogenesis. In mice, endogenous IL-10 does not appear to regulate peritoneal healing[159] but does reduce adhesion formation.[160]

Mesenchymal Stem Cell (MSC) Seeding

Mesothelial compromise is a primary event in adhesiogenesis. Because MSC differentiate into mesothelial cells, the hypothesis that MSC seeded onto peritoneal defects could reduce adhesiogenesis was demonstrated in a dose-dependent manner in rats.[161] Dead cells, irrelevant (smooth muscle) cells, and late passage cells failed to reduce adhesiogenesis.

Systemically Active Drugs

Systemically and orally active specific inhibitors of adhesiogenesis are the goal of pharmaceutical research. These might serve to "prime" a patient before surgery, or might be taken throughout the immediate postoperative period. Ideally they may also have an effect on existing adhesions, either "softening" them and facilitating lysis, or by stimulating autolytic pathways. Although no drug is known to match these descriptions, several drugs in development may meet some of these criteria, including halofuginone, a drug with multiple cellular effects[162] and small molecules (FibroGen Inc.) that is targeted at connective tissue growth factor.

Conclusion

Significant strides have been made in the science and business of adhesion prevention. Chief among the challenges that remain is efficacy. Despite the many advances, it is unlikely that a single product will be marketed in the near future that is able to completely abolish adhesions.

Basic research into the mechanisms of adhesiogenesis is providing clues as to the role of mesothelial cells and macrophages in adhesion formation and yielding information about new opportunities for therapeutic intervention. Advances in biomaterials have resulted in improvements in efficacy over earlier products. These advances have placed us in the position of being able to reconstitute serosal membranes by "tissue engineering" or to deliver specific and effective drugs to sites at risk of adhesiogenesis. We are also beginning to understand the correlations between animal and clinical studies (see Chapter 38, this volume). Other challenges relate to the widespread use of adhesion prevention products in different surgical indications such as abdominal, spinal, tendon, and heart surgery. Lessons learned in one arena cannot but advance efforts in another surgical arena. Last, noninvasive methods of imaging adhesions and methods for collecting data with clinical (e.g., pain, fertility, and bowel obstruction) and economic (cost of adhesions) endpoints must be established.

It is little more than 100 years since the first agents were proposed for use in adhesion prevention. It is difficult not to speculate how the pioneers of the past would view the answers this century has provided to the challenges that they set. I would suspect that they would share our satisfaction with the advances that have been made, our frustration that significant challenges remain, and our optimism that sometime "past the future" we can indeed achieve adhesion-free surgery.

Acknowledgments

It is a pleasure to thank Rabbis David Shawel and BenTzion Epstein for their illuminating discussions on adhesions in the Talmud.

References

1. Richardson EH. Studies on peritoneal adhesions. Ann Surg 1911;54:758–797.
2. Boys F. The prophylaxis of peritoneal adhesions. Surgery (St. Louis) 1942;11:118–168.
3. Krook SS. Obstruction of the small intestine due to adhesion bands. Acta Chir Scand 1947;95(suppl 125).
4. Connolly JE, Smith JW. The prevention and treatment of intestinal adhesions. Int Abs Surg 1960;110:417–431.
5. Ellis H. The cause and prevention of postoperative intraperitoneal adhesions. Surg Gynecol Obstet 1971;133: 497–511.
6. Malcolm JD. On the importance of the practice of washing out the peritoneal cavity as a means of securing a natural disposition of the intestines after an abdominal section. Lancet 1890;i:75–76.
7. Senn N. An experimental contribution to intestinal surgery with special reference to the treatment of intestinal obstruction. Ann Surg 1888;7:171–186.
8. Hertzler AE. Trans West Surg Gynecol Assoc, 1904.
9. Craig AB, Ellis AG. An experimental and histological study of Cargile membrane. Ann Surg 1905;41:810–822.
10. Claypool JR, Vance BM, Robertson PR, Field CW. A study in the prevention of adhesions. J Am Med Assoc 1910; 55:312.
11. Ochsner A, Storck A. Prevention of peritoneal adhesions by papain. Ann Surg 1936;104:736–747.
12. Johnson HL. Observations on the prevention of postoperative peritonitis and abdominal adhesions. Surg Gynecol Obstet 1927;45:612–619.
13. Lehman EP, Boys F. Heparin in the prevention of peritoneal adhesions; report of progress. Ann Surg 1940;112: 969–974.
14. Davidson MM. Systemic administration of heparin and dicumarol for postoperative adhesions. Arch Surg 1949; 59:300–325.
15. James DC, Ellis H, Hugh TB. The effect of streptokinase on experimental intraperitoneal adhesion formation. J Pathol Bacteriol 1965;90:279–287.
16. Swolin K. Die Einwirkung von grossen, intraperitonealen Dosen Glukokortikoid auf die Bildung von postoperativen Adhäsionen. Klinische Studien mit Hilfe des Laparoskopes an operierten Extrauteringraviditäten. Acta Obstet Gynecol Scand 1967;46:204–218.
17. Larsson B, Lalos O, Marsk L, et al. Effect of intraperitoneal instillation of 32% dextran 70 on postoperative adhesion formation after tubal surgery. Acta Obstet Gynecol Scand 1985;64:437–441.
18. Adhesion Study Group. Reduction of postoperative pelvic adhesions with intraperitoneal 32% dextran 70: a prospec-

tive, randomized clinical trial. Fertil Steril 1983;40: 612–619.
19. Rosenberg SM, Board JA. High-molecular weight dextran in human infertility surgery. Am J Obstet Gynecol 1984; 148:380–385.
20. Jansen RP. Failure of intraperitoneal adjuncts to improve the outcome of pelvic operations in young women. Am J Obstet Gynecol 1985;153:363–371.
21. Wiseman DM, Trout JR, Franklin RR, Diamond MP. Meta-analysis of safety and efficacy of an absorbable adhesion barrier (Interceed TC7) in laparotomy. J Reprod Med 1999;44:325–331.
22. Rodgers KE, Johns DB, Girgis W, Campeau J, diZerega GS. Reduction of adhesion formation with hyaluronic acid after peritoneal surgery in rabbits. Fertil Steril 1997;67: 553–558.
23. Lo H, Maier KH, Anderson JM, Zupon MA. Inhibition of postoperative pelvic adhesions by a bioresorbable carbohydrate solution (ADCON-P). Fertil Steril 1998;(Prog suppl):S25.
24. Myomectomy Adhesion Multicenter Study Group. An expanded polytetrafluoroethylene barrier (Gore-Tex Surgical Membrane) reduces post-myomectomy adhesion formation. Fertil Steril 1995;63:491–493.
25. Diamond MP. Reduction of adhesions after uterine myomectomy by Seprafilm membrane (HAL-F): a blinded, prospective, randomized, multicenter clinical study. Seprafilm Adhesion Study Group. Fertil Steril 1996;66:904–910.
26. Becker JM, Dayton MT, Fazio VW, et al. Prevention of postoperative abdominal adhesions by a sodium hyaluronate-based bioresorbable membrane: a prospective, randomized, double-blind multicenter study. J Am Coll Surg 1996; 183:297–306.
27. Burns JW, Colt MJ, Burgess LS, Skinner KC. Preclinical evaluation of Seprafilm bioresorbable membrane. Eur J Surg (Suppl) 1997:40–48.
28. Diamond MP, Sepracoat Adhesion Study Group. Reduction of de novo postsurgical adhesions by intraoperative precoating with Sepracoat (HAL-C) solution: a prospective, randomized, blinded, placebo-controlled multicenter study. The Sepracoat Adhesion Study Group. Fertil Steril 1998;69:1067–1074.
29. Thornton MH, Johns DB, Campeau JD, Hoehler F, diZerega GS. Clinical evaluation of 0.5% ferric hyaluronate adhesion prevention gel for the reduction of adhesions following peritoneal cavity surgery: open-label pilot study. Hum Reprod (Oxf) 1998;13:1480–1485.
30. Johns DB, Rodgers KE, Donahue WD, Kiorpes TC, diZerega GS. Reduction of adhesion formation by postoperative administration of ionically cross-linked hyaluronic acid. Fertil Steril 1997;68:37–42.
31. Leach RE, Burns JW, Dawe EJ, Smith Barbour MD, Diamond MP. Reduction of postsurgical adhesion formation in the rabbit uterine horn model with use of hyaluronate/carboxymethylcellulose gel. Fertil Steril 1998;69:415–418.
32. Haney AF, Doty E. A barrier composed of chemically cross-linked hyaluronic acid (Incert) reduces postoperative adhesion formation. Fertil Steril 1998;70:145–151.
33. De Iaco PA, Stefanetti M, Pressato D, et al. A novel hyaluronan-based gel in laparoscopic adhesion prevention: preclinical evaluation in an animal model. Fertil Steril 1998;69:318–323.
34. Wiseman DM, Kamp LF, Saferstein L, Linsky CB, Gottlick LE, Diamond MP. Improving the efficacy of INTERCEED Barrier in the presence of blood using thrombin, heparin or a blood insensitive barrier, modified INTERCEED (nTC7). Prog Clin Biol Res 1993;381:205–212.
35. Rodgers K, Cohn D, Hotovely A, Pines E, Diamond MP, diZerega G. Evaluation of polyethylene glycol/polylactic acid films in the prevention of adhesions in the rabbit adhesion formation and reformation sidewall models. Fertil Steril 1998;69:403–408.
36. Okuyama N, Rodgers KE, Wang CY, et al. Prevention of retrosternal adhesion formation in a rabbit model using bioresorbable films of polyethylene glycol and polylactic acid. J Surg Res 1998;78:118–122.
37. Wang CY, Rose EA, Okuyamo N, et al. A novel transparent bioresorbable film reduces postoperative retrosternal adhesions. J Heart Lung Transplant 1998;17:50 (Abstract 28).
38. Diamond MP, Rodgers K, Stern T, Cohn D, Pines E, diZerega G. Resolve TM. A solution approach to reduce postoperative adhesions in the rabbit double uterine horn model. Presented at Annual Regional int. soc. gynaecologic endoscopy (ISGE) Meeting, Amsterdam, 1998.
39. Hill-West JL, Chowdhury SM, Sawhney AS, Pathak CP, Dunn RC, Hubbell JA. Prevention of postoperative adhesions in the rat by in situ photopolymerization of bioresorbable hydrogel barriers. Obstet Gynecol 1994;83: 59–64.
40. Leach RE, Henry RL. Reduction of postoperative adhesions in the rat uterine horn model with poloxamer 407. Am J Obstet Gynecol 1990;162:1317–1319.
41. Kennedy R, Costain DJ, McAlister VC, Lee TD. Prevention of experimental postoperative peritoneal adhesions by *N,O*-carboxymethyl chitosan. Surgery (St. Louis) 1996; 120:866–870.
42. Dobbie JW. Separation of peritoneal surfaces through the maintenance of an artificial ascites as a preventative of peritoneal adhesions. In: International Congress of Peritoneal Tissue Repair, Gothenburg, Sweden, 1997:61.
43. de Tribolet N, Porchet F, Lutz TW, et al. Clinical assessment of a novel antiadhesion barrier gel: prospective, randomized, multicenter, clinical trial of ADCON-L to inhibit postoperative peridural fibrosis and related symptoms after lumbar discectomy. Am J Orthop 1998;27:111–120.
44. Merle M, Foucher G, Egloff DV. Peritendinous and perineural scar and adhesions—treatment with a new anti-adhesion barrier gel ADCON T/N. In: Hand Surgery Frankfurt International Hand Surgery Conference, November 1996, Frankfurt, Germany. Stuttgart: Thieme, 1997:33–40.
45. Strandell A, Thorburn J, Tronstad SE, et al. Effectiveness and safety of a bioresorbable carbohydrate solution for prevention of post-operative adhesions in pelvic surgery. Fertil Steril 1998;Prog Suppl:S412.
46. Malm T, Bowald S, Bylock A, Busch C. Prevention of postoperative pericardial adhesions by closure of the pericardium with absorbable polymer patches. An experimental study. J Thorac Cardiovasc Surg 1992;104:600–607.
47. Urry DW, Pattanaik A, Accavitti MA, et al. Transductional elastic and plastic protein-based polymers as potential

medical devices. In: Domb A, Kost Y, Wiseman DM, eds. Handbook of Biodegradable Polymers. Amsterdam: Harwood, 1997:367–386.

48. Capello J. Genetically engineered protein polymers. In: Domb A, Kost Y, Wiseman DM, eds. Handbook of Biodegradable Polymers. Amsterdam: Harwood, 1997: 387–414.
49. Sherman N, Zlotowitz M, Mishnah Chullin. Sefer Kodashim IIa. Brooklyn, New York: Mesorah Publications, 1989:82–84.
50. Carson HW. The evolution of the modern treatment of septic peritonitis. Lancet 1923;i:1035–1037.
51. Morris RT. Peritoneal adhesions. Am J Obstet 1906;54: 764–770.
52. Vogel K. Clinical and experimental study of peritoneal adhesion occurring after laparotomy. Deutsche Zeit Chir ixiii:296 (cited in Ann Surg 1902;36:961–962).
53. Wright LT, Smith DH, Rothman M, Quosh ET, Metzger WI. Prevention of postoperative adhesions in rabbits with streptococcal metabolites. Proc Soc Exp Biol Med 1950; 75:602–604.
54. Johnson HL. Amniotic fluid concentrate in the prevention of adhesions. N Engl J Med 1928;199:661–664.
55. Hill-West JL, Dunn RC, Hubbell JA. Local release of fibrinolytic agents for adhesion prevention. J Surg Res 1995; 59:759–763.
56. Larsson B. Prevention of postoperative formation and reformation of pelvic adhesions. In: Treutner KH, Schumpelick V, eds. Peritoneal Adhesions. Berlin: Springer, 1997:331–334.
57. Dmytryk ET. Peritoneal reaction to oxidized cellulose. Arch Surg 1948;56:386–397.
58. Frantz VK. Absorbable cotton, paper and gauze (oxidized cellulose). Ann Surg 1943;118:116–126.
59. Larsson B, Nissell H, Grandberg I. Surgicel: an absorbable hemostatic material in prevention of peritoneal adhesion in rats. Acta Chir Scand 1978;44:375–378.
60. Raftery A. Absorbable hemostatic materials and intraperitoneal adhesion formation. Br J Surg 1980;67:57–58.
61. Hixson C, Swanson LA, Friedman CI. Oxidized cellulose for preventing adnexal adhesions. J Reprod Med 1986;31: 58–60.
62. Shimanuki T, Nishimura K, Montz FJ, Nakamura RM, diZerega GS. Localized prevention of postsurgical adhesion formation and reformation with oxidized regenerated cellulose. J Biomed Mater Res 1987;21:173–185.
63. Linsky CB, Diamond MP, Cunningham T, Constantine B, DeCherney AH, diZerega GS. Adhesion reduction in the rabbit uterine horn model using an absorbable barrier, TC-7. J Reprod Med 1987;32:17–20.
64. Azziz R. Microsurgery alone or with INTERCEED Absorbable Adhesion Barrier for pelvic sidewall adhesion reformation. the INTERCEED (TC7) Adhesion Barrier Study Group II. Surg Gynecol Obstet 1993;177:135–139.
65. Wiseman DM. Hazards and prevention of postsurgical pericardial adhesions. In: Treutner KH, Schumpelick V, eds. Peritoneal Adhesions. Berlin: Springer, 1996:240–254.
66. Burns JW, Skinner K, Colt J, et al. Prevention of tissue injury and postsurgical adhesions by precoating tissues with hyaluronic acid solutions. J Surg Res 1995;59:644–652.
67. Hagberg L. Exogenous hyaluronate as an adjunct in the prevention of adhesions after flexor tendon surgery: a controlled clinical trial. J Hand Surg (Am) 1992;17: 132–136.
68. Hagberg L, Gerdin B. Sodium hyaluronate as an adjunct in adhesion prevention after flexor tendon surgery in rabbits. J Hand Surg (Am) 1992;17:935–941.
69. Nagelschmidt M, Saad S. Influence of polyethylene glycol 4000 and dextran 70 on adhesion formation in rats. J Surg Res 1997;67:113–118.
70. Nyska M, Porat S, Nyska A, Rousso M, Shoshan S. Decreased adhesion formation in flexor tendons by topical application of enriched collagen solution—a histological study. Arch Orthop Trauma Surg 1987;106:192–194.
71. Edwards GA, Glattauer V, Nash TJ, et al. In vivo evaluation of a collagenous membrane as an absorbable adhesion barrier. J Biomed Mater Res 1997;34:291–297.
72. Lindenberg S, Lauritsen JG. Prevention of peritoneal adhesion formation by fibrin sealant. An experimental study in rats. Ann Chir Gynaecol 1984;73:11–13.
73. De Iaco P, Costa A, Mazzoleni G, Pasquinelli G, Bassein L, Marabini A. Fibrin sealant in laparoscopic adhesion prevention in the rabbit uterine horn model. Fertil Steril 1994;62:400–404.
74. de Virgilio C, Dubrow T, Sheppard BB, et al. Fibrin glue inhibits intra-abdominal adhesion formation. Arch Surg 1990;125:1378–1381.
75. Tulandi T. Effects of fibrin sealant on tubal anastomosis and adhesion formation. Fertil Steril 1991;56:136–138.
76. Takeuchi H, Awaji M, Hashimoto M, Nakano Y, Mitsuhashi N, Kuwabara Y. Reduction of adhesions with fibrin glue after laparoscopic excision of large ovarian endometriomas. J Am Assoc Gynecol Laparosc 1996;3:575–579.
77. van den Tol MP, van Stijn I, Bonthuis F, Marquet RL, Jeekel J. Reduction of intraperitoneal adhesion formation by use of non-abrasive gauze. Br J Surg 1997;84:1410–1415.
78. Wiseman DM, Trout JR, Diamond MP. The rates of adhesion development and the effects of crystalloid solutions on adhesion development in pelvic surgery. Fertil Steril 1998;70:702–711.
79. Bhatia DS, Allen JE. The prevention of experimentally induced postoperative adhesions. Am Surg 1997;63:775–777.
80. Tilton EB. Instrumentation for laparoscopic insertion and application of sheet like surgical material. U.S. Patent 5,503,623, 1996.
81. Tilton EB. Instrumentation for surgical endoscopic insertion and application of liquid and gel material. U.S. Patent 5,766,157, 1998.
82. Klein HM, Klosterhalfen B, Töns C, Steinau G, Günther RW. Conventional radiography and cross-sectional imaging modalities in the diagnosis of intestinal adhesions. In: Treutner KH, Schumpelick V, eds. Peritoneal Adhesions. Berlin: Springer, 1996:172–178.
83. Duvernoy O, Malm T, Thuomas KA, Larsson SG, Hansson HE. CT and MR evaluation of pericardial and retrosternal adhesions after cardiac surgery. J Comput Assist Tomogr 1991;15:555–560.
84. Makanjuola D. Computed tomography compared with small bowel enema in clinically equivocal intestinal obstruction. Clin Radiol 1998;53:203–208.

85. Uberoi R, D'Costa H, Brown C, Dubbins P. Visceral slide for intraperitoneal adhesions? A prospective study in 48 patients with surgical correlation. J Clin Ultrasound 1995;23:363–366.
86. Caprini JA, Arcelus JA, Swanson J, et al. The ultrasonic localization of abdominal wall adhesions. Surg Endosc 1995;9:283–285.
87. Conze J, Truong S, Schumpelick V. Value of ultrasonography in diagnosis of pelvic adhesions. In: Treutner KH, Schumpelick V, eds. Peritoneal Adhesions. Berlin: Springer, 1996:163–171.
88. Guerriero S, Ajossa S, Lai MP, Mais V, Paoletti AM, Melis GB. Transvaginal ultrasonography in the diagnosis of pelvic adhesions. Hum Reprod (Oxf) 1997;12:2649–2653.
89. Hoban LD, Pierce M, Quance J, et al. Use of polypentapeptides of elastin to prevent postoperative adhesions: efficacy in a contaminated peritoneal model. J Surg Res 1994;56:179–183.
90. Wiseman DM. Polymers for the prevention of surgical adhesions. In: Domb AJ, ed. Polymeric Site-Specific Pharmacotherapy. Chichester: Wiley, 1994:369–421.
91. Malm T, Bowald S, Bylock A, Saldeen T, Busch C. Regeneration of pericardial tissue on absorbable polymer patches implanted into the pericardial sac. An immunohistochemical, ultrastructural and biochemical study in the sheep. Scand J Thorac Cardiovasc Surg 1992;26:15–21.
92. Wiseman DM, Johns DB. Anatomical synergy between sodium hyaluronate (HA) and INTERCEED barrier in rabbits with two types of adhesions. Fertil Steril 1993;Prog Suppl:S25.
93. Hockel M, Ott S, Siemann U, Kissel T. Prevention of peritoneal adhesions in the rat with sustained intraperitoneal dexamethasone delivered by a novel therapeutic system. Ann Chir Gynaecol 1987;76:306–313.
94. Jansen RP. Failure of peritoneal irrigation with heparin during pelvic operations upon young women to reduce adhesions. Surg Gynecol Obstet 1988;166:154–160.
95. Diamond MP, Linsky CB, Cunningham T, et al. Synergistic effects of INTERCEED (TC7) and heparin in reducing adhesion formation in the rabbit uterine horn model. Fertil Steril 1991;55:389–394.
96. Diamond MP, Linsky CB, Cunningham T, et al. Adhesion reformation: reduction by the use of INTERCEED R (TC7) plus heparin. J Gynecol Surg 1991;7:1–6.
97. Reid RL, Hahn PM, Spence JE, Tulandi T, Yuzpe AA, Wiseman DM. A randomized clinical trial of oxidized regenerated cellulose adhesion barrier (Interceed, TC7) alone or in combination with heparin. Fertil Steril 1997;67:23–29.
98. Lehman EP, Boys F. The prevention of peritoneal adhesions with heparin. Ann Surg 1940;111:427–435.
99. Knightly JJ, Agostino D, Cliffton EE. The effect of fibrinolysin and heparin on the formation of peritoneal adhesions. Surgery (St. Louis) 1962;52:250–258.
100. Fukasawa M, Girgis W, diZerega GS. Inhibition of postsurgical adhesions in a standardized rabbit model. II. Intraperitoneal treatment with heparin. Int J Fertil 1991; 36:296–301.
101. Noishiki Y, Miyata T. Antiadhesive collagen membrane with heparin slow release. J Bioact Compat Polymers 1987;2:325–333.
102. Lu JH, Chang Y, Sung HW, Chiu YT, Yang PC, Hwang B. Heparinization on pericardial substitutes can reduce adhesion and epicardial inflammation in the dog. J Thorac Cardiovasc Surg 1998;115:1111–1120.
103. Wiseman DM, Kamp L, Linsky CB, Jochen RF, Pang RH, Scholz PM. Fibrinolytic drugs prevent pericardial adhesions in the rabbit. J Surg Res 1992;53:362–368.
104. Doody KJ, Dunn RC, Buttram VC Jr. Recombinant tissue plasminogen activator reduces adhesion formation in a rabbit uterine horn model. Fertil Steril 1989;51:509–512.
105. Montz FJ, Fowler JM, Wolff AJ, Lacey SM, Mohler M. The ability of recombinant tissue plasminogen activator to inhibit post-radical pelvic surgery adhesions in the dog model. Am J Obstet Gynecol 1991;165:1539–1542.
106. Orita H, Fukasawa M, Girgis W, diZerega GS. Inhibition of postsurgical adhesions in a standardized rabbit model: intraperitoneal treatment with tissue plasminogen activator. Int J Fertil 1991;36:172–177.
107. Dargenio R, Cimino C, Ragusa G, Garcea N, Stella C. Pharmacological prevention of postoperative adhesions experimentally induced in the rat. Acta Eur Fertil 1986; 17:267–272.
108. Ozogul Y, Baykal A, Onat D, Renda N, Sayek I. An experimental study of the effect of aprotinin on intestinal adhesion formation. Am J Surg 1998;175:137–141.
109. Raftery AT. Noxythiolin (Noxyflex), aprotinin (Trasylol) and peritoneal adhesion formation: an experimental study in the rat. Br J Surg 1979;66:654–656.
110. O'Leary JP, Wickbom G, Cha SO, Wickbom A. The role of feces, necrotic tissue, and various blocking agents in the prevention of adhesions. Ann Surg 1988;207:693–698.
111. Arumugam K, Yip YC. De novo formation of adhesions in endometriosis: the role of iron and free radical reactions. Fertil Steril 1995;64:62–64.
112. Beati CA, De Carlis L, Samori G, Calzoni DA. Vitamin C prevents induced peritoneal adhesions in rats. Med Sci Res 1992;20:683–684.
113. Hemadeh O, Chilukuri S, Bonet V, Hussein S, Chaudry IH. Prevention of peritoneal adhesions by administration of sodium carboxymethyl cellulose and oral vitamin E. Surgery (St. Louis) 1993;114:907–910.
114. Tsimoyiannis EC, Tsimoyiannis JC, Sarros CJ, et al. The role of oxygen-derived free radicals in peritoneal adhesion formation induced by ileal ischaemia/reperfusion. Acta Chir Scand 1989;155:171–174.
115. Galili Y, Ben-Abraham R, Rabau M, Klausner J, Kluger Y. Reduction of surgery-induced peritoneal adhesions by methylene blue. Am J Surg 1998;175:30–32.
116. Tsimoyiannis EC, Lekkas ET, Paizis JB, Boulis SA, Page P, Kotoulas OB. Prevention of peritoneal adhesions in rats with trimetazidine. Acta Chir Scand 1990;156:771–774.
117. Portz DM, Elkins TE, White R, Warren J, Adadevoh S, Randolph J. Oxygen free radicals and pelvic adhesion formation. I. Blocking oxygen free radical toxicity to prevent adhesion formation in an endometriosis model. Int J Fertil 1991;36:39–42.
118. KE Rodgers, Girgis W, St Amand K, Campeau J, diZerega GS. Reduction of adhesion formation in rabbits by intraperitoneal administration of lazaroid formulations. Hum Reprod (Oxf) 1998;13:2443–2451.

119. Soybir G, Koksoy F, Ekiz F, Yalcin O, Ozseker A, Cokneseli B. Effect of mangan-desferrioxamin in the prevention of peritoneal adhesions. J R Coll Surg Edinb 1998;43:26–28.
120. Suh H, Wadhwa NK, Peresleni T, McNurlan M, Garlick P, Goligorsky MS. Decreased L-arginine during peritonitis in ESRD patients on peritoneal dialysis. Adv Perit Dial 1997;13:205–209.
121. Ketteler M, Cetto C, Kirdorf M, Jeschke GS, Schafer JH, Distler A. Nitric oxide in sepsis-syndrome: potential treatment of septic shock by nitric oxide synthase antagonists. Kidney Int Supplt 1998;64:S27–S30.
122. Maxwell AJ, Cooke JP. Cardiovascular effects of L-arginine. Curr Opin Nephrol Hypertens 1998;7:63–70.
123. Kim SJ, Bang OS, Lee YS, Kang SS. Production of inducible nitric oxide is required for monocytic differentiation of U937 cells induced by vitamin E-succinate. J Cell Sci 1998;111:435–441.
124. Sinha B, Eigler A, Baumann KH, Greten TF, Moeller J, Endres S. Nitric oxide downregulates tumour necrosis factor in mRNA in RAW 264.7 cells. Res Immunol 1998;149: 139–150.
125. Dakak N, Husain S, Mulcahy D, et al. Contribution of nitric oxide to reactive hyperemia: impact of endothelial dysfunction. Hypertension 1998;32:9–15.
126. Kaleli B, Ozden A, Aybek Z, Bostanci B. The effect of L-arginine and pentoxifylline on postoperative adhesion formation. Acta Obstet Gynecol Scand 1998;77:377–380.
127. Gean KF, Messinger JA, Poiani GG, Riley DJ, Kohn J. New polymeric carriers of *cis*-hydroxy-L-proline: potential agents for the inhibition of excess collagen synthesis. Polymer Preprints 1992;33:51–52.
128. Treutner KH, Bertram P, Schumpelick V. Experimental prevention of peritoneal adhesions in general surgery. In: diZerega GS, DeCherney AH, Diamond MP, et al., eds. Pelvic Surgery: Adhesion Formation and Prevention. New York: Springer-Verlag, 1997:71–78.
129. Bengmark S. Peritoneal conditioning: the role of the supply of natural membrane lipids. In: diZerega GS, DeCherney AH, Diamond MP, et al., eds. Pelvic Surgery: Adhesion Formation and Prevention. New York: Springer-Verlag, 1997:103–113.
130. Hubbell JA, Hill-West JL, Drumheller PD, Sanghamitra C, Sawhney A. Multifunctional organic polymers. U.S. Patent 5,462,990, 1995.
131. Wiseman DM, Huang WJ, Johns DB, Rodgers KE, diZerega GS. Time-dependent effect of tolmetin sodium in a rabbit uterine adhesion model. J Invest Surg 1994;7: 527–532.
132. Nishimura K, Nakamura RM, diZerega GS. Ibuprofen inhibition of postsurgical adhesion formation: a time and dose response biochemical evaluation in rabbits. J Surg Res 1984;36:115–124.
133. Bakkum EA, Emeis JJ, Dalmeijer RA, van Blitterswijk CA, Trimbos JB, Trimbos-Kemper TC. Long-term analysis of peritoneal plasminogen activator activity and adhesion formation after surgical trauma in the rat model. Fertil Steril 1996;66:1018–1022.
134. Porter JM, Ball AP, Silver D. Mesothelial fibrinolysis. J Cardiovasc Surg 1971;62:725–730.
135. diZerega GS, Rodgers KE. The Peritoneum. New York: Springer-Verlag, 1992.
136. Ar'Rajab A, Dawidson I, Sentementes J, Sikes P, Harris R, Mileski W. Enhancement of peritoneal macrophages reduces postoperative peritoneal adhesion formation. J Surg Res 1995;58:307–312.
137. Rodgers K, Ellefson D, Girgis W, diZerega GS. Protease and protease inhibitor secretion by postsurgical macrophages following in vitro exposure to tolmetin. Agents Actions 1992;36:248–256.
138. Reddy S, Santanam N, Reddy PP, Rock JA, Murphy AA, Parthasarathy S. Interaction of Interceed oxidized regenerated cellulose with macrophages: a potential mechanism by which Interceed may prevent adhesions. Am J Obstet Gynecol 1997;177:1315–1320.
139. Tietze L, Elbrecht A, Schauerte C, et al. Modulation of pro- and antifibrinolytic properties of human peritoneal mesothelial cells by transforming growth factor $beta_1$ (TGF-$beta_1$), tumor necrosis factor alpha (TNF-alpha) and interleukin 1_{beta} (IL-1_{beta}). Thromb Haemostasis 1998;79: 362–370.
140. Haney AF, Doty E. Comparison of the peritoneal cells elicited by oxidized regenerated cellulose (Interceed) and expanded polytetrafluoroethylene (Gore-Tex Surgical Membrane) in a murine model. Am J Obstet Gynecol 1992;166:1137–1146.
141. Dethlefsen SM, Nickersen CJ, Garlick DS, et al. The effect of Seprafilm™ and Interceed® (TC7) adhesion barriers on the early phases of peritoneal wound repair. Fertil Steril 1997;(Prog Suppl):S65–S66.
142. Watt PW, Harvey W, Lorimer E, Wiseman D. Use of oxidized cellulose and complexes thereof for chronic wound healing. Patent Application WO 98/00180, 1998.
143. Wiseman DM, Saferstein L, Wolf S. Bioresorbable medical devices from oxidized polysaccharides. Patent Application EP 0815 879 A2, 1998.
144. Copeland D, Konz R, Reynolds S, et al. The intraperitoneal cellular response to Seprafilm™ and Interceed ® (TC7) adhesion barriers. Fertil Steril 1997; Prog Suppl: S66.
145. Idell S, Pendurthi U, Pueblitz S, Koenig K, Williams T, Rao LV. Tissue factor pathway inhibitor in tetracycline-induced pleuritis in rabbits. Thromb Haemostasis 1998; 79:649–655.
146. Witz CA, Montoya-Rodriguez IA, Miller DM, Schneider BG, Schenken RS. Mesothelium expression of integrins in vivo and in vitro. J Soc Gynecol Invest 1998;5:87–93.
147. Rodgers KE, Girgis W, Campeau JD, diZerega GS. Reduction of adhesion formation by intraperitoneal administration of RGD containing peptides. Fertil Steril 1998;Prog Suppl:S498.
148. Wiczyk HP, Grow DR, Adams LA, O'Shea DL, Reece MT. Pelvic adhesions contain sex steroid receptors and produce angiogenesis growth factors. Fertil Steril 1998;69: 511–516.
149. Sharpe-Timms KL, Zimmer RL, Jolliff WJ, Wright JA, Nothnick WB, Curry TE. Gonadotropin-releasing hormone agonist (GnRH-a) therapy alters activity of plasminogen activators, matrix metalloproteinases, and their

inhibitors in rat models for adhesion formation and endometriosis: potential GnRH-a-regulated mechanisms reducing adhesion formation. Fertil Steril 1998;69: 916–923.

150. Grow DR, Coddington CC, Hsiu JG, Mikich Y, Hodgen GD. Role of hypoestrogenism or sex steroid antagonism in adhesion formation after myometrial surgery in primates. Fertil Steril 1996;66:140–147.
151. Krause TJ, Goldsmith NK, Ebner S, Zazanis GA, McKinnon RD. An inhibitor of cell proliferation associated with adhesion formation is suppressed by N,O-carboxymethyl chitosan. J Invest Surg 1998;11:105–113.
152. Wiseman DM, Polverini PJ, Kamp DW, Leibovich SJ. Transforming growth factor-beta (TGF-beta) is chemotactic for human monocytes and induces their expression of angiogenic activity. Biochem Biophys Res Commun 1988; 157:793–800.
153. Leibovich SJ, Polverini PJ, Shepard HM, Wiseman DM, Shively V, Nuseir N. Macrophage-induced angiogenesis is mediated by tumour necrosis factor-alpha. Nature (Lond) 1987;329:630–632.
154. Ma C, Tarmizzer RW, Chegini N. Modulation of matrix metalloproteinases and tissue inhibitor of MMPs expression in human myometrial smooth muscle cell, mesothelial cell and macrophages by transforming growth factor β_1. Fertil Steril 1998;Prog Suppl:S49–S50.
155. Chegini N, Zhao Y, Kotseos K, et al. Comparative analysis of matrix metalloproteinase (MMP-1) tissue inhibitor (TIMP-1) and MMP-1/TIMP-1 complex expression in intraperitoneal environment and their relation to adhesion development. Fertil Steril 1998;Prog Suppl:S26–S27.
156. Chegini N. The role of growth factors in peritoneal healing: transforming growth factor beta (TGF-beta). Eur J Surg (Suppl) 1997:17–23.
157. Lucas PA, Warejcka DJ, Young HE, Lee BY. Formation of abdominal adhesions is inhibited by antibodies to transforming growth factor-beta$_1$. J Surg Res 1996;65:135–136.
158. Saltzman AK, Olson TA, Mohanraj D, Carson LF, Ramakrishnan S. Prevention of postoperative adhesions by an antibody to vascular permeability factor/vascular endothelial growth factor in a murine model. Am J Obstet Gynecol 1996;174:1502–1506.
159. Holschneider CH, Cristoforoni PM, Ghosh K, Punyasavatsut M, Abed E, Montz FJ. Endogenous versus exogenous IL-10 in postoperative intraperitoneal adhesion formation in a murine model. J Surg Res 1997;70:138–143.
160. Montz FJ, Holschneider CH, Bozuk M, Gotlieb WH, Martinez-Maza O. Interleukin 10: ability to minimize postoperative intraperitoneal adhesion formation in a murine model. Fertil Steril 1994;61:1136–1140.
161. Lucas PA, Warejcka DJ, Zhang LM, Newman WH, Young HE. Effect of rat mesenchymal stem cells on development of abdominal adhesions after surgery. J Surg Res 1996; 62:229–232.
162. Nagler A, Rivkind AI, Raphael J, et al. Halofuginone—an inhibitor of collagen type I synthesis—prevents postoperative formation of abdominal adhesions. Ann Surg 1998;227:575–582.

Section 7
Developing Technology

36

Transperitoneal Pharmacokinetics

Michael F. Flessner

CONTENTS

The peritoneal cavity is a major portal of entry into the body for drugs, parental fluids, and even cellular materials. Because of the extensive system of lymphatics in the diaphragm,[1,2] which accept particles up to 25 μm in diameter,[3] the cavity has even been used in the past for neonatal blood transfusions.[4,5] Because intravenous (i.v.) administration is superior to intraperitoneal (i.p.) for systemic administration and for the attainment of a given peak concentration, the systemic circulation is rarely the target of i.p. therapy. i.p. administration is more appropriate for regional therapy within the cavity or in the surrounding tissue or for the purpose of gaining access to such systems as the thoracic lymphatics that drain the cavity. To treat locally metastatic neoplasms, for example, i.p. chemotherapy often takes advantage of the relatively slow absorption of drugs from the cavity to establish toxic levels of an agent in the cavity while the systemic concentrations are one to two orders of magnitude lower.[6,7] Agents designed to minimize or prevent postsurgical adhesions between opposing surfaces of the peritoneum likely are better applied directly to serosa to maximize the local effect in the target tissue. Because of the orientation of this volume, the peritoneal cavity-to-tissue direction of transport is emphasized throughout this chapter.

Pharmacokinetic Advantage

Pharmacokinetics is the science that defines the rates of transfer between the point of entry and a given target. The pharmacokinetics of a particular drug are based on the transport physiology of the region in which it is administered as well as pharmacokinetic processes in the rest of the body. If a drug is infused at a constant rate into a fixed volume of fluid in the peritoneal cavity until steady state is achieved, the regional pharmacokinetic advantage is[8]

$$R_{IP} = \left(\frac{C_P}{C_B}\right)_{ip} \text{ or } R_{IP} = \left(\frac{AUC_P}{AUC_B}\right)_{ip} \quad (1)$$

where C_P is the concentration in the peritoneal cavity, C_B is the concentration in the systemic circulation, *AUC* is the area under the curve of the concentration versus time curve for the i.p.-injected agent in the peritoneal cavity (P) or blood (B), and the subscripts (ip) indicate the route of administration.

The regional pharmacokinetic advantage for a drug such as cisplatin has been estimated to be 26.[9] A more general equation that permits assessment of the i.p. route versus the i.v. route is provided by the pharmacokinetic advantage (R_d), which at steady state can be defined by[8]

$$R_d = \frac{\left(\frac{C_P}{C_B}\right)_{ip}}{\left(\frac{C_P}{C_B}\right)_{iv}} \quad (2)$$

Equations 1 and 2 define the advantage in terms of i.p. and i.v. concentration, which is clearly appropriate when the target is within the cavity, such as malignant cells, or at the peritoneal surface. However, the desired target may be not only the mesothelial lining but deeper in the submesothelial tissue. Here, depending on the location of the desired target with respect to the peritoneal surface and the specific agent, there may or may not be an advantage to i.p. administration. To predict the pharmacokinetic advantage, the rates of transport from the cavity to the target must be known as well as the systemic elimination rates; these will differ depending on the agent used and its properties of lipid solubility and molecular size. Other major factors that may have a significant impact on the success of a treatment are the area of the peritoneum in contact with the solution in the cavity, the capillary permeability and perfused area within the tissues, the blood flow through the tissue, binding of the agent to the tissue, and metabolism of the drug within the tissue. Each of these topics is discussed here.

This chapter briefly reviews the highlights of peritoneal anatomy and physiology, which have been discussed in depth in previous chapters. Emphasis is placed on those factors which affect transport. If the purpose of the i.p. therapy is exchange between the blood and a solution in the cavity (as in peritoneal dialysis), the appropriate pharmacokinetic model might be a simple two-compartment concept. If, however, the target of the therapy is the mesothelium and the underlying tissue that contains a multitude of different cells, then a more complex model of transport across the peritoneum must be utilized to predict the location of the solute versus time and what effect the therapy might have on the overall system. The diffusive transport of small, water-soluble agents (<6000 daltons) is best understood, and relatively simple theoretical concepts have been used to quantify the transport. Considerably less research has been performed on the transport of novel drugs such as monoclonal antibodies (MAbs) or viral vectors that contain splices of gene products. New experimental forms of therapy must be tested with in vivo experimentation to define the concentrations necessary for the solution of Eqs. 1 and 2. In the delivery of these macromolecular agents, where gaps exist in our quantitative knowledge, the salient points that may affect drug delivery are discussed.

Transport Model Concepts

Compartmental Models: Peritoneal Dialysis

Figure 36.1 displays the classic view of peritoneal dialysis. Transport occurs across a peritoneal barrier between two well-mixed compartments, which are typically designated the Body compartment and the Peritoneal Cavity. The volume of the cavity (V_P) equals the volume of the solution in the cavity and the concentration (C_P) equals the solute concentration in the dialysis solution. In the body compartment, the concentration (C_B) is typically equated to plasma concentration in the mixed venous sample, and the volume (V_B) is equal to the volume of distribution in the body for the solute under study. If urea is the solute, for example, V_B would equal total body water. Although the model depicted in Fig. 36.1 is adequate to portray the therapy of peritoneal dialysis, it tells us nothing of the underlying mechanisms of transport through the tissue space. The transport barrier is treated as a "black box," in which several barriers are lumped together and represented in the mass transfer-area coefficient (MTAC), the coefficient that governs the solute mass transfer across the peritoneum. Many clinicians believe that the anatomic peritoneum is in fact the peritoneal barrier or "peritoneal membrane." The anatomic peritoneum, made up of a single layer of mesothelial cells overlying five or six layers of connective tissue,[10] is extremely important for host defense and for secretion of substances that cause the viscera to slide smoothly against the parietal portion of the peritoneum. Both these topics have been reviewed in detail earlier in this volume.

Despite its important roles in the biology of the peritoneal cavity, the peritoneum is not a selective barrier to solute transport. Macromolecules pass without impediment from the cavity into the subperitoneal interstitium at a rate directly proportional to the hydrostatic pressure-driven fluid flux.[11] The peritoneal barrier is not equivalent to that of the capillary endothelium but characterized as similar to the interstitium of the underlying subperitoneal tissue. Therefore, the barrier in transperitoneal transport is not the anatomic peritoneum but can be considered to be a combination of the tissue interstitium and the blood capillary endothelium. To estimate the rate of drug delivery and the drug effects to the tissue space surrounding the peritoneum, a better conceptual model is needed than that depicted in Fig. 36.1.

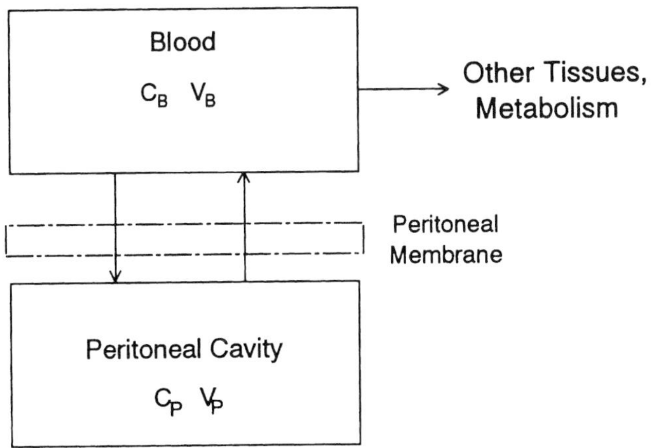

Fig. 36.1. Compartmental model concept of intraperitoneal drug delivery in which transport occurs between the cavity and the body compartment across the "peritoneal membrane," which lumps all the actual barriers into a single entity. *C*, concentration; *V*, volume of the compartment. Subscripts *B* and *P* refer to the body compartment and peritoneal cavity, respectively.

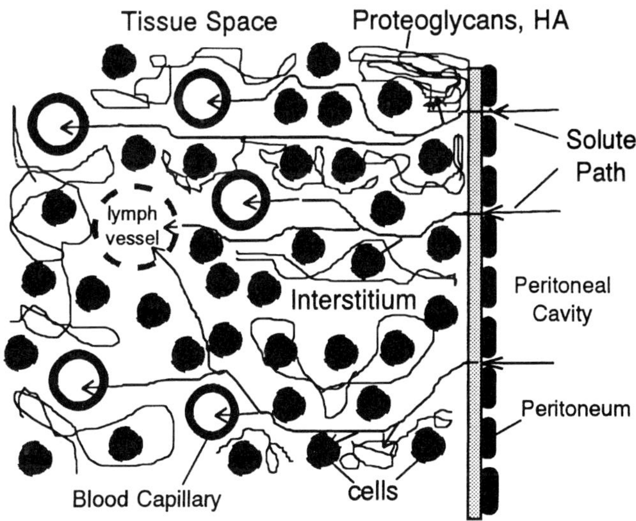

Fig. 36.2. Distributed model concept in which blood flows through exchange capillaries, which are distributed uniformly in the tissue surrounding the peritoneal cavity. Drugs introduced into the peritoneal cavity are transported into the surrounding tissue interstitium. From the tissue interstitium, the solutes transfer into either blood capillaries (small molecules) or lymphatic capillaries (the pathway for macromolecules). Solutes may also be taken up and metabolized by cells in the tissue or bound to the extracellular matrix, which is made up of proteoglycans and hyaluronan (HA).

Distributed Model Concept: Anatomic Barriers to Transport

Figure 36.2 illustrates an idealized cross section of tissue through which substances transport from the peritoneal cavity to targeted cells or extracellular matrix or are removed from the tissue by lymphatics or by blood capillaries. The lymphatics are the chief route of removal for macromolecules (>20,000 daltons) while the more important route for smaller solutes (<10,000 daltons) is the system of blood capillaries. The concept illustrated in Fig. 36.2 is often termed "the distributed model" because the blood and lymphatic capillary systems are distributed throughout the subperitoneal tissue space. In this model, drugs in solution in the cavity transport across the peritoneum and into the tissue space via diffusion and convection (solvent drag). Once in the interstitium, the solute continues to diffuse passively in accordance with its concentration gradient and is subject to convection by the solvent flow present. As each substance moves through the interstitium, uptake and metabolism by cells may occur.

Solutes may also interact with the extracellular matrix, which is made up of a collagen framework with hyaluronan (HA) bound to or associated with the framework and glycoaminoglycans bound to the HA. As they transport through the tissue space, solutes not taken up into cells or bound in the extracellular space transport into blood or lymphatic capillaries and are return to the central venous system. Although the blood and lymph capillaries are illustrated as uniformly distributed in the tissue space, there is considerable variation among the different tissues. Lymphatics, for example, tend to be located in the tissue planes between layers of muscle; in contrast, they are more diffusely located in the wall of the gut.[12]

Peritoneum

The peritoneum itself does not present any more barrier than the equivalent thickness of the cellular and interstitial layer that underlies it. A recent review detailed several studies of transmesenteric permeability.[13] The mesentery is essentially a double-walled fold of peritoneum with a small amount of connective tissue and vessels between the layers, and it has been used as a surrogate for the peritoneum, which is difficult to dissect from the surrounding tissues. Unfortunately, in vitro permeabilities tend to be unreliable because mesothelial cells degrade quickly in vitro and detach from the remainder of the peritoneum.[14] However, the permeability of the peritoneum can be assessed indirectly. Zink and Greenway[15] were the first to demonstrate that solutions containing 8% serum albumin are readily absorbed without change in protein concentration in the cavity.[15] Absorption of solutions containing immunoglobulin G occurs in the same way without sieving of the protein at the peritoneum.[16] In the past there have been proposals[17] that protein is transported across via vesicles. However, other histologic studies have demonstrated intermesothelial gaps of approximately 50 nm,[18] which would offer little resistance to the passage of macromolecules. Functional studies[19] have shown that labeled iron coupled to transferrin transports across the mesothelium without dissociation. Because dissociation of the iron from the apoprotein would occur if the protein were taken up in an acidic compartment of the vesicle, it is unlikely that this transport occurs via endocytic vesicles.

Because of the large intercellular gaps, the mesothelium also does not present a barrier to the osmotic agent glucose. Therefore, the same osmotically induced transport mechanism that occurs across renal epithelium cannot be invoked for the peritoneum, because there is no retardation of the transmesothelial transport of the glucose. This concept is further supported by the fact that interstitial hydrostatic pressures adjacent to the peritoneum are not negative as one would anticipate if water were extracted by osmosis across a membrane.[20] Our laboratory has just completed a set of unpublished experiments in which the peritoneum is mechanically removed and osmotic water flow is induced with a hypertonic solution containing 4% mannitol; the removal of the peritoneum did not influence the rate of positive flow out of the tissue toward the cavity. As the anatomic peritoneum is not a significant barrier to transport, this leaves the blood capillary endothelium and the interstitium as the major resistances to transport.

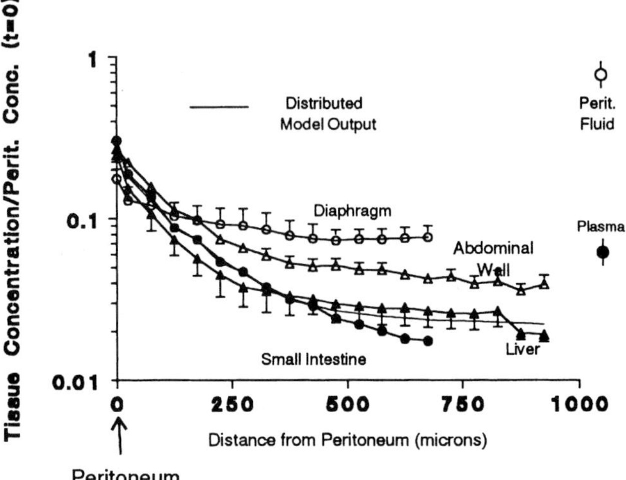

FIG. 36.3. Tissue concentration profiles of ^{14}C-EDTA (342 daltons) in tissues surrounding the peritoneal cavity after a 60-min dwell of a solution at an i.p. pressure of 3–4 cm H_2O. Tissue levels at $x = 0$ (the peritoneal edge) are lower than the peritoneal concentration because of the exclusion of the solute from the cells and a portion of the extracellular space. The model used to fit the data took into account diffusion through the tissue and simultaneous capillary uptake. (Data from Flessner et al.[21])

Interstitium

After transporting across the peritoneum, the solute enters the tissue interstitium, through which it must move toward the blood or lymph capillaries (see Fig. 36.2). Studies in rats that employed quantitative autoradiography to measure tissue concentration profiles have demonstrated that the tissue concentration of ^{14}C-EDTA (approximately the molecular size of sucrose), which is injected i.p. and allowed to diffuse into the surrounding tissue for 60 minutes, does not approach the plasma concentration until at a distance of 500 to 800 mm from the peritoneum (Fig. 36.3).[21] As the rat peritoneum is 25 mm thick, the finding that the concentration profile extends to hundreds of microns suggests that a large number of the capillaries contained within the underlying tissue are actively involved with the transport. Because individual capillaries are located at variable distances from the cavity, the barrier presented by the interstitium will vary depending on the location of the capillary with respect to the peritoneum.

Studies of gas transfer from the cavity support the principle that the interstitial barrier is significant. If inert gases in the peritoneal cavity equilibrate with the blood flowing in capillaries, their rate of transfer should be the same and proportional to the rate of local blood flow, if the interstitium is an insignificant part of the barrier. Collins[22] measured the simultaneous clearance of several inert gases from the peritoneal cavity of piglets and found a threefold range of gas transfer rate. The clearance rate of each gas was proportional to its diffusivity in water, which implied that gas transport was limited by diffusional barriers of the interstitium in conjunction with the blood capillary wall.

The interstitial barrier among peritoneal tissues depends on the density of the cells and of the extracellular matrix and varies with the pressure forces on the tissue. During its transit through the interstitium, the solute is excluded from much of the tissue space by cells, collagen fibers, and large molecular weight interstitial matrix proteins, called glycosaminoglycans. Small solutes such as sucrose (360 daltons) are restricted to as little as 20% of the extravascular space.[23,24] Large solutes such as albumin (58,000 daltons) are excluded from approximately 90% of the extravascular space.[24] This tissue exclusion results in proportionate decreases in the rate of diffusion. Added to this is the tortuous path of the solute, which has been estimated to be two to three times the linear distance between two points[25,26] and causes further reduction of rates of transport. Depending on the solute charge, it may be further retarded in its progress through the matrix maze. The result of the exclusion phenomena, the tortuosity, and the charge effect is a decrease in the rate of diffusion by one to two orders of magnitude. The effective diffusivity, or *D*, is defined by the product of the diffusivity within the interstitium times the nonexcluded fraction of tissue that is available to solute. Figure 36.4 displays the estimated diffusivities in tissue in the interstitium versus molecular weight from a variety of studies.[13] The diffusivities in water are plotted for comparison.

With significant amounts of fluid in the cavity (>1000 mL in human adults), the hydrostatic pressure rises in the cavity (Fig. 36.5).[27,28] The pressure varies within the tissue space, depending on the tissue and on distance from the peritoneum; this is most pronounced in the abdominal wall, where the full hydrostatic pressure inside the cavity is exerted across the tissue (Fig. 36.6). Figure 36.7 displays the interstitial hydrostatic pressure profile in the abdominal wall in a rat in which the i.p. pressure is held constant at 6 mm Hg.[20] Note that the curves are the same whether the solution in the cavity is isotonic or hypertonic (450 mosm/kg with 4% mannitol). If the peritoneum were a significant barrier to mannitol or dextrose, the tissue pressure adjacent to the peritoneum would be well below zero for the first few hours after introducing the hypertonic solution.[29] That the curves are the same adds further evidence that the mesothelium–peritoneum is not an osmotic barrier to small solutes such as dextrose.

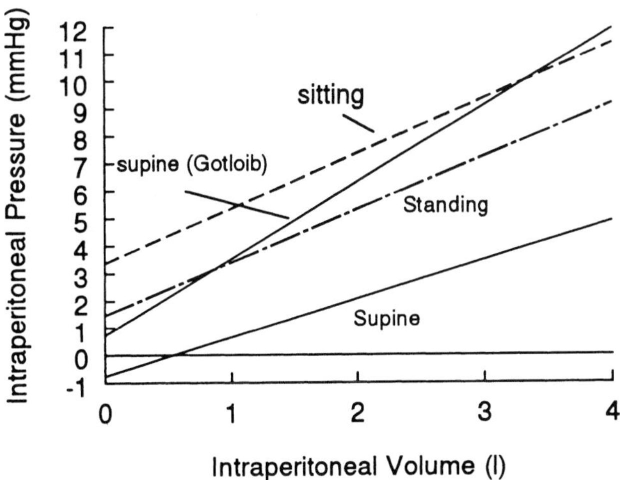

FIG. 36.5. Hydrostatic pressure (i.p.) measured in dialysis patients in various positions (derived from Gotloib et al.,[27] curve is labeled; or Twardowski et al.,[28] curves unlabeled). The major difference between the supine curves of the two studies was that Gotloib's patients[27] likely had larger residual volumes in their peritoneal cavity and this was not accounted for in the volume data. The figure demonstrates how the i.p. pressure rises with i.p. volume.

Figure 36.8 displays data from a study in rats[11] in which isotonic solution containing labeled immunoglobulin G was placed into the peritoneal cavity; the catheter into the cavity was connected to a reservoir that was raised and lowered to exert a constant hydrostatic pressure referenced to the right side of the heart. After 3 hours the animals were killed and volume absorbed during the 3 hours was determined. In addition, the concentration of the protein in the cavity, plasma, and abdominal wall tissue was measured. The protein concentration in the cavity was constant throughout the experiment, as observed by Zink[15] in cats. As the i.p. pressure was increased, the rate of volume flow from the cavity rose proportionately. The deposition of the protein into the abdominal wall muscle paralleled the flow rate curve, implying that the flow of protein into this tissue is unhampered by the

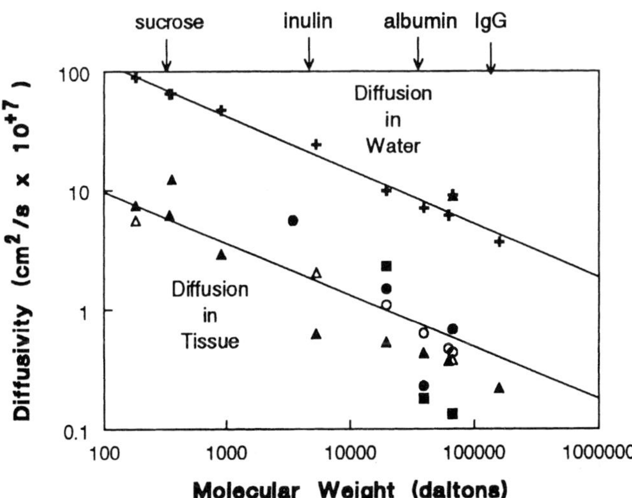

FIG. 36.4. Diffusivity (coefficient in the diffusion equation) versus molecular weight. Solutes are water soluble. The plot demonstrates that the diffusion in tissue is at least an order of magnitude smaller than the diffusion in water alone. (Data from Flessner.[13])

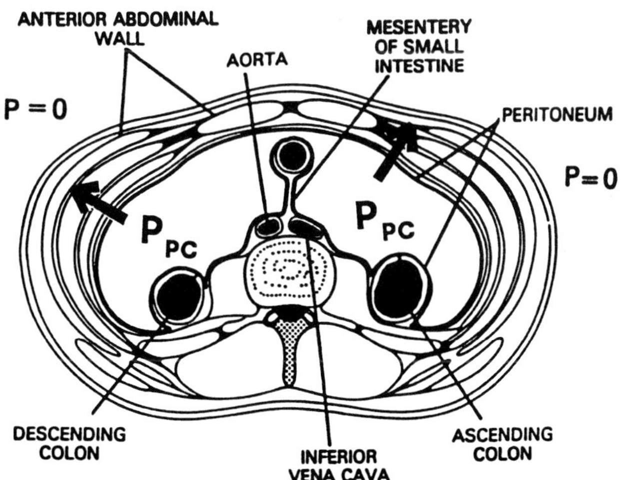

FIG. 36.6 Cross section of the cavity below the transverse colon. With the presence of fluid in the cavity, a pressure gradient is set up from the cavity into all surrounding tissue and is of greatest magnitude across the abdominal wall. This pressure gradient causes large solutes and water to flow into the surrounding tissue.

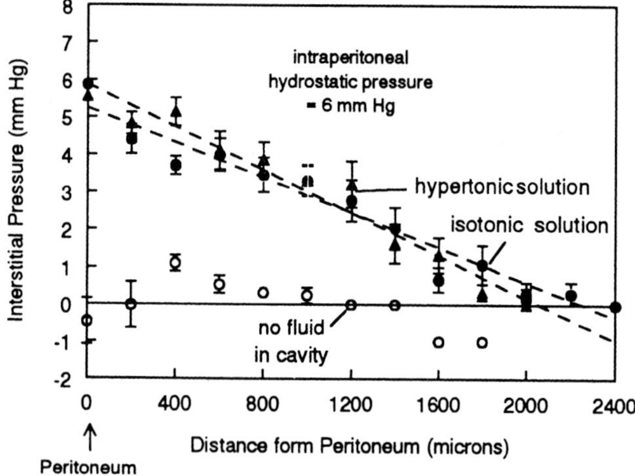

FIG. 36.7. Hydrostatic pressure gradients in the abdominal wall of rats at 0 and 6 mmHg i.p. pressure. Note that the pressure gradient is nearly identical with either an isotonic or hypertonic solution (450 mOsm/kg). (Data replotted from Flessner.[20])

peritoneum and is primarily dependent on the pressure gradient in the tissue that was generated by the i.p. pressure. Analogous studies in stable peritoneal dialysis patients have demonstrated that protein is absorbed from the cavity with 2-L dwells, which should exert i.p. pressures of 2 to 10 mmHg (see Fig. 36.5), at a rate of 60 to 90 mL/hour.[30–32]

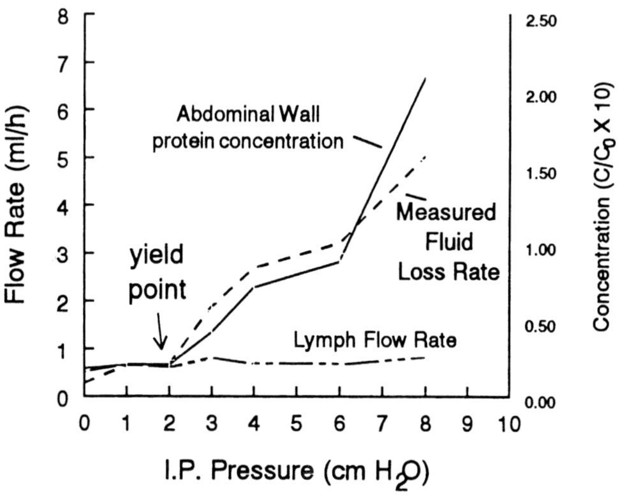

FIG. 36.8. Data from rat experiments in which the fluid in the cavity was held at constant pressure and the fluid loss rate from the cavity was determined.[11] A portion of this loss results from lymphatic removal, which does not appear to be affected by the i.p. pressure. The pressure was referenced to the right heart and demonstrated a "yield point" at 2 cm H_2O. Above this pressure, the fluid entry into the tissue overwhelms the ability of the lymphatics to remove it. Protein deposition in the abdominal wall signifies fluid transport into the tissue and appears to parallel the overall flow rate from the cavity. Results for hypertonic solutions paralleled the results for isotonic solutions.

Blood Capillary

The blood capillary endothelium with its basement membrane is the major size-selective barrier in the transport system between the peritoneal cavity and the blood. The capillary barrier depends on the tissue type, which determines the capillary density (surface area per unit volume of tissue) and the capillary permeability. Although the liver has a capillary permeability times area density of nearly 40 fold that of skeletal muscle[33] and capillaries of the gut mucosa are much more permeable that those of muscle,[33] most of the exchange between the intracavitary solution and the surrounding tissue is with muscle capillaries. The subserosal, outer layers of the gut are made up of muscle, as are the diaphragm and abdominal wall, which are attached to parietal peritoneum. Muscle capillaries, therefore, appear to be the dominant capillary exchange element, as most of the parietal tissue is equivalent to skeletal muscle (retroperitoneum, abdominal wall, and diaphragm) and most of the visceral tissue is made up of the gastrointestinal tract with smooth muscle in the outer layers adjacent to the peritoneum.

The three-pore theory[34,35] of transcapillary transport has been applied to the peritoneal transport system. Figure 36.9 illustrates the essence of the theory, which attempts to account for the observed size discrimination and water flux of the peritoneal barrier. Imagine that we are looking at the capillary endothelium with the lumen to the right and the tissue interstitium on the left. The protein content (large circles) within the capillary is usually greater than in the interstitium while in peritoneal

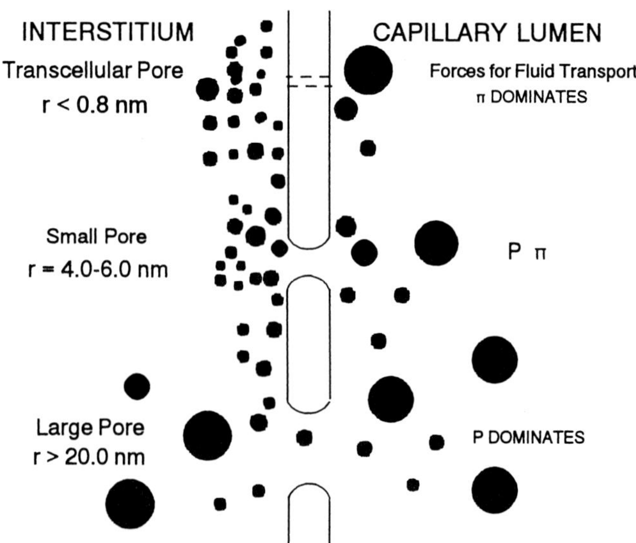

FIG. 36.9. Three-pore model of blood capillary transport. *r*, pore radius; *P*, hydrostatic pressure; π, osmotic pressure.

interstitium the concentration of dextrose or other small solutes (small circles) can be higher than in the capillary lumen.

If we focus on the very small pore at the top of the diagram, termed the transcellular pore, we see that no solutes but only water can pass through. All solutes exert the full potential osmotic pressure across the pore. The radius of this pore is of the order of 0.2 to 0.4 nm. Even if only 1% to 2% of the pores are of this type, as much as 40% of the filtration induced by a hypertonic glucose solution in the peritoneal cavity can occur across these pores because they function as a true semipermeable membrane. The morphologic equivalent of the "water-only" pore is a new class of "aquaporin." The existence of this structure was found by Agre and his colleagues in the red cell membrane and termed the CHIP-28 molecule.[36] CHIP-28 is also located in the mammalian kidney (proximal tubule and the descending thin limb of the nephron), in the eye (ciliary and lens epithelium, corneal endothelium), in the gastrointestinal tract (hepatic bile duct, gallbladder epithelium), in eccrine sweat glands, in lymphatic endothelium, and in nonfenestrated endothelia.[36]

The next pore to discuss is the "small" pore that allows passage of small substances (molecular radius, <1.3 nm, up to the size of molecules such as inulin) but severely restricts proteins. Here, a small part of the osmotic pressure of the small solutes and the full oncotic pressure is exerted across these pores, as well as the hydrostatic pressure. The intercellular junction is the morphologic equivalent of the small pore and has a radius of 4 to 6 nm.[37] Approximately 90% to 93% of the total pore area is likely made up of the small pores, and they are responsible for the majority of fluid transport.

The large pore (radius >20 nm) at the bottom of Fig. 36.9 is responsible for most of the protein transport out of the circulation. Gunnar Grotte, a Swedish physiologist, was the first to propose in 1956 that the capillary endothelia had to possess large leaks or pores that would allow passage of large proteins and dextrans.[38] Others proposed that this transport occurred by vesicular transport. Jens Frokhar-Jensen[39] subsequently carried out rigorous electron microscopic studies in which he sequentially sectioned capillary endothelia in 7.5-nm sections from the interstitium to the lumen. He found that so-called vesicular transporters were in fact blind invaginations into the cell, which appeared to be circular "vesicles" on cross section. However, a few of these (1/50,000) could be observed to fuse together to form a large pore. These pores offer no resistance to the passage of small solutes and minimal resistance to large solutes, and they account for 3% to 5% of the total pore area.

There is essentially no osmotic or oncotic force across the pore and therefore hydrostatic pressure dominates in the Starling relationship. Typical capillary hydrostatic pressures vary from 9.5 mmHg in the rat[40] to 18 mmHg in the human.[39] The interstitial pressures are typically −0.4 to −0.5 mmHg[41,42] for both species. Therefore, transport is one way out of the capillary because there is almost always a 10-mmHg hydrostatic pressure gradient out of the capillary. Because their transport is dominated by convection under normal conditions, large proteins pass from the circulation to the interstitium but do not return. The chief role for lymphatics within the tissue is the return of this protein and fluid from the interstitium to the general circulation. Although fluid and small solutes are carried out with the protein in the convection through the large pore, the total solute or fluid flow is small compared with that through the other two pores.[35]

To estimate the relative contribution of the capillary wall and the interstitium to the total peritoneal transport resistance during steady-state conditions, we define the following relationship for small solutes (<5000 daltons), which transport primarily by diffusion:[43]

$$R_{total} = \frac{1}{P_{capillary}} + \frac{diffusion\ length}{D} \tag{3}$$

where $p_{capillary}$ is the permeability of the capillary, and the diffusion distance is the distance between the capillary and the peritoneal cavity. Using $p_{capillary} = 3.2 \times 10^{-4}$ cm/min,[33] and $D = 4 \times 10^{-6}$ cm²/min for a solute of the size of sucrose,[23] estimates of the total transport resistance that is caused by the interstitium have been calculated for various distances from the peritoneum.[43] At a minimal distance of 50 μm, the interstitial contribution to the total resistance is 29%, at 100 μm, 44%; at 300 μm, 71%; and at 600 μm, 83%. For small solutes, therefore, the interstitium presents a significant barrier. Estimates of the interstitial barrier for larger solutes, such as proteins, are complicated by the fact that their transport may be a combination of diffusion and convection coupled with binding to constituents in the tissue. As discussed later, there are limited data with which to model and calculate the transport of large molecules.

Lymphatics

The lymph system is important for the return of macromolecules from the tissue interstitium to the blood. As seen from Fig. 36.8, lymph flow, which is calculated from the clearance of protein from the cavity to the blood, was not affected by hydrostatic pressure. Note should be made of the "yield point" of 2 cm H_2O, at which the flow rate increases at a significantly higher rate and exceeds the ability of the lymph to carry away the incoming fluid. Beyond the yield point, the tissue interstitium must expand because of the influx and retention of fluid not passed immediately to the lymph. Other tissues, such as the rabbit knee synovium, also display the property that flow through the tissue increases considerably when a certain threshold pressure is passed.[44] Studies in peritoneal dialysis patients have also displayed a similar pattern of rates of absorption (60–90 mL/h) of protein that are significantly greater than the calculated rate of lymph flow (10–20 mL/h)[30,31] Even with hypertonic solutions (500 mOsm/kg), which cause a net increase in fluid volume in the peritoneal cavity, the deposition of protein in the abdominal wall and the rates of lymph flow were not different from those in Fig. 36.8.[11]

Pharmacokinetic Models

A general mathematical expression, which incorporates several elements affecting transport through the tissue space, is given by

$$\textit{Rate of mass transfer} = R_{diffusion} + R_{convection} - R_{binding} - R_{metabolism} - R_{capillary} \quad (4)$$

where R_i is the specific rate expression governing the process within the tissue space specified in the subscript. Diffusion is the movement of molecules from areas of high concentration to areas of lower concentration. The typical mathematical expression consists of a diffusivity multiplied by the concentration gradient in the tissue or a mass transfer coefficient times a concentration difference. Convection is the process by which the solute moves or is "dragged" by the flow of the solvent, which in the body is water. It does not depend on concentration gradients but is driven by pressure gradients in the tissue that result in the flow. Most mathematical expressions incorporate some form of Darcy's law, which relates the fluid flow (Q) to the hydraulic conductivity of the tissue (K), the cross-sectional area of the tissue (A), and the pressure gradient in the tissue (dP_T/dx):[44]

$$Q = KA\frac{dP_T}{dx} \quad (5)$$

To find $R_{convection}$, Q would be multiplied by the concentration in the tissue space and a coefficient to account for slowing of the solute relative to the solvent as it moves through the tissue. The processes of binding, metabolism (which can be intracellular or extracellular), and capillary uptake (either blood capillaries or lymphatics) are all processes by which the solute is removed from the state of free transport through the tissue. Each of these processes of removal may have the effect of accelerating the process of diffusion by decreasing the concentration in the tissue and thereby increasing the concentration gradient of the free solute. On the other hand, if most of the agent is removed in the first few cell layers in the tissue, then more remote regions may not receive the agent. If the target is located deeper in the tissue, then there may in effect be an additional barrier of metabolism, capillary uptake, binding, or some combination of these processes that prevents the agent from reaching its goal. The goal of the following discussion is not the presentation of mathematical details of these expressions, which are better left to those who specialize in this area. Rather, the purpose of the following paragraphs are to make the reader aware of the factors during i.p. therapy that can influence the transport process.

Small Solute Transport: Combining the Membrane and Distributive Approaches

The conceptual model in Fig. 36.1 or "membrane" model is appropriate if the goal is the prediction of compartmental concentrations. In its simplest mathematical form, the rate of transfer across the barrier is defined by a diffusive model that employs a mass transfer-area coefficient (MTAC) times the concentration difference:

$$\textit{Rate of mass transfer} = MTAC(C_P - C_B) \quad (6)$$

where t is time. Certain assumptions are implied in this equation: (a) that there is no limitation by blood flow to the peritoneal tissues; (b) that all the transfer across the peritonuem can be lumped into the one parameter, MTAC; and (c) that there is no binding, metabolism, or transfer to the intracellular compartment. If the MTAC is known for a particular drug or is endogenous, the rate of transfer can be calculated with Eq. 6. For solutes with molecular weight less than 10,000, Eq. 6 can be used to calculate the transfer in either direction of transport, that is, either plasma to peritoneal cavity or peritoneal cavity to plasma. This model is most useful for the prediction of concentrations in either compartment, once the MTAC is specified.

Transport of small substances from the peritoneal cavity can also be viewed as a process of diffusion from the fluid in the cavity into the adjacent tissues, followed by absorption from the tissue extracellular space into blood in the exchange vessels (see Fig. 36.2). Convection generally does not play a quantitatively significant role for small solutes, and lymphatic uptake is negligible compared with removal from the tissue by the blood flowing in capillaries. The result is that a concentration profile is established within the tissue (see Fig. 36.3). At steady state, the rate of diffusion down the profile at any location is exactly balanced by the removal by flowing blood. For a solute that undergoes no metabolism in the tissue but is taken up by a uniformly distributed capillary network, the rate of uptake into blood perfusing the tissue may be calculated from the following equation, which is written for a specific "tissue":[45]

$$\textit{Rate of mass transfer to tissue} = \sqrt{D_{tissue}(pa)_{tissue}}\, A_{tissue}(C_P - C_B) \quad (7)$$

where the net rate of uptake of the solute into the tissue is in μg/min, D_{tissue} is the the effective diffusivity of the solute in the tissue (cm^2/min), $(pa)_{tissue}$ is the the product of the intrinsic permeability of the blood capillaries times the capillary surface area per unit tissue volume

($cm^3\ min^{-1}\ cm^{-3}$), A_{tissue} is the the superficial surface area of the tissue exposed to peritoneal fluid (cm^2), C is the the free solute concentration ($\mu g/cm^3$), and the subscripts P and B refer to peritoneal fluid and blood (or plasma), respectively. The effective diffusivity is equal to the diffusivity in the tissue interstitial space multiplied by the tissue fractional interstitial space, which is available to the solute.

A number of observations may be made about Eq. 7. First, the rate of solute transfer is proportional to the square root of the effective diffusivity, the capillary permeability, and the capillary surface area; doubling of the capillary permeability, for example, would be expected to be associated with only a 41% increase in mass transfer ($2^{1/2} = 1.41$). Second, the net transport rate is directly proportional to the superficial area of the tissue in contact with the fluid. A doubling of the surface area of the tissue will result in a doubling of the total amount of mass transfer. Third, the rate of transport is proportional to the difference in the free concentration of solute between the peritoneal fluid and blood.

Equation 7 serves as the basis for the definition of an equivalent MTAC of the tissue. In practice, the area in contact with the fluid is not known, but if it were, then $MTAC = MTC \times A_{tissue}$. Comparison of Eqs. 6 and 7 shows that the equivalent tissue MTC can be calculated from

$$MTC_{tissue} = \sqrt{D_{tissue}(pa)_{tissue}} \tag{8}$$

Either Eq. 6 or Eq. 7 can be used to calculate the rate of absorption of a drug from the peritoneal cavity into the blood because they are equivalent. Equations similar to Eqs. 6 and 7 can be written for as many types of peritoneal tissue as desirable. Because uptake rates into the various tissue types are parallel processes, the equations may be summed to calculate the overall rate of mass transfer. The distributed model concept of the tissue offers certain advantages because it provides some insight into the underlying transport mechanisms and how these might be altered by pathologic processes or pharmacologic manipulations. It also serves as a natural link to the literature on capillary physiology and provides a natural framework to incorporate this into descriptions and predictions of peritoneal transport rates. Further, it predicts that a concentration profile extends a finite depth into the tissue, and tissue penetration is an important consideration if the goal of intraperitoneal therapy is to treat disease in the tissue or disease of finite thickness such as peritoneal carcinomatosis on serosal surfaces. Explicitly, the concentration profile is given by[45]

$$\frac{C_{tissue} - C_B}{C_P - C_B} = \exp - \sqrt{\frac{(pa)_{tissue}}{D_{tissue}}}\, x \tag{9}$$

where x is the distance from the serosal surface.

The "A_{tissue}" of Eq. 7 is not equal to the topologic surface area of the peritoneum but to the area in contact with the fluid contained in the cavity. Chagnac and colleagues recently developed a new technique that utilizes stereologic methods combined with computed tomographic scanning of the peritoneal cavity filled with dialysate containing contrast fluid,[46] and their determinations in three patients produced a mean of 0.58 m^2; this is much less than the determinations of dissected tissue area that approach the total body area.[47]

Parameters for Calculation of Small Solute Transport

Variation of MTAC with Molecular Weight and Body Size

The value of MTAC has been calculated in numerous studies of peritoneal dialysis. The best data, therefore, exist for urea and creatinine, the common indicators of azotemia and physiologic markers that have been measured in these studies of anephric patients. Figure 36.10 shows some values of MTAC plotted against molecular weight.[48] The data vary approximately as the inverse of the square root of molecular weight. This result would be expected from the penetration model if the capillary permeability varies with the −0.63 power of molecular weight (Fig. 36.11) and the diffusivity in tissue varies with the −0.45 power of molecular weight observed for diffusion in water.[13] From this correlation, MTAC for sucrose would equal 8.5 cm/min; the MTAC for inulin would be 2.8 ml/min. Rubin et al.[49] measured the MTAC for inulin to be 3.3 mL/min in humans. Rubin's calculation, however, likely includes the convective component of blood-to-peritoneal cavity transport, and this would produce a higher value than that caused by diffusion alone.

Figure 36.12 shows the MTAC for urea and inulin for the rat, rabbit, dog, and human; these species cover a body weight range from 200 g to 70 kg.[8] The parameter increases as the 0.62 to 0.74 power of body weight for in-

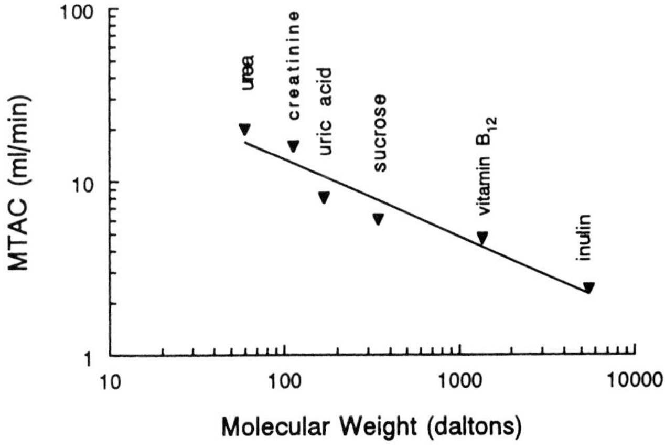

FIG. 36.10. Peritoneal mass transfer area coefficient (MTAC) versus molecular weight from human dialysis patients. (Adapted from Dedrick et al.[48])

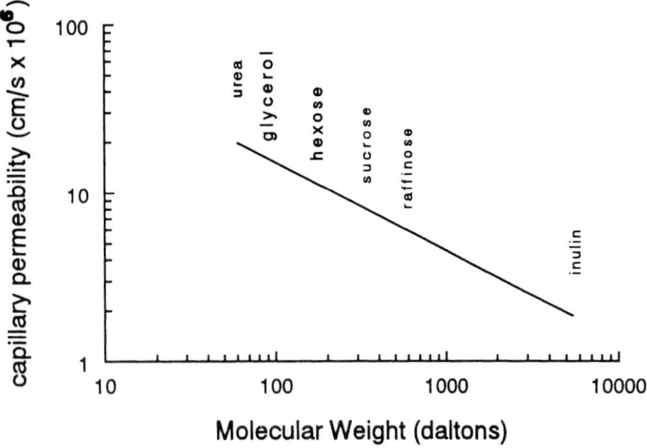

FIG. 36.11. Capillary permeability versus molecular weight. (Adapted from Dedrick et al.[45])

ulin and urea, respectively. The average of these two values is very close to the 2/3 expected for body surface area scaling. In a study of 10 patients with body surface areas ranging from 1.4 to 2.3 m². Keshaviah and colleagues[50] recently demonstrated a linear correlation between the volume at which MTAC was maximum and the body surface area. As the characteristic time for absorption from the peritoneal cavity is equal to V_p/MTAC, similar time scales can be achieved in humans and experimental animals if the volume is scaled as the 2/3 power of the body weight. For example, 2 L in the peritoneal cavity of the 70-kg human patient (29 mL/kg) would be equivalent to 40 ml in a 200-g rat (200 mL/kg) because $(200/70{,}000)^{2/3}(2000) = 40$. These scaling criteria permit the design of experiments that more accurately reflect in small animals intraperitoneal therapy which is carried out in humans.

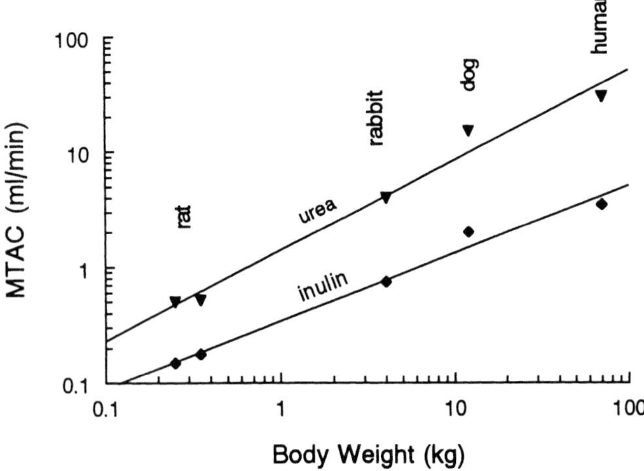

FIG. 36.12. Peritoneal mass transfer-area coefficient (MTAC) for urea and inulin versus body weight. (Adapted from Dedrick et al.[45])

Regional Values for MTC: Justification for Combining All Regions

Most peritoneal transport investigations are carried out as whole-cavity experiments, in which the cavity is filled with a solution and the rate of mass transfer is determined along with the concentrations in the cavity and the blood. The MTAC is calculated by dividing the rate of mass transfer by the concentration difference between the cavity and the blood. The area of contact of the fluid is unknown, and therefore the MTC cannot be separated from the A and the transfer coefficient is called the MTAC. To determine MTC values for specific tissues, isolation of the transport process to a specific area of the tissue must be carried out. To do this, experiments were carried out in anesthetized rats whose peritoneum was exposed surgically by laparotomy. Plastic chambers were affixed to portions of the peritoneum overlying the liver, cecum, stomach, and abdominal wall. The chamber was filled with an isotonic solution, which could be sampled during the experiment and the volume of which could be determined. Labeled mannitol was infused continuously i.v. or was mixed with the solution in the chamber. By measuring the volume in the chamber and the mannitol concentration versus time, the rate of appearance of mannitol into the chamber or the rate of disappearance from the chamber could be calculated. By determining the mannitol concentration in the plasma and after substituting the chamber and plasma concentrations and area of the base of the chamber for C_P, C_B, and A_{tissue} in Eq. 6, MTC could be calculated.

The results demonstrated no significant difference among the four tissues and no dependence on the direction of transport (overall average = $2.14 \pm 0.37 \times 10^{-3}$ cm/min);[51] analogous results have been found for urea.[52] While the equivalence of transport directions (peritoneal cavity to blood and blood to peritoneal cavity) was anticipated, the equivalence of transport across the surface of diverse tissues was not. Subsequent studies of the tissue concentration profiles of these substances have demonstrated very similar results in each tissue (unpublished observations). If it is assumed that the human peritoneum is similar in its physiologic properties to the rat, then, where appropriate, these data justify the lumping of the surfaces together into one MTAC = $\Sigma_{all\ tissues}\ MTC \bullet A$. It also implies that the critical variable in determination of MTAC is the area which is in contact with the solution in the cavity.

Role of Capillary Permeability

Figure 36.10 shows that the MTAC for a 250-dalton hydrophilic drug in a human would be expected to be about 10 mL/min. If the peritoneal surface area is approximately 6000 cm², as has been discussed, then the average equivalent peritoneal permeability would be 1.7×10^{-3} cm/min. Figure 36.11 shows that the intrinsic permeability, p, of mammalian muscle capillaries is 10^{-5} cm/sec or 0.6×10^{-3} cm/min. The similarity between the values for *MTC* and p is probably fortuitous. Peritoneal transport appears to derive its selectivity partly from the properties of the capillaries; however, the quantitative contribution of the capillaries must be interpreted in conjunction with diffusion into the tissues as shown in Eqs. 7 and 9.

Lipid Solubility

Lipid solubility of a drug is a major factor in the rate of transfer of a drug from the cavity into the surrounding tissue and the blood. Torres et al.[53] measured the absorption of model compounds dissolved in 50 mL of saline in the rat. As the heptane–water partition coefficient (K_{hep}) increased above 0.001, they found that the rate of absorption increased significantly. Barbital with a K_{hep} of 0.001 was observed to have an absorption of 57% at the end of 1 hour. On the other hand, thiopental, with a K_{hep} of 3.3, had an absorption of 96% at the end of 1 hour. Other studies with the lipid-soluble drugs hexamethylmelamine in the mouse[54] and thioTEPA in human subjects[55] have demonstrated peritoneal clearances about an order of magnitude greater than would be expected for hydrophilic drugs. Unfortunately, capillary permeabilities and tissue diffusivities are not available for these compounds.

Blood Flow: Does It Limit Transperitoneal Transport?

Current estimates of the effective blood flow in the tissue surrounding the peritoneal cavity suggest that transport between the blood and the cavity is not limited by the supply of blood. Physiologists have attempted to determine the "effective" blood flow by measuring the clearances of various gases from the peritoneal cavity, assuming that these were limited by blood flow only. Gas clearances of hydrogen[56,57] and CO_2[58] have been measured in small mammals and observed to equal 4% to 7% of the cardiac output. However, this method of determining the effective peritoneal blood flow may actually underestimate the true blood flow. As was discussed earlier, Collins[22] studied absorption of several inert gases from peritoneal gas pockets in pigs and found almost a threefold range in clearance, which correlated with the gas diffusivity in water. The clearance of each gas would have been the same if the transport of these gases was limited by blood flow. Because the transport of these gases is not limited by blood flow, diffusion in the tissue is a significant portion of the total resistance. Therefore, gas clearance data underestimate the true peritoneal blood flow, and the conclusion, based on lumped clearance data, would be that blood flow limitation in the peritoneal cavity is unlikely.

Findings based on the lumped clearance data, however, does not rule out specific limitations in a portion of the peritoneal cavity, which may be offset by another set of tissues. To investigate the possibility of blood flow limitation of transport across specific surfaces of the peritoneum, the chamber technique (discussed earlier under Regional Values for MTCs) was utilized to answer the question of "local" limitations of blood flow on urea transport across the liver, stomach, cecum, and abdominal wall. Urea was chosen because it is a small molecule that should diffuse rapidly because of its small molecular weight and which would be more likely to demonstrate blood flow limitations. The mass transfer rates of urea were measured under conditions of control blood flow, blood flow reduced by 50% to 80%, and no blood flow (postmortem); the blood flow was monitored simultaneously with laser Doppler flowmetry.

While all four tissues demonstrated marked decreases in urea transport after cessation of blood flow, only the liver displayed a decrease in the rate of transfer during periods of reduced blood flow. Further studies with the chamber technique tested the effects of blood flow on osmotically induced water flow from the same four tissues; small but statistically nonsignificant decreases in water flow in the cecum, stomach, and abdominal wall were observed.[59] Analogous to the solute data, the liver demonstrated a significant drop in water transfer with reduced blood flow. Thus transport of both solute and water across the surface of the liver is limited by blood flow. This restriction however does not appear to affect the overall transperitoneal transport, because the elimination of the surface area of the liver has been recently shown to have only a small effect on the overall transport.[60] These data support and extend earlier studies of peritoneal dialysis in dogs during conditions of shock,[61] and support the use of peritoneal dialysis for solute or fluid removal during periods of low systemic blood pressure in which blood perfusion of the organs surrounding the peritoneal cavity is likely to be low.

Contact Surface Areas Available for Transport

In studies in which the peritoneal tissues were dissected from cadavers and their area determined by planimetry, the peritoneal surface area of the adult human has been estimated to be of the order of 1 to 2 m^2.[47,62,63] Of this value, the surface of the liver constitutes about 6% to 13% (range of averages from the two references), the diaphragm 4% to 8%, and the peritoneal walls, 11% (anterior abdominal wall, 7%). Corresponding percentages for the 595 cm^2 surface area of the adult rat were liver, 16%; diaphragm, 3%; and peritoneal walls, 19%.[51,62] From Eq. 7, the rate of transfer depends directly on the actual area in contact with the dialysis fluid. In studies with rodents,[51] the MTCs for different surfaces were determined as well as the dissected areas (presumed to equal the maximum area available to the dialysis fluid) of the entire peritoneum. When the values for MTC were multiplied by the corresponding dissected areas and summed, the resulting number was three to four times the MTAC obtained with a volume corresponding to 2000 mL in a human (40–50 mL in 200- to 300-g rats).

Separate animals were dialyzed with solution containing an intensely staining dye to detect which surfaces were in contact with the fluid. Large parts of the peritoneum had no staining, including one side of the cecum, one side of the stomach, and large parts of the abdominal wall and diaphragm.[51] Independent investigators[64,65] measured the rate of transport of urea, creatinine, and glucose in rats at rest or vigorously agitated and found a three- to fourfold increase in MTAC with vigorous movement; the authors presumed that the agitation was breaking up "unstirred layers." If it is assumed that the experimental maneuvers to increase the MTAC do not change MTC, these studies all imply that only 25% to 30% of the anatomic peritoneum is available to the dialysis solution during quiescent conditions. The single study in humans,[46] from which the wetted area in three patients was estimated to be 0.6 m^2, would appear to agree with the principle that wetted area is significantly less than that of the dissected area.

The volume in the cavity and the body size are major determinants of wetted area. In the study by Keshaviah and colleagues[50] in 10 patients in which the MTACs for urea, creatinine, and glucose were determined for different dwell volumes varying from 500 to 3000 mL, a nearly linear relationship was found between MTAC and dialysate volume until a peak at 2500 to 3000 mL of "true dialysate volume." Although there was no way to separate *MTC* from *A*, the authors attributed the correlation to an increase in *A* with increasing peritoneal volume.

Contact with the entire peritoneal area is a major problem in cancer chemotherapy within the peritoneal cavity. Presumably, metastatic disease can occur anywhere on the surface, but there is no guarantee that the area of contact between the fluid containing the therapeutic agent and the area of the metastatic lesion will overlap. As reviewed recently,[66] studies adequate to define the difference between the functional surface area and the anatomic surface area in human subjects have not been conducted. To increase the functional surface area and better expose targeted disease on serosal surfaces, a recent trial was conducted of continuous hyperthermic peritoneal perfusion with carboplatin in six patients with small-volume residual ovarian cancer.[67] Pharmacokinetic data adequate to calculate MTAC that were obtained from four patients demonstrated values which were approximately four times the value expected from published studies of conventional intraperitoneal carboplatin administration, consistent with the laboratory studies described earlier. Immediately after surgical debulking of the primary tumor, two peritoneal catheters were placed into the cavity. The perfusion technique involved rapid recirculation (1.5 L/min) of drug-containing solution through the peritoneal cavity by means of the two-catheter system combined with vigorous manual shaking of the abdomen. Temperature uniformity was documented with three probes. Because the solution temperature was maintained consistently greater than 40°C, an important effect of the elevated temperature on transport was not definitively excluded, but the authors argued that elevated temperature alone was unlikely to be the cause of the large increase in MTAC.

Macromolecular Transport Across the Peritoneum

Diagnosis and intraperitoneal treatment of metastatic carcinoma with monoclonal antibodies (MAbs) to the tumor have been areas of fertile investigation in the past.[68–70] Diagnosis of a tumor nodule is possible with surface adherence of the marker. However, treatment of a nodule that is several millimeters thick is challenging because the macromolecule will likely have to penetrate to all parts of the tumor to eliminate it. Other types of macromolecular agents may be required to penetrate deeper inside the tissue as well. Because diffusion of these large molecules is very slow, appreciable penetration into the tissue can only be obtained with convection. More than 90% of the tissue space is not available to these substances, and the interstitial matrix excludes these molecules from much of the interstitial space. Molecules such as immunoglobulins may bind to specific or nonspecific receptors or they may be taken up by cells and metabolized. Techniques of determination of the concentration in the tissue space rarely differentiate between whether a MAb is free to transport to a site or is bound within the tissue. Depending on the target of the therapy, the additional barriers of metabolism and binding may greatly affect the result of therapy.

Convection: The Major Mode of Macromolecular Transport

From Figs. 37.6 through 37.8 and Eq. 5, hydrostatic pressure is the major driving force for convection, the transport that is often called "solvent drag" and which is driven by water flow. IgG concentrations in the major tissues attached to the peritoneum in experiments in which i.p. pressure was maintained at 3 to 4 cm H_2O are shown in Fig. 36.13.[16] These data demonstrate the dependency of this deposition on time but relative independence of osmolality. The lack of dependence on solution osmolality means that standard dialysis solutions can be used to introduce the agent into the cavity without greatly affecting the deposition of drug. The rela-

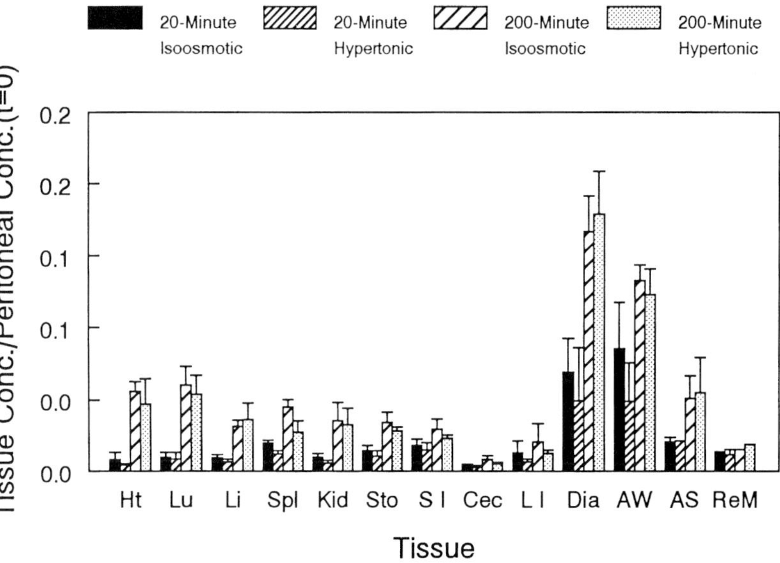

FIG. 36.13. Mean concentration of immunoglobulin G (IgG) in tissues surrounding the peritoneal cavity and in tissues outside the cavity. The IgG was dissolved in either an isotonic or hypertonic solution (initial osmolality, 450 mOsm/kg) and allowed to dwell in the peritoneal cavity of rats for 20 min or 200 min at an i.p. pressure of 3–4 cm H_2O. *Ht,* heart; *Lu,* lung; *Li,* liver; *Spl,* spleen; *Kid,* kidney; *Sto,* stomach; *SI,* small intestine; *Cec,* cecum; *LI,* large intestine; *Dia,* diaphragm; *AW,* anterior abdominal wall muscle; *AS,* skin overlying AW; *ReM,* retroperitoneal muscle.

tively high concentrations of protein in the abdominal wall are likely the result of the pressure gradient exerted by the pressure inside the cavity across the wall ($P_{IP} - 0$). Likewise the high concentrations in the diaphragm probably result from the pressure gradient and to the presence of the extensive subdiaphragmatic lymphatic system, which is made up of stomata that open during expiration and which allow fluid, solutes, and cells to flow into lacunae within the diaphragmatic parenchyma.[1,2] Upon inspiration, the diaphragm contracts, which closes the stomata and forces the initial lymph chiefly into the parasternal lymphatics, which drain to the right lymph duct and to the thoracic duct.[71]

The limited data on the effects of i.p. pressure on transport in patients appear to support the data from animal studies. In one set of experiments, the intraabdominal pressure of patients who were administered 2 L of dialysis fluid i.p. was increased by tightening a girdle that encircled the abdomen.[72] The pressure was raised from 8 to 18 mm Hg and the flow from the cavity increased from 64 mL/h to 112 mL/h. In another set of experiments, the pressure in the cavity was manipulated by changing the i.p. volume of solution and determination of the net fluid recovery versus i.p. pressure.[73] Because dialysis solutions are made hypertonic to withdraw water from the patient's body, the net fluid flow is usually toward the cavity. As has been discussed, animal experiments have shown that the hydrostatic pressure-driven flow from the cavity into the body is not affected by the osmotically induced flow outward from the tissue to the cavity.[11] Figure 36.14 displays the data from 33 patients in whom a 3.86% dextrose solution was allowed to dwell for 2 hours; it clearly demonstrates that the net fluid removal (often called net ultrafiltration by nephrologists) decreases as the i.p. pressure is raised.[73]

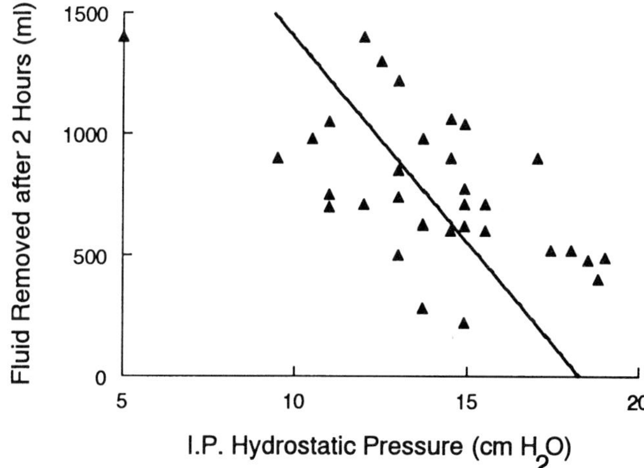

FIG. 36.14. Fluid removed after a 2-hour dwell of dialysis solution containing 3.86% glucose (400 mOsm/kg) in 33 patients. The hypertonic solution typically results in fluid removal from the patient. The negative slope versus i.p. pressure indicates that increased i.p. pressures decrease the fluid removed from the patient, presumably because of the phenomenon discussed in Fig. 37.8. (Data replotted from Durand et al.[73])

As has been discussed (see Fig. 36.8), the flow from the cavity at i.p. pressures above the threshold pressure (2 cm H_2O in rats) exceeds the ability of the lymphatic system to carry fluid from the tissue. Without radical alteration in the Starling forces, the fluid will accumulate in the tissue and the interstitial space will expand. Data from a study in rats (Fig. 36.7)[20] have demonstrated that the pressure profiles do not change sufficiently to explain the marked increase in fluid flow into the tissue as the i.p. pressure increases (Fig. 36.8). As noted in Eq. 5, Darcy's law relates the fluid flow (Q) to the hydraulic conductivity of the tissue (K), the cross-sectional area of the tissue (A), and the pressure gradient in the tissue (dP_T/dx).[44] Figure 36.15 displays in vivo data that were obtained in the rat abdominal wall,[72] a model tissue which our lab has used to explore the phenomena of convection in the interstitium. The overall pressure gradient across the wall was set by the level of i.p. pressure. At each pressure level, the hydraulic conductivity of the tissue or the interstitial space was determined. The volume flux into the tissue (flow rate divided by the peritoneal area in contact with the fluid) is plotted as well. The threshold pressure of 2 cm H_2O now not only signifies a point at which the flow into the tissue exceeds the lymph flow draining the tissue (see Fig. 36.8) but is also the transition point in the tissue space with simultaneous increases in the hydraulic conductivity, which governs the rate of water flow through tissue.

The fraction of space that is interstitium (θ_{if}) was calculated from the equilibrium distribution of labeled mannitol and is also plotted in Fig. 36.15. The expansion of the interstitium occurs at the same threshold pressure as that for hydraulic conductivity, and θ_{if} doubles between 2 and 4 cm H_2O. Because K depends on θ_{if}, it was anticipated that both variables would parallel each other in Fig. 36.15. However, θ_{if} levels off without further increase despite the continued rise in K (see following further discussion). The pressure gradients across the hollow viscera and solid organs that are within the peritoneal cavity are unknown. However, the pressures that are normally seen in peritoneal dialysis (PD) are well above the threshold pressure of 2 cm H_2O and likely cause considerable expansion in all tissue which is in

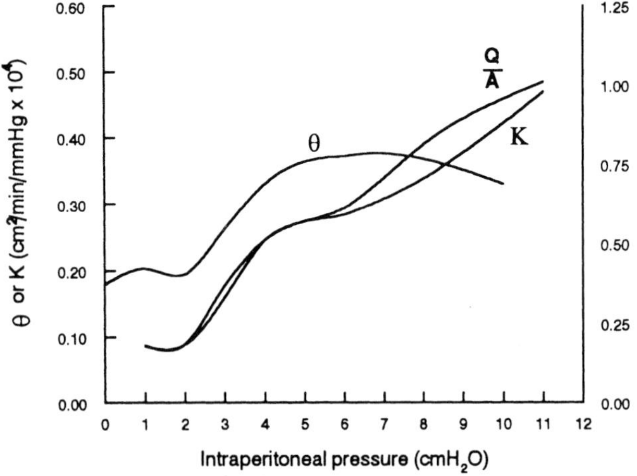

FIG. 36.15. Fluid under pressure in the rat peritoneal cavity results in swelling of the interstitial volume fraction (θ, mL/g tissue) and a marked increase in the fluid flux (Q/A) out of the cavity and the hydraulic conductivity of the tissue space (K). These changes in the tissue space occur at the yield point of i.p. pressure = 2 cm H_2O which was plotted in Fig. 37.8. Curves were derived from data in Zakaria et al.[74]

contact with the solution. If we can assume that human tissue responds to pressure in a similar fashion as does rat tissue, then the subperitoneal tissue during a large volume dwell is in an expanded state that facilitates penetration of large and small solutes into the tissue space. Because the transport coefficient for both diffusion and convection depend on θ_{if}, the interstitial resistance to diffusion and convection (solvent drag) is therefore variable depending on the interstitial pressure.

Not only does the hydrostatic pressure-driven fluid flow into the tissue result in expansion of the interstitial space but may cause changes in the extracellular matrix. K theoretically depends on both θ_{if} and the concentration of the matrix macromolecules in the interstitial space. Because of the discrepancy between the rise in hydraulic conductivity and that of θ_{if} in Fig. 36.15, experiments in rats were carried out to investigate the role of this convection on the concentration of an interstitial matrix component called hyaluronan (HA), which has a major role in tissue conductivity and a portion of which is mobile in the tissue.[75] The concentration of HA was determined in the abdominal wall in control rats, with no fluid in the peritoneal cavity, and in animals whose abdominal wall was exposed to an isotonic solution under a constant pressure of 6 cm H_2O for 2 hours. At the end of the experiment, portions of the abdominal wall immediately adjacent to the fluid were separated from the outer layers and the subcutaneous space. The inner layer of the anterior abdominal wall muscle was dissected free from the outer layer of muscle; the inner portion demonstrated a greater decrease in HA contents from 487 ± 16 μg/g dry tissue to 265 ± 40 μg/g dry tissue than the outer layer of abdominal wall muscle, which is decreased to only 349 ± 67 μg/g after dialysis at P_{ip} = 6 mmHg. The HA content in the full-thickness anterior abdominal muscle (AAM) specimen was reduced from 487 ± 16 μg/g dry tissue (n = 4) to 360 ± 27 μg/g dry tissue (n = 4; $p < 0.05$), and increased from 528 ± 72 μg/g dry tissue (n = 8) to 1050 ± 136 μg/g dry tissue (n = 4; $p < 0.001$) in the subcutaneous tissue. This result demonstrates an apparent movement of HA from the innermost part of the abdominal wall toward the subcutaneous space.[74]

Because HA is a major resistive element in the interstitium, its disappearance from the tissue will cause an increase in the rate of solute and water flow through the tissue space. Whether this effect on interstitial HA occurs in humans is unknown. Part of the problem is the lack of data on the in vivo metabolism of HA in tissue and the effects of pressure or the presence of sterile fluid on HA synthesis by the mesothelial cells or by fibroblasts within the tissue space. As outlined in a previous chapter (see Chapter 5), mesothelial cells in tissue culture have been observed to respond to inflammation by increasing their synthesis of HA. How this metabolism affects the underlying tissue or its transport properties is unknown.

From the previous discussion, we can now return to our tissue model (see Fig. 36.2). Not only is the basic structural unit of the peritoneal transfer system more complicated than the simple membrane model of Fig. 36.1, but there is now an overlying problem of variability of the tissue space with the pressure imposed by the fluid in the cavity. If the interstitial space swells with the flow of water into the tissue, the space available for solutes will increase. Therefore, rates of both diffusion and convection will be significantly affected by not only the driving forces (gradients of concentration and pressure) but also by the degree of tissue swelling caused by the presence of a large volume of solution in the cavity.

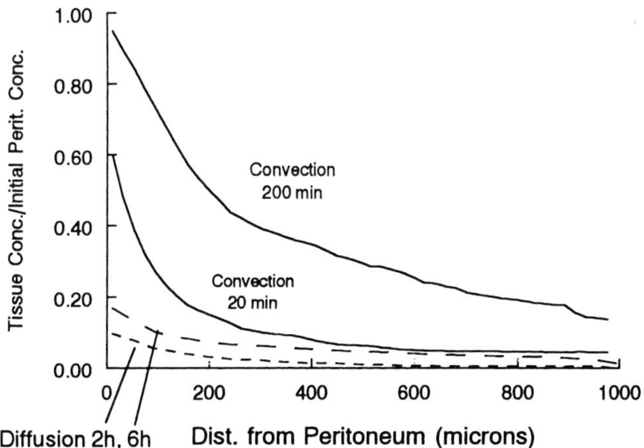

FIG. 36.16. Tissue concentration profiles of IgG in the rat abdominal wall. The peritoneum is at $x = 0$. Curves labeled *diffusion* resulted from experiments in which the solution was in contact with the tissue for 2 or 6 hours and there was no pressure in the cavity; curves labeled *convection* resulted from experiments in which the solution pressure was 3–4 cm H_2O and contact between the fluid and the tissue was maintained for 20 or 200 min. The large difference in magnitude illustrates how pressure-driven convection of large proteins dominates over diffusion. Curves were derived from data in Flessner et al.[77]

Diffusion Versus Convection of Macromolecules

The interstitial barrier includes exclusion of solute and water by the matrix macromolecules. Because of the effects of solutions under pressure in the cavity, the surrounding tissue interstitium may be considerably expanded during intraperitoneal chemotherapy or during dialysis. In addition, chronic exposure to fluids under pressure may also result in changes within the interstitium, which may influence the barrier characteristics. All these changes, which come about with large-volume solutions and the accompanying increased hydrostatic pressure, promote penetration of large molecular weight solutes. Aside from the fact that smaller volumes may provide less coverage of the peritoneal surface,[50] the difference between a low-volume–low i.p. pressure and a higher volume–higher pressure technique comes down to the mechanism of transport of the macromolecule. Figure 36.16 illustrates the resulting tissue concentration profiles for experiments in which a solution containing labeled IgG was introduced into the cavity either at 0 pressure, which should theoretically result in pure diffusion, or at 3 to 4 cm H_2O, which would produce convection in addition to diffusion. The solution was allowed to dwell in the cavity for periods ranging from 20 minutes to 6 hours. The curves from the zero i.p. pressure experiments are labeled diffusion only and are of lower magnitude at 6 hours than those at 20 minutes, with convection resulting from a relatively small amount of hydrostatic pressure-driving force. The curves resulting from primarily diffusive transport represent a rate of transport of approximately 10% of the convective rate.[76,77] These data clearly demonstrate the effect of convection on large solute transport.

Effects of Binding

Binding of the macromolecular agent, particularly immunoglobulins, must be considered to be a possibility whenever high concentrations are found in tissue. For example, in Fig. 36.16, the actual volume of distribution of IgG (volume in which IgG is free to transport divided by total tissue volume) in abdominal wall muscle has been determined to be 0.04 to 0.05 mL/g tissue.[77] Even in an expanded state at an i.p. pressure of 3 to 4 cm H_2O, the fraction of the tissue available to IgG is likely no more that 0.10 mL/g tissue. The high concentration of tracer observed in the tissue (any concentration $>0.05-0.1$) can only result from accumulation caused by convection or binding of the tracer to sites in the tissue. In the case of the diffusion curves, this apparent accumulation must be the result of binding. Using an in vitro technique, the binding of the IgG (which had been chosen for the experiments because of its lack of specific binding to rat tissue) was found to account for the apparent accumulation of tracer in the tissue.[77]

Much of the concentration observed in the diffusion plus convection curves is also caused by binding. In tracer concentrations, the IgG was found to bind to the abdominal wall tissue in a nonspecific, nonsaturable fashion with a binding coefficient of 0.0065 min^{-1} multiplied by the duration of the exposure of the tissue to the immunoglobulin. If an overabundance of IgG was added, the binding constant becomes time independent and equals 0.042.[77] Theoretical predictions of the effects of binding in the tissue have demonstrated that a type of "binding-site" barrier actually impedes the transport of antibodies through the tissue.[78,79] This type of binding is often not accounted for in papers that report penetration data after many hours of tissue exposure to a solution containing a biologic agent. Failure to account for the binding may lead to the wrong conclusion that there is an overabundance of IgG or other macromolecular agent that is free to move about in the interstitium.

Metabolism in the Tissue

An aspect of transperitoneal pharmacokinetics, which has not received much attention, is metabolism of the agent in the tissue. Dextrose, for example, is used as an osmotic solute in peritoneal dialysis. As it diffuses into the tissue space, it is taken up not only by blood capillaries but also the muscle cells making up most of the subperitoneal tissue. Although rates of metabolism of dextrose in the tissue have not been formally determined, there is abundant evidence in the form of advanced glycosylation products that the dextrose is metabolized.[80] Indeed, a recent abstract reported that blockade of the glucose transporter by phlorizin caused a 20% decrease in transport of glucose out of the cavity.[81] A molecule of the size of glucose, which does not undergo cellular uptake and metabolism, transports rapidly through the peritoneum, interstitium, and across blood capillaries, and this transport should not have been changed by the presence of phlorizin. However, as glucose transports through tissue, it is taken up by cells via glucose transporter(s). Therefore, a decrease in the transport of dextrose with the blockade of the transporter implies that a major site of dextrose removal within the tissue space has been eliminated and that the rate of diffusion will slow because the concentration gradient that drives the process has a lower absolute magnitude.

In the same fashion, other drugs that are taken up into cells and metabolized will affect the free and apparent total concentrations in the tissue and the depth of penetration of the agent. Researchers who measure the total label of a drug as a surrogate marker for the drug might observe an increase of concentration at the site of metabolism, but the concentration of free drug in the extracellular compartment would be less than the total. For small molecular weight solutes, which transport primarily by diffusion, the free concentration will not increase beyond that which would have resulted for a molecule of similar size but that was not taken up by cells. Cellular uptake would therefore increase the slopes of the total drug concentration profiles of Figures 36.3 and 36.16.

Gene Therapy with Transformed Mesothelial Cells

A new and exciting method of drug delivery is the in vitro manipulation of mesothelial cells harvested from the peritoneum and their reintroduction into the peritoneal cavity. Recent animal experiments have tested mesothelial cells as producers and delivery devices for cytokines such as IL-10.[82] Gene products, which encode the desired product, have been introduced in vitro into mesothelial cells that have been harvested from the peritoneal cavity of small animals. The transformed cells, which secrete the product, are then reintroduced into the cavity and proliferate to cover the surface. The location of the cells on the peritoneal surface places the source at the surface, similar to the use of a solution containing an agent, and the agent would then transport from the surface to deeper layers in the subperitoneal interstitium. This transport would mimic the transport of an agent of similar molecular size introduced in a large volume of solution into the cavity. The advantage of this form of therapy is that the agent is produced locally and will be present in the tissue for the life of the transformed cells. The inability to directly control the actual concentration of the agent in the tissue and the necessity to harvest, infect, and reimplant mesothelial cells may make this therapeutic technique impractical for short-term application.

Summary

The use of the peritoneal cavity for the introduction of therapeutic agents is usually advantageous when the target is within the peritoneal cavity or in the adjacent tissue. The pharmacokinetic advantage of i.p. versus i.v. administration can be quantified if concentrations at the target and at the site of injection are known. Depending on the location of the target of the therapy, different transport models may be used in quantifying the transport. The membrane model lumps all resistance between the peritoneal compartment and the blood (the body compartment) into a single barrier. In contrast, the distributed approach attempts to model the tissue space by distributing capillaries uniformly within a tissue space, which is made up of cells surrounded by interstitium. The transperitoneal transport of small solutes (<10,000 daltons) is dominated by diffusion; both models adequately simulate this transport for water-soluble solutes. Factors such as lipid solubility, local cellular metabolism, or binding to cells or to the interstitial matrix will alter the transport process and must be taken into account to properly estimate drug delivery to the target.

Blood flow does not appear to limit transport, even under conditions of shock, and transport is not altered in a significant way except across the surface of organs such as the liver and spleen. That the portion of peritoneal area in contact with the therapeutic solution may only be a fraction of the dissected area presents a major limitation of i.p. therapy; techniques need to be devised to perfuse the entire area to ensure treatment of all targeted areas. Macromolecules move through tissue chiefly by convection, a process that has not been studied to the same extent as diffusion. i.p. hydrostatic pressure, which correlates with the size of the volume in the cavity, determines the rates of convective transport. Binding, cellular uptake and metabolism, lymph drainage, interstitial expansion, and solute exclusion by the interstitial matrix are variables that have major impacts on macromolecular transport. Data gaps continue to appear in the transport of new macromolecular biologic agents, including antibodies, viruses, and transfected cells.

Acknowledgment

The author was supported in this work by NIH grant DK48479.

References

1. Leak LB, Rahil K. Permeability of the diaphragmatic mesothelium: the ultrastructural basis for "stomata." Am J Anat 1978;151:557–594.
2. Bettendorf U. Lymph flow mechanism of the subperitoneal diaphragmatic lymphatics. Lymphology 1978;11: 111–116.
3. Allen L. On the penetrability of the lymphatics of the diaphragm. Anat Rec 1956;124:639–658.
4. Cole WCC, Montgomery JC. Intraperitoneal blood transfusion. Am J Dis Child 1929;37:497–510.
5. Clausen J. Studies on the effects of intraperitoneal blood transfusion. Acta Paediatr Stockholm 1940;27:24–31.
6. Markmann M, Hakes T, Reichmann B, Hoskins W, Rubin S, Lewis JL Jr. Intraperitoneal versus intravenous cisplatin-based therapy in small-volume residual refractory ovarian cancer: evidence supporting an advantage for local drug delivery. Reg Cancer Treat 1990;3:10–12.
7. Alberts DS, Liu PY, Hannigan EV, et al. Intraperitoneal cisplatin plus intravenous cyclophosphamide versus intravenous cisplatin plus intravenous cyclophosphamide for stage III ovarian cancer. N Engl J Med 1996;335: 1950–1955.
8. Dedrick RL. Interspecies scaling of regional drug delivery. J Pharm Sci 1986;75:1047–1052.
9. Goel R, Cleary SM, Horton C, et al. Effect of sodium thiosulfate on the pharmacokinetics and toxicity of cisplatin. J Natl Cancer Inst 1989;81:1552–1560.
10. Baron MA. Structure of the intestinal peritoneum in man. Am J Anat 1941;69:439–445.
11. Flessner MF, Schwab A. Pressure threshold for fluid loss from the peritoneal cavity. Am J Physiol 1996;F377–F390.
12. Barrowman JA. Physiology of the Gastro-Intestinal Lymphatic System. Cambridge: Cambridge University Press, 1978.
13. Flessner MF. Peritoneal transport physiology: insights from basic research. J Am Soc Nephrol 1991;2:122–135.
14. Tesi D, Detraz P, Forssmann WC. Permeability studies with the interstitial tissue of the rat mesentery. I. Technical description. Pfluegers Arch 1971;322:183–187.
15. Zink J, Greenway CV. Control of ascites absorption in anesthetized cats: effects of intraperitoneal pressure, protein, and furosemide diuresis. Gastroenterology 1973;73: 1119–1124.
16. Flessner MF, Dedrick RL, Reynolds JC. Bidirectional peritoneal transport of immunoglobulin in rats: compartmental kinetics. Am J Physiol 1992;262:F275–F287.
17. Shostak A, Gotloib L, Jaichenko J, Galdi P, Fudin R. Transcytosis of intraperitoneally injected albumin in mice peritoneum (abstract). J Am Soc Nephrol 1990;1:392.
18. Pfeiffer CJ, Pfeiffer DC, Mistra HP. Enteric serosal surface in the piglet. A scanning and transmission electron microscopic study of the mesothelium. J Submicrosc Cytol 1987;19:237–246.
19. Regoeczi E, Zaimi O, Chindemi PA, Charlwood PA. Absorption of plasma proteins from peritoneal cavity of normal rats. Am J Physiol 1989;256:E447–E452.
20. Flessner MF. Osmotic barrier of the parietal peritoneum. Am J Physiol 1994;267:F861–F870.
21. Flessner MF, Fenstermacher JD, Dedrick RL, Blasberb RG. A distributed model of peritoneal-plasma transport: tissue concentration gradients. Am J Physiol 1985;248: F425–F435.
22. Collins JM. Inert gas exchange of subcutaneous and intraperitoneal gas pockets in piglets. Respir Physiol 1981; 46:391–404.
23. Schultz JS, Armstrong W. Permeability of interstitial space of muscle (rat diaphragm) to solutes of different molecular weights. J Pharm Sci 1978;67:696–700.
24. Bell DR, Watson PD, Renkin EM. Exclusion of plasma proteins in interstitium of tissues from the dog hind paw. Am J Physiol 1980;239:H532–H538.
25. Brookes N, Mackay D. Diffusion of labelled substances through isolated rat diaphragm. Br J Pharmacol 1971;47: 367–378.
26. Page E, Bernstein RS. Cat heart muscle in vitro. V. Diffusion through a sheet of right ventricle. J Gen Physiol 1964; 47:1129–1140.
27. Gotloib L, Mines M, Garmizo L, Varla I. Hemodynamic effects of increasing intra-abdominal pressure in peritoneal dialysis. Perit Dial Bull 1981;1:41–43.
28. Twardowski ZJ, Prowant BF, Nolph KD. High volume, low frequency continuous ambulatory peritoneal dialysis. Kidney Int 1983;23:64–70.
29. Seames EL, Moncrief JW, Popovich RP. A distributed model of fluid and mass transfer in peritoneal dialysis. Am J Physiol 1990;258:R958–R972.
30. Daugirdas JT, Ing TS, Gandhi VC, Hano JE, Chen WT, Yuan L. Kinetics of peritoneal fluid absorption in patients with chronic renal failure. J Lab Clin Med 1980;85: 351–361.
31. Rippe B, Stelin G, Ahlmen J. Lymph flow from the peritoneal cavity in CAPD patients. In: Maher JF, Winchester JF, eds. Frontiers in Peritoneal Dialysis. New York: Field, Rich 1986:24–30.
32. Mactier RA, Khanna R, Twardowski Z, Nolph KD. Role of peritoneal cavity lymphatic absorption in peritoneal dialysis. Kidney Int 1987;32:165–174.
33. Crone C. The permeability of capillaries in various organs as determined by use of the "indicator diffusion" method. Acta Physiol Scand 1963;58:292–305.
34. Rippe B, Haraldsson B. Fluid and protein fluxes across small and large pores in the microvasculature. Application

of two-pore equations. Acta Physiol Scand 1987;131: 411–428.
35. Rippe B, Stelin G, Haraldsson B. Computer simulations of peritoneal fluid transport in CAPD. Kidney Int 1991;40: 315–325.
36. Agre P, Preston GM, Smith BL, et al. Aquaporin CHIP: the archetypal molecular water channel. Am J Physiol 1993; 265:F463–F476.
37. Perry MA. Capillary filtration and permeability coefficients calculated from measurements of interendothelial cell junctions in rabbit lung and skeletal muscle. Microvasc Res 1980;19:142–157.
38. Grotte G. Passage of dextran molecules across the blood-lymph barrier. Acta Chir Scand Suppl 1956;211:1–84.
39. Frokjaer-Jensen J. Three-dimensional organization of plasmalemmal vesicles in endothelial cells. An analysis by serial sectioning of frog mesenteric capillaries. J Ultrastruct Res 1980;73:9–20.
40. Hargens AR, Akeson WH, Mubarak S, Hogan JS, Tucker BJ, Peters R. Fluid balance within the canine anterolateral compartment and its relationship to compartment syndromes. J Bone Joint Surg 1978;60A:499–505.
41. Hargens AR, Cologne JB, Menninger FJ, et al. Normal transcapillary pressures in human skeletal muscle and subcutaneous tissues. Microvasc Res. 1981;22:177–189.
42. Reed RK. Interstitial fluid volume, colloid osmotic and hydrostatic pressure in rat skeletal muscle. Effect of venous stasis and muscle activity. Acta Physiol Scand 1981;112: 7–17.
43. Flessner MF. The importance of the interstitium in peritoneal transport. Perit Dial Int 1996;16:S76–S79.
44. Levick JR. Flow through interstitium and fibrous matrices. Q J Exp Physiol 1987;72:409–438.
45. Dedrick RL, Flessner MF, Collins JM, Schultz JS. Is the peritoneum a membrane? Am Soc Artif Intern Organs (ASAIO) 1982;5:1–8.
46. Chagnac A, Herkovitz P, Weinstein T, et al. The peritoneal membrane in peritoneal dialysis patients: estimation of its functional surface area by applying stereological methods to CT scans. J Am Soc Nephrol 1999;10:342–346.
47. Putiloff PV. Materials for the study of the laws of growth of the human body in relation to the surface areas of different systems; the trial on Russian subjects of planigraphic anatomy as a means for exact anthropometry-one of the problems of anthropology. Report of Dr. P.V. Putiloff at the meeting of the Siberian Branch of the Russian Geographic Society, October 29th, 1884, Omsk, 1886.
48. Dedrick RL, Myers CE, Bungay PM, DeVita VT. Pharmacokinetic rationale for peritoneal drug administration in the treatment of ovarian cancer. Cancer Treat Rep 1978;61: 1–11.
49. Rubin JA, Reed V, Adair C, Bower J, Klein E. Effect of intraperitoneal insulin on solute kinetics in CAPD: insulin kinetics in CAPD. Am J Med Sci 1986;291:81–87.
50. Keshaviah P, Emerson PF, Vonesh EF, Brandes JC. Relationship between body size, fill volume, and mass transfer area coefficient in peritoneal dialysis. J Am Soc Nephrol 1994;4:1820–1826.
51. Flessner MF. Small solute transport across specific peritoneal tissue surfaces in the rat. J Am Soc Nephrol 1996;7: 225–233.
52. Kim M, Lofthouse J, Flessner MF. Blood flow limitations of solute transport across the visceral peritoneum. J Am Soc Nephrol 1997;8:1946–1950.
53. Torres IJ, Litterst CL, Guarino AM. Transport of model compounds across the peritoneal membrane in the rat. Pharmacology (Basel) 1978;17:330–340.
54. Wikes AD, Howell SB. Pharmacokinetics of hexamethylmelamine administered via the ip route in an oil emulsion vehicle. Cancer Treat Rep 1985;69:657–662.
55. Lewis C, Lawson N, Rankin EM, et al. Phase I and pharmacokinetic study of intraperitoneal thioTEPA in patients with ovarian cancer. Cancer Chemother Pharmacol 1990; 26:283–287.
56. Aune S. Transperitoneal exchange. II. Peritoneal blood flow estimated by hydrogen gas clearance. Scand J Gastroenterol 1970;5:99–104.
57. Flessner MF. Transport of water soluble solutes between the peritoneal cavity and the plasma in the rat. Dissertation, Department of Chemical Engineering, University of Michigan, Ann Arbor, 1981.
58. Grzegorzewska AE, Moore HL, Nolph KD, Chen TW. Ultrafiltration and effective peritoneal blood flow during peritoneal dialysis in the rat. Kidney Int 1991;39:608–617.
59. Demissachew H, Lofthouse J, Flessner MF. Tissue sources and blood flow limitations of osmotic water flow across the peritoneum. J Am Soc Nephrol 1999;103:347–353.
60. Zakaria ER, Carlsson O, Rippe B. Liver is not essential for solute transport during peritoneal dialysis. Kidney Int 1996;50:298–303.
61. Erb RW, Greene JA Jr, Weller JM. Peritoneal dialysis during hemorrhagic shock. J Appl Physiol 1967;22:131–135.
62. Rubin J, Clawson M, Planch A, Jones Q. Measurements of peritoneal surface area in man and rat. Am J Med Sci 1988;295:453–458.
63. Esperanca MJ, Collins DL. Peritoneal dialysis efficiency in relation to body weight. J Pediatr Surg 1966;1:162–169.
64. Levitt MD, Kneip JM, Overdahl MC. Influence of shaking on peritoneal transfer in rats. Kidney Int 1989;35: 1145–1150.
65. Zakaria ER, Carlsson O, Rippe B. Limitation of small-solute exchange across the visceral peritoneum: effects of vibration. Perit Dial Int 1996;17:72–79.
66. Dedrick RL, Flessner MF. Pharmacokinetic problems in peritoneal drug administration: tissue penetration and surface exposure. J Natl Cancer Inst 1997;89:480–487.
67. Steller MA, Egorin MJ, Trimble EL, et al. A pilot phase I trial of continuous hyperthermic peritoneal perfusion (CHPP) with high-dose carboplatin (CBDCA) as primary treatment of patients with small volume residual ovarian cancer. Cancer Chemother Pharmacol 1999;43: 106–114.
68. Ward BG, Mather SJ, Hawkins LR, et al. Localization of radioiodine conjugated to the monoclonal antibody HMFG2 in human ovarian carcinoma: assessment of intravenous and intraperitoneal routes of administration. Cancer Res 1987;47:4719–4723.
69. Dedrick RL, Flessner MF. Pharmacokinetic considerations on monoclonal antibodies. In: Immunity to Cancer, Vol. II. New York: Liss, 1989:429–438.
70. Griffin TW, Collins J, Bokhari F, et al. Intraperitoneal immunoconjugates. Cancer Res 1990;50:1031s–1038s.

71. Olin T, Saldeen T. The lymphatic pathways from the peritoneal cavity: a lymphangiographic study in the rat. Cancer Res 1964;24:1700–1711.
72. Imholz ALT, Koomen GCM, Struijk DG, Arisz L, Krediet RT. Effect of an increased intraperitoneal pressure on fluid and solute transport during CAPD. Kidney Int 1993; 44:1078–1085.
73. Durand P-Y, Chanliau J, Gamberoni J, Hestin D, Kessler M. Intraperitoneal hydrostatic pressure and ultrafiltration volume in CAPD. Adv Perit Dial 1993;9:44–48.
74. Zakaria E-L, Lofthouse J, Flessner MF. In vivo effects of hydrostatic pressure on interstitial space of muscle. Am J Physiol 1999;276:14517–14529.
75. Price FM, Levick JR, Mason RM. Changes in glycosaminoglycan concentration and synovial permeability at raised intra-articular pressure in rabbit knees. J Physiol (Lond) 1996;495:821–833.
76. Flessner MF, Dedrick RL, Reynolds JC. Bidirectional peritoneal transport of immunoglobulin in rats: tissue concentration profiles. Am J Physiol 1992;263:F15–F23.
77. Flessner MF, Lofthouse J, Zakaria E-R. In vivo diffusion of immunoglobulin G in muscle: effects of binding, solute exclusion, and lymphatic removal. Am J Physiol 1998; 273:H2783–H2793.
78. Fujimori K, Covell DB, Fletcher JE, Weinstein JN. A modeling analysis of monoclonal antibody percolation through tumors: a binding-site barrier. J Nucl Med 1990;31: 1191–1198.
79. van Osdol W, Fujimori K, Weinstein JN. An analysis of monoclonal antibody distribution in microscopic tumor nodules: consequences of a "binding site barrier." Cancer Res 1991;51:4776–4784.
80. Dawney A. Advanced glycation end products in peritoneal dialysis. Perit Dial Int 1996;16:S50–S53.
81. Wang T, Heimburger, Cheng H, Waniewski J, Berstrom J, Lindholm B. Glucose transporter inhibitor decreases peritoneal glucose abssorption (abstract). J Am Soc Nephrol 1998;9:194a.
82. Hoff CM, Inman KL, Piscopo D, Shockley TR. Mesothelial cells genetically modified to produce IL-10 inhibit LPS-induced macrophage MCP-1 and MMP-9 production (abstract). J Am Soc Nephrol 1998;9:283a.

37

Developing Pharmacologic Agents for Adhesion Prevention

Kathleen E. Rodgers and Gere S. diZerega

CONTENTS

Various approaches for the prevention of adhesion formation have been actively explored.[1–6] It is well known that good surgical technique is important in reducing adhesion formation. However, adjuncts to good techniques are needed for adhesion prevention. Physical barriers have been used in an attempt to prevent adhesion formation by limiting tissue apposition during the critical period of peritoneal healing, thereby minimizing the development of fibrin matrix between tissue surfaces.[2,7,8] Studies have indicated that placement of an absorbable barrier of oxidized regenerated cellulose [Interceed® (TC7) Absorbable Adhesion Barrier; Ethicon, Somerville, NJ, USA], expanded polytetrafluoroethylene (Preclude® Surgical Membrane; W.L. Gore & Associates, Flagstaff, AZ, USA), or hyaluronic acid/carboxymethylcellulose (Seprafilm® Bioresorbable Membrane; Genzyme, Cambridge, MA, USA)[9] between injury sites, or addition of a viscous solution (Intergel® ferric cross-linked hyaluronic acid; Ethicon)[10] to the peritoneal cavity during or after surgery may reduce postoperative adhesion formation. In the case of Interceed, Preclude, or Seprafilm, the surgeon must predict potential sites of adhesion formation to determine placement site and optimize barrier benefit. Interest therefore continues in the development of an intraperitoneal device that functions more broadly as a postsurgical adhesion prophylactic.

Understanding the physiology of adhesion formation and peritoneal repair after surgery provides insight into the rational selection of pharmacologically active agents for adhesion prevention. This chapter describes two animal models that were used to screen drug candidates for adhesion prevention as well as an approach to selection of a clinically useful vehicle. Examples of a number of different pharmacologic agents with a variety of putative mechanisms of action are provided. In these animal models, compounds with potentially distinct mechanisms of action were tested that could block or enhance sites within the cascade of adhesion formation.

The compounds screened in these models included all-*trans* retinoic acid, quinacrine, dipyridamole, anti-inflammatory peptides (anti-inflammin), hirudin analogs, and lazaroids. The data derived from these screening studies, together with the theoretical mechanisms of action based upon the published literature, are discussed; the preclinical development of one of these compounds is further described. Finally, the animal data and preclinical development together with mechanistic studies to elucidate the site of action for nonsteroidal antiinflammatory drugs are reviewed.

Surgical Models

The sidewall model and double uterine horn models were used with delivery of the materials via Alzet pump to screen for the efficacy of the pharmaceuticals described here.

Sidewall Model

This model of adhesion formation in rabbits has been described in detail elsewhere.[11,12] Following a midline laparotomy, a 3 cm × 5 cm area of peritoneum and transversus abdominis muscle was removed on the right lateral abdominal wall. The cecum and bowel were exteriorized, and digital pressure was exerted to create subserosal hemorrhages over all surfaces. The damaged intestine was then lightly abraded with sterile gauze until punctuate bleeding was observed. The cecum and bowel were then returned to their normal anatomic position. After injury, a miniosmotic pump was placed in the subcutaneous space with a catheter attached to the end of the pump. The pump delivered material at a rate of 10 μL/hour for 7 days. The catheter was run from the pump in the subcutaneous space to the site of injury (sidewall excision or between the bladder and the uterine horns). The tube was attached to the sidewall with suture to immobilize it to the desired delivery site. The pumps placed in the control rabbits contained vehicle only.

After 7 days, the rabbits were killed and the percentage of the area of the sidewall injury that was involved in adhesions was determined by two blinded and independent observers. In addition, the tenacity of the adhesions was scored using the following system:

0, no adhesions
1, mild, easily dissectable adhesions
2, moderate adhesions; nondissectable, does not tear the organ
3, dense adhesions; nondissectable, tears organ when removed

A reduction in either the area or the tenacity of the adhesions was considered to be beneficial.

Double Uterine Horn Model

This model was previously shown to form severe adhesions after surgery.[11–14] A midline laparotomy was performed and both uterine horns were traumatized by abrasion of the serosal surface with gauze until punctate bleeding developed. Ischemia of both uterine horns was induced by removal of the collateral blood supply. The remaining blood supply to the uterine horns was the ascending branch of the uterovaginal arterial supply of the myometrium. After injury, a miniosmotic pump was placed to deliver the medication and the abdominal wall was closed in two layers. To deliver the compounds to the site of injury, a tube was attached to a miniosmotic pump that was placed in a subcutaneous pocket next to the midline incision. The pump delivered material at a rate of 10 μL/hour for 7 days. The tube was run from the attachment site to the pump in the subcutaneous space to the site of injury (sidewall excision or between the bladder and the uterine horns). The tube was attached to the sidewall with Ethilon suture to immobilize it to the desired delivery site.

The pumps placed in the control rabbits contained vehicle appropriate for the drug. In kinetic studies, the tube leading from the pump to the intraperitoneal space was disconnected through a small skin incision at the times indicated. After 7 days, the rabbits were killed and the degree of adhesion formation was determined. In this model, an initial score, which incorporated the organs involved and the tenacity and extent of adhesions, was given. The percentage of the horn that faced a given organ involved in adhesions to adjacent organs (including itself, the contralateral horn, bowel, small intestine, and bladder) was noted. After 7 days, the rabbits were terminated and the degree of adhesion formation was determined. In this model, an initial score to represent the overall extent of adhesions was given.[15,16] The percentage of the surface of the horn involved in adhesions to various organs (including bowel, bladder, itself, and the contralateral horn) was also noted.

Pharmaceuticals Screened in These Models

Retinoic Acid

One of the compounds tested was all-*trans* retinoic acid, one member of the retinoid family. Retinoids are a group of natural and synthetic vitamin A analogs whose principal effects on target cells are growth inhibition and induction of cellular differentiation. Retinoids have also been shown to have immunomodulatory and antiinflammatory activities, as well as other activities that may be of benefit in the prevention of adhesion formation. For example, retinoids reduce the formation of tumor necrosis factor (TNF), a proinflammatory cytokine that could conceivably increase adhesion formation.[17] Further, retinoids reduced interleukin-1 (IL-1)-induced IL-6 production.[18] Like TNF, IL-6 is a proinflammatory cytokine that may contribute to adhesion formation.

Retinoids also increase the potential fibrinolytic enzyme activity in several systems. Specifically, retinoids increased phorbol ester-induced plasminogen activator production as well as the expression of urokinase receptors.[19-23] Schuster et al.[19] however, also noted an increase in plasminogen activator inhibitors. Retinoids also modulate thrombomodulin, tissue factor, and procoagulant activity in such a way as to increase fibrinolytic activity.[24-26] This potential increase in fibrinolytic activity may, in turn, reduce the amount of fibrin deposited. As fibrin serves as a scaffold for adhesion formation, a reduction in the amount of fibrin deposited for a prolonged period of time may be one mechanism by which retinoids reduce adhesion formation.

The ability of retinoic acid to reduce adhesion formation in the rabbit sidewall model was tested (Fig. 37.1); Administration of retinoic acid to the site of sidewall injury for 7 days postoperatively dramatically reduced the formation of adhesions in this model. Initial studies were then conducted in which retinoic acid was administered to the site of injury for 7 days after abrasion and devascularization of both uterine horns (Table 37.1; Fig. 37.2). Administration of both doses of retinoic acid resulted in a significant reduction in the overall adhesions (Table 37.1). In addition, the number of sites without adhesions was also altered by administration of retinoic acid (Fig. 37.2).

Studies were then conducted to determine whether the effects of administration of retinoic acid for 1, 2, or 3 days reduced adhesion formation. At various times after

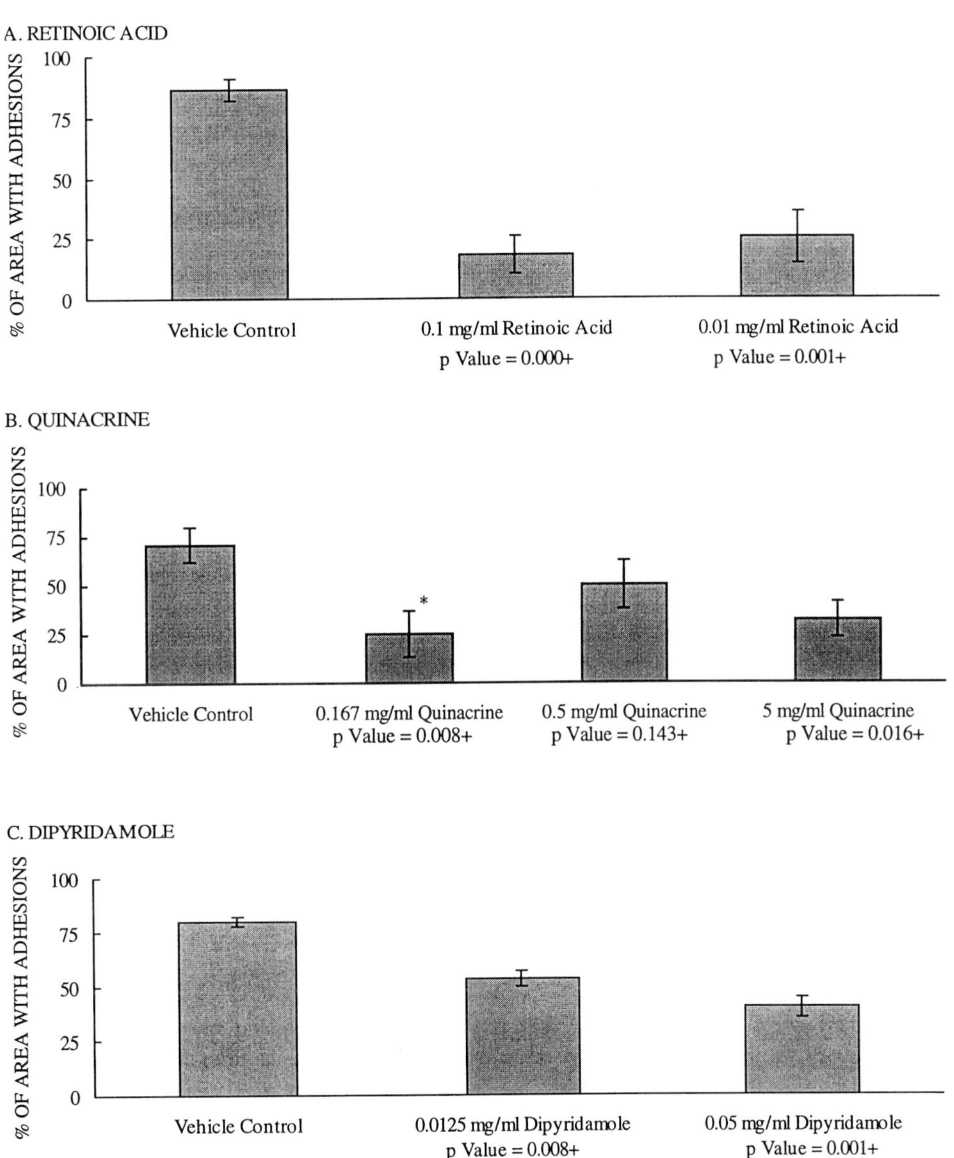

FIG. 37.1 Effects of administration of various medicaments on the formation of adhesions in the sidewall model. **A,** Retinoic acid; **B,** quinacrine; **C,** dipyridamole. The *p*-value is the value for comparing the treated group with the vehicle control areas. *, Quinacrine precipitated at the site of sidewall injury in 2 of 6 animals. Reproduced with permission from *J Invest Surg* 1998 Sep–Oct;11(5):327–329.

TABLE 37.1. Effect of continuous administration for 7 days of three medicaments on the overall adhesion score in the double uterine horn model.

Group	Rank (Mean ± SEM)	p-value (compared to control)
Vehicle control	15.5 ± 1.4	
Retinoic acid:		
0.1 mg/mL	5.1 ± 2.1	0.000
0.01 mg/mL	8.0 ± 3.5	0.000
Vehicle control	15.5 ± 1.6	
Quinacrine:		
0.056 mg/mL	5.42 ± 2.89	0.012
0.167 mg/mL	7.58 ± 3.211	0.052
Vehicle control	15.0 ± 1.7	
Dipyridamole:		
0.0125 mg/mL	7.25 ± 4.4	0.002
0.05 mg/mL	6.25 ± 2.9	0.000

TABLE 37.2. Effect of three compounds administered for various times on the rank order analysis of the overall score in the double uterine horn model.

	Rank (mean ± SEM): hours postoperatively tube disconnected		
Group	24	48	72
Vehicle control			38.5 ± 1.1
Retinoic Acid:			
0.01 mg/mL	22.4 ± 9.7	15.8 ± 8.3	15.8 ± 8.3
0.1 mg/mL	16.1 ± 7.9	18.7 ± 9.1	14.2 ± 12.7
Vehicle control			38.9 ± 1.0
Quinacrine:			
0.056 mg/mL	12.1 ± 5.1	15.1 ± 1.8	22.9 ± 5.0
0.167 mg/mL	19.1 ± 3.2	20.8 ± 3.5	21.8 ± 2.9
Vehicle control			37.3 ± 1.9
Dipyridamole:			
0.0125 mg/mL	16.2 ± 4.7	16.6 ± 8.3	20.3 ± 9.3
0.05 mg/mL	20.2 ± 10.0	18.8 ± 11.8	14.4 ± 9.4

initiation of treatment, the pumps were disconnected from the tube to stop treatment to the injury site. The results of these studies are shown in Table 37.2 and Fig. 37.3.

Quinacrine

A second compound tested was quinacrine, commonly used as an antimalarial drug.[27,28] Quinacrine inhibits of phospholipase A_2 (PLA_2) in platelets and other cell types.[29–32] Coinjection of quinacrine with PLA_2 reduced the inflammogenic potential of the latter by 64%, suggesting that quinacrine has some antiinflammatory activity.[33] Arachidonic acid is released from the plasma membrane through the action of PLA_2.[32] Therefore, quinacrine may reduce the amount of arachidonic acid available for metabolism by cyclooxygenase and lipooxygenase to lipid inflammatory mediators, such as prostaglandins and leukotrienes. Quinacrine reduces the secretion of leukotrienes, lipooxygenase metabolites of arachidonic acid, by macrophages.[34] Arachidonic acid metabolites, such as prostaglandin E_2, are proinflammatory[35] and when administered into the peritoneal cavity increase postoperative adhesion formation.[36,37]

Quinacrine also acts to inhibit platelet aggregation and the subsequent release of alpha-granule.[38] Because platelet aggregation accelerates the coagulation process and subsequent fibrin deposition, inhibition of platelet aggregation by quinacrine may inhibit the deposition of fibrin. Prolonged or excessive deposition of fibrin is thought to be involved in adhesion formation.[39] If the fibrin is not cleared by the time healing begins, it will act as a scaffold for mesothelial cell chemotaxis and proliferation.

The administration of quinacrine, an antimalarial drug, administered for a relatively short period of time after surgery reduced the formation of peritoneal adhesions (see Figs. 37.1 and 37.2). Further, the efficacy of

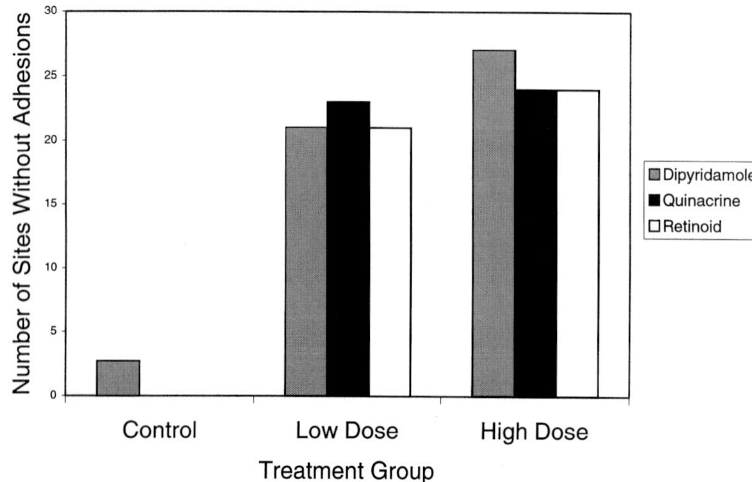

FIG. 37.2 The number of sites evaluated (8 per rabbit) that did not form adhesions to the uterine horns after surgery. The highest concentration of compound given was 0.1 mg/nL (retinoic acid, *light bars*), 0.167 mg/mL (quinacrine, *black bars*), and 0.05 mg/mL (dipyridamole, *gray bars*). The lowest concentration of compound given was 0.01 mg/mL (retinoic acid), 0.056 mg/mL (quinacrine), and 0.0125 mg/mL (dipyridamole). These data are a summary of some of the information (that is, the number of possible sites that the uterine horns could adhere to that were adhesion free) presented in Table 38.2. Reproduced with permission from *J Invest Surg* 1998 Sep–Oct; 11(5):327–329.

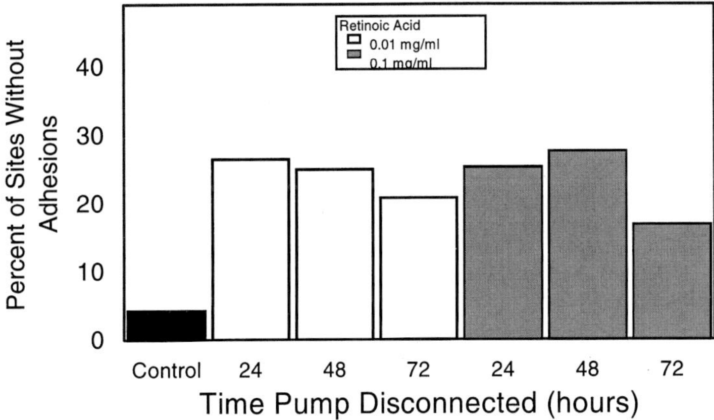

FIG. 37.3 The percentage of sites evaluated (8 per rabbit) that did not form adhesions to the uterine horns after surgery. The concentration of retinoic acid administered and the time that the pump was disconnected are noted on the figure. Reproduced with permission from *J Invest Surg* 1998 Sep–Oct;11(5): 327–329.

quinacrine was dramatically increased when the fibrotic side effects noted in the literature after high-dose treatment with quinacrine are avoided by administration of lower concentrations for shorter periods of time.[40] Administration of quinacrine for various lengths of time also reduced adhesion formation (see Tables 37.1 and 37.2; Fig. 37.4). Although administration of both doses of quinacrine at all time points resulted in a significant reduction in adhesion score, there was a greater reduction in adhesion formation at the 24-hour than at the 72-hour time point. This observation is consistent with results from the sidewall studies (see Fig. 37.1).

Dipyridamole

The third compound tested was dipyridamole, a drug used clinically to reduce postoperative thromboembolism.[41] There are several possible mechanisms by which dipyridamole may reduce adhesion formation including modulation of fibrin deposition and removal. Studies have shown that prolonged deposition of fibrin contributes to the formation of postoperative adhesions.[39,42] Dipyridamole has been shown to have a number of activities that would reduce the amount or time of fibrin deposition. Dipyridamole has been shown to reduce thromboembolism after surgery through inhibition of platelet aggregation in response to adenosine and increased production of prostacyclin.[43–45] Prostacyclin is also a potent inhibitor of platelet aggregation.[46] Platelet aggregation accelerates coagulation and the deposition of fibrin. As fibrin acts as a scaffold for adhesion formation, inhibition of platelet aggregation may reduce fibrin deposition and, subsequently, adhesion formation.

Dipyridamole has also been suggested to have beneficial effects in disorders characterized by extravascular fibrin deposition. Dipyridamole was shown to decrease the expression of tissue thromboplastin activity while concurrently stimulating production and release of urokinase.[47] In addition, dipyridamole may prevent fibrin accumulation at sites of inflammation through direct effects on macrophages.[48] Therefore, dipyridamole may prevent fibrin accumulation at sites of inflammation through direct effects on macrophage function. Dipyridamole has also been shown to modify the throm-

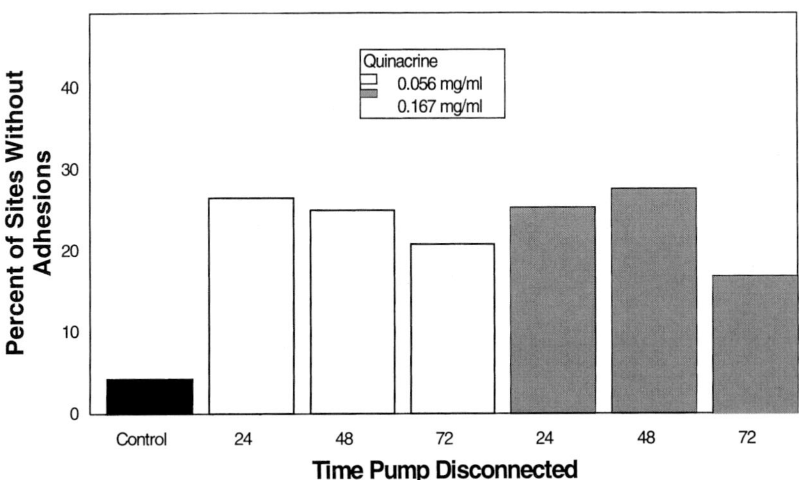

FIG. 37.4 The percentage of sites evaluated (8 per rabbit) that did not form adhesions to the uterine horns after surgery. The concentration of quinacrine administered and the time that the pump was disconnected are noted on the figure. Reproduced with permission from *J Invest Surg* 1998 Sep–Oct; 11(5):327–329.

bogenic properties of the extracellular matrix produced by endothelial cells.[49]

Dipyridamole, in relatively low doses, was also shown to be antiinflammatory. Dipyridamole was previously shown to reduce macrophage secretion of TNF (a proinflammatory cytokine) and the synthesis of leukotrienes (proinflammatory lipid mediators) by polymorphonuclear neutrophils.[50] Dipyridamole also inhibits the production of superoxide anion, a microbiocidal product of the respiratory burst system, by neutrophils and mononuclear cells.[48,51,52]

Administration of dipyridamole, a compound that reduces platelet aggregation in response to adenosine and increases the production of prostacyclin, significantly reduced the formation of postoperative adhesions. Administration of higher concentrations of dipyridamole increased the inflammatory reaction at the site of injury as assessed by the gross appearance of tissue. Administration of dipyridamole to the site of sidewall injury for 7 days postoperatively dramatically reduced the formation of adhesions in this model. (see Fig. 37.1). Studies were then conducted in which dipyridamole was administered to the site of injury for 7 days after abrasion and devascularization of both uterine horns (see Table 37.1 and Fig. 37.2). Administration of both doses of dipyridamole resulted in a significant reduction in the overall adhesion score (Table 37.1). Administration of dipyridamole to the site of injury significantly reduced the formation of adhesions to various organs. In addition, the number of sites without adhesions was also altered by administration of dipyridamole (Fig. 37.2).

Administration of dipyridamole for various lengths of time also reduced adhesion formation (Table 37.2; Fig. 37.5). Administration of both doses of dipyridamole at all time points resulted in a significant reduction in the overall adhesion score. However, at the lower concentration of dipyridamole, there was a greater reduction in adhesion formation at the 72-hour than at the 24-hour time point.

Antiinflammatory Peptide 2 (Anti-inflammin)

Lipocortins are a group of proteins that have been proposed as mediators of the antiinflammatory actions of glucocorticolds in some peripheral tissues.[53,54] Fragments of the lipocortin proteins have been shown to be antiinflammatory.[53,55–57] The action of these fragments may be through inhibition of PLA activity.[53] PLA_2 is an enzyme involved in the release of arachidonic acid from the lipid membrane.[32] Metabolites of arachidonic acid, such as prostaglandins, are proinflammatory.[35] In addition, prostaglandin of the E series has been shown to increase adhesion formation.[36,37] Reduction of the availability of the substrate for enzymes that metabolize arachidonic acid will reduce the formation of these metabolites. Therefore, inhibitors of PLA are antiinflammatory. Specifically, the fragment screened for antiadhesion activity, antiinflammatory peptide 2 (anti-inflammin), suppressed PLA activity, and carrageenan-induced rat paw edema but not arachidonic acid- or phorbol ester-induced ear edema.[53,58,59] Anti-inflammin may reduce adhesion formation through a reduction in the inflammatory responses that occur after surgery. This reduction in inflammation may reduce the amount of fibrin deposited or alter the activity of peritoneal leukocytes in such a way as to increase fibrinolytic activity.[60–62] If this occurs, the deposited fibrin is cleared more quickly, thereby reducing the amount of fibrin available to act as bridges for adhesion formation.

The ability of anti-inflammin to reduce the formation of intraperitoneal adhesions in two rabbit models of adhesion formation was also tested. In the sidewall model, anti-inflammin was administered via Alzet miniosmotic pump for the entire postoperative interval, and there was a dose-dependent reduction in the area of the sidewall injury that was involved in adhesions to the cecum and the bowel (Fig. 37.6). In the double uterine horn model, anti-inflammin was administered via Alzet miniosmotic pump to the area of injury for either 1, 2, 3, or 7

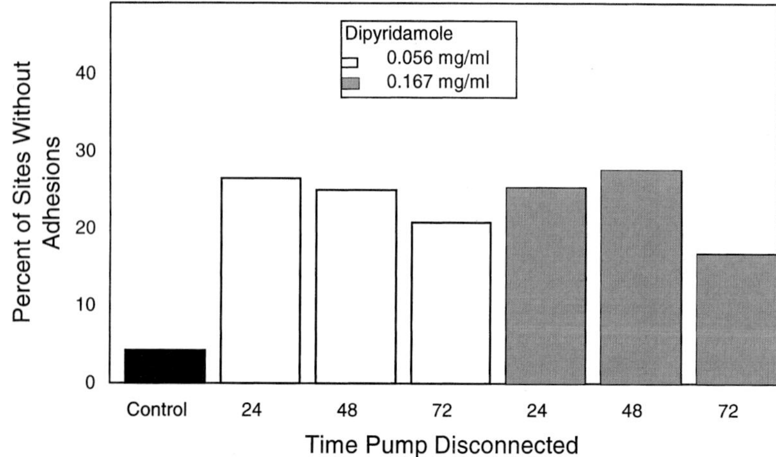

FIG. 37.5 The percentage of sites evaluated (8 per rabbit) that did not form adhesions to the uterine horns after surgery. The concentration of dipyridamole administered and the time that the pump was disconnected are noted on the figure. Reproduced with permission from *J Invest Surg* 1998 Sep–Oct;11(5):327–329.

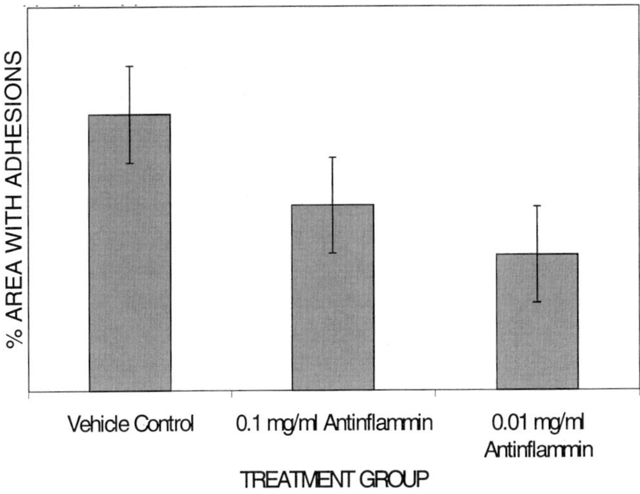

FIG. 37.6 Effects of anti-inflammin on the formation of adhesion in rabbits. Reproduced with permission from ref. 12.

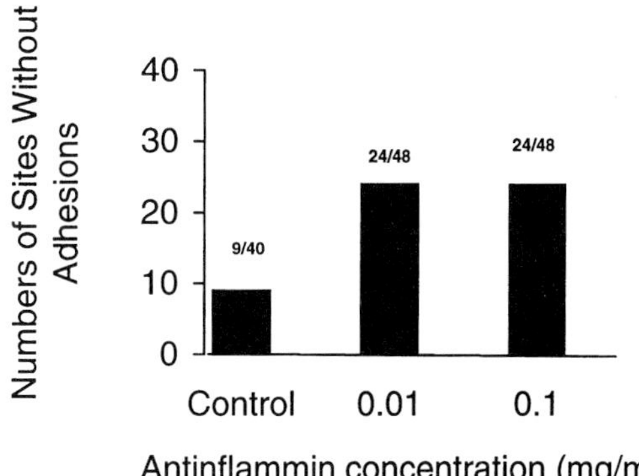

FIG. 37.7 The effect of continous administration of anti-inflammin on the incidence of adhesion formation, showing the number of sites evaluated (8 per rabbit) that did not form adhesions to the uterine horns after surgery. Reproduced with permission from ref. 12.

days (Tables 37.3 and 37.4; Fig. 37.7 and 37.8). Administration of anti-inflammin for as little as 24 hours after surgery significantly reduced the extent of adhesion formation (Table 37.4). Administration of the peptide for longer periods of time did not further increase the reduction in adhesion formation. These studies clearly demonstrate that postoperative administration of anti-inflammin to the site of injury reduced the formation of postoperative adhesions in two animal models.

TABLE 37.3. Effect of continuous administration of anti-inflammin on the overall adhesion score in individual animals in the double uterine horn model.

	Anti-inflammin (mg/mL)		
	Vehicle control	0.01	0.1
Overall score	2.5+	1.5+	2.0+
	2.5+	1.0+	1.5+
	2.5+	1.5+	1.0+
	3.5+	1.5+	1.0+
	3.5+	1.0+	1.0+
		1.5+	1.5+
Rank (mean ± SEM)	15.0 ± 1.2	6.7 ± 2.6	6.3 ± 3.5
p-value	—	0.000	0.000

Hirudin

The procoagulant thrombin is the activation product of prothrombin in the blood and has central bioregulatory action in thrombosis and hemostasis, various disease states, and healing.[62–64] In addition, thrombin causes the aggregation and activation of platelets as part of the coagulation cascade. The interaction of thrombin with biologic substrates involves various structural domains, including a catalytic site and two flanking accessory binding sites that are bound by hirudin.[65] Thrombin is a procoagulant protein that is central to the coagulation cascade and hemostasis. Thrombin also tightly binds to the formed fibrin and thereby proteolytically activates platelets and cleaves fibrinogen.[65] Thrombin, therefore, is involved in the restoration of hemostatic homeostasis through the deposition of fibrin. During surgery, the ability to remove this fibrin is reduced as a result of the trauma. Studies have shown that trauma and ischemia reduce the fibrinolytic activity of peritoneal peritoneum. Raftery determined that the changes in peritoneal fibrinolytic activity decreased immediately and continued to decrease at 24 hours after three different types of trauma (excision, grafting, and ischemia).[39] The prolonged de-

TABLE 37.4. Effect of anti-inflammin administered for various times on the overall adhesion score in individual animals in the double uterine horn model.

		Anti-inflammin (0.01 mg/mL)			Anti-inflammin (0.1 mg/mL)		
	Vehicle control	24 h	48 h	72 h	24 h	48 h	72 h
Overall score	3.0+	3.5+	2.5+	2.0+	2.0+	1.5+	1.0+
	3.0+	0.5+	2.5+	2.0+	2.0+	1.5+	1.0+
	2.5+	1.5+	2.5+	1.5+	1.0+	2.0+	1.5+
	3.0+	1.5+	2.5+	1.0+	2.0+	1.5+	2.0+
	3.0+	2.5+	2.0+	1.5+	1.5+	1.5+	1.5+
	3.5+	2.0+	3.5+	2.0+		1.5+	
Rank	3.4 ± 1.9	21.6 ± 12.9	26.0 ± 8.6	19.0 ± 8.7	19.0 ± 19.0	16.6 ± 4.7	16.2 ± 10.8
p-value		0.019	0.000	0.000	0.001	0.000	0.001

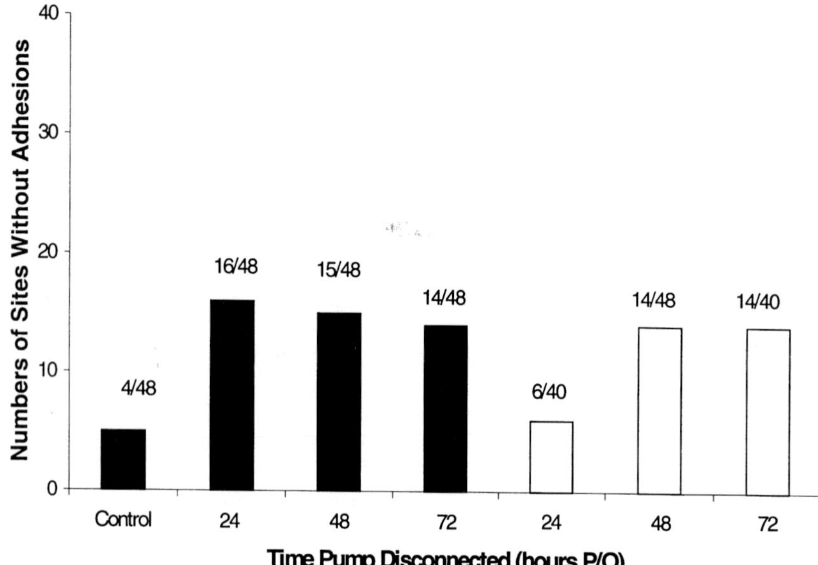

FIG. 37.8 The number of sites evaluated (8 per rabbit) that did not form adhesion to the uterine horns after surgery. *Black bars,* 0.01 mg/mL anti-inflammin; *light bars,* 0.1 mg/mL anti-inflammin. Reproduced with permission from ref. 12.

position of fibrin in turn makes fibrin available to act as a bridge for adhesion formation.

Hirudin, a 65-amino-acid protein originally isolated from the medicinal leech, is a potent natural inhibitor of thrombin.[66] Hirudin and segments of hirudin that bind to the catalytic site of thrombin (hirulogue) have been shown to prolong clotting time, reduce thrombosis formation after laser injury, and accelerate thrombolysis by tissue plasminogen activator.[67–69] RecHirudin, an analog of hirudin and an inhibitor of thrombin, was tested for its ability to reduce adhesion formation when administered to the site of injury in the two screening models already described. RecHirudin may reduce adhesion formation through its ability to inhibit thrombin. Bleeding was not noted in the animals treated postoperatively with RecHirudin, but bleeding or increased risk of hemorrhage is a possible complication of the therapeutic use of this protein.

RecHirudin was shown to significantly reduce adhesion formation in two animal models of adhesion formation (Table 37.5; Fig. 37.9). This result indicates that the administration of a compound that inhibits thrombin activity during the entire postoperative interval dramatically reduces the formation of peritoneal adhesions.

TABLE 37.5. Effects of continuous administration of RecHirudin on the overall adhesion score in the double uterine horn model.

	Vehicle	RecHirudin 0.03 mg/mL	RecHirudin 0.3 mg/mL
Score	3	2	1.5
	3	2	1.5
	3.5	1.5	1.5
	3	2	1.5
	3.5	2	1
	3.5	1.5	1.5
Rank	15.5 ± 1.5	8.7 ± 2.6	4.3 ± 1.5

Lazaroids

Lazaroids are a unique group of 21-aminosteroid (steroidal lazaroids) and 2-methylaminochroman (nonsteroidal lazaroids) compounds that exert a protective effect against tissue damage or ischemia.[70,71] In several models of traumatic and ischemic injury to the central nervous system, lazaroids have been shown to prevent secondary tissue injury associated with oxidative cell damage.[71] The protective effects of lazaroids have been attributed to their ability to inhibit lipid peroxidation reactions as well as to reduce the production of reactive oxygen metabolites by leukocytes and monocytes.[72–78] Based upon the ability of lazaroids to reduce tissue damage secondary to traumatic ischemic injury, the effect of various lazaroid formulations on the formation of adhesions was examined in three animal models.

The effect of two lazaroids, PNU83,836E (a nonsteroidal compound) or PNU74006F (a steroidal compound), on the formation of intraperitoneal adhesions was studied. PNU83,836E was shown to significantly reduce adhesion formation in the two screening models of adhesion formation. In addition, administration of the compound for as little as 24 hours reduced the formation of adhesions, although administration for longer periods of time further increased the efficacy of the compound (Table 37.6). Further, administration of lazaroids in various formulations at the end of surgery was also efficacious in the reduction of adhesion formation (Table 37.7). Pretreatment with the steroidal lazaroid PNU74006F before the initiation of surgery followed by a bolus of drug at the conclusion of surgery was

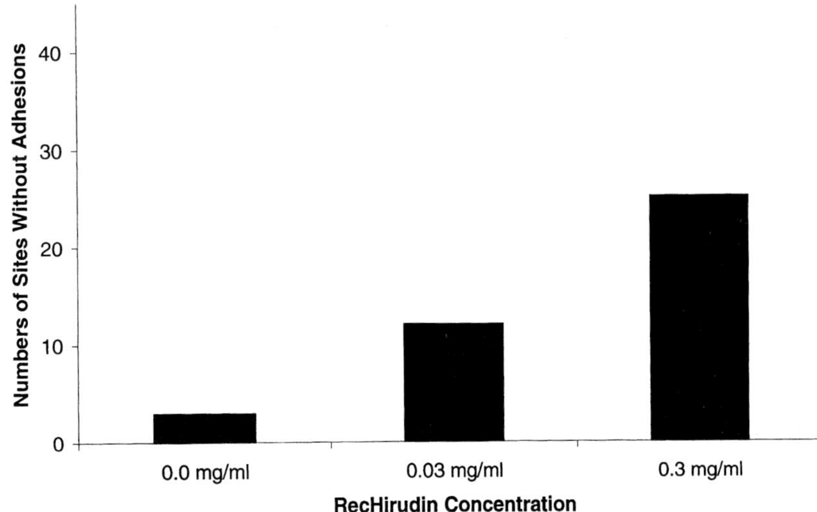

FIG. 37.9 The number of sites evaluated (8 per rabbit) that did not form adhesions to the uterine horns after surgery at various RecHiradin concentrations. Reproduced with permission from ref. 11.

TABLE 37.6. Effect of PNU83,836E administered for various times on the site-specific formation of adhesion in the double uterine horn model.

		PNU83,836E concentration:					
		0.06 mg/mL			0.6 mg/mL		
	Control	24 h	48 h	72 h	24 h	48 h	72 h
Right horn to:							
Bowel	46.7 ± 8.4	26.0 ± 10.3	5.0 ± 3.4*	3.3 ± 2.1*	25.0 ± 15.7	6.7 ± 3.7*	1.7 ± 1.7*
Bladder	50.0 ± 14.1	12.0 ± 7.4	16.7 ± 4.2*	3.7 ± 3.3*	15.0 ± 7.2	21.7 ± 4.8	1.7 ± 1.7*
Itself	36.7 ± 3.3	34.0 ± 2.5	20.0 ± 5.8*	8.3 ± 4.8*	30.0 ± 6.8	33.3 ± 4.2	18.3 ± 4.0*
Left horn	45.0 ± 9.9	14.0 ± 5.1*	0 ± 0*	0 ± 0*	6.7 ± 3.3*	6.7 ± 3.3*	11.7 ± 4.8*
Left horn to:							
Bowel	46.7 ± 8.4	22.0 ± 9.7	5.0 ± 3.4*	3.3 ± 2.1*	25.0 ± 15.7	6.7 ± 6.7*	1.7 ± 1.7*
Bladder	50.0 ± 14.1	12.0 ± 7.4	13.3 ± 3.3*	6.7 ± 3.3*	15.0 ± 7.2	18.3 ± 6.0	1.7 ± 1.7*
Itself	36.7 ± 4.9	18.0 ± 7.4	6.7 ± 2.1*	18.3 ± 4.0*	11.7 ± 4.8*	13.3 ± 4.9*	16.7 ± 3.3*
Right horn	45.0 ± 9.9	14.0 ± 5.1*	0 ± 0*	0 ± 0*	6.7 ± 3.3*	6.7 ± 3.3*	11.7 ± 4.8*

Data are % organ involvement.
*p-value ≤0.05 compared with controls.

TABLE 37.7. Effect of administration of lazaroids (1 mg/mL) at the end of surgery on the site-specific formation of adhesions in the double uterine horn model.

	Citrate buffer	PNU83,836E in citrate buffer	Cyclodextrin	PNU74006F in cyclodextrin	Lipid emulsion	PNU74006F in lipid emulsion
Right horn to:						
Bowel	44.3 ± 5.3	21.4 ± 3.4	40.0 ± 0.0	12.9 ± 5.2*	35.7 ± 3.7	14.3 ± 4.8*
Bladder	30.0 ± 2.2	0.0 ± 0.0*	8.6 ± 4.6	1.4 ± 4*	14.3 ± 4.8	4.3 ± 3.0
Itself	42.9 ± 8.7	27.1 ± 4.1	38.6 ± 4.0	28.6 ± 4.0	35.7 ± 3.0	27.1 ± 2.9
Left horn	24.3 ± 6.9	17.1 ± 4.7	38.6 ± 4.6	20.0 ± 4.4*	45.7 ± 4.8	22.9 ± 2.9*
Left horn to:						
Bowel	44.3 ± 5.3	21.4 ± 3.4*	40.0 ± 0.0	12.9 ± 5.2*	35.7 ± 3.7	14.3 ± 4.8*
Bladder	30.0 ± 2.2	0.0 ± 0.0*	5.7 ± 4.3	1.4 ± 1.4*	14.3 ± 4.8	2.9 ± 2.9*
Itself	50.0 ± 5.4	27.1 ± 4.1*	34.3 ± 3.0	30.0 ± 3.8	41.4 ± 8.3	24.3 ± 3.0
Right horn	24.3 ± 6.9	17.1 ± 4.7	38.6 ± 4.6	20.0 ± 4.4*	45.7 ± 4.8	22.9 ± 2.9*

Data are % organ involvement.
*p-value ≤0.05 compared with controls.

TABLE 37.8. Effect of administration of lazaroids (1 mg/mL) at the end of surgery on the site-specific formation of adhesions in the double uterine horn model.

	Placebo (Pre)	Placebo (Pre/Post)	PNU74006F (mg/mL)			
			1 (Pre)	1 (Pre/Post)	5 (Pre)	5 (Pre/Post)
Right horn to:						
Bowel	35.0 ± 3.4	22.9 ± 5.7	21.7 ± 3.3	12.9 ± 4.7	18.6 ± 4.6*	5.7 ± 4.3*
Bladder	28.3 ± 3.1	14.3 ± 6.9	3.3 ± 3.3*	2.9 ± 2.9	1.4 ± 1.4*	2.9 ± 1.8
Itself	35.0 ± 3.4	34.3 ± 2.0	23.3 ± 3.3*	27.1 ± 3.6	27.1 ± 3.6	21.4 ± 3.4*
Left horn	36.7 ± 2.1	34.3 ± 2.0	18.3 ± 4.0*	10.0 ± 4.4*	5.7 ± 2.0*	15.7 ± 4.8*
Left horn to:						
Bowel	35.0 ± 3.4	28.8 ± 5.2	21.7 ± 3.3	12.9 ± 4.7*	15.7 ± 5.3*	5.7 ± 4.3*
Bladder	28.3 ± 3.1	14.3 ± 6.9	3.3 ± 3.3*	5.7 ± 3.7	2.9 ± 1.8*	2.9 ± 1.8
Itself	40.0 ± 4.5	34.3 ± 2.0	23.3 ± 3.3*	21.4 ± 5.1*	25.7 ± 6.1	20.0 ± 3.1*
Right horn	34.9 ± 1.6	34.3 ± 2.0	18.3 ± 4.0*	10.1 ± 4.4*	5.7 ± 2.0*	15.7 ± 4.8*

Pre, preoperative; Post, postoperative.
Data are % organ involvement.
* p-value ≤0.05 compared with controls.

the most effective in reducing adhesion formation. Further, pre- and postoperative administration of lazaroid reduced the incidence of adhesion reformation (Table 37.8). Administration of as little as 3 mg (1.5 mg before and 1.5 mg after) PNU 75006F, as a total dose, maximally reduced adhesion formation (Table 37.9). This result indicates that the administration of compounds that will reduce inflammation and lipid peroxidation during the first 3 days after surgery can reduce the formation of peritoneal adhesions.

The steroidal lazaroid PNU74006F, because of its lipophilicity (calculated log partition = 8), is expected to deposit into lipid and be released slowly from the site of administration. This hypothesis is supported by several pharmacokinetic studies that show a prolonged beta half-life (of the order of 60–120 hours) for this compound after administration via a variety of routes. This characteristic of the compound would allow the abdominal tissues (e.g., omentum and other fat deposits) to act as a slow release depot in a manner analogous to the miniosmotic pumps during the early (5 days) postoperative interval.

The 21-aminosteroid lazaroids (e.g., PNU74006F) were developed as antioxidant steroids that reduce inflammation without the immunosuppressive effects or modulation of pituitary stimulation of glucocorticoids. The initial series of 21-aminosteroids (steroidal lazaroids; PNU74006F) were shown to be effective in the reduction of secondary tissue damage in several traumatic and ischemic injury models, particularly models of central nervous system disease.[79–81] The protective effects of lazaroids from this series have been attributed to their ability to inhibit lipid peroxidation reactions as well as the production of reactive oxygen metabolites (e.g., hydrogen peroxide and free radicals) by leukocytes and monocytes.[72–77] In the second generation of lazaroids, the steroid modality of the molecule was substituted with a methylaminochroman, resulting in a series of nonsteroidal lazaroid compounds (PNU83,836E).[71] These compounds were selected for their ability to inhibit lipid peroxidation.

One compound from each generation of lazaroids was shown to reduce adhesion formation, presumably through the reduction of lipid peroxidation and tissue damage secondary to trauma and ischemia. Studies have shown that trauma and ischemia reduce the fibrinolytic activity of parietal peritoneum.[42] Raftery determined that peritoneal fibrinolytic activity decreased immedi-

TABLE 37.9. Effect of various doses of PNU74006F on the site of specific formation of adhesion (%) in the double uterine horn model.

	Placebo	0.3 mg	1.0 mg	3.0 mg	10 mg	50 mg
Right horn to:						
Bowel	32.0 ± 4.8	27.0 ± 6.0	18.9 ± 7.4	7.0 ± 2.1*	11.1 ± 3.5*	9.0 ± 4.6
Bladder	27.0 ± 5.8	19.0 ± 6.2	7.8 ± 2*	1.0 ± 1.0*	3.0 ± 1.7	4.0 ± 2.2*
Itself	41.0 ± 3.5	40.0 ± 4.2	28.9 ± 5.9	18.0 ± 3.6*	15.6 ± 2.4*	20.0 ± 3.7
Left horn	35.0 ± 2.2	34.0 ± 3.4	22.0 ± 3.6*	9.0 ± 1.8*	13.3 ± 3.7*	9.0 ± 2.3*
Left horn to:						
Bowel	32.0 ± 4.8	27.0 ± 6.0	26.0 ± 7.5	6.0 ± 2.2*	11.1 ± 3.5*	5.0 ± 4.0*
Bladder	27.0 ± 5.8	19.0 ± 6.2	7.8 ± 3.2*	2.0 ± 1.3*	3.3 ± 1.7*	4.0 ± 2.2*
Itself	42.0 ± 2.5	37.0 ± 4.0	32.2 ± 4.0	23.0 ± 3.4	7.8 ± 4.0*	15.0 ± 4.0*
Right horn	35.0 ± 2.2	34.0 ± 3.4	24.4 ± 3.2*	9.0 ± 1.8	13.3 ± 3.7*	9.0 ± 2.3*

* p-value ≤0.05 compared with controls.

ately and continued to decrease at 24 hours after three different types of trauma (excision, grafting, and ischemia)[39]; this suggests that secondary damage occurs after these acute injuries that further reduces fibrinolytic activity. As lazaroids reduce secondary damage that occurs after acute trauma and ischemia, it is conceivable that they act to ameliorate the inhibition of fibrinolysis which occurs in our surgical model. If this occurs, the deposited fibrin would be more rapidly cleared, thereby reducing the amount of fibrin available for adhesion formation.

Nonsteroidal Antiinflammatory Drugs

Nonsteroidal antiinflammatory drugs (NSAIDs) are a class of compounds that alter the metabolism of arachidonic acid in a variety of tissues and thereby alter the endogenous balance of the cyclooxygenase, lipoxygenase, and epoxygenase enzyme systems and formation of their end products. Arachidonic acid metabolites are produced by the polymorphonuclear leukocytes (PMNs) and macrophages present at the site of inflammation or may result from platelet aggregation and thereby mediate inflammatory events. Labeled arachidonic acid metabolized by peritoneal exudate cells forms metabolites by the lipoxygenase and cyclooxygenase pathways including prostaglandins, thromboxane, and hydroxyeicosatetraenoic acid (HETE).[82] An increase in 15-HETE and di-HETE, and a decrease in 5-HETE formation, beginning 24 hours after surgical injury, were observed in rabbits. In addition, there was an increase in thromboxane B and in prostaglandin E_2 (PGE_2) throughout the study interval (2–10 days postoperatively). These arachidonic acid metabolites mediate some aspects of the postsurgical inflammatory response. PGs are involved in events that occur during the generation of inflammation including leukocyte infiltration, edema formation, and endothelial cell procoagulant activities.[35] Golan et al.[36,37] found that addition of prostaglandins F_2 and E_2 into the peritoneal cavity of rats enhanced the formation of adhesions to the injury site. NSAIDs inhibit the formation of arachidonic acid metabolites through suppression of cyclooxygenase and lipoxygenase pathways, and thus lead to a reduction in inflammation mediated by these metabolites.[83,84]

NSAIDs in Reduction of Adhesion Formation

NSAIDs were shown to reduce formation of peritoneal adhesions in a variety of animal models (Table 37.10).[85–92] However, not all studies demonstrated adhesion reduction with NSAIDs.[85] Most studies were conducted using systematic administration of these agents. Oxyphenbutazone, administered perioperatively in rats and monkeys, reduced postoperative adhesion formation.[92–94] Siegler et al.[88] and Bateman et al.[90] observed a marked reduction in adhesion formation following systemic administration of 7 and 10 mg/kg of ibuprofen, respectively, during the perioperative interval. Nishimura et al.[95] found that administration of two doses of ibuprofen after the completion of surgery did not affect adhesion formation. However, a significant reduction in adhesion formation was noted after five doses (including preoperative dosing) of ibuprofen (70 mg/kg) when administered systemically.[96,97]

Further studies were conducted with NSAIDs administered intraperitoneally in an attempt to reduce adhesion

TABLE 37.10. Summary of representative experimental studies of nonsteroidal antiinflammatory drugs (NSAIDs) on postoperative adhesion formation.

Experimental model	NSAID (dose)	Treatment regimen	Results[a]	Reference
Rabbit ileum trauma	Piroxicam (PIR) (10 mg/kg/day/i.m.)	2 h or immediately presurgery and daily postop for 7 days	PIR > Control	86
Rat uterine horn reanastomosis	Ibuprofen (IBU) (12.5 mg/kg i.p.)	30 min presurgery and q8h postop for 2 days	IBU = Control IBU > Dexamethasone	87
Rabbit uterine horn reanastomosis	Ibuprofen (IBU) (7 mg/kg i.v.)	30 min presurgery and q8h postop for 2 days	IBU = Control IBU > Dexamethasone	88
Rabbit uterine horn reanastomosis	Ibuprofen (IBU) (75 mg i.v.) Flurbiprofen (FLUR) (12.5 mg i.v.)	Immediately presurgery and q6h postop for 2 days	IBU = Control FLUR > Control	89
Rabbit uterine horn trauma	Ibuprofen (IBU) (10 mg/kg i.m.)	30 min presurgery and q8h postop for 4 days	IBU = Control	90
Rabbit uterine adhesiolysis	Ibuprofen (IBU) (12.5 mg/kg i.m.)	15 min presurgery and q12h postop for 3 days	IBU = Control	85
Guinea pig uterine horn reanastomosis	Ibuprofen (IBU) (12.5 mg/kg i.m.) Indomet hacin (INDO) (1 mg/kg i.m.)	3 min presurgery and q8h postop for 3 days	IBU = Control INDO > Control	91
Rabbit cecum trauma	Oxyphenbutazone (OXY) (10 mg/kg)[b]	6 days[b]	OXY > Control	92

[a]Results of statistical analysis of treated versus control groups.
[b]Unspecified route of administration and dosing frequency.

formation. However, not all studies demonstrated adhesion reduction with NSAIDs.[85] Intraperitoneal administration of ibuprofen through a miniosmotic pump, in hydron polymer, or in a liposome carrier reduced adhesion formation following abrasion of the parietal peritoneum and serosal surface of the colon.[16,82] Tolmetin, another NSAID, reduced adhesion formation at low concentrations when administered in miniosmotic pumps.[15] Tolmetin, in a series of micellar (5% Tween 80) and vesicle (multilaminar liposomes) preparations, significantly reduced adhesion formation in a variety of animal models.[15,16] Tolmetin reduced adhesion formation in animals models when placed in a high molecular weight carrier, which may act as a viscoelastic barrier in conjunction with the pharmacologic effects of tolmetin.[98] These data suggest that inhibitors of arachidonic acid metabolism, such as ibuprofen and tolmetin, effectively reduce postoperative adhesion formation.

NSAID Mechanisms of Action

There are several possible mechanisms by which NSAIDs reduce adhesion formation following peritoneal surgery. First, adhesion formation may be reduced through diminished PG synthesis, which would subsequently reduce inflammatory events mediated by PGs.[35] A decrease in leukocyte infiltration and coagulation (which follows platelet aggregation) may decrease the formation of matrix necessary for fibroblast organization. Alternatively, macrophages secrete plasminogen activator (PA),[99–101] which activates the fibrinolytic enzyme plasmin. Tolmetin-enhanced secretion of PA by postsurgical macrophages would lyse clots and reduce the formation of fibrinous bands that would support fibroblast organization.

A decrease in PA synthesis coincides with the initiation of inflammation-induced differentiation of macrophages.[102] Many macrophage functions that are modulated during inflammation are suppressed in resident macrophages by PG.[102] Therefore, a decrease in PG synthesis through chemical intervention could allow a more rapid differentiation of resident and infiltrating leukocytes in response to inflammatory signals such as complement and bacterial endotoxin following surgery. If stimulation of differentiation by NSAIDs occurred, any potential infection present would be cleared more rapidly and would therefore be less stimulatory to leukocytes.

Macrophages and PMNs are centrally involved in the initial clearance of bacteria and damaged tissue. Macrophages and PMNs increase capacities including phagocytosis,[103] superoxide anion (O_2^-) release,[104] and tumoricidal/microbiocidal[105] activity following inflammatory and other stimuli, which, in turn, allows for the rapid clearance of infectious agents. Because many of these functions that are enhanced during inflammation may be regulated by PGs, administration of an NSAID, which inhibits PG synthesis,[106] may modulate these enhanced leukocytic cell functions.

Modulation of Macrophage Function by Tolmetin

After rat surgery, administration of tolmetin significantly elevated respiratory burst-activating release at postoperative days 3 and 5, phagocytic capability at days 7 and 14, and tumoricidal activity at day 3 (Fig. 37.10). Differential staining and microscopic analysis revealed increases in PMN numbers with tolmetin doses of 3 and 10 mg.[107] PGs modulate PMN chemotaxis during inflammation.

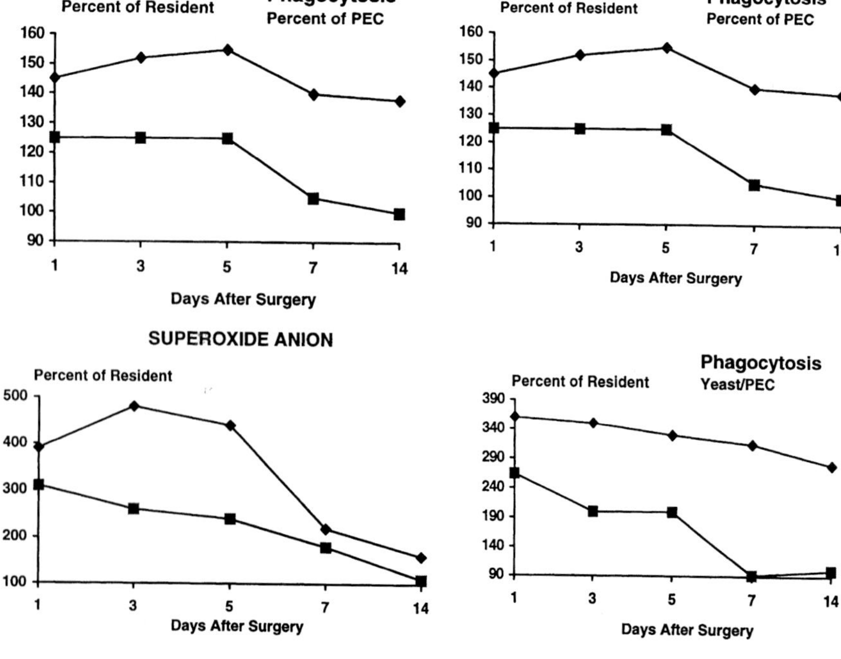

FIG. 37.10 The effect of peritoneal trauma with (*diamonds*) and without (*squares*) the administration of tolmetin, (3 mg/rat) at the end of surgery on peritoneal exudative cell (PEC) function. The functions examined include phagocytosis, respiratory burst, and tumoricidal activities, which are important in the clearance of bacteria. These data are presented as the percentage of resident peritoneal cell function. All parameters examined were increased at early postoperative time points and further elevated by the acute administration of tolmetin (Rodgers et al. 1988).[107]

PG synthesis and release initially decrease during inflammation followed by a concomitant increase in neutral protease secretion by macrophages.[99,108] These findings suggest that PG synthesis by macrophages is necessary to maintain the resident differentiative state of the macrophage. As a result, inhibition of PG synthesis by NSAIDs may provide the necessary signal(s) to initiate macrophage (and perhaps PMN) differentiation.

Protease Activity

NSAIDs may reduce adhesion formation by increasing the expression of fibrinolytic activity either through modulation of protease and protease inhibitor secretion or reduction of protease inhibitor activity in wound fluid.[60,98] Following peritoneal surgery, the level of neutral proteases secreted by peritoneal macrophages increases. Exposure of postsurgical rabbit macrophages to tolmetin in vitro suppresses collagenase and elevates elastase activities at early time points after surgery (Table 37.11). In contrast, the level of PA inhibitory (PAI) activity in cultures of postsurgical macrophages harvested within 48 hours after surgery is reduced by in vitro exposure of postsurgical macrophages to tolmetin. These data suggest that NSAIDs modify the ability of postsurgical macrophages to remodel and clear debris from the site of trauma.

Collagenase activity is reduced in macrophage-conditioned media up to 48 hours after surgery after exposure to tolmetin (Table 37.11). Wahl and Lampel[109] found that indomethacin (a PG synthesis inhibitor) decreased the level of collagenase secreted by human monocytes. They proposed that collagenase secretion contains a PG-dependent step.[110] Up to 48 hours after surgery, peritoneal macrophages appear to be susceptible to modulation by tolmetin.[60,98]

Elastase secretion by postsurgical macrophages is also elevated by in vitro exposure to tolmetin (Table 37.11). Previous studies by Werb et al.[111] showed that purified macrophage elastase could cleave elastin as well as fibronectin, laminin, fibrinogen, proteoglycan, and matrix secreted by rat smooth muscles. In the peritoneal cavity, elastase may be important for the clearance of fibrin clots and tissue debris after surgery. The increase in elastase secretion observed after in vitro exposure to tolmetin suggests an additional mechanism by which tolmetin reduces adhesion formation.

A decrease in the level of PAI activity found in postsurgical macrophage-conditioned media may increase fibrinolytic activity in the peritoneal cavity after surgery. In vitro exposure of peritoneal macrophages to tolmetin for up to 48 hours after surgery reduces the amount of PAI activity in macrophage-conditioned media.[60,98] Because adhesion formation may be dependent upon fibrin deposition to support fibroblast organization, an increase in fibrinolysis would decrease adhesion formation.

TABLE 37.11. Modulation of protease activity in macrophage-conditioned media by tolmetin.

Hours after surgery	Collagenase	Elastase	PAI
0	71 ± 6*	272 ± 4**	45 ± 4*
6	49 ± 9*	129 ± 1**	83 ± 2*
12	50 ± 10*	113 ± 4	65 ± 3*
24	68 ± 4*	95 ± 6	78 ± 3*
48	60 ± 12*	101 ± 4	81 ± 2*
72	74 ± 21	99 ± 7	98 ± 10
96	141 ± 17**	94 ± 1	106 ± 4

PAI, plasmogen-activator inhibitor.
Macrophages were harvested from rabbits at various times after surgery, placed in culture for 4 days with 2 mg/mL tolmetin, and the protease or protease inhibitor activity in the supernatant measured. Data are presented as percent of surgical control (Rodgers et al. 1990[15]).
* Significantly ($p < 0.05$) suppressed compared to control.
** Significantly ($p < 0.05$) elevated compared to control.

Conclusion

Previous studies demonstrated that systemic administration of medicaments did not significantly reduce adhesion formation, whereas intraperitoneal administration of the same agents was effective. This disparity may be caused by a limitation in drug delivery. Anatomic sites supplied by blood that are distal to vascular occlusion after surgical injury (clamped, cut, ligated, or fulgurated) are the primary sites for adhesion formation. Accordingly, a drug delivered via the systemic circulation is prevented from arriving at the site where it is most needed.

In this chapter, animal models were described with an intraperitoneal delivery system that allows screening of pharmaceuticals that may reduce adhesion formation. Through implantation of a miniosmotic pump, it was possible to maintain sustained delivery of a therapeutic concentration of medicament at the site of injury. Because the pump can be disconnected at various postoperative intervals, this model allows for both dose–response and time–response studies to characterize the parameters for optimal delivery of the drug. These data can be used to identify a vehicle system appropriate to sustain intraperitoneal concentrations of the drug for the time needed for a single intraoperative administration at the time of surgery.

References

1. diZerega G, Rodgers KE. Prevention of postoperative adhesions. In: The Peritoneum. New York: Springer-Verlag, 1992:307–370.
2. diZerega GS. Contemporary adhesion prevention. Fertil Steril 1994;61:219–235.
3. Adhesion Study Group. Reduction of postoperative pelvic adhesions with intraperitoneal 32% dextran 70: a pro-

spective, randomized clinical trial. Fertil Steril 1983;40: 612–619.

4. diZerega GS. Use of adhesion prevention barriers in ovarian surgery, tuboplasty, ectopic pregnancy, endometriosis, adhesiolysis, and myomectomy. Curr Opin Obstet Gynecol 1996;8:230–237.
5. Thornton MH, Campeau JD, diZerega GS. Use of adhesion prevention barriers in gynecological surgery. In: Treutner KH Schumpelick VS, eds. Peritoneal Adhesions. New York: Springer-Verlag, 1997:370–377.
6. diZerega GS. Use of adhesion prevention barriers in pelvic reconstructive and gynecologic surgery. In: diZerega GS, DeCherney AH, Diamond MP, et al., eds. Pelvic Surgery. New York: Springer-Verlag, 1997:188–209.
7. Thornton M, diZerega GS. Use of barriers in adhesion prevention. Contemp Obstet Gynecol 1996;41:107–124.
8. Treutner KH, Bertram P, Loser L, et al. Prophylaxe und therapie intraabdomineller adhasionen—Eine umfrage an 1200 Kliniken in Deutschland. Chirurg 1995;66:398–403.
9. Diamond M. Precoating with Seprafilm. Abstract presented at the 43rd Annual Meeting of the Society for Gynecologic Investigations, Philadelphia, PA, March 1996.
10. Thornton MH, Johns DB, Campeau JD, et al. Clinical evaluation of 0.5% ferric hyaluronate adhesion prevention gel for the reduction of adhesions following peritoneal cavity surgery: open-label pilot study. Hum Reprod (Oxf) 1998;13(6):1480–1485.
11. Rodgers KE, Girgis W, Campeau JD, et al. Reduction of adhesion formation by intraperitoneal administration of a recombinant hirudin analog. J Invest Surg 1996;9: 388–391.
12. Rodgers KE, Girgis W, Campeau JD, et al. Reduction of adhesion formation by intraperitoneal administration of anti-inflammatory peptide. 2. J Invest Surg 1997;10:31–36.
13. Rodgers KE, Johns D, diZerega GS. Prevention of adhesion formation after intraperitoneal administration of tolmetin and hyaluronic acid. J Invest Surg 1997;10:367–373.
14. Nishimura K, Shimanuki T, diZerega GS. The use of ibuprofen for the prevention of postoperative adhesions in rabbits. Am J Med 1984;77:102–106.
15. Rodgers KE, Girgis W, Johns D, diZerega GS. Intraperitoneal tolmetin prevents postsurgical adhesion formation in rabbits. Int J Infertil 1990;35:40–45.
16. Rodgers KE, Bracken K, Cox G, Richer L, Girgis W, diZerega GS. Inhibition of post surgical adhesions by liposomes containing anti-inflammatory drugs. Int J Fertil 1990;35(5):315.
17. Mehta K, McQueen T, Tucker S, Pandita R, Aggarwal BB. Inhibition by all-trans-retinoic acid of tumor necrosis factor and nitric oxide production by peritoneal macrophages. J Leukocyte Biol 1994;44:336–342.
18. Zitnik Kotloff RM, Latifpour J, Schwalb J, Zheng T, Whiting NL, Elias JA. Retinoic acid inhibition of IL-1 induced IL-6 production by human lung fibroblasts. J Immunol 1994;152:1419–1427.
19. Schuster AT, Medcalf RL, Kruithof EKO. Retinoic acid potentiates phorbol ester-mediated induction of urokinase and plasminogen activator inhibitor type 2 in human myeloid leukemic cell lines. Endocrinology 1993;133: 1724–1730.
20. Immonen CS, Siren V, Stephens RW, Liesto K, Vaheri A. Retinoids increase urokinase-type plasminogen activator production by human retinal pigment epithelial cells in culture. Invest Ophthal Visual Sci 1993;34:2062–2067.
21. Van Giezen JJJ, Boon GIA, Jansen JWCM, Bouma BN. Retinoic acid enhances fibrinolytic activity in vivo by enhancing tissue type plasminogen activator (tPA) activity and inhibits venous thrombosis. Thromb Haemostasis 1993;69:381–386.
22. Medh RD, Santell L, Levin EG. Stimulation of tissue plasminogen activator production by retinoic acid: synergistic effect on protein kinase C-mediated activation. Blood 1992;80(4):981–987.
23. Van Bennekum AM, Emeis JJ, Kooistra T, Hendriks HF. Modulation of tissue type plasminogen activator by retinoids in rat plasma and tissues. Am J Physiol 1993;264: R931–R937.
24. Conese M, Montemurro P, Fumarulo R, et al. Inhibitory effects of retinoids on the generation of procoagulant activity by blood mononuclear phagocytes. Thromb Haemostasis 1991;66:662–665.
25. Horie S, Kizaki K, Ishii H, Kazama M. Retinoic acid stimulates expression of thrombomodulin, a cell surface anticoagulant glycoprotein, on human endothelial cells. Biochem J 1993;281:149–154.
26. Ishii H, Horie S, Kizaki K, Kazama M. Retinoic acid counteracts both the downregulation of thrombomodulin and the induction of tissue factor in human endothelial cells exposed to tumor necrosis factor. Blood 1992;80: 2556–2562.
27. Olansky AJ. Antimalarials and ophthalmologic safety. J Am Acad Dermatol 1982;6:19–23.
28. Fitch CD. Mode of action of antimalarial drugs. CIBA Found Symp 1983;94:222–232.
29. Beckman A, Seferynska F. Possible involvement of phospholipase activation in erythroid progenitor cell proliferation. Exp Hematol 1989;17:309–312.
30. White SR, Strek ME, Kulp GV, et al. Regulation of human eosinophil degranulation and activation by endogenous phospholipase A2. J Clin Invest 1993;91:2118–2125.
31. Stacey NH, Klaassen CD. Effects of phospholipase A2 inhibitors on diethyl maleate-induced lipid peroxidation and cellular injury in isolate rat hepatocytes. J Toxicol Environ Health 1982;9:439–450.
32. O'Rourke AM, Mescher MR, Apgar JR. IgE receptor-mediated arachidonic acid release by rat basophilic leukemia (RBL-2H3) cells: possible role in activating degranulation. Mol Immunol 1992;29:1299–1308.
33. Moreno JJ, Ferrer X, Ortega E, Carganico G. PLA2-induced oedema in rat skin and histamine release in rat mast cells. Evidence for involvement of lysophospholipids in the mechanism of action. Agents Actions 1992;36: 258–263.
34. Foeldes AJ, Filep RE. Mepacrine inhibits fMLP-induced activation of human neutrophil granulocytes, leukotrienes B4 formation and fMLP binding. J Leukocyte Biol 1992; 52:545–550.
35. Randall RW, Eakins KE, Higgs GA. Inhibition of arachidonic acid cyclooxygenase and lipo-oxygenase activities by indomethacin and compound BW755. Agents Actions 1980;10:553–555.
36. Golan A, Bernstein T, Wexler S, Neuman M, Bukovsky I, David MP. The effect of prostaglandins and aspirin: an in-

hibitor of prostaglandin synthesis on adhesion formation in rats. Human Reprod (Oxf) 1991;6:251–254.
37. Golan A, Stolik O, Wexler S, Lander R, Ber A, David MP. Prostaglandins—a role in adhesion formation. An experimental study. Acta Obstet Gynecol Scand 1990;69: 339–341.
38. Prowse C, Pepper D, Dawes J. Prevention of the platelet alpha-granule reaction by membrane active drugs. Thromb Res 1982;25:219–227.
39. Raftery AT. Effect of peritoneal trauma on peritoneal fibrinolytic activity and intraperitoneal adhesion formation. Eur Surg Res 1981;13:397–401.
40. Mumford D, Kessel SJ. Sterilization needs in the 1990s: the case for quinacrine nonsurgical female sterilization. Am J Obstet Gynecol 1992;167:1203–1207.
41. Mammen EF. An overview of dipyridamole. Thromb Res Suppl 1990;XIII:1–10.
42. Buckman RF, Buckman PD, Hufnagel HV, Gervin AS. A physiologic basis for the adhesion-free healing of deperitonealized surfaces. J Surg Res 1976;21:67–76.
43. Tzanakakis GN, Agarwal KC, Vezeredis MP. Prevention of human pancreatic cancer cell-induced hepatic metastasis in nude mice by dipyridamole and its analog RA-233. Cancer (Phila) 1993;71:2466.
44. Costantini V, Talpacci A, Bastino ML, et al. Increased prostacyclin production from human veins by dipyridamole: an in vitro and ex vitro study. Biomed Biochim Acta 1990;49(4):263–271.
45. Saniabadi AR, Fisher TC, McLaren M, Belch JF, Forbes CD. Effect of dipyridamole alone and in combination with aspirin on whole blood platelet aggregation, PGI2 generation, and red cell deformability ex vivo in man. Cardiovasc Res 1991;25:177.
46. Gryglewski RJ. Prostaglandins, platelets, and atherosclerosis. CRC Crit Rev Biochem 1980;7(4):291–338.
47. Hasday JD, Sitrin RJ. Dipyridamole stimulates urokinase production and suppresses procoagulant activity of rabbit alveolar macrophages: a possible mechanism of antithrombotic action. Blood 1987;69:660.
48. Colli S, Tremoli E. Multiple effects of dipyridamole on neutrophils and mononuclear leukocytes: adenosine-dependent and adenosine-independent mechanisms. J Lab Clin Med 1991;118:126.
49. Aznar-Salatti J, Bastida E, Escolar G, et al. Dipyridamole induces changes in the thrombogenic properties of extracellular matrix produced by endothelial cell in culture. Thromb Res 1991;64:341–345.
50. LeVraux V, Chen YL, Masson I, et al. Inhibition of human monocyte TNF production by adenosine receptor agonists. Life Sci 1993;52:1917.
51. Bronza JP, et al. Dipyridamole inhibits superoxide anion release and expression of tissue factor activity by peripheral blood monocytes stimulated with lipopolysaccharide. Thromb Res 1990;60:141.
52. Suzuki S, Sugai K, Sato H, Sakatume M, Arakawa M. Inhibition of active oxygen generation by dipyridamole in human polymorphonuclear leukocytes. Eur J Pharmacol 1992;227:395.
53. Miele L, Cordella-Miele E, Facchiano A, Mukherjee AN. Novel antiinflammatory peptides from the region of highest similarity between uteroglobin and lipocortin 1. Nature (Lond) 1988;335:726–730.
54. Carey F, Forder R, Edge MD, et al. Lipocortin I fragment modifies pyrogenic activity of cytokines in rats. Am J Physiol 1990;259:R266–R269.
55. Perretti M, Ahluwalia A, Harris JG, Goulding NJ, Flower RJ. Lipocortin 1 fragments inhibit neutrophil accumulation and neutrophil-dependent edema in the mouse: a qualitative comparison with an anti-CD1 lb monoclonal antibody. J Immunol 1993;151:4306–4314.
56. Perretti M, Becherucci C, Mugridge KG, Solito E, Silvestri S, Parente L. A novel anti-inflammatory peptide from human lipocortin 5. Br J Pharmacol 1991;103:1327–1332.
57. Caideraro V, Parrillo C, Giovane A, et al. Antinflammins suppress the A23187- and arachidonic acid-dependent chloride secretion in rabbit distal colonic mucosa. J Pharmacol Exp Ther 1992;263:579–587.
58. Cirino G, Cicala C, Sorrentino L, et al. Anti-inflammatory actions of an N-terminal peptide from human lipocortin 1. Br J Pharmacol 1993;108:573–574.
59. Lloret S, Moreno JJ. Effect of nonapeptide fragments of uteroglobin and lipocortin on oedema and mast cell degranulation. Eur J Pharmacol 1994;264:379–384.
60. Rodgers KE, Ellefson DD, Girgis W, diZerega GS. Protease and protease inhibitor secretion by postsurgical macrophages following in vitro exposure to tolmetin. Agents Actions 1992;36:248–256.
61. Rodgers KE, Abe H, Campeau JD, Ellefson D, Girgis W, diZerega GS. In vivo administration of tolmetin in hyaluronic acid modulates protease levels in post-surgical macrophage conditioned media. J Invest Surg 1992;5: 285–293.
62. Rodgers KE, Ellefson DD, Girgis W, et al. Modulation of postsurgical cell infiltration and fibrinolytic activity by tolmetin in two species. J Surg Res 1994;56:314–325.
63. Fenton JW, Ofosu FA, Moon DG, Maraganore JM. Thrombin and hemostasis. Blood Coagul Fibrinolysis 1991;2: 69–75.
64. Fenton JW. Seminars in thrombosis. Hemostasis 1988;14: 265–268.
65. Kelly AB, Maraganore JM, Bourdon P, Hanson SR, Harker LA. Antithrombotic effects of synthetic peptides targeting various functional domains of thrombin. Proc Natl Acad Sci USA 1992;89:6040–6044.
66. Bourdon P, Jablonski JA, Chao BH, Maraganore JM. Structure-function relationships of hirulog peptide interactions with thrombin. FEBS 1991;294:163–166.
67. Klement P, Borm A, Hirsch J, Maraganore J, Wilson G, Weitz J. The effect of thrombin inhibitors on tissue plasminogen activator induced thrombolysis in a rat model. Thromb Haemostasis 1992;68:64–68.
68. Krupinski K, Breddin HK, Markwardt F, Haarmann W. Antithrombotic effects of three thrombin inhibitors in a rat model of laser-induced thrombosis. Haemostasis 1989; 19: 74–82.
69. Ofosu FA, Fenton JW, Maraganore J, et al. Inhibition of the amplification reactions of blood coagulation by site-specific inhibitors of alpha-thrombin. Biochem J 1992; 283:893–897.
70. Thomas PD, Mao GD, Rabinovitch A, et al. Inhibition of superoxide-generating species NADPH oxidase of human neutrophils by lazaroids (21-aminosteroids and 2-methylaminochromans. Biochem Pharmacol 1993;45:241–251.

71. Hall ED. Novel inhibitors of iron-dependent lipid peroxidation for neurodegenerative disorders. Ann Neurol 1992; 32(suppl):137–142.
72. Braughler JM, Pregenzer JF. The 21-aminosteroid inhibitors of lipid peroxidation reactions with lipid peroxyl and phenoxyl radicals. Free Radical Biol Med 1989;7: 125–139.
73. Braughler JM, Pregenzer JF, Chase RL, et al. Novel 21-amino steroids as potent inhibitors of iron-dependent lipid peroxidation. J Biol Chem 1987;262:10438–10440.
74. Shappell SM, Smith RJ, McGuire GM, et al. Inhibition of neutrophil beta-2-integrin-mediated hydrogen peroxide production by lazaroids U75412 and U78517. FASEB J 1994;14:A1428.
75. Fisher AA, Levine PH, Doyle EM, et al. A 21-aminosteroid inhibits stimulated monocyte hydrogen peroxide and chemiluminescence measurements from MS patients and controls. Neurology 1991;41:297–299.
76. Fisher AA, Levine PH, Cohen RA. A 21-aminosteroid reduces hydrogen peroxide generation by and chemiluminescence of stimulated human leukocytes. Stroke 1990;21: 1435–1438.
77. McCall JM. The discovery and pharmacology of tirilazad mesylate. In: Lemasters JJ, Oliver C, eds. Cell Biology of Trauma. Boca Raton: CRC Press, 1995.
78. Kalra J, Mantha SV, Kumar, P, et al. The protective effects of lazaroids against oxygen free radicals induced lysosomal damage. Mol Cell Biochem 1994;136:125–129.
79. Braughler JM, Hall ED. Central nervous system trauma and stroke. I. Biochemical considerations for oxygen radical formation and lipid peroxidation. Free Radical Biol Med 1989;6:289–301.
80. Aoki N, Lefer AM. Protective effects of a novel non-glucocorticoid 21-aminosteroid (U74006F) during traumatic shock in rats. J Cardiovasc Pharmacol 1996;15:205–219.
81. Choi M, Ehrlich HP. U75412E, a lazaroid, prevents progressive burn ischemia in a rat burn model. Am J Pathol 1993;142:519–528.
82. Shimanuki T, Nakamura RM, diZerega GS. A kinetic analysis of peritoneal fluid cytology and arachidonic acid metabolism after abrasion and reabrasion of rabbit peritoneum. J Surg Res 1986;41:245–251.
83. Vane JR. Inhibition of prostaglandin synthesis as a mechanism of action for aspirin-like drugs. Nat New Biol 1971; 231:232–235.
84. Flower R, Gryglewski R, Herbaczynska-Cedro K, Vane JR. Effects of anti-inflammatory drugs on prostaglandin biosynthesis. Nat New Biol 1972;238:104–106.
85. Holtz G. Failure of a non-steroidal anti-inflammatory agent (ibuprofen) to inhibit peritoneal adhesion reformation after lysis. Fertil Steril 1982;37:582–583.
86. Maurer JH, Bonventura LM. The effect of aqueous progesterone on operative adhesion formation. Fertil Steril 1983;39:485–489.
87. Luciano A, Hauser K, Benda J. Evaluation of commonly used adjuvants in the prevention of postoperative adhesion. Am J Obstet Gynecol 1983;146:88–92.
88. Siegler AM, Kontopoulos V, Wang CF. Prevention of postoperative adhesions in rabbits with ibuprofen, a nonsteroidal anti-inflammatory agent. Fertil Steril 1980;34:46–49.
89. Jarett J, Darwood M. Adhesion formation and uterine tube healing in the rabbit: a controlled study of the effects of ibuprofen and flurbiprofen. Am J Obstet Gynecol 1986;155(6):1186–1192.
90. Bateman BG, Nunley WC, Kitchen JD. Prevention of postoperative peritoneal adhesion: an assessment of ibuprofen. Fertil Steril 1982;38:107–115.
91. DeLeon FD, Toledo AA, Sanfilippo JS, et al. The prevention of adhesion formation by nonsteroidal anti-inflamatory drugs: an animal study comparing ibuprofen and indomethacin. Fertil Steril 1984;41:639–642.
92. Kapur BML, Gulati SM, Talwar JR. Prevention of reformation of peritoneal adhesions: effect of oxyphenbutazone, proteolytic enzymes for carcia papaya and extran 40. Arch Surg 1972;105:761–764.
93. Kapur BML, Talwar JR, Gulati SM. Oxyphenbutazone: anti-inflammatory agent in prevention of peritoneal adhesions. Arch Surg 1969;98:301–302.
94. Larsson B, Svanberg SG, Swolin K. Oxyphenbutazone—an adjuvant to be used in prevention of adhesion in operations for fertility. Fertil Steril 1977;28:807–808.
95. Nishimura K, Shimanuki T, diZerega GS. Ibuprofen in the prevention of experimentally induced postoperative adhesions. Am J Med 1984;77:102–106.
96. Nishimura K, Nakamura RM, diZerega GS. Biochemical evaluation of postsurgical wound repair: prevention of intraperitoneal adhesion formation with ibuprofen. J Surg Res 1983;34:219–226.
97. Nishimura K, Nakamura RM, diZerega GS. Ibuprofen inhibition of postsurgical adhesion formation: a time- and dose-response biochemical evaluation in rabbits. J Surg Res 1984;36:115–124.
98. Rodgers KE. Nonsteroidal anti-inflammatory drugs (NSAIDs) in the treatment of postsurgical adhesion. In: diZerega GS, Malinak LR, Diamond MD, Linsky CP, eds. Treatment of Adhesions. New York: Wiley-Liss, 1990: 119–130.
99. Unkeless JC, Gordon S, Reich S. Secretion of plasminogen activator by stimulated macrophages. J Exp Med 1974; 139: 834–850.
100. Chapman HA, Vavrin Z, Hibbs JB. Macrophage fibrinolytic activity: identification of two pathways of plasmin formation by intact cells of a plasminogen activator inhibitor. Cell 1982;28:653–662.
101. Orita H, Gale J, Campeau JD, et al. Differential secretion of plasminogen activator by post-surgical activated macrophages. J Surg Res 1986;41:569–573.
102. Bonney RJ, Davies P. Possible autoregulatory functions of the secretory products of monouclear phagocytes. Contemp Top Immunol 1984;10:199–223.
103. Ratzan KR, Musher DM, Keusch GT, et al. Correlation of increased metabolic activites resistance to infection, enhanced phagocytosis and inhibition of bacterial growth by macrophages from listeria and BCG-infected mice. Infect Immunol 1972;5:499–503.
104. Johnston RB, Godzik CA, Cohn ZA. Increased superoxide anion production by immunologically activated and chemically elicited macrophages. J Exp Med 1978;142: 115–122.
105. Hibbs JB, Chapman HA, Weinberg JB. The macrophage as an antineoplastic surveillance cell: biological perspective. J Reticuloendothel Soc 1978;24:549–556.
106. Taylor RJ, Salata JJ. Inhibition of prostaglandin synthetase by tolmetin (Tolection, NcN-2559), a new non-steroidal

anti-inflammatory agent. Biochem Pharmacol 1976;25: 2479–2484.

107. Rodgers K, Ellefson D, Girgis W, et al. Effects of tolmetin sodium dihydrate on normal and postsurgical peritoneal cell function. Int J Immunopharmacol 1988;10:111–120.

108. Humes JL, Burger G, Galavage, et al. The diminished production of arachidonic acid oxygenation products by elicited mouse peritoneal macrophages: possible mechanism. J Immunol 1980;124:2110–2116.

109. Wahl LM, Lampel LL. Regulatoin of human peripheral blood monocyte collagenase by prostaglandins and anti-inflammatory drugs. Cell Immunol 1987;105:411–422.

110. Wahl LM, Winter CC. Regulation of guinea pig macrophage collagenase by dexamethasome and colchicine. Arch Biochem Biophys 1984;230:661–667.

111. Werb Z, Banda MJ, Jones PA. Degradation of connective tissue by macrophages: I. Protoelysis of elastin, glycoproteins and collagen by proteinases isolated from macrophages. J Exp Med 1980;152:13440–13457.

38

Animal Adhesion Models: Design, Variables, and Relevance

David M. Wiseman

CONTENTS

What Result Would You Like?

Perhaps the most commonly asked question in adhesions research is "Which is the best animal model of adhesions?" The reply "What result are you looking for?" is not intended as a facetious retort, but rather as a suggestion to the questioner to consider carefully the objectives for a particular inquiry (Table 38.1). Thus, models in which a favorable result is easy to obtain ("permissive models") are suitable for early stages of research, whereas more challenging models are required for later stages. The mismatch of models and objectives can lead to costly disappointments on the part of patients, investigators, and pharmaceutical companies alike.

Although there is no "standard adhesion model," the careful selection of an animal model to accomplish the objectives of a particular stage in research will facilitate rational decisions about the choice of candidate, optimization of its formulation, and the allocation of resources to fund and staff its development. Most models of postsurgical adhesions involve the same basic design. The animal is prepared for aseptic surgery and the organ of interest exposed and injured. Some animals are treated with the test article. Animals are allowed to recover for up to 4 weeks and adhesions assessed by quantitative and qualitative criteria using gross or histologic methods. Details of this basic design and its relevance to clinical practice are elaborated upon in this chapter.

General Considerations

Animal Welfare Issues

The use of animals in biomedical science is a matter upon which an investigator must reflect seriously, not just at the beginning of a project or at the submission of a protocol to an ethics committee to use animals, but with the use of each animal. The scientist must question how that animal will be used with dignity to advance science and the resolution of an important medical prob-

TABLE 38.1. Choice of animal model is governed by research objectives.

Objective	Type of model
To screen for candidates with at least minimum efficacy	Permissive
To obtain evidence to support a patent application	Permissive
To optimize formulation variables	Challenging, with clinical correlates
To support regulatory submissions	Challenging, with clinical correlates
To justify investment in clinical development	Challenging, with clinical correlates
To develop improved versions of the product	More challenging: low efficacy for products with good clinical efficacy
To investigate basic mechanisms of adhesiogenesis	Permissive/challenging
To investigate efficacy under special conditions	Superimposition of special condition (e.g., bleeding, ischemia, contamination)

lem. Having internalized these matters personally, the investigator must obey the law. In the United States of America, the use of animals is regulated federally by the Animal Welfare Act, which requires prior approval by an Institutional Animal Care and Use Committee (IACUC). The "Guide for the Care and Use of Laboratory Animals"[1] defines standards, and is an excellent resource for all aspects of animal research. IACUC approval requires assurances from an investigator that the use of animals in general and surgery in particular are necessary for the proposed research. Together with assurances concerning consultation with a veterinarian and the use of literature searches to avoid duplication of research, these statements help the investigator focus his or her research, critically designing each experiment to yield the most useful data.

Consistency, Reliability, and Reproducibility

The literature is replete with studies that have been performed without any effort to ensure that a model is consistent, reliable, or reproducible. This practice raises animal welfare and cost issues, leads to erroneous product development decisions, and results in the recording of obfuscating data in the permanent scientific record. Fortunately, a number of laboratories have provided fine examples of how to conduct models that are consistent, reliable, and reproducible.

Consistency

Before any test article is administered to an animal, the consistency of the model must be established. A surgeon must be thoroughly familiar with the dissection technique. It should be practiced in animals euthanized for other reasons and then in live animals to ensure that sufficiently extensive and severe adhesions are obtained consistently from one experiment to the next. The method of assessing adhesions must be also well defined before an agent is tested.

Reliability

Once consistency is achieved, the reliability of the model must be assessed. Ultimately, this refers to the ability to rely on the results obtained from a model to make correlations with clinical outcomes, under specific surgical situations. An animal model should be validated with both positive and negative controls (see "Correlations Between Animal and Human Studies") from clinical experience. A model should not be so severe that no agent reduces adhesions, nor too permissive such that all agents are efficacious, although "challenging" and "permissive" models have their uses (see Table 38.1). Positive and negative controls are also reference standards that ensure consistency and calibrate a model for high and low levels of adhesion formation.

Reproducibility

Reproducibility refers to the ability of one investigator to replicate the results of another. The consistency and reliability of the model must be reproduced for each surgeon in a laboratory[2] using positive and negative controls. Reproducibility should also be checked periodically as models may "drift" even with the same surgeon. Similar precautions must be taken when a model is established in a new laboratory. Merely copying a protocol from a published report may not yield success. Although authors do not generally withhold experimental details, seemingly unnecessary minutiae omitted for the sake of brevity can become critical. If possible, a visit to the originating laboratory and direct observation of every procedure are recommended. Even with the use of a mechanical abrasion device to minimize operator variability[2] variation between laboratories can be considerable, although trends are essentially similar[3] (Table 38.2).

Teamwork

The importance of teamwork should not be underestimated in such a socially intense activity as surgery. The most diligent surgery is worthless without a well-functioning team to prepare and recover animals efficiently; to operate and supply equipment and materials; to oversee the assignment of treatments; and to record intraoperative notes accurately. This comment may seem rather obvious, but malfunctioning equipment, an inadequately prepared operating room, delays in deliver-

TABLE 38.2. Variation between laboratories for a rat cecal abrasion model.

Group	Lab #1	Lab #2	Lab #3
No coating	56	92	90
PBS	79	88	70
0.10% HA	40	40	64
0.25% HA	36	24	62
0.40% HA	12	12	50

Using a mechanical abrasion device, a rat cecal abrasion model was performed using the test articles indicated in three different laboratories. The percent of animals with "significant adhesions" (score ≥2) is shown.
From Burns et al.[3]

ing animals to the operating room, and problems in recovering animals are all distractions that result in the loss of momentum critical to achieving consistency, reliability, and reproducibility.

It is also essential that team members, including technicians, observe at first hand the type of human surgery they are attempting to model. The more they know about the problem, the better equipped they are to contribute to the research program. Fundamental errors in judgment have been made because researchers had never availed themselves of this invaluable experience.

Environmental Variables

A number of environmental factors have been known to influence the outcome of animal studies in adhesions.

Animal Supply

Animals must be purchased from reliable and licensed suppliers and acclimated. Maturity, sex, housing, light–dark cycle, season, and feed can affect the hormonal status and responsiveness of animals to surgery and treatment. Should a change in supplier be necessary, revalidation of a model may be necessary. Intraspecies differences may exist in the propensity to form adhesions or in responsiveness to treatment, as has been observed empirically in mice (A. Kaplun, personal communication), and in a tendon adhesion model in chickens.[4] In another study, gnotobiotic rats formed intestinal adhesions less readily than their conventional counterparts, suggesting a role for bacterial translocation[5] or other factors related to the immunologic status of bacteriologically experienced animals. Certainly conclusions must be drawn with caution when animals with known defects in macrophage function (e.g., C3H/HeN mice) are used.[6]

Feed and Water Supply

Changes in feed and quality of water supply can also affect animals undergoing adhesions studies. Should responses to positive and negative controls suddenly differ from historical data, contamination of the water supply might be suspected.

Ambient Humidity

We have observed that ambient humidity may affect the performance of some materials. For example, Seprafilm® becomes plasticized in relatively humid conditions and appears to perform well. On drier days, the product is more brittle, fractures more readily on placement, and does not perform well in certain models.

Foreign Bodies and Intraperitoneal Anesthesia

Surgical glove powder adhesiogenesis (see Chapter 11) and gauze lint[7] are both known to elicit foreign-body reactions and to contribute to adhesion formation. The same brand of gloves and gauze and type of sutures should be used in all experiments to ensure consistency. Gloves should also be washed before surgery. Drugs should not be administered intraperitoneally for anesthesia or euthanasia because these may evoke tissue responses that interfere with the study.

Choice of Species, Site, and Adhesiogenic Stimulus

Choice of Species

Historically, animal species have been chosen for adhesions studies on empirical grounds. Mice and rats are readily available and inexpensive. With proper validation, mice may be particularly useful for drug screening or mechanistic studies.[8] Unlike rodents, the size and internal geometry of rabbits permits the implantation of devices with dimensions that approach more reasonably those which would be used in humans. Cost and logistics factors restrict the use of larger species (primates,[9–11] dogs, pigs, and cattle). Because of their known propensity to adhesive bowel disease, horses have been studied in several adhesion models.[12,13]

Geometric Considerations

For barrier devices, minimum quantities are required to cover body surfaces, leading to likely[14] artifacts in small animals. Interceed Barrier, although shown to be effective in humans,[15] caused peritoneal injury[6,16] and increased adhesion formation in mice.[17] The amount of fabric (1–2 cm^2) appears appropriate to cover a given area of the abdominal wall. However, the volume and buffer capacity of murine peritoneal fluid appears insufficient to neutralize the acidity of a material used in an amount equivalent to approximately 50 to 70 times that used in humans on a weight basis. Furthermore the large remnants of material observed indicate that phagocytic and hydrolytic processes were inadequate to handle such a large amount of material.

The relative thickness of the peritoneum and subperitoneal musculature, and the presence of submesothelial fibroelastic tissue, may also determine the ability of tissue to withstand and recover from insult. In the mouse, the thickness of the entire abdominal wall is approximately equivalent to that of the first muscle layer in the rat. Similarly, the entire thickness of the rat wall is equivalent to the first muscle layer in the rabbit, which has a similar relationship with the dog. Thus, a given unit area of Interceed Barrier will "erode" a given depth of tissue, representing a significant fraction of the entire layer in the mouse and geometrically diminishing fractions in rats, rabbits, and dogs (and humans). The problem may be large enough to explain why Interceed Barrier was ineffective in some rat models[18] but not in others.[19] Because a barrier is placed on damaged tissue in clinical use, this "damage" becomes all the more insignificant.

Pharmacokinetic Differences Between Species

A number of anatomic and physiologic factors contribute to interspecies variations in the persistence of drugs or devices in the abdominal cavity. The peritoneal cavity is not merely an empty vessel in which fluids and solutes are free to move from one part to another; there is a definite pattern of fluid circulation.[20] Anatomic and postural differences between species will influence this circulation as well as the approximation of organs.

Generally accepted to be similar to the surface area of skin,[21] peritoneal surface area relative to body weight is higher in small animals than in large animals (Table 38.3). Thus, the volume of fluid required to coat surfaces in smaller animals is disproportionately higher. The extensive absorption across the peritoneum[22,23] is also dependent on its surface area. The elimination of molecules from the peritoneal cavity thus will be faster in smaller animals, given that the intrinsic ability of the peritoneum to transport molecules appears similar among mammals.[24–26] Absorption may also occur by pinocytosis and lymphatic drainage, which may also vary between species.

Pharmacodynamic Differences Between Species

Pharmacodynamic differences between species obviously affects our ability to extrapolate drug data from animals to humans. Less obvious is the impact such differences may have on devices, as it is only recently that biologic mechanisms for "passive" devices have been suggested.[29–33] Most of the sparse data on pharmacodynamic differences between species relate to the fibrinolytic system. Using a fibrin slide method, Myhre-Jensen et al.[34] examined serosal, vascular, and synovial tissues in rats, guinea pigs, and rabbits. Most active were rat tissues, followed by guinea pig tissues. Barely trace levels of fibrinolytic activity were found in the rabbit tissues studied.

Responses to streptokinase, both the activation of fibrinolysis and the reduction of adhesions, were lower in rats than in rabbits. The effect of streptokinase on human blood was similar to that on rabbit blood.[35] Another report[36] suggested that streptokinase neither reduced adhesions nor activated serum in the dog. Biochemical changes in peritoneal fluid during the menstrual cycle that may affect adhesion formation or its treatment include changes in fibrinolytic activity,[37] hormone levels,[38] and other proteins.[39] Interspecies differences in the types of ovulatory cycles thus provide an additional source of variation.

Choice of Anatomic Site

Shape, position, motility, and blood supply distinguish one anatomic site from another. Sites are selected to facilitate extrapolations to the equivalent human site and to justify embarking on a clinical study from surgical, ethical, investment, or regulatory aspects. Posture may influence interspecies variation in adhesiogenesis by altering the relationship between one organ and another.

TABLE 38.3. Peritoneal surface area in different species.

	Weight	Rel wt[a]	Height[b]	SA[c]	SA/wt[d]	Coat vol[e]	Coat vol/wt[f]
Mouse	0.025	0.00036	0.05	0.005	0.195	0.45	18.1
Rat	0.25	0.0036	0.15	0.029	0.115	2.6	10.7
Rabbit	2.5	0.036	0.61	0.209	0.084	19.4	7.7
Dog	25	0.36	0.91	0.745	0.030	69.1	2.8
Human	70	1	1.70	1.81	0.026	167	2.4

[a]Weight relative to humans, typical weight (kg) selected.
[b]Height in meters.
[c]Surface area (m^2) calculated from Dubois and Dubois[27]:
$SA = weight^{0.425} \times height^{0.725} \times 0.2025$. An alternative method of $SA = (weight/70)^{0.67} \times 1.8$, gives close agreement. Both methods are approximate and apply to similarly shaped bodies.
[d]Surface area/body weight.
[e]Minimum volume of fluid required to coat the peritoneal surface (mL).[28] Coating volume = SA × 92.7 mL/m^2.
[f]Minimum volume of fluid required to coat the peritoneal surface/weight (mL/kg).

The erect posture of humans either sitting or standing is very different from the posture of quadrupeds. In the immediate postoperative period, critical for adhesion formation, humans tend to recline in a supine position, but laboratory animals are mostly prone. The duration of this period may also influence adhesiogenesis, the recovery of animals from surgery (laparotomy) being typically faster than for humans.

Uterus

Adhesiogenic trauma to the "uterine horns" (UH) is widely used to model pelvic surgery. Other than primates, most laboratory species possess a bicornuate uterus. The contralateral UH may be used as a control[40,41] but with caution, because crossover effects may occur, especially in small animals. Although mice,[42] rats,[40,43–46] and hamsters[47] have all been used, the "rabbit uterine horn" model is perhaps the most popular. Note that rabbit UH models may share little except a name (Table 38.4).

We have observed empirically that the larger the size of the uterus, the more difficult it is to induce adhesions. For this reason we only use animals whose uterus measures between 8 and 16 on the French catheter scale.[63]

Bowel

The cecum of rodents and rabbits provides a well-defined surface area for adhesion formation[3,52,64,65] and a model for intestinal surgery. Unlike that in humans, the cecum in these species is well developed for digestion and will support a film or membrane barrier placed against the sidewall. The anatomy and biology of the intestine of larger animals approximates more closely to that of humans. Although the diet and microflora of the omnivorous swine is more like that of a human, only the small intestine is usable because of the spiral arrangement of its colon. The small and large bowel of the dog resemble more closely the human intestine in anatomy and vascular supply.[66] Models involving canine bowel may be used to assess adhesiogenesis as well as the effect of an agent on wound healing in a contaminated field.[67] Similar models have been reported in rats[68] and monkeys.[10]

Sidewall

The abdominal sidewall provides a definable surface to model abdominal or gynecologic surgery. Surface areas are readily estimated, although wound contraction may be variable. The two sides are not equivalent and cannot be used pairwise to assess test and control articles. Although performed alone,[8,69] sidewall injuries are often combined with abrasion injuries to the cecum in rats[3,18,46,64] and rabbits.[46,64,70] Excisions,[18,46,52,64,65,71,72] ligations,[35,73] and flaps[74–76] have been made to induce adhesions to neighboring organs. The variability in the development of adhesions observed in rats and rabbits after sidewall excision can be improved by circumferential suturing.[64]

Biologic Basis for Anatomic Variation

Just as little is known about what biologic factors contribute to variation in adhesion formation between species, even less is known about what differences exist between tissues. Differences in fibrinolytic activity have been documented between whole tissues in animals[77] and humans.[78] Fibrinolytic activity determined from human surgical biopsies of serosal tissue was nearly four times greater in the omentum than the gallbladder, which had the lowest activity.[79] Although most other sections of bowel had similar activities, the sigmoid colon had slightly more.

Ultrastructurally there appears to be little difference in the healing of (rat) parietal and visceral peritoneum.[80] Fibrinolytic activity is higher in uninjured visceral than in parietal peritoneum in rats,[81] but about the same after injury. Again in rats, the same injury induced more adhesions in visceral than in parietal tissue.[82] The ovary is not covered by mesothelium, but does have endogenous fibrinolytic activity. A common site for adhe-

TABLE 38.4. Rabbit uterine horn (UH) models of adhesion development.

Type	Description	Assessment	References
A: Simple abrasion	Abrasion, 5 cm	Composite score	48,49
A: Simple abrasion	Abrasion, 5 cm	Extent (cm)	50,51,52
A: Simple abrasion	Abrasion, 5 cm	Composite score	53
B: Reformation	Reformation after lysis	Score/extent	54
C: Abrasion/devascularization	Abrasion + mesenteric stripping	Overall grade	45,46,55,56
D: Reformation	Reformation after cautery	Incidence	57
E: Abrasion/cautery	1-cm resection + cautery	Descriptive	58
F: Cautery/excision	Excision of 2 × 2 cm cauterized lesion	Descriptive	59
Devascularization	Devascularization of 3 cm by cautery	Area	60,61
Abrasion/cautery	Abrasion, cautery	Area	62

Letters A–F identify models described in Fig. 38.1.

sion formation, periovarian adhesions cause infertility and pain. Despite their importance, surprisingly few studies have attempted to model periovarian adhesions directly.[83–86]

Adhesiogenic Stimulus

Primary Methods

The type and extent of adhesiogenic stimulus (Table 38.5) employed affects the healing response, the period and intensity of inflammation, the formation of adhesions, and the ability to reduce them. There is no single "correct" method to use, provided that it results in consistent, reproducible, and reliable data. The basic rule is that the more damage (abrasion < excision < ischemia/free grafts), the more adhesions. Reports comparing the ability of several methods to induce adhesions are worth reviewing.[46,74,87–89]

Commonly used, abrasion (e.g., gauze, scalpel, brush) is perhaps the most difficult method to standardize. Templates may ensure that a consistent area is abraded.[3,64] Devices consisting of a spring-loaded punch[90] or a circular polishing tool[2,3] can standardize the duration and degree of the abrasive injury. Crush injuries are often made with standard surgical instruments at defined locations, for a defined time, and closed to a defined ratchet position.[76,91] Power settings and distance and duration of exposure can be controlled for electrocautery[42] and laser cautery.[92] For electrocautery, care must be taken to exert a constant pressure on tissue. A thermostatically controlled device was used to create a standard thermal injury in mice.[93]

Results of using chemical adhesiogenic stimuli are likely to reflect the diversity of the mechanisms through which they act. Practically, it may be difficult to distinguish between quantitative or qualitative differences between stimuli, as in a study in which abrasion, nitrogen mustard, formalin, and phenol had different effects on peritoneal fibrinolytic activity.[94] Tetracycline and cefazolin[95] and several antineoplastic drugs[96] induce adhesion formation after intraperitoneal administration and have been used in animal models of adhesions.

Foreign bodies (e.g., starch, talc, gauze) are effective adhesiogenic stimuli[97,98] that persist so long as the foreign body is present. Thus, this method is generally restricted to studies of powder adhesiogenesis. Nonabsorbable intraperitoneal meshes for hernia repair are associated with adhesion formation, which has been studied in mice,[14] rats,[99,100] rabbits,[33] and pigs.[101]

TABLE 38.5. Types of adhesiogenic stimulus used in adhesion models.

Stimulus	Additional variables
Abrasion	Bleeding
Crushing	Ischemia
Desiccation (air or alcohol)	Contamination–infection
Incision	Anastomosis
Excision	Other pathology (endometriosis, cancer)
Electrocautery	Formation vs. reformation
Laser injury	Laparoscopy vs. laparotomy
Thermal injury	
Chemical injury	
Radiation injury	
Foreign body–tissue irritation	

Additional Variables

A number of factors add pathologic complexity to adhesiogenesis by intensifying, prolonging, or extending the scope of the peritoneal response to injury. Other operational factors provide additional challenges.

Adhesion Reformation

Articulated by the classification[102,103] of adhesions into types 1a, 1b, 2a, and 2b, adhesion reformation is believed to pose a greater challenge to an antiadhesion agent than primary adhesion formation. In a reformation model, adhesions are induced as in a primary model, lysed 1 to 4 weeks later, at which time test and control articles are applied. Only those animals that have formed adhesions to a certain stated extent or degree of severity should be included.[54] These studies[10,11,42,69] should not be undertaken lightly because a second operative procedure often raises animal welfare concerns.

Bleeding

Active bleeding provides the fibrin needed for the initial adhesion of two surfaces. The amount of residual bleeding will differ according to the intrinsic vascularity of the tissue, the angiogenesis (and disease) dependent density of leaky blood vessels, and the difficulty in locating and controlling all bleeders. Perception of what constitutes "meticulous" or "adequate" hemostasis differs among surgeons. An ideal antiadhesion agent must therefore function when hemostasis is less than "meticulous," a quality lacking in the prototypical Interceed Barrier.[104] To study this, we superimposed two levels of bleeding in a rabbit UH model[63] to simulate the low and high limits of "acceptable" bleeding. At the low end we allowed the abraded UH to "ooze." For high levels of bleeding, four medium-sized mesouterine vessels were nicked that would soon stop bleeding spontaneously but which would normally be controlled by conventional means. As a negative control, Interceed Barrier was shown to be ineffective. In another model,[69] no attempt was made to achieve hemostasis after cecal abrasion. Other workers[104] have injected a standard volume of fresh blood at the surgical site rather than permit active bleeding.

Ischemia

Ischemia induces injury that may result in tissue death. Ligation,[35,73] free-flap grafts,[75,76] devascularization by stripping,[55,56,85] circumferential suturing,[69] creation of ischemic buttons,[35,105] temporary intestinal vascular obstruction,[106] creation of isolated intestinal segments,[64,107] and cautery[43,60] have been used. The effect of ischemia can be assessed by comparing two almost identical rabbit UH models.[55,63] When ischemia by devascularization is added to abrasion, adhesions form to the uterus as well as to organs remote from the primary injury.[55] With abrasion alone, adhesions are restricted to the uterus,[63] suggesting that ischemia results in the release of mediators able to induce injury at secondary sites.

Extensive Dissection

Most animal models of adhesions involve focal and relatively small injuries. To mimic large dissections in humans, a radical pelvic dissection model was developed in dogs[108] and pigs.[109] There is one report of a hysterectomy and bilateral salpingo-oophorectomy model in rabbits.[110]

Adhesion Formation in a Contaminated or Infected Field

Bacterial and fecal contamination that commonly occur in bowel surgery are potent stimuli of adhesiogenesis[107] and are additional challenges for antiadhesion agents. This problem has been addressed in a limited number of studies.[97,111] There is considerable regional and interspecies variation in microbial intestinal ecology.[112] Whether these differences modulate the efficacy of an adhesion product is still unknown. The additional challenge that infection provides may be caused by lipopolysaccharide (LPS, endotoxin), which increases the adhesivity and permeability of mesothelial cells in vitro. Tumor necrosis factor (TNF), a mediator that is not specific to infection, was unable to induce this response.[113] Pelvic inflammatory disease is also associated with adhesion formation and has been studied in a model involving gonococcus-induced adhesions in rabbits.[114]

Adhesion Formation in Endometriosis

Endometriosis is a painful and often debilitating disease associated with adhesions and inflammation that may provide an additional challenge for an antiadhesion agent. Although animal models of endometriosis[115,116] have been developed, this issue has not been studied extensively in animals.

Endoscopic Surgery

Endoscopic surgery may impose additional constraints on an antiadhesion agent. A pneumoperitoneum exerts enough pressure to cause the tamponade of small vessels; thus, hemostasis should be checked by reducing the pressure before placement of an antiadhesion agent. The FDA has determined that laparoscopy and laparotomy are sufficiently different and require separate clinical demonstrations of safety and efficacy. Manufacturers should indeed show that their product is compatible with endoscopic access in "handling studies," but available evidence suggesting that there are biologic[117] and clinical[103] differences between the two access methods do not support the regulatory distinction. Endoscopic versions of adhesion models in pigs[101,118] and rabbits[119–121] have nonetheless been reported.

Approximation

To increase the baseline incidence and extent of adhesions and to standardize the location and area of adhesion formation, investigators have approximated two injured surfaces such as the UH of mice,[42,122] the abraded uterus and a sidewall excision in rabbits[71,72] and rats,[40,123] and the lacerated UH to the small intestine in rats.[44,124] An elegant use of this technique is the standardization of the area of adhesions before adhesiolysis in a rat UH model.[125]

Double Injury

Adhesions of several types (1a, 1b, 2a, 2b) may form simultaneously and may be modeled by creating two injury types in the same animal. This method allows assessment of the effect of one agent alone, or two agents in combination on different adhesion types. In rabbits the cecum was abraded and a sidewall patch excised to model severe and localized adhesions (e.g., type 1b). For diffuse and less severe adhesions (type 1a), UH were abraded and devascularized. Accordingly, we showed the benefit of a site-specific agent (Interceed) to reduce the more severe adhesions, combined with hyaluronic acid solution, which reduced less severe, more diffuse adhesions.[126]

Functionality Studies

Before regulatory approval is granted, a battery of standard toxicology and safety studies is required. Other studies that are neither "safety" nor "efficacy" studies may be required for regulatory or other reasons. These "functionality studies" address various aspects of a product's performance such as ergonomics, application procedure, compatibility with other procedures, or positional stability.

Handling Studies

The most elegant product will fail unless it can be delivered in a simple and rapid manner. This is especially true for endoscopic surgery. In handling studies, the appropriate quantity and method of delivery[127] can be established in a suitably large animal. It is advisable to employ a practicing surgeon who can anticipate problems. If necessary, specific instrumentation should be designed to deliver the product in the most ergonomic and economic manner.

Positional Stability

Despite impressive efficacy data in laboratory animals, at least one product has failed in clinical study because, as was later discovered, it did not remain in place for a sufficiently long time. With perfect hindsight, this failure may have been averted had a "positional stability" study been performed. Using large animals (e.g., swine), the product is placed at several identifiable locations in the abdomen with or without simple abrasion. The persistence of this material may be determined by laparoscopic observation several times during the next 4 days. Because remesothelialization requires 3 to 7 days, barrier products that detach within hours clearly may be inadequate.

Adhesion Formation and Wound Healing

Because wound healing and adhesiogenesis are similar processes, the effect of an antiadhesion agent on critical wounds such as incisions or anastomoses should be determined. Incisional wound strength may be assessed tensiometrically in rats or rabbits.[70] For anastomotic healing, rats,[128] rabbits,[70,129,130] dogs,[131] and monkeys[10] have all been used. The colon is preferred because this is regarded as the site most susceptible to dehiscence. Other models may be useful for the study of adhesions and wound healing in the presence of infection.[68,132,133]

Infection Potentiation

The enhancement of bacterial infectivity in the presence of a foreign material[134] is well known. Assurance is needed that a material does not potentiate infection before clinical use of a product is attempted in contaminated fields. At a given level of mortality (e.g., 30%–50%) or morbidity (e.g., abscess formation), bacteria are introduced into the abdomen of rats or rabbits by "controlled" intestinal puncture,[73,111] injection of a defined inoculum,[135] or insertion of a capsule containing a cocktail of feces and other adjuvants such as barium sulfate.[136] This method is the most popular and was used recently to show that certain hyaluronic acid and ferric hyaluronate formulations enhanced infectivity in rats.[137] These models are difficult to conduct and require expert assistance.

Statistics and Assessment

The statistical design must ensure that study objectives can be met. It is advisable to consult reviews[138] on this subject as well as an experienced biostatistician. Statistical outcomes can only complement judgments made with the perspective of extensive experience of the behavior of a particular animal model and its relationship to other models.

Study Size

Study size depends largely on whether data are to be used for "screening" ("vectorial") or "definitive" purposes. A definitive study to demonstrate efficacy marks the end of one research phase and the beginning of another. It may also be used for regulatory purposes, for publication, or to justify a research grant or venture capital investment. The number of animals per group should provide sufficient power (e.g., 80%) to show a stated reduction in adhesions from controls at a stated p value (e.g., ≤ 0.05). In "typical" adhesion studies, with reductions of 50% in the primary efficacy parameter, 10 to 15 animals are required per group. Definitive studies should always include untreated controls and possibly other controls or reference groups. Several methods may be used to calculate sample size.[139]

In a screening study, several candidates and their delivery methods are evaluated to determine which deserve further study. Information about the variability of the response is used in power calculations for definitive studies. By limiting group size ($n = 3-8$), the investigator is effectively stating that they are willing to accept that a difference is statistically significant at a higher p (e.g., 0.1–0.2) value and lower power (e.g., 60%). Combined with one's experience of that model, decisions can be made about the direction of further research.

Randomization and Control of Bias

Randomization is used in an attempt to protect a study from known and unknown confounding variables. Even experienced surgeons fatigue; their technique may "drift," and a "(re)learning curve" may be present. More rarely, equipment may fail or climatic conditions may vary. Thus, block randomization should be considered to ensure that treatments are not unevenly distributed within or between the several surgical sessions, each of which may last half a day or more.

The randomization schedule is prepared in advance by a person other than the surgeon, and a protocol for marking the administration of treatment is established. The surgeon(s) must be unaware of the group assignment until administration of treatment is necessary. In a trial involving a physical barrier and an untreated control, "blinding" ceases at this point. Where several candidates have a similar form (e.g., solutions, gels), a certain degree of blinding can remain. Similarly, during evaluation, group assignments should be concealed if possible. In definitive studies, the randomization code should only be broken after all the analyses have been performed. In "screening" studies it is sometimes helpful for the evaluator to know the group assignment after all notes have been recorded but before proceeding to the next animal. This method permits an overall impression to be gained about the efficacy and degradation characteristics of individual candidates.

Assessment of Adhesions

Many of the following remarks also relate to the clinical assessment of adhesions.

Time to Assessment

A model must be stable over time. In a rabbit UH model,[49] adhesion formation was consistent at 2, 4, and 8 weeks. Sufficient time should elapse to allow an agent to degrade and temporary filmy adhesions to undergo autolysis.

Efficacy Parameters

Clear, measurable, and reproducible efficacy parameters must be established.

Fertility

Endpoints that measure adhesion formation are strictly "surrogates" for clinically meaningful but elusive outcomes such as fertility or bowel obstruction. In one of the few studies to measure "outcomes" in animals, Interceed reduced adhesions and increased the nidation index (embryos/corpus luteum) after a bisecting electrosurgical injury to the ovary in rabbits.[83]

Incidence of Adhesions/Adhesion-Free Outcome

Simply put, are adhesions present or absent? Incidence of adhesions can be reported on a per site or per animal basis. In studies involving multiple anatomic locations, the former precludes an animal being "failed" because of an adhesion at a single site. The incidence of adhesions at particular sites of interest, such as the ovary or bowel, should still be reported. Adhesion-free outcome is the converse of incidence and expresses a result in clinically meaningful terms. For tubular organs, care must be taken to identify all adhesions between the tube and its mesentery. Also, anatomic familiarity is essential to avoid mistaking normal attachments for adhesions (e.g., rabbit/rat UH; porcine spiral colon; cecal/intestinal mesentery of the rabbit).

Extent of Adhesions

The overall involvement of a particular organ with adhesions is assessed, for example, the length of abraded uterus, the length of an incision line (bowel, uterus, or abdominal wall), or the area of an excised sidewall patch.

Data should be recorded in absolute and relative terms (% of total area or length available). Lengths should be measured with a ruler and areas by planimetry. In practice, this is rarely done. Even if tissues were linear and planar structures, they are often distorted in handling and adhesions do not occur in continuous blocks. Therefore, lengths are measured to the nearest 5 mm and percent areas are measured to the nearest quartile or decile. That this method is somewhat imprecise and the source of intra- and interobserver variability has been discussed for clinical studies.[140–142] Such variability can be minimized by having two independent operators simultaneously observe the same animal; agreement is generally obtained.[2]

Tenacity of Adhesions

The tenacity of an adhesion refers to the ease with which it is dissected. The tenacity of adhesions may be graded on a three-point or four-point (Table 38.6) scale. For organs having areas of varying tenacity, the highest score should be recorded. This subjective parameter is surprisingly reproducible and understandable among different investigators (personal observation).

Severity of Adhesions

The need to describe the picture of adhesions in an animal using a single number has led to a plethora of grading systems that attempt to grade what are judged to be progressively more severe cases of organ involvement. (e.g., Table 38.7). The more descriptive a system, the more prone it is to intra- and interobserver variability. Two observers viewing the same tissue can agree on a grade and later visualize the appearance that a grade projects outside the laboratory. However, anyone outside this enlightened circle cannot readily appreciate the significance of a single grade of this kind. This problem is amplified when descriptive statistics are transformed by ranking to facilitate comparative analysis.

TABLE 38.6. Typical four-point scale for assessing tenacity of adhesions.

0	Adhesions absent
1	Filmy adhesions, requiring blunt dissection
2	Tenacious, requiring aggressive blunt or moderate sharp dissection
3	Dense vascularized adhesions requiring sharp dissection at risk of damaging organ

TABLE 38.7. Typical system for assessing overall adhesion grade.

Grade	Description
0.0	No adhesions
0.5	Easily separable, filmy pelvic adhesions involving only the bladder; typically only one or two small adhesions
1.0	Easily separable, filmy adhesions, not extensive, although slightly more extensive than 0.5
1.5	Adhesions slightly more extensive and tougher than a 1.0 rating
2.0	More tenacious adhesions, a little more extensive, one UH having filmy adhesions and the other having adhesions between either the bowel or the bladder, but not both
2.5	Same as 2.0, except that adhesions to the UH are not filmy
3.0	Tougher adhesions than 2.0 (requiring sharp dissection), more extensive, both horns attached to either the bladder or bowel; some movement of the uterus possible
3.5	Same as 3.0, but both UH attached to both bladder and bowel
4.0	Severe adhesions, both UH attached to both bladder and bowel; unable to move the uterus without tearing the adhesions

UH, uterine horn.
Adapted from Wiseman et al.[55]

With perfect hindsight it is obvious that despite technically sound and reproducible work, such systems can lead to costly errors in product development. Agents such as hyaluronic acid[56] that reduce adhesions by several grades have proven to have limited clinical effectiveness.[143] It is thus essential that the grading system be fully understood before relying on data of this kind. This problem is partly overcome by integrating extent and tenacity scores into an overall score, facilitating statistical manipulation and dissection of individual score components. One method[49] involves the addition of an extent (0, 1 = 0%–25%; 2 = 26%–50%; 3 ≤ 50%) and tenacity score (0, 0.5 = filmy; 1 = cohesive). Refining this further,[53] a three-component system combines extent (0–4 by quadrant involvement), severity (0–3; none/filmy/vascular/cohesive), and degree (0–3; none/gentle traction/moderate traction/sharp dissection). These and other examples are certainly reproducible. Practically, some components of these systems are duplicative; in other words, a "cohesive adhesion" is likely to require moderate traction or sharp dissection.

Quantifiable Measurements of Adhesions

Although tedious and subject to tracing errors, planimetric estimation of an area involved with adhesions[90] is one of a few methods that have been used to more objectively assess adhesions and to reduce inter- and intraobserver variability. Other workers have used tensiometry to determine the strength of adhesion attachment at a defined locus.[18] These methods may allow fine distinctions to be made between prototypes or they may facilitate deductions to be made about mechanisms of action or pathogenesis. However, it is unclear whether this degree of precision is needed if our goal is complete adhesion prevention.

Significant and Nonsignificant Adhesions

In the absence of complete adhesion prevention, the concept has arisen of significant and nonsignificant adhesions, in which filmy adhesions are regarded as "acceptable" because they are easy to lyse at laparoscopy. This concept has been used in animal models by comparing the distribution of "significant" and "nonsignificant" adhesions in control and treatment groups.[69,144]

Segregation by Adhesion Types

Because of the different rates of development, care should be taken in studying models in which several adhesion types are present (e.g., 1a, 1b, 2a, 2b). In a UH abrasion and devascularization model, adhesions between sites with direct, indirect, or completely incidental trauma[145] were analyzed independently.

Histologic Evaluation

Tedious and expensive, histology often appears to slow the pace of adhesions research. Light[146,147] and electron[80,148] microscope studies provide important details that, combined with immunohostochemical[149] and in situ hybridization techniques,[150] are likely to play important roles in the elucidation of cellular mechanisms and the identification of novel targets for therapeutic intervention.

Statistical Analysis

Summary Statistics and Comparisons

Incidence of adhesions can be summarized by totaling the number of adhesion-free sites or animals in each group and then comparing them using a test such as Fisher's exact test,[151] a χ^2 test, or a test for proportions. Where multiple sites (e.g., ischemic buttons, cautery burn sites, etc.) are involved, interanimal variability can be considered by calculating the average number of sites per animal for each group and comparing them with a suitable test such as Student's *t*-test.

The median and range are given to summarize nonparametric data such as tenacity or overall adhesion severity or score. Extent data based on quartiles (e.g., 0; >0%–25%; 26%–50%; 51%–75%; 76%–100%) are obviously nonparametric and should be compared using appropriate tests such as Wilcoxon's rank sum test.

Purists will object, but the honoring of statistical rules more by their breach than their observance is possibly forgiven by the crystallization of a result into a single visualizable number (mean) rather than by an abstract statistic (e.g., rank sum). Toleration of such a "mean" ends when "standard deviations" are calculated and Student's *t*-tests performed. This practice has certainly led individuals, physicians, and entire corporations to devote considerable resources erroneously to the development of antiadhesion agents. Slightly more excusable is the application of this practice to "quasi"-parametric data such as extent data estimated to the nearest decile or 5 mm. Caution must nonetheless be applied in these cases.

Multiple Comparisons

Statistically equivalent to fishing with several rods to increase the chances of a catch, several agents are often tested in a single study. Depending on whether the agents are compared with each other[152,153] or only with controls,[154] the test statistic or the level of required statistical significance should be adjusted.[155,156] Caution is still in order because "the experimenter may find himself provided with an exact measure of the uncertainty of a proposition he does not fully comprehend."[155]

Multiple Comparisons of Nonparametric Data: Rank Transformations

Well-known methods exist to compare two nonparametric data sets, but there are no good methods to incorporate adjustments for multiple comparisons. One solution is to transform nonparametric data[157,158] by arranging adhesion scores for all animals in ascending rank order, assigning the average rank for animals whose scores tie. These ranks follow normal (and related distributions). Mean rank positions are calculated for each group and compared using parametric methods, with adjustment for multiple comparisons. This method lacks a descriptive statistic that can be used to compare data obtained in different studies. For this reason, a median and range can be shown for display purposes.

The Simultaneous Reduction of Incidence, Extent, and Severity of Adhesions

The statement "substance X reduces the incidence, extent, and severity of adhesions" has become a cliché in adhesions research. Such a statement, while possibly true, implies that substance X *simultaneously* modulates all three parameters. The inclusion of observations with zero incidence of adhesions in calculations for extent or severity lowers the average extent or severity for the entire group. By omitting these observations, an estimate of the ability of the agent to reduce extent or severity even when adhesions do develop is obtained. The following example illustrates this:

In a clinical evaluation[113] of a barrier after adhesiolysis, adhesion-free outcome was 24% in control sidewalls and 51% in treated sidewalls. Reductions in extent of adhesion reformation (% area) were 55.6% and 75.6%, respectively. The conclusion was drawn that the treatment reduced "*the incidence, extent and severity of . . . adhesion re-formation.*" Excluding adhesion-free sites, the reduction in extent only at sites which reformed adhesions is 41.7% for controls and 50.5% for treated sidewalls, a difference that is no longer as large or clinically significant.

This is more than an exercise in semantics. The (near) equality in the extent of adhesions at sites where adhesions did form suggests that the product either functioned or failed, with little in between. Such a conclusion enables researchers to find the reasons for this failure and to make improvements. The alternative conclusion conceals a possible failure mode and impedes progress.

These conclusions affect pharmacoeconomic analyses and the decisions reliant upon them. An agent that reduces incidence *and* extent of adhesions may benefit more patients than one which only reduces incidence. These conclusions will also determine the claims a manufacturer may make about its product.

Correlations Between Animal and Human Studies

Heard among congregations (coherences?) of adhesiologists is a mantra that bemoans the inability to predict a clinical outcome from animal data. Heretofore this may have reflected the status quo, but with the availability of clinical data for different agents, the sounds of this mantra are becoming muffled.

An attempt has been made to construct what is perhaps the first correlation between animal and clinical data in adhesions research (Fig. 38.1). The largest series of data exists for the rabbit UH simple abrasion model, which have been aggregated based on personal involvement or knowledge of the studies and their conduct. The method can be criticized on a number of grounds, but nonetheless serves as the basis for future refinements. Although it deviates from the line of equality, the surprisingly good correlation between animal and clinical data for pelvic surgery has certain predictive value. This correlation however may only hold true for device-type products in pelvic surgery. With the exception of heparin, pharmaceuticals are as yet untested. Furthermore, we do not have enough data points at low levels of adhesion formation (<30% relative to control) in humans.

The dearth of data for other rabbit UH models limits the conclusions that can be made; however, two points are noteworthy. The rabbit UH simple abrasion model appears to be too permissive, in the case of Interceed in polycystic ovary disease (PCOD) surgery (A10 in Fig. 38.1). Because we have other correlates for Interceed, this may reflect biologic differences inherent in PCOD surgery rather than in the model. Conversely, in the abrasion–devascularization model, the permissivity for hyaluronic acid (HA) is a reflection of the model rather than in the clinical surgery as we have other correlates

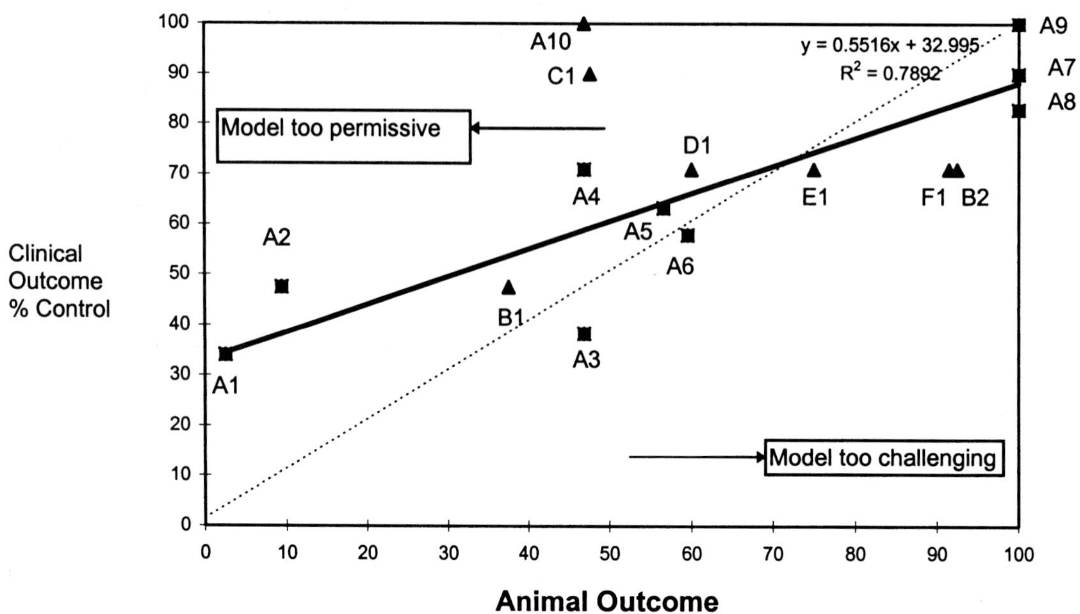

Data point	Agent	Animal data	Clinical data
A1	ADCON P	Extent[51]	Area reduction[159]
A2	Interceed + Heparin	Extent[50]	Area at 2LL[160]
A3	Interceed, laparoscopy	Extent[50]	Incidence[82,161–163]
A4	Interceed, laparotomy	Extent[50]	Incidence[15,164–170]
A5	Intergel	Extent[171]	Incidence[172]
A6	Seprafilm	Extent*	Adherent sites[173]
A7	Hyaluronic acid	Extent[52]	Presumed efficacy[143]
A8	Hyskon (Dextran 70)	Adhesion score[174]	Various[175–178]
A9	Heparin i.p.	Adhesion score[179]	Incidence change[180]
A10	Interceed, PCOD	Extent[50]	Incidence[181,182]
B1	Interceed + Heparin	R/F extent[54]	Area at 2LL[180]
B2	Interceed	R/F extent[54]	Incidence[164]
C1	Hyaluronic acid	Rank score[56]	Presumed efficacy[143]
D1	Interceed	R/F incidence[57]	Incidence[164]
E1	Interceed	Incidence[58]	Incidence[164]
F1	Interceed	Score[59]	Incidence[164]

R/F, reformation model.
From Wiseman; average data from four studies, unpublished.
Regression data (*solid line*) are shown for the simple abrasion model ($p < 0.01$), excluding the outlying point A10. The *dotted line* indicates an ideal 1:1 correlation.

FIG. 38.1. Correlation of data from rabbit uterine horn models with clinical data. Data were extracted regarding the efficacy of the agents indicated below. Where possible, parametric measurements were used and normalized against the result for the control population: 100% = no efficacy; 0% = complete absence of adhesions. Minimum responses were censured at 100%. Variants of the UH model (letters A–F) are as described in Table 38.4. Where more than one reference is shown, averages have been taken.

for pelvic surgery. An examination of the scoring system (see Table 38.7)[55] reveals that a reduction in adhesions to tissues that were not directly traumatized reduces the overall score to about 50% of the control score.

The variety of data available for rat[3,18,64,69] and rabbit[52,64,65] models involving sidewall injury, often with cecal abrasion, suggests that these models are generally permissive. In other models of pelvic surgery (e.g., rabbit ovary,[85,86] mice,[42] rats,[40,44,92,124] pigs,[109] monkeys[11]) data are insufficiently diverse to permit general conclusions to be drawn. Specific observations such as the apparent efficacy of Ringer's lactate in a rat UH model[46] are worthy of mention.

Conclusion

More than a century of investigation in animals and humans has provided a plethora of information about the choice and design of adhesion prevention models. In the quest for the most representative species and surgical model are a number of often forgotten fundamentals, which include establishment of consistent, reliable, and reproducible models, basic statistical design and analysis, and clear definition of usable and understandable efficacy parameters. Once these basics are attended to, the more complex task of model selection can begin. Despite advances in the understanding of adhesiogenesis, we remain largely ignorant of species and anatomic differences that should govern model selection. Nonetheless, empirically derived correlations between animal and clinical data now can be made that, to some degree and on a rational basis, can match a model with the objectives for a particular inquiry.

No animal can of course fully replicate all the conditions present in human surgery and the cautionary statement that "past performance is no guarantee of future success" must be invoked. The correlations so far established may only hold for materials acting through similar mechanisms (e.g., barriers), and in elective pelvic surgery. Where pharmacologic mechanisms are involved, interspecies pharmacodynamic and pharmacokinetic variation may reduce the strength of these correlations. Furthermore, correlations are still needed to study adhesions after bowel surgery, including the severe and extensive cases involving constant pain and frequent bowel obstruction.

It is hoped that the construction of correlations between animal and clinical data attempted herein will yield valuable clues about the mechanisms of adhesiogenesis as well as the differences between species and models. By provoking thought about the tools that we use to study the pathology of adhesiogenesis and the materia medica of its prevention, those tools may be sharpened to facilitate solutions to an important medical problem in a timely and cost-effective manner.

References

1. National Research Council. Guide for the Care and Use of Laboratory Animals. Washington, DC: National Academy Press, 1996.
2. Burgess LS, Rose RL, Colt JC, Skinner KC, Burns JW. An evaluation of operator variability in a rat cecal abrasion model for the formation of abdominal models. In: diZerega GS, DeCherney AH, Diamond MP, et al., eds. Pelvic Surgery: Adhesion Formation and Prevention. New York: Springer-Verlag, 1997:242–243.
3. Burns JW, Skinner K, Colt J, et al. Prevention of tissue injury and postsurgical adhesions by precoating tissues with hyaluronic acid solutions. J Surg Res 1995;59:644–652.
4. Manske PR, Jones GT, Wiseman DM. Comment on "A biomechanical study of tendon adhesion reduction using a biodegradable barrier in a rabbit model." J Appl Biomater 1990;1:255.
5. Bothin C, Midtvedt T. The role of the gastrointestinal microflora in postsurgical adhesion formation—a study in germfree rats. Eur Surg Res 1992;24:309–312.
6. Haney AF, Doty E. Comparison of the peritoneal cells elicited by oxidized regenerated cellulose (Interceed) and expanded polytetrafluoroethylene (Gore-Tex Surgical Membrane) in a murine model. Am J Obstet Gynecol 1992; 166:1137–1146.
7. van den Tol MP, van Stijn I, Bonthuis F, Marquet RL, Jeekel J. Reduction of intraperitoneal adhesion formation by use of non-abrasive gauze. Br J Surg 1997;84: 1410–1415.
8. Montz FJ, Holschneider CH, Bozuk M, Gotlieb WH, Martinez-Maza O. Interleukin 10: ability to minimize postoperative intraperitoneal adhesion formation in a murine model. Fertil Steril 1994;61:1136–1140.
9. Seitz HM, Schenker JG, Epstein S, Garcia CR. Postoperative intraperitoneal adhesions: a double-blind assessment of their prevention in the monkey. Fertil Steril 1973;24: 935–940.
10. Glucksman DL, Warren WD. The effect of topically applied corticosteroids in the prevention of peritoneal adhesions. An experimental approach with a review of the literature. Surgery (St. Louis) 1966;60:352–360.
11. Grow DR, Seltman HJ, Coddington CC, Hodgen GD. The reduction of postoperative adhesions by two different barrier methods versus control in cynomolgus monkeys: a prospective, randomized, crossover study. Fertil Steril 1994;61:1141–1146.
12. Mueller PO, Hunt RJ, Allen D, Parks AH, Hay WP. Intraperitoneal use of sodium carboxymethylcellulose in horses undergoing exploratory celiotomy. Vet Surg 1995;24: 112–117.
13. Baxter GM, Jackman BR, Eades SC, Tyler DE. Failure of calcium channel blockade to prevent intra-abdominal adhesions in ponies. Vet Surg 1993;22:496–500.
14. Baykal A, Onat D, Rasa K, Renda N, Sayek I. Effects of polyglycolic acid and polypropylene meshes on postoperative adhesion formation in mice. World J Surg 1997; 21:579–582.
15. Wiseman DM, Trout JR, Franklin RR, Diamond MP. Metaanalysis of safety and efficacy of an adhesion barrier in (INTERCEED TC7) in laparotomy. J Reprod Med 1998; 43:1999;44;325–331.
16. Haney AF, Doty E. The peritoneal response to expanded polytetrafluoroethylene and oxidized regenerated cellulose surgical adhesion barriers. Artif Cells Blood Substit Immobil Biotechnol 1996;24:121–141.
17. Haney AF, Doty E. Murine peritoneal injury and de novo adhesion formation caused by oxidized-regenerated cellulose (Interceed [TC7]) but not expanded polytetrafluoroethylene (Gore-Tex Surgical Membrane). Fertil Steril 1992;57:202–208.
18. Harris ES, Morgan RF, Rodeheaver GT. Analysis of the kinetics of peritoneal adhesion formation in the rat and evaluation of potential antiadhesive agents. Surgery (St. Louis) 1995;117:663–669.
19. Ryan CK, Sax HC. Evaluation of a carboxymethylcellulose sponge for prevention of postoperative adhesions. Am J Surg 1995;169:154–159.
20. Levison ME, Pontzer RE. Peritonitis and other intraabdominal infections. In: Mandell GL, Douglas RG, Ben-

nett JE, eds. Principles and Practice of Infectious Diseases, 2nd Ed. New York: Wiley, 1979:476–503.
21. Esperanca MJ, Collins DL. Peritoneal dialysis efficiency in relation to body weight. J Pediatr Surg 1966;1:162–169.
22. diZerega GS, Rodgers KE. The Peritoneum. New York: Springer-Verlag, 1992.
23. Flessner MF. Peritoneal transport physiology: insights from basic research. J Am Soc Nephrol 1991;2:122–135.
24. Dedrick RL. Interspecies scaling of regional drug delivery. J Pharm Sci 1986;75:1047–1052.
25. Dedrick RL, Bischoff KB. Species similarities in pharmacokinetics. Fed Proc 1980;39:54–59.
26. Dedrick RL, Flessner MF, Collins JM, Schultz JS. A distributed model of peritoneal transport. In: Maher JF, Winchester JF, eds. Frontiers in Peritoneal Dialysis. New York: Field, Rich, 1986:31–35.
27. Dubois D, Dubois E. A formula to estimate the approximate surface area if height and weight be known. Arch Intern Med 1916;17:863–871.
28. Cromack DT, Cromack TR, Pretorius G, DeMeules JE. Development of a predictive value equation for the minimum fluid volume to completely coat the intraperitoneal surface of rodents. Surg Forum 1985;36:477–478.
29. Krause TJ, Goldsmith NK, Ebner S, Zazanis GA, McKinnon RD. An inhibitor of cell proliferation associated with adhesion formation is suppressed by N,O-carboxymethyl chitosan. J Invest Surg 1998;11:105–113.
30. Wiseman DM, Saferstein L, Wolf S. Bioresorbable Medical Devices from Oxidized Polysaccharides Patent Application: EP 0815 879 A2, 1998.
31. Reddy S, Santanam N, Reddy PP, Rock JA, Murphy AA, Parthasarathy S. Interaction of Interceed oxidized regenerated cellulose with macrophages: a potential mechanism by which Interceed may prevent adhesions. Am J Obstet Gynecol 1997;177:1315–1320.
32. Watt PW, Harvey W, Lorimer E, Wiseman D. Use of Oxidized Cellulose and Complexes Thereof for Chronic Wound Healing. U.S. Patent Application WO 98/00-180, 1998.
33. Bellon JM, Contreras LA, Bujan J, Jurado F. Effect of phosphatidylcholine on the process of peritoneal adhesion following implantation of a polypropylene mesh prosthesis. Biomaterials 1996;17:1369–1372.
34. Myhre-Jensen O, Larsen SB, Astrup T. Fibrinolytic activity in serosal and synovial membranes. Rats, guinea pigs, and rabbits. Arch Pathol 1969;88:623–630.
35. James DC, Ellis H, Hugh TB. The effect of streptokinase on experimental intraperitoneal adhesion formation. J Pathol Bacteriol 1965;90:279–287.
36. Wright LT, Smith DH, Rothman M, Quosh ET, Metzger WI. Prevention of postoperative adhesions in rabbits with streptococcal metabolites. Proc Soc Exp Biol Med 1950;75: 602–604.
37. Bouckaert PX, van Wersch JW, Schellekens LA, Evers JL, Rolland R. Haemostatic and fibrinolytic properties of peritoneal fluid in the menstrual cycle. Br J Obstet Gynaecol 1984;91:256–259.
38. Bouckaert PX, Evers JL, Doesburg WH, Schellekens LA, Rolland R. Patterns of changes in glycoproteins, polypeptides, and steroids in the peritoneal fluid of women during the periovulatory phase of the menstrual cycle. J Clin Endocrinol Metab 1986;62:293–299.
39. Bouckaert PX, Evers JL, Doesburg WH, Schellekens LA, Brombacher PH, Rolland R. Patterns of changes in proteins in the peritoneal fluid of women during the periovulatory phase of the menstrual cycle. J Reprod Fertil 1986; 77:329–336.
40. Montgomery-Rice V, Shanti A, Moghissi KS, Leach RE. A comparative evaluation of Poloxamer 407 and oxidized regenerated cellulose (Interceed [TC7]*) to reduce postoperative adhesion formation in the rat uterine horn model. Fertil Steril 1993;59:901–906.
41. Arora M, Jaroudi KA, Hamilton CJ, Dayel F. Controlled comparison of Interceed and amniotic membrane graft in the prevention of postoperative adhesions in the rabbit uterine horn model. Eur J Obstet Gynecol Reprod Biol 1994;55:179–182.
42. Haney AF, Doty E. Expanded-polytetrafluoroethylene but not oxidized regenerated cellulose prevents adhesion formation and reformation in a mouse uterine horn model of surgical injury. Fertil Steril 1993;60:550–558.
43. West JL, Chowdhury SM, Sawhney AS, Pathak CP, Dunn RC, Hubbell JA. Efficacy of adhesion barriers. Resorbable hydrogel, oxidized regenerated cellulose and hyaluronic acid. J Reprod Med 1996;41:149–154.
44. Ortega-Moreno J. Effects of TC7 associated to 32% dextran 70, heparin and carboxymethylcellulose in adhesion prevention in the rat. Arch Gynecol Obstet 1993;253: 27–32.
45. Pagidas K, Tulandi T. Effects of Ringer's lactate, Interceed (TC7) and Gore-Tex Surgical Membrane on postsurgical adhesion formation. Fertil Steril 1992;57:199–201.
46. LeGrand EK, Rodgers KE, Girgis W, et al. Efficacy of tolmetin sodium for adhesion prevention in rabbit and rat models. J Surg Res 1994;56:67–71.
47. Best CL, Rittenhouse D, Sueldo CE. A comparison of TC7 and 32% dextran 70 for prevention of postoperative adhesions in hamsters. Obstet Gynecol 1991;78:858–860.
48. Linsky CB, Cunningham T, Diamond MP, Constantine B, DeCherney AH, diZerega GS. Development of a uterine horn model of adhesions in the rabbit. Infertility 1987; 10:71–85.
49. Linsky CB, Diamond MP, Cunningham T, Constantine B, DeCherney AH, diZerega GS. Adhesion reduction in the rabbit uterine horn model using an absorbable barrier, TC-7. J Reprod Med 1987;32:17–20.
50. Wiseman DM, Kamp LF, Saferstein L, Linsky CB, Gottlick LE, Diamond MP. Improving the efficacy of Interceed Barrier in the presence of blood using thrombin, heparin or a blood insensitive barrier, modified Interceed (nTC7). Prog Clin Biol Res 1993;381:205–212.
51. Lo H, Maier KH, Anderson JM, Zupon MA. Inhibition of postoperative pelvic adhesions by a bioresorbable carbohydrate solution (ADCON-P). Fertil Steril 1998; (Prog Suppl):S25.
52. Johns DB, Rodgers KE, Donahue WD, Kiorpes TC, diZerega GS. Reduction of adhesion formation by postoperative administration of ionically cross-linked hyaluronic acid. Fertil Steril 1997;68:37–42.
53. Leach RE, Burns JW, Dawe EJ, Smith Barbour MD, Diamond MP. Reduction of postsurgical adhesion formation in the rabbit uterine horn model with use of hyaluronate/ carboxymethylcellulose gel. Fertil Steril 1998;69:415–418.

54. Diamond MP, Linsky CB, Cunningham T, et al. Adhesion reformation: reduction by the use of INTERCEED R (TC7) plus heparin. J Gynecol Surg 1991;7:1–6.
55. Wiseman DM, Huang WJ, Johns DB, Rodgers KE, diZerega GS. Time-dependent effect of tolmetin sodium in a rabbit uterine adhesion model. J Invest Surg 1994;7:527–532.
56. Rodgers KE, Johns DB, Girgis W, Campeau J, diZerega GS. Reduction of adhesion formation with hyaluronic acid after peritoneal surgery in rabbits. Fertil Steril 1997;67: 553–558.
57. Steinleitner A, Lopez G, Suarez M, Lambert H. An evaluation of Flowgel as an intraperitoneal barrier for prevention of postsurgical adhesion reformation. Fertil Steril 1992;57:305–308.
58. Maxson WS, Herbert CM, Oldfield EL, Hill GA. Efficacy of a modified oxidized cellulose fabric in the prevention of adhesion formation. Gynecol Obstet Invest 1988;26: 160–165.
59. Best CL, Rittenhouse D, Vasquez C, Norng T, Subias E, Sueldo CE. Evaluation of Interceed(TC7) for reduction of postoperative adhesions in rabbits. Fertil Steril 1992;58: 817–820.
60. Dunn RC, Mohler M. Effect of varying days of tissue plasminogen activator therapy on the prevention of postsurgical adhesions in a rabbit model. J Surg Res 1993;54: 242–245.
61. Dunn RC, Steinleitner AJ, Lambert H. Synergistic effect of intraperitoneally administered calcium channel blockade and recombinant tissue plasminogen activator to prevent adhesion formation in an animal model. Am J Obstet Gynecol 1991;164:1327–1330.
62. Doody KJ, Dunn RC, Buttram VC Jr. Recombinant tissue plasminogen activator reduces adhesion formation in a rabbit uterine horn model. Fertil Steril 1989;51:509–512.
63. Wiseman DM, Gottlick LE, Diamond MP. Effect of thrombin-induced hemostasis on the efficacy of an absorbable adhesion barrier. J Reprod Med 1992;37:766–770.
64. Burns JW, Skinner K, Colt MJ, Burgess L, Rose R, Diamond MP. A hyaluronate based gel for the prevention of postsurgical adhesions: evaluation in two animal species. Fertil Steril 1996;66:814–821.
65. Wiseman DM, Gottlick-Iarkowski L, Kamp L. Prevention of bowel adhesions using two barriers of Oxidized Regenerated Cellulose (ORC). J Invest Surg 1999, in press.
66. Swindle MM. Swine as replacements for dogs in the surgical teaching and research laboratory. Lab Anim Sci 1984;34:383–385.
67. Gomez NA, Leon CJ, Iniquez SA. Use of TC7 in the prevention of adhesions in handsewn and stapled colonic anastomoses. Dis Colon Rectum 1994;37:512–513.
68. Snoj M, Ar'Rajab A, Ahren B, Bengmark S. Effect of phosphatidylcholine on postoperative adhesions after small bowel anastomosis in the rat. Br J Surg 1992;79:427–429.
69. Burns JW, Colt MJ, Burgess LS, Skinner KC. Preclinical evaluation of Seprafilm bioresorbable membrane. Eur J Surg (Suppl) 1997:40–48.
70. Menzies D, Ellis H. The role of plasminogen activator in adhesion prevention. Surg Gynecol Obstet 1991;172: 362–366.
71. Diamond MP, Linsky CB, Cunningham T, Constantine B, diZerega GS, DeCherney AH. A model for sidewall adhesions in the rabbit: reduction by an absorbable barrier. Microsurgery 1987;8:197–200.
72. Boyers SP, Diamond MP, DeCherney AH. Reduction of postoperative pelvic adhesions in the rabbit with Gore-Tex surgical membrane. Fertil Steril 1988;49:1066–1070.
73. Snoj M, Ar'Rajab A, Ahren B, Larsson K, Bengmark S. Phospholipase-resistant phosphatidylcholine reduces intraabdominal adhesions induced by bacterial peritonitis. Res Exp Med (Berl) 1993;193:117–122.
74. Ar'Rajab A, Ahren B, Rozga J, Bengmark S. Phosphatidylcholine prevents postoperative peritoneal adhesions: an experimental study in the rat. J Surg Res 1991;50:212–215.
75. Ar'Rajab A, Dawidson I, Sentementes J, Sikes P, Harris R, Mileski W. Enhancement of peritoneal macrophages reduces postoperative peritoneal adhesion formation. J Surg Res 1995;58:307–312.
76. Buckman RF, Woods M, Sargent L, Gervin AS. A unifying pathogenetic mechanism in the etiology of intraperitoneal adhesions. J Surg Res 1976;20:1–5.
77. Albrechtsen OK. The fibrinolytic activity of animal tissues. Acta Physiol Scand 1957;39:284–290.
78. Albrechtsen OK. The fibrinolytic activity of human tissues. Br J Haematol 1957;3:284–291.
79. Merlo G, Fausone G, Barbero C, Castagna B. Fibrinolytic activity of the human peritoneum. Eur Surg Res 1980; 12:433–438.
80. Raftery AT. Regeneration of parietal and visceral peritoneum: an electron microscopical study. J Anat 1973;115: 375–392.
81. Raftery AT. Method for measuring fibrinolytic activity in a single layer of cells. J Clin Pathol 1981;34:625–629.
82. Wallwiener D, Meyer A, Bastert G. Adhesion formation of the parietal and visceral peritoneum: an explanation for the controversy on the use of autologous and alloplastic barriers? Fertil Steril 1998;69:132–137.
83. Marana R, Catalano GF, Caruana P, Margutti F, Muzii L, Mancuso S. Postoperative adhesion formation and reproductive outcome using Interceed after ovarian surgery: a randomized trial in the rabbit model. Hum Reprod (Oxf) 1997;12:1935–1938.
84. Magro B, Mita P, Bracco GL, Coccia E, Scarselli G. Expanded polytetrafluoroethylene surgical membrane in ovarian surgery on the rabbit. Biocompatibility, adhesion prevention properties and ability to preserve reproductive capacity. J Reprod Med 1996;41:73–78.
85. Wiskind AK, Rice VM, Dudley AG. Evaluation of adhesion formation using Interceed (TC7) absorbable adhesion barrier on ovarian surgical wounds in the rabbit model. Obstet Gynecol 1993;81:1025–1028.
86. Hill-West JL, Chowdhury SM, Dunn RC, Hubbell JA. Efficacy of a resorbable hydrogel barrier, oxidized regenerated cellulose, and hyaluronic acid in the prevention of ovarian adhesions in a rabbit model. Fertil Steril 1994; 62:630–634.
87. Rozga J, Ahren B, Bengmark S. Prevention of adhesions by high molecular weight dextran in rats. Re-evaluation in nine experiments. Acta Chir Scand 1990;156:763–769.
88. Elkins TE, Stovall TG, Warren J, Ling FW, Meyer NL. A histologic evaluation of peritoneal injury and repair: implications for adhesion formation. Obstet Gynecol 1987;70: 225–228.

89. Ellis H. The cause and prevention of postoperative intraperitoneal adhesions. Surg Gynecol Obstet 1971;133: 497–511.
90. Treutner KH, Bertram P, Lerch MM, et al. Prevention of postoperative adhesions by single intraperitoneal medication. J Surg Res 1995;59:764–771.
91. Nagelschmidt M, Saad S. Influence of polyethylene glycol 4000 and dextran 70 on adhesion formation in rats. J Surg Res 1997;67:113–118.
92. Urman B, Gomel V, Jetha N. Effect of hyaluronic acid on postoperative intraperitoneal adhesion formation in the rat model. Fertil Steril 1991;56:563–567.
93. Kaplun A, Griffel B, Halperin B, Aronson M. A model for adhesion formation by thermal injury in the abdominal cavity of the mouse. Eur Surg Res 1984;16:131–135.
94. Porter JM, Ball AP, Silver D. Mesothelial fibrinolysis. J Cardiovasc Surg 1971;62:725–730.
95. Rappaport WD, Holcomb M, Valente J, Chvapil M. Antibiotic irrigation and the formation of intraabdominal adhesions. Am J Surg 1989;158:435–437.
96. Rodgers KE, Girgis W, diZerega GS. Effect of tolmetin sodium dihydrate on adhesion formation by intraperitoneal administration of antineoplastic agents. Cancer Chemother Pharmacol 1992;29:248–256.
97. Lehman EP, Boys F. The prevention of peritoneal adhesions with heparin. Ann Surg 1940;111:427–435.
98. Reikeras O, Nordstrand K. Use of dextran to prevent intraperitoneal adhesions caused by maize starch powder. Eur Surg Res 1985;17:251–253.
99. Farmer L, Ayoub M, Warejcka D, Southerland S, Freeman A, Solis M. Adhesion formation after intraperitoneal and extraperitoneal implantation of polypropylene mesh. Am Surg 1998;64:144–146.
100. Naim JO, Pulley D, Scanlan K, Hinshaw JR, Lanzafame RJ. Reduction of postoperative adhesions to Marlex mesh using experimental adhesion barriers in rats. J Laparoendosc Surg 1993;3:187–190.
101. Fitzgibbons RJ Jr, Salerno GM, Filipi CJ, Hunter WJ, Watson P. A laparoscopic intraperitoneal onlay mesh technique for the repair of an indirect inguinal hernia. Ann Surg 1994;219:144–156.
102. Diamond MP, Nezhat F. Adhesions after resection of ovarian endometriomas. Fertil Steril 1993;59:934–935.
103. Wiseman DM, Trout JR, Diamond MP. The rates of adhesion development and the effects of crystalloid solutions on adhesion development in pelvic surgery. Fertil Steril 1998;70:702–711.
104. Linsky CB, Diamond MP, DeCherney AH, diZerega GS, Cunningham T. Effect of blood on the efficacy of barrier adhesion reduction in the rabbit uterine horn model. Infertility 1988;11:273–280.
105. Evans DM, McAree K, Guyton DP, Hawkins N, Stakleff K. Dose dependency and wound healing aspects of the use of tissue plasminogen activator in the prevention of intraabdominal adhesions. Am J Surg 1993;165:229–232.
106. Tsimoyiannis EC, Tsimoyiannis JC, Sarros CJ, et al. The role of oxygen-derived free radicals in peritoneal adhesion formation induced by ileal ischaemia/reperfusion. Acta Chir Scand 1989;155:171–174.
107. O'Leary JP, Wickbom G, Cha SO, Wickbom A. The role of feces, necrotic tissue, and various blocking agents in the prevention of adhesions. Ann Surg 1988;207:693–698.
108. Montz FJ, Wheeler JH, Lau LM. Inability of polyglycolic acid mesh to inhibit immediate postradical pelvic surgery adhesions. Gynecol Oncol 1990;38:230–233.
109. Montz FJ, Monk BJ, Lacy SM. Effectiveness of two barriers at inhibiting post-radical pelvic surgery adhesions. Gynecol Oncol 1993;48:247–251.
110. Gallup D, Wheelock T, Plouffe L, Metheny W. Assessment of the efficacy of INTERCED after hysterectomy in preventing adhesion formation in the rabbit model. Gynecol Oncol 1993;50:265–266.
111. Hoban LD, Pierce M, Quance J, et al. Use of polypentapeptides of elastin to prevent postoperative adhesions: efficacy in a contaminated peritoneal model. J Surg Res 1994;56:179–183.
112. Williams-Smith H. Observations on the flora of the alimentary tract of animals and factors affecting its composition. J Pathol Bact 1965;89:95–122.
113. Toh H, Torisu M, Shimura H, et al. In vitro analysis of peritoneal adhesions in peritonitis. J Surg Res 1996;61: 250–255.
114. Marcovici I, Rosenzweig BA, Brill AI, Scommegna A. Colchicine and post-inflammatory adhesions in a rabbit model: a dose-response study. Obstet Gynecol 1993;82: 216–218.
115. Dunselman GA, Willebrand D, Land JA, Bouckaert PX, Evers JL. A rabbit model of endometriosis. Gynecol Obstet Invest 1989;27:29–33.
116. Wright JA, Sharpe-Timms KL. Gonadotropin-releasing hormone agonist therapy reduces postoperative adhesion formation and reformation after adhesiolysis in rat models for adhesion formation and endometriosis. Fertil Steril 1995;63:1094–1100.
117. Taskin O, Buhur A, Birincioglu M, et al. The effects of duration of CO_2 insufflation and irrigation on peritoneal microcirculation assessed by free radical scavengers and total glutathion levels during operative laparoscopy. J Am Assoc Gynecol Laparosc 1998;5:129–133.
118. Chen MD, Teigen GA, Reynolds HT, Johnson PR, Fowler JM. Laparoscopy versus laparotomy: an evaluation of adhesion formation after pelvic and paraaortic lymphadenectomy in a porcine model. Am J Obstet Gynecol 1998;178:499–503.
119. Marana R, Luciano AA, Muzii L, Marendino VE, Mancuso S. Laparoscopy versus laparotomy for ovarian conservative surgery: a randomized trial in the rabbit model. Am J Obstet Gynecol 1994;171:861–864.
120. Fielder EP, Guzick DS, Guido R, Kanbour-Shakir A, Krasnow JS. Adhesion formation from release of dermoid contents in the peritoneal cavity and effect of copious lavage: a prospective, randomized, blinded, controlled study in a rabbit model. Fertil Steril 1996;65:852–859.
121. De Iaco PA, Stefanetti M, Pressato D, et al. A novel hyaluronan-based gel in laparoscopic adhesion prevention: preclinical evaluation in an animal model. Fertil Steril 1998;69:318–323.
122. Haney AF, Doty E. The formation of coalescing peritoneal adhesions requires injury to both contacting peritoneal surfaces. Fertil Steril 1994;61:767–775.

123. Kaleli B, Ozden A, Aybek Z, Bostanci B. The effect of L-arginine and pentoxifylline on postoperative adhesion formation. Acta Obstet Gynecol Scand 1998;77:377–380.
124. Ortega-Moreno J, Caballero-Gomez JM. Postoperative adhesion after uterine horn surgery in the rat, with the use of TC7. Eur J Obstet Gynecol Reprod Biol 1993;48:51–59.
125. Korell M, Scheidel P, Hepp H. Experimental animal model for readhesion formation study. J Invest Surg 1994;7:409–415.
126. Wiseman DM, Johns DB. Anatomical synergy between sodium hyaluronate (HA) and INTERCEED barrier in rabbits with two types of adhesions. Fertil Steril 1993;Prog Suppl:S25.
127. Diamond MP, Cunningham T, Linsky CB, DeCherney AH. Laparoscopic application of Interceed (TC7) in the pig. J Gynecol Surg 1989;5:145–148.
128. Jibhorn H, Ahonen J, Zederfeldt B. Bursting strength of the colon after left colon resection and anastomosis. Am J Surg 1978;136:587–594.
129. Hesp FLEM, Hendriks T, Lubbers JC, de Boer HHM. Wound healing in the intestinal wall. A comparison between ileal and colonic anastomoses. Dis Colon Rectum 1984;27:99–104.
130. Medina M, Paddock HN, Connolly RJ, Schwaitzberg SD. Novel antiadhesion barrier does not prevent anastomotic healing in a rabbit model. J Invest Surg 1995;8:179–186.
131. Wise L, McAlister W, Stein T, Schuck P. Studies on the healing of anastomoses of small and large intestines. Surg Gynecol Obst 1975;141:190–194.
132. Houston KA, McRitchie DI, Rotstein OD. Tissue plasminogen activator reverses the deleterious effect of infection on colonic wound healing. Ann Surg 1990;211: 130–135.
133. Hesp FLEM, Hendriks T, Lubbers JC, de Boer HHM. Wound healing in the intestinal wall. Effects of infection on experimental ileal and colonic anastomoses. Dis Colon Rectum 1984;27:462–467.
134. Edlich RF, Panek PH, Rodeheaver GT, Turnbull VG, Kurtz LD, Edgerton MT. Physical and chemical configuration of sutures in the development of surgical infection. Ann Surg 1973;177:679–688.
135. Dunn DL, Rotstein OD, Simmons RL. Fibrin in peritonitis. IV. Synergistic intraperitoneal infection caused by *Escherichia coli* and *Bacteroides fragilis* within fibrin clots. Arch Surg 1984;119:139–145.
136. Bartlett JG, Gorbach S. An animal model of intra-abdominal sepsis. Scand J Infect Dis Suppl 1979;19:26–29.
137. Miller RJ, Tzianabos A, Dethlefsen S, Gershkovich J, Burns JW, Onderdonk A. The effect of bacterial species on the infection propagation with adhesion reduction products in vivo. Fertil Steril 1998;Prog Suppl:S26.
138. Hsiang YN. Application of appropriate statistical methods in experimental surgery. J Invest Surg 1991;4:415–421.
139. Cohen J; Statistical Power Analysis for the Behavioral Sciences, 2nd Ed. Hillsdale, NJ: Lawrence Erlbaum, 1988.
140. Bowman MC, Li TC, Cooke ID. Inter-observer variability at laparoscopic assessment of pelvic adhesions. Hum Reprod (Oxf) 1995;10:155–160.
141. Corson SL, Batzer FR, Gocial B, Kelly M, Gutmann JN, Maislin G. Intra-observer and interobserver variability in scoring laparoscopic diagnosis of pelvic adhesions. Hum Reprod (Oxf) 1995;10:161–164.
142. Adhesion Scoring Group. Improvement of interobserver reproducibility of adhesion scoring systems. Fertil Steril 1994;62:984–988.
143. Lifecore Biomedical Inc. Quarterly report form 10K. Chaska, MN. September 5, 1996.
144. Yaacobi Y, Israel AA, Goldberg EP. Prevention of postoperative abdominal adhesions by tissue precoating with polymer solutions. J Surg Res 1993;55:422–426.
145. Burns J, Colt MJ, Skrabut E, Wiseman D. Evaluation of de novo adhesion prevention in a rabbit model by precoating with a tissue protective hyaluronate solution. Fertil Steril 1997;Prog Suppl:S66.
146. Milligan DW, Raftery AT. Observations on the pathogenesis of peritoneal adhesions: a light and electron microscopical study. Br J Surg 1974;61:274–280.
147. Raftery AT. Regeneration of parietal and visceral peritoneum. A light microscopical study. Br J Surg 1973;60: 293–299.
148. Schade DS, Williamson JR. The pathogenesis of peritoneal adhesions: an ultrastructural study. Ann Surg 1968; 167:500–510.
149. Chegini N, Simms J, Williams RS, Masterson BJ. Identification of epidermal growth factor, transforming growth factor-alpha, and epidermal growth factor receptor in surgically induced pelvic adhesions in the rat and intraperitoneal adhesions in the human. Am J Obstet Gynecol 1994;171:321–327.
150. Whawell SA, Wang Y, Fleming KA, Thompson EM, Thompson JN. Localization of plasminogen activator inhibitor-1 production in inflamed appendix by in situ hybridization. J Pathol 1993;169:67–71.
151. McKinney WP, Young MJ, Hartz A, Lee MB. The inexact use of Fisher's Exact Test in six major medical journals. JAMA 1989;261:3430–3433.
152. Tukey JW. Comparing individual means in the analysis of variance. Biometrics 1949;5:99–114.
153. Duncan DB. Multiple range and multiple F tests. Biometrics 1955;2:1–42.
154. Dunnett CW. New tables for multiple comparisons with a control. Biometrics 1964;20:482–491.
155. Box GEP, Hunter WG, Hunter JS. Statistics for Experiments. New York: Wiley, 1978:203–207.
156. Godfery K. Comparing the means of several groups. N Engl J Med 1985;313:1450–1456.
157. SAS. Users Guide: Statistics Version 5. Cary, NC: SAS Institute, 1985:651.
158. Conover WJ, Iman RL. Rank transformations as a bridge between parametric and non-parametric statistics. Am Statist 1981;35:124–128.
159. Strandell A, Thorburn J, Tronstad SE, et al. Effectiveness and safety of a bioresorbable carbohydrate solution for prevention of post-operative adhesions in pelvic surgery. Fertil Steril 1998;Prog Suppl:S412.
160. Reid RL, Lie K, Spence JE, Tulandi T, Yuzpe A. Clinical evaluation of the efficacy of heparin-saturated Interceed for prevention of adhesion reformation in the pelvic sidewall of the human. Prog Clin Biol Res 1993;381:261–264.
161. Mais V, Ajossa S, Marongiu D, Peiretti RF, Guerriero S, Melis GB. Reduction of adhesion reformation after laparoscopic endometriosis surgery: a randomized trial with

an oxidized regenerated cellulose absorbable barrier. Obstet Gynecol 1995;86:512–515.

162. Mais V, Ajossa S, Piras B, Guerriero S, Marongiu G, Melis GB. Prevention of de novo adhesion formation after laparoscopic myomectomy: a randomized trial to evaluate the effectiveness of an oxidized regenerated cellulose absorbable barrier. Hum Reprod (Oxf) 1995;10: 3133–3135.
163. Keckstein J, Ulrich U, Sasse V, Roth A, Tuttlies F, Karageorgieva E. Reduction of postoperative adhesion formation after laparoscopic ovarian cystectomy. Hum Reprod (Oxf) 1996;11:579–582.
164. Azziz R. Microsurgery alone or with INTERCEED Absorbable Adhesion Barrier for pelvic sidewall adhesion reformation. The INTERCEED (TC7) Adhesion Barrier Study Group II. Surg Gynecol Obstet 1993;177:135–139.
165. Li TC, Cooke ID. The value of an absorbable adhesion barrier, Interceed, in the prevention of adhesion reformation following microsurgical adhesiolysis. Br J Obstet Gynaecol 1994;101:335–339.
166. Franklin RR. Reduction of ovarian adhesions by the use of Interceed. Ovarian Adhesion Study Group. Obstet Gynecol 1995;86:335–340.
167. Sekiba K. Use of Interceed (TC7) absorbable adhesion barrier to reduce postoperative adhesion reformation in infertility and endometriosis surgery. The Obstetrics and Gynecology Adhesion Prevention Committee. Obstet Gynecol 1992;79:518–522.
168. Nordic Adhesion Prevention Study Group. The efficacy of Interceed (TC7)* for prevention of reformation of postoperative adhesions on ovaries, fallopian tubes, and fimbriae in microsurgical operations for fertility: a multicenter study. Fertil Steril 1995;63:709–714.
169. Surrey M. Postoperative adhesion formation following myomectomy. Fertil Steril 1992;(Prog Suppl):78S–79S.
170. Van Geldorp H, Trimbos-Kemper T. INTERCEED® (TC7) Absorbable Adhesion Barrier reduces the formation of postsurgical adhesions after ovarian surgery. Fertil Steril 1994;Prog Suppl:P273 [and Johnson & Johnson Medical Protocol 3067:11C/1311.00].
171. Huang WJ, Johns DB, Kronenthal RL. Ionically Cross-linked Carboxyl-Containing Polysaccharides for Adhesion Prevention. U.S. Patent 5,532,221, 1996.
172. Thornton MH, Johns DB, Campeau JD, Hoehler F, di-Zerega GS. Clinical evaluation of 0.5% ferric hyaluronate adhesion prevention gel for the reduction of adhesions following peritoneal cavity surgery: open-label pilot study. Hum Reprod (Oxf) 1998;13:1480–1485.
173. Diamond MP. Reduction of adhesions after uterine myomectomy by Seprafilm membrane (HAL-F): a blinded, prospective, randomized, multicenter clinical study. Seprafilm Adhesion Study Group. Fertil Steril 1996;66: 904–910.
174. Diamond MP, DeCherney AH, Linsky CB, Cunningham T, Constantine B. Assessment of carboxymethylcellulose and 32% dextran 70 for prevention of adhesions in a rabbit uterine horn model. Int J Fertil 1988;33:278–282.
175. Adhesion Study Group. Reduction of postoperative pelvic adhesions with intraperitoneal 32% dextran 70: a prospective, randomized clinical trial. Fertil Steril 1983; 40:612–619.
176. Larsson B, Lalos O, Marsk L, et al. Effect of intraperitoneal instillation of 32% dextran 70 on postoperative adhesion formation after tubal surgery. Acta Obstet Gynecol Scand 1985;64:437–441.
177. Rosenberg SM, Board JA. High-molecular weight dextran in human infertility surgery. Am J Obstet Gynecol 1984; 148:380–385.
178. Jansen RP. Failure of intraperitoneal adjuncts to improve the outcome of pelvic operations in young women. Am J Obstet Gynecol 1985;153:363–371.
179. Diamond MP, Linsky CB, Cunningham T, et al. Synergistic effects of INTERCEED(TC7) and heparin in reducing adhesion formation in the rabbit uterine horn model. Fertil Steril 1991;55:389–394.
180. Jansen RP. Failure of peritoneal irrigation with heparin during pelvic operations upon young women to reduce adhesions. Surg Gynecol Obstet 1988;166:154–160.
181. Saravelos H, Li TC. Post-operative adhesions after laparoscopic electrosurgical treatment for polycystic ovarian syndrome with the application of Interceed to one ovary: a prospective randomized controlled study. Hum Reprod (Oxf) 1996;11:992–997.
182. Greenblatt EM, Casper RF. Adhesion formation after laparoscopic ovarian cautery for polycystic ovarian syndrome: lack of correlation with pregnancy rate. Fertil Steril 1993;60:766–770.

39

Adhesion Prevention: The Role of Fibrin Glue

Matthias Korell

CONTENTS

The formation of adhesions is very common after intraabdominal surgery. It represents one of the major complications, especially in reproductive surgery, which may lead to infertility and abdominal symptoms going so far as the ileus.[1,2] Following myomectomy or reconstructive tubal surgery in particular the incidence of postoperative adhesions reaches more than 90%.[3]

To prevent postoperative adhesions, several methods have been described however without significant clinical success.[4,5] Merely covering the damaged peritoneal surface was shown to reduce adhesion formation substantially. Two barriers—Interceed TC7 and Gore-Tex SM—are commercially available and have been used in clinical practice with proven effectiveness.[6–9] With these barriers, we could demonstrate a reduction of adhesions following myomectomy. The proportion of patients without adhesions was comparable with the use of Interceed TC7 (54.5%) or Gore-Tex SM (56.3%), but significantly higher compared without any prophylaxis (21.4%).[10] In addition, the use of fibrin glue is also recommended for the prevention of adhesions. Clinical and experimental data concerning its use and impact on the formation of adhesions are presented and discussed next.

Characteristics of Fibrin Glue

Fibrin glue is a derivative of human and animal blood serum. The main components consist of fibrinogen, plasminogen, factor XIII, thrombin, and calcium chloride (Table 39.1). The commercially available product is delivered in two syringes to prevent a premature biochemical reaction and must be stored frozen to maintain the quality. In Fig. 39.1 is shown the system of reaction that converts fibrin to fibrinogen. Depending on the conditions (temperature, concentration, etc.), several minutes are required to achieve the optimum adhesive capacity.

Fibrin glue is used in many different specialties such as neurosurgery, orthopedics, vascular surgery, pediatrics, and otorhinolaryngology for a wide spectrum of indications.[11–15] In open heart surgery, the application of fibrin glue reduces the incidence of adhesions and leads to easier reoperations.[16] The aim of the application of fibrin glue, however, is not only the prevention of adhesions. The treatment of intraabdominal injury requires an effective hemostatic agent such as fibrin glue to stop the acute bleeding.[17] Here, the laparoscopic injection of fibrin glue helps to arrest parenchymal hemorrhage, especially in liver and spleen injuries. In general surgery, fibrin glue is used as a hemostatic and adhesive agent. It is effective in increasing the resistance of bowel anastomosis to intraluminal pressure, but cannot reduce the incidence of postoperative adhesions.[18–20]

The Gynecologic Use of Fibrin Glue

In gynecology, fibrin sealant is mainly used for bleeding control, for gluing of tubal anastomoses, and for recon-

TABLE 39.1. Content of fibrin glue (Tissucol®, IMMUNO, Heidelberg, Germany).

First syringe, 2 mL, deep-frozen	
Human plasma protein fraction including fibrinogen	160–240 mg
Factor XIII	140–220 mg
Fibronectin	20–100 U
Plasminogen	4–18 mg
Aprotinin (bovine)	0.04–0.16 mg
Second syringe, 2 mL, deep-frozen	
Thrombin (human)	1000 IU
Calcium chloride • $2H_2O$	11.76 mg

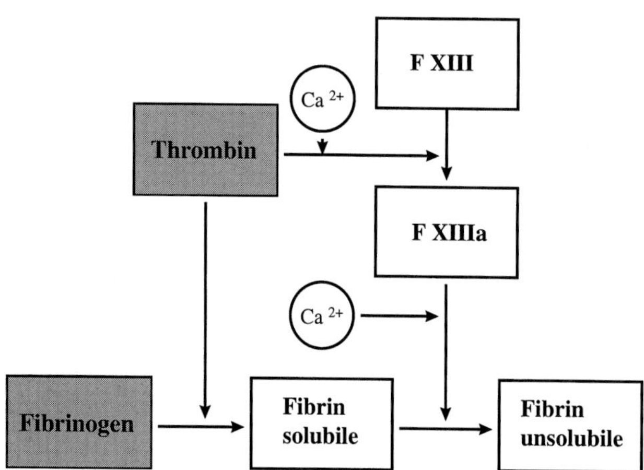

FIG. 39.1. Reaction to convert fibrinogen to fibrin.

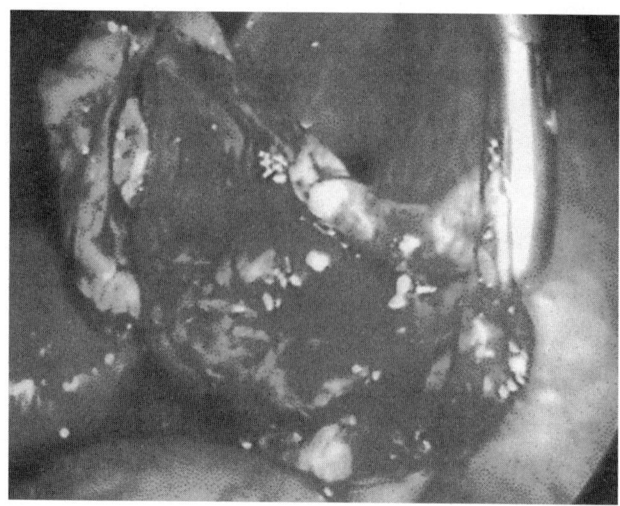

FIG. 39.3. Wide-open capsule after excision of ovarian cyst. *Please see insert for color reproduction of this figure.*

struction of ovaries following cystectomy.[21–28] The extirpation of an ovarian cyst leads to an open capsule with a wide wound surface (Figs. 39.2 and 39.3). Here, suturing is required to achieve results comparable to those after laparotomy. The fibrin glue can be used to close and reform the ovary (Fig. 39.4). For endoscopic use, an application system is available with a 5-mm introduction sheet (Fig. 39.5). Especially in large endometriomas, there was a significant reduction of postoperative adhesions compared with no suturing.[22,29] The decrease of adhesions was most marked in patients with ovarian cysts of more than 5 cm and for those with preoperative adhesions.

The standard of comparison in respect to postoperative quality, however, must be the suture. In tubal surgery the results were better using microsurgical sutures to approximate the oviduct.[30,31] In the rat uterine horn model, the tubal patency rate was 60% with fibrin glue compared to 90% with sutures, and the adhesion score was significantly higher (1.7 versus 1.4).[32] These data were confirmed also by other authors.[21,27] According to these data, the application of fibrin glue is helpful in the reconstruction of the ovary and in microsurgery but could not attain the operative quality of microsutures.

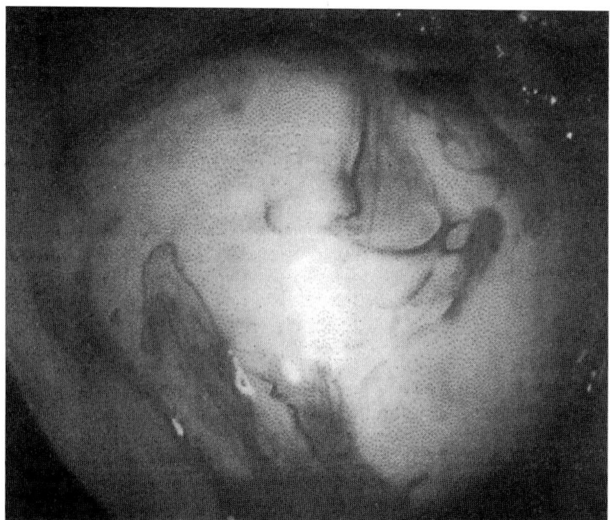

FIG. 39.2. Large endometrioma at right side. *Please see insert for color reproduction of this figure.*

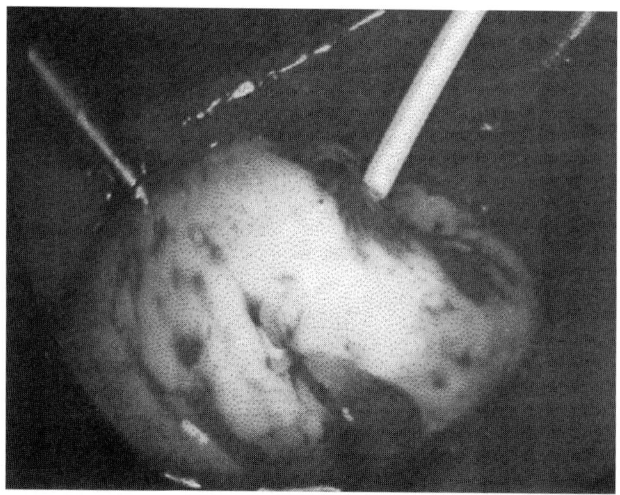

FIG. 39.4. Endoscopic application of fibrin glue to close the ovary. *Please see insert for color reproduction of this figure.*

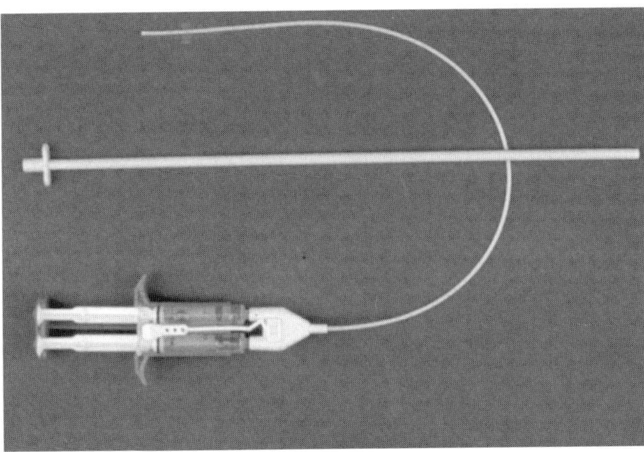

FIG. 39.5. Application set for endoscopic use of fibrin glue.

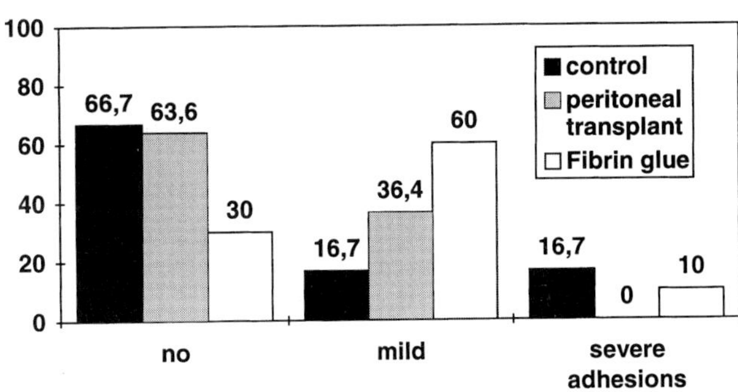

FIG. 39.7. Adhesions following defects on pelvic sidewall in rats. Comparison of fibrin glue and peritoneal sidewall versus control. (From Korell et al. 1994,[43] with permission.)

Fibrin Glue for the Reduction of Adhesions

The starting point of every adhesion is a peritoneal trauma.[4] Various studies have been undertaken to evaluate the effects of multiple agents on adhesion formation but have failed to demonstrate a clear benefit.[5] On the contrary, covering the traumatized peritoneal surface—the so-called barrier methods—provides exclusively effective adhesion prophylaxis.[33-36] The fibrin glue provides a layer that shields the traumatized area from other organs. It must cover the defect until the superficial healing is completed, which lasts about 1 week. Fibrin is applied like Interceed TC7, although the resorption time is much shorter.

Many experimental studies on adhesion prevention showed no significant beneficial effect of fibrin glue.[31,37,38] In contrast, other authors have described inhibition of intraabdominal adhesion formation.[23,26,39-41] In defects on the abdominal walls of rats, the use of fibrin glue could reduce the severity of adhesions and increase the number of animals without adhesions (Fig. 39.6).[41] In the rabbit uterine horn model, the use of fibrin glue significantly reduced the incidence of adhesions, from 70% to 25%.[42]

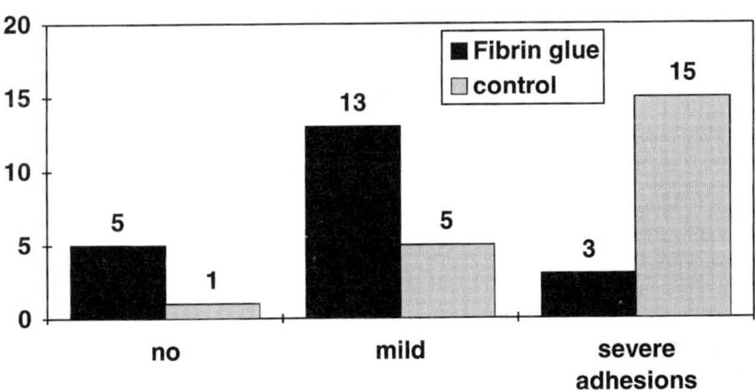

FIG. 39.6. Number of animals with adhesions following defects on abdominal wall in rats. (From Sheppard et al. 1993,[41] with permission.)

We have studied the efficacy of fibrin glue and peritoneal transplant in the pelvic sidewall model in rats.[43] Here, the incidence of adhesions was comparable between the use of peritoneal transplants and the control group (Fig. 39.7). However, the covering of the peritoneal defect with fibrin glue led to more adhesions.

Adhesion Prophylaxis: The Role of Fibrin Glue?

The real value of fibrin glue for preventing postoperative adhesions remains unclear because the results of experimental animal studies are conflicting. Although some authors showed better results with fibrin use, other investigators could not demonstrate a beneficial effect. In addition, clinical studies were rare and mostly neither controlled nor randomized.

There are various reasons for the conflicting results. It is known from experimental and clinical experience that the location of the peritoneal trauma induces a different incidence and severity of adhesions. It seems that the visceral peritoneum (ovary, fallopian tube, uterus, and bowel) reacts more intensely to every trauma than does the parietal peritoneum (pelvic or abdominal wall). We found an 84% adhesion rate in uterine horns after uncovered defects compared to 33% at the pelvic sidewall.[43] Intensive search of publications regarding the use of fibrin glue supports the hypothesis that it is effective in case of extensive adhesion formation. In a model in which 13 of 15 control animals develop adhesions, the use of fibrin glue can reduce the incidence to 3 of 15 in the treatment group.[39] The more risk of postoperative adhesion exists, the better a prophylactic agent could work. Besides the different locations of peritoneal

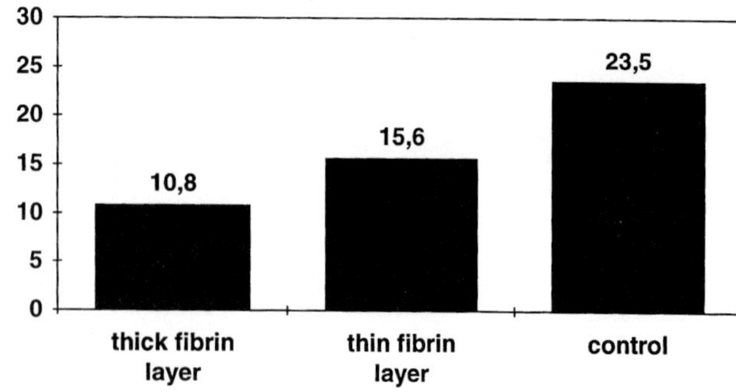

FIG. 39.8. Length of adhesions (mm) in relation to treatment of the peritoneal defect at the abdominal wall in rats. (From Lindenberg et al. 1985,[44] with permission.)

trauma, the various animal species used can determine the outcome in terms of adhesion rate and efficacy of fibrin glue.

Also, the method of application has an influence.[44] A dose-dependent effect is possible because a thick layer of fibrin glue gives better results compared to a thin layer and the control (Fig. 39.8). Thus, indication and application of fibrin glue are decisive to achieve the optimum postoperative result. Provided that it is applied correctly, the use of fibrin glue does not lead to more adhesions. The required waiting time can be hard for some eager surgeons. However, the efficacy of fibrin glue as adhesion prophylaxis is certainly limited. One can expect effectiveness similar to that of artificial ascites. For example, fibrin glue is equieffective in prevention of adhesions compared to Ringer's lactate but significant better than the control group on the abdominal walls of rats.[45]

It is questionable whether the efficacy of other barrier methods can be reached. The incidence of postoperative adhesions following myomectomy is extremely high; the use of Interceed TC7 can reduce the number of adhesion-free patients from 12% to 60%.[34] Here, not only the barrier function is important; it is also important how intensely the agent affects the reparative wound regeneration. With fibrin glue, the induction of peritoneal activity was more compared with Interceed TC7 but less than with the use of catgut.[46] The least peritoneal activity was produced by Prolene sutures.

Summary

Fibrin glue has an important role for gluing in many different operative indications. In addition, it is helpful as an effective hemostatic agent in case of acute bleeding. In ovarian surgery, the use of fibrin glue is helpful to close the organ, specially in case of large endometriomas.

The value of fibrin glue in adhesion prevention however is questionable (Table 39.2). In some cases, like the excision of large ovarian endometrioma, it is better compared to not suturing, but the use of microsutures leads to better results. In summary, fibrin glue does not have proven efficacy for adhesion prevention to recommend it for routine use.

TABLE 39.2. Evaluation of fibrin glue.

Advantages	Disadvantages
Easy to handle	Expensive
Gluing and Hemostatic capacity	Effective in adhesion prevention?

References

1. Monk B, Berman M, Montz F. Adhesions after extensive gynecologic surgery: clinical significance etiology and prevention. Am J Obstet Gynecol 1994;170:1396–1403.
2. Stone K. Adhesions in gynecologic surgery. Curr Opin Obstet Gynecol 1993;5:322–327.
3. Tulandi T, Murray C, Guralnik M. Adhesion formation and reproductive outcome after myomectomy and second look laparoscopy. Obstet Gynecol 1993;82:213–215.
4. diZerega G. Comtemporary adhesion prevention. Fertil Steril 1994;61:219–235.
5. Holtz G. Prevention and management of peritoneal adhesions. Fertil Steril 1984;41:497–511.
6. Boyers S, Diamond M, DeCherney A. Reduction of postoperative pelvic adhesions in the rabbit with Gore-Tex Surgical Membrane. Fertil Steril 1988;49:1066–1070.
7. Interceed Adhesion Barrier Study Group. Prevention of postsurgical adhesions by Interceed (TC7), an absorbable adhesion barrier: a prospective, randomized study. Fertil Steril 1989;51:933–938.
8. Linsky C, Diamond M, Cunningham T, et al. Adhesion reduction in the rabbit uterine horn model using an resorbable barrier, TC7. J Reprod Med 1987;32:17–20.
9. Surgical Membrane Study Group. Prophylaxis of pelvic sidewall adhesions with Gore-Tex surgical membrane: a multicenter clinical investigation. Fertil Steril 1992;57: 921–923.
10. Korell M. Adhesion prophylaxis in gynecology. In: Treutner KH, Schumpelick V, eds. Peritoneal Adhesions. Heidelberg: Springer, 1996:325–330.
11. Alleyne CH, Cawley CM, Barrow DL, et al. Efficacy and biocompatibility of a photopolymerized, synthetic, absorbable hydrogel as a dural sealant in a canine craniotomy model. J Neurosurg 1998;88(2):308–313.
12. Frykman E, Jacobsson S, Widenfalk B. Fibrin sealant in prevention of flexor tendon adhesions: an experimental study in the rabbit. J Hand Surg 1993;18(1):68–75.
13. Dickson CS, Magovern JA. The effect of fibrin glue on the formation of perivascular adhesions. Vasc Surg 1993;27 (1):15–18.
14. Brands W, Diehm TH, Lockbuhler H, Konig M, Stock M. The use of fibrin glue in the prophylaxis and therapy of intraabdominal adhesions. Chirurg 1990;61(1):22–26.
15. Zohar Y, Shwilli Y, Schimberg R, Buler N. Human fibrin glue in head and neck surgery. Harefuah 1994;126(10): 567–570, 628.

16. Boris WJ, Gu J, McGrath LB. Effectiveness of fibrin glue in the reduction of postoperative intrapericardial adhesions. J Invest Surg 1996;9(4):327–333.
17. Salvino CK, Esposito TJ, Smith DK, et al. Laparoscopic injection of fibrin glue to arrest intraparenchymal abdominal hemorrhage: an experimental study. J Trauma 1991; 35(5):762–766.
18. Shinohara K, Kobayashi E, Yoshida T, et al. Effect of fibrin glue on small and large bowel anastomoses in the rat. Eur Surg Res 1998;30(1):8–12.
19. van der Ham AC, Kort WJ, Wejma IM, van den Ingh HFGM, Jeekel J. Effect of fibrin sealant on the healing colonic anastomosis in the rat. Br J Surg 1991;78:49–53.
20. Hulkko OA, Haukipuro KA, Laitinen ST. Fibrin glue protection of primary anastomosis in the obstructed left colon. An experimental study on the rat. Acta Chir Scand 1988;154(1):49–52.
21. Haberal A, Turgut F, Oral S, Demirhan B, Batioglu S. Comparison of microsurgery and cyanoacrylate for tubal anastomosis: an experimental study in the rat. J Gynecol Surg 1996;12(4):261–265.
22. Takeuchi H, Awaji M, Hashimoto M, Nakano Y, Mitsuhashi N, Kuwabara Y. Reduction of adhesions with fibrin glue after laparoscopic excision of large ovarian endometriomas. J Am Assoc Gynecol Laparosc 1996;3(4):575–579.
23. Takeuchi HU, Toyonari Y, Mitsuhashi N, Kuwabara Y. Effects of fibrin glue on postsurgical adhesions after uterine or ovarian surgery in rabbits. J Obstet Gynaecol Res 1997; 23(5):479–484.
24. Ozeren S, Corakci A, Erk A, Yucesoy G, Yucesoy J, Karabacak O. The effects of human amniotic membrane and fibrin sealant in the prevention of postoperative adhesion formation in the rabbit ovary model. Aust NZ J Obstet Gynaecol 1998;38/2:207–209.
25. Adamyan LV, Myinbayev OA, Kulakov VI. Use of fibrin glue in obstetrics and gynecology: a review of the literature. Int J Fertil 1991;36(2):76–77, 81–88.
26. Adamyan LV, Myinbayev OA, Ishrat J, Kulakov VI. Comparative effects of different methods of anastomosis on rat uterine horn. Int J Fertil 1992;37(6):368–372.
27. Gauwerky JFH, Klose RP, Vierneisel P, Bastert G. Fibrin glue for reanastomosis of the fallopian tube in the rabbit: adhesions and fertility. Hum Reprod (Oxf) 1992;7(9): 1274–1277.
28. Gauwerky JFH, Klose RP, Forssmann WG. Fibrin glue for anastomosis of the fallopian tube: morphology. Hum Reprod (Oxf) 1993;8(12):2108–2114.
29. Donnez J, Nisolle M. Laparoscopic management of large ovarian endometrial cyst: use of fibrin sealant. J Gynecol Surg 1991;7(3):163–166.
30. Adamyan LV, Kulakov VI, Myinbayev OA, Jahan I. Reproductive function after reconstructive surgery on rat uterine horns. Int J Fertil Menopaus Stud 1994;39(4): 229–233.
31. Bilgin T, Cengiz C, Demir U. Postoperative adhesion formation following ovarian reconstruction with fibrin glue in the rabbit. Gynecol Obstet Invest 1995;39(3):186–187.
32. Kamaci M, Zorlu CG, Suludere Z, Can C. Comparison of microsurgery and fibrin sealant in reanastomosis of the uterine horns of rats. J Gynecol Surg 1997;3(3):125–129.
33. diZerega GS. Use of adhesion prevention barriers in ovarian surgery, tubalplasty, ectopic pregnancy, endometriosis, adhesiolysis and myomectomy. Curr Opin Obstet Gynecol 1996;8:230–237.
34. Larsson B. Efficacy of Interceed in adhesion prevention in gynecologic surgery: a review of 13 clinical studies. J Reprod Med 1996;41:27–34.
35. Li TC, Cooke ID. The value of an absorbable adhesion barrier, Interceed, in the prevention of adhesion reformation following microsurgical adhesiolysis. Br J Obstet 1994; 101:335–339.
36. Mais V, Ajossa S, Piras B, Guerriero S, Marongiu D, Melis GB. Prevention of de novo adhesion formation after laparoscopic myomectomy: a randomized trial to evaluate the effectiveness of an oxidiced regenerated cellulose absorbable barrier. Hum Reprod (Oxf) 1995;10:3133–3135.
37. Evrard VA, De Bellis A, Boeckx W, Brosens IA. Peritoneal healing after fibrin glue application: a comparative study in a rat model. Hum Reprod (Oxf) 1996;11(9):1877–1880.
38. Marana R, Muzii L, Catalano G, Caruana U, Mancuso L. Use of fibrin sealant for reproductive surgery: a randomized study in the rabbit model. Gynecol Obstet Invest 1996;41(3):199–202.
39. De Virgilio C, Dubrow T, Sheppard BB, et al. Fibrin glue inhibits intra-abdominal adhesion formation. Arch Surg 1990;125(10):1378–1382.
40. Muzii L, Marana R. Prevention of postoperative adhesion formation in reproductive surgery. Ital J Gynaecol Obstet. 1996;8(1):36–42.
41. Sheppard BB, De Virgilio C, Bleiweis M, Milliken JC, Robertson JM. Inhibition of intra-abdominal adhesions: fibrin glue in a long term model. Am Surg 1993;59:786–790.
42. De Iaco P, Costa A, Mazzoleni G, Pasquinelli G, Bassein L, Marabini A. Fibrin sealant in laparoscopic adhesion prevention in the rabbit uterine horn model. Fertil Steril 1994;62:400–404.
43. Korell M, Scheidel P, Hepp H. An animal experimental model for adhesion reformation study. J Invest Surg 1994; 7:409–415.
44. Lindenberg S, Steentoft P, Sorensen SS, Olesen HP. Studies on prevention of intra-abdominal adhesion formation by fibrin sealant. Acta Chir Scand 1985;151:525–527.
45. Caballero J, Tulandi T. Effects of Ringer's lactate and fibrin glue on postsurgical adhesions. J Reprod Med Obstet Gynecol 1992;37(2):141–143.
46. Myinbayev OA, Rubliova KI. Use of chemiluminescent method for evaluation of postoperative adhesion formation after reproductive pelvic surgery: an experimental study. Am J Reprod Immunol 1996;36(4):238–241.

40

Bioadhesive Polymers That Reduce Adhesion Formation

Stig Bengmark

CONTENTS

Biological Interphases and Surface Protection

Tissue surfaces need protection depending on the type and extent of wearing that normally occurs. Most tissues in the body are, for that reason, covered by a monolayer mainly consisting of lipids and proteins that in the case of alveolar surfaces have been called the surfactant layer. The surface tissues (mucosa) of respiratory, gastrointestinal, and to some extent the genitourinary tracts, normally exposed to a rather "hostile" environment, are also covered by a layer of a viscoelastic gel with very strong protective abilities consisting of polysaccharides and glucoproteins and given the name mucus. Endothelium has no protective layer at all, which renders it vulnerable to inflammatory reactions and to development of its sequelae, atherosclerosis. Tissues such as synovia and mesothelium, which under normal conditions are not exposed to wear of the same magnitude as the mucosa, do not have a mucus protection, making these tissues especially vulnerable to infection and trauma, especially so in the modern age when these tissues are increasingly exposed to treatments such as surgical operations, dialysis, or administration of various pharmaceuticals.

The thin film covering mesothelium and synovia consists of a mixture of glucose aminoglucans such as hyaluronic acid (HA) and an outer monolayer of polar lipids, mainly phospholipids (PL). The dominating lipids are dipalmitoylphosphatidylcholine, phosphatidylethanolamine, and sphingomyelin, but several other lipids are also involved, although in smaller concentrations. The film is rich in biologically active cells,[1,2] such as mast cells, lymphocytes, macrophages, polymorphs, and free mesothelial cells, which produce lytic enzymes, oxidative free radicals (intended to eliminate invading microorganisms), angiogenesis factors, prostaglandins, cytokines, growth factors, and many other active substances. These various compounds are basically meant for protection of the tissues but if "overproduced" during the acute-phase reaction—the inflammatory response to trauma and infection—also constitute a potential threat to the tissues. Other ingredients in the film are macromolecules such as albumin, globulins, lipoproteins, and cholesterol.

The mesothelial cells, the largest cell population of uninfected peritoneal, pleural, and pericardial cavities, are more biologically active than thought in the past. They constitute by themselves a first line of defense, and play a significant role in the activation, amplification, and control of inflammatory processes.[3] The fact that the mesothelial cells secrete molecules such as IL-6[4] and synthesize arachidonic acid metabolites[5] supports the assumption that their primary role is to control rather than only initiate inflammation.[3]

Peritoneal Dialysis Experience

The expanding treatment of end-stage renal disease using repeated peritoneal dialysis brought the production of phospholipids (PL) by the peritoneal membrane into focus. The recognizion of the role of hyaluronic acid/hyaluronan (HA) as active in the protection and lubrication of the peritoneum is slightly more recent. As a consequence of this rather new knowledge, external supply of both substances has in recent years been tried rather extensively, experimentally but also clinically, with the aim to enforce protection and thereby hopefully minimize the effects of injury and prevent the development of late sequelae to injury such as adhesion formation.

This main aim of this chapter is to provide a comprehensive summary and discussion of these points:

1. Efforts made to supply "autologous" molecules such as phospholipids and hyaluronic acid and their analogs
2. Possibilities of and attempts made to use other bioactive polymers, which normally are not synthesized by either eukaryotic or bacterial cells, to develop better surface protection than so far has been possible through the use of "autologous" molecules
3. The acute-phase response and the importance for understanding its complex mechanisms to develop efficient treatments for the future

Of crucial importance to a strong and lasting protective effect is the ability of the substance to "glue to," or adhere to, the surfaces and thereby produce an effective and durable protection and lubrication layer. For use on mesothelium-covered surfaces, such a layer should be expected to remain at the surface for at least 36 to 48 hours. Both natural and synthetic macromolecules are known under certain conditions to adhere to biologic tissues,[6] a phenomenon usually refered to as bioadhesion. To increase the bioadhesivity of the protecting molecule, attempts have been made to enforce its effect using a variety of different chemical strategies. One such new approach is to use oppositely charged polymers with ability to separate tissues through electrostatic repulsion, which is extensively discussed here (see following).

Phospholipids

Phospholipids Thought to Have Great Potential

From studies during the early 1930s it was generally believed that PLs are fibrogenic, that is, they induce growth of connective tissue components,[7,8] a view further supported by the observation that intraperitoneal injection of phospholipids recovered from silicotic lesions results in vigorous connective tissue reaction.[9] Observations during the early development of repeat peritoneal dialysis as a treatment did dramatically change this opinion. It is well known today that mesothelial cells synthesize PLs such as phosphatidylcholine (PC) in quantities similar to that produced by the lung.[10] The amphiphilic nature and surface tension-reducing properties of this complex mixture of PLs are very similar to those of pulmonary surfactants.[11,12] Intraperitoneal administration of PC, when used in continuous ambulatory peritoneal dialysis (CAPD) systems, was shown 10 to 15 years ago to reduce cumulative lymphatic absorption from the peritoneum and enhance ultrafiltration.[13]

Unsuccessful Attempts with Nonsoluble Phospholipids

It was the observation by Grahame et al.[11] in 1985 of surprisingly large amounts of surface-active material in the peritoneal effluent from patients maintained on CAPD that evoked our interest to study an eventual adhesion preventive role of surface-active material (SAM). A drastic increase in the content of PL in the effluent of CAPD patients having problems with reduced ultrafiltration or peritonitis, and significant improvement of ultrafiltration by supplementing the dialysate with PC were reported.[13,14] These findings led to the suggestion that PC could be excellent to protect the mesothelium and improve its healing and thus should routinely be added to commercially produced and marketed dialysate bags.

Our first experimental attempts to prevent adhesions in animal experiments, made with nonsoluble egg yolk PC (Sigma, St. Louis, MO, USA), were unsuccessful.[15] Three different classical experimental models were tried:

Model 1: Abrasion of the cecum with a dry gauze, carried out until petechial subserosal hemorrhages are observed

Model 2: Abrasion of intestines for 10 minutes with gauze soaked with either PC or saline (controls)

Model 3: Surgical extirpation of the serosa (visceral peritoneum) of ileum for a distance of four vascular arcades, approximately 1.5 cm proximal to the ileocecal junction. The operation was performed using an operation microscope and microsurgical instruments.

Either 1% PC or saline, 2 mL each, was administered intraperitoneally to all animals on closure of the abdomen and repeated on the second and third day. All postoperative evaluations were carried out after 7 days. The extent of adhesion formation was significantly more extensive in all the PC-treated animals, irrespective of model tried.

Peritoneal phagocytes are known to play a crucial role in the defense of the peritoneum. One of the mechanisms used by macrophages to control invading microorganisms is to produce reactive oxygen species,[16] essential for killing of invading microorganisms.[17] We observed during in vitro studies that the viability of peritoneal macrophages incubated with PC was uninfluenced (controls, 95 ± 3; 0.5% PC, 97 ± 5; 1% PC, 95 ± 4) but their ability for superoxide production was totally abolished (after 2 h: controls, 21.87 ± 3.06; 0.5% PC, 0.70 ± 0.70; 1% PC, 0 ± 0). It was thus obvious that nonsoluble egg yolk PC is not only ineffective but shows negative effects when attempting to protect surfaces such as the peritoneum.

Success with Solublized PC

Solublized PC (Lipostabil®; A. Nattermann & Cie, GbmH, Köln, Germany) was used in our next attempts.[18] The amount of PC given intraperitoneally was 20 mg per rat and per injection and intravenously either 20 or 50 mg per rat and per injection. As in the previous set of experiments the treatment was repeated on the second and third postoperative days. All evaluations were carried out after 7 days. Four different experimental models were now used.

Model 1: Resection and retransplantation of a 2 × 2 cm area of parietal peritoneum (ischemic graft)

Model 2: Resection of a 1 × 3.5 cm area of perietal peritoneum subsequently closed by continuous sutures

Model 3: Abrasion of the cecum with dry gauze until petechial subseral hemorrhages occurred

Model 4: Surgical extirpation of the ileal serosa to the extent of four vascular arcades (~1.5 cm) and about 25% of the circumference made just proximal to the ileocecal junction

The amount of adhesions was assessed using a five-grade scoring scale for models 1 and 3 and a three-grade scale for model 4. In model 2, the degree of adhesions to the suture line was assessed and reported as percent of suture line involved with adhesions. Solublized PC administered intraperitoneally reduced the degree of adhesions (reduction with 56%, 79%, 62%, and 78%, respectively, for models 1 to 4), all effects being statistically significant. No effects were obtained by intravenous administration, not even when given in a dose as high as 50 mg/rat. It seemed now obvious to us that solublized PC can effectively prevent adhesion development, but it was still not clear if this effect could also be obtained in connection with anastomoses of the intestines. And most important, would such treatment not impair healing and increase the rate of leakage and wound dehiscence?

Therefore, in the next set of experiments various doses of PC were tried following small-bowel anastomoses in rats.[19] Three different doses were tested: 20 mg, 40 mg, and 60 mg per treatment, both administered as a single and repeated dose over 3 days. We found that 20 mg PC administered at the end of the operation did significantly, and without any side effects, decrease the formation of adhesions. The maximal length of ileum entrapped in adhesions (expressed in mm) decreased after a single dose and use of continuous sutures with 46% compared with the controls (PC-treated, 12.0 ± 2.4; control, 22.3 ± 4; $p < 0.01$), and single-dose and interrupted sutures with 44% (PC-treated, 12.3 ± 1.9; controls, 22.1 ± 6.1; $p < 0.001$). The binding to/involvement with adhesions to other intestinal segments decreased significantly irrespective of suture technique used. However, the adhesion preventive effects could only be slightly augmented (~10%) by repetition of the treatment on the subsequent 2 days (continuous sutures, 12.0 ± 2.4; interrupted sutures, 10.7 ± 3.5). Use of larger doses did not further improve adhesion prevention, but the rate of anastomotic dehiscence and leakage increased significantly (40 mg, 10%; 60 mg, 40%), indicating that the safety margin with PC treatment, if repeated, could be narrow.

Is Phospholipase-Resistant PC More Effective?

All studies thus far were only performed with the L-form of of PC. It is likely, however, that not only endogenously but also exogenously supplied PC is hydrolyzed in the body to a considerable degree by activated phospholipases, released as a part of the reaction of the inflammatory response in infection and trauma. Leukocytes are known to produce phospholipase A_2, and phospholipase A_2 activity has been demonstrated in peritoneal neutrophils and inflammatory fluids.[20] Verapamil, a calcium channel blocker, but also a phospholipase inhibitor, has been shown to significantly reduce primary postoperative adhesions in rabbits.[21] For this reason, we decided in the next set of experiments to study the preventive effects of phospholipase-resistant phosphatidylcholine.[21] The D-form is resistant to enzymatic degrading, while the L-form of PC (L-PC) is known to be degraded by phospholipases. We thought that DL-α-phosphatidylcholine didodecyl (DL-PC), a substance 50% resistant to enzymatic degradation, could offer an attractive alternative.

Peritonitis was induced by an established experimental method consisting of cecal ligation and puncture, with cecotomy performed after 15 hours.[22] All animals were during 3 consecutive days treated either with saline, L-PC, or DL-PC. The mortality in peritonitis was similar for the groups treated with saline (25%) and DL-PC (30%) but three times as high when treated with L-PC (75%). All surviving animals were killed on the seventh day and the degree of adhesions evaluated using a seven-point score system. The adhesion score was reduced by 58% in L-PC-treated animals (1.80 ± 0.45 vs. controls, 4.24 ± 0.86; $p < 0.05$) and by 55% in DL-PC-treated animals (1.93 ± 0.47 vs. controls, 4.24 ± 0.86; $p < 0.01$). As the local increase of phospholipase A_2 activity is known to occur mainly during the first few hours after induction of inflammation (maximum reached after 13 hours),[23] we considered it an interesting alternative to delay for 24 hours the administration of L-PC with the hope of minimizing its deleterious effects. When the animals were administered saline on day 1 followed by L-PC on days 2 and 3, the mortality also did decrease to about the same level as the nontreated controls (i.e., from 75% to 30%), but the antiadhesion effect (35%) was also significantly less (2.76 ± 0.72 vs. controls, 4.24 ± 0.86; $p < 0.01$).

Phosphatidylinositol Has a Special Potentiating Effect?

Phosphatidylinositol (PI), a constituent of the human peritoneal membrane, normally occurs in much smaller amounts than PC. Diacylglycerol (DAG), a vital second messenger involved in signal transduction and growth, is released by hydrolysis of inositol phospholipids in the body.[24] As we had previously observed when studying the effects of different phospholipids in an experimental colitis model,[25] that PI has somewhat stronger preventive effects than L-PC, we judged it to be of the greatest interest to compare the effects of PI with those of L-PC and DL-PC. Two models were tried[26]:

Model 1: Resection of a 1 × 3.5 cm area of parietal peritoneum, subsequently closed by continuous sutures
Model 2: Resection and retransplantation of a 2 × 2 cm area of parietal peritoneum (ischemic graft)

Both a single dose and repeat dose over 3 days were tried. A single dose of 20 mg/rat did not show any significant effect irrespective of phospholipid used, but significant differences in effect were seen with administration of 40 mg of both PI and DL-PC, the strongest effect (75% reduction) being observed after administration of 20 mg PI repeatedly over 3 days (adhesion scores for PI, 0.7 ± 0.2; control, 2.8 ± 0.3; $p < 0.05$).

PI from egg yolk is rich in polyunsaturated omega-3 fatty acids, and it cannot be excluded that its strong effects, at least to some extent, result from inhibition of the activity of plasminogen activator inhibitors (PAI-1), an important amyloid β-protein precursor (APP) increased during the acute inflammatory response. PAI-1 is, at least partly, responsible for the inhibition of fibrin degradation, which is essential for production of adhesions. PLs provide unique lubrication, and the strong preventive effect observed could simply be mechanical, that is, the result of production of a lubricant film to cover the injured peritoneum during the 36 to 48 hours after trauma when adhesions are initiated, and preventing attraction between opposing surfaces. It is known that polar lipids are deeply involved in acute phase response (APR) but whether they participate in its modulation is not known, although this should be object of future investigations.

Supporting Studies on PL-Induced Peritoneal Protection

Adhesion formation was effectively prevented in a British experimental study[27] in which PC was administered during an unusually long period, 8 days before and 7 days after induction of adhesions. Adhesions were induced by a 5-minute-long intraperitoneal irrigation with saline heated to 40°C. A German study[28] compared the adhesion prevention effects of PC, sphingolipids (SL), and galactolipids (GL) and found a pronounced reduction in adhesion formation when primary adhesions were induced by a standard abrasion of the peritoneum, but also a reduction in redevelopment of adhesions following adhesiolysis. No differences could be observed in the ability of the three lipids to prevent primary adhesions, but GL exhibited slightly stronger ability to prevent reformation of adhesions.[29]

Hyaluronic Acid

HA Reduces Connective Tissue Growth and Prevents Adhesions

Hyaluronic acid (hyaluronan, HA) is produced by endothelial and mesothelial cells, but also by other cells such as fibroblasts and synovial cells. It is a rather recent finding that the peritoneal mesothelial cells are among the most important sources of HA in the body,[30,31] and that significant amounts of HA are present in the effluent of CAPD patients, especially when signs of peritonitis are present.[32] Several cytokines have been shown to upregulate the HA synthetase activity and HA production. Among these are transforming growth factor-β (TGF-β) and platelet-derived growth factor (PDGF)[33,34] but also IL-1.[35] HA is known to be present in high concentrations in most tissues undergoing remodeling and morphogenesis, where it seems to act as a support for cell adhesion and locomotion. There are indications that HA supports epithelial growth over connective tissue growth.[35] HA is reported to be the crucial factor accelerating healing with minimal growth of connective tissue and scar formation,[36] and is also the main factor behind scarless healing in fetuses.[37] It is also suggested to play an important role in the balance of parenchymal and connective tissue elements of importance to the development of liver fibrosis and cirrhosis. HA is also shown to act as an important scavenger, decrease release of free radicals by macrophages,[38] and inhibit release of proteases from peritoneal leukocytes.[39]

Increased serum levels of HA have been observed in a variety of acute and chronic inflammatory and neoplastic conditions: rheumatoid arthritis, psoriatic arthropathy, and systematic scleroderma,[40] liver disease,[41] and inflammatory processes of the lung, skin, middle ear, and intestine.[42] Serum HA is significantly elevated in peritonitis and in CAPD patients.[43] Serum HA, a sensitive marker of of infection, is known to be elevated in sepsis,[44] most likely because of increased HA synthesis. So far, no systematic studies have been performed in elective, nonseptic surgical patients, but studies in pigs show a sharp increase in serum HA levels after surgery and trauma.[45] It has also been observed in humans that the highest concentrations of circulating HA seen postoperatively are obtained in the most seriously ill patients.[46] Observation in a patient undergoing peripheral vascular surgery indicates that only minimal HA changes occur after peripheral surgery,[47] while substantial increases are seen after larger operations such as human organ transplantion (kidney, intestine, and heart),[48,49] and during rejection in experimental animals.[50,51]

Urman et al.[52] seemed to be the first to try the adhesion preventive effects of externally supplied HA; 0.25% and 0.4% solutions of HA were administered before induction of laser-induced peritoneal lesions[52] and after adhesiolysis.[53] The two concentrations were effective to reduce primary adhesions[52] (0.4% HA, 2.35 ± 2.7 mm^2; controls, 6.9 ± 5.4 mm^2 $p < 0.05$), but only the 0.4% solution could reduce secondary adhesions.[53] Burns et al. reported a large study[55] in which the effects of precoating the peritoneum with HA were investigated in an experimental model based on cecal abrasion. The mean cecal adhesion score decreased by 56% (treated, 0.7 ± 0.09; controls, 1.6 ± 0.11; $p < 0.001$) and the number of animals with cecal adhesions almost as large (from 89% to 50%) following administration of 0.4% HA solution. Slightly better results (75% reduction) were obtained on pericardial and epicardial surfaces (adhesion score: treated, 3.3 ± 0.4; controls, 0.8 ± 0.3; $p < 0.0001$) in dogs after surface abrasion.[55] The six animals treated with HA showed no adhesions or only filmy and transparent adhesions, which were described to be significantly less severe than in the untreated controls. HA has also been shown in rabbit experiments to effectively prevent adhesions to the sheets of flexor tendons.[56]

Both PL and HA Are Unsatisfactory for Single-Dose Prevention

It can be estimated that during the coming 10 years there will be a need for adhesion prevention in about 20% of all surgical operations, which means more than 1 million operations annually on each of the continents of North America, Europe, and Asia. To this should be added the need of the numerous patients on CAPD. It reasonable to assume that such a prophylaxis, although most desirable, will at least in the case of surgery only receive more general acceptance if it is reasonably inexpensive and can be administered as a one-dose treatment in connection with the operation. Furthermore, such a treatment must be safe and very effective. It is clear that 100% elimination of adhesions should not be expected, as such a treatment would most likely also impair healing of anastomoses and lead to complications such as GI leakage with subsequent increased morbidity. Elimination of 80% to 90% of adhesions, leaving 10% to 15% of loose adhesions, is as close to optimum as one can expect to arrive.

Although considerable success have been obtained in experimental studies using both PLs and HA, the effects so far observed are at the best about 50% reduction and only achieved by a 3-day repeat treatment, which is far from satisfactory for a product intended for general prophylactic treatment and expected to be applied in all surgical operations involving body cavities or tendon sheets. HA as such, but also PLs, are characterized by a too rapid absorption, which is incompatible with the residence time necessary for effective single-dose adhesion prevention, as the protection layer needs, for the barrier to be effective, to remain for a minimum of 36 hours.[57] It is true that phosphatidylinositol (PI) with a 75% reduction of adhesions is extraordinarily effective, but this strong effect is only obtained after repeat treatment over 3 days. Thus, it appears as unsuitable for surgery but might prove useful in CAPD. This compound is, like most pure HA and PL compounds, very expensive and and also for that reason unlikely to be accepted for mass prophylaxis. Products based on pure HA and pure PL, especially if the treatment is to be repeated, will also be regarded as troublesome to handle as intracavitary catheters must be applied and injections given during the 3 days following surgery. Furthermore, application of comparatively large amounts of the substance to each patient will be necessary, at least when applied to larger mesothelial surfaces such as the peritoneum. Another possible disadvantage observed, especially with natural HA, is that it cannot be processed in such a way that it can be transformed into biomaterial forms.

Polyanionic Polysaccharides Tried Are HA Analogs

All these as well as other reasons have induced increased interest in the use of various other natural or modified natural polymers, molecules not normally existing in eukaryotic or microbial cells. Most of the attempts have so far concentrated on substances related to HA, that is, various polyanionic polysaccharides, also called glucans. To this family belong substances such as carboxymethylcellulose (CMC), carboxymethylamylose, chondroitin-6-sulfate, dermatan sulfate, heparin, heparine sulfate, and heparan sulfate. To overcome their various disadvantages, prolong their disappearance, and make it possible to process HA into various physical forms a variety of HA esters and cross-linked derivates of HA (part of carboxy groups are modified) have been developed and also, at least to some extent, tried in animal experiments. A recent such development is based on benzyl esters of HA or internally cross-linked derivates of HA.[58] These are claimed to have strong antiadhesion properties, but no studies have yet been published making it possible to compare them to other modalities of treatment. A recent patent[59] suggests the use of various hydrophobic bioabsorbable polymers attached to various polyanionic polysadcharides, but so far no experimental studies supporting its effects have been presented.

Sodium carbomethylcellulose (NaCMC; 350,000 mol wt) is an anionic substituted natural polysaccharide which in 2% solution is clear and semigelatinous and known to have slow peritoneal absorption. When applied in experimental systems, it causes some adhesion reduction,[60,61] but the effect seems not to be superior to that which can be obtained with PL and HA. Two NaCMC solutions of different viscosity were tried with the hope that a higher viscosity would improve the effect,[61] but increased viscosity (>1000 centipoise) and higher molecular weight (>700,000) made no difference. It was, however, observed that the volume of the applied solution is important and that the preventive effects increase significantly with increasing volumes administered, an observation also supported by other studies. Attempts were made to combine NaCMC with other polymers such as low molecular weight heparin (LMWH).[62] Although the adhesion scores fell 18% with only NaCMC (treated, 2.8 ± 1.15; controls, 3.4 ± 0.89; $p < 0.05$), they did fall 53% with the combination of NaCMC and LMWH (treated, 1.6 ± 1.18; controls, 3.4 ± 0.89; $p < 0.001$), indicating that the effect was most likely mainly caused by heparin. It is not unlikely, however, that the LMWH effect is potentiated by adding NaCMC as it might act as an effective slow-release agent. It is also well known that heparin stimulates plasminogen activator activity, which enhances fibrinolysis.[63] The fibrinolytic activity of LMWH is also known to be superior to that of unfractionated heparin and its effect to last longer (up to 24 h).[64,65] In addition, heparin is suggested to further stimulate the secretion of plasminogen activator by postsurgically activated macrophages.[66] The combination of LMWH with NaCMC, and more so, with other bioactive polymers, is worth further exploration.

Cationic Polymers: A More Effective Approach?

The driving force behind the tendency of surfactants to stick to surfaces and to form micelles is the hydrophobic attraction.[67] The surfactant concentration needed for onset of formation of micelles is rather well defined.[68] Biosurfaces consist of a negatively charged layer of lipids. Two basically different approaches—two models—have been suggested for holding the layers apart during the healing process:

1. The kinetic model: attempts are made to reduce the speed of the movements by supplying compounds with viscosity-increasing characteristics. Water-soluble polymers with high molecular weights are regarded as the most effective. HA is a good example of such molecules. It is desirable to stay in the so-called semidiluted stage, which starts in the range of 0.1% to 1%, depending on the molecular weight of the polymer. Most of the attempts in the past to inhibit formation of adhesions have been according to this model.

2. The thermodynamic model: the purpose of treatment according to this model is to make it energetically unfavorable to for two surfaces to approach each other. Anchoring of long water-soluble polymer chains to the surfaces make it disadvantageous for the surfaces to adhere to each other, which is why they stay repelled at a certain distance from each other. This so-called steric repulsion is based on what has been called an entropic (osmotic) effect, the built-in "desire" of the chains to stay hydrated. We have tried this "new" model in our most recent attempts to prevent adhesions by cationic hydrophobized polymers.

Hydrophobically modifed polymers (HM polymers) have both polymer and surfactant characteristics. They consist of a hydrophilic backbone to which a low number (usually less than 5 mol%) of hydrophobic side chains have been attached.[69] Such polymers can be produced by hydrophobic modification of several molecules including hyaluronans, chitosans, and celluloses. Solutions of hydrophobically modified polymers are also found to have higher viscosities than the solutions of their unmodified analogs,[69,70] a feature supposed to further contribute to the ability to mechanically separate adjoining traumatized surfaces.

It is known[69] that addition of small amounts of anionic polymers to a cationic polymer solution will significantly increase its viscosity effects. LM-200 is a typical example of an ionic associating polymer that can act as an efficient thickener. In a mixture of hydrophobically modified anionic and cationic polymers, a three-dimensional network can be very efficient because both electrostatic and hydrophobic interactions cooperate.

Another aspect of using a mixture of two oppositely charged polymers is to enhance adsorption. It is known that the adsorption of a polyelectrolyte can be limited by electrostatic repulsion between polymer chains and considerably reduced by even relatively small amounts of an oppositely charged polymer. Among other obvious advantages of using the available cationic polymers in adhesion prevention should also be mentioned that they have no or little toxicity, are cheap to produce, and have documented much stronger clinical effects than other polymers, including the anionic.

Few Studies Using Chitosans

As far as I am aware no studies as to the adhesion preventive effects have been performed using hydrophobized HA. All studies so far are our own, and have been performed using either hydrophobized chitosan (Falk et al., in manuscript, a) or hydrophobized celluloses such as HM-EHEC and LM-200[71] (and Falk et al., in manuscript, a, b). Both are hydrophobically modified water-soluble polymers. Because LM-200 is positively charged, it will exhibit strong attachment to surfaces, not only through hydrophobic association but also through electrostatical association. It has been suggested by others[72] that cationic polymers by reason of their bioadhesion should offer advantages, at least as carriers of drugs and vaccines to biologic surfaces, a function suggested to be especially strong in a neutral or slightly alkaline environment where the mucoadhesive properties are shown to be optimal.

Chitosan is a typical cationic polymer, with an adhesivity mediated on cell surfaces through ionic interaction between positively charged amino groups and negatively charged siliac acid residues.[73] Polysaccharides containing amino sugars, such as chitosan or derivates thereof, have unique potentials as slowly biodegradable, absorbable polymers, ideal for adhesion prevention,[74] not only because of their strong ability to adhere to surfaces but also because of their lack of toxicity. In vitro studies[75] have shown that chitosans with 35% degree of acetylation and 170 kDa have ideal properties at least as biocarriers: early onset of action, very low toxicity, and a flat dose–absorption response. *N,O*-Carbomethyl chitosan (NOCC) is a novel agent with claimed structural similarities to HA. The addition of carboxymethyl groups renders this otherwise positively charged polymer negatively charged. It is, depending on nature and extent of cross-linking, available in a variety of forms, which usually are hydrophilic, lubricious, and viscoelastic. A recent experimental study[76] based on two different animal models showed also significant antiadhesion effects. When a 2% NOCC solution was tried in a so-called uterine horn adhesion model the extent of adhesions fell 62% (treated, 1.30 ± 0.68; controls, 3.38 ± 0.48; $p < 0.001$), and similar results were obtained with a small-bowel suture model. We are presently trying hydrophobized chitosan in our experimental models, but it is too early to draw any definite conclusions.

Cationic Hydrophobized Celluloses Are Most Effective

Our early intention with the hydrophobized polymers was to use them together with lipid surfactants with the hope that this combination would reduce the absorption and enzymatic destruction of the lipid, widen the therapeutic spectrum, and make a single treatment enough for an effective adhesion prevention. If successful it would open the way to a routine prophylaxis, ideally consisting in only one single intracavitary administration of a liquid, or more likely a gel, most likely on conclusion of the operation.

Celluloses consist in linear polymers of glucose residues. Binding of water leads to the formation of a gel. Hydrophobic modified molecules such as surfactant polyquarternium-24 (LM-200), and derivates of the ethyl (hydroxyethyl) cellulose (EHEC) add to these substances an affinity for an lipid–water interface at cellular surfaces, including the sites of injury. HM-EHEC (obtained from Akzo Nobel Surface Chemistry, Stenungsund, Sweden) is a nonionic polymer with about five hydrophobic tails, and LM-200 (obtained from Bionord, Gothenburg, Sweden) is a cationic polymeric ammonium salt of hydroxyethylcellulose with a hydrophilic backbone and lipophilic pendant groups. The two polymers were tried as a 1% solution in water.[71] All animals received a 0.75-mL (0.25 mg/g body weight) injection intraperitoneally immediately on closure of the abdomen. The administration was repeated in some groups of animals after 24 (day 2) and 48 hours (day 3). A standard defect of 2×15 mm was produced on each side of the parietal peritoneum to induce adhesion formation. It was immediately closed with five separate 5/0 silk sutures. The percentage of sutured peritoneal defect covered with adhesions was as standard calculated on the seventh day. Both the polymers reduced significantly the adhesion percentage: single-treatment HM-EHEC by 31% (treated, 48.1 ± 5.1; controls, 69.7 ± 6.7, $p = 0.012$, and LM-200 by 37% (treated, 44.2 ± 6.3; controls, 69.7 ± 6.7; $p = 0.013$) and repeat treatment (during 3 days): HM-EHEC 56% (treated, 47.6 ± 6.5; controls, 84.5 ± 6.2), and LM-200 by 71% (treated, 24.4 ± 5.3; controls, 84.5 ± 6.2). We concluded from these studies that both polymers were able to significantly reduce adhesion formation, but the enhanced effect was only achieved by repeat treatment when LM-200 was used (single-treatment, 44.2 ± 6.3; repeat treatment, 24.4 ± 6.3; $p = 0.032$).[71]

Our goal, to develop a single-treatment prophylaxis eliminating at least 80% to 90% of the adhesions, was now almost, but not fully, reached when using LM-200. With the hope that the effects of the polymers could be further improved, in the next set of experiments (Falk et al., in manuscript, b) we tried HM-EHEC in combination with both a surfactant lipid (phosphatidylglycerol) and hyaluronic acid (Genzyme, Cambridge, MA, USA). None of the formulations were, however, able to dramatically reduce the adhesion percentage: HM-EHEC plus phosphatidylglycerol by 25% (46.1 ± 6.6; $p = 0.0438$), and HM-EHEC + phosphatidylglycerol + HA by 29% (43.6 ± 3.7; $p = 0.0062$), HM-EHEC alone by 26% (45.5 ± 3.2; $p = 0.0042$) compared to controls (61.5 ± 2.8).[75] So far studies combining LM-200 with polar lipids or HA, which have the potential of being more effective, have not been concluded. Instead LM-200 was successfully tried in another combination.

Polyacrylic Acid Has Strong Potentiating Effects

As discussed, significant adhesion prevention was obtained when LM-200 was used. Based on the synergistic effects of mixed cationic-anionic polymer systems discussed here with respect both to rheology and to adsorption to charged surfaces, it seemed to us logical to try to further increase the effect of LM-200 by adding small amounts of an anionic polymer. Polyacrylate was chosen as our first alternative.

Polyacrylic acid (HPA) is in different forms known to be highly bioadhesive,[77,78] which is why it has been tried experimentally in controlled drug delivery systems.[79,80] Sodium acrylate (NaPA) has been claimed to be mucosa protective.[81] We decided to study the effects of an 1% solution of LM-200 to which 0.125% wt of NaPa/HPA was added. The NaPA/HPA solution was prepared by dissolving HPA in water and then neutralized with NaOH until a pH of approximately 7.0 was reached. At this pH the relationship between NaPA and HPA was 3:1.

The approach turned out to be extraordinarily successful, and the LM-200–NaPA/HPA combination brought a major breakthrough to our efforts to develop a unique polymer-based single-treatment adhesion prevention. No single substance or combination of substances so far tried have been able to reduce the adhesion percentage more than at best 50% to 60%. With the LM-200–NaPA/HPA combination, a reduction of no less than 82% was obtained (treated, 10.9 ± 3.4; controls, 60.9 ± 2.2; $p < 0.0001$), a reduction probably close to ideal. Furthermore, 5 of 15 animals studied (33.3%) were totally free of adhesions, and the number of adhesions to omentum/pelvic fat bodies and to the bowel was significantly lower compared to controls ($p < 0.0001$).

These studies have shown that the combination of cationic polymers and anionic polymers have a great potential to prevent adhesion formation. However, it remains to be shown which anionic polymer in combination with which cationic polymer will at the end prove to be the most effective to prevent adhesions. Apart from a cationic polymer such as cellulose various starches and chitosans can also be tried. Good alternatives to acrylates can be alginates, heparin and karageenans. These various combinations are presently under study in our laboratory.

It is clear that about half the suture line, or at the best one-third, remains covered by adhesions after the the various treatment earlier presented: PLs, HA, CMCs, and even LM-EHEC. With the LM-200–NaPA/HPA combination only about 10% of the suture line still held adhesions. One should bear in mind that the whole suture line is almost never totally covered by adhesions. The adhesion percentage of the controls seems to vary from experiment to experiment, normally ranging from about 60% to 80%. Why some individuals do not develop adhesions, or only limited adhesions, has not been addressed sufficiently. It is an old clinical observations that some patients are simply strong "adhesion builders," which often makes adhesiolysis unsuccessful. Nobody has been able to provide explanations for and mechanisms behind this phenomenon, but age, sex, stage in menstrual cycle, season of year, consumption of trophical factors and hormones, antioxidants, and other nutritional factors are certain to play a role. A recent observation reports a significant reduction peritoneal fibrinolytic capacity in persons with greater propensity to develop adhesions,[82] suggesting that these persons have a different acute-phase response to trauma.

Could Inositol Be as Effective?

An attractive idea is to potentiate the effects of hydrophobized celluloses by combining them with different inositol phosphates. As discussed, the strongest effect obtained with PLs was obtained with phosphatidylinositol (PI).[26] It cannot be excluded that the inositol part of the molecule has in itself strong tissue protective abilities. There are observations suggesting that within the cell the choline moiety of PC is exchanged for free inositol, a process in which temporarily PI is formed.[83] This PI is, however, soon phosphorylated and hydrolyzed to produce DAG and inositol triphosphate, a process that most likely is supported by exogenous supply of inositol phosphates.

Some natural inositolphosphates are in contrast to PI relatively inexpensive, which was one of the reasons we decided to further explore the effects of combined treatment with natural inositol phosphates and hydrophobized polymers. Inositol hexaphosphate ($InsP_6$) is an ubiquitous compound, abundant in plants, and especially rich in foods such as cereals and legumes, where it exists under the name of phytic acid. $InsP_6$, its lower phosphorylated forms, and free inositol are all present in most mammalian cells, where they play an important role in the cellular signal transduction.[84] External supply of phytic acid is known to have strong biologic effects including anticell proliferative and antineoplastic functions.[85-88] It is possible that most of the effects are achieved by lower phosphorylated inositol phosphates, as $InsP_6$ to a large extent is within the body dephosphorylated by exogenous phytases (phosphatases). Phytic acid is a recognized strong chelator of molecules such as iron, which molecule is known to have a strong accelerating effect on the acute-phase reaction following trauma. For further information on the effects of $InsP_6$ in health and disease, see the review by Shamsuddin et al.[89]

Traumas such as abdominal operations induce acute inflammation of the peritoneum as does CAPD, which induces a state of chronic inflammation. Leukocytes activated during this stage release large amounts of free radicals into the peritoneal cavity,[90] a generation that can be prevented by administration of antioxidants such as vitamin E,[91] but also by various macromolecules which in themselves are free radical scavengers. One such molecule is chondroitin sulfate.[92] It is not unlikely that molecules such as inositol but also biologically active polymers, in addition to the tissue separating and lubricating ability, also act as powerful scavengers. Much support is provided in that as an example the HA molecule modulates peritoneal inflammation by inhibiting release of proteases from peritoneal leucocytes,[93] decreasing the release of free radicals from the macrophages,[94,95] or direct scavenging of the radicals. These observations make it reasonable to assume the various polymers in addition to their separating and lubricating effects also directly influence the acute-phase response.

Acute-Phase Response

Understanding the Acute-Phase Response Is Essential

There is no doubt that adhesion formation is an integral part of the acute-phase response (APR) and that several so-called acute-phase proteins (APPs) are intimately involved in the adhesion formation process. The development of adhesions is intimately related to the reaction of the body to trauma, the acute-phase response, its extent and duration. An extensive and detailed knowledge about these various functions is undoubtedly necessary to make further progress with prevention programs. It is most likely that future antiadhesion products will be based on pharmaceutical compositions of polymers in combination with other molecules, a composition which in addition its strong ability to tissue separation and lubrication also exhibits a strong inhibitory effect on the local APR.

Although a new definition, APR has been known as a clinical phenomenon for millennia. The ancient Greeks observed an increased sedimentation of blood erythrocytes in severely ill patients, a phenomenon today known to be caused by increased plasma concentrations of fibrinogen and other so-called acute-phase proteins (APPs). It is only 25 years since it was suggested that this reaction is induced by the liver and through blood-borne mediators.[96] Soon clear evidence was presented that C-reactive protein (CRP) is synthesized and secreted by the hepatocytes.[97] Since then a long list of factors produced by the liver and involved in the acute-phase response has been identified. Among the conditions leading to APR are microbial invasion, allergic reactions, surgical operations, physical trauma, burn, tissue ischemia, tissue infarction, and strenuous exercise, but also childbirth.

Development of adhesions should be regarded as a late phenomenon of or sequelae to APR. APR consists basically of two types of adaptive early response: (1) hypothalamus-induced alterations in temperature setpoint and generation of febrile response, and (2) alteration in gene regulation and metabolism in the liver,[98,99] which initiates all the metabolic changes in the body through synthesis of acute-phase proteins (APPs). It is mainly the second response that directly affects adhesion formation. Several liver-produced APP molecules such as fibrinogen, different complements, and plasminogen activator inhibitor 1 (PAI-1) are known to be involved in the core pathogenesis of adhesions. The APPs are, based on the magnitude of response, divided into three different groups: group 1, increase about 0.5 fold—ceruloplasmin, complement C3, complement C4; group 2, increase 2- to 4-fold—orosomucoid, α_1-antitrypsin, α_1-antichymotrypsin, haptoglobin, fibrinogen; and group 3, increase up to 1000 fold—C-reactive protein, serum amyloid A.

Acute-Phase Response and Activation of Immune Cells

APR is primarily induced at the local site of injury through various mediators or cytokines. Mobile cells such as macrophages, monocytes, T cells, and NK cells produce such cytokines but also fixed cells including intestinal and bronchial epithelial cells, endothelial cells, fibroblasts, and Kupffer cells. All these various cells are continuously involved in a highly sophisticated chemical surveillance of the body, ready to institute a state of alarm in case of threat of trauma or infection. The rapidly emerging information on the signaling mechanisms between the different eukaryotic and bacterial cells will not only provide a detailed understanding of disease, but also provide the basis for new therapeutic strategies. Cytokine production is commonly believed to be harmful and associated with disease, but a basal, physiologic cytokine production is of the greatest importance and essential to a healthy life.[100] There are indications that IL-6 and IL-6-like molecules are the main mediators of APR, but IL-1, TNF, and glucocorticoids are also involved. Higher levels of peritoneal fluid IL-6 activity have been observed in patients with pelvic adhesions,[101] in patients 4 to 24 hours after onset of CAPD,[102] and in patients with endometriosis.[103]

Conventional T cells, which have major regulatory activities essential for optimal function of the immune system, are mediated by cytokines, mainly from eukaryotic cells but also from bacterial cells. It has been suggested that the balance between Th1 lymphocytes, primarily associated with cellular immunity, and Th2 lymphocytes, mainly associated with humoral immunity should be of special importance to our health and well-being.[104,105] It has been observed that profound immunologic changes occur within the peritoneum soon after the initiation of CAPD.[102] It has also been shown that the peritoneal macrophages during a 1-year period of repeat CAPD treatment become increasingly immature, which explains a significant alteration in ability to secrete inflammatory cytokines and prostaglandins.[106] The constitutive levels of peritoneal fluid cytokines such as IL-1 and IL-6 are reported to increase significantly, while the levels of prostaglandins such as PGE_2 and 6-keto-$PGF_{1\alpha}$ remain unchanged.

The intracellular pathways leading to activation of the acute-phase genes are poorly understood, but lipases such as phospholipase A_2, phosphatases, proteinkinase C (PKC), and various proteases are clearly involved. Much evidence supports that dysregulation in macrophage function to a large extent is responsible for the loss of peritoneal membrane function seen in long-term CAPD treatment.[106] Steroidal and nonsteroidal antiinflammatory drugs, which are known to prevent leukocyte migration, have also been used with some success to prevent adhesions,[107,108] which is why it was recently suggested that induction of neutropenia might reduce the formation of peritoneal adhesions.[109] Adherence of polymorphonuclear leukocytes (PMNs) to the endothelial (mesothelial) cells is a prerequisite for migration of PMNs into the tissue in response to a stimulus,[111] and PMN adherence and migration can successfully be inhibited by monoclonal antibodies against CD11/CD18. Consequently, anti-CD11 and anti-CD18 antibodies can be expected to increase the PMN endothelial cell adherence and stimulate development of increased amounts of adhesions, a hypothesis recently tried in two experimental adhesion models in rabbits[112] in which administration of anti-CD-18 significantly increased the development of adhesions. Whether this observation will open new pathways for control of adhesions remains to be seen.

Oral Nutrition Modulates Immune Response

Not only the invading flora, but also the commensal flora, influence significantly the early acute-phase reactions. This influence is modulated through production of various enzymes but also through secretion of molecules such as cytokine-like molecules, often referred to as bacteriokines.[112] Lactic acid bacteria (LAB) are especially known to modulate immune activities. As an example, the depression of T-cell function seen in tumor-bearing mice can be effectively abolished by oral administration of *Lactobacillus casei,*[113] and most likely also many other LAB so far untried. This T-cell activation is associated with pronounced changes in the cytokine pattern.[114] Human intake of *Lactobacillus acidophilus* is known to result in an increase in IgA response of more than fourfold when challenged by Salmonella typhi.[115,116] Similarly, the mononuclear activity of 2′-5′ synthetase, an expression of IFN-γ, is significantly increased 24 hours after a LAB-containing meal.

So far the influence of the intestinal flora in peritoneal protection and healing has not been the object of any studies. Little attention has been given to the influence of enteral nutritrion on prevention of formation of adhesions, despite the fact that it is well known that enteral nutrition exhibits a strong influence on the immune response. It has been observed that rats on a high-fat diet generally express a higher T-2 helper cell activity, but also show higher levels of PGE_2, known to be critical to both cytokine production and macrophage function.[117] It has not received enough attention that enteral feeding immediately after surgery has a strong impact on the acute-phase response and preservation of visceral protein metabolism, most likely through downregulation of the splanchnic cytokine response.[118] Unfortunately, direct immunologic parameters are rarely studied in connection with trauma and surgical operation, but several studies report a reduced morbidity and mortality in patients receiving early enteral nutrition following trauma or surgery.[119–121]

Significant changes in different immune parameters in patients with severe acute pancreatitis were recently observed and related to the mode of nutrition.[122] While the sickness score (APACHE II) fell significantly in enterally fed patients, it remained unchanged in patients on parenteral nutrition, and while c-reactive protein (CRP) decreased from a mean of 156 to 84 mg/L in patients of enteral nutrition, it remained unchanged in the parenterally fed patients. Furthermore, the antioxidant score increased by an average of 33% in the enterally fed group while it decreased by 28% in the patients on parenteral nutrition, and endotoxin antibodies expressed as IgM EndoCAb remained unchanged in the enteral group but increased by 29% in the parenterally fed group. Furthermore, 5 of 12 patients in the parenteral group developed multiple organ failure (MOF) in contrast to none among the enterally fed patients, and 2 of 12 in the parenteral group but 0 of 11 in the enteral group died. Similar observations have recently been reported in connection with early enteral nutrition after liver resections.[123] These observations strongly support the assumption that enteral feeding modulates the acute inflammatory response in physical stress. It was also recently observed in liver transplant patients[124] that early enteral feeding not only reduces morbidity and mortality but significantly reduces the rate of early rejection. Experimental studies performed in animals with experimental peritonitis have also demonstrated strong immunomodulatory effects, also within the peritoneum, from oral supplementation of substances such as omega fats,[125] arginine,[126] and glutamin,[127] but also from a supply of *Lactobacillus plantarum* and oat fiber (Nobaek S et al. in manuscript). Based on the observations discussed here and various other observations, it is not unreasonable to assume that the extent of adhesion development depends on nutrition and most likely can be modulated by an aggressive enteral nutrition, parallel to the installed local treatment. Further support to this assumption is given by the observation that people living in rural areas and who have more plant fibers and lactobacilli in their daily diet produce softer jelly-like clots and exhibit longer coagulation times than those living in urban areas[128] and by the observation that fiber consumption reduces the incidence of venous thrombosis.[129,130] This concept is further supported by a recent study[131] showing that 6% soy fiber and pure cellulose added to food significantly reduces serum fibrinogen and prolongs clotting time. More support is given by the observation that high oral intake of vitamin E to a large extent prevented adhesions in rats following intraperitoneal glove powder instillation.[132]

Future Progress Through Multimodality Treatment?

It is unquestionable that both polar lipids and the polymers we have tried so far exhibit strong antiadhesive and lubricating effects. Near total freedom from adhesion formation is obtained when the polycationic polymer LM-200 is combined with the polyanionic polyacrylic acid. It cannot be excluded that some of the polymers, in addition to their ability to separate and lubricate tissues, also are able to modulate the cytokine reaction and the acute phase and immune responses and affect both the release of cytokines and the production of fibrinogen, PAI-1, and other APPs involved. The different polar lipids and polymers are known to be effective carriers of molecules, making them suitable also as biocarriers in various slow-release delivery systems. This unique ability can most likely be utilized to further enhance their antiadhesion properties. Potential candidates for such combinations, molecules that enhance fibrin degradation, are plasminogen activator (tPA), urokinase plasminogen activator (uPA), inhibitors of plasminogen-activating inhibitors (PAIs), and other drugs that affect the inflammatory response and cytokine production, various growth factors, antioxidants, steroids, and nonsteroidal anti-inflammatory drugs.[133] So far, such combinations have not been tried.

A new treatment concept needs extensive clinical evaluation in humans. After phase 1 studies aimed to assure that the treatment is safe, most often several phase 2 studies are performed with the aim to optimize the treatment before the final phase 3 studies are performed to finally document the clinical efficiency of the treatment. Such studies are always designed as true randomized clinical trials. There are many obstacles to performing such studies with a product in which the clinical advantages (reduced rate of adhesions, reduced incidence of intestinal obstruction, reduced rate of female infertility) are often not seen until several years have passed. An alternative could be, as in experimental animals, to perform a second-look operation during the postoperative period, or alternatively to try to evaluate the extent of adhesions by laparoscopy. Both these alternatives are expensive and also, at least the first alternative, ethically questionable.

For practical purpose such studies have so far been restricted to patients for whom a second-look operation is a clinical necessity, which no doubt in the past has restricted both the number of trials and the number of patients involved. Diamond et al.[134] recently reported, however, an excellent multicenter study involving 23 North American institutions and no fewer than 277 patients for safety evaluation and 245 patients for efficacy studies. Laparoscopy on about the 40th day proved valuable to assess incidence, severity, and extent of de novo adhesions at 23 intraabdominal sites. This approach should open new possibilities for an early and more effective evaluation of new treatment concepts relating to adhesion prevention in closed body cavities. This in turn offers hope that it will not be long before potent drugs designed for global prevention of adhesions will be available.

References

1. Miserocchi G, Agostino E. Contents of the pleural space. Appl Physiol 1971;30:208–213.
2. Topley N, Mackenzie RK, Williams JD. Macrophages and mesophelial cells in bacterial peritonitis. Immunobiology 1996;195:563–573.
3. Topley N, Williams JD. Effect of peritoneal dialysis on cytokine production by peritoneal cells. Blood Purif 1996; 14:188–197.
4. Topley N, Jörres A, Luttmann W, et al. Human peritoneal mesothelial cells synthesize IL-6: induction by IL-1β and TNF-α. Kidney Int 1993;43:226–233.
5. Steinhauer HB, Schollmeyer P. Prostaglandin mediated loss of proteins during peritonitis in continuous ambulatory peritoneal dialysis. Kidney Int 1986;29:584–590.
6. Peppas NA, Buri PA. Surface, interfacial and molecular aspects of bioadhesion. J Controlled Release 1985;2: 257–275.
7. Sabin FR. Cellular reactions to fractions isolated from tubercle bacilli. Physiol Rev 1932;12:141–165.
8. Anderson RJ. Chemistry of lipoids of tubercle bacilli. Physiol Rev 1932;12:166–189.
9. Fallon JT. Specific tissue reaction to phospholipids: a suggested explanation for the similarity of the lesions of silicosis and pulmonary tuberculosis. Can Med Assoc J 1937; 36:223–228.
10. Dobbie JW, Pavlina T, Lloyd J, Johnson R. Phosphatidylcholine synthesis by peritoneal mesotheium. Its implication for peritoneal dialysis. Am J Kidney Dis 1988;12: 31–36.
11. Grahame GR, Torchia MG, Dankewich KA, Ferguson IA. Surface active material in peritoneal effluent of CAPD patients. Bull Perit Dial 1985;5:109–111.
12. Ziegler C, Torchia M, Grahame GR, Ferguson IA. Peritoneal surface-active material in continuous ambulatory peritoneal dialysis (CAPD) patients. Perit Dial Int 1898;9: 47–49.
13. Mactier RA, Khanna R, Twardowski ZJ, et al. Influence of phosphatidylcholine on lymphatic absorption during peritoneal dialysis. Perit Dial Int 1988;8:179–186.
14. DiPaolo N, Bouncristiani U, Capotondo L et al. Phosphatidylcholine and peritoneal transport during peritoneal dialysis. Nephron 1986;44:365–370.
15. Rozga J, Andersson R, Srinivas U, et al. Influence of phosphatidylcholine on intraabdominal adhesion formation and peritoneal macrophages. Nephron 1990;54:134–138.
16. Babior BM. Oxidants from phagocytes: agents of defence and destruction. Blood 1984;64:959–964.
17. Elsbach P, Weiss J. A re-evaluation of the role of O_2 independent microbiocidal systems of phagocytes. Rev Infect Dis 1983;5:843–853.
18. Ar Rajab A, Ahrén B, Rozga J, Bengmark S. Phosphatidylcholine prevents postoperative peritoneal adhesions: an experimental study in the rat. J Surg Res 1991;50:212–215.
19. Snoj M, Ar Rajab, Ahrén B, Bengmark S. Effect of phosphatidylcholine on postoperative adhesions after small bowel anastomosis in the rat. Br J Surg 1992;79:427–429.
20. Kennedy SP, Becker EL. Ectophospholipase A_2 activity of the rabbit peritoneal neutrophil. Int Arch Allergy Appl Immunol 1987;83:239–246.
21. Steinleiter A, Lampert H, Kazensky C, et al. Reduction of primary postoperative adhesion formation under calcium channel blockade in the rabbit. J Surg Res 1990;48: 42–45.
22. Snoj M, Ar Rajab A, Ahrén B, Larsson K, Bengmark S. Phospholipase-resistant phosphatidylcholine reduces intraabdominal adhesions induced by bacterial peritonitis. Res Exp Med 1993;193:117–122.
23. Wright GW, Ooi CE, Weiss J, Elsbach P. Purification of cellular (granulocyte) and extracellular serum phospholipase A_2 that participate in the destruction of *E. coli* in rabbit inflammatory exudate. J Biol Chem 1990;265:6675–6681.
24. Misra S, Ghosh A, Varticovski L. Naturally occurring ether-linked phosphatidylcholine activates phosphatidylinositol 3-kinase and stimulates cell growth. J Cell Biochem 1994; 55:146–153.
25. Fabia R, Ar Rajab A, Willén R, et al. Effects of phosphatidylcholine and phosphatidylinositol on acetic-acid-induced colitis in the rat. Digestion 1992;53:35–44.
26. Ar Rajab A, Snoj M, Larsson K, Bengmark S. Exogenous phospholipid reduces postoperative peritoneal adhesions in rats. Eur J Surg 1995;161:341–345.
27. Kappas AM, Barsoum GH, Ortiz JB, Keighley MRB. Prevention of peritoneal adhesions in rats with verapamil, hydrocortisone sodium succinate and phosphatidylcholine. Eur J Surg 1992;158:33–35.
28. Treutner KH, Bertram P, Klimaszewski M, Schumpelick V. Prevention of adhesions in rabbits by intrabdominal application of lipid compounds. In: Treutner KH, Schumpelick V, eds. Peritoneal Adhesions. Berlin: Springer, 1994: 344–351.
29. Treutner KH, Bertram P, Schumpelick V. Experimental prevention of peritoneal adhesions in general surgery. In: diZerega GS, DeCherney AH, Dunn RC, Haney AF, Tulardi T, Diamond MP, Goldberg EP, Rock JA, Rodgers KE, eds. Pelvic Surgery: Adhesion Formation and Prevention. New York: Springer-Verlag, 1997:71–78.
30. Yung S, Coles GA, Williams JD, Davis M. The source and possible significance of hyaluronan in the peritoneal cavity. Int Soc Nephrol 1994;46:527–533.

31. Ohaski Y, Honda A, Iwai T, et al. Stimulatory effect of vanadate on hyaluronic acid synthesis in mesothelial cells from rabbit peritoneum. Biochem Int 1988;16:293–302.
32. Pannekeet MM, Zemel D, Koomen GC, et al. Dialysate markers of peritoneal tissue during peritonitis and in stable CAPD. Perit Dial Int 1995;15:217–225.
33. Honda A, Iwai T, Mori Y. Insulin-like growth factor-I (IGF-I) enhances hyaluronic acid synthesis in rabbit pericardium. Biochim Biophys Acta 1989;1014:305–312.
34. Heldin P, Asplund T, Yttgerberg D, et al. Characterization of the molecular mechanism involved in the activation of hyaluronan synthetase by platelet-derived growth factor in human mesothelial cells. Biochem J 1992;283:165–170.
35. Breborowics A, Korybalski K, Grzybowski, et al. Synthesis of hyaluronic acid by human peritoneal mesothelial cells: effect of cytokines and dialysate. Perit Dial 1996;16: 374–378.
36. Weigel PH, Fuller GM, LeBoeuf RD. A model for the role of hyaluronic acid and fibrin in the early events during the inflammatory response and wound healing. J Theor Biol 1986;119:219–226.
37. Adzick NS, Longaker MT. Scarless fetal healing. Therapeutic implications. Ann Surg 1992;215:3–7.
38. Suzuki Y, Yamaguchi T. Effects of hyaluronic acid on macrophage phagocytosis and active oxygen release. Agents Actions 1993;38:32–37.
39. Akatsaku M, Yamamoto Y, Tobetto K, et al. Suppressive effects of hyaluronic acid and fibrin in early events during the inflammatory response and wound healing. Pharm Pharmacol 1993;45:110–114.
40. Engström-Laurent A, Feltelius N, Hallgren R, Waterson P. Elevated serum hyaluronate in systematic scleroderma. An effect of growth factor induced activation of connective tissue cells. Ann Rheum Dis 1985;44:614–620.
41. Engström-Laurent A. Changes in hyaluronic acid in tissue and body fluids in disease states In: Whelan ED, Chichester J, eds. The Biology of Hyaluronan. Ciba Foundation Symposium. 143 New York: Wiley, 1989:233–247.
42. Engström-Laurent A, Laurent T. Hyaluronan as a clinical marker. In: Lindh E, Thorell JI. Clinical Impact of Bone and Connective Tissue Markers. London: Academic Press, 1989.
43. Honkanen E, Froseth B, Gronhagen-Riska C. Serum hyaluronic acid and precollagen III amino terminal propeptide in chronic renal failure. Am J Nephrol 1991;11: 201–206.
44. Berg S. Hyaluronan turnover in relation to infection and sepsis. J Int Med 1997;242:73–77.
45. Berg S, Jansson I, Hesselvik FJ, et al. Hyaluronan: relationship to hemodynamics and survival in porcine injury and sepsis. Crit Care Med 1992;20:1315–1321.
46. Berg S, Brodin B, Hesselvik F, et al. Elevated levels of plasma hyaluronan in septicaemia. Scand J Clin Lab Invest 1988;48:727–732.
47. Berg S, Hesselvik JF, Laurent TC. Influence of surgery on serum concentgrations of hyaluronan. Crit Care 1994;22: 810–814.
48. Wells AF, Larsson E, Tengblad A, et al. The localization of hyaluronan in normal and rejected rat kidney graft. Transplantation (Baltimore) 1990;50:240–243.
49. Hallgren G, Gerdin B, Tengblad A, Tufveson G. Accumulation of hyaluronan (hyaluronic acid) in myocardial interstitial tissue parallels development of transplantation edema in heart allografts in rats. J Clin Invest 1990;85:668–673.
50. Ronchetti F, Colombo D, Taino PA, et al. Mucosal hyaluronic acid quantification in small bowel transplantation in pigs. Transplant Proc 1996;28:2558–2559.
51. Mueller AR, Platz KP, Heckert et al. The extracellular matrix: an early target of preservation/reperfusion injury and acute rejection after small bowel transplantation. Transplantation (Baltimore) 1998;27:770–776.
52. Urman B, Gomel V, Jetha N. Effect of hyaluronic acid on postoperative intraperitoneal adhesion formation in the rat model. Fertil Steril 1991;56:563–567.
53. Urman B, Gomel V. Effect of hyaluronic acid on postoperative intraperitoneal adhesion formation and reformation in the rat model. Fertil Steril 1991;56:568–570.
54. Burns JW, Skinner K, Colt J, et al. Prevention of tissue injury and postsurgical adhesions by precoating tissues with hyaluronic acid solutions. J Surg Res 1995;59:644–652.
55. Mitchell JD, Lee R, Hodakowski GT, et al. Prevention of postoperative pericardial adhesions with a hyaluronic acid coating solutions. J Thorac Cardiovasc Surg 1994;107: 1481–1488.
56. Hagberg L, Gerdin B. Sodium hyaluronate as an adjunct in adhesion prevention after flexor tendon surgery in rabbits. J Hand Surg 1992;17A:935–941.
57. Harris ES, Morgan RF, Rodehaever GT. Analysis of the kinetics of peritoneal adhesion formation in the rat and evaluation of potential antiadhesive agents. Surgery (St. Louis) 1995;117:663–669.
58. Pressato D, Pavesio A, Callegaro L. Biomaterials for preventing postsurgical adhesions comprised of hyaluronic acid derivates. PTC patent WO97/07833, March 6, 1997.
59. Burns JW, Greenwalt KE. Compositions containing polyanionic polysacharides and hydrophobic bioabsorbable polymers. EP patent 0705878 A2, April 10, 1996.
60. Elkins TE, Bury R, Ritter J, et al. Adhesion prevention by solutions of sodium carboxymethylcellulose in the rat. I. Fertil Steril 1984;41:926–928.
61. Elkins TE, Bury R, Ritter J, et al. Adhesion prevention by solutions of sodium carboxymethylcellulose in the rat. II. Fertil Steril 1984;41:929–932.
62. Sahin Y, Saglam A. Synergistic effects of caroxymethylcellulose and low molecular weight heparin in reducing adhesion formation in the rat uterine horn model. Acta Obstet Gynecol Scand 1994;73:70–73.
63. Andrade-Gordon P, Strickland S. Interaction of heparin with plasminogen activators and plasminogen: effects on the activation of plasminogen. Biochemistry 1986;25: 4033–4040.
64. Stassen JM, Juhan-Vague I, Alessi MC, et al. Potentiation by heparin fragments of thrombosis induced human tissue-type plasminogen activator of human single-chain urokinase-type plasminogen activator. Thromb Haemostasis 1987;58: 947–950.
65. Friedman MD, Leese P, Prasad P, Hayden D. An evaluation of the biologic response to fraxiparine (a low molecular weight heparin) in the healthy individual. J Clin Pharmacol 1990;30:720–727.
66. Orita H, Campeau JD, Gale JA, Nakamura RM, diZerega GS. Differential secretion of plasminogen activator activity

by postsurgical activated macrophages. J Surg Res 1986; 41:569–573.

67. Tanford C. The Hydrophobic Effect: Formation of Micelles and Biological Membranes, 2nd Ed. New York: Wiley, 1980.
68. Lindman B, Wennerström H. Micelles. Amphiphile aggregation in aqueous solution. Top Curr Chem 1980;87:1–83.
69. Thuresson K. Solution properties of hydrophobically modified polymers. Ph.D. Thesis, Lund University, Lund, Sweden, 1996.
70. Thuresson K. Polyelectrolyte composition. Swedish patent application 9504257-8; PTC application made 1997. Akzo Nobel Chemistry AB, Sweden.
71. Falk K, Holmdahl L, Halvarsson M, et al. Polymers that reduce intraperitoneal adhesion formation. Br J Surg 1998; 85:1153–1156.
72. Rental CO, Lehr CM, Bouwstra JA. Enhanced peptide absorption by the mucoadhesive polymers polycarbophil and chitosan. Proc Int Symp Control Release Soc 1993;20: 446–447.
73. Lehr CM, Bouwstra JA, Schacht EH, Junginger HE. In vitro evaluation of mucoadhesive properties of chitosan and some other natural polymers. Int J Pharm (Amst) 1992;78:43–48.
74. Hingham PA. Composition containing derivates of chitin for preventing adhesions. European patent EP 426 268 A2, 1990.
75. Schipper NGM, Vårum KM, Artursson P. Pharm Res 1996; 13:1686–1692.
76. Kennedy R, Costain DJ, McAlister VC, et al. Prevention of experimental postoperative peritoneal adhesions by *N,O*-carboxymethylchitosan. Surgery (St. Louis) 1996;120: 866–870.
77. Anlar S, Capan Y, Hincal AA. Physicochemical and bioadhesive properties of polyacrylic acid polymers. Pharmazie 1993;48:285–287.
78. Hassan EE, Gallo JM. A simple rheological method for the in vitro assessment of mucin-polymer bioadhesive bond strength. Pharm Res 1990;7:491–495.
79. Bottenberg P, Cleymaet R, de Muynck, et al. Development and testing of bioadhesive, fluoride-containing slow-release tablets for oral use. J Pharm Pharmacol 1991;43: 457–464.
80. Longer MA, Ch'ng HS, Robinson JR. Bioadhesive polymers for oral controlled drug delivery III: oral delivery of chlorothiazide using a bioadhesive polymer. J Pharm Sci 1985;74:406–411.
81. Nakamura K, Ozawa Y, Furuta Y, Miyasaki H. Effects of sodium polyacrfylate (pANa) on acute esophagitis by gastric juice in rats. Jpn J Pharmacol 1982;32:445–456.
82. Ivarsson M-L, Bergström M, Eriksson E, et al. An investigation of tissue markers as predictors of post-surgical adhesions. Br J Surg 1998;85:1549–1554.
83. Nishizuka Y. Intracellular signalling by hydrolysis of phospholipids and activation of protein kinase C. Science 1992;258:607–614.
84. Berridge MJ. Inositol triphosphate and calcium signalling. Nature (Lond) 1993;361:315–325.
85. Shamsuddin AM, Yang G-U. Inositol hexaphosphate inhibits growth and induces differentiation of PC-3 human prostate cancer cells. Carcinogenesis (Oxf) 1995;16: 1975–1979.
86. Kamp DW, Israbian VA, Yeldandi AV, et al. Phytic acid, an iron chelator, attenuates pulmonary inflammation and fibrosis in rats after intratracheal instillation of asbestosis. Toxic Pathol 1995;23:689–695.
87. Carrington AL, Calcutt NA, Ettlinger CB, et al. Effects of treatment with myoinositol or its 1,2,6-triphosphate (PP56) on nerve conduction in streptozotocin-diabetes. Eur J Pharmacol 1993;237:257–263.
88. Shamsuddin AM, Yung G-Y, Vucenik I. Novel anti-cancer functions of IP_6: growth inhibition and differentiation of human mammary cancer cell lines in vitro. Anticancer Res 1996;16:3287–3292.
89. Shamsuddin AM, Vucenik I, Cole KE. IP_6: a novel anti-cancer agent. Life Sci 1997;61:343–354.
90. Zhou JR, Erdman JW Jr. Phytic acid in health and disease. Clin Rev Food Sci Nutr 1995;35:495–508.
91. Broberowics A. Free radicals in peritoneal dialysis: agents of damage. Perit Dial Int 1992;12:194–198.
92. Breborowics A, Witowski J, Wieczorowska K, et al. Toxicity of free radicals to mesothelial cells and peritoneal membranes. Nephron 1993;65:62–66.
93. Breborowics A, Wieczorowska K, Martis L, Oreopoulos DG. Glycosaminoglucan chondroitin sulphate prevents loss of ultrafiltration during peritoneal dialysis in rats. Nephron 1994;67:346–350.
94. Akatsuku M, Yamamoto Y, Tobetto K, et al. Suppressive effects of hyaluronic acid on elastase release from the rat peritoneal leukocytes. J Pharm Pharmacol 1993;45: 110–114.
95. Suzuki Y, Yamaguchi T. Effects of hyaluronic acid on macrophage phagocytosis and active oxygen release. Agents Action 1993;38:32–37.
96. Koj A. Acute phase reactants. Their synthesis, turnover and biological significance. In: Allison AC, ed. Structure and Function of Acute Phase Proteins, Vol. I. London: Plenum Press, 1974:73–125.
97. Trautwein C, Böker K, Manns MP. Hepatocyte and immune system: acute phase reaction as a contribution to early defence mechanisms. Gut 1994;35:1163–1166.
98. Kushner I, Rzewnicki DL. The acute phase response: general aspects. Baillière's Clin Rheumatol 1994;8:513–530.
99. Mackiewics A. Acute phase proteins and transformed cells. Int Rev Cytol 1997;170:225–300.
100. Bocci V. The physiological interferon response. In: Baron S, Baron S Dianzani F Stanton GJ, Fleischmann WR, et al., eds. The Interferon System. A Current Review. Austin: University of Texas Press, 1987:177–186.
101. Buyalos RP, Watson JM, Funari VA, et al. Elevated interleukin-6 levels in peritoneal fluid of patients with pelvic adhesions. Fertil Steril 1992;58:302–306.
102. Holmes C, Lewis S. Host defence mechanisms in the peritoneal cavity of continuous ambulatory peritoneal dialysis patients. Perit Dial Int 1991;11:112–117.
103. Ho HN, Wu MY, Yang YS. Peritoneal cell immunity and endometriosis. AJRI 1997;38:400–412.
104. Liblau RS, Singer SM, McDevitt HO. Th1 and Th2 CD4+ T cells in the pathogenesis of organ-specific autoimmune diseases. Immunol Today 1995;16:34–38.

105. Katz JD, Benoist Ch, Mathis D. T-helper cell subsets in insulin-dependent diabetes. Science 1995;268:1185–1188.
106. Gregor SJ, Topley N, Jörres A, et al. Longitudinal evaluation of peritoneal macrophage function and activation during CAPD: maturity, cytokine synthesis and arachidonic acid metabolism. Kidney Int 1996;49:523–533.
107. Siegler AM, Kontopoulos V, Wang CF. Prevention of postoperative adhesions in rabbits with ibuprofen, a nonsteroidal anti-inflammatory agent. Fertil Steril 1980;34: 46–49.
108. Replogle RL, Johnson R, Gross RE. Prevention of postoperative intestinal adhesions with combined promethazine and dexamethasone therapy: experimental and clinical studies. Ann Surg 1966;163:580–588.
109. Braslow L. Neutrophilia, oxygen free radicals, and abominal adhesions. Arch Surg 1992;127:747.
110. Harlan JM, Schwartz BR, Wallis WJ, Pohlman TH. The role of neutrophil membrane proteins in neutrophil emigration. In: Movat HZ, ed. Leukocyte Emigration and Its Sequelae. Basel: Karger Verlag, 1987.
111. Ar'Rajab A, Meleski W, Sentementes JT, et al. The role of neutrophils in peritoneal adhesion formation. J Surg Res 1996;61:143–146.
112. Henderson B, Poole S, Wilson M. Review article: Microbial/host interactions in health and disease: who controls the cytokine network? Immunopharmacology 1996;35: 1–21.
113. Kato I, Endo K, Yokokura T. Effects of oral administration of *Lactobacillus casei* on antitumor responses induced by tumor resection in mice. Int J Immunopharmacol 1994; 16:29–36.
114. Matzusaki T, Shimizu Y, Yokokura T. Augmentation of antimetastatic effects on Lewis lung carcinoma (3LL) in C57BL/6 mice by priming with *Lactobacillus casei*. Med Microbiol Immunol 1990;179:161–168.
115. Solis-Pereyra B, Aattouri N, Lemonnier D. Role of food in the stimulation of cytokine production. Am J Clin Nutr 1997;66:S521–S525.
116. Rangavajhyala N, Shahani KM, Sridevi G, Srikumaran S. Nonlipopolysaccharide component(s) of *Lactobacillus acidophilus* stimulate(s) the production of interleukin-1α and tumor necrosis factor-α by murine macrophages. Nutr Cancer 1997;28:130–134.
117. Lin B-F, Huang C-C, Chiang B-L, Jeng S-J. Dietary fat influences antigen expression, cytokines and prostaglandin E_2 production of immune cells in autoimmune-prone NZBxNZW F1 mice. Br J Nutr 1996;75:711–722.
118. Kudsk KA, Minard G, Wojtysiac SL, et al. Visceral protein response to enteral versus parenteral nutrition and sepsis in patients with trauma. Surgery (St. Louis) 1994;116: 516–523.
119. Moore FA, Feliciano DF, Minard G, et al. Early enteral feeding compared with parenteral reduces postoperative septic complications: the results of a metaanalysis. Ann Surg 1991;216:172–183.
120. Kudsk KA, Groce MA, Fabian TC, et al. Enteral versus parenteral feeding: effects on septic morbidity after blunt and penetrating abdominal trauma. Ann Surg 1992;215: 503–513.
121. Senkal M, Mumme A, Eickhoff U, et al. Crit Care Med 1997;25:1489–1496.
122. Windsor ACJ, Kanwar S, Li AGK, et al. Compared with parenteral nutrition, enteral feeding attenuates the acute phase response and improves disease severity in acute pancreatitis. Gut 1998;42:431–435.
123. Shirabe K, Matsumata T, Shimada M, et al. A comparison of parenteral hyperalimentation and early entral feeding regarding systemic immunity after major hepatic resection—the results of a randomized prospective study. Hepato-Gastroenterologica 1997;44:205–209.
124. Sharpe MD, Pikul J, Lowndes R, et al. Early enteral feeding (EEF) reduces incidence of early rejection following orthotopic liver transplantation (abstract). Joint Congress of Liver Transplantation, London, 1995.
125. Peck MD, Ogla CK, Alexander JW. Composition of fat in enteral diets can influence outcome in experimental peritonitis. Ann Surg 1991;214:74–82.
126. Gianotti L, Alexander JW, Pyles T, Fukushima R. Arginine-supplemented diets improve survival in gut-derived sepsis and peritonitis by modulating bacterial clearance. The role of nitric oxide. Ann Surg 1993;217:644–654.
127. Furukawa S, Saito H, Inaba T, et al. Glutamin-enriched enteral diet enhances bacterial clearance in protracted bacterial peritonitis, regardless of glutamin form. J Parenter Enteral Nutr 1997;21:208–214.
128. Malhotra SL. Studies in blood coagulation, diet and ischaemic heart disease in two population groups in India. Br Heart J 1968;30:303–308.
129. Latto C, Wilkinson RW, Gilmore OJ. Diverticular disease and varicose veins. Lancet 1973;1:1089–1090.
130. Frohn MJ. Left-leg varicose veins and deep-vein thrombosis. Lancet 1976;11:1019–1020.
131. Wang C, Zhao L, Chen Y. Hypolipidemic action of soy fiber and its effects on platelet aggregation and coagulation time in rats. Chin J Prev Med 1996;30:205–208.
132. Shenoy HD. Formation and prevention of peritoneal adhesion—an experimental study on a rat model. J Kuwait Med Coll 1997;29:172–179.
133. Bengmark S, Larsson K, Lindman B, Holmdahl L. Compositions for lubricating and separating tissues and biological membranes. Swedish patent application SE-9702693-3, PTC/SE98/01371.
134. Diamond MP, Sepracoat Study Group. Reproduction of de novo postsurgical adhesions by intraoperative precoating with Sepracoat (HAL-C) solution: a prospective, randomized, blinded, placebo-controlled multicenter study. Fertil Steril 1998;69:1067–1074.

41

Polymer Solutions and Films as Tissue-Protective and Barrier Adjuvants

Lynn S. Peck and Eugene P. Goldberg

CONTENTS

This chapter is primarily devoted to a discussion of two very different concepts for development of polymeric compositions designed to inhibit postoperative adhesion formation in all types of surgery. One concept, which has received the least attention and which we therefore consider in more detail, is that of tissue protection during surgery by the use of polymer solutions as tissue coatings intended to minimize manipulative and desiccation trauma in the surgical field. The second concept, which has been the primary focus of research in this field for the past 20 years, is that of barrier coatings or films designed to be placed, at the end of surgery, over tissues that have been damaged during surgery. Such coatings or films may thereby act as barriers to the bridging of apposite damaged tissues with unwanted internal scar tissue (adhesions).

Tissue Protection During Surgery

Tissue protection may be regarded as a prophylactic approach to adhesion prevention that is intended to reduce trauma to tissue surfaces during surgical procedures. In most surgeries, considerable tissue damage may normally occur adjacent to and beyond the primary site of necessary unavoidable cutting and manipulation (i.e., incision, cautery, suture sites). Manipulative and desiccative trauma adjacent to and beyond the primary site is an unwanted adjunct to the surgery. We therefore prefer the term "adjunctive trauma" to describe this surgical tissue damage. Although adjunctive trauma has been generally accepted as an unavoidable consequence of normal surgical procedures, some pioneering surgeons (most notably Dr. K. Swolin[1] beginning more than 30 years ago) have been advocates for "gentle surgery"; that is, procedures that are quicker, simpler, involve less tissue handling, and use gloves which are free of talc or starch. However, in view of the practical limitations of the "gentle surgery" philosophy alone, the development of surgical devices or solutions that might afford protection to tissues during surgery has become an important and challenging field of research which is emphasized in this chapter.

Barrier adjuvants (either solutions or "solid" devices, as described in the "Postsurgical Barrier Solutions" and "Barrier Films" sections of this chapter) are used to physically separate damaged tissue surfaces at the end of surgery. Bioactive agents that modify the sequelae of biochemical or cellular events leading to adhesion formation after serosal injury are also used at the end of surgery. In contrast, tissue protective adjuvants are applied at the beginning of surgery and during surgical manipulations to help reduce or prevent serosal injury. We believe that this important distinction, that of defining the function of adhesion prevention adjuvants in terms of their biophysical behavior and the timing of their use in surgery, has not been adequately discussed or appreciated. In short, tissue protective adjuvants are intended to reduce the generalized or nonspecific trauma that occurs during surgery in the highly complex geometry of the surgical field. This trauma leads to adhesion formation at sites adjacent to or beyond the necessary primary surgical insult. Protective tissue coating solutions therefore represent a unique class of adhesion prevention adjuvants that work by inhibiting adjunctive trauma.

Mechanistic Aspects of Tissue Protection by Hydrophilic Coatings

The general concepts for achieving tissue protective surfaces and interfaces originally stemmed from studies at the University of Florida on damage to fragile ocular tissues such as the corneal endothelium during cataract surgery with intraocular lens (IOL) insertion.[2] Acrylic IOL surfaces are hydrophobic: that is, they tend to repel water and cause water droplets to "bead" up, rather than spread to a thin layer as occurs with hydrophilic surfaces. Scanning electron microscopy (SEM) revealed that fragile ocular tissues, such as the corneal endothelium, adhered to the hydrophobic IOL surface with sufficient strength to denude cells and tear cell membranes when even very gentle tissue-IOL contacts were made. Subsequent observations indicated that cell membranes adhere to most hydrophobic surfaces.

Many materials commonly used in surgery (i.e., gloves, plastic instruments, and polymeric or metallic implants and devices) may have hydrophobic surfaces and exhibit similar damaging hydrophobic tissue adherence. Tissue damage from this adhesive surface interaction has been regarded as different from simple abrasion[2] and can exacerbate abrasive trauma caused by rubbing various surgical materials across the endothelial or peritoneal surfaces (e.g., contact of latex gloves with the bowel surface).[3,4] However, when hydrophilic polymers were placed at the tissue-material interface (either aqueous polymer solutions or permanent chemically grafted hydrophilic polymer surface modifications), no such "sticking" or associated damage to endothelium or bowel serosal surfaces occurred.

Hydrophobic and/or electrostatic biophysical interactions are known to be involved in a variety of bioadhesive phenomena, such as the binding of serum albumin to implant surfaces and to drugs. Aqueous solutions of hydrophilic, high molecular weight polymers such as polyvinylpyrrolidone (PVP; povidone) interposed between tissues such as the endothelium and various materials, however, inhibited damaging surface interactions by creating a lubricious protective nonadherent interface.[2] Other studies have since shown that a boundary layer of high molecular weight (MW) hyaluronic acid (HA) or other polymers can also protect the corneal endothelium from injury during abrasion,[3] constant force mechanical trauma,[5] or sonication.[6–8] This protection appears to be a function of polymer concentration,[9] molecular structure, MW, and thickness of the surface coating.[3]

Like the fragile corneal endothelial cell monolayer, the peritoneal mesothelium is susceptible to damage from contacts with surgical instrument and device materials[4,10] as well as from other forms of trauma.[11–15] Ultrastructural SEM studies have shown that mesothelial cells are arranged as a somewhat loosely connected single-layer structure. Numerous long microvilli greatly increase the exposed surface area of individual cells and make the mesothelium vulnerable to adhesive and abrasive contact damage.[10,16,17] Such trauma can result in desquamation or denudation of the serosa with exposure of the basement membrane, with release of cytokines, fibrin deposition, other chemotactic and inflammatory events, and collagen deposition by fibroblasts, etc., all processes now recognized as important to the formation of postoperative adhesions. Denudation alone is a sufficient insult to cause fibrin deposition and may be of significantly more import than previously realized in the formation of adhesions.[10,15,16]

"Adjunctive" Surgical Trauma

Although we have briefly defined what we mean by the inadvertent adjunctive tissue trauma that accompanies virtually all surgery, more detailed discussion of this complication is important to understanding strategies for mitigating such trauma. Many different traumatic events occur during a surgical procedure, some of which are a direct, unavoidable, and inherent part of the procedure itself. For example, unavoidable direct damage occurs by cutting injury during a myomectomy or resection, by electrocautery, and by thermal injury when a laser excision is performed. We term this *primary trauma* to clearly differentiate it from adjunctive trauma.

Adjunctive trauma occurs, often nonspecifically, concomitant with the surgical procedure but often apart from the actual site or focus of the procedure. It has also been termed indirect,[16] unintentional,[12] accidental,[15] and inadvertent or incidental.[18] Adjunctive trauma may be generalized in the surgical field, that is, as the result of excessive irrigation[15] or elevated irrigating solution temperature.[19] It may also be localized or discrete, for example, from holding or blotting tissues with a sponge. It may occur in a more passive way than primary trauma, as in desiccation from exposure to air (or to CO_2 in laparoscopic procedures). Adjunctive trauma and its effects also increase with operating time.[20,21] This etiologic distinction between these two types of trauma, primary and adjunctive, is essential to understanding the purpose and applications of tissue protective solutions.

Occurrence of Adjunctive Trauma in a Typical Bowel Resection Procedure

Extensive adjunctive trauma occurs in many different ways during a single surgical procedure. A brief, simplified, step-by-step description of a bowel resection and anastomosis procedure is presented as a typical example to highlight the numerous steps that produce adjunctive trauma.

An incision is made, opening the peritoneal cavity; this is primary trauma. Rapidly circulating dry air in the operating room immediately rushes into the abdomen initiating desiccation of tissues (desiccative trauma).[12,13,15,22] Retractors are placed (with adhesive contact and abrasive trauma[4] resulting in local ischemia[23]) along the incision line. The surgeon reaches for a loop of bowel with a gloved finger (adhesive contact and abrasive trauma[4,17]) and works along the length of bowel to locate the obstructed site (manipulative abrasion). Once it is located, the surgeon isolates the area by exteriorizing it (enhancing desiccation), holding it with a sponge (further adhesive contact and manipulative damage[4,24–26] to the often drier, more sticky, and less elastic tissue surfaces). The rest of the bowel is packed off with a warm saline-moistened towel (contact adhesion; further manipulative abrasion; initiation of a foreign-body reaction to textile fibers[27]).

Although the surgeon wears so-called "powder-free" gloves, these are not necessarily "particulate-free."[28] Handling the wet towels is likely to bring glove powders that are still used as manufacturing release agents to the surface of the gloves.[28] A touch of the surgeon's hand may thereby deposit a small amount of particulate matter onto the tissues and instruments (eliciting a particulate foreign-body reaction[28–30]). Additionally, surgical assistants may don powdered gloves nearby, resulting in airborne powder.[31–33] Electrostatic deposition of particulates may also occur, especially on drier tissues. Such particulate foreign material also induces release of growth factors[34] and cytokines,[30,35] leading to increased inflammation and delayed wound healing.

As the surgery proceeds, bleeders are cauterized (resulting in carbon deposits[36] and thermal injury[36]) or clamped (with traumatic crushing) to keep the surgical field free of blood. The bowel is clamped (with crushing damage and local ischemia). The pathologic tissue section is resected (with primary cutting trauma coupled with adjunctive manipulative damage) and healthy tissue anastomosed (with primary and adjunctive trauma from suturing or stapling, including manipulative damage and local ischemia along the suture/staple line[37]). During this process, heat from surgical lamps exacerbates desiccation of the exposed bowel surfaces (adjunctive thermal and/or desiccative trauma). Warm saline or lactated Ringer's solution at 40°C may be used periodically to keep towels and tissues moist and to rinse away debris and contaminants (resulting in thermal and mechanical trauma). Some irrigation fluid accumulates in the peritoneal cavity, where it may produce cytotoxic effects.[38] Soluble chemical residues accumulating in the irrigation solution from the surgeon's gloves may also kill mesothelial cells after only a few minutes of exposure.[39] Starch particles and chemical residues washed from the gloves can also prove toxic to macrophages and mesothelial and other cell types[30,40] and stimulate cytokine release from peritoneal macrophages.[30,34,35]

About 30 minutes after the beginning of the procedure, peritoneal tissue plasminogen activator (tPA) activity has also fallen by about 50% (because of surgical injury and local ischemia).[41] After the anastomosis is examined for leaks (with traumatic pressure and abrasive manipulation), a final thorough irrigation may be performed (which can produce thermal, mechanical, and pH-related trauma.[14,15]) The incisions are closed (with both primary trauma and adjunctive trauma from tissue manipulation and suture or staple placement.[42])

At least 15 different traumatic surgical events that produce adjunctive trauma to the parietal and visceral peritoneum have occurred in this relatively simple procedure (as summarized in Table 41.1). The damage is widely and irregularly distributed and, for the most part, is grossly undetectable at the time of surgery. However, the impact of this adjunctive trauma is highly significant in terms of adhesiogenesis and may ultimately prove more important than the "primary" trauma (Fig. 41.1). The various adjunctive trauma events have caused damage or destruction of mesothelium,[4,15] reduced peritoneal fibrinolytic capacity,[15,23] and increased production of cytokines[30,35,38] and growth factors,[34] which can stimulate adhesion formation. Furthermore, visceral peritoneum, which may be more vulnerable to forming adhesions than parietal peritoneum,[43,44] has received a much greater assortment of adjunctive insults during this, and perhaps most, procedures. This multiplicity of sources and distribution of sites of adjunctive damage may be uniquely important, because surgical injury to multiple peritoneal surfaces can dramatically increase adhesion formation in animal models when compared with injury to a single surface.[45] The most significant point to be made here is that much of this broad-ranging adjunctive tissue damage, which is not confined to the primary surgical site, may be preventable through the routine use of tissue protective solutions during surgery.

Tissue Protective Solutions

Further Mechanistic Aspects of Tissue Protection

Our early studies at the University of Florida suggested that hydrophobic or electrostatic interactions were the basis for adhesive contacts between cells and surgical materials resulting in tissue damage.[4] Hydrophilic coatings and solutions provide a nonadherent surface and also diminish possible electrostatic interactions. Hydrophilic solutions also form a lubricating boundary layer that reduces friction and shearing forces and consequent tissue damage.[4] This boundary layer provides a specific, local, protective effect that requires a minimal volume of a coating solution, and the protective effect does not appear to be significantly enhanced by using large volumes of solution.[46]

Tissue protective solutions, then, may be generically categorized as aqueous hydrophilic solutions of either natural or synthetic macromolecules (e.g., hyaluronic acid [HA], proteins, phospholipids; polyvinylpyrroli-

TABLE 41.1. Sources of primary and adjunctive surgical trauma.

Primary surgical trauma	Adjunctive surgical trauma
Scalpel incision/puncture entry	Desiccation/exposure
Sharp or blunt dissection	OR environment
Cutting/coagulation electrocautery:	CO_2 in laparoscopic surgery
Thermal injury	Manual manipulation of tissue:
Carbon deposits	Adhesive contact and abrasive trauma from glove or instrument surface
Laser injury	Retraction
Tissue clamps/hemostats/ligatures/clips:	Local ischemia,
Crushing injury	Adhesive/abrasive trauma
Local ischemia	Use of sponges (woven/nonwoven):
Resection	Adhesive/abrasive trauma
Anastomosis: (staples or sutures)	Introduction of foreign bodies (fibers, lint)
Puncture injury	Packing:
Local ischemia	Adhesive/abrasive trauma
Closing: sutures, staples	Introduction of foreign bodies (fibers, lint)
	Glove powders/release agents:
	Particulate foreign bodies
	Cytotoxic effects (mesothelium)
	Increased inflammation via release of cytokines and growth factors
	Irrigating solutions:
	Cytotoxic effects
	Thermal trauma if warmed above 40°C
	Mechanical trauma from rinsing
	Carrier for soluble cytotoxic residues from surgeons' gloves

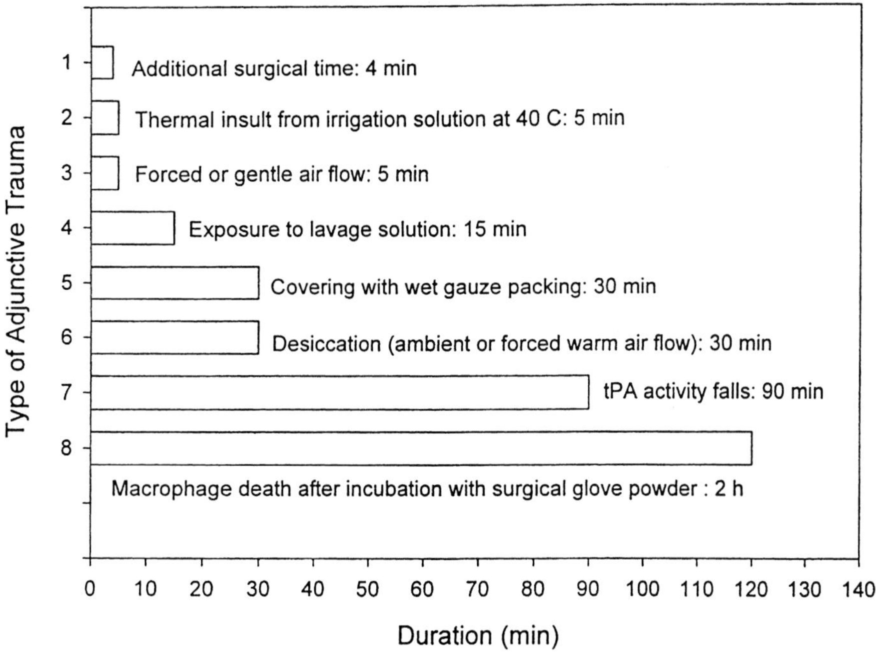

Notes and Sources for Types of Trauma

1. Increasing surgeries from 8 to 12 min (rodent model) [20].
2. Rodent model [19].
3. Forced air flow: [13]; gentle air flow + added blood: [15].
4. Mesothelial cells incubated in lavage solution had significant rise in plasminogen activator inhibitor (PAI-1) activity [38].
5. Saline or RL used for wetting; with 2 mL blood added before closing (rodent model) [15].
6. Desiccation after gauze abrasion (canine pericardial model) [12,65].
7. Wound tPA activity fell to near zero after 90 min of surgery [23].
8. 2 to 5 h incubation with glove powder led to macrophage death [30].

FIG. 41.1. Adjunctive surgical trauma: type and duration of insults sufficient to cause mesothelial damage leading to adhesion formation.

done [povidone, PVP], modified cellulosics such as carboxymethylcellulose [CMC], and water-soluble polyethers such as polyethylene glycols [PEGs]). The ionicity of these polymers (anionic or cationic) and their affinity for specific cell-surface receptor sites (i.e., CD44 binding of HA) may also be important with respect to possible electrostatic interactions, surface binding, and their role in inhibiting trauma and adhesion formation. In this regard, a recent paper by Falk et al.[47] has also suggested some beneficial effects for hydrophobic and cationic modifications of cellulosic polymers.

Possible Role of Tissue Surface Electrical Potential

The omentum is an important tissue in adhesion formation because of its ready adherence to traumatized areas of peritoneum, with likelihood of resulting adhesions. In "almost forgotten" rabbit studies reported by Cantacuzene and Soru in 1931, injury to peritoneal surfaces was shown to significantly alter the electrical potential of the peritoneum, resulting in a large potential difference relative to the intact omentum as compared with healthy undamaged peritoneum.[48] Such electrical potential gradients may enhance adherence of the omentum to damage sites and are also likely to influence chemotactic events and electrostatic tissue interactions that may be involved in the formation of adhesions.[49] In these early rabbit studies, manipulation of the electrical potential gradient by the use of positively or negatively charged dyes that bind to the omentum, was found to enhance or prevent the formation of adhesions. Increasing the potential difference between mesothelium and omentum was associated with adhesion formation. In contrast, reducing the electrical potential gradient resulted in adhesion-free animals.

Studies of wound healing and tissue electrical potentials have also indicated that normal, intact tissue surfaces tend to be negatively charged and that damaged tissue develops a positive electrical potential shortly after injury.[50-52] This potential gradient then slowly declines as wound healing progresses.[50] Together, these studies suggest that when the mesothelial layer of peritoneum (negatively charged when intact) is damaged severely enough to expose deeper tissue layers (positively charged), electrostatic interactions can occur with negatively charged metabolites and polymers. These electrostatic interactions, in combination with specific receptor affinity, can promote binding of anionic polysaccharides such as HA or CMC at sites of injury during the initial period of wound healing. At very high anionic polymer concentrations, electrostatic interactions may also influence thrombus formation,[53] which suggests another possible mechanism for adhesion reduction via inhibition of local fibrin deposition. Additionally, solutions of anionic polyelectrolytes used as tissue coatings may uniformly distribute a negative surface charge throughout the abdominal cavity and thereby inhibit intimate contact with other negatively charged (i.e., intact) tissue surfaces, including the omentum. Concurrently, other adverse electrostatic chemotactic processes may be affected. In this context, tissue surface charge has also been shown to induce directional migration of neutrophils, macrophages, and fibroblasts.[54]

Viscosity and Polymer Molecular Weight Effects

Studies at the University of Florida and elsewhere have shown that solutions that are moderately to highly viscous and of high molecular weight (>500,000) are more efficacious than less viscous or lower molecular weight solutions (Fig. 41.1[55,56] and unpublished data). However, solution viscosity appears to be a more dominant factor than MW. For example, we have recently shown that chemical modification of very low MW hydrophilic polymers with hydrophobic (perfluoroaklyl) groups increases solution viscosity, apparently because of hydrophobic molecular associations in aqueous solution. This modification produces tissue protective compositions with MW less than the normal kidney glomerulus clearance MW of about 40,000, yet which effectively inhibit adhesion formation. However, for most conventional polymers, high MW is important in favoring higher viscosities at lower solution concentrations because of the direct relationship between MW and solution viscosity. Higher MW solutions also tend to form boundary layers that are not so readily solvated, diluted, or wiped off, and may be more slowly cleared from the peritoneum, leading to longer residence times.[57] A longer residence time also provides an opportunity for potential clinical applications using medicated or drug-containing polymer solutions. Such solutions could function as both a protective tissue coating during surgery and as a prolonged drug release device for delivery of antiinflammatory, fibrinolytic, or other bioactive agents after surgery.

Because tissue protective solutions are designed for use at the beginning of surgery and throughout the surgical procedure, they must also have excellent handling characteristics. Solutions that are "sticky," very viscous, or cause excessive slipperiness of tissue and glove or instrument surfaces would be less readily accepted for clinical use. High MW polyelectrolytes and polymers that tend to associate in solution are generally likely to prove most useful because they can provide adequate viscosity even at low or very low concentrations (e.g., 0.1%–0.4% solutions for HA), thereby minimizing some of the adverse handling characteristics that may occur at higher concentrations. Polymers with broad MW distributions and those which have to be used at higher concentrations (above 5%) tend to be more "sticky" in their handling characteristics, and therefore are less favorable for clinical use. Other factors to be considered in developing and using tissue protective solutions include biocompatibility, iso-osmolality, and lack of suitability as a substrate for bacterial growth.

Hydrophilic Polymers for Tissue Protection

Sodium Hyaluronate (Hyaluronic Acid, Hyaluronan)

Biophysical Effects

Hyaluronic acid (HA) is a naturally occurring, anionic polysaccharide that is found in virtually all mammalian tissues and body fluids. It is a primary lubricant in synovial fluid and is also a component of the vitreous. Composed of repeating *N*-acetylglucosamine and glucuronate disaccharide units, the natural polymer ranges from several hundred thousand to several million daltons. Free of protein and other contaminants, that is, highly purified, HA from a variety of sources has been found to be highly biocompatable. Fibroblasts can synthesize HA of 5 to 6×10^6 MW and extrude it into the extracellular matrix (ECM). As a component of the ECM, HA is thought to play a role in regulating (a) the movement of cells, (b) the water content of tissues, and (c) the exclusion of large molecules via its physicochemical properties (i.e., rigid steric space-occupying molecular structure and negative charge).[58,59]

HA solutions, as the sodium salt, have remarkable pseudoplastic viscoelastic properties: solutions become much less viscous when forced to flow at high shear rates (e.g., during injection through a syringe), and then quickly return to the original higher viscosity when the high shear flow is stopped. This property led to the first major clinical application in the early 1980s for ophthalmic surgery as an injectable highly viscous fluid device (Healon™; Pharmacia) for tissue separation and to maintain the shape of the anterior chamber of the eye during ophthalmic surgery.[3,60] For this purpose HA of more than 10^3 kDa, as a 1% aqueous solution with viscosity of 40,000 to 80,000 centipoise (cps) at low shear, was used. More recently, HA solutions have been evaluated at various concentrations and molecular weights in animal and human clinical studies as both a tissue protective adjuvant during surgery and as a barrier tissue coating applied at the end of surgery.[11,61–64]

Insofar as tissue protection during surgery is concerned, numerous animal model studies, which evaluated the incidence and severity of adhesion formation and tissue histology after surgical manipulation with abrasion[12,13,65] and desiccation,[12,13,60,65] have clearly shown that HA solutions reduced tissue trauma and formation of adhesions. Protection has also been afforded for laser injuries,[11] particulate foreign-body reactions[66] (and our unpublished data), and in experiments involving constant-force mechanical trauma.[5] These studies have been conducted using many different animal models: rodent and rabbit cecal[13,46,67,68] and uterine,[11,61,69,70] dog pericardial,[12,65,71] and rabbit ocular muscle.[72,73] HA has also been reported to reduce corneal endothelial damage during ophthalmic surgical procedures,[3,5–8,74] including those using sonication or phacoemulsification.[6,7,74]

An analysis of our data at the University of Florida during a 5-year period using a rat cecal abrasion model showed that use of HA as a tissue protective solution reduced the incidence of clinically significant adhesions (grade 2 on a 0 to 4 scale[75]) from 71% for animals receiving phosphate buffered saline (PBS; $n = 404$) to 44% for animals receiving HA ($n = 153$; two-tailed $p < 0.0001$). The incidence of animals that were free of adhesions increased from 16% for PBS controls to 41% for those receiving HA.[67]

Tissue precoating with HA in a rat uterine devascularization and serosal cautery model reduced the incidence of adhesions from 73% (controls) to 44%.[69] In some models of more severe primary tissue trauma, however, it appeared that HA was of less benefit.[64,76] This finding is consistent with the concept of tissue protection directed at reducing adjunctive, rather than primary, trauma. Various HA formulations have also been tested in animal experiments as a postoperative barrier with conflicting results, some suggesting adhesion reduction[61–63] and other studies indicating no effect[11,64] (and our data; refer also to the section in this chapter on "Barrier Solutions").

A randomized, blinded, placebo-controlled, multicenter human clinical study[77] using a 0.4% aqueous HA sodium salt formulation (Sepracoat™; Genzyme Corporation) indicated, at second-look laparoscopy (SLL) about 40 days postoperatively, that HA was effective in reducing the number and severity of adhesions at sites of adjunctive trauma. In this study, 245 women undergoing gynecologic procedures via laparotomy received either PBS or Sepracoat at opening, after irrigation, and at 30-minute intervals during surgery. At SLL, 13.1% of Sepracoat patients and 4.6% of control patients were free of de novo adhesions. Patients receiving Sepracoat also had a significant reduction overall in the extent and severity of de novo adhesions at 23 intraabdominal sites evaluated in this study.

Possible Biochemical Effects

In addition to highly favorable biophysical properties for tissue coating during surgery, there have been a variety of reports concerning possible biologic activity for HA that could also favorably affect wound healing and inhibit adhesion formation. HA has been reported to reduce inflammatory response by reducing platelet aggregation, increasing the time to onset of aggregation, and inhibiting the release of platelet-derived growth factor (PDGF).[61] Inhibition of elastase release (a proteolytic enzyme) from stimulated rat peritoneal leukocytes has also been reported.[78] In fibroblast cultures, there have been conflicting data regarding the inhibition or proliferation of cells and stimulation of collagen synthesis.[61,79] Postsurgical fibroblast metabolism, as measured by [^{3}H] thymidine uptake, was indicated to decrease on exposure to HA in culture but increase in mixed fibroblast–macrophage cultures.[80] Exposure to HA in an in vitro system suggested increased production of tumor necrosis factor-alpha (TNF-α) by human macrophages with decreased collagen synthesis by fibroblasts.[81] In mice, HA appeared to stimulate the migration of inflammatory cells and recruitment of activated macrophages,[82] whereas in a rabbit study aggregation of neutrophils was inhibited.[83]

At least some of the reported effects of HA appear to be modulated by MW and concentration[83] as well as by timing of administration. In a rat study, high molecular weight HA apparently inhibited the growth of blood vessels in ocular muscle tissue during the first postoperative week after strabismus surgery.[76] A similar inhibitory effect on vascular ingrowth in an in vivo rat ear model was reported when HA (3.9×10^6 daltons) was administered daily for 1 week. Curiously, an opposite stimulatory effect was seen when HA was administered intermittently.[84] Unfortunately, the correlation of these (and other) in vitro and in vivo studies concerning possible bioactivity for HA with the behavior of HA solutions as tissue protective agents during surgery or for adhesion-inhibiting barriers remains unclear at this time.

Carboxymethylcellulose

Carboxymethylcellulose (CMC), generally used as the sodium salt (CMC, methylcellulose gum), is an anionic, water-soluble polymer derived from natural cellulose.

The repeat disaccharide unit has a molecular structure that is somewhat similar to that of HA. Purified CMC is available in a wide range of MW, from about 90,000 to greater than 900,000 daltons (Aqualon). Solutions can be prepared with lubricating and viscoelastic properties similar to those of HA solutions and synovial fluids.[85] CMC exhibits good biocompatibility, for example, no adverse reactions observed when injected into the rabbit "knee" joint or vitreous.[85] Ponies given CMC intraabdominally at the end of surgery showed only 1 aberration of about 20 blood chemistry and electrolyte values during the first 5 days postoperatively that might be attributable to the CMC; an elevated serum calcium concentration 24 hours postoperatively, which returned to a normal range within 72 hours.[86] CMC exhibits a longer intraabdominal residence time in rats than HA (5 days for CMC vs. 2 days for HA) and lower MW CMC (about 70,000 with a radiolabel) was found to clear the renal system in less than 30 days (unpublished data, University of Florida and Genzyme).

Compared to HA, there have been far fewer studies of possible CMC biologic activity. Ryan and Sax[87] found that CMC did not affect transforming growth factor-beta (TGF-β) expression in rat fibroblasts and endothelial cells collected on day 3 and day 10 after surgery. CMC-treated animals showed marked suppression of serosal fibroblast growth and large numbers of CMC-containing macrophages. Peritoneal macrophage secretion products, which contain modulators of fibroblast growth, differentiation, and activity, were unaffected. In another study in which a lyophilized CMC-coated polypropylene mesh barrier was successfully used to reduce visceral adhesion formation in a rat incisional hernia model, histology suggested impaired proliferation of fibroblasts and decreased collagen accumulation compared with controls 7 days postoperatively.[88] CMC has also been reported to be a poor substrate for bacterial growth. *E. coli* growth cultures did not grow in media in which CMC was provided as the sole source of carbon-containing nutrient.[89]

In most published reports, CMC has been evaluated as a postoperative barrier coating (see "Barrier Solutions"). However, CMC exhibits excellent adhesion inhibition efficacy when tested as a tissue protective coating solution during surgery. Our cumulative 5-year data using a rat cecal adhesion model with 1% aqueous CMC solution (MW >700,000 indicate a reduction in clinically significant (grade 2 on a 0 to 4 scoring scale) adhesion incidence, from 71% for PBS controls ($n = 404$) to 32% for CMC-treated animals ($n = 87$; two-tailed $p < 0.0001$). Also observed was an increase in the incidence of rats with no adhesions for CMC treatment (52%), compared to 16% for PBS controls (16%). Statistical significance of these data was indicated by chi-square analysis; two-tailed $p < 0.0001$.[67]

In these CMC studies, adhesion reduction was directly related to solution concentration, viscosity, and molecular weight. For solutions prepared with CMC of high MW (>700,000 daltons) at concentrations of 0.3% (w/v) to 2.0%, increasing viscosity resulted in an increase in the number of animals having no adhesions (our unpublished data; Fig. 41.2). At concentrations of 1.0% or less, there was a strong first-order relationship ($r^2 = 0.997$) between the number of animals with grade 2 adhesions or higher and increasing concentration (Fig. 41.3). Even a small increase in concentration produced a noticeable decrease in the incidence of adhesions. The number of adhesion-free animals remained relatively constant at concentrations below 0.5%, but increased significantly (as does the viscosity) at 1.0% CMC concentration

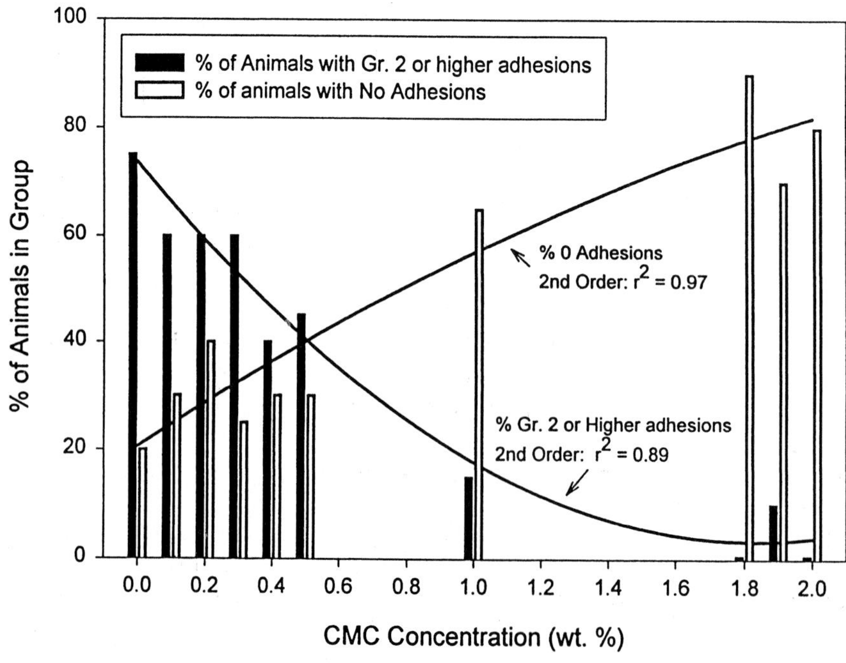

FIG. 41.2. Tissue protection with carboxymethylcellulose (CMC) solutions: effect of concentration.

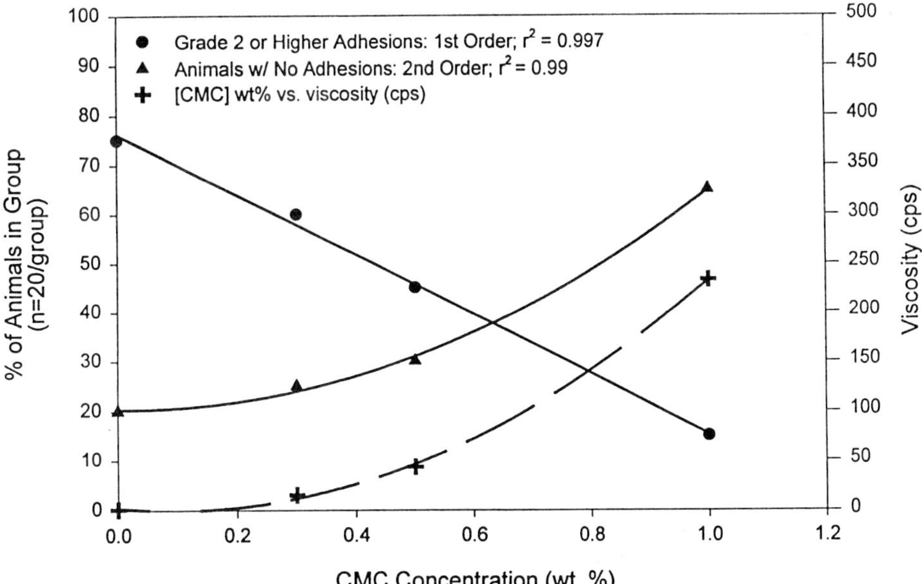

FIG. 41.3. Tissue protection: effect of CMC concentration and viscosity on adhesion formation.

(second-order relationship; $r^2 = 0.99$), suggesting a threshold viscosity above which tissue protection is optimal. Further increases in concentration that produced very viscous solutions did not result in a corresponding increase in tissue protective efficacy (Fig. 41.2).

In other studies testing solutions of CMC with different MW at comparable concentrations, high MW CMC solutions were significantly more efficacious than medium (~250 kDa) or low (~90 kDa) MW, as indicated by results showing 70% of animals with no adhesions for high MW, compared to 10% for medium MW and 0% for low MW (chi-square analysis: two-tailed $p < 0.005$; with groups of $n = 10$). The idea that this effect is only related to viscosity was negated by a study comparing solutions of various MW prepared at different CMC concentrations to afford equivalent viscosities. At similar viscosities, the high MW solutions proved more efficacious: 70% with no adhesions for high MW versus 20% (medium MW) and 30% (low MW). Chi-square analysis, two-tailed, gave $p = 0.054$ for groups of $n = 10$ (unpublished data).

Our studies have also indicated that the volume of CMC solution used as a tissue protective coating during surgery does not appear to be a primary determinant of efficacy. Minimal coating of tissues before traumatic insult appears to be sufficient to inhibit adhesion formation. This effect was not enhanced when large volumes of fluid were instilled intraperitoneally.[46] In contrast, a very different effect was seen when CMC was used as a postsurgical barrier coating. When used as a barrier coating, adhesion prevention efficacy was found to be related to solution volume[55] (see "Clinical Considerations").

CMC solutions were also shown to be effective for protection of pericardial tissues in animal models of open heart surgery that normally produce very extensive adhesions which seriously compromise resternotomies. In a canine pericardial abrasion/desiccation model, 1% CMC was comparable in efficacy to 0.4% HA.[65] Mean pericardial adhesion scores (0 to 4 scale) were 0.6 for animals treated with 0.4% HA or 1% CMC, compared to 2.3 for animals treated with Ringer's lactate (RL; $p < 0.05$, Duncan's ANOVA). Only 20% of animals treated with HA or CMC solutions had clinically significant (grade 2) adhesions whereas 80% of animals treated with RL had significant adhesions. (The term "clinically significant" used here and elsewhere in this chapter denotes adhesions that, because of extent or strength of attachment at time of evaluation, appear unlikely to resolve without surgical intervention, and so indicate greater potential risk of clinically important pathologic consequences.)

Other Tissue-Protective Polymer Solutions

In our studies at the University of Florida, various polymer solutions and lipids have been investigated for tissue protection efficacy, including PVP (polyvinylpyrrolidone, "povidone") of various MW, dextran, polyethylene glycol (PEG), polypropylene glycol copolymers (Pluronics), fluorocarbon-modified PEG, proteins, and phospholipids. Solutions of lower MW PVP (40 kDa) at 25% and 30% (w/w) have been studied in canine intestinal abrasion[4] and pericardial abrasion/desiccation[12] models. Dextran (200–300 kDa) was also studied at 25% in the canine bowel abrasion model. Although the very concentrated PVP solutions were effective in reducing adhesions (average score, 0.3 [0 to 4 scale] for PVP-treated vs. 2.5 for dry controls; $n = 3$ and $n = 4$, respectively), poor handling characteristics (instrument and glove surfaces became very "sticky"), and questions concerning renal clearance made serious consideration of clinical use unlikely. Dextran was less effective than PVP as a tissue protective solution in these experiments (average score, 1.3; $n = 4$), and also caused "stickiness" in handling. In a rat cecal abrasion study, a 32% dextran 70 solution (MW 70,000; Hyskon, Pharmacia) afforded no benefit compared to PBS controls (our unpublished data). In addition, dextran may be problematic in view of reports of ascites, pleural effusion,[90] possible immunosuppression,[91] and other effects associated with its use[90] (also reviewed in ref. 92, pp. 323–328).

Insoluble phospholipids, as dispersions (0.5% lecithin; 0.1% dilauroyl phosphate, and 0.1% dipalmitoyl phosphate), were ineffective as tissue protective solutions in a rat cecal model (our unpublished data). Similar findings were reported by investigators in Sweden with insoluble phospholipids as postoperative barrier coating solutions in several different animal models.[93] However, partially soluble phospholipids and phospholipase-resistant phospholipids were reported to be effective as postoperative barrier coatings in reducing adhesion formation.[94,95] Phosphatidylcholine administered intraperitoneally after surgery in a single 20-mg dose or in three separate doses totaling 20 mg per rat also reduced adhesions in a bowel anastomosis model. Higher doses (40 or 60 mg/rat) increased the incidence of anastomotic dehiscence leading to peritonitis.[96] However, phospholipid solutions and dispersions have not yet been studied in detail as tissue-coating adjuvants to prevent adjunctive surgical trauma.

Chemical modification of water soluble polymers may also be a useful approach to improving properties for more practical clinical use (i.e., increased viscosity at low MW and/or low concentration). Because low MW (<40 kDa) facilitates renal clearance, we have examined unique fluorocarbon-modified PEG of low MW (~35 kDa) as tissue protective solutions during surgery with very encouraging results. In a rat cecal abrasion study, 68% of animals (13/19) were adhesion free using a fluoromodified PEG (F-PEG) compared to 20% adhesion free (4/20; $p = 0.0036$) for PBS controls. Mean adhesion incidence for F-PEG solutions was 0.4 ± 0.6 versus 2.1 ± 1.9 ($\bar{X} \pm SD$) for controls ($p = 0.003$).

Modified chitosan, as *N,O*-carboxymethylchitosan (NOCC), has been reported as an adhesion-reducing adjuvant.[63,97] NOCC is a water-soluble, long-chain polysaccharide derived from chitosan by hydrolysis of chitin (a crab shell constituent) followed by carboxymethylation. It is anionic, hydrophilic, and can be formulated as a pseudoplastic solution or cross-linked hydrogel.[63] Animal studies in several different rodent models suggest efficacy of NOCC solutions as tissue protective adjuvants during surgery as well as in postsurgical barrier coating applications.[63,97]

Clinically Important Factors for Tissue Protection

Optimal clinical use of tissue protective solutions requires an understanding of their purpose (to reduce adjunctive trauma from manipulation, desiccation, and other insults), their physical and biochemical properties (rheology, tissue-surface affinity, lubricity, ionicity, stability, and renal clearance), and other factors that may influence their effectiveness. These factors include simplicity and timing of use (application and reapplication during surgery), volume of solution required, and the effect of combined use with standard irrigating solutions such as Ringer's lactate, normal saline, or PBS.

Timing of Application and Reapplication of Tissue Protective Solutions

As previously discussed, tissue protective polymer solutions are intended to be applied to tissue surfaces immediately at the beginning of the surgical procedure. For abdominal or pelvic procedures, a volume of solution sufficient to coat all the tissues should be instilled into the peritoneal cavity as soon as the entry incision is made. Where appropriate, manual manipulation of tissues with the surgeon's gloved fingers coated with solution may help to distribute solution to fully coat less accessible tissues.

For most procedures in which exposure, desiccation, significant manipulation, and occasional irrigation/aspiration are involved, periodic reapplication of solution is indicated. In a canine pericardial abrasion and desiccation model, Kaelin et al.[22] observed that solutions of 0.1% or 0.4% HA or 1.0% CMC substantially reduced clinically significant pericardial adhesions (grade 2 or higher) when applied before pericardial abrasion and before and after 30 minutes of desiccation by exposure to room air ($p < 0.05$ for all test groups compared to Ringer's lactate controls). In a similar but more severe canine pericardial adhesion model in which desiccation was accomplished by a 2-hour period of forced warm air flow, Mitchell et al.[71] found that reapplication of 0.4% HA solution at 20-minute intervals during the desiccation/abrasion procedure resulted in few adhesions in treated animals at 8 weeks after surgery. Mean adhesion scores were 0.8 ± 0.3 (0 to 4 severity scale) for each HA- or CMC-treated group ($n = 6$/group). In contrast, animals receiving PBS or no irrigation had multiple, dense adhesions (mean adhesions score, 3.3 ± 0.2 and 3.2 ± 0.4, respectively; $p < 0.001$ for PBS controls vs. HA).

Periodic coating during surgery with tissue protective solutions therefore appears to be generally indicated. The volume of solution and the timing of reapplication are at the judgment of the surgeon, dependent upon the size and geometry of the surgical field, duration of surgery, extent of tissue manipulation, bleeding, and amount of irrigation required.

Protective Solution Volume

A volume adequate to amply coat all tissue surfaces is clearly required. However, a large volume of solution, for example, to substantially fill the intraperitoneal space in pelvic surgery, does not appear to be necessary or desirable. Our research, using a rat cecal abrasion model with 0, 2, 5, or 7 mL of 0.5% CMC solution instilled i.p. in addition to a 2-mL cecal coating applied before the abrasive insult, has shown that cecal precoating alone afforded sufficient tissue protection to reduce adhesion formation to the same degree observed when additional volumes of solution were used. For CMC-treated animals the incidence of adhesions of grade 2 decreased from 70% for PBS controls to 20% for animals receiving 0, 2, or 5 mL CMC i.p. ($p < 0.01$; $n = 10$/group) and to 40% for animals receiving 7 mL. The number of adhesion-free animals was also virtually identical for all treatment groups, regardless of the amount of additional solution volume (40%–50% adhesion free for all test groups vs. 20% for controls; two-tailed $p = 0.16$, chi-square). Similar insensitivity to solution volume was observed in a parallel study using 0.4% HA solution.[46]

Although increasing the volume of CMC solutions beyond the small amount required to coat tissues during surgery may have little value in inhibiting adhesions, efficacy as a postsurgical barrier coating does appear to exhibit volume dependence. In a rabbit uterine horn model, a 50-mL volume of 2% CMC reduced adhesion formation to a greater extent than smaller volumes of 20 to 40 mL ($p < 0.01$).[55]

Irrigation

It is reasonable to consider that irrigation with a standard lavage solution such as RL or PBS after applying a tissue protective polymer coating solution may dilute the polymer solution (e.g., HA or CMC) and thereby reduce tissue protection. To examine this question, we have used a rat cecal abrasion model in the following manner with 0.4% HA solution: 2 mL instilled i.p. and 2 mL applied as a cecal precoating (1 mL per side), followed by cecal lavage with RL (4 mL per side), with or without subsequent reapplication of HA (2 mL per side). Ceca were then abraded under controlled conditions. The RL irrigation group (irrigation without reapplication of HA; $n = 10$/group) showed some increase in the mean incidence of adhesions and a small decrease in the number of adhesion-free animals (neither reaching statistical significance) as compared with the precoated but not irrigated control group. Reapplication of HA solution following irrigation largely restored the protective effect. It should be noted that all groups receiving HA solution, even those with irrigation, exhibited highly significant reduction in adhesion formation compared with the control group (Fig. 41.4).

Postsurgical Barrier Coating Solutions

Many polymer solutions have been investigated as postsurgical barrier coatings in a number of animal models and in human clinical trials. Used in this way at the end of surgery, any adhesion-inhibiting effects have usually been attributed to one of two mechanisms, "siliconization" or "hydroflotation." Siliconization is an interesting term that has been used to refer to the possible lubricating effect of viscous solutions to make tissue surfaces more slippery and thereby allow damaged tissue surfaces to slide more easily past one another instead of adher-

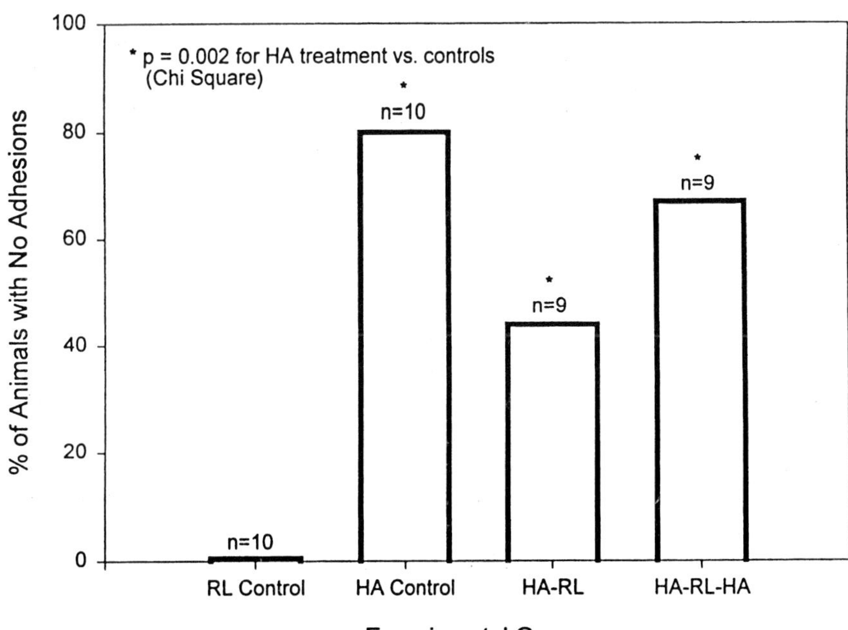

Fig. 41.4. HA tissue protection: effect of irrigation with RL on the incidence of adhesion-free animals.

ing.[55] Hydroflotation usually refers to the introduction of large amounts of fluid into the peritoneal cavity, either through intraperitoneal instillation of irrigation-type solutions postoperatively (i.e., RL), or by drawing fluid into the peritoneal cavity through the use of hyperosmolar polymer solutions (e.g., Hyskon; 32% dextran 70). The resultant "bathing" of the damaged tissue surfaces is thought to remove fibrin and separate tissue surfaces.[55,98] A third proposed mechanism is based on the idea that viscous polymeric postsurgical barrier solutions may help to "trap" fibrinolytic agents such as tPA at the surface of damaged tissues so that high local concentrations can promote increased local fibrinolytic activity.[44,99]

It is important to emphasize that these barrier solutions are applied only after tissue injury has occurred. The strategy is therefore to prevent damaged tissue contacts and possibly to modulate the cellular and biochemical sequence of events that have already been initiated through primary and adjunctive tissue injury. This approach can involve both mechanical (i.e., physical barrier) effects and biological activity of the polymer solutions. In contrast to tissue protective solutions used during surgery, however, the degree of tissue damage, particularly adjunctive damage, will be greater and may involve a more extensive area when only barrier solutions are used. As a consequence, the effectiveness of barrier solutions (which do not inhibit trauma during surgery) may be inherently more limited.

Hyaluronic Acid (HA)

HA has been studied as a postsurgical barrier coating solution in several animal models with varying results.[11,61] Investigations by us and others[11] have consistently found 0.4% HA solution to be of much greater efficacy when used during surgery for tissue protection than when used as a postoperative barrier solution. However, some studies have suggested adhesion-reducing efficacy when used at the end of surgery.[61,62] One recent study, in which a rat cecal puncture and ligation model was used to induce bacterial peritonitis, found that animals given 0.4% HA solution i.p. 24 hours postoperatively had reduced adhesion formation 7 days after surgery (5/11 animals with grade 3 or 4 adhesions [0–4 scale] vs. 11/12 for normal saline controls; $p < 0.05$). At 21 days postoperatively, 2 of 11 animals had grade 3 or 4 adhesions compared to 9 of 12 for normal saline controls. Furthermore, animals receiving HA had fewer intraabdominal abscesses than did controls. At 7 days, 0 of 11 had abscesses more than 2 cm in diameter, compared with 6 of 12 for controls ($p < 0.01$); at 21 days after surgery, 0 of 11 were abscessed, compared with 4 of 12 for controls).[100] These results are provocative and should stimulate further research into possible uses of HA solutions for postsurgical application where there is danger of peritonitis or other complications from infection.

Carboxymethylcellulose

CMC has been studied as a postsurgical barrier coating solution by a number of investigators, most of whom have reported efficacy when used in large volumes with relatively concentrated (2%–3%), highly viscous solutions.[55,56,86,98,101–103] Fredericks et al.[56] found that the efficacy of CMC used in this way was highly concentration dependent and thus viscosity dependent ($r^2 = 0.97$). In our own studies, CMC was most efficacious as a barrier coating solution in a rat cecal abrasion model when used in very high viscosity/high concentration solutions (1.8%–2%) and with relatively large solution volumes[104] (Fig. 41.5). In the rat cecal model, however, even under these conditions CMC was less effective as a barrier in preventing adhesions than when used at lower concentrations and smaller volumes as a tissue protective coating during surgery.

CMC solutions used at the end of surgery have been reported to draw significant volumes of fluid into the abdominal cavity, that is, a "hydroflotation" effect.[98] In a rat study, significant fluid volumes were found i.p. at 24 and 48 hours but not at 7 days postoperatively.[102] A second study by the same investigator reported moderate amounts (<3 mL) of CMC solution (concentration not given) still present in the abdomen of rats 2 weeks postoperatively.[98] Our studies have indicated increased fluid in the peritoneal cavity on postoperative days 1 and 2 with very viscous, gel-like, highly concentrated CMC solutions (3%–11%) of low (90 kDa) and medium (250 kDa) MW. By day 3 the fluid had largely resolved. Because the solutions were iso-osmolar and prepared in PBS, the reason for this fluid accumulation is unclear; however, it, may be hydrogen bonding interactions of the polyanionic polyelectrolyte with water as the gel-like viscous solution hydrates, coupled with temporary mechanical obstruction of stomata through which peritoneal fluid enters the lymphatic circulation,[105] and possible trauma-induced postoperative changes in peritoneal permeability.

Chitosan and *N,O*-Carboxymethyl Chitosan

N,O-Carboxymethyl chitosan (NOCC), a water-soluble, long-chain anionic polysaccharide derived from chitosan (see "Tissue Protective Solutions"), has been reported to reduce adhesion formation in several different rodent models when applied either as a 2% postsurgical barrier coating solution or as a cross-linked gel. In an aortic anastomosis model,[63,97] 20% to 30% of treated animals formed adhesions to the liver compared to 100% for untreated controls. The largest effect was observed for the combination of solution and gel. Administration as a tissue precoating in addition to postoperative application appeared to be slightly beneficial (but not statistically significant). The use of NOCC was reported to have no effect on the strength of bowel anastomoses and skin in wound healing models.

Other Barrier Solution Polymers

Solutions of the sodium salt of a carboxylated derivative of hydroxyethyl starch (hetastarch, a commonly used volume expander) have recently been reported to reduce adhesions in a rabbit uterine horn/bowel/sidewall model.[106] Chondroitin sulfate, a naturally occurring unbranched glycosaminoglycan up to 250 kDa,[107] Poloxamer 407,[108–110] and 32% dextran 70[55,111–113] (also reviewed in ref. 92, pp. 323–328, and ref. 114) have also been suggested to be useful as barrier coating solutions used at the end of surgery. (These have all been adequately described previously.) An apparently carboxylated and hydrocarbon-modified hydroxyethylcellulose and a hydrocarbon-modified quarternary polymer "polyquarternium-24 (LM-200)," both of uncertain molecular structure and both water-soluble derivatives of cellulose, have also been reported to exhibit adhesion prevention properties for barrier solutions. Added benefit was suggested for the LM-200 when given on 3 consecutive days postoperatively.[47]

Very Viscous Solutions

Very viscous solutions (VVS) may be regarded as a special subgroup of postsurgical barrier coatings. These are solutions that are gel like in viscosity (>1000 cps) but, unlike hydrogels, are not chemically cross-linked. The absence of chemical cross-linking makes VVS more quickly soluble than chemically cross-linked compositions and therefore more readily cleared from the site of application (e.g., the abdominal cavity for pelvic surgery). Examples of VVS include solutions of CMC of high MW at concentrations greater than about 2.0% or gel-like high MW (>1 million daltons) HA solutions at concentrations greater than about 1.0% (see Fig. 41.5). Our recent research at the University of Florida suggests that VVS prepared from CMC of low MW (~90 kDa) and medium MW (250 kDa), at concentrations of 3% to 11%, may also exhibit useful barrier properties.

In addition, gel-like polymer solutions that are ionically cross-linked, for example, based on anionic polysaccharide mixtures such as HA-CMC, also have promise as adhesion barrier materials for use at the end of surgery. Because such cohesive gel-like materials, unlike barrier films, can be applied to all tissue surfaces in very complex surgical field geometries and are more easily introduced following laparoscopy (and other minimally invasive procedures), there is considerable future promise for further research on VVS materials. Ionically cross-linked examples of VVS compositions that have been recently developed and intensively studied include Sepragel (Genzyme Corp.; HA/CMC mixture) and Intergel (Lifecore), a ferric chloride cross-linked HA. A comprehensive review of adhesion-inhibiting gel materials is found in another chapter in this volume.

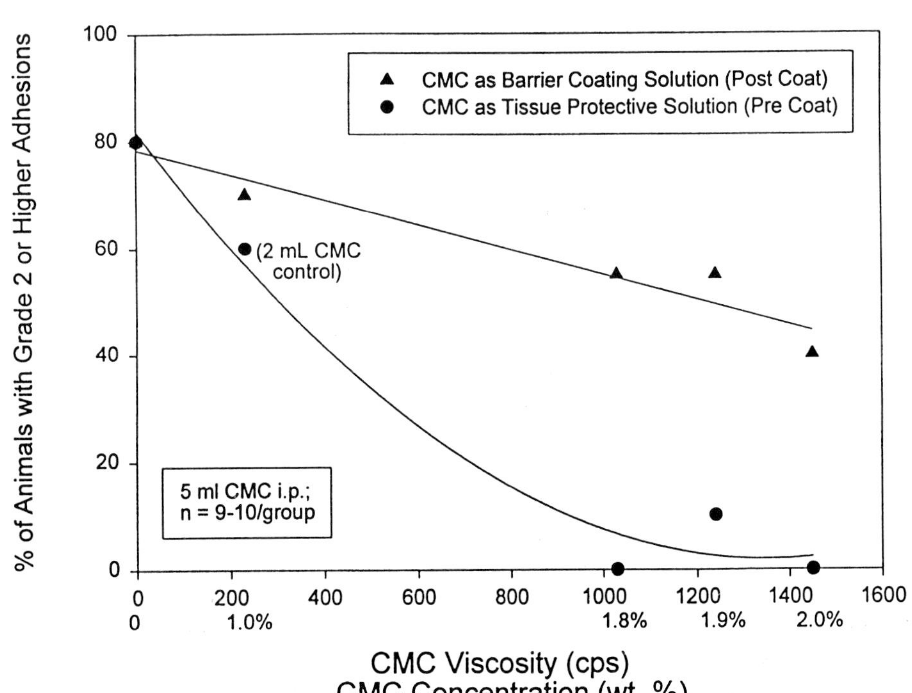

FIG. 41.5. Very viscous CMC solutions: efficacy for tissue protection vs. barrier coating.

Polymer Barrier Films

Polymer barrier films are applied to sites of trauma at the end of a surgical procedure and are intended thereby to physically separate injured tissue surfaces during wound healing and so prevent formation of adhesions. These solid physical barriers are most effective at sites of primary rather than adjunctive surgical trauma where the areas of tissue injury are discrete and easily identifiable, for example, at sites of resection/anastomosis, incisions, suture lines, electrocautery, and adhesion lysis. Barrier films that are used clinically are of two principal types: (1) biostable, which do not resorb and therefore remain in place permanently or must be removed surgically; and (2) bioresorbable, which degrade in vivo over a period of time following surgical placement.

The most studied example of a biostable polymer barrier film is Gore-Tex Surgical Barrier made of polytetrafluoroethylene (Teflon, PTFE), a film with a porous foamed or expanded microstructure (ePTFE). Adhesion inhibition using this biostable device has been widely studied with both highly favorable and some unfavorable clinical results.[114–116] Conceptually, if such adhesion-inhibiting barriers are to be of widespread clinical application, they must elicit no adverse long-term effects as they are in fact permanent implants. On the other hand, if required, removal of biostable barriers necessitates another surgery, with attendant risks and the potential for creating new sites of trauma and the consequent possibility of forming new adhesions. Some materials that have been used for fistula and peritoneal defect repair (i.e., polypropylene, Dacron polyester, and polyethylene mesh) have been investigated for use as substrates for coatings which may also act as adhesion prevention barriers. These have been discussed elsewhere.[87]

Partially biodegradable polyurethane films have also been described.[117] These adhesion barriers are two-layer compositions with a polyesterurethane (which is biodegradable) on a biostable polydimethylsiloxane (PDMS) polymer graft. The bilayer construction affords the potential for one side to be adherent to tissue surfaces for secure placement, whereas the other side provides a slippery outer surface. However, there are questions concerning the potential for inflammation by polyurethane degradation products and by complications or the need for surgical removal associated with the silicone film substrate for such barriers.

Bioresorbable barrier films have been much more extensively studied. There are two currently available films for clinical use that biodegrade or bioresorb during the first week following surgery. They are hydrophilic and quickly hydrate to a gel-like state. This highly hydrated gel-like tissue coating then slowly dissolves, acting as a tissue-separating barrier during the critical postoperative wound healing period of 1 to 7 days. The two devices are Interceed Absorbable Adhesion Barrier (an oxidized regenerated cellulose that is available clinically as a 3 × 4 in. membrane; Johnson & Johnson), and Seprafilm Bioresorbable Membrane (a chemically modified sodium hyaluronate/carboxymethylcellulose composition that is insolubilized by ionic cross-linking and is clinically available as a 5 × 6 in. membrane; Genzyme).

Reports of clinical results for Interceed range from excellent adhesion inhibition to marginal performance and some adverse adhesiogenic properties, especially if used in surgical settings where hemostasis and a blood-free surgical field are difficult to achieve. Efforts to improve Interceed performance in the presence of blood, involving changes in pH and modification with heparin, have apparently not been successful. The clinical use and performance of Interceed have been thoroughly reviewed elsewhere in some detail[118] and are not discussed further here.

Chemically Modified HA/CMC Bioresorbable Membrane (Seprafilm™)

One of the most recently developed resorbable barrier membranes, Seprafilm, is now in general clinical use. Because it is relatively new, it warrants more consideration here of some important property and performance characteristics. Seprafilm is a colorless, transparent, flexible, nontoxic, nonmutagenic, nonimmunogenic, nonpyrogenic, nonirritating, biocompatible polysaccharide film prepared by ionic cross-linking of a mixture of HA and CMC.[119] It hydrates within 1 to 2 days to a hydrophilic gel-like material that may remain in the abdominal cavity up to 7 days. It is completely excreted within 28 days, primarily through renal excretion (Seprafilm product literature). When applied at the conclusion of surgery, Seprafilm adheres well to tissues and other moist surfaces without need for suturing. For ease of handling, it must be kept dry until placement, as it may adhere to some degree to glove or instrument surfaces if wet. The dry film is somewhat rigid and may fracture if sharply folded. However, an improved formulation (Seprafilm 2) is more flexible, and can be easily folded, rolled, or manipulated without breaking, a property that is of particular value for use in laparoscopic insertion and placement. Of considerable importance is the fact that, unlike Interceed, the adhesion-inhibiting properties of Seprafilm appear to be unaffected by the presence of blood or moderately large volumes of irrigating solutions such as saline.[119]

In preclinical studies using a rat cecal abrasion model, Seprafilm significantly reduced the mean incidence of adhesions (0.2 vs. 1.9 adhesions for controls), and greatly increased the number of adhesion-free animals (32 of 40 adhesion free for Seprafilm vs. 3 of 39 for controls; $p < 0.0001$ for both). In an ischemic, peritoneum-stripped sidewall rat model, 70% of Seprafilm-treated animals were reported to be adhesion free, compared with only 20% of controls ($p < 0.001$). When used following adhesiolysis, 72% of Seprafilm-treated rats were reported to be adhesion free 7 days after lysis, compared with 28% of untreated controls ($p = 0.007$).[119] In bowel anastomosis studies using a rabbit model, Seprafilm applied at the anastomosis site did not reduce anastomotic bursting pressure when tested 7 or 14 days after surgery, compared with untreated controls.[121] In another interesting experiment, Seprafilm was reported to significantly inhibit adhesions to a polypropylene mesh ($p = 0.0008$) when used in a rat hernia repair model in which the film was placed over the viscera as a barrier to prevent adhesions to the mesh.[120]

Many favorable human clinical studies with Seprafilm have been reported. Multicenter clinical trials in patients undergoing restorative proctocolectomy and ileal J-pouch anastomosis with ileostomy showed Seprafilm to be very effective in inhibiting adhesion formation. For 91 patients treated with Seprafilm, 51% were free of adhesions at second-stage laparoscopy for ileostomy closure 8 to 12 weeks later, compared with a control group of 92 patients (who did not receive Seprafilm) in which only 6% were adhesion free ($p < 0.0001$). Adhesions that did form were also reduced in severity with Seprafilm (15% grade 3 adhesions on a 0 to 3 severity scale, vs. 58% for controls ($p < 0.0001$). No adverse clinical effects were observed for this resorbable barrier film in this study.[122] Additional clinical studies for barrier films are discussed in other chapters in this volume and therefore are not reviewed here.

Seprafilm Evaluation in New and More Severe Animal Adhesion Models

In an attempt to develop more stringent animal models for adhesion formation as a basis for evaluating surgical adjuvants with superior adhesion-inhibiting properties, our research at the University of Florida has in part been devoted to the development of two new "more severe" adhesion models, using either (1) talc powder (anhydrous magnesium silicate) or (2) recombinant human transforming growth factor-β_2 (TGF-β_2). These are clinically relevant adhesiogenic agents which, when applied directly to the cecum after controlled abrasion, significantly increase adhesion formation.[66] It was shown that these agents increase the mean incidence of adhesions by two- to threefold compared to a conventional rat cecal abrasion model, and thereby afford more demanding tests of adhesion prevention efficacy (unpublished data).

In our studies, using the more severe talc model with cecal abrasion, Seprafilm was placed on sites of primary trauma at the end of surgery, resulting in a mean adhesion incidence of 1.2 ± 0.4 compared with. 2.9 ± 0.7 for controls at day 7 reoperation ($p < 0.05$ for groups of $n = 9$ and $n = 10$, respectively). Test groups of the same size examined at 28-day reoperation provided a most interesting and apparently much more discriminating outcome. Mean adhesion incidence was 1.3 ± 0.5 for the Seprafilm group versus 4.5 ± 0.8 for controls ($p = 0.003$). In the very adhesiogenic TGF-β_2 model, adhesion incidence was 2.1 ± 0.4 using Seprafilm compared with 3.5 ± 0.7 for controls ($n = 9$ and $n = 10$, respectively) when examined at 7 days post surgery.

Polyethylene Oxide–Polylactic Acid Copolymer Barrier Films (REPEL)

Films of polyethylene glycol (EO)/polylactic acid (LA) copolymers (REPEL; Life Medical Sciences) of varying EO/LA ratios have recently been reported to act as resorbable barriers for inhibiting both de novo adhesions and adhesion reformation. [123] Repel is an opaque film with an EO/LA ratio of 3.0 and must be sutured in place. It is resorbed within 1 to 2 days after placement and is considered to exhibit acceptable tissue compatibility. Changes in the EO/LA ratio change the resorption time as well as film strength.

De novo adhesion formation was studied in a rabbit peritoneal sidewall, cecum, and bowel injury model with or without the addition of blood to the material after placement. All Repel-treated animals ($n = 9$/group) were free of adhesions at necropsy approximately 30 days postoperatively. The incidence of adhesions for control animals ($n = 10$) was 70%. In the presence of blood, no reduction in efficacy was reported for films having a 3.7 EO/LA ratio (15 of 15 rabbits were free of adhesions at necropsy compared with 7 of 15 animals with adhesions using Interceed barrier films with added blood). A study of efficacy in an adhesion lysis and reformation model indicated that Repel-treated animals reformed adhesions with a mean area of less than 5% of the initial adhesiolysis area, compared with a mean reformed area of 72% for controls ($n = 34$/group). Both groups had comparable (60%–70%) sidewall injury area covered by adhesions before lysis.[123] These studies suggest that Repel may be a promising barrier material for reducing adhesion formation.

Prevention of Adhesions Following Adhesiolysis

Most research on surgical adjuvants designed to prevent adhesion formation has been devoted to de novo, or new, adhesion formation involving tissues that have not previously been injured. However, once postoperative adhesions have formed, surgical lysis, often performed by laparoscopy, may be required and can be effective in reducing the number of adhesions and associated complications.[124–126] Nevertheless, because adhesiolytic surgery may itself prove traumatic, adhesions can reform after lysis, especially when lysis is performed by more tissue-damaging electrocautery as opposed to blunt dissection.[75,124] The general concepts for tissue protection during surgery and the application of barrier coatings or films to sites of tissue trauma that have been discussed are also applicable to surgical adhesiolysis to inhibit adjunctive trauma and provide barrier protection to the sites of adhesion lysis. Inhibition of adhesions following adhesiolysis is particularly challenging because of the need to prevent formation of de novo adhesions as well as adhesion reformation at sites of lysis.

Use of Tissue-Protective Solutions During Adhesiolysis

Few studies have been published concerning the use of tissue-protective solutions during adhesiolysis surgery, that is, applied before adhesion lysis to prevent reformation of adhesions. Although 0.4% HA solution has not been shown to be of significant benefit as a prelysis coating for reducing adhesion reformation,[69,70,75] CMC solutions have shown some efficacy in this application. Our studies at the University of Florida[75] have compared PBS, 0.4% HA, and 0.5% and 1.0% CMC solutions in an experiment involving solution application before blunt dissection adhesion lysis in a rat cecal adhesion model. The reduction observed in the incidence of grade 2 or higher adhesions (0 to 4 scoring scale) 7 days after lysis was 31% for PBS and 33% for 0.4% HA, versus 71% and 56%, respectively, for the CMC solutions ($n = 19–20$/group, with adhesion incidence similar for all groups at time of lysis). Statistical analysis of these data showed a highly significant decrease in the overall incidence of cecal adhesions (all grades) after lysis for animals receiving 0.5% or 1.0% CMC (from 2.3 ± 1.3 to 0.4 ± 0.9 for 0.5% CMC, and from 2.4 ± 1.3 to 0.95 ± 1.1 for 1.0% CMC; mean ± SD, two-tailed $p < 0.003$). There were trends toward adhesion reduction for both PBS ($p = 0.12$) and HA ($p = 0.13$) groups, suggesting that lysis alone was of benefit for reducing adhesions in this study.

This efficacy in adhesiolysis experiments observed for CMC solutions did not clearly correlate with solution viscosity, because the fewest adhesions were observed with the less viscous 0.5% CMC. This solution had the lowest viscosity of the three polymer treatment solutions (50 cps compared with 92 cps for HA and 295 cps for 1.0% CMC). The greater biostability and longer i.p. residence time of CMC may be an important factor in this observation, suggesting a barrier-type mechanism of action.

Dextran 70 (32%) has also been studied as a tissue protective solution for adhesion lysis procedures. In a study comparing pre- or postlysis application during adhesiolysis in a rabbit uterine horn, ovary, and peritoneal sidewall model, 25 mL of dextran was instilled i.p. either immediately upon abdominal opening (tissue precoating) or following microsurgical lysis (as a barrier coating). No differences were reported for the two treatments at evaluation 3 weeks post lysis. Mean adhesion scores (0 to 3 severity scale) increased from about 2.5 at time of lysis to 5.5 ± 2.9 (mean + SD) for dextran administered before lysis and 5.1 ± 2.5 for dextran administered post lysis ($n = 9–10$/group). Unfortunately, no surgical control animals were included in this adhesion lysis/reformation study for assessing the efficacy of lysis alone.[111]

Post-Lysis Barrier Solutions

CMC has been reported to reduce adhesion reformation when applied to tissue surfaces after adhesion lysis (post-lysis), apparently functioning as an adhesion barrier solution.[68,101] Best results have been obtained using larger solution volumes. This volume-dependent effect was observed with both a 1% CMC solution[68] and with a more viscous 2% CMC solution.[101] In contrast, relatively small volumes of very viscous 1.8% to 2.0% CMC solutions (2 mL cecal coating plus 2 mL i.p. instillation) failed to inhibit adhesions after adhesiolysis compared to control animals in a rat cecal adhesion study.[75] This observation is consistent with the volume effect previously discussed for postsurgical barrier applications of very viscous solutions for prevention of de novo adhesions.

A low MW (4000 daltons) water-soluble polyethylene glycol (PEG-4000) has been reported to help prevent adhesion reformation when used in moderate volumes (5 mL).[127] HA,[128] CMC,[129,130] PEG,[127] and dextran[131] solutions containing pharmacologically active agents are also of considerable interest and may, in the future, prove to be valuable in preventing postlysis adhesion reformation. This possibility has been suggested for solutions containing plasminogen activator in post-operative applications[128,131] (see "Medicated Solutions and Films").

Post-Lysis Barrier Films

Barrier films applied to sites of trauma after surgical lysis of adhesions can function mechanistically in the same way as they do for the inhibition of adhesions at primary sites of tissue damage in initial surgical procedures: that is, they provide a physical separation between the lysed adhesion sites (which have been damaged by scalpel, laser, or cutting electrocautery) and the surrounding tissues. The use of barrier films at the end of adhesiolysis surgery permits selective placement at identifiable sites of injury, and will usually afford a longer intraabdominal residence time than barrier solutions. However, barrier films may not be as versatile in completely covering the intricate geometries of organ structures and will be more difficult to place by laparoscopic insertion. Although positive results reported for Seprafilm[119] and Repel[123] encourage clinical use of such bioresorbable films in adhesiolytic procedures, it is likely that there will also be an important role in such surgery for barrier solutions and gels.

Medicated Solutions and Films

Tissue protective solutions and barrier coating solutions and films are of growing interest as drug delivery vehicles to provide prolonged local release of bioactive compounds to areas of trauma. In this way, the viscoelastic tissue protective and barrier separation properties can be supplemented by pharmacologic activity during the critical 1- to 7-day postoperative wound healing period. Drugs and bioactive agents can be dissolved in irrigating or tissue coating solutions, dispersed in such media by encapsulation in liposomes or protein-based microspheres to ensure prolonged drug release or phagocytic uptake by macrophages to modulate inflammatory processes, or incorporated into resorbable barrier films for prolonged activity as the film dissolves. Bioerodable polymer films are also potentially valuable for the local delivery of bioactive agents to sites of tissue trauma. A wide variety of pharmaceuticals may be readily incorporated into such barrier membranes for prolonged and controlled drug delivery. However, these "medicated devices," which may be regarded as second-generation adhesion-inhibiting surgical adjuvants, will probably be subject to more severe regulatory constraints, requiring more extensive clinical evaluation for regulatory approval.

The pharmaceuticals most commonly considered for such applications, especially for administration intraabdominally, include heparin (usually in irrigating solutions[56,112,132] but also in HA[133] or CMC[134] solutions), corticosteroids,[112] nonsteroidal antiinflammatory drugs,[135–138] and antibiotics.[112,139] Many other agents intended to mediate inflammation, fibrinolysis, collagen synthesis, or other aspects of the healing process have also been studied for intraperitoneal administration. Because they have generally been given topically at the time of surgery or postoperatively by injection (with consequent relatively short-lived activity), there has been very limited clinical success. Such drugs include plasminogen activators,[128,129,131,140–144] halofuginone (an inhibitor of collagen synthesis),[145] the antithrombin agent, recombinant hirudin analog,[146] interleukin-10 (an antiinflammatory cytokine),[147,148] disodium cromoglycate (cromolyn sodium, a mast cell stabilizer and inhibitor of degranulation),[149] antiinflammatory peptide 2 (a phospholipase A_2 inhibitor),[150] aprotinin (an antiinflammatory/antifibrinolytic agent),[151] and anti-TGF-β, antibodies.[152] Pharmacologic interventions are discussed in more detail in various other chapters in this volume.

Conclusions

This chapter substantially updates and expands on our review of tissue protective solutions and films for adhesion prevention published in 1997.[18] There have been many additional biomaterials research studies and clinical experience since that time with water-soluble polymer solutions for use during surgery to protect tissues and with hydrophilic resorbable adhesion barrier films for application to areas of trauma at the end of surgery to inhibit formation of postoperative adhesions. As we have suggested before, such solutions and films may be regarded as first-generation surgical device concepts that may be more readily introduced clinically than pharmaceutical products, particularly from a regulatory standpoint.

Recent research suggests that solutions and films will also be augmented by gel-like polymer compositions (discussed in another chapter in this volume). Additionally, ongoing wound healing research will undoubtedly soon lead to the use of biochemical agents designed to favorably intervene in the complex mix of postoperative processes involving cytokine and growth factor production, chemotactic events, fibrinolysis, macrophage and fibroblast mobilization, collagen synthesis, and neovascularization. In most instances, these bioactive agents will probably be most effective when used locally with controlled and prolonged release from solutions, gels, and films such as those discussed in this chapter. Second-generation adhesion-inhibiting adjuvants may therefore be best described as "medicated devices" and, depending upon the novelty of the pharmaceutical agents employed, may require more rigorous proof of safety and efficacy than previously. However, it is reasonable to believe that the incorporation into solutions, gels, and films of agents such as heparin, rtPA, steroids, antioxidants, and antibacterials (for which there are well-established pharmacologic data) will lead to "1.5-generation" adjuvants for facilitated regulatory approvals and more rapid clinical introduction.

Although we believe that the basic conclusions presented in our 1997 review of solutions and films for adhesion prevention remain valid,[18] new product developments and new insights derived from surgical experience suggest some changes in our point of view in prescribing the following "best approach" for inhibiting adhesions in initial surgeries and for surgical adhesiolysis:

1. Use tissue-protective polymer solutions at the start of and during surgery to minimize desiccation and mechanical tissue trauma; that is, to reduce adjunctive tissue damage near the sites of primary injury and throughout the intricate tissue structure of the surgical field.
2. Use resorbable barrier polymer compositions at the end of surgery to inhibit formation of adhesions at

sites of unavoidable primary trauma. Although barrier films will continue to be valuable to cover obvious areas of surgical trauma (e.g., at anastomoses and suture lines), gels will also become increasingly important as barrier materials because of (a) their ability to conform to and coat complex tissue geometries and (b) their relative ease of application in laparoscopic and other minimally invasive surgical procedures.

References

1. Swolin K. Beitrage zur operativen Behandlung der weiblichen Sterilitat: experimentelle und klinische Studien. Acta Obstet Gynecol Scand 1967;46(suppl 4).
2. Kaufman HE, Katz J, Valenti J, et al. Corneal endothelium damage with intraocular lenses: contact adhesion between surgical materials and tissue. Science 1977;198:525–527.
3. Hammer ME, Burch TG. Viscous corneal protection by sodium hyaluronate, chondroitin sulfate, and methylcellulose. Invest Ophthalmol Visual Sci 1984;25(11): 1329–1332.
4. Goldberg EP, Sheets JW, Habal MB. Peritoneal adhesions. Arch Surg 1980;115:776–780.
5. Miyauchi S, Iwata S. Biochemical studies on the use of sodium hyaluronate in the anterior eye segment. IV. The protective efficacy of the corneal endothelium. Curr Eye Res 1984;3(8):1063–1067.
6. Pedersen OO. Comparison of the protective effects of methylcellulose and sodium hyaluronate on corneal swelling following phacoemulsification of senile cataracts. J Cataract Refractive Surg 1990;16(5):594–596.
7. Koch DD, Liu JF, Glasser DB, et al. A comparison of corneal endothelial changes after use of Healon or Viscoat during phacoemulsification. Am J Ophthalmol 1993;115 (2):188–201.
8. Miyauchi S, Horie K, Morita M, et al. Protective efficacy of sodium hyaluronate on the corneal endothelium against the damage induced by sonication. J Ocular Pharmacol Ther 1996;12(1):27–34.
9. Guthoff R, Wendl U, Bohnke M, et al. [Endothelial cell protective effect of high viscosity substances in cataract surgery]. Ophthalmologe 1992;89(4):310–312.
10. Watters WB, Buck RC. Scanning electron microscopy of mesothelial regeneration in the rat. Lab Invest 1972;26: 604–609.
11. Urman B, Gomel V, Jetha N. Effect of hyaluronic acid on postoperative intraperitoneal adhesion formation in the rat model. Fertil Steril 1991;56(3):563–567.
12. Duncan DA, Yaacobi Y, Goldberg EP, et al. Prevention of postoperative pericardial adhesions with hydrophilic polymer solutions. J Surg Res 1988;45:44–49.
13. Burns JW, Skinner K, Colt J, et al. Prevention of tissue injury and postsurgical adhesions by precoating tissues with hyaluronic acid solutions. J Surg Res 1995;59:644–652.
14. Yaacobi Y, Goldberg EP, Habal MB. Effect of Ringer's lactate irrigation on the formation of postoperative abdominal adhesions. J Invest Surg 1991;4:31–36.
15. Ryan GB, Grobety J, Majno G. Mesothelial injury and recovery. Am J Pathol 1973;71(1):93–112.
16. Ellis H. The clinical significance of adhesions: focus on intestinal obstruction. Eur J Surg 1997; Suppl 577:5–9.
17. diZerega GS. Biochemical events in peritoneal tissue repair. Eur J Surg 1997; Suppl 577:10–16.
18. Goldberg EP. Tissue-protective solutions and films for adhesion prevention. In: Pelvic Surgery: Adhesion Formation and Prevention, Proceedings of 3rd International Congress on Pelvic Surgery and Adhesion Prevention, 1997, San Diego, CA.
19. Kappas AM, Fatouros M, Papadimitriou K, et al. Effect of intraperitoneal saline irrigation at different temperatures on adhesion formation. Br J Surg 1988;78:854–856.
20. Ordonez JJ, Dominguez J, Edvard V, et al. The effect of training and duration of surgery on adhesion formation in the rabbit model. Hum Reprod (Oxf) 1997;12(12): 2654–2657.
21. Tsukada K, Katoh H, Shiojima M, et al. Concentrations of cytokines in peritoneal fluid after abdominal surgery. Eur J Surg 1993;159(9):475–479.
22. Kaelin LD, Seeger JM, Staples EM, et al. Prevention of postoperative pericardial adhesions in a canine model by tissue precoating with hyaluronic acid solutions. In: Proceedings for the 48th Annual Sessions of the Forum on Fundamental Surgical Problems, 1992 Clinical Congress. New Orleans, LA: American College of Surgeons, 1992.
23. Holmdahl L, Eriksson E, Eriksson BI, et al. Depression of peritoneal fibrinolysis during operation is a local response to trauma. Surgery (St. Louis) 1998;123(5):539–544.
24. Down RH, Whitehead R, Watts JM. Do surgical packs cause peritoneal adhesions? Aust N Z J Surg 1979;49(3): 379–382.
25. Down RH, Whitehead R, Watts JM. Why do surgical packs cause peritoneal adhesions? Aust N Z J Surg 1980;50(1): 83–85.
26. van den Tol MP, van Stijn I, Bonthius F, et al. Reduction of intraperitoneal adhesion formation by use of non-abrasive gauze. Br J Surg 1997;84(10):1410–1415.
27. Luijendijk RW, de Lange DC, Wauters CC, et al. Foreign material in postoperative adhesions. Ann Surg 1996;223 (3):242–248.
28. Tolbert TW, Brown JL. Surface powders on surgical gloves. Arch Surg 1980;115:729–732.
29. Holmdahl L, al-Jabreen M, Xia G, et al. The impact of starch-powdered gloves on the formation of adhesions in rats. Eur J Surg 1994;160(5):257–261.
30. Renz H, Schmidt A, Hofmann P, et al. Tumor necrosis factor-alpha, interleukin 1, eicosanoid, and hydrogen peroxide release from macrophages exposed to glove starch particles. Clin Immunol Immunopathol 1993;68(1):21–28.
31. Swanson MC, Bubak ME, Hunt LW, et al. Quantification of occupational latex aeroallergens in a medical center. J Allergy Clin Immunol 1994;94:445–451.
32. Bauer X, Ammon J, Chen Z, et al. Health risk in hospitals through airborne allergens for patients presensitised to latex. Lancet 1993;342:1148–1149.
33. Newsome SWB, Shaw P. Airborne particles from latex gloves in the hospital environment. Eur J Surg 1997; Suppl 579:31–33.
34. Tang X, Chegini N, Rossi MJ, et al. The effect of surgical glove powder on proliferation of human skin fibroblast and monocyte/macrophage. J Gynecol Surg 1994;10(3): 139–150.
35. Rong H, Tang X-M, Zhao Y, et al. Postsurgical intraperitoneal exposure to glove powders modulates inflamma-

tory and immune-related cytokine production. Wound Repair Regen 1997;5:89–96.
36. Rappaport WD, Hunter GC, Allen R, et al. Effect of electrocautery on wound healing in midline laparotomy incisions. Am J Surg 1990;160:618–620.
37. Myllarniemi H. Healing and adhesion formation of peritoneal wounds. An angio-, histoangiographic, and ultrastructural study. Acta Chir Scand 1973;139(3):258–263.
38. Westreenen MV, Pronk A, Papendrecht AAGMHv, et al. Peritoneal responses to perioperative lavage: in vitro and in vivo observations (abstract). In: International Congress on Peritoneal Tissue Repair, The 4th Peritoneum and Peritoneal Access Meeting, 1997, Gothenburg, Sweden.
39. McEntee GP, Stuart RC, Byrne PJ, et al. Experimental study of starch-induced intraperitoneal adhesions [see comments]. Br J Surg 1990;77(10):1113–1114.
40. Sharefkin JB, Fairchild KD, Albus RA, et al. The cytotoxic effect of surgical glove powder particles on adult human vascular endothelial cell cultures: implications for clinical uses of tissue culture techniques. J Surg Res 1986;41(5):463–472.
41. Holmdahl L, Eriksson E, Al-Jabreen M, et al. Fibrinolysis in human peritoneum during surgery. Surgery 1996;119:701–705.
42. Holmdahl L, Al-Jabreen M, Risberg B. Experimental models for quantitative studies on adhesion formation in rats and rabbits. Eur Surg Res 1994;26:248–256.
43. Wallwiener D, Meyer A, Bastert G. Adhesion formation of the parietal and visceral peritoneum: an explanation for the controversy on the use of autologous and alloplastic barriers? Fertil Steril 1998;69:132–137.
44. Holmdahl L. The role of fibrinolysis in adhesion formation. Eur J Surg (Suppl) 1997;577:24–31.
45. Haney AF, Doty E. The formation of coalescing peritoneal adhesions requires injury to both contacting peritoneal surfaces. Fertil Steril 1994;61(4):767–775.
46. Peck LS, Quigg JM, Farnworth ST, et al. Effect of solution volume on prevention of surgical adhesions using hyaluronic acid and carboxymethylcellulose tissue precoating solutions (abstract). J Invest Surg 1991;4:387.
47. Falk K, Holmdahl L, Halvarsson M, et al. Bioadhesive polymers that reduce intraperitoneal adhesion formation. Br J Surg 1998;85:1153–1156.
48. Cantacuzene J, Soru E. [The mechanism of adhesions of the omentum to damaged tissues of the peritoneal cavity electrostatic interactions]. Arch Roum Pathol Exp Microbiol 1931;4:173.
49. Kloth LC. Physical modalities in wound management: UVC, therapeutic heating and electrical stimulation. Ostomy Wound Manage 1995;41(5):18–20, 22–24, 26–27.
50. Barnes TC. Healing rate of human skin determined by measurement of the electrical potential of experimental abrasions: a study of treatment with petrolatum and with petrolatum containing yeast and liver extracts. Am J Surg 1945;69(1):82–88.
51. Foulds IS, Barker AT. Human skin battery potentials and their possible role in wound healing. Br J Dermatol 1983;109(5):515–522.
52. Chiang M, Robinson KR, Vanable JW Jr. Electrical fields in the vicinity of epithelial wounds in the isolated bovine eye. Exp Eye Res 1992;54(6):999–1003.
53. Helmus MN, Gibbons DF, Jones RD. The effect of surface charge on arterial thrombosis. J Biomed Materials Res 1984;18:165–183.
54. Orida N, Feldman JD. Directional protrusive pseudopodial activity and motility in macrophages induced by extracellular electric fields. Cell Motil 1982;2(3):243–255.
55. Diamond MP, DeCherney AH, Linsky CB, et al. Assessment of carboxymethylcellulose and 32% dextran 70 for prevention of adhesions in a rabbit uterine horn model. Int J Fertil 1988;33(4):278–282.
56. Fredericks CM, Kotry I, Holtz G, et al. Adhesion prevention in the rabbit with sodium carboxymethylcellulose solutions. Am J Obstet Gynecol 1986;155:667–670.
57. Flessner MF, Dedrick RL, Schultz JS. Exchange of macromolecules between peritoneal cavity and plasma. Am J Physiol 1985;248(1 pt 2):H15–H25.
58. Fraser JR, Laurent TC, Laurent UB. Hyaluronan: its nature, distribution, functions and turnover. J Intern Med 1997;242(1):27–33.
59. Toole BP. Hyaluronan in morphogenesis. J Intern Med 1997;242(1):35–40.
60. Kerr Muir MG, Sherrard ES, Andrews V, et al. Air, methylcellulose, sodium hyaluronate and the corneal endothelium. Endothelial protective agents. Eye (Lond) 1987;1(pt 4):480–486.
61. Shusan A, et al. Mor-Yosef S, Avgar A, Hyaluronic acid for preventing experimental postoperative intraperitoneal adhesions. J Reprod Med 1994;39:398–402.
62. Rodgers KE, Johns DB, Girgis W, et al. Reduction of adhesion formation with hyaluronic acid after peritoneal surgery in rabbits. Fertil Steril 1997;67(3):553–558.
63. Kennedy R, Costain DJ, McAllister VC, et al. Prevention of experimental postoperative peritoneal adhesions by *N,O*-carboxymethyl chitosan. Surgery (St. Louis) 1996;120:866–870.
64. Hill-West JL, Chowdhury SM, Dunn RC, et al. Efficacy of a resorbable hydrogel barrier, oxidized regenerated cellulose, and hyaluronic acid in the prevention of ovarian adhesions in a rabbit model. Fertil Steril 1994;62(3):630–634.
65. Seeger JM, Kaelin LD, Staples EM, et al. Prevention of postoperative pericardial adhesions using tissue-protective solutions. J Surg Res 1997;68:63–66.
66. Peck LS, Skrabut E, Kiribuchi K, et al. Development of a severe adhesion model using talc or TGF-β2: efficacy of Seprafilm and Sepracoat in reducing postoperative adhesion formation (abstract). In: International Congress on Peritoneal Tissue Repair: 4th Peritoneum and Peritoneal Access Meeting, 1997, Gothenburg, Sweden.
67. Peck LS, Goldberg EP, Burns JW. A rat cecal abrasion model for evaluating surgical adhesions: retrospective analysis of tissue protection studies using HA and CMC solution precoating (abstract). In: Academy of Surgical Research: Tenth Annual Scientific Session, 1994, Orlando, FL.
68. Wurster SH, Bonet V, Mayberry A, et al. Intraperitoneal sodium carboxymethylcellulose administration prevents reformation of peritoneal adhesions following surgical lysis. J Surg Res 1995;59(1):97–102.
69. West JL, Chowdhury SM, Sawhney AS, et al. Efficacy of adhesion barriers: resorbable hydrogel, oxidized regenerated cellulose and hyaluronic acid. J Reprod Med 1996;41:149–154.

70. Urman B, Gomel V. Effect of hyaluronic acid on postoperative intraperitoneal adhesion formation and reformation in the rat model. Fertil Steril 1991;56(3):568–570.
71. Mitchell JD, Lee R, Hodakowski GT, et al. Prevention of postoperative pericardial adhesions with a hyaluronic acid coating solution. J Thorac Cardiovasc Surg 1994;107(6): 1481–1488.
72. Yaacobi Y, Hamed LM, Kaul KS, et al. Reduction of postoperative adhesions secondary to strabismus surgery in rabbits. Ophthal Surg 1992;23(2):123–128.
73. Oh SO, Lee J. Reduction of postoperative adhesions in strabismus surgery. Korean J Ophthalmol 1992;6(2):76–82.
74. Ravalico G, Tognetto D, Baccara F, et al. Corneal endothelial protection by different viscoelastics during phacoemulsification. J Cataract Refractive Surg 1997;23(3):433–439.
75. Peck LS, Quigg JM, Fossum GT, et al. Evaluation of CMC and HA solutions for adhesiolysis. J Invest Surg 1995;8:337–348.
76. Fulga V, Koren R, Ezov N, et al. Sodium hyaluronate as a tool in strabismus surgery in rabbits. Ophthalmic Surg Lasers 1996;27(3):228–233.
77. Diamond MP. Reduction of de novo postsurgical adhesions by intraoperative precoating with Sepracoat (HAL-C) solutions: a prospective, randomized, blinded, placebo-controlled multicenter study. Sepracoat Adhesion Study Group. Fertil Steril 1998;69(6):1067–1074.
78. Akatsuka M, Yamamoto Y, Tobetto K, et al. Suppressive effects of hyaluronic acid on elastase release from rat peritoneal leucocytes. J Pharm Pharmacol 1993;45(2):110–114.
79. Mast BA, et al. Hyaluronic acid modulates proliferation, collagen and protein synthesis of cultured fetal fibroblasts. Matrix 1993;13:441–446.
80. Klein ES, Asculai SS, Ben-Ari GY. Effects of hyaluronic acid on fibroblast behavior in peritoneal injury. J Surg Res 1996;61:473–476.
81. Boyce DE, Thomas A, Hart J et al. Hyaluronic acid induces tumour necrosis factor-alpha production by human macrophages in vitro. Br J Plast Surg 1997;50(5):362–368.
82. Ponzin D, Vecchia P, Toffano G, et al. Characterization of macrophages elicited by intraperitoneal injection of hyaluronate. Agents Actions 1986;18(5–6):544–549.
83. Toole BP, Knudson CB, Goldberg RL, et al. Hyaluronate-cell interactions in morphogenesis and tumorigenesis. In: Wolff JR, Sievers J, Berry M, eds. Mesenchymal-Epithelial Interactions in Neural Development. Berlin: Springer, 1987:267–278.
84. Lebel L, Gerdin B. Sodium hyaluronate increases vascular ingrowth in the rabbit ear chamber. Int J Exp Pathol 1991; 72(2):111–118.
85. Homsy CA, Stanley RF, King JW. Pseudosynovial fluids based on sodium carboxymethylcellulose. In: Gabelnick HL, Litt M, eds. Rheology of Biological Systems. Springfield: Thomas, 1973:278.
86. Moll HD, Schumacher J, Wright JC, et al. Evaluation of sodium carboxymethylcellulose for prevention of experimentally induced abdominal adhesions in ponies. Am J Vet Res 1991;52(1):88–91.
87. Ryan CK, Sax HC. Evaluation of a carboxymethylcellulose sponge for prevention of postoperative adhesions. Am J Surg 1995;169:154–160.
88. Alponat A, Lakshminarasappa SR, Teh M, et al. Effects of physical barriers in prevention of adhesions: an incisional hernia model in rats. J Surg Res 1997;68:126–132.
89. Hunt RJ, Wilson B, Moore JN, et al. In vitro evaluation of sodium carboxymethylcellulose on bacterial growth (abstract). Center for Continuing Education, University of Georgia: Symposium Abstracts, Fourth Equine Colic Research Symposium, 1991, p. 51.
90. Gauwerky JF, Heinrich D, Kubli F. Complications of intraperitoneal dextran application for prevention of adhesions. Biol Res Pregnancy Perinatol 1986;7:93–97.
91. Rein MS, Hill JA. 32% dextran 70 (Hyskon) inhibits lymphocyte and macrophage function in vitro: a potential new mechanism for adhesion prevention. Fertil Steril 1989;52(6):953–957.
92. diZerega GS, Rodgers KE. The Peritoneum. New York: Springer-Verlag, 1992:378.
93. Rozga J, Andersson R, Srinivas U, et al. Influence of phosphatidylcholine on intra-abdominal adhesion formation and peritoneal macrophages. Nephron 1990;54(2):134–138.
94. Snoj M, Ar'Rajab A, Ahren B, et al. Phospholipase-resistant phosphatidylcholine reduces intra-abdominal adhesions induced by bacterial peritonitis. Res Exp Med 1993;193(2):117–122.
95. Ar'Rajab A, Ahren B, Rozga J, et al. Phosphatidylcholine prevents postoperative peritoneal adhesions: an experimental study in the rat. J Surg Res 1991;50(3):212–215.
96. Snoj M, Ar'Ajab A, Ahren B, et al. Effect of phosphatidylcholine on postoperative adhesions after small bowel anastomosis in the rat. Br J Surg 1992;79(5):427–429.
97. Costain DJ, Kennedy R, Ciona C, et al. Prevention of postsurgical adhesions with *N,O*-carboxymethyl chitosan: examination of the most efficacious preparation and the effect of *N,O*-carboxymethyl chitosan on postsurgical healing. Surgery (St. Louis) 1997;121:314–319.
98. Elkins TE, Ling FW, Ahokas RA, et al. Adhesion prevention by solutions of sodium carboxymethylcellulose in the rat. II. Fertil Steril 1984;41(6):929–932.
99. Mayer M, Yedgar S, Hurwitz A. Effect of viscous macromolecules on peritoneal plasminogen activator activity: a potential mechanism for their ability to reduce postoperative adhesion prevention. Am J Obstet Gynecol 1988; 159:957–963.
100. Reijnen MMPJ, Meis J, Postma VA, et al. Prevention of intra-abdominal abscesses and adhesions by a hyaluronate based solution (Sepracoat) in a rat peritonitis model (abstract). In: International Congress on Peritoneal Tissue Repair: The 4th Peritoneum and Peritoneal Access Meeting, 1997, Gothenburg, Sweden.
101. Diamond MP, DeCherney AH, Linsky CB, et al. Adhesion reformation in the rabbit uterine horn model. I. Reduction with carboxymethylcellulose. Int J Fertil 1988;33(5): 372–375.
102. Elkins TE, Bury RJ, Ritter JL, et al. Adhesion prevention by solutions of sodium carboxymethylcellulose in the rat. I. Fertil Steril 1984;41:926–928.
103. Heidrick GW, Pippitt CH, Jr, Farnworth ST, et al. Efficacy of intraperitoneal sodium carboxymethylcellulose in preventing postoperative adhesion formation. J Reprod Med 1994;39(8):575–578.
104. Peck LS, Quigg JM, Farnworth ST, et al. Effect of solution volume and viscosity on surgical adhesion prevention using CMC in pre- and post-abrasion tissue coating models (abstract). J Invest Surg 1992;5(3):277.

105. diZerega GS, Rodgers KE. Peritoneal Fluid. In: The Peritoneum. New York: Springer-Verlag, 1992:34–38.
106. Gist RS, Lu PP, Raj HG, et al. Use of sodium hetastarch (Hespan) solution for reduction of postoperative adhesion formation in rabbits. J Invest Surg 1996;9(5):369–373.
107. Graebe RA, Oelsner G, Cornelison TL, et al. An animal study of different treatments to prevent postoperative pelvic adhesions. Microsurgery 1989;10(1):53–55.
108. Steinleitner A, Lumbert H, Kazensky C, et al. Poloxamer 407 as an intraperitoneal barrier material for the prevention of postsurgical adhesion formation and reformation in rodent models for reproductive surgery. Obstet Gynecol 1991;77(1):48–52.
109. Reigel DH, Bozmi B, Shih SR, et al. A pilot investigation of poloxamer 407 for the prevention of leptomeningeal adhesions in the rabbit. Pediatr Neurosurg 1993;19(5):250–255.
110. Leach RE, Henry RL. Reduction of postoperative adhesions in the rat uterine horn model with poloxamer 407. Am J Obstet Gynecol 1990;162(5):1317–1319.
111. Frishman GN, Peluso JJ, Kratka SA, et al. Preoperative versus postoperative dextran 70 for preventing adhesion formation. J Reprod Med 1991;36(10):707–710.
112. Cohen BM, Heyman T, Mast D. Use of intraperitoneal solutions for preventing pelvic adhesions in the rat. J Reprod Med 1983;28(10):649–653.
113. Singer ER, Livesey MA, Barker IK, et al. Utilization of the serosal scarification model of postoperative intestinal adhesion formation to investigate potential adhesion-preventing substances in the rabbit. Can J Vet Res 1996; 60(4):305–311.
114. diZerega GS. Contemporary adhesion prevention. Fertil Steril 1994;61(2):219–235.
115. diZerega GS. Use of adhesion prevention barriers in ovarian surgery, tubalplasty, ectopic pregnancy, endometriosis, adhesiolysis, and myomectomy. Curr Opin Obstet Gynecol 1996;8(3):230–237.
116. Saravelos HG, Li TC. Physical barriers in adhesion prevention. J Reprod Med 1996;41(1):42–51.
117. Rehman IU. Biodegradable polyurethanes: biodegradable low adherence films for the prevention of adhesions after surgery. J Biomater Appl 1996;11(2):182–257.
118. Larsson B. Efficacy of Interceed in adhesion prevention in gynecologic surgery: a review of 13 clinical studies. J Reprod Med 1996;41(1):27–34.
119. Burns JW, Colt MJ, Burgees LS, et al. Preclinical evaluation of Seprafilm bioresorbable membrane. Eur J Surg (Suppl) 1997;577:40–48.
120. Medina M, Paddock HN, Connolly RJ, et al. Novel antiadhesion barrier does not prevent anastomotic healing in a rabbit model. J Invest Surg 1995;8(3):179–186.
121. Alponat A, Lakshminarasoppa SR, Yavuz N, et al. Prevention of adhesions by Seprafilm, an absorbable adhesion barrier: an incisional hernia model in rats. Am Surg 1997;63(9):818–819.
122. Beck DE. The role of Seprafilm bioresorbable membrane in adhesion prevention. Eur J Surg (Suppl) 1997;577: 49–55.
123. Rodgers K, Cohn D, Hotovely A, et al. Evaluation of polyethylene glycol/polylactic acid films in the prevention of adhesions in the rabbit adhesion formation and reformation sidewall models. Fertil Steril 1998;69(3):403–408.
124. Hershlag A, Diamond MP, DeCherney AH. Adhesiolysis. Clin Obstet Gynecol 1991;34(2):395–402.
125. Holtz G, Kling OR. Effect of surgical technique on peritoneal adhesion reformation after lysis. Fertil Steril 1982; 37(4):494–496.
126. Diamond MP, Daniell JF, Feste J, et al. Adhesion reformation and de novo adhesion formation after reproductive pelvic surgery. Fertil Steril 1987;47(5):864–866.
127. O'Sullivan D, O'Riordain M, O'Conneil RP, et al. Peritoneal adhesion formation after lysis: inhibition by polyethylene glycol 4000. Br J Surg 1991;78:427–429.
128. Menzies D, Ellis H. The role of plasminogen activator in adhesion prevention. Surg Gynecol Obstet 1991;172(5): 362–366.
129. Vipond MN, Whawell SA, Scott-Coombes DM, et al. Experimental adhesion prophylaxis with recombinant tissue plasminogen activator. Ann R Coll Surg Engl 1994;76(6): 412–415.
130. Gehlbach DL, O'Hair KC, Parks AL, et al. Combined effects of tissue plasminogen activator and carboxymethylcellulose on adhesion reformation in rabbits. Int J Fertil Menopausal Stud 1994;39(3):172–176.
131. Doody KJ, Dunn RC, Buttram JVC. Recombinant tissue plasminogen activator reduces adhesion formation in a rabbit uterine horn model. Fertil Steril 1989;51(3): 509–512.
132. Jansen RP. Failure of peritoneal irrigation with heparin during pelvic operations upon young women to reduce adhesions. Surg Gynecol Obstet 1988;166(2):154–160.
133. Basbug M, Aygen E, Tayyar M, et al. Hyaluronic acid plus heparin for improved efficacy in prevention of adhesion formation in rat uterine horn model. Eur J Obstet Gynecol Reprod Biol 1998;78(1):109–112.
134. Sahin Y, Saglam A. Synergistic effects of carboxymethylcellulose and low molecular weight heparin in reducing adhesion formation in the rat uterine horn model. Acta Obstet Gynecol Scand 1994;73(1):70–73.
135. LeGrand EK, Rodgers KE, Girgis W, et al. Efficacy of tolmetin sodium for adhesion prevention in rabbit and rat models. J Surg Res 1994;56(1):67–71.
136. LeGrand EK, Rodgers KE, Girgis W, et al. Comparative efficacy of nonsteroidal anti-inflammatory drugs and antithromboxane agents in a rabbit adhesion-prevention model. J Invest Surg 1995;8(3):187–194.
137. Rodgers KE, Johns DB, Girgis W, et al. Prevention of adhesion formation with intraperitoneal administration of tolmetin and hyaluronic acid. J Invest Surg 1997;10: 367–373.
138. Yilmazlar T, Kaya E, Gurpinar E, et al. Efficacy of tenoxicam on intra-abdominal adhesion prevention in a rat model. J Int Med Res 1996;24(4):352–357.
139. Rappaport WD, Holcomb M, Valente J, et al. Antibiotic irrigation and the formation of intraabdominal adhesions. Am J Surg 1989;158:435–437.
140. Orita H, Fukasawa M, Girgis W, et al. Inhibition of postsurgical adhesions in a standardized rabbit model: intraperitoneal treatment with tissue plasminogen activator. Int J Fertil 1991;36(3):172–177.
141. Dunn RC, Mohler M. Effect of varying days of tissue plasminogen activator therapy on the prevention of postsurgi-

cal adhesions in a rabbit model. J Surg Res 1993;54: 242–245.

142. Gehlbach DL, O'Hair KC, Parks AL, et al. Combined effects of tissue plasminogen activator and carboxymethylcellulose on adhesion reformation in rabbits. Int J Fertil Menopausal Stud 1994;39(3):172–176.

143. Hill-West JL, Dunn RC, Hubbell JA. Local release of fibrinolytic agents for adhesion prevention. J Surg Res 1995; 59:759–763.

144. Menzies D, Ellis H. Intra-abdominal adhesions and their prevention by topical tissue plasminogen activator. J R Soc Med 1989;82(9):534–535.

145. Nagler A, Rivkind AI, Raphael J, et al. Halofuginone—an inhibitor of collagen type I synthesis—prevents postoperative formation of abdominal adhesions. Ann Surg 1998; 227(4):575–582.

146. Rodgers KE, Girgis W, Campeau JD, et al. Reduction of adhesion formation by intraperitoneal administration of a recombinant hirudin analog. J Invest Surg 1996; 9(5):385–391.

147. Montz FJ, Holschneider CH, Bozuk M, et al. Interleukin 10: ability to minimize postoperative intraperitoneal adhesion formation in a murine model. Fertil Steril 1994; 61(6):1136–1140.

148. Holschneider CH, Cristoforoni PM, Ghosh K, et al. Endogenous versus exogenous IL-10 in a postoperative intraperitoneal adhesion formation in a murine model. J Surg Res 1997;70(2):138–143.

149. Vural B, Mercan R, Corakci A, et al. A trial of reducing adhesion formation in a uterine horn model. Gynecol Obstet Invest 1998;45:58–61.

150. Rodgers KE, Girgis W, Campeau JD, et al. Reduction of adhesion formation by intraperitoneal administration of anti-inflammatory peptide. 2. J Invest Surg 1997;10 (1–2):31–36.

151. Ozogul Y, Boykal A, Onat D, et al. An experimental study of the effect of aprotinin on intestinal adhesion formation. Am J Surg 1998;175(2):137–141.

152. Lucas PA, Worejcka DJ, Young HE, et al. Formation of abdominal adhesions is inhibited by antibodies to transforming growth factor-beta 1. J Surg Res 1996;65(2): 135–138.

Index